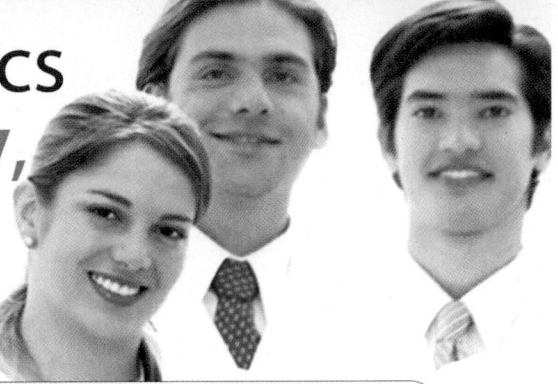
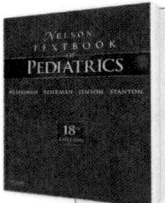
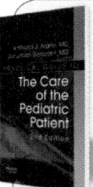
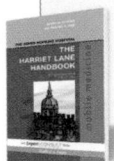
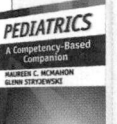
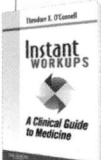
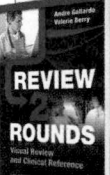
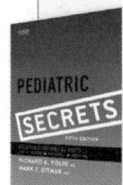
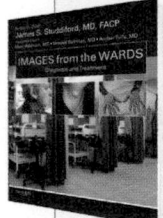

# NELSON

# Essentials of Pediatrics

## SIXTH EDITION

**Karen J. Marcdante, MD**
Professor and Vice Chair of Education
Department of Pediatrics
Medical College of Wisconsin
Children's Hospital of Wisconsin
Milwaukee, Wisconsin

**Robert M. Kliegman, MD**
Professor and Chair
Department of Pediatrics
Medical College of Wisconsin
Pediatrician-in-Chief
Pamela and Leslie Muma Chair in Pediatrics
Children's Hospital of Wisconsin
Milwaukee, Wisconsin

**Hal B. Jenson, MD**
Chief Academic Officer, Baystate Health
Springfield, Massachusetts
Professor of Pediatrics and Dean for Baystate Medical Center
Tufts University School of Medicine
Boston, Massachusetts

**Richard E. Behrman, MD**
Emeritus Professor of Pediatrics and Dean
Case Western Reserve University
Clinical Professor of Pediatrics, University of California, San Francisco,
California, and George Washington University
Washington, DC

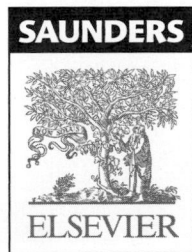

SAUNDERS

ELSEVIER

## SAUNDERS
ELSEVIER

1600 John F. Kennedy Blvd.
Ste 1800
Philadelphia, PA 19103-2899

Nelson Essentials of Pediatrics, Sixth Edition ISBN-13: 978-1-4377-0643-7

*Acquisitions Editor:* James Merritt
*Developmental Editor:* Barbara Cicalese
*Project Manager:* Mary Stermel
*Design Direction:* Steven Stave

Printed in Canada

Last digit is the print number:  9  8  7  6  5  4  3

*This book is dedicated to the faculty and learners*
*(both medical students and residents)*
*who share their enthusiasm and passion*
*as they provide excellent care*
*to the children we are*
*honored to serve.*

# Contributors

**Joel J. Alpert, MD**
Professor and Chairman of Pediatrics Emeritus; Professor of Public Health (Health Law) Emeritus, Boston University School of Medicine; Director of Pediatrics, Honorary, Boston Medical Center, Boston, Massachusetts
*The Profession of Pediatrics*

**Warren P. Bishop, MD**
Professor of Pediatrics, Roy J. and Lucille A. Carver College of Medicine, University of Iowa; Director, Division of Gastroenterology, Department of Pediatrics, University of Iowa Children's Hospital, Iowa City, Iowa
*The Digestive System*

**Kim Blake, MD, MRCP, FRCPC**
Associate Professor, Department of Pediatrics, Division of Medical Education, Dalhousie University; Professor of Pediatrics, Department of Pediatrics, IWK Health Centre, Halifax, Nova Scotia, Canada
*Adolescent Medicine*

**Nathan J. Blum, MD**
Associate Professor of Pediatrics, The University of Pennsylvania School of Medicine; Director, Section of Behavioral Pediatrics, Division of Child Development, Rehabilitation, and Metabolic Disease, The Children's Hospital of Philadelphia, Philadelphia, Pennsylvania
*Psychosocial Issues*

**Edward R. Carter, MD**
Associate Professor of Pediatrics, University of Washington School of Medicine, Seattle; Director of Clinical Services, Pulmonary Division, Seattle Children's Hospital, Seattle, Washington
*The Respiratory System*

**Cindy W. Christian, MD**
Associate Professor of Pediatrics, The University of Pennsylvania School of Medicine; Chair, Child Abuse and Neglect Prevention, The Children's Hospital of Philadelphia, Philadelphia, Pennsylvania
*Psychosocial Issues*

**Victoria Davis, MD, FRCSC, IFEPAG**
Staff, Obstetrics and Gynecology, Scarborough Grace Hospital, Scarborough, Ontario, Canada
*Adolescent Medicine*

**Ramsay L. Fuleihan, MD**
Associate Professor, Northwestern University Feinberg School of Medicine; Attending Physician; Director, Primary Immunodeficiency Clinical Services, Children's Memorial Hospital, Chicago, Illinois
*Immunology*

**Sheila Gahagan, MD, MPH**
Professor and Chief, Division of Child Development and Community Health, Martin T. Stein Endowed Chair in Developmental-Behavioral Pediatrics, University of California San Diego, San Diego, California; Research Professor, University of Michigan, Ann Arbor, Michigan
*Behavioral Disorders*

**Rick Goldstein, MD**
Assistant Professor of Pediatrics, Boston University Medical Center; Associate Program Director, Boston Combined Residency Program in Pediatrics, Boston, Massachusetts
*The Profession of Pediatrics*

**Clarence W. Gowen Jr., MD**
Associate Professor of Pediatrics; Vice-Chair for Education, Eastern Virginia Medical School; Director of Medical Education, Children's Hospital of The King's Daughters, Norfolk, Virginia
*Fetal and Neonatal Medicine*

**Larry A. Greenbaum, MD, PhD**
Division Director, Pediatric Nephrology, Emory University, Atlanta; Children's Healthcare of Atlanta, Atlanta, Georgia
*Fluids and Electrolytes*

**Hilary M. Haftel, MD, MHPE**
Associate Professor of Pediatrics, Internal Medicine, and Medical Education; Associate Chair and Director of Pediatric Education, University of Michigan Medical School; Attending Physician, University of Michigan Health System, Ann Arbor, Michigan
*Rheumatic Diseases of Childhood*

**Kelly Hetherington, MD**
Allergy Fellow, Department of Pediatrics/Internal Medicine, University of Washington School of Medicine; Allergy Fellow, Children's Hospital and Regional Medical Center, Seattle, Washington
*Allergy*

**Nicholas Jospe, MD**
Professor of Pediatrics; Chief, Pediatric Endocrinology, University of Rochester, Rochester, New York
*Endocrinology*

**Nancy F. Krebs, MD, MS**
Professor of Pediatrics, University of Colorado Denver, Aurora; Medical Director, Department of Nutrition, The Children's Hospital, Aurora, Colorado
*Pediatric Nutrition and Nutritional Disorders*

**Mary V. Lasley, MD**
Clinical Assistant Professor, Department of Pediatrics, University of Washington School of Medicine; Private Practice, Northwest Asthma and Allergy Center, Seattle, Washington
*Allergy*

**K. Jane Lee, MD, MA**
Assistant Professor, Pediatrics (Critical Care) and Population Health (Bioethics), Medical College of Wisconsin; Associate Director PICU, Children's Hospital of Wisconsin, Milwaukee, Wisconsin
*The Acutely Ill or Injured Child*

**David A. Levine, MD**
Chief, Division of Predoctoral Education; Associate Professor of Clinical Pediatrics, Department of Pediatrics, Morehouse School of Medicine, Atlanta Georgia
*Growth and Development*

**Paul A. Levy, MD, FAAP, FACMG**
Assistant Professor of Pediatrics and Pathology, Albert Einstein College of Medicine; Assistant Professor of Pediatrics and Pathology, Children's Hospital of Montefiore, Bronx, New York
*Human Genetics and Dysmorphology*

**Donald W. Lewis, MD, FAAP, FAAS**
Professor and Chairman, Department of Pediatrics, Eastern Virginia Medical School; Senior Vice President for Academic Affairs, Children's Hospital of The King's Daughters, Norfolk, Virginia
*Neurology*

**Valerie B. Lyon, MD**
Assistant Professor, Departments of Dermatology and Pediatrics, Medical College of Wisconsin, Pediatric Dermatologic Surgery and Skin Oncology, Children's Hospital of Wisconsin, Milwaukee, Wisconsin
*Dermatology*

**John D. Mahan, MD**
Professor of Pediatrics, Vice Chairman for Education, The Ohio State University College of Medicine; Program Director, Pediatric Residency and Pediatric Nephrology Fellowship Programs, Nationwide Children's Hospital, Columbus, Ohio
*Nephrology and Urology*

**Karen J. Marcdante, MD**
Professor and Vice Chair of Education, Department of Pediatrics, Medical College of Wisconsin; Children's Hospital of Wisconsin, Milwaukee, Wisconsin
*The Acutely Ill or Injured Child*

**Robert W. Marion, MD**
Ruth L. Gottesman Professor of Developmental Pediatrics, Pediatrics, Obstetrics, Gynecology, and Women's Health, Albert Einstein College of Medicine; Chief, Divisions of Genetics and Developmental Medicine, Children's Hospital at Montefiore, Bronx; Director of Genetics, Blythedale Children's Hospital, Valhalla, New York
*Human Genetics and Dysmorphology*

**Susan G. Marshall, MD**
Associate Dean for Curriculum, University of Washington School of Medicine; Attending Physician, Pediatric Pulmonary Division, Seattle Children's Hospital; Associate Professor of Pediatrics, University of Washington School of Medicine, Seattle, Washington
*The Respiratory System*

**Thomas W. McLean, MD**
Associate Professor of Pediatrics, Wake Forest University School of Medicine; Department of Pediatrics, Brenner Children's Hospital, Winston-Salem, North Carolina
*Oncology*

**Julie A. Panepinto, MD, MSPH**
Associate Professor of Pediatrics, Medical College of Wisconsin and The Children's Research Institute of the Children's Hospital of Wisconsin, Milwaukee, Wisconsin
*Hematology*

**Laura E. Primak, RD, CNSD**
Professional Research Assistant, University of Colorado Denver, Aurora, Colorado
*Pediatric Nutrition and Nutritional Disorders*

**Russell Scheffer, MD**
Chair, Department of Psychiatry and Behavioral Sciences; Professor, Department of Pediatrics, University of Kansas School of Medicine—Wichita; Medical Director, Behavioral Health, Via Christi Hospitals, Wichita, Kansas
*Psychiatric Disorders*

**Daniel S. Schneider, MD**
Associate Professor of Pediatrics, University of Virginia; Director, Pediatric Cardiology Noninvasive Laboratory, Children's Hospital Heart Center, University of Virginia, Charlottesville, Virginia
*The Cardiovascular System*

**J. Paul Scott, MD**
Professor of Pediatrics, Medical College of Wisconsin; Attending Physician, Children's Hospital of Wisconsin, Milwaukee, Wisconsin
    *Hematology*

**Margretta R. Seashore, MD, FAAP, FACMG**
Professor, Genetics, Department of Genetics, Yale University School of Medicine; Attending Physician, Yale-New Haven Hospital, New Haven, Connecticut
    *Metabolic Disorders*

**Benjamin S. Siegel, MD**
Professor of Pediatrics and Psychiatry, Boston University School of Medicine; Attending Physician, Boston Medical Center, Boston, Massachusetts
    *The Profession of Pediatrics*

**Sherilyn Smith, MD**
Associate Professor of Pediatrics, University of Washington, Department of Pediatrics, Division of Infectious Disease, Children's Hospital and Regional Medical Center, Seattle, Washington
    *Infectious Diseases*

**Kevin D. Walter, MD, FAAP**
Assistant Professor, Department of Orthopedics and Department of Pediatrics, Medical College of Wisconsin; Program Director, Pediatric and Adolescent Primary Care Sports Medicine, Children's Hospital of Wisconsin, Milwaukee, Wisconsin
    *Orthopedics*

**Marcia M. Wofford, MD**
Associate Professor of Pediatrics, Wake Forest University School of Medicine; Associate Professor of Hematology/Oncology, Brenner Children's Hospital, Winston-Salem, North Carolina
    *Oncology*

# Preface

The continuing discovery of medical knowledge is resulting in amazing improvements in our ability to diagnose, treat, and prevent diseases in children. We must learn from the many investigators who have delineated the pathophysiology and who continue pursuing the mechanisms of diseases to help us provide excellent care to our patients. As educators and authors, our goal is to deliver these new advances, as well as classic pediatrics, in a readable and concise text for medical students and residents.

This new edition has been updated with the advances that have occurred in the last 5 years. We are honored to have many of these outstanding contributions written by clerkship directors with expertise in pediatrics and pediatric subspecialties, as well as others who were selected for their roles in teaching, administration, and research. As in previous editions of this very successful and well-used textbook, we focus our attention on the learner and what is expected of him or her during his or her medical training.

We emphasize the common and classic pediatric disorders in a time-honored, logical format to help the student and resident acquire knowledge and apply that knowledge to their patients. The student and resident will gain the knowledge and skills necessary to succeed both in caring for patients and in preparing for clerkship or in-service examinations.

We hope this revised edition will continue to serve the thousands of learners who rotate through pediatrics as well as those who will become new providers of pediatric care in the years to come.

KAREN J. MARCDANTE, MD

ROBERT M. KLIEGMAN, MD

HAL B. JENSON, MD

RICHARD E. BEHRMAN, MD

# Acknowledgments

The editors could never have published this edition without the assistance and attention to detail of James Merritt and Barbara Cicalese. In addition, we are grateful, once again, to Carolyn Redman for her outstanding editing, suggestions, organization, and initiative in making this book a reality.

# Contents

# THE PROFESSION OF PEDIATRICS

**Benjamin S. Siegel, Joel J. Alpert, and Rick Goldstein**

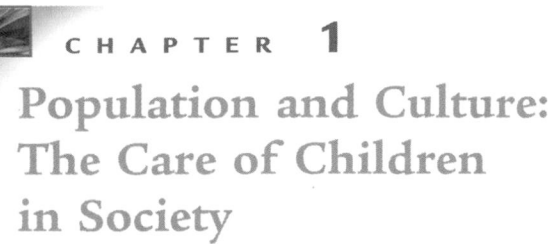

CHAPTER **1**

# Population and Culture: The Care of Children in Society

Health care professionals need to appreciate the interactions between medical conditions and social, economic, and environmental influences associated with the provision of pediatric care. New technologies and treatments help improve morbidity, mortality, and the quality of life for children and their families, but the costs may exacerbate disparities in medical care. The challenge for pediatricians is to deliver care that is socially equitable; integrates psychosocial, cultural, and ethical issues into practice; and ensures that health care is available for all children.

## CURRENT CHALLENGES

Currently, many challenges affect children's health outcomes. These include access to health care; health disparities; supporting their social, cognitive, and emotional lives in the context of families and communities; and addressing environmental factors, especially poverty.

Many scientific advances have an impact on the role of pediatricians because they must incorporate the use of newer genetic technologies that allow the diagnosis of diseases at the molecular level and provide information on the prognosis of some diseases. Prenatal diagnosis and newborn screening improve the accuracy of early diagnosis of a variety of conditions, allowing for earlier treatment even when a cure is impossible. Functional magnetic resonance imaging allows a greater understanding of psychiatric and neurologic problems, such as dyslexia and attention-deficit/hyperactivity disorder.

Challenges persist. The incidence and prevalence of chronic illness has increased in recent decades. Chronic illness is now the most common reason for hospital admissions for children (excluding trauma and newborn admissions). From middle school on, mental illness is the main non-childbirth–related reason for hospitalization for children. Pediatricians must also address the

increasing concern about environmental toxins and the prevalence of physical, emotional, and sexual abuse as well as violence. Since the September 11, 2001, destruction of the World Trade Center, fear of terrorism in the United States has increased the level of anxiety for many families and children.

Pediatricians must practice as part of a health care team. Many pediatricians already practice collaboratively with psychiatrists, psychologists, nurses, and social workers. Team composition can change depending on location and patient needs. Some pediatric programs have incorporated lawyers into the full-time staff to address the legal issues of school placement for special needs students and housing and immigration issues, reflecting the challenges seen in an urban, underserved, and diverse population. Although school health and school-based health clinics have improved access and outcomes for many common childhood and adolescent conditions, the shortage of available general pediatricians and family physicians has led to the development of retail medical facilities in pharmacies and retail stores.

Childhood antecedents of adult health conditions, such as alcoholism, depression, obesity, hypertension, and hyperlipidemias, are increasingly being recognized. Maternal health status can affect the fetus. Infants who are smaller size and relatively underweight at birth because of maternal malnutrition have increased rates of coronary heart disease, stroke, type 2 diabetes mellitus, obesity, the metabolic syndrome, and osteoporosis in later life. Because of improved neonatal care, a greater percentage of preterm, low birth weight, or very low birth weight newborns survive, increasing the number of children with chronic medical conditions and developmental delays with lifelong implications.

## LANDSCAPE OF HEALTH CARE FOR CHILDREN IN THE UNITED STATES

Complex health, economic, and psychosocial challenges greatly influence the well-being and health outcomes of children. These issues include the following:

- **Health insurance coverage.** Of the more than 92 million children 21 years of age or younger (2006), 8.8% had no health insurance coverage for a full year. In addition, another 13%, (approximately 12 million), went without health insurance for some period during the year. In addition, an estimated 10 to 20 million were very likely underinsured. Many children, despite public sector insurance, did not have coverage for recommended immunizations. (In 2006, 40% of states in the United States did not cover the meningococcal vaccine, and 17% of the states did not cover the pneumococcal vaccine.) Employer-provided insurance in the workplace decreased significantly from 1984 to 2006. Although Medicaid and the State Child Health Insurance Program (SCHIP) increased during this period, covering nearly 72% of children below 100% of poverty and 9% of children whose family income was 200% of poverty, approximately 1.7 million children were unable to get needed medical care because the family could not afford it. In addition, medical care was delayed for an additional 2.5 million children because of worry about costs. Twenty-three percent of all uninsured children had unmet dental needs compared with 4% of children with private insurance and 7% of children with Medicaid or other public coverage.

The United States has the highest percentage of children living in poverty in the industrialized world (26%).

● **Access to primary care.** The American Academy of Pediatrics proposes that all children have a medical home where their pediatrician and medical team provide needed preventive and curative services. Unfortunately, many pediatric offices, whether large or small, are not equipped to provide the full spectrum of services recommend by the medical home concept. Children without health insurance are more likely not to have seen a physician over a two-year period.

● **Prenatal and perinatal care.** Eighty-four percent of all women (85.4% white, 77.5% Latina, and 76.4% African American) received prenatal care in the first trimester. Smoking during pregnancy has declined from 19.5% in 1989 to 1991 to 16.4% of pregnant women in 2007. Approximately 5.2% of pregnant woman used illicit drugs (7.2% of women 18 to 25 years of age), and 11.6% used alcohol. Binge drinking occurs in 3.7% of all pregnant women, and 6.6% reported binge drinking during the first trimester.

● **Births.** In 2006, there were approximately 4 million births. Thirty-eight percent of births were to unmarried women. The number of births to Hispanic women was greater than 1 million, up from 15% of total births in 1990; this represents the largest increase of any ethnic group.

● **Cesarean sections.** These surgeries have increased to 31% of all births, which is a 33% increase since 1996. There is little difference in the Cesarean section rates for whites, African Americans, or Latina women.

● **Preterm births.** The incidence of **preterm births** (<37 weeks) has been increasing since the 1980s (11.7% in whites, 18.4% in African Americans, and 12.4% in Latinas). There has been an increase in low birth weight infants (≤2500 g [8.3% of all births]) and a steady rate of very low birth weight infants (≤1500 g [1.5% of all births]) since the 1990s.

● **Birth rate in adolescents.** The national birth rate among adolescents has been steadily dropping since 1990 before rising in 2006. The youngest adolescent population (10 to 14 years) experienced a slight decrease in birth rate from 0.7 per 1000 to 0.6 per 1000 from 2005 to 2006.

● **Adolescent abortions.** In 2004, 1,222,000 abortions were performed, down from a peak of 1,609,000 abortions in 1990. In 2005 to 2006, for adolescents younger than 15 years of age, the abortion rate was 70.8 per 100 live births, down from a peak of 139.7 per 100 live births in 1980. From 2000 to 2005, 575,000 women used mifepristone for medical abortions. There has also been increasing contraception use in women 15 to 19 years of age (24% of adolescents in 1982 and 31% in 2002).

● **Infant mortality.** There has been a 74% decline in infant mortality since 1960, with equal declines in the rates for white and nonwhite populations. However, the disparity among the ethnic groups has not changed. In 2006, the infant mortality rates per 1000 live births were white, 5.57; Latina, 5.49; and African American, 13.35. In 2004, the United States ranked 29th in infant mortality. Marked variations in infant mortality also exist by state. In 2004, Massachusetts (4.80 per 1000 live births) and Vermont (4.60 per 1000 live births) had the lowest infant mortality rates in the United States. Mississippi (10.32 per 1000 live births) and the District of Columbia (11.42 per 1000 live births) had the highest rates, comparable to developing countries.

● **Initiation and maintenance of breastfeeding**: Seventy-four percent of women initiate breastfeeding following the birth of their infants. Women with bachelor's degrees are more likely to initiate breastfeeding (80%), whereas adolescents are much less likely to do so (51%). Breastfeeding rates vary by ethnicity (81% of Latina women, 77% of white women, and 61% of African-American women). Only 42% of women continue breastfeeding for 6 months, with 21% continuing at 12 months.

● **Cause of death in U.S. children.** The overall causes of death in all children (1 to 19 years of age) in the United States in 2005, in order of frequency, were accidents (unintentional injuries), assaults (homicide), malignant neoplasms, suicide, and congenital malformations (Table 1-1). There was a slight improvement in the rate of death from all causes. Sixty-one percent of these deaths were caused by violence, and about 33% were related to injuries, 11% to homicide, and 7% to suicide. Many deaths are associated with alcohol abuse. Two thirds of child passengers (≤14 years of age) die in automobile crashes in association with a drunk driver.

● **Hospital admissions for children and adolescents.** Forty-five percent of all admissions are nonemergent, and 44% of children are admitted from an emergency department. Asthma is the most common reason for nonelective hospital admissions in 3- to 5- and 6- to 12-year-old children. Mental illness accounts for 7.3% of all hospital admissions and is the most common cause of admissions for children 13 to 17 years of age.

● **Significant adolescent health challenges: substance use and abuse.** There was considerable substance use and abuse in U.S. high school students. Fifty percent of high school students reported trying cigarettes in 2005; nearly 11% smoke more than 10 cigarettes/day. More than 33% of high school students have tried marijuana; 43% alcohol (25% admit to more than five drinks

| TABLE 1-1 Causes of Death by Age in the United States, 2005 | |
|---|---|
| **Age Group (yr)** | **Causes of Death in Order of Frequency** |
| 1–4 | Accidents (unintentional injuries) |
| | Congenital malformations, deformations, and chromosomal abnormalities |
| | Malignant neoplasms |
| | Homicide |
| | Heart disease |
| 5–9 | Accidents (unintentional injuries) |
| | Malignant neoplasms |
| | Congenital malformations, deformations, and chromosomal abnormalities |
| | Homicide |
| | Heart disease |
| 10–14 | Accidents (unintentional injuries) |
| | Malignant neoplasms |
| | Suicide |
| | Homicide |
| | Congenital malformations, deformations, and chromosomal abnormalities |
| 15–19 | Accidents (unintentional injuries) |
| | Homicide |
| | Suicide |
| | Malignant neoplasms |
| | Heart disease |

Data from U.S. Centers for Disease Control and Prevention/NCHS: *National Vital Statistics Report System: Mortality, 2005.*

per month); 12% have tried inhalants; 8.5% hallucinogens; 6.3% Ecstasy (MDMA); 6% methamphetamine; 2% heroin; and 2% injectables.

- **Children in foster care.** Currently, there are about 500,000 children in the foster care system. Approximately 25,000 of these children must leave the child welfare system each year. Of those who leave, 25% to 50% experience homelessness and/or joblessness and will not graduate from high school. These children have a high incidence of mental health problems, substance abuse, and early pregnancy for females with an increased likelihood of having a low birth weight baby.

## OTHER HEALTH ISSUES THAT AFFECT CHILDREN IN THE UNITED STATES

- **Obesity.** Within the past decade, there has been a huge increase in the prevalence of obesity. The prevalence of **overweight** children 6 to 11 years of age and 12 to 19 years of age has increased more than fourfold from 4% in 1965 to 17% in 2004. Currently, it is estimated that 32% of children 2 to 19 years of age have a body mass index above the 85th percentile. There are 300,000 deaths a year and at least $117 billion in health care costs associated with the 66% of Americans who are overweight.
- **Sedentary lifestyle.** Among high school students, 72.2% of girls and 56.2% of boys did not engage in

recommended amounts of moderate or vigorous physical activity. Twenty-one percent of high school students played video or computer games more than 3 hours per school day, and 37% of students watched TV more than 3 hours on an average school day.

- **Motor vehicle accidents and injuries.** In 2004, 1638 children 14 years of age or younger died in motor vehicle crashes, and 214,000 were injured. Other causes of childhood injury included drowning, child abuse, and poisonings. It is estimated that the costs of all childhood injuries is $46 billion per year. A significant percentage of injuries are associated with alcohol use.
- **Children in protective services programs.** In 2003, an estimated 2.9 million referrals to child protective services involved 5.5 million children. Of these, 30% were for psychological maltreatment, 26% percent were for neglect, and another 26% were for sexual abuse. Only 27% were reported by medical personnel; 22% were reported by the education system and 21% by the law enforcement/justice system.
- **Juvenile challenges, crime, and the juvenile justice system.** There was a 44% drop in the number of juveniles killed from 1993 (a peak of 2800) to 2002 (1600), with African-American youth being killed four times more frequently than white youth. Teenagers, in general, are two to three times more likely than adults to be victims of rape, robbery, and aggravated assault. Nationwide, 1.7 million youth were runaways or pushed out of their homes, with a large percentage ending up working for sexual predators and selling their bodies on the streets. About 2.2 million teens younger than 18 years of age were arrested; about half the arrests were for larceny, theft, simple assault, drug abuse or liquor laws violation, and disorderly conduct. There were more female arrests than male arrests. In 2003, there were 97,000 juvenile offenders in juvenile residential faculties, with the rate of African-American youth of 754/100,000, American Indian 496/100,000, Latina 348/100,000, white 190/100,000, and Asian 113/100,000.
- **Current social and economic stress on the U.S. population.** There are considerable societal stresses affecting the health and mental health of children, including rising unemployment associated with the economic slowdown, financial turmoil, and the high price of oil. Millions of families have lost their homes or are at risk for losing their homes after defaulting on mortgage payments.
- **Adverse child events leading to adult health challenges.** Beginning before the current economic crisis (2008), even adults in a higher socioeconomic status experienced a great deal of stress in childhood. More than 60% had at least one significant stressor (abuse, neglect, and household dysfunction) as a child (26% had one stressor, 25% had two to three stressors, and 13% had four or more stressors). The greater the number of stressors in childhood, the worse the outcomes as adults. The adverse outcomes included an increased likelihood of suicide attempt; increased risk of teen pregnancy, marrying an alcoholic, or having marital problems; and increased likelihood of substance abuse and interpersonal violence.
- **Military deployment and children.** The wars in Iraq and Afghanistan have affected millions of adults and

their children. There are an estimated 2.3 million active duty and National Guard/Reserve servicemen and women with 1.8 million children up to 23 years of age. Since October of 2001, there have been approximately 1.64 million troops (parents to >700,000 children) deployed to Iraq and Afghanistan. An estimated 31% of troops returning from Iraq and Afghanistan have a mental health condition (alcoholism, depression, and post-traumatic stress disorder) or report experiencing a traumatic brain injury. Approximately 300,000 members of the armed forces currently suffer from post-traumatic stress disorder or a major depression. Their children are affected by their morbidities, as well as the psychological affects of deployment on children of all ages. Child maltreatment was 42% higher in families of U.S. enlisted soldiers during combat deployment than in nondeployed soldiers.

## HEALTH DISPARITIES IN HEALTH CARE FOR CHILDREN

Health disparities are the differences that remain after taking into account patients' needs, preferences, and the availability of health care. Social conditions, social inequity, discrimination, social stress, language barriers, and poverty are antecedents to and associated causes of health disparities. The disparities in infant mortality relate to poor access to prenatal care during pregnancy and the lack of access and appropriate heath services for women, such as preventive services, family planning, and appropriate nutrition and health care, throughout their life span.

- Infant mortality increases as the mother's level of education decreases.
- Poorer children are less likely to be immunized at 4 years of age and less likely to receive dental care.
- Rates of hospital admission are higher for people who live in low-income areas.
- Children of ethnic minorities and children from poor families are less likely to have physician office or hospital outpatient visits and more likely to have hospital emergency department visits.
- Children with Medicaid/public coverage are less likely to be in excellent health than children with private health insurance.
- Access to care for children is easier for whites and for children of higher income families than for minority and low-income families.

## CHANGING MORBIDITY: THE SOCIAL/EMOTIONAL ASPECTS OF PEDIATRIC PRACTICE

- **Changing morbidity** reflects the relationship among environmental, social, emotional, and developmental issues; child health status; and outcome. These observations are based on significant interactions of **biopsychosocial** influences on health and illness. Poverty and access to health care should be a major concern of pediatricians. These health issues include the following: school problems, learning disabilities, and attention problems; child and adolescent mood and anxiety disorders;

adolescent suicide and homicide; firearms in the home; school violence; human immunodeficiency virus (HIV); effects of media violence, obesity, and sexual activity; and substance use and abuse by adolescents.

- Currently, 20% to 25% of children are estimated to have some mental health problems; 5% to 6% of these problems are severe. Pediatricians are estimated to identify only 50% of mental health problems. The overall prevalence of psychosocial dysfunction of preschool and school-age children is 10% and 13%, respectively. Children from poor families are twice as likely to have psychosocial problems as children from higher income families. Nationwide, there is a lack of adequate mental health services for children. It will take the training of an adequate number of clinicians to address mental health services as well as requiring that insurance programs cover mental health as they do physical health services.

Important influences on children's health, in addition to poverty, include homelessness, single-parent families, parental divorce, domestic violence, both parents working, and inadequate child care. Related pediatric challenges include improving the quality of health care, social justice, equality in health care access, and improving the public health system. For adolescents, there are special concerns about sexuality, sexual orientation, pregnancy, substance use and abuse, violence, depression, and suicide.

## CULTURE

Culture is an active, dynamic, and complex process of the way people interact and behave in the world. Culture encompasses the concepts, beliefs, values (including nurturing of children), and standards of behavior, language, and dress attributable to people that give order to their experiences in the world, offer sense and purpose to their interactions with others, and provide meaning for their lives. Culture requires an attempt to understand, from the patient and family perspective, questions such as:

What is the nature of health?
What is the nature of illness? Where does it come from?
What is the approach to treatment?
What is the expected outcome?

An appropriate inquiry that addresses this realm includes open-ended questions, such as: "What *worries* (concerns) you the most about your child's illness?" or "What do you *think* has caused your child's illness?" These questions facilitate a discussion of parents' thoughts and feelings about the illness and its causes. Cultural understanding also includes concepts and beliefs about how one interacts with health professionals. The spiritual and religious aspects of health and health care can also be viewed from this perspective. These differences in perspectives, values, or beliefs may result in differences between the pediatrician and the patient and family. Significant conflicts may arise because religious or cultural practices may lead to the possibility of child abuse and neglect. In this circumstance, the pediatrician is required by law to report the suspected child abuse and neglect to the appropriate social service authorities (see Chapter 22).

Complementary and alternative medicine (CAM) practices constitute a part of the broad cultural perspective. It is estimated that 20% to 30% of all children and 50% to 75% of adolescents use CAM. Of children with chronic illness, 30% to 70% use CAM therapies, especially for asthma and cystic fibrosis, although only 30% to 60% of children and families tell their physicians about their use of CAM. Therapeutic modalities for CAM include biochemical, lifestyle, biomechanical, and bioenergetic treatments, as well as homeopathy. Some modalities may be effective, whereas others may be ineffective or even dangerous.

By 2023, half of U.S. children will be nonwhite. In many states, this shift already has occurred. Rapidly changing demographic shifts in populations make it likely that the pediatrician will encounter many different cultural identities. Understanding patient and family health beliefs and practices will enable pediatricians to practice better health care.

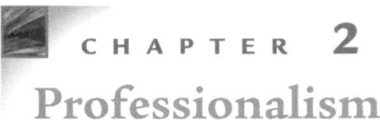

## CHAPTER 2
# Professionalism

## CONCEPT OF PROFESSIONALISM

Society provides a profession with economic, political, and social rewards. Professions have specialized knowledge and the potential to maintain a monopoly on power and control, remaining relatively autonomous. The profession's autonomy can be limited by societal needs. A profession exists as long as it fulfills its responsibilities for the social good.

Today, the activities of medical professionals are subject to explicit public rules of accountability. Governmental and other authorities grant limited autonomy to the professional organizations and their membership. City and municipal government departments of public health establish and implement heath standards and regulations. At the state level, boards of registration in medicine establish the criteria for obtaining and revoking medical licenses. The federal government regulates the standards of services, including Medicare, Medicaid, and the Food and Drug Administration. The Department of Health and Human Services regulates physician behavior in conducting research with the goal of protecting human subjects. The Health Care Quality Act of 1986 authorized the federal government to establish the National Practitioner Data Bank, which contains information about physicians (and other health care practitioners) who have been disciplined by a state licensing board, professional society, hospital, or health plan. Practitioners who have been named in medical malpractice judgments or settlements also are included. Hospitals are required to review information in this data bank every 2 years as part of clinician recredentialing. There are accrediting agencies for medical schools (Liaison Committee on Medical Education) and postgraduate training (Accreditation Council for Graduate Medical Education [ACGME]). The ACGME includes committees that review subspecialty training programs.

Historically, the most privileged professions have depended for their legitimacy on serving the public interest. The public trust of physicians is based on the physician's commitment to altruism. Many medical schools include variations on the traditional Hippocratic oath as part of the commencement ceremonies as a recognition of a physician's responsibility to put the interest of others ahead of self-interest.

The core of professionalism is embedded in the daily healing work of the physician and encompassed in the patient-physician relationship. Professionalism includes an appreciation for the cultural and religious/spiritual health beliefs of the patient, incorporating the ethical and moral values of the profession, and the moral values of the patient. The inappropriate actions of a few practicing physicians, physician investigators, and physicians in positions of power in the corporate world have created a societal demand to punish those involved and have led to the erosion of respect for the medical profession.

The American Academy of Pediatrics (AAP), the American Board of Pediatrics, the American Board of Internal Medicine, the Liaison Committee on Medical Education, the Medical Student Objectives Project of the Association of American Medical Colleges, and the ACGME in their Outcomes Project have called for increasing attention to professionalism in the practice of medicine and in the education of physicians.

## PROFESSIONALISM FOR PEDIATRICIANS

The American Board of Pediatrics adopted professional standards in 2000, and the AAP updated the policy statement and technical report on professionalism in 2007, as follows:

- **Honesty/integrity** is the consistent regard for the highest standards of behavior and the refusal to violate one's personal and professional codes. Maintaining integrity requires awareness of situations that may result in conflict of interest or that may result in personal gain at the expense of the best interest of the patient.
- **Reliability/responsibility** includes accountability to one's patients and their families, to society to ensure that the public's needs are addressed, and to the profession to ensure that the ethical precepts of practice are upheld. Inherent in this responsibility is reliability in completing assigned duties or fulfilling commitments. There also must be a willingness to accept responsibility for errors.
- **Respect for others** is the essence of humanism. The pediatrician must treat all persons with respect and regard for their individual worth and dignity, be aware of emotional, personal, family, and cultural influences on a patient's well-being, rights, and choices of medical care and respect appropriate patient confidentiality.

- **Compassion/empathy** is a crucial component of medical practice. The pediatrician must listen attentively, respond humanely to the concerns of patients and family members, and provide appropriate empathy for and relief of pain, discomfort, and anxiety as part of daily practice.
- **Self-improvement** is the pursuit of and commitment to providing the highest quality of health care through lifelong learning and education. The pediatrician must seek to learn from errors and aspire to excellence through self-evaluation and acceptance of the critiques of others.
- **Self-awareness/knowledge of limits** includes recognition of the need for guidance and supervision when faced with new or complex responsibilities. The pediatrician also must be insightful regarding the impact of his or her behavior on others and cognizant of appropriate professional boundaries.
- **Communication/collaboration** is crucial to providing the best care for patients. Pediatricians must work cooperatively and communicate effectively with patients and their families and with all health care providers involved in the care of their patients.
- **Altruism/advocacy** refers to unselfish regard for and devotion to the welfare of others. It is a key element of professionalism. Self-interest or the interests of other parties should not interfere with the care of one's patients and their families.

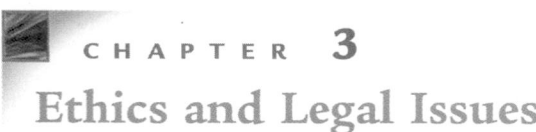

CHAPTER **3**

# Ethics and Legal Issues

## ETHICS IN HEALTH CARE

The ethics of health care are embedded in the process whereby patients, family members, and clinicians engage in medical decision making by balancing personal, family, cultural/religious/spiritual, and professional values. These values lead to choices about medical care. Ethical decision making relies on values to determine what kinds of decisions are best or appropriate for all. Sometimes ethical decision making in medical care is a matter of choosing the least harmful option for a patient among many adverse alternatives. In the day-to-day practice of medicine, although all clinical encounters may have an ethical component, major ethical challenges are infrequent.

The legal system defines the minimal standards of behavior required of physicians and the rest of society through the legislative, regulatory, and judicial systems. The role of the law is to provide for social order and adjudicate disputes, not to address ethical concerns. An example is a teenager who seeks birth control information and a prescription and would like to keep this information confidential. The laws are clear and support the principle of **confidentiality** for teenagers who are competent to decide about such issues. Using the concept of **limited confidentiality**, parents, teenagers and the pediatrician may all agree to openly discuss serious health challenges, such as suicidal ideation

and pregnancy. This reinforces the long-term goal of supporting the autonomy and identity of the teenager while encouraging appropriate conversations with parents.

Ethical problems derive from **value differences** among patients, families, and clinicians about choices and options in the provision of health care. Resolving these value differences involves several important ethical principles. **Autonomy**, which is based on the principle of **respect for persons**, means that competent adult patients can make choices about health care that they perceive to be in their best interests, after being appropriately informed about their particular health condition and the risks and benefits of alternatives of diagnostic tests and treatments. **Paternalism** challenges the principle of autonomy and involves the clinician deciding what is best for the patient based on how much information is provided. Paternalism, under certain circumstances, may be more appropriate than autonomy. These circumstances are usually emergency situations, when a patient has a serious life-threatening medical condition or a significant psychiatric disorder threatening oneself or others. Weighing the values of autonomy and paternalism can challenge the clinician. Other important ethical principles are those of **beneficence** (doing good), **nonmaleficence** (doing no harm or as little harm as possible), and **justice** (the values involved in the equality of the distribution of goods, services, benefits, and burdens to the individual, family, or society). In end-of-life decision making, the quality of life and how much suffering is too much become important considerations for the provision of palliative and hospice care (see Chapter 4). These principles apply to competent patients, who have the capacity for decision making and engage in the process of informed consent.

## ETHICAL PRINCIPLES RELATED TO INFANTS, CHILDREN, AND ADOLESCENTS

Children vary from being totally dependent on parents or guardians to meet their health care needs to being more independent. Infants and young children do not have the capacity for making medical decisions. Paternalism by parents and pediatricians in these circumstances is appropriate. Adolescents (<18 years of age), if competent, have the legal right to make medical decisions for themselves. Children 8 to 9 years old can understand how the body works and the meaning of certain procedures, and by age 14 to 15, young adolescents may be considered autonomous through the process of being designated a mature or emancipated minor or by having certain medical conditions. It is ethical for pediatricians to involve children in the decision-making process with information appropriate to their capacity to understand. The process of obtaining the **assent** of a child is consistent with this goal.

The principle of shared decision making is appropriate, but this process may be limited because of issues of confidentiality in the provision of medical care. A parent's concern about the side effects of immunization raises a conflict between the need to protect and support the health of the individual and the public with the rights of the individual and involves ethical issues of distributive justice in regard to the costs and distribution of the vaccinations and responsibility for side effects.

## LEGAL ISSUES

All competent patients of an age defined legally by each state (usually ≥18 years of age) are considered autonomous with regard to their health decisions. To have the capacity to decide, patients must:

- Understand the nature of the medical interventions and procedures, understand the risks and benefits of these interventions, and be able to communicate their decision.
- Reason, deliberate, and weigh the risks and benefits using their understanding about the implications of the decision on their own welfare.
- Apply a set of personal values to the decision-making process and show an awareness of the possible conflicts or differences in values as applied to the decisions to be made.

These requirements need to be placed within the context of medical care and applied to each case with its unique characteristics. Most young children are not able to meet the requirements for competency and need others, usually the parent, to make decisions for them. Legally, parents are given great discretion in making decisions for their children. This discretion is legally limited when there is child abuse and neglect, which triggers a further legal process in determining the best interests of the child.

Because laws vary by state, it is important to become familiar with the state laws. State, not federal, law determines when an adolescent can consent to medical care and when parents may access confidential adolescent medical information. The Health Insurance Portability and Accountability Act of 1996 (HIPAA), which became effective in 2003, requires a minimal standard of confidentiality protection. The law confers less confidentiality protection to minors than to adults. It is the pediatrician's responsibility to inform minors of their confidentiality rights and help them exercise these rights under the HIPAA regulations.

Under special circumstances, nonautonomous adolescents are granted the legal right to consent under state law when they are considered mature or emancipated minors or because of certain public health considerations, as follows:

- **Mature minors.** Some states have legally recognized that many adolescents age 14 and older can meet the cognitive criteria and emotional maturity for competence and may decide independently. The Supreme Court has decided that pregnant, mature minors have the constitutional right to make decisions about abortion without parental consent. Although many state legislatures require parental notification, pregnant adolescents wishing to have an abortion do not have to seek parental consent. The state must provide a judicial procedure to facilitate this decision making for adolescents.
- **Emancipated minors.** Children who are legally emancipated from parental control may seek medical treatment without parental consent. The definition varies from state to state, but generally includes children who have graduated from high school, are members of the armed forces, married, pregnant, runaways, are parents, live apart from their parents, and are financially independent, or are declared emancipated by a court.
- **Interests of the state (public health).** State legislatures have concluded that minors with certain medical conditions, such as sexually transmitted infections and other contagious diseases, pregnancy (including

prevention with the use of birth control), certain mental illnesses, and drug and alcohol abuse, may seek treatment for these conditions autonomously. States have an interest in limiting the spread of disease that may endanger the public health and in eliminating barriers to access for the treatment of certain conditions.

## ETHICAL ISSUES IN PRACTICE

Most often, the parent or guardian is the decision maker for young children. From an ethical perspective, clinicians should engage children and adolescents, based on their developmental capacity, in discussions about medical plans so that they have a good understanding of the nature of the treatments and alternatives, the side effects, and expected outcomes. There should be an assessment of the patient's understanding of the clinical situation, how the patient is responding, and the factors that may influence the patient's decisions. Pediatricians should always listen to and appreciate patients' requests for confidentiality and their hopes and wishes. The ultimate goal is to help nourish children's capacity to become as autonomous as is appropriate to their developmental stage.

### Confidentiality

Confidentiality is crucial to the provision of medical care and is an important part of the basis for a trusting patient-family-physician relationship. Confidentiality means that information about a patient should not be shared without consent. If confidentiality is broken, patients may experience great harm and may not seek needed medical care. Patient-physician confidentiality is an important value of the medical profession. See Chapter 67 for discussion of confidentiality in the care of adolescents.

### Ethical Issues in Genetic Testing and Screening in Children

The goal of **screening** is to identify diseases when there is no clinically identifiable risk factor for disease. Screening should take place only when there is a treatment available or when a diagnosis would benefit the child. **Testing** usually is performed when there is some clinically identifiable risk factor. Genetic testing and screening present special problems because test results have important implications. Some genetic screening (sickle cell anemia or cystic fibrosis) may reveal a carrier state, which may lead to choices about reproduction or create financial, psychosocial, and interpersonal problems (guilt, shame, social stigma, and discrimination in insurance and jobs). Confidentiality, beneficence, and the best interests of the child are the ethical principles involved in such decision making. Collaboration with, or referral to, a clinical geneticist is appropriate in helping the family with the complex issues of genetic counseling when a genetic disorder is detected or likely to be detected.

Newborn screening should not be used as a surrogate for parental testing. Examples of diseases that can be diagnosed by genetic screening, even though the manifestations of the disease process do not appear until later in life, are polycystic kidney disease; Huntington disease; certain cancers, such as breast cancer in some ethnic populations; and hemochromatosis. Parents may pressure the pediatrician to order genetic tests when the child is still young, for the parents' purposes. Testing for these disorders should be delayed until the child has the capacity for informed consent or assent and is competent to make decisions, unless there is a direct benefit to the child at the time of testing.

## Religious Issues and Ethics

When religious tenets interfere with the health and well-being of the child, the pediatrician is required to act in the best interests of the child. Freedom of religion does not justify children being harmed. When an infant or child whose parents have a religious prohibition against a blood transfusion needs a transfusion to save his or her life, the courts always have intervened to allow a transfusion. In contrast, parents with strong religious beliefs under some state laws may refuse immunizations for their children. However, state governments can mandate immunizations for all children during disease outbreaks or epidemics. By requiring immunization of all, including individuals who object on religious grounds, the state government is using the principle of **distributive justice,** which states that all members of society must share in the burdens and the benefits to have a just society.

## Children as Human Subjects in Research

The goal of research is to develop new and generalized knowledge. Parents may give informed permission for children to participate in research under certain conditions. Children cannot give consent but may assent or dissent to research protocols. Special federal regulations have been developed to protect child and adolescent participants in human investigation. These regulations provide additional safeguards beyond the safeguards provided for adult participants in research, while still providing the opportunity for children to benefit from the scientific advances of research.

Many parents with seriously ill children hope that the research protocol will have direct benefit for their particular child. The greatest challenge for researchers is to be clear with parents that research is not treatment. This fact should be addressed as sensitively and compassionately as possible.

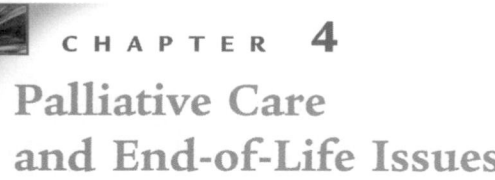

CHAPTER **4**

# Palliative Care and End-of-Life Issues

The death of a child is one of life's most difficult experiences. The **palliative care** approach to a child's medical care should be instituted when medical diagnosis, intervention, and treatment cannot reasonably be expected to affect the imminence of death. In these circumstances, the goals of care focus on improving the quality of life, maintaining dignity, and ameliorating the suffering of the seriously ill child. Central to this approach is the willingness of clinicians to look beyond the traditional medical goals of curing disease and preserving life. They need to look toward enhancing the lives of the child and working with family members and close friends when the child's needs are no longer met by curative goals. High-quality palliative care is an expected standard at the end of life.

Palliative care in pediatrics is not simply end-of-life care. There are conditions where death is not predictably imminent, and a child's needs are best met by the palliative care approach. Children needing palliative care have been described as falling into four basic groups (Table 4-1). These conditions present different timelines and different models of medical intervention. Yet they all share the need to attend to concrete elements, which affect the quality of a child's death, mediated by medical, psychosocial, cultural, and spiritual concerns.

| TABLE 4-1 Conditions Appropriate for Pediatric Palliative Care* |
| --- |
| **CONDITIONS FOR WHICH CURATIVE TREATMENT IS POSSIBLE BUT MAY FAIL** |
| Advanced or progressive cancer or cancer with a poor prognosis |
| Complex and severe congenital or acquired heart disease |
| **CONDITIONS REQUIRING INTENSIVE LONG-TERM TREATMENT AIMED AT MAINTAINING THE QUALITY OF LIFE** |
| Human immunodeficiency virus infection |
| Cystic fibrosis |
| Severe gastrointestinal disorders or malformations, such as gastroschisis |
| Severe epidermolysis bullosa |
| Severe immunodeficiencies |
| Renal failure in cases in which dialysis, transplantation, or both are not available or indicated |
| Chronic or severe respiratory failure |
| Muscular dystrophy |
| **PROGRESSIVE CONDITIONS IN WHICH TREATMENT IS EXCLUSIVELY PALLIATIVE AFTER DIAGNOSIS** |
| Progressive metabolic disorders |
| Certain chromosomal abnormalities, such as trisomy 13 or trisomy 18 |
| Severe forms of osteogenesis imperfecta |
| **CONDITIONS INVOLVING SEVERE, NONPROGRESSIVE DISABILITY, CAUSING EXTREME VULNERABILITY TO HEALTH COMPLICATIONS** |
| Severe cerebral palsy with recurrent infection or difficult-to-control symptoms |
| Extreme prematurity |
| Severe neurologic sequelae of infectious disease |
| Hypoxic or anoxic brain injury |
| Holoprosencephaly or other severe brain malformations |

*Premature death is likely or expected with many of these conditions.
From Himelstein BP, Hilden JM, Morstad Boldt A, Weissman D: Pediatric palliative care, *N Engl J Med* 350:1752–1762, 2004. Copyright ©2004 Massachusetts Medical Society. All rights reserved.

The sudden death of a child also requires elements of the palliative care approach, although conditions do not allow for the full spectrum of involvement. Many of these deaths involve emergency medicine caregivers and first responders in the field, and they may involve dramatic situations where no relationship may exist between caregivers and the bereaved family. Families who have not had time to prepare for the tragedy of an unexpected death require considerable support. Palliative care can make important contributions to the end-of-life and bereavement issues families face in these circumstances. This may become complicated in circumstances where the cause of the death must be fully explored. The need to investigate the possibility of child abuse or neglect subjects the family to intense scrutiny and may create guilt and anger directed at the medical team.

## PALLATIVE AND END-OF-LIFE CARE

Palliative treatment is directed toward the relief of symptoms as well as assistance with anticipated adaptations that may cause distress and diminish the quality of life of the dying child. Elements of palliative care include pain management; expertise with feeding and nutritional issues at the end of life; and minimizing nausea and vomiting, bowel obstruction, air hunger, and fatigue. Psychological elements of palliative care have a profound importance and include sensitivity to bereavement, a developmental perspective of a child's understanding of death, helping clarify the goals of care, and ethical issues. Curative care and palliative care can coexist; aggressive pain medication may be provided while curative treatment is continued in the hopes of a remission or improved health status. Palliative care is delivered with a multidisciplinary approach, giving a broad range of expertise to patients and families as well as providing a supportive network for the caregivers. Caregivers involved may be pediatricians, nurses, mental health professionals, social workers and pastoral care.

A model of integrated palliative care rests on the following principles:

- *Respect for the dignity of patients and families.* The clinician should respect and listen to patient and family goals, preferences, and choices. School-age children can articulate preferences about how they wish to be treated. Adolescents, by the age of 14, can engage in decision making (see Section 12). The pediatrician should assist the patient and the family in understanding the diagnosis, treatment options, and prognosis; help clarify the goals of care; promote informed choices; allow for the free flow of information; and listen to and discuss the social-emotional concerns. **Advanced care** (advance directives) should be instituted with the child and parents, allowing discussions about what they would like as treatment options as the end of life nears. Differences of opinion between the family and the pediatrician should be addressed by identifying the multiple perspectives, reflecting on possible conflicts, and altruistically coming to agreements that validate the patient and family perspectives, yet reflect sound practice. **Hospital ethics committees** and consultation services

are important resources for the pediatrician and family members.
- *Access to comprehensive and compassionate palliative care.* The clinician should address the physical symptoms, comfort, and functional capacity, with special attention to pain and other symptoms associated with the dying process, and respond empathically to the psychological distress and human suffering, providing treatment options. Respite care should be available at any time during the illness to allow the family caretakers to rest and renew.
- *Use of interdisciplinary resources.* Because of the complexity of care, no one clinician can provide all the needed services. The team members may include primary and subspecialty physicians, nurses in the hospital/facility or for home visits, the pain management team, psychologists, social workers, pastoral care, schoolteachers, friends of the family, and peers of the child. The child and family should be in a position to decide who should know what during all phases of the illness process.
- *Acknowledging and providing support for caregivers.* The death of a child is difficult to accept and understand. The primary caregivers of the child, family, and friends need opportunities to address their own emotional concerns. Siblings of the child who is dying react emotionally and cognitively based on their developmental level. Opportunities to have team meetings to address thoughts and feelings of team members are crucial. Soon after the death of the child, the care team should review the experience with the parents and family and share their reactions and feelings. Institutional support may include time to attend funerals, counseling for the staff, opportunities for families to return to the hospital, and scheduled ceremonies to commemorate the death of the child.
- *Commitment to quality improvement of palliative care through research and education.* Hospitals should develop support systems and staff to monitor the quality of care continually, assess the need for appropriate resources, and evaluate the responses of the patient and family members to the treatment program. Issues often arise over less than completely successful attempts to control the dying child's symptoms or differences between physicians and family members in the timing of the realization that death is imminent. Consensus results in better palliative care from the medical and psychosocial perspective.

**Hospice care** is a treatment program for the end of life, providing the range of palliative care services by an interdisciplinary team, including specialists in the bereavement and end-of-life process. Many insurance companies do not provide coverage for these services; children younger than 17 years of age make up only 0.4% of hospice admissions. Typically, hospice uses the adult Medicare model, requiring a prognosis of death within 6 months and the cessation of curative efforts for children to receive hospice services. Recently, some states have developed alternative pediatric models where curative efforts may continue while the higher level of coordinated end-of-life services may be applied.

# BEREAVEMENT

**Bereavement** refers to the process of psychological and spiritual accommodation to death on the part of the child and the child's family. **Grief** has been defined as the emotional response caused by a loss, including pain, distress, and physical and emotional suffering. It is a normal adaptive human response to death. Palliative care attends to the grief reaction. Assessing the coping resources and vulnerabilities of the affected family before death takes place is central to the palliative care approach.

Parental grief is recognized as being more intense and sustained than other types of grief. Most parents work through their grief. Complicated grief, a pathologic manifestation of continued and disabling grief, is rare. Parents who share their problems with others during the child's illness, who have had access to psychological support during the last month of their child's life, and who have had closure sessions with the attending staff, are more likely to resolve their grief.

A particularly difficult issue for parents is whether to talk with their child about the child's imminent death. Although evidence suggests that sharing accurate and truthful information with a dying child is beneficial, each individual case presents its own complexities based on the child's age, cognitive development, disease, timeline of disease, and parental psychological state. Parents are more likely to regret not talking with their child about death than having done so. Among those who did not talk with their child about death, parents who sensed their child was aware of imminent death, parents of older children, and mothers more than fathers were more likely to feel regretful.

# COGNITIVE ISSUES IN CHILDREN AND ADOLESCENTS: UNDERSTANDING DEATH AND DYING

The pediatrician should communicate with children about what is happening to them, while respecting the cultural and personal preferences of the family. A developmental understanding of children's concepts of health and illness helps frame the discussion with children and can help parents understand how their child is grappling with the situation. Piaget's theories of cognitive development, which help illustrate children's concepts of death and disease, are categorized as sensorimotor, preoperational, concrete operations, and formal operations.

For very young children, up to 2 years of age (sensorimotor), death is seen as separation, and there is probably no concept of death. The associated behaviors in grieving children of this age usually include protesting and difficulty of attachment to other adults. The degree of difficulty depends on the availability of other nurturing people with whom the child has had a good previous attachment.

Children from 3 to 5 years of age (preoperational) (sometimes called the magic years) have trouble grasping the meaning of the illness and the permanence of the death. Their language skills at this age make understanding their moods and behavior difficult. Because of a developing sense of guilt, death may be viewed as punishment.

If the child's younger sibling suddenly died and the child previously wished the infant to have died, the reality of a sibling's death may be seen psychologically as being caused by the child's wishful thinking. They can feel overwhelmed when confronted with the strong emotional reactions of their parents.

In children age 6 to 11 years of age (late preoperational to concrete operational), the finality of death gradually comes to be understood. Magical thinking gives way to a need for detailed information to gain a sense of control. Older children in this range have a strong need to control their emotions by compartmentalizing and intellectualizing.

In adolescents (>12 years of age) (formal operations), death is a reality and is seen as universal and irreversible. Adolescents handle death issues at the abstract or philosophical level and can be realistic. They may also avoid emotional expression and information, instead relying on anger or disdain. Adolescents can discuss withholding treatments. Their wishes, hopes, and fears should be attended to and respected.

# CULTURAL, RELIGIOUS, AND SPIRITUAL CONCERNS ABOUT PALLIATIVE CARE AND END-OF-LIFE DECISIONS

Understanding the family's religious/spiritual or cultural beliefs and values about death and dying can help the pediatrician work with the family to integrate these beliefs, values, and practices into the palliative care plan. Cultures vary regarding the roles family members have, the site of treatment for dying people, and the preparation of the body. Some ethnic groups expect the clinical team to speak with the oldest family member or only to the head of the family outside the patient's presence. Some families involve the entire extended family in decision making. For some families, dying at home can bring the family bad luck, whereas others believe that the patient's spirit will become lost if the death occurs in the hospital. In some traditions, the health care team cleans and prepares the body, whereas in others, family members prefer to complete this ritual. Religious/spiritual or cultural practices may include prayer, anointing, laying on of the hands, an exorcism ceremony to undo a curse, amulets, and other religious objects placed on the child or at the bedside. Families differ in the idea of organ donation and the acceptance of autopsy. Decisions, rituals, and withholding of palliative or lifesaving procedures that could harm the child or are not in the best interests of the child should be addressed. Quality palliative care attends to this complexity and helps parents and families through the death of a child while honoring the familial, cultural, and spiritual values.

# ETHICAL ISSUES IN END-OF-LIFE DECISION MAKING

Before speaking with a child about death, the caregiver should assess the child's age, experience, and level of development; the child's understanding and involvement in end-of-life decision making; the parents' emotional acceptance of death; their coping strategies; and their philosophical, spiritual, and cultural views of death. These may change over time, and the use of open-ended questions to repeatedly assess these areas contributes to the end-of-life process. The care of a dying child can create **ethical dilemmas** involving **autonomy, beneficence** (doing good), **nonmaleficence** (not initiating and eliminating or mitigating harm, pain, and suffering), truth telling, confidentiality, or the physician's duty. It is extremely difficult for parents to know when the burdens of continued medical care are no longer appropriate for their child. Pediatricians, patients, and family members may differ on when this time has come, depending on their beliefs and values of what constitutes quality of life, when life ceases to be worth living, and their religious/ spiritual, cultural, and philosophical beliefs. The most important ethical principle is what is in the **best interest** of the child as determined through the process of **shared decision making**, **informed permission/consent** from the parents, and **assent** from the child. Sensitive and meaningful communication with the family, in their own terms, is essential. The physician, patient, and family must **negotiate** the goals of continued medical treatment while recognizing the burdens and benefits of the medical intervention plan. There is no ethical or legal difference between withholding treatment and withdrawing treatment, although many parents and physicians see the latter as more challenging. Family members and the patient should agree about what are appropriate **do not resuscitate (DNR)** orders. Forgoing some measures does not preclude other measures being implemented, based on the needs and wishes of the patient and family. When there are serious differences among parents, children, and physicians on these matters, the physician may consult with the **hospital ethics committee** or, as a last resort, turn to the legal system by filing a report about potential abuse or neglect.

## SUGGESTED READING

American Academy of Pediatrics, Committee on Bioethics: Professionalism in pediatrics: Statement of principles, *Pediatrics* 120:895–897, 2007.

American Academy of Pediatrics, Committee on Psychosocial Aspects of Child and Family Health: The new morbidity revisited: A renewed commitment to the psychosocial aspects of pediatric care, *Pediatrics* 108:1227–1230, 2001.

Bloom B, Cohen RA: Summary Health Statistics for U.S. Children: National Health Interview Survey, 2006, National Center for Health Statistics, *Vital Health Stat* 10(234), 2007.

Flores G, Tomany-Korman SC: Racial and ethnic disparities in medical and dental health, access to care and use of health services in U.S. children, *Pediatrics* 121: e286–e298, 2008.

Gluckman PD, Hanson MA, Cooper C, et al: Effect on in-utero and early-life considerations on adult health and disease, *N Engl J Med* 359:61–73, 2008.

Hamilton BE, Martin JA, Ventura SJ: Births: Preliminary Data for 2006, *Nat Vital Stat Rep* 56(7):2007.

National Center for Health Statistics: *Health, United States: With Chartbook on Trends in the Health of Americans,* Hyattsville, MD, 2007.

# GROWTH AND DEVELOPMENT

David A. Levine

## THE HEALTH MAINTENANCE VISIT

The frequent office visits for health maintenance in the first 2 years of life are more than *physicals*. Although a somatic history and physical examination are important parts of each visit, many other issues are discussed, including nutrition, development, safety, and behavior.

Disorders of growth and development are often associated with chronic or severe illness or may be the only symptom of parental neglect or abuse. Although normal growth and development does not eliminate a serious or chronic illness, in general, it supports a judgment that a child is healthy except for acute, often benign, illnesses that do not affect growth and development.

The processes of growth and development are intertwined. However, it is convenient to refer to **growth** as the increase in size and **development** as an increase in function of processes related to body and mind. Being familiar with normal patterns of growth and development allows those practitioners who care for children to recognize and manage abnormal variations.

The genetic makeup and the physical, emotional, and social environment of the individual determine how a child grows and develops throughout childhood. One goal of pediatrics is to help each child achieve his or her individual potential through periodically monitoring and screening for the normal progression or abnormalities of growth and development. The American Academy of Pediatrics recommends routine office visits in the first week of life (depending on timing of nursery discharge): at 2 weeks; at 2, 4, 6, 9, 12, 15, and 18 months; at 2 years, 2½ years, at 3 years, then annually up to age 6; and every 2 years between age 6 and adolescence. During adolescence, a complete health maintenance visit is recommended every 2 years, with an annual risk-assessment visit every year (see Fig. 9-1).

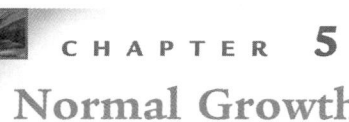

## CHAPTER 5

## Normal Growth

Deviations in growth patterns may be nonspecific or may be important indicators of serious and chronic medical disorders. An accurate measurement of length/height, weight, and head circumference should be obtained at every health supervision visit. Table 5-1 summarizes several convenient benchmarks to evaluate normal growth. Growth should be measured and compared with statistical norms in a standard fashion on growth charts. Serial measurements are much more useful than single measurements to detect deviations from a particular child's growth pattern even if the value remains within statistically defined normal limits (percentiles). Following the trend helps define whether growth is within acceptable limits or warrants further evaluation.

### TABLE 5-1 Rules of Thumb for Growth

#### WEIGHT

1. Weight loss in first few days: 5%–10% of birth weight
2. Return to birth weight: 7–10 days of age
   Double birth weight: 4–5 mo
   Triple birth weight: 1 yr
   Quadruple birth weight: 2 yr
3. Average weights:
   3.5 kg at birth
   10 kg at 1 yr
   20 kg at 5 yr
   30 kg at 10 yr
4. Daily weight gain:
   20–30 g for first 3–4 mo
   15–20 g for rest of the first yr
5. Average annual weight gain: 5 lb between 2 yr and puberty (spurts and plateaus may occur)

#### HEIGHT

1. Average length: 20 in at birth, 30 in at 1 yr
2. At age 3 yr, the average child is 3 ft tall
3. At age 4 yr, the average child is 40 in tall (double birth length)
4. Average annual height increase: 2–3 in between age 4 yr and puberty

#### HEAD CIRCUMFERENCE (HC)

1. Average HC: 35 cm at birth (13.5 in)
2. HC increases: 1 cm/mo for first yr (2 cm/mo for first 3 mo, then slower); 10 cm for rest of life

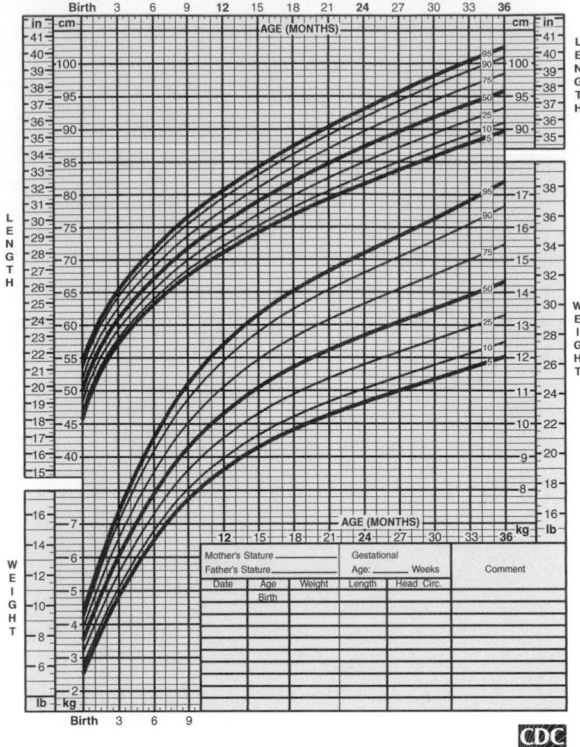

**FIGURE 5-1**

**Length-by-age and weight-by-age percentiles for boys, birth to 36 months of age.** Developed by the National Center for Health Statistics in collaboration with the National Center for Chronic Disease Prevention and Health Promotion. *(From Centers for Disease Control and Prevention, Atlanta, Ga, 2000. Available at http://www.cdc.gov/growthcharts.)*

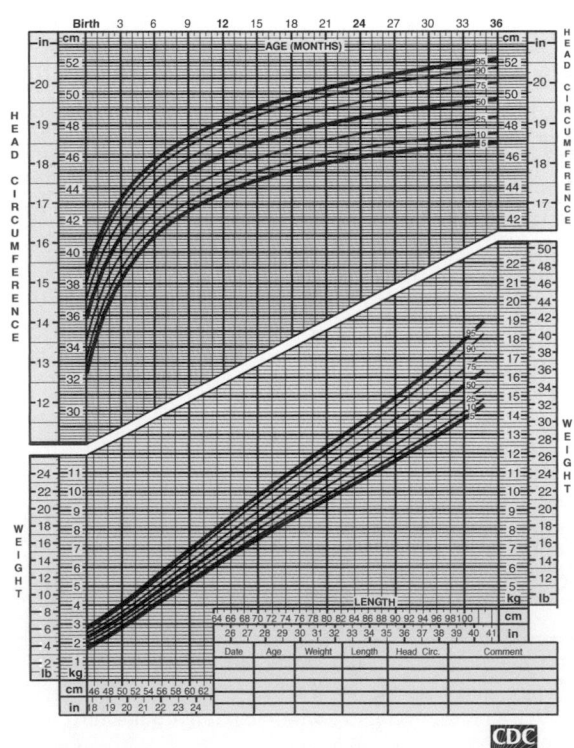

**FIGURE 5-2**

**Head circumference and weight-by-length percentiles for boys, birth to 36 months of age.** Developed by the National Center for Health Statistics in collaboration with the National Center for Chronic Disease Prevention and Health Promotion. *(From Centers for Disease Control and Prevention, Atlanta, Ga, 2000. Available at http://www.cdc.gov/growthcharts.)*

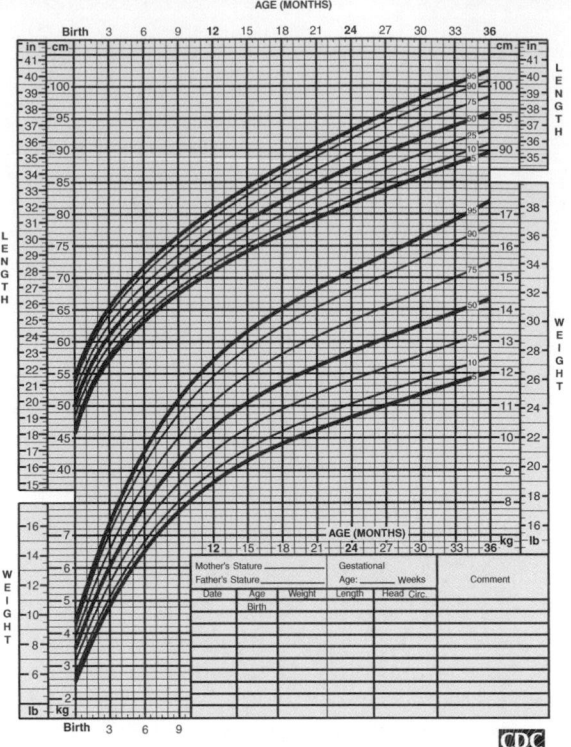

**FIGURE 5-3**

**Stature-for-age and weight-for-age percentiles for girls, 2 to 20 years of age.** Developed by the National Center for Health Statistics in collaboration with the National Center for Chronic Disease Prevention and Health Promotion. *(From Centers for Disease Control and Prevention, Atlanta, Ga, 2000. Available at http://www.cdc.gov/growthcharts.)*

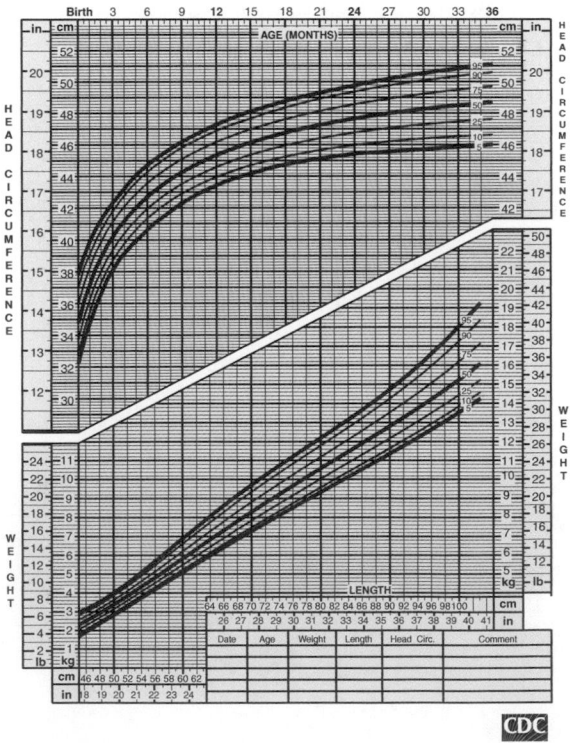

**FIGURE 5-4**

**Body mass index–for-age percentiles for girls, 2 to 20 years of age.** Developed by the National Center for Health Statistics in collaboration with the National Center for Chronic Disease Prevention and Health Promotion. *(From Centers for Disease Control and Prevention, Atlanta, Ga, 2000. Available at http: //www.cdc.gov/growthcharts.)*

Growth is assessed by plotting accurate measurements on growth charts and comparing each set of measurements with previous measurements obtained at health maintenance visits or at other visits if there is a concern over the child's growth pattern. Please see examples in Figures 5-1 to 5-4. Complete charts can be found at http://www.cdc.gov/growthcharts. The body mass index is defined as body weight in kilograms divided by height in meters squared. The body mass index is an index for classifying adiposity and is recommended as a screening tool for children and adolescents to determine whether an individual is overweight or at risk for being overweight (see Chapter 29).

Because growth charts are based on a population sample, they make it seem that children grow in a smooth, continuous fashion. However, normal growth patterns have spurts and plateaus, so some shifting on percentile graphs can be expected. Large shifts in percentiles warrant attention, as do large discrepancies in height, weight, and head circumference percentiles. When caloric intake is inadequate, the weight percentile falls first, then the height, and, lastly, the head circumference. Caloric intake may be poor as a result of inadequate feeding or because the child is not receiving adequate attention and stimulation (*nonorganic* failure to thrive [see Chapter 21]).

Caloric intake also may be inadequate because of increased caloric needs. Children with chronic illnesses, such as heart failure or cystic fibrosis, may require a significantly higher caloric intake to sustain growth. An increasing weight percentile in the face of a falling height percentile suggests hypothyroidism. Head circumference may be disproportionately large when there is familial megalocephaly, hydrocephalus, or merely *catch-up* growth in a neurologically normal premature infant. A child is considered microcephalic if head circumference is less than the third percentile, even if length and weight measurements also are proportionately low. Serial measurements of head circumference are crucial during infancy, a period of rapid brain development, and should be plotted regularly until the child is 3 years of age. Any suspicion of abnormal growth warrants at least close follow-up, further evaluation, or both.

## CHAPTER 6
# Disorders of Growth

The most common reasons for deviant measurements are technical (i.e., faulty equipment and human errors in measurement or plotting). Repeating a deviant measurement should be the first step. Separate growth charts are available for very low birth weight infants (weight <1500 g) and for children of various nationalities and those with Turner syndrome, Down syndrome, achondroplasia, and various other dysmorphology syndromes.

Variability in body proportions occurs from fetal to adult life. Newborns' heads are significantly larger in proportion to the rest of their body. This difference gradually disappears as the child gets older. Differences in body proportions depend on variations in the growth rates of parts of the body or organ systems. Certain growth disturbances result in characteristic changes in the proportional sizes of the trunk, extremities, and head. Patterns requiring further assessment are summarized in Table 6-1.

Evaluating a child over time often elucidates the growth pattern as normal or abnormal. This evaluation of the growth pattern should be coupled with a careful history and physical examination. Parental heights may be useful when deciding whether to observe or proceed with a further evaluation.

For a girl, midparental height is calculated as follows:

$$\frac{\text{Paternal height (inches)} + \text{Maternal height (inches)}}{2} - 2.5$$

For a boy, midparental height is calculated as follows:

$$\frac{\text{Paternal height (inches)} + \text{Maternal height (inches)}}{2} + 2.5$$

Midparental height determination is only a gross approximation. Actual growth depends on too many variables to make an accurate prediction for every child. The growth pattern of a child with low weight, length, and head circumference is commonly associated with **familial short stature** (see Chapter 173). These children are genetically normal but are smaller than most children. A child who, by age, is preadolescent or adolescent and who starts puberty later than others may have the normal variant called **constitutional short stature** (see Chapter 173). These children should be examined closely for abnormalities of pubertal development, although most are normal. Girls are considered normal if there is any development of secondary sexual characteristics (e.g., breast budding) on or before the 14th birthday and menarche occur by 16 years of age. Girls who do not start menstruation until 16 years of age usually are smaller than their peers at 12 and 13 years of age. Similar patterns are observed in boys who start puberty later (see Chapter 174).

In many children, growth moves to lower percentiles during their first year of life. These children often start out in high growth percentiles, but between 6 and 18 months they assume a lower percentile until they match their genetic programming, and then begin to grow along new, lower percentiles. They usually do not decrease more than two major percentiles. They have normal developmental, behavioral, and physical examination. These children with *catch-down growth* should be followed closely, but no further evaluation is warranted.

Children recovering from neonatal illnesses often exhibit *catch-up growth*. Infants who were born small for gestational age or prematurely ingest more breast milk or formula, unless there are complications that require extra calories, usually catch up in the first six months. Families should be taught to feed these infants on demand and provide as much as they want unless they are vomiting (not just spitting up [see Chapter 128]). Some of these infants may benefit from a higher caloric content formula if they are formula-fed. Many risk factors that may have led to the infant being born small or early are the same psychosocial risks that may contribute to nonorganic failure to thrive (see Chapter 21).

**TABLE 6-1  Specific Growth Patterns Requiring Further Evaluation**

| Pattern | Representative Diagnoses to Consider | Further Evaluation |
| --- | --- | --- |
| Weight, length, head circumference all <5th percentile | Familial short stature | Midparental heights |
| | Constitutional short stature | Evaluation of pubertal development |
| | Intrauterine insult | Examination of prenatal records |
| | Genetic abnormality | Chromosome analysis |
| Discrepant percentiles (e.g., weight 5th, length 5th, head circumference 50th, or other discrepancies) | Normal variant (familial or constitutional) | Midparental heights |
| | Endocrine growth failure | Thyroid hormone |
| | Caloric insufficiency | Growth factors, provocative growth hormone testing |
| | | Evaluation of pubertal development |
| Declining percentiles | *Catch-down growth* | Complete history and physical examination |
| | | Dietary and social history |
| | | Failure to thrive evaluation |

Growth of the nervous system is most rapid in the first 2 years, correlating with increasing physical, emotional, behavioral, and cognitive development. There is rapid change again during adolescence. Osseous maturation (bone age) is determined from radiographs on the basis of the number and size of calcified epiphyseal centers; the size, shape, density, and sharpness of outline of the ends of bones; and the distance separating the epiphyseal center from the zone of provisional calcification.

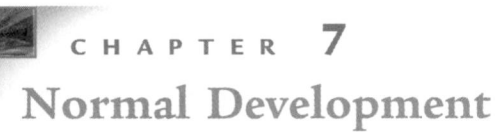

# CHAPTER 7

# Normal Development

## PHYSICAL ASSESSMENT

Parallel to the changes in the developing brain (cognition, language, behavior) are changes in the physical development of the body.

## NEWBORN PERIOD

Primitive neonatal reflexes are unique in the newborn period. Any asymmetry, increase, or decrease in tone elicited by passive movement may indicate a significant central nervous system abnormality and requires further evaluation. Similarly, a delay in the expected disappearance of the reflexes may warrant an evaluation of the central nervous system. The most important reflexes to assess during the newborn period are as follows:

The **Moro reflex** is elicited by allowing the infant's head gently to move back suddenly (from a few inches off the mattress). This results in abduction and upward movement of the arms followed by adduction and flexion.

The **rooting reflex** is elicited by touching the corner of the infant's mouth, resulting in lowering of the lower lip on the same side with tongue movement toward the stimulus. The face may turn to the stimulus.

The **sucking reflex** occurs with almost any object placed in the newborn's mouth. The infant responds with vigorous sucking. The sucking reflex is replaced later by voluntary sucking.

The **grasp reflex** occurs when placing an object, such as a finger, onto the infant's palm (palmar grasp) or sole (plantar grasp). The infant responds by flexing fingers or curling the toes.

The **asymmetric tonic neck reflex** is elicited by placing the infant supine and turning the head to the side. This placement results in ipsilateral extension of the arm and the leg into a "fencing" position. The contralateral side flexes as well.

See Sections 11 and 26 for additional information on the newborn period.

## LATER INFANCY

With the development of gross motor skills, the infant is first able to control his or her posture, then proximal musculature, and lastly distal musculature. As the infant progresses through these developmental stages, the parents may notice orthopedic deformities (see Chapters 201 and 202). The infant also may have deformities that are related to intrauterine positioning. Physical examination should indicate whether the deformity is fixed or is able to be moved passively into the proper position. When the infant positions a joint in an abnormal fashion, but the examiner is able to move the extremity passively into the proper position, this deformity has a high likelihood of resolving with the progression of gross motor development. Fixed deformities warrant immediate pediatric orthopedic consultation (see Section 26).

Evaluation of vision and ocular movements is important to prevent the serious outcome of strabismus. The cover test and light reflex should be performed at every health maintenance visit (see Chapter 179).

## LATE SCHOOL-AGE PERIOD/EARLY ADOLESCENCE

Older school-age children, who begin to participate in competitive sports, should have a comprehensive sports history and physical examination, including evaluation of the cardiovascular system. The American Academy of Pediatrics sports preparticipation form is excellent for documenting cardiovascular and other risks. Before the examination, the patient and parent should be interviewed to assess cardiovascular risk. Any history of heart disease or a murmur must be referred for evaluation by a pediatric cardiologist. Similarly, a child with a history of dyspnea or chest pain on exertion, irregular heart rate (skipped beats, palpitations), or syncope should be referred to a pediatric cardiologist for further evaluation. A family history of a primary (immediate family) or secondary (immediate family's immediate family) atherosclerotic disease (myocardial infarction or cerebrovascular disease) before 50 years of age or sudden unexplained death at any age also requires additional assessment.

Children interested in contact sports should be assessed for special vulnerabilities. Similarly, vision should be assessed as a crucial part of a comprehensive history and physical examination before participation in sports.

## ADOLESCENCE

Adolescents need a comprehensive health assessment to ensure that they progress through puberty without major problems (see Chapters 67 and 68). Other issues in physical development include scoliosis, obesity, and trauma (see Chapters 29 and 202). Most scoliosis is mild and requires only observation for progression. Obesity may first become manifest during childhood and is an issue for many adolescents. Orthopedic problems may arise from trauma to developing joints and bones (see Chapter 198).

Sexual maturity is another important issue in adolescents. All adolescents should be assessed to determine the sexual maturity rating (see Chapter 67). Monitoring the progression through sexual maturity rating stages provides an ongoing evaluation of puberty.

## DEVELOPMENTAL MILESTONES

The use of milestones to assess development focuses on discrete behaviors that the clinician can observe or accept as present by parental report. This approach is based on comparing the patient's behavior with that of many normal children whose behaviors evolve in a uniform sequence within specific age ranges (see Chapter 8). The development of the neuromuscular system, similar to that of other organ systems, is determined first by genetic endowment and then molded by environmental influences.

Although a sequence of specific, easily measured behaviors can adequately represent some areas of development (**gross motor**, **fine motor**, and **language**), other areas, particularly social and emotional development, are not adequately assessed. Easily measured developmental milestones are well established only through 6 years of age. Other types of assessment (intelligence tests, achievement tests, school performance, personality profiles, and neurodevelopmental assessments) that expand the developmental milestone approach beyond the 6 years of age are available for older children. These tests generally require time and expertise in administration and interpretation that are not available in the primary care setting.

## PSYCHOSOCIAL ASSESSMENT

### Bonding and Attachment in Infancy

The terms bonding and attachment describe the affective relationships between parents and infants. **Bonding** occurs shortly after birth and reflects the feelings of the parents toward the newborn (unidirectional). **Attachment** involves reciprocal feelings between parent and infant and develops gradually over the first year. Effective bonding in the postpartum period may enhance the development of attachment.

Attachment of infants outside of the newborn period is crucial for optimal development. Infants who receive *extra* attention, such as parents responding immediately to any crying or fussiness, show less crying and fussiness at the end of the first year. **Stranger anxiety** develops between 9 and 18 months of age, when infants normally become insecure about separation from the primary caregiver. The infant's new motor skills and attraction to novelty may lead to headlong plunges into new adventures that result in fright or pain followed by frantic efforts to find and cling to the primary caregiver. The result is dramatic swings from stubborn independence to clinging dependence that can be frustrating and confusing to parents. With a secure attachment, this period of ambivalence may be shorter and less tumultuous.

### Developing Autonomy in Early Childhood

Toddlers build on attachment and begin developing autonomy that allows separation from parents. In times of stress, toddlers often cling to their parents, but in their usual activities they may be actively separated (frequently saying "No!" to their parents). Ages 2 to 3 years are a time of major accomplishments in fine motor skills, social skills, cognitive skills, and language skills. The dependency of infancy yields to developing independence, and the "I can do it myself" age. Limit setting is essential to balance the child's emerging independence.

### School Readiness

When a toddler has achieved autonomy and independence, school readiness should be assessed. Readiness for preschool depends on the development of autonomy and the ability of the parent and the child to separate for hours at a time. Preschool experiences help 3- to 4-year-old children develop socialization skills; improve language; increase skill building in areas such as colors, numbers, and letters; and increase problem solving (puzzles).

Readiness for school (kindergarten) requires emotional maturity, peer group and individual social skills, cognitive abilities, and fine and gross motor skills (Table 7-1). Other issues include chronologic age and gender. Although not a perfect association, children do better in kindergarten if their fifth birthday is at least 4 to 6 months before the

**TABLE 7-1 Evaluating School Readiness**

**PHYSICIAN OBSERVATIONS**
**(BEHAVIORS OBSERVED IN THE OFFICE)**

Ease of separation of the child from the parent
Speech development and articulation
Understanding of and ability to follow complex directions
Specific preacademic skills
Knowledge of colors
Counts to 10
Knows age, first and last name, address, and phone number
Ability to copy shapes
Motor skills
Stand on one foot, skip, and catch a bounced ball
Dresses and undresses without assistance

**PARENT OBSERVATIONS**
**(QUESTIONS ANSWERED BY HISTORY)**

Does the child play well with other children?
Does the child separate well, such as a child playing in the backyard alone with occasional monitoring by the parent?
Does the child show interest in books, letters, and numbers?
Can the child sustain attention to quiet activities?
How frequent are toilet-training *accidents*?

beginning of school. In addition, girls usually are ready earlier than boys. Knowledge of the prior developmental status also helps. If the child is in less than the average developmental range, he or she should not be forced into early school. Holding a child back for reasons of developmental delay, in the false hope that the child will catch up, can also lead to difficulties. The child should enroll on schedule, and educational planning should be initiated to address any deficiencies. Pushing a child into an environment for which he or she is not prepared can contribute to school refusal, poor school achievement, and behavioral problems.

Physicians should be able to identify children at risk for school difficulties, such as those who have developmental delays or physical disabilities. These children may require specialized school services. Federal law mandates these services for children who qualify; services may include speech-language therapy, occupational therapy, or physical therapy (see Chapter 10).

## Adolescence

Although the Society for Adolescent Medicine defines adolescence as 10 to 25 years of age, adolescence is characterized better by developmental stages (*early, middle,* and *late* adolescence) that all teens must negotiate to develop into healthy, functional adults. Different behavioral and developmental issues characterize each stage. The age at which each issue becomes manifest and the importance of these issues vary widely among individuals, as do the rates of cognitive, psychosexual, psychosocial, and physical development.

During **early adolescence**, attention is focused on the present and on the peer group. Concerns are primarily related to the body's physical changes and normality. Strivings for independence are ambivalent. These young adolescents are difficult to interview because they often respond with short, clipped conversation and may have little insight. They are just becoming accustomed to abstract thinking.

**Middle adolescence** can be a difficult time for adolescents and the adults who have contact with them. Cognitive processes are more sophisticated. Through abstract thinking, middle adolescents can experiment with ideas, consider things as they might be, develop insight, and reflect on their own feelings and the feelings of others. As they mature cognitively and psychosocially, these adolescents focus on issues of identity not limited solely to the physical aspects of their body. They explore their parents' and the culture's values, and they may do this by expressing the contrary side of the dominant value. Many middle adolescents explore these values only in their minds; others do so by challenging their parents' authority. Many engage in high-risk behaviors, including unprotected sexual intercourse, substance abuse, or dangerous driving. The strivings of middle adolescents for independence, limit testing, and need for autonomy are often distressing to their families, teachers, or other authority figures. These adolescents are at higher risk for morbidity and mortality from accidents, homicide, or suicide.

**Late adolescence** usually is marked by formal operational thinking, including thoughts about the future (educational, vocational, and sexual). Late adolescents are usually more committed to their sexual partners than are middle adolescents. Unresolved separation anxiety from previous developmental stages may emerge at this time as the young person begins to move physically away from the family of origin to college or vocational school, a job, or military service.

## MODIFYING PSYCHOSOCIAL BEHAVIORS

Child behavior is determined by heredity and by the environment. Behavioral theory postulates that behavior is primarily a product of external environmental determinants and that manipulation of the environmental antecedents and consequences of behavior can be used to modify maladaptive behavior and to increase desirable behavior (operant conditioning). The four major methods of operant conditioning are positive reinforcement, negative reinforcement, extinction, and punishment. Many common behavioral problems of children can be ameliorated by these methods.

**Positive reinforcement** increases the frequency of a behavior by following the behavior with a favorable event. Praising a child for his or her excellent school performance and rewarding an adolescent with a later curfew hour are examples. **Negative reinforcement** increases the frequency of a behavior by following the behavior with the removal, cessation, or avoidance of an unpleasant event. Conversely, sometimes, this reinforcement may occur unintentionally, increasing the frequency of an undesirable behavior. A toddler may purposely try to stick a pencil in a light socket to obtain attention, be it positive or negative. **Extinction** occurs when there is a decrease in the frequency of a previously reinforced behavior because the reinforcement is withheld. Extinction is the principle behind the common advice to ignore such behavior as crying at bedtime or temper tantrums, which parents may unwittingly reinforce through attention and comforting.

**Punishment** decreases the frequency of a behavior through unpleasant consequences. Positive reinforcement has been proved to be more effective than punishment. Punishment is more effective when combined with positive reinforcement. A toddler who draws on the wall with a crayon may be punished, but he or she learns much quicker when positive reinforcement is given for proper use of the crayon, on paper, not the wall. Interrupting and modifying behaviors are discussed in detail in Section 3.

## TEMPERAMENT

Significant individual differences exist within the normal development of temperament (behavioral style). Temperament must be appreciated because, if an expected pattern of behavior is too narrowly defined, normal behavior may be inappropriately labeled as abnormal or pathologic. There are three common constellations of temperamental characteristics:

1. The **easy child** (about 40% of children) is characterized by regularity of biologic functions (consistent, predictable times for eating, sleeping, and elimination), a positive approach to new stimuli, high adaptability to change, mild or moderate intensity in responses, and a positive mood.
2. The **difficult child** (about 10%) is characterized by irregularity of biologic functions, negative withdrawal from new stimuli, poor adaptability, intense responses, and a negative mood.
3. The **slow to warm up child** (about 15%) is characterized by a low activity level, withdrawal from new stimuli, slow adaptability, mild intensity in responses, and a somewhat negative mood.

The remaining children have more mixed temperaments. The individual temperament of a child has important implications for parenting and for the advice a pediatrician may give in anticipatory guidance or behavioral problem counseling.

Although temperament may be, to some degree, hardwired (*nature*) in each child, the environment (*nurture*) in which the child grows has a strong effect on the child's adjustment. Social and cultural factors can have marked effects on the child through differences in parenting style, educational approaches, and behavioral expectations.

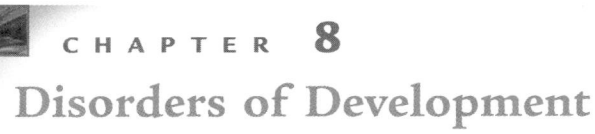

CHAPTER **8**

# Disorders of Development

## DEVELOPMENTAL SURVEILLANCE AND SCREENING

Developmental and behavioral problems are more common than any category of problems in pediatrics except acute infections and trauma. Approximately 15% to 18% of children in the United States have developmental or behavioral disabilities. As many as 25% of children have serious psychosocial problems. Parents often neglect to mention these problems because they think the physician is uninterested or cannot help. It is necessary to monitor development and screen for the presence of such problems at health supervision visits, particularly in the preschool years, when the pediatrician may be the only professional to evaluate the child.

**Development surveillance,** done at every office visit, is an informal process comparing skill levels to lists of milestones. If suspicion of developmental or behavioral issues recurs, further evaluation is warranted (Table 8-1)

**Developmental screening** involves the use of standardized screening tests and a brief evaluation comparing the developmental skills of a particular child with a population of children to identify children who require further diagnostic assessment. The American Academy of Pediatrics recommends the use of validated standardized screening tools at three of the health maintenance visits—9 months, 18 months, and 30 months. Clinics and offices that serve a higher risk patient population (children living in poverty) often perform a screening test at *every* health maintenance visit. A failed developmental screening test requires more comprehensive evaluation. Developmental evaluations for children with suspected delays and intervention services for children with diagnosed disabilities are available free to families. A combination of U.S. state and federal funds provide these services.

Screening tests can be categorized as general screening tests that cover all behavioral domains or as targeted screens that focus on one area of development. Some may be administered in the office by professionals, and others may be completed at home (or in a waiting room) by parents. Good developmental/behavioral screening instruments have sensitivity of 70% to 80% to detect suspected problems and specificity of 70% to 80% to detect normal development. Although 30% of children screened may be *over-referred*, this group also includes children whose skills are below average and who may benefit from definitive testing that may help address relative developmental deficits. The 20% to 30% of children who have disabilities that are not detected by the single administration of a screening instrument are likely to be identified on repeat screening at subsequent health maintenance visits.

The **Denver Developmental Screening Test II** is commonly used by general pediatricians (Figs. 8-1 and 8-2). The Denver II assesses the development of children from birth to 6 years of age in four domains:

1. Personal-social
2. Fine motor–adaptive
3. Language
4. Gross motor

Items on the Denver II are carefully selected for their reliability and consistency of norms across subgroups and cultures. The Denver II is a useful screening instrument, but it cannot assess adequately the complexities of socioemotional development. Children with *suspect* or *untestable* scores must be followed carefully.

| | | TABLE 8-1 Developmental Milestones | | | |
|---|---|---|---|---|---|
| Age | Gross Motor | Fine Motor–Adaptive | Personal-Social | Language | Other Cognitive |
| 2 wk | Moves head side to side | | Regards face | Alerts to bell | |
| 2 mo | Lifts shoulder while prone | Tracks past midline | Smiles responsively | Cooing<br>Searches for sound with eyes | |
| 4 mo | Lifts up on hands<br>Rolls front to back<br>If pulled to sit from supine, no head lag | Reaches for object<br>Raking grasp | Looks at hand<br>Begins to work toward toy | Laughs and squeals | |
| 6 mo | Sits alone | Transfers object hand to hand | Feeds self<br>Holds bottle | Babbles | |
| 9 mo | Pulls to stand<br>Gets into sitting position | Starting to pincer grasp<br>Bangs 2 blocks together | Waves bye-bye<br>Plays pat-a-cake | Says Dada and Mama, but nonspecific<br>2-syllable sounds | |
| 12 mo | Walks<br>Stoops and stands | Puts block in cup | Drinks from a cup<br>Imitates others | Says Mama and Dada, specific<br>Says 1–2 other words | |
| 15 mo | Walks backward | Scribbles<br>Stacks 2 blocks | Uses spoon and fork<br>Helps in housework | Says 3–6 words<br>Follows commands | |
| 18 mo | Runs<br>Kicks a ball | Stacks 4 blocks | Removes garment<br>"Feeds" doll | Says at least 6 words | |
| 2 yr | Walks up and down stairs<br>Throws overhand | Stacks 6 blocks<br>Copies line | Washes and dries hands<br>Brushes teeth<br>Puts on clothes | Puts 2 words together<br>Points to pictures<br>Knows body parts | Understands concept of *today* |
| 3 yr | Walks steps alternating feet<br>Broad jump | Stacks 8 blocks<br>Wiggles thumb | Uses spoon well, spilling little<br>Puts on T-shirt | Names pictures<br>Speech understandable to stranger 75%<br>Says 3-word sentences | Understands concepts of *tomorrow* and *yesterday* |
| 4 yr | Balances well on each foot<br>Hops on one foot | Copies O, maybe +<br>Draws person with 3 parts | Brushes teeth without help<br>Dresses without help | Names colors<br>Understands adjectives | |
| 5 yr | Skips<br>Heel-to-toe walks | Copies □ | | Counts<br>Understands opposites | |
| 6 yr | Balances on each foot 6 sec | Copies Δ<br>Draws person with 6 parts | | Defines words | Begins to understand *right* and *left* |

The pediatrician asks questions (items labeled with an "R" may be asked of parents to document the task "by report") or directly observes behaviors. On the scoring sheet, a line is drawn at the child's chronologic age. All tasks that are entirely to the left of the line that the child has not accomplished are considered delayed (at least 90% of the population accomplished the task). If the test instructions are not followed accurately or if items are omitted, the validity of the test becomes much poorer. To assist physicians in using the Denver II, the scoring sheet also features a table to document confounding behaviors, such as interest, fearfulness, or apparent short attention span. Repeat screening at subsequent health maintenance visits often detects abnormalities that a single screen was unable to detect.

Other developmental screening tools include parent-completed Ages and Stages Questionnaires, Child

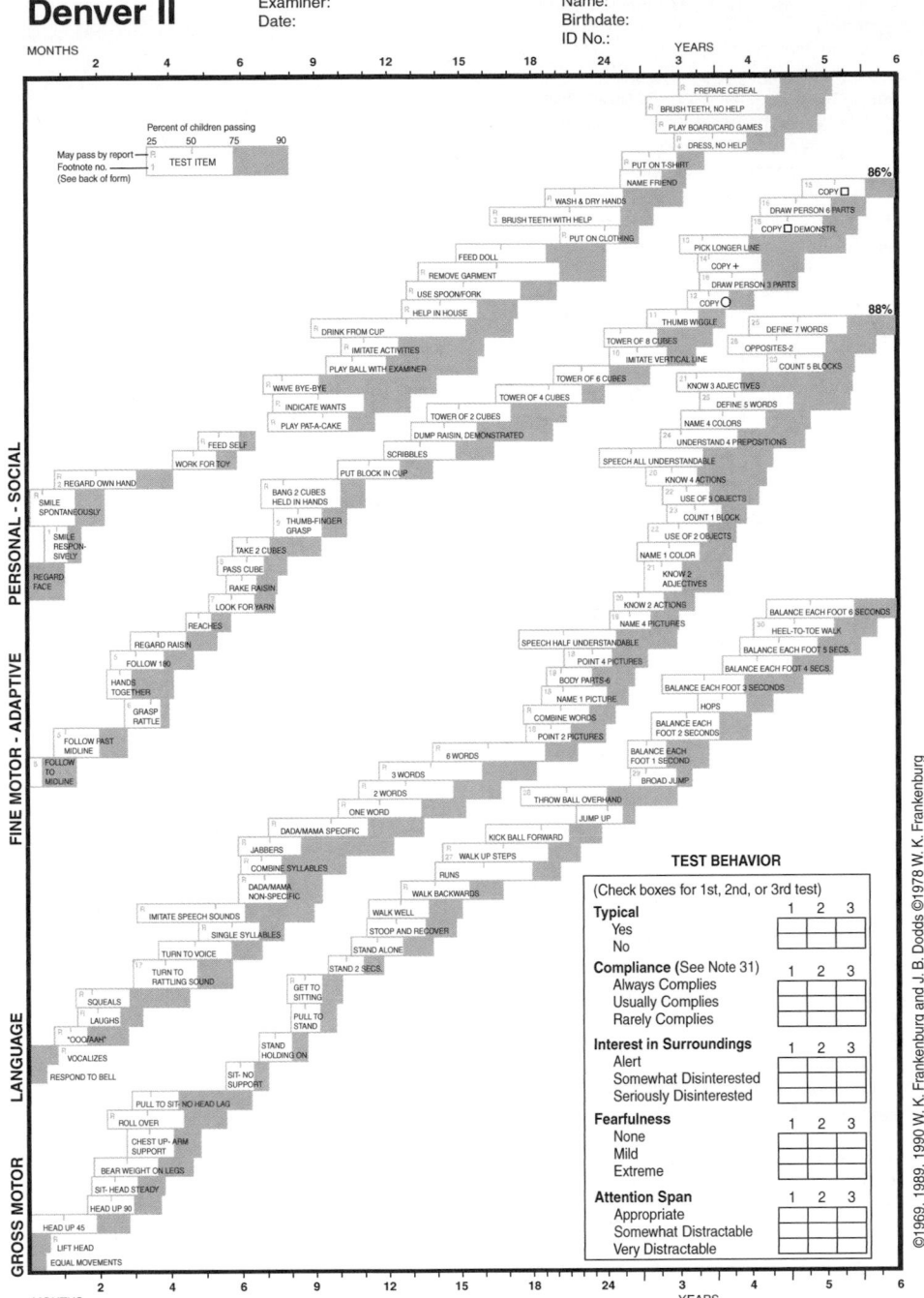

**FIGURE 8-1**

**Scoring form for Denver II.** (From Frankenburg WK: Denver II Developmental Screening Test Training Manual, 2nd ed, Denver, *Denver Developmental Materials*, 1992.)

Development Inventories, and Parents' Evaluations of Developmental Status. The last is a simple, 10-item questionnaire that parents complete between birth and 8 years. Parent-reported screens have good validity compared with office-based screening measures. In addition to these full screens, there may be a concern about only one area of development identified by parents or by an abnormal screen on the Denver II or other standardized screening tool.

**Autism screening** is recommended for all children at 18 and 24 months of age. Although there are several tools, many pediatricians use the Modified Checklist for Autism in Toddlers (M-CHAT). M-CHAT is an office-based questionnaire that asks parents about 23 typical behaviors, some of which are more predictive than others for autism or other pervasive developmental disorders. If the child demonstrates more than two predictive or three total behaviors, further assessment with an interview algorithm is indicated to distinguish normal variant behaviors from those children needing referral for definitive testing (see Chapter 20).

**Language screening** correlates best with cognitive development in the early years. Table 8-2 provides some

1. Try to get child to smile by smiling, talking or waving. Do not touch him/her.
2. Child must stare at hand several seconds.
3. Parent may help guide toothbrush and put toothpaste on brush.
4. Child does not have to be able to tie shoes or button/zip in the back.
5. Move yarn slowly in an arc from one side to the other, about 8" above child's face.
6. Pass if child grasps rattle when it is touched to the backs or tips of fingers.
7. Pass if child tries to see where yarn went. Yarn should be dropped quickly from sight from tester's hand without arm movement.
8. Child must transfer cube from hand to hand without help of body, mouth, or table.
9. Pass if child picks up raisin with any part of thumb and finger.
10. Line can vary only 30 degrees or less from tester's line. |/
11. Make a fist with thumb pointing upward and wiggle only the thumb. Pass if child imitates and does not move any fingers other than the thumb.

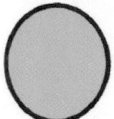   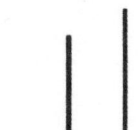   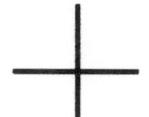   

12. Pass any enclosed form. Fail continuous round motions.

13. Which line is longer? (Not bigger.) Turn paper upside down and repeat. (pass 3 of 3 or 5 of 6)

14. Pass any lines crossing near midpoint.

15. Have child copy first. If failed, demonstrate.

When giving items 12, 14, and 15, do not name the forms. Do not demonstrate 12 and 14.

16. When scoring, each pair (2 arms, 2 legs, etc.) counts as one part.
17. Place one cube in cup and shake gently near child's ear, but out of sight. Repeat for other ear.
18. Point to picture and have child name it. (No credit is given for sounds only.)
    If less than 4 pictures are named correctly, have child point to picture as each is named by tester.

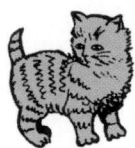   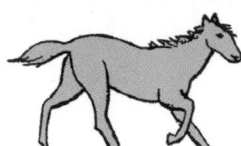   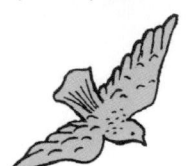   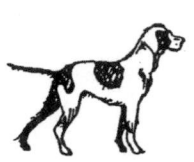   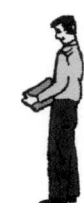

19. Using doll, tell child: Show me the nose, eyes, ears, mouth, hands, feet, tummy, hair. Pass 6 of 8.
20. Using pictures, ask child: Which one flies?... says meow?... talks?... barks?... gallops? Pass 2 of 5, 4 of 5.
21. Ask child: What do you do when you are cold?... tired?... hungry? Pass 2 of 3, 3 of 3.
22. Ask child: What do you do with a cup? What is a chair used for? What is a pencil used for? Action words must be included in answers.
23. Pass if child correctly places <u>and</u> says how many blocks are on paper. (1, 5).
24. Tell child: Put block **on** table; **under** table; **in front of** me, **behind** me. Pass 4 of 4. (Do not help child by pointing, moving head or eyes.)
25. Ask child: What is a ball?... lake?... desk?... house?... banana?... curtain?... fence?... ceiling? Pass if defined in terms of use, shape, what it is made of, or general category (such as banana is fruit, not just yellow). Pass 5 of 8, 7 of 8.
26. Ask child: If a horse is big, a mouse is __? If fire is hot, ice is __? If the sun shines during the day, the moon shines during the __? Pass 2 of 3.
27. Child may use wall or rail only, not person. May not crawl.
28. Child must throw ball overhand 3 feet to within arm's reach of tester.
29. Child must perform standing broad jump over width of test sheet (8 1/2 inches).
30. Tell child to walk forward, ⊂⊃⊂⊃⊂⊃⊂⊃➤ heel within 1 inch of toe. Tester may demonstrate. Child must walk 4 consecutive steps.
31. In the second year, half of normal children are non-compliant.

**OBSERVATIONS:**

**FIGURE 8-2**

**Instructions for the Denver II.** Numbers are coded to scoring form (see Fig. 8-1). *Suspect* is defined as two or more delays (failure of an item passed by 90% at that age) in two or more categories or two or more delays in one category with one other category having one delay and an age line that does not intersect one item that is passed. (From Frankenburg WK: Denver II Developmental Screening Test Training Manual, 2nd ed, Denver, *Denver Developmental Materials*, 1992.)

rules of thumb for language development that focus on speech production (expressive language). Although expressive language (speech) is the most obvious language element, the most dramatic changes in language development in the first years involve recognition and understanding (receptive language).

Whenever there is a language delay, a **hearing deficit** must be considered. The implementation of universal newborn hearing screening detects many, if not most, of these children in the newborn period, and appropriate early intervention services may be provided. Conditions that present a high risk of an associated hearing deficit

| TABLE 8-2 Rules of Thumb for Speech Screening | | | |
|---|---|---|---|
| Age (yr) | Speech Production | Articulation (Amount of Speech Understood by a Stranger) | Following Commands |
| 1 | 1–3 words | | One-step commands |
| 2 | 2- to 3-word phrases | ½ | Two-step commands |
| 3 | Routine use of sentences | ¾ | |
| 4 | Routine use of sentence sequences; conversational give-and-take | Almost all | |
| 5 | Complex sentences; extensive use of modifiers, pronouns, and prepositions | Almost all | |

### TABLE 8-3 Conditions Considered High Risk for Associated Hearing Deficit

Congenital hearing loss in first cousin or closer relative
Bilirubin level of ≥20 mg/dL
Congenital rubella or other nonbacterial intrauterine infection
Defects in the ear, nose, or throat
Birth weight of ≤1500 g
Multiple apneic episodes
Exchange transfusion
Meningitis
5-minute Apgar score of ≤5
Persistent fetal circulation (primary pulmonary hypertension)
Treatment with ototoxic drugs (e.g., aminoglycosides and loop diuretics)

### TABLE 8-4 Context of Behavioral Problems

#### CHILD FACTORS

Health (past and current)
Developmental status
Temperament (e.g., difficult, slow to warm up)
Coping mechanisms

#### PARENTAL FACTORS

Misinterpretations of stage-related behaviors
Mismatch of parental expectations and characteristics of child
Parental characteristics (e.g., depression, lack of interest, rejection, overprotectiveness)
Coping mechanisms

#### ENVIRONMENTAL FACTORS

Stress (e.g., marital discord, unemployment, personal loss)
Support (e.g., emotional, material, informational, child care)

#### PARENT-CHILD INTERACTIONS

The common pathway through which the listed factors interact to influence the development of a behavior problem
The key to resolving the behavior problem

are listed in Table 8-3. Dysfluency (*stuttering*) is common in 3- and 4-year-olds. Unless the dysfluency is severe, is accompanied by tics or unusual posturing, or occurs after 4 years of age, parents should be counseled that it is normal and transient and to accept it calmly and patiently.

After the child's sixth birthday and until adolescence, developmental assessment is initially done by inquiring about school performance (academic achievement and behavior). Inquiring about concerns raised by teachers or other adults who care for the child (after-school program counselor, coach, religious leader) is prudent. Formal developmental testing of these older children is beyond the scope of the primary care pediatrician. Nonetheless, the health care provider should be the coordinator of testing and evaluation performed by other specialists (e.g., psychologists, educational professionals).

## OTHER ISSUES IN ASSESSING DEVELOPMENT AND BEHAVIOR

Ignorance of the environmental influences on child behavior may result in ineffective or inappropriate management (or both). Table 8-4 lists some contextual factors that should be considered in the etiology of a child's behavioral or developmental problem.

Building rapport with the parents and the child is a prerequisite for obtaining the often-sensitive information that is essential for understanding a behavioral or developmental issue. Rapport usually can be established quickly if the parents sense that the clinician respects them and is genuinely interested in listening to their concerns. The clinician develops rapport with the child by engaging the child in developmentally appropriate conversation or play, providing toys while interviewing the parents, and being sensitive to the fears the child may have. Too often, the child is ignored until it is time for the physical examination. Similar to their parents, children feel more comfortable if they are greeted by name and involved in pleasant interactions before they are asked sensitive questions or threatened with examinations. Young children can be engaged in conversation on the parent's lap, which provides security and places the child at the eye level of the examiner.

With adolescents, emphasis should be placed on building a physician-patient relationship that is distinct from the relationship with the parents. The parents should not be excluded; however, the adolescent should have the opportunity to express concerns to and ask questions of the physician in confidence. Two intertwined issues must be taken into consideration—consent and confidentiality. Although laws vary from state to state, in general, adolescents who are able to give informed consent (mature minors) may consent to visits and care related to high-risk behaviors (i.e., substance abuse; sexual health, including prevention, detection, and treatment of sexually transmitted infections; and pregnancy). Pediatricians should become familiar with the governing law in the state where they practice (see http://www.guttmacher.com/statecenter/ updates/index.html). Most physicians who regularly work with adolescents believe that confidentiality is crucial to providing adolescents with optimal care (especially for obtaining a history of risk behaviors). States vary in the law governing confidentiality rights for adolescents, although most states support the physician who wishes the visit to be confidential. When assessing development and behavior, confidentiality can be achieved by meeting with the adolescent alone for at least part of each visit. However, parents must be informed when the clinician has significant concerns about the health and safety of the child. Often the clinician can convince the adolescent to inform the parents directly about a problem or can reach an agreement with the adolescent about how the parents will be informed by the physician.

## EVALUATING DEVELOPMENTAL AND BEHAVIORAL ISSUES

In an initial health supervision visit, the time to assess development is often short, and the assessment usually is only part of what needs to be accomplished during that office visit. Therefore, it may be best to explore developmental and behavioral problems during subsequent visits, when more comprehensive information and observations can be obtained. Responses to open-ended questions often provide clues to underlying, unstated problems and identify the appropriate direction for further, more directed questions. Histories about developmental and behavioral problems are often vague and confusing; to reconcile apparent contradictions, the interviewer frequently must request clarification, more detail, or mere repetition. By summarizing an understanding of the information at frequent intervals and by recapitulating at the close of the visit, the interviewer and patient and family can ensure that they understand each other.

If the clinician's impression of the child differs markedly from the parent's description, there may be a crucial parental concern or issue that has not yet been expressed either because it may be difficult to talk about (e.g., marital problems), because it is unconscious, or because the parent overlooks its relevance to the child's behavior. Alternatively the physician's observations may be atypical, even with multiple visits. The observations of teachers, relatives, and other regular caregivers may be crucial in sorting out this possibility. The parent also may have a distorted image of the child, rooted in parental psychopathology. A sensitive, supportive, and noncritical approach to the parent is crucial to appropriate intervention.

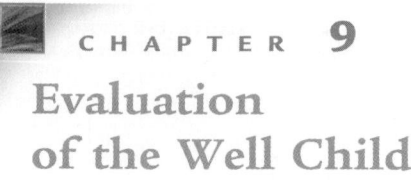

CHAPTER **9**

# Evaluation of the Well Child

Health maintenance or supervision visits should consist of a comprehensive assessment of the child's health and of the parent's/guardian's role in providing an environment for optimal growth, development, and health. **Bright Futures** standardizes each of the health maintenance visits and provides resources for working with the children and families of different ages (http://brightfutures.aap.org). Elements of each visit include evaluation and management of parental concerns; inquiry about any interval illness since the last physical, growth, development, and nutrition; anticipatory guidance (including safety information and counseling); physical examination; screening tests; and immunizations (Table 9-1). Figure 9-1 indicates the ages that specific prevention measures should be undertaken (by testing, such as vision and hearing; by physician history and physical examination; or by laboratory screening, such as the neonatal metabolic screening test or lead screening).

## SCREENING TESTS

Children usually are quite healthy, especially after 1 year of age, and only the following screening tests are recommended: newborn metabolic screening with hemoglobin electrophoresis, hearing and vision evaluation, anemia and lead screening, and tuberculosis testing. Children born to families with dyslipidemias or early heart disease also may be screened for lipid disorders. (Items marked by a *star* in Figure 9-1 should be performed if a risk factor is found.) Sexually experienced adolescents should be screened for sexually transmissible infections. When an infant or child begins care after the newborn period, the pediatric provider should perform any missing screening tests and immunizations.

### Newborn Screening

#### Metabolic Screening

Every state in the United States mandates newborn metabolic screening. Phenylketonuria (PKU) is the prototypic illness to be screened for and prevented. However, if PKU is detected early, a modified diet (a highly specialized phenylalanine-free formula) can be provided, and the disease-related developmental and growth problems can be prevented. Each state determines its own priorities and procedures, but the following diseases are usually included in metabolic screening: PKU, galactosemia, congenital hypothyroidism, and maple sugar urine disease (see Section 10). Many states have instituted screening programs for cystic fibrosis using a screening test of immunoreactive trypsinogen (IRT). If that test is positive, then DNA analysis for cystic fibrosis mutations is performed.

| TABLE 9-1 Topics for Health Supervision Visits |
| --- |
| **FOCUS ON THE CHILD** |
| Concerns (parent's or child's) |
| Past problem follow-up |
| Immunization and screening test update |
| Routine care (e.g., eating, sleeping, elimination, and health habits) |
| Developmental progress |
| Behavioral style and problems |
| **FOCUS ON THE CHILD'S ENVIRONMENT** |
| *Family* |
| Caregiving schedule for caregiver who lives at home |
| Parent-child and sibling-child interactions |
| Extended family role |
| Family stresses (e.g., work, move, finances, illness, death, marital and other interpersonal relationships) |
| Family supports (relatives, friends, groups) |
| *Community* |
| Caregivers outside the family |
| Peer interaction |
| School and work |
| Recreational activities |
| *Physical Environment* |
| Appropriate stimulation |
| Safety |

## Hemoglobin Electrophoresis

Children with hemoglobinopathies are at higher risk for infection and complications from anemia. Early detection may prevent or ameliorate these complications. Infants with sickle cell disease are begun on oral penicillin prophylaxis to prevent sepsis, the major cause of mortality in these infants (see Chapter 150).

## Hearing Evaluation

Because speech and language are central to a child's cognitive development, hearing screening is performed before discharge from the newborn nursery. An infant's hearing is tested by placing headphones over the infant's ears and electrodes on the head. Standard sounds are played, and the transmission of the impulse to the brain is documented. If this screening test is abnormal, a further evaluation is indicated, using evoked response technology of sound transmission, similar to an electroencephalogram.

## Hearing and Vision Screening of Older Children

### Infants and Toddlers

Inferences about hearing are drawn from asking parents about responses to sound and speech and by examining speech and language development closely. Inferences about vision may be made by examining gross motor milestones (children with vision problems may have a delay) and by physical examination of the eye. Parents should be queried as to any concerns about vision until the child is 3 years of age and about hearing until the child is 4 years of age. If there are concerns, definitive testing should be arranged. Hearing can be screened by auditory evoked responses as mentioned for infants. For toddlers and older children who cannot cooperate with formal audiologic testing with headphones, behavioral audiology may be used. Sounds of a specific frequency or intensity are provided in a standard environment within a sound-proof room, and responses are assessed by a trained audiologist. Vision may be assessed by referral to a pediatric ophthalmologist and by visual evoked responses.

### Children 3 Years of Age and Older

At various ages, hearing and vision should be screened objectively using standard techniques. In Figure 9-1, any age marked *O* requires objective screening and *S* denotes that a subjective assessment is adequate at that age. Asking the family and child about any concerns or consequences of poor hearing or vision accomplishes subjective evaluation. At 3 years of age, children are screened for vision for the first time if they are developmentally able to be tested. Many children at this age do not have the interactive language or interpersonal skills to perform a vision screen; these children should be re-examined at a 3- to 6-month interval to ensure that vision is normal. Because most of these children do not identify letters yet, using a Snellen eye chart with standard shapes is recommended. When a child is able to identify letters, the more accurate letter-based chart should be used. Audiologic testing of sounds with headphones and children identifying sounds heard should be begun on the fourth birthday (although Head Start requires that pediatricians attempt hearing screening at 3 years of age). Any suspected audiologic problem should be evaluated by a careful history and physical examination, and the child should be referred for comprehensive testing. Children who have a documented vision problem, failed screening, or parental concern should be referred, preferably to a pediatric ophthalmologist. However, many communities do not have access, so a general ophthalmologist is consulted.

### Anemia Screening

After the newborn period, when hemoglobin electrophoresis is used to detect inherited abnormalities, children are screened for anemia at ages when there is a higher incidence of iron deficiency anemia. Anemic infants do not perform as well on standard developmental testing. Infants are screened at birth and again at 4 months if there is a documented risk, such as low birth weight or prematurity. Healthy term infants usually are screened at 12 months of age because this is when a high incidence of iron deficiency is noted. Children are assessed at other visits for risks or concerns related to anemia (denoted by a star in Fig. 9-1). Any abnormalities detected should be evaluated for etiology. When iron deficiency is strongly suspected, a therapeutic trial of iron may be used (see Chapter 150).

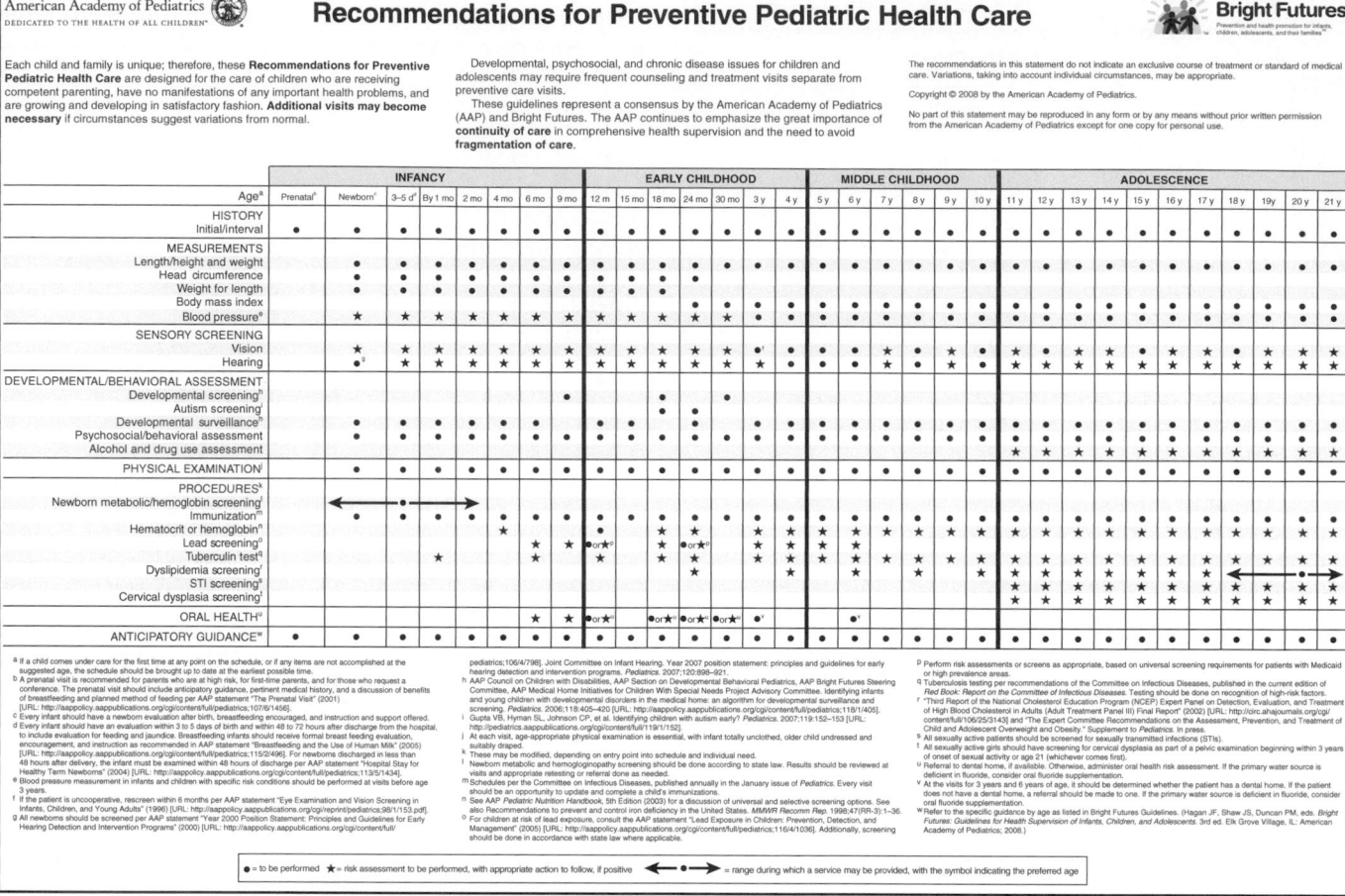

**FIGURE 9-1**

**Recommendations for preventive pediatric health care**. (From the Committee on Practice and Ambulatory Medicine: Recommendations for Preventive Pediatric Health Care, *Pediatrics* 120(6): 1376, 2007.)

## Lead Screening

Lead intoxication may cause developmental and behavioral abnormalities that are not reversible even if the hematologic and other metabolic complications are treated. Although the Centers for Disease Control and Prevention (CDC) recommends environmental investigation at blood lead levels of 20 μg/dL on a single visit or persistent 15 μg/dL over a 3-month period, levels of 5 to 10 μg/dL may cause learning problems. Risk factors for lead intoxication include living in older homes with cracked or peeling lead-based paint, industrial exposure, use of foreign remedies (e.g., a diarrhea remedy from Mexico), and use of pottery with lead paint glaze. Because of the significant association of lead intoxication with poverty and the numerous children living in poverty, the CDC recommends blood lead screening at 12 and 24 months. In addition, standardized screening questions for risk of lead intoxication should be asked for all children between 6 months and 6 years of age (Table 9-2). Any positive or suspect response is an indication for obtaining a blood lead level. Because capillary blood sampling may produce false-positive results, a venous blood sample should be obtained. County health departments and private

### TABLE 9-2 Lead Poisoning Risk Assessment Questions to Be Asked Between 6 Months and 6 Years

Does the child spend any time in a building built before 1960 (e.g., home, school, barn) that has cracked or peeling paint?

Is there a brother, sister, housemate, playmate, or community member being followed or treated (or even rumored to be) for lead poisoning?

Does the child live with an adult whose job or hobby involves exposure to lead (e.g., lead smelting and automotive radiator repair)?

Does the child live near an active lead smelter, battery recycling plant, or other industry likely to release lead?

Does the family use home remedies or pottery from another country?

companies provide lead inspection and detection services to determine the source of the lead. Standard decontamination techniques should be used to remove the lead while avoiding aerosolizing the toxic metal that a child might breathe or creating dust that a child might ingest (see Chapters 149 and 150).

## Tuberculosis Testing

The prevalence of tuberculosis is increasing, largely as a result of the adult human immunodeficiency virus (HIV) epidemic, and children often present with serious and multisystem disease (miliary tuberculosis). All children should be assessed for tuberculosis at health maintenance visits, especially after 1 year of age. The high-risk groups, as defined by the CDC, are listed in Table 9-3. In general, the standardized purified protein derivative (PPD) intradermal test is used. Because parents may misinterpret the test, a health care provider must evaluate the test 48 to 72 hours after injection. The size of induration, not the color of any mark, denotes a positive test. For most patients, 10 mm of induration is a positive test. For HIV-positive patients, those with recent tuberculosis contacts, patients with evidence of old healed tuberculosis on chest film, or immunosuppressed patients, 5 mm is a positive test (see Chapter 124). The CDC has approved (in adults) the QuantiFERON-TB Gold Test, which has the advantage of needing only one office visit.

## Cholesterol

Children and adolescents who have a family history of cardiovascular disease or have at least one parent with a high blood cholesterol level are at increased risk of having high blood cholesterol levels as adults and increased risk of coronary heart disease. The American Academy of Pediatrics (AAP) recommends dyslipidemia screening in the context of regular health care for at-risk populations (Table 9-4) by a fasting lipid profile. The recommended screening levels are the same for all children 2 to 18 years. Total cholesterol of less than 170 mg/dL is normal, 170 to 199 mg/dL is borderline, greater than 200 mg/dL is elevated.

## Sexually Transmitted Infection Testing

Annual office visits are recommended for adolescents, at least in ones older than 12 years of age. A full adolescent psychosocial history should be obtained in confidential fashion, with the parent excused from the examination room and confidential matters discussed. Part of this evaluation is a comprehensive sexual history. Often adolescents must be questioned creatively to elicit information on sexual activity. Not all adolescents identify oral sex as sex, and some adolescents misinterpret the term *sexually active* to mean that one has many sexual partners or is very vigorous during intercourse. The questions "Are you having sex?" and "Have you ever had sex?" should be asked. Any child or adolescent who has had any form of sexual intercourse should have at least an annual evaluation (more often if there is a history of high-risk sex) for sexually transmitted diseases by physical examination (genital warts, genital herpes, and pediculosis) and laboratory testing (chlamydia, gonorrhea, syphilis, and HIV) (see Chapter 116). Adolescent girls should be assessed for human papillomavirus and precancerous lesions by Papanicolaou smear 3 years after beginning vaginal intercourse or at 21 years of age.

# IMMUNIZATIONS

Immunization records should be checked at each office visit, regardless of the reason. Appropriate vaccinations should be administered (see Chapter 94).

# DENTAL CARE

Many families in the United States, particularly poor families and ethnic minorities, underuse dental health care. Pediatricians may identify gross abnormalities, such as large caries, gingival inflammation, or significant malocclusion. All children should have a dental examination by a dentist at least annually and a dental cleaning by a dentist or hygienist every 6 months. Dental health care visits should include instruction about preventive care practiced at home (brushing and flossing). Other prophylactic methods shown to be effective at preventing caries are fluoride topical treatments and acrylic sealants on the molars provided by dentists. Pediatric dentists recommend beginning visits at age 1 year to educate families and to screen for milk bottle caries. Some recommend that pediatricians apply dental varnish to the children's teeth, especially in communities that do not have pediatric dentists. Fluoridation of water or fluoride supplements in communities that do not have fluoridation is important in prevention of cavities (see Chapter 127).

# NUTRITIONAL ASSESSMENT

Plotting a child's growth on the standard charts is a vital component of the nutritional assessment. A dietary history should be obtained because the content of the diet may suggest a risk of nutritional deficiency (see Chapters 27 and 28).

---

**TABLE 9-3  Groups at High Risk for Tuberculosis**

Close contact with persons known or suspected to have tuberculosis (TB)—do you or your child know anyone with TB, with a positive TB test, or suspected to have TB

Foreign-born persons from areas with high TB rates (Asia, Africa, Latin America, Eastern Europe, Russia)

Health care workers

High-risk racial or ethnic minorities or other populations at higher risk (Asian, Pacific Islander, Hispanic, African American, Native American, groups living in poverty [e.g., Medicaid recipients], migrant farm workers, homeless persons, substance abusers)

Infants, children, and adolescents exposed to adults in high-risk categories

---

**TABLE 9-4  Cholesterol Risk Screening Recommendations**

1. Children and adolescents who have a family history of high cholesterol or heart disease
2. Children whose family history is unknown
3. Children who have other personal risk factors—obesity, high blood pressure, or diabetes

## ANTICIPATORY GUIDANCE

Anticipatory guidance is information conveyed to parents verbally or in written materials (or even directing parents to certain websites on the Internet) that is meant to assist them in facilitating optimal growth and development for their children. Figure 9-1 calls for discussions in four areas: injury prevention, violence prevention, sleep position counseling (until 6 months of age), and nutrition counseling. Table 9-5 summarizes representative issues that might be discussed within the four areas and a fifth area, fostering optimal development and behavior. It is important to review briefly the safety topics previously

### TABLE 9-5  Anticipatory Guidance Topics Suggested by Age

| Ages | Injury Prevention | Violence Prevention | Sleep Position | Nutritional Counseling | Fostering Optimal Development |
|---|---|---|---|---|---|
| Birth | Crib safety<br>Hot water heaters <120°F<br>Car safety seats<br>Smoke detectors | Assess bonding and attachment<br>Identify family strife, lack of support, pathology<br>Educate parents on nurturing | Back to sleep<br>Crib safety | Exclusive breastfeeding encouraged<br>Formula as a second-best option | Discuss parenting skills<br>Refer for parenting education |
| 2 wk | Falls | Reassess<br>Discuss sibling rivalry<br>Assess if guns in the home | Back to sleep | Assess breastfeeding and offer encouragement, problem solving | Recognize and manage postpartum blues<br>Child care options |
| 2 mo | Burns/hot liquids | Reassess<br>Firearm safety | Back to sleep | | Parent getting enough rest and managing returning to work |
| 4 mo | Infant walkers<br>Choking/suffocation | Reassess | Back to sleep | Introduction of solid foods | Discuss central to peripheral motor development<br>Praise good behavior |
| 6 mo | Changing car seats<br>Burns/hot surfaces | Reassess | | Assess status | Consistent limit-setting versus "spoiling" an infant<br>Praise good behavior |
| 9 mo | Water safety<br>Home safety review<br>Ingestions/poisoning | Assess parents' ideas on discipline and "spoiling" | | Assess anemia, discuss iron-rich foods | Assisting infants to sleep through the night if not accomplished<br>Praise good behavior |
| 12 mo | Firearm hazards<br>Auto-pedestrian safety | Discuss timeout versus corporal punishment<br>Avoiding media violence<br>Review firearm safety | | Introduction of whole cow's milk (and constipation with change discussed) | Avoiding walkers<br>Safe exploration<br>Proper shoes<br>Praise good behavior |
| 15 mo | Review and reassess topics | Encourage nonviolent punishments (timeout or natural consequences) | | Discuss decline in eating with slower growth<br>Assess food choices and variety | Fostering independence<br>Reinforce good behavior<br>Ignore annoying but not unsafe behaviors |
| 18 mo | Review and reassess topics | Limit punishment to high yield (not spilled milk!)<br>Parents consistent in discipline | | Discuss food choices, portions, "finicky" feeders | Preparation for toilet training<br>Reinforce good behavior |

**TABLE 9-5 Anticipatory Guidance Topics Suggested by Age—cont'd**

| Ages | Injury Prevention | Violence Prevention | Sleep Position | Nutritional Counseling | Fostering Optimal Development |
|------|-------------------|---------------------|----------------|------------------------|------------------------------|
| 2 yr | Falls—play equipment | Assess and discuss any aggressive behaviors in the child | | Assess body proportions and consider low-fat milk<br>Assess family cholesterol and atherosclerosis risk | Toilet training and resistance |
| 3 yr | Review and reassess topics | Review, especially avoiding media violence | | Discuss optimal eating and the food pyramid<br>Healthy snacks | Read to child<br>Socializing with other children<br>Head Start if possible |
| 4 yr | Booster seat versus seat belts | | | Healthy snacks | Read to child<br>Head Start or pre-K options |
| 5 yr | Bicycle safety<br>Water/pool safety | Developing consistent, clearly defined family rules and consequences<br>Avoiding media violence | | Assess for anemia<br>Discuss iron-rich foods | Reinforcing school topics<br>Read to child<br>Library card<br>Chores begun at home |
| 6 yr | Fire safety | Reinforce consistent discipline<br>Encourage nonviolent strategies<br>Assess domestic violence<br>Avoiding media violence | | Assess content, offer specific suggestions | Reinforcing school topics<br>After-school programs<br>Responsibility given for chores (and enforced) |
| 7–10 yr | Sports safety<br>Firearm hazard | Reinforcement<br>Assess domestic violence<br>Assess discipline techniques<br>Avoiding media violence<br>Walking away from fights (either victim or spectator) | | Assess content, offer specific suggestions | Reviewing homework and reinforcing school topics<br>After-school programs<br>Introduce smoking and substance abuse prevention (concrete) |
| 11–13 yr | Review and reassess | Discuss strategies to avoid interpersonal conflicts<br>Avoiding media violence<br>Avoiding fights and walking away<br>Discuss conflict resolution techniques | | Junk food versus healthy eating | Reviewing homework and reinforcing school topics<br>Smoking and substance abuse prevention (begin abstraction)<br>Discuss and encourage abstinence; possibly discuss condoms and contraceptive options<br>Avoiding violence<br>Offer availability |
| 14–16 yr | Motor vehicle safety<br>Avoiding riding with substance abuser | Establish new family rules related to curfews, school, and household responsibilities | | Junk food versus healthy eating | Review school work<br>Begin career discussions and college preparation (PSAT)<br>Review substance abuse, sexuality, and violence regularly |

*Continued*

| | | | Sleep | | Fostering Optimal |
|---|---|---|---|---|---|
| Ages | Injury Prevention | Violence Prevention | Position | Nutritional Counseling | Development |
| | | | | | Discuss condoms, contraception options, including emergency contraception |
| | | | | | Discuss sexually transmitted diseases, HIV |
| | | | | | Providing no-questions-asked ride home from at-risk situations |
| 17–21 yr | Review and reassess | Establish new rules related to driving, dating, and substance abuse | | Heart healthy diet for life | Continuation of above topics |
| | | | | | Off to college or employment |
| | | | | | New roles within the family |

HIV, human immunodeficiency virus; PSAT, Preliminary Scholastic Aptitude Test.

discussed at other visits for reinforcement. Age-appropriate discussions should occur at each visit. **Bright Futures** is an AAP project to standardize and improve issues in anticipatory guidance for pediatricians and other health care providers (see http://brightfutures.aap.org).

## Safety Issues

The most common cause of death for infants 1 month to 1 year of age is motor vehicle crashes. No newborn should be discharged from a nursery unless the parents have a functioning and properly installed car seat. Many automobile dealerships offer services to parents to ensure that safety seats are installed properly in their specific model. Most states have laws that mandate safety seats until the child reaches 4 years of age or 40 pounds in weight or even heavier. Repeat offenses may lead to suspension of driving privileges. The following are age-appropriate recommendations for car safety.

- Infants younger than 1 year of age and weighing less than 20 lb—use a rear-facing infant seat.
- Children older than 1 year of age and 20 to 40 lb—use a front-facing infant seat.
- Children 4 to 8 years of age and 40 to 80 lb—use a booster seat (for as long as the child fits comfortably).
- If the shoulder belt lies across the child's neck or the lap belt is across the abdomen, the child is not ready for seat belts.
- Children 12 years of age and younger should always be in the back seat, with the seat belt buckled 100% of the time. Front seat air bags are dangerous for younger and smaller children.

The **Back to Sleep** initiative has reduced the incidence of sudden infant death syndrome (SIDS). Before the initiative, infants routinely were placed prone to sleep. Since

1992, when the AAP recommended this program, the annual SIDS rate has decreased by more than 50%. Another initiative is aimed at day care providers, because 20% of SIDS deaths occur in day care settings.

## Fostering Optimal Development

See Figure 9-1 and Table 9-5 for presentation of age-appropriate activities that the pediatrician may advocate for families.

**Discipline** means to teach, not merely to punish. The ultimate goal is the child's self-control. Overbearing punishment to control a child's behavior interferes with the learning process and focuses on external control at the expense of the development of self-control. Parents who set too few reasonable limits may be frustrated by children who cannot control their own behavior. Discipline should teach a child exactly what is expected by supporting positive behaviors and responding appropriately to negative behaviors with proper limits. It is more important to reinforce good behavior than to punish bad behavior.

Commonly used techniques to control undesirable behaviors in children include scolding, physical punishment, and threats. These techniques have potential adverse effects on children's sense of security and self-esteem. The effectiveness of scolding diminishes the more it is used. Scolding should not be allowed to expand from an expression of displeasure about a specific event to derogatory statements about the child. Scolding also may escalate to the level of psychological abuse. It is important to educate parents that they have a *good child who does bad things from time to time*, so parents do not think and tell the child that he or she is "bad."

Frequent mild physical punishment (corporal punishment) may become less effective over time and tempt the parent to escalate the physical punishment, increasing the risk of child abuse. Corporal punishment teaches a child that in certain situations it is proper to strike another person. Commonly, in households that use spanking, older children who have been raised with this technique are seen responding to younger sibling behavioral problems by hitting their siblings.

Threats by parents to leave or to give up the child are perhaps the most psychologically damaging ways to control a child's behavior. Children of any age may remain fearful and anxious about loss of the parent long after the threat is made; however, many children are able to see through *empty* threats. Threatening a mild loss of privileges (no video games for 1 week or *grounding* a teenager) may be appropriate, but the consequence must be enforced if there is a violation.

Parenting involves a dynamic balance between **setting limits** on the one hand and allowing and encouraging freedom of expression and exploration on the other. A child whose behavior is out of control improves when clear limits on their behavior are set and enforced. Children find comfort and security in clear limits. However, parents must agree on where the limit will be set and how it will be enforced. The limit and the consequence of breaking the limit must be clearly presented to the child. Enforcement of the limit should be consistent and firm. Too many limits are difficult to learn and may thwart the normal development of autonomy. The limit must be reasonable in terms of the child's age, temperament, and developmental level. To be effective, both parents (and other adults in the home) must enforce limits. Otherwise, children may effectively *split* the parents and seek to test the limits with the more indulgent parent. In all situations, to be effective, punishment must be brief and linked directly to a behavior. More effective behavioral change occurs when punishment also is linked to praise of the intended behavior.

**Extinction** is an effective and systematic way to eliminate a frequent, annoying, and relatively harmless behavior by ignoring it. First, parents should note the frequency of the behavior to appreciate realistically the magnitude of the problem and to evaluate progress. It also is important to help parents determine what reinforces the child's behavior and what needs to be consistently eliminated. An appropriate behavior is identified to give the child a positive alternative that the parents can reinforce. Parents should be warned that the annoying behavior usually increases in frequency and intensity (and may last for weeks) before it decreases when the parent ignores it (removes the reinforcement). A child who has an attention-seeking temper tantrum should be ignored or placed in a secure environment. This action may anger the child more, and the behavior may get louder and angrier. Eventually, as the child realizes that there is no audience for the tantrum, the tantrums decrease in intensity and frequency. In each specific instance, when the child has begun to play with a favorite toy in a quiet and appropriate fashion, he or she should be praised, and extra attention should be given. This is an effective technique for early toddlers, before their capacity to understand and adhere to a timeout.

The **timeout** consists of a short period of isolation *immediately* after a problem behavior is observed. Timeout interrupts the behavior and immediately links it to an unpleasant consequence. This method requires considerable effort by the parents because the child does not wish to be isolated. A parent may need to hold the child physically in timeout. In this situation, the parent should become *part of the furniture* and should not respond to the child until the timeout period is over. When established, a simple isolation technique, such as making a child stand in the corner or sending a child to his or her room, may be effective. If such a technique is not helpful, a more systematic procedure may be needed. One effective protocol for the timeout procedure involves interrupting the child's play when the behavior occurs and having the child sit in a dull, isolated place for a brief period, measured by a portable kitchen timer (kitchen timers are valuable because the clicking noises document that time is passing and the bell alarm at the end signals the end of the punishment; this obviates responding to the inevitable question, "Is time up yet?") Timeout is simply punishment and is not a time for a young child to *think* about the behavior (because these children do not possess the capacity for abstract thinking) or a time to de-escalate the behavior. The amount of timeout should be appropriate to the child's short attention span. One minute per year of a child's age is recommended. This inescapable and unpleasant consequence of the undesired behavior motivates the child to learn to avoid the behavior.

CHAPTER **10**

# Evaluation of the Child with Special Needs

Children with disabilities (cerebral palsy), severe chronic illnesses (diabetes or acquired immunodeficiency syndrome [AIDS]), congenital defects (cleft lip and palate), and health-related educational and behavioral problems (attention-deficit/hyperactivity disorder or a learning disability) are **children with special health care needs**. Many of these children share a broad group of experiences and encounter similar problems, such as school difficulties and family stress. The term *children with special health care needs* defines these children noncategorically, without regard to specific diagnoses, in terms of increased service needs. Approximately 18% of children in the United States younger than 18 years of age have a physical, developmental, behavioral, or emotional condition requiring services of a type or amount beyond that required by children generally. If the definition of chronic illness is restricted to a condition that lasts or is expected to last more than 3 months and limits age-appropriate social functioning, such as school performance or recreational activities, about 6% of children are affected in the United States.

The goal in managing a child with special health care needs is to maximize the child's potential for productive adult functioning by treating the primary diagnosis and by helping the patient and family deal with the stresses and secondary impairments incurred because of the disease or disability. Whenever a chronic disease is diagnosed, family members typically grieve, show anger, denial, negotiation (in an attempt to forestall the inevitable), and depression. Because the child with special health care needs is a constant reminder of the object of this grief, it may take family members a long time to accept the condition. A supportive physician can facilitate the process of acceptance by education and by allaying guilty feelings and fear. To minimize denial, it is helpful to confirm the family's observations about the child. The family may not be able to absorb any additional information initially, so written material and the option for further discussion at a later date should be offered. Parents often recount that they did not remember anything after the pediatrician shared the devastating news.

The primary pediatrician should provide a **medical home** to maintain close oversight of treatments and subspecialty services, provide preventive care, and facilitate interactions with school and community agencies. The family is the one constant in a child's life, whereas service systems and support personnel within those systems fluctuate. A major goal of *family-centered care* is for the family and child to feel in control. Although the medical management team usually directs treatment in the acute health care setting, the locus of control should shift to the family as the child moves into a more routine, home-based life. Treatment plans should be organized to allow the greatest degree of normalization of the child's life. As the child matures, self-management programs that provide health education, self-efficacy skills, and techniques such as symptom monitoring help promote good long-term health habits. These programs should be introduced at 6 or 7 years of age, or when a child is at a developmental level to take on chores and benefit from being given responsibility. Self-management minimizes *learned helplessness* and the *vulnerable child syndrome*, both of which occur commonly in families with chronically ill or disabled children.

## MULTIFACETED TEAM ASSESSMENT OF COMPLEX PROBLEMS

When developmental screening and surveillance suggest the presence of significant developmental lags, the pediatrician should take responsibility for coordinating the further assessment of the child by the team of professionals and provide continuity in the care of the child and family. The physician should become aware of the facilities and programs for assessment and treatment in the local area. If the child is at high risk because of prematurity or another identified illness that might have long-term developmental effects, a structured follow-up program to monitor the child's progress may already exist. Under federal law, children are entitled to developmental assessments regardless of income if there is a suspected developmental delay or a risk factor for delay (e.g., prematurity, failure to thrive, and parental mental retardation). Up to 3 years of age, special programs are developed by states to

implement this policy. Developmental interventions are arranged in conjunction with third-party payers (insurance companies, Medicaid, state children's health insurance program) with the local program funding the cost only when there is no insurance coverage. After 3 years of age, development programs usually are administered by school districts. Federal laws also mandate that special education programs be provided for all children with developmental disabilities from birth through 21 years of age.

Children with special needs may be enrolled in pre-K programs with a therapeutic core, including visits to the program by therapists to work on challenges in the context of the pre-K schedule. Children who are of traditional school age (kindergarten through secondary school) should be evaluated by the school district and provided an **individualized educational plan (IEP)** to address any deficiencies. An IEP may feature individual tutoring time (resource time), placement in a special education program, placement in classes with children with severe behavioral problems, or other strategies to address deficiencies. As part of the comprehensive evaluation of developmental/behavioral issues, all children should receive a thorough medical assessment. A variety of other specialists may assist in the assessment and intervention, including subspecialist pediatricians (e.g., neurology, orthopedics, psychiatry, developmental/behavioral), therapists (e.g., occupational, physical, oral-motor), and others (e.g., psychologists, early childhood development specialists).

### Medical Assessment

The physician's main goals in team assessment are to identify the cause of the developmental dysfunction, if possible (often a specific cause is not found), and identify and interpret other medical conditions that have a developmental impact. The comprehensive history (Table 10-1) and physical examination (Table 10-2) include a careful graphing of growth parameters and an accurate description of dysmorphic features. Many of the diagnoses are rare or unusual diseases or syndromes. Many of these diseases and syndromes are discussed further in Sections 9 and 24.

### Motor Assessment

The comprehensive neurologic examination is an excellent basis for evaluating motor function, but it should be supplemented by an adaptive functional evaluation (see Chapter 179). Watching the child at play aids assessment of function. Specialists in early childhood development and therapists (especially occupational and physical therapists who have experience with children) can provide excellent input into the evaluation of age-appropriate adaptive function.

### Psychological Assessment

Psychological assessment includes the testing of cognitive ability (Table 10-3) and the evaluation of personality and emotional well-being. The IQ and mental age scores, taken in isolation, are only partially descriptive of a person's functional abilities, which are a combination of cognitive, adaptive, and social skills. Tests of achievement are

**TABLE 10-1 Information to Be Sought During the History Taking of a Child with Suspected Developmental Disabilities**

| Item | Possible Significance |
|---|---|
| **Parental Concerns** | Parents are quite accurate in identifying development problems in their children |
| **Current Levels of Developmental Functioning** | Should be used to monitor child's progress |
| **Temperament** | May interact with disability or may be confused with developmental delay |
| **PRENATAL HISTORY** | |
| Alcohol ingestion | Fetal alcohol syndrome; an index of caretaking risk |
| Exposure to medication, illegal drug, or toxin | Development toxin (e.g., phenytoin); may be an index of caretaking risk |
| Radiation exposure | Damage to CNS |
| Nutrition | Inadequate fetal nutrition |
| Prenatal care | Index of social situation |
| Injuries, hyperthermia | Damage to CNS |
| Smoking | Possible CNS damage |
| HIV exposure | Congenital HIV infection |
| Maternal PKU | Maternal PKU effect |
| Maternal illness | Toxoplasmosis, rubella, cytomegalovirus, herpesvirus infections |
| **PERINATAL HISTORY** | |
| Gestational age, birth weight | Biologic risk from prematurity and small for gestational age |
| Labor and delivery | Hypoxia or index of abnormal prenatal development |
| Apgar scores | Hypoxia, cardiovascular impairment |
| Specific perinatal adverse events | Increased risk of CNS damage |
| **NEONATAL HISTORY** | |
| Illness—seizures, respiratory distress, hyperbilirubinemia, metabolic disorder | Increased risk of CNS damage |
| Malformations | May represent syndrome associated with developmental delay |
| **FAMILY HISTORY** | |
| Consanguinity | Autosomal recessive condition more likely |
| Mental functioning | Increased hereditary and environmental risks |
| Illnesses (e.g., metabolic disease) | Hereditary illness associated with developmental delay |
| Family member died young or unexpectedly | May suggest inborn error of metabolism or storage disease |
| Family member requires special education | Hereditary causes of developmental delay |
| **SOCIAL HISTORY** | |
| Resources available (e.g., financial, social support) | Necessary to maximize child's potential |
| Educational level of parents | Family may need help to provide stimulation |
| Mental health problems | May exacerbate child's conditions |
| High-risk behaviors (e.g., illicit drugs, sex) | Increased risk for HIV infection; index of caretaking risk |
| Other stressors (e.g., marital discord) | May exacerbate child's conditions or compromise care |
| **OTHER HISTORY** | |
| Gender of child | Important for X-linked conditions |
| Developmental milestones | Index of developmental delay; regression may indicate progressive condition |
| Head injury | Even moderate trauma may be associated with developmental delay or learning disabilities |
| Serious infections (e.g., meningitis) | May be associated with developmental delay |
| Toxic exposure (e.g., lead) | May be associated with developmental delay |
| Physical growth | May indicate malnutrition; obesity, short stature associated with some conditions |
| Recurrent otitis media | Associated with hearing loss and abnormal speech development |
| Visual and auditory functioning | Sensitive index of impairments in vision and hearing |
| Nutrition | Malnutrition during infancy may lead to delayed development |
| Chronic conditions such as renal disease | May be associated with delayed development or anemia |

CNS, central nervous system; HIV, human immunodeficiency virus; PKU, phenylketonuria.
From Liptak G: Mental retardation and developmental disability. In Kliegman RM, editor: Practical Strategies in Pediatric Diagnosis and Therapy, Philadelphia, 1996, *WB Saunders.*

**TABLE 10-2 Information to Be Sought During the Physical Examination of a Child with Suspected Developmental Disabilities**

| Item | Possible Significance |
| --- | --- |
| **General Appearance** | May indicate significant delay in development or obvious syndrome |
| **STATURE** | |
| Short stature | Williams syndrome, malnutrition, Turner syndrome; many children with severe retardation have short stature |
| Obesity | Prader-Willi syndrome |
| Large stature | Sotos syndrome |
| **HEAD** | |
| Macrocephaly | Alexander syndrome, Sotos syndrome, gangliosidosis, hydrocephalus, mucopolysaccharidosis, subdural effusion |
| Microcephaly | Virtually any condition that can retard brain growth (e.g., malnutrition, Angelman syndrome, de Lange syndrome, fetal alcohol effects) |
| **FACE** | |
| Coarse, triangular, round, or flat face; hypotelorism or hypertelorism, slanted or short palpebral fissure; unusual nose, maxilla, and mandible | Specific measurements may provide clues to inherited, metabolic, or other diseases such as fetal alcohol syndrome, cri du chat syndrome (5p− syndrome), or Williams syndrome |
| **EYES** | |
| Prominent | Crouzon syndrome, Seckel syndrome, fragile X syndrome |
| Cataract | Galactosemia, Lowe syndrome, prenatal rubella, hypothyroidism |
| Cherry-red spot in macula | Gangliosidosis ($GM_1$), metachromatic leukodystrophy, mucolipidosis, Tay-Sachs disease, Niemann-Pick disease, Farber lipogranulomatosis, sialidosis III |
| Chorioretinitis | Congenital infection with cytomegalovirus, toxoplasmosis, or rubella |
| Corneal cloudiness | Mucopolysaccharidosis I and II, Lowe syndrome, congenital syphilis |
| **EARS** | |
| Pinnae, low set or malformed | Trisomies such as 18, Rubinstein-Taybi syndrome, Down syndrome, CHARGE association, cerebro-oculofacial-skeletal syndrome, fetal phenytoin effects |
| Hearing | Loss of acuity in mucopolysaccharidosis; hyperacusis in many encephalopathies |
| **HEART** | |
| Structural anomaly or hypertrophy | CHARGE association, CATCH-22, velocardiofacial syndrome, glycogenosis II, fetal alcohol effects, mucopolysaccharidosis I; chromosomal anomalies such as Down syndrome; maternal phenylketonuria; chronic cyanosis may impair cognitive development |
| **LIVER** | |
| Hepatomegaly | Fructose intolerance, galactosemia, glycogenosis types I to IV, mucopolysaccharidosis I and II, Niemann-Pick disease, Tay-Sachs disease, Zellweger syndrome, Gaucher disease, ceroid lipofuscinosis, gangliosidosis |
| **GENITALIA** | |
| Macro-orchidism | Fragile X syndrome |
| Hypogenitalism | Prader-Willi syndrome, Klinefelter syndrome, CHARGE association |
| **EXTREMITIES** | |
| Hands, feet, dermatoglyphics, and creases | May indicate specific entity such as Rubinstein-Taybi syndrome or be associated with chromosomal anomaly |
| Joint contractures | Sign of muscle imbalance around joints (e.g., with meningomyelocele, cerebral palsy, arthrogryposis, muscular dystrophy; also occurs with cartilaginous problems such as mucopolysaccharidosis) |

## TABLE 10-2 Information to Be Sought During the Physical Examination of a Child with Suspected Developmental Disabilities—cont'd

| Item | Possible Significance |
|------|----------------------|
| **SKIN** | |
| Café au lait spots | Neurofibromatosis, tuberous sclerosis, Bloom syndrome |
| Eczema | Phenylketonuria, histiocytosis |
| Hemangiomas and telangiectasia | Sturge-Weber syndrome, Bloom syndrome, ataxia-telangiectasia |
| Hypopigmented macules, streaks, adenoma sebaceum | Tuberous sclerosis, hypomelanosis of Ito |
| **HAIR** | |
| Hirsutism | de Lange syndrome, mucopolysaccharidosis, fetal phenytoin effects, cerebro-oculofacial-skeletal syndrome, trisomy 18 |
| **NEUROLOGIC** | |
| Asymmetry of strength and tone | Focal lesion, cerebral palsy |
| Hypotonia | Prader-Willi syndrome, Down syndrome, Angelman syndrome, gangliosidosis, early cerebral palsy |
| Hypertonia | Neurodegenerative conditions involving white matter, cerebral palsy, trisomy 18 |
| Ataxia | Ataxia-telangiectasia, metachromatic leukodystrophy, Angelman syndrome |

CATCH-22, cardiac defects, abnormal face, thymic hypoplasia, cleft palate, hypocalcemia, defects on chromosome 22; CHARGE, coloboma, heart defects, atresia choanae, retarded growth, genital anomalies, ear anomalies (deafness).

From Liptak G: Mental retardation and developmental disability. In Kliegman RM, Greenbaum LA, Lye PS, editors: Practical Strategies in Pediatric Diagnosis and Therapy, ed 2, Philadelphia, 2004, *WB Saunders*, p 540.

## TABLE 10-3 Tests of Cognition

| Test | Age Range | Special Features |
|------|-----------|------------------|
| **INFANT SCALES** | | |
| Bayley Scales of Infant Development (2nd ed) | 2–42 mo | Mental, psychomotor scales, behavior record; weak intelligence predictor |
| Cattell Infant Intelligence Scale | Birth–30 mo | Used to extend Stanford-Binet downward |
| Gesell Developmental Schedules | Birth–3 yr | Used by many pediatricians |
| Ordinal Scales of Infant Psychological Development | Birth–24 mo | Six subscales; based on Piaget's stages; weak in predicting later intelligence |
| **PRESCHOOL SCALES** | | |
| Stanford-Binet Intelligence Scale (4th ed) | 2 yr–adult | Four area scores, with subtests and composite IQ score |
| McCarthy Scales of Children's Abilities | 2½–8 yr | 6–18 subtests; good at defining learning disabilities; strengths/weaknesses approach |
| Wechsler Primary and Preschool Test of Intelligence–Revised (WPPSI-R) | 3–6½ yr | 11 subtests; verbal, performance IQs; long administration time; good at defining learning disabilities |
| Merrill-Palmer Scale of Mental Tests | 2–4½ yr | General test for young children |
| Differential Abilities Scale | 2½ yr–adult | Special nonverbal composite; short administration time |
| **SCHOOL-AGE SCALES** | | |
| Stanford-Binet Intelligence Scale (4th ed) | 2 yr–adult | See above |
| Wechsler Intelligence Scale for Children (4th ed) (WISC IV) | 6–16 yr | See comments on WPPSI-R |
| Leiter International Performance Scale | 2 yr–adult | No verbal abilities needed |
| Wechsler Adult Intelligence Scale–Revised (WAIS-R) | 16 yr–adult | See comments on WPPSI-R |
| Differential Abilities Scale | 2½ yr–adult | See above |
| **ADAPTIVE BEHAVIOR SCALES** | | |
| Vineland Adaptive Behavior Scale | Birth–adult | Interview/questionnaire; typical persons and blind, deaf, developmentally delayed and retarded |
| American Association on Mental Retardation (AAMR) Adaptive Behavioral Scale | 3 yr–adult | Useful in mental retardation, other disabilities |

subject to variability based on culture, educational exposures, and experience and must be standardized for social factors. Projective and nonprojective tests are useful in understanding the child's emotional status. Although a child should not be labeled as having a problem solely on the basis of a standardized test, such tests do provide important and reasonably objective data for evaluating a child's growth within a particular educational program.

## Educational Assessment

Educational assessment involves the evaluation of areas of specific strengths and weaknesses in reading, spelling, written expression, and mathematical skills. Schools routinely screen children with group tests to aid in problem identification and program evaluation. For the child with special needs, this screening ultimately should lead to individualized testing and the development of an IEP that would enable the child to progress comfortably in school. Diagnostic teaching, in which the child's response to various teaching techniques is assessed, also may be helpful.

## Social Environment Assessment

Assessment of the environment in which the child is living, working, playing, and growing is important in understanding the child's development. A home visit by a social worker, community health nurse, or home-based intervention specialist can provide valuable information about the child's social milieu. If there is a suspicion of inadequate parenting and, especially, if there is a suspicion of neglect or abuse (including emotional abuse), the child and family must be referred to the local child protection agency. Information about reporting hotlines and local child protection agencies usually is found inside the front cover of local telephone directories (see Chapter 22).

## MANAGEMENT OF DEVELOPMENTAL PROBLEMS

### Intervention in the Primary Care Setting

The clinician must decide whether a problem requires referral for further diagnostic workup and management or whether management in the primary care setting is appropriate. Counseling roles required in caring for these children are listed in Table 10-4. When a child is young,

---

**TABLE 10-4 Primary Care Counseling Roles**

Allow ventilation
Facilitate clarification
Support patient problem solving
Provide specific reassurance
Provide education
Provide specific parenting advice
Suggest environmental interventions
Provide follow-up
Facilitate appropriate referrals
Coordinate care and interpret reports after referrals

---

much of the counseling interaction takes place between the parents and the clinician, and as the child matures, direct counseling shifts increasingly toward the child.

The assessment process may be therapeutic in itself. By assuming the role of a nonjudgmental, supportive listener, the clinician creates a climate of trust in which the family feels free to express difficult or painful thoughts and feelings. Expressing emotions may allow the parent or caregiver to move on to the work of understanding and resolving the problem.

Interview techniques also may facilitate clarification of the problem for the family and for the clinician. The family's ideas about the causes of the problem and descriptions of attempts to deal with it can provide a basis for developing strategies for problem management that are much more likely to be implemented successfully because they emanate in part from the family. The clinician shows respect by endorsing the parent's ideas when appropriate; this can increase self-esteem and sense of competency.

Educating parents about normal and aberrant development and behavior may prevent problems through early detection and anticipatory guidance. Such education also communicates the physician's interest in hearing parental concerns. Early detection allows intervention before the problem becomes entrenched, and associated problems develop.

The severity of developmental and behavioral problems ranges from variations of normal, to problematic responses to stressful situations, to frank disorders. The clinician must try to establish the severity and scope of the patient's symptoms so that appropriate intervention can be planned.

### Counseling Principles

Behavioral change is difficult in any situation. For the child, behavioral change must be learned, not simply imposed. It is easiest to learn when the lesson is simple, clear, and consistent and presented in an atmosphere free of fear or intimidation. Parents often try to impose behavioral change in an emotionally charged atmosphere, most often at the time of a behavioral *violation*. Clinicians often try to *teach* parents with hastily presented advice when the parents are distracted by other concerns or not engaged in the suggested behavioral change.

Apart from management strategies directed specifically at the problem behavior, regular times for positive parent-child interaction should be instituted. Frequent, brief, affectionate physical contact over the day provides opportunities for positive reinforcement of desirable child behaviors and for building a sense of competence in the child and the parent.

Most parents feel guilty when their children have a developmental/behavioral problem. This guilt may be caused by the assumption or fear that the problem was caused by inadequate parenting or guilt about previous angry responses to the child's behavior. If possible and appropriate, the clinician should find ways to alleviate guilt, which may be a serious impediment to problem solving.

### Interdisciplinary Team Intervention

In many cases, a team of professionals is required to provide the breadth and quality of services needed to appropriately serve the child who has developmental problems.

The primary care physician should monitor the progress of the child and continually reassess that the requisite therapy is being accomplished.

**Educational intervention** for a young child begins as home-based infant stimulation, often with an early childhood educator; nurse; or occupational, speech, or physical therapist providing direct stimulation for the child and training the family to provide the stimulation. As the child matures, a center-based nursery program may be indicated. For the school-age child, special services may range from extra attention given by the classroom teacher to a self-contained special education classroom.

**Psychological intervention** may be parent or family directed or may become, with an older child, primarily child directed. Examples of therapeutic approaches are guidance therapies, such as directive advice giving, counseling the family and child in their own solutions to problems, psychotherapy, behavioral management techniques, psychopharmacologic methods, and cognitive therapy.

**Motor intervention** may be performed by a physical or occupational therapist. *Neurodevelopmental therapy* (NDT), the most commonly used method, is based on the concept that nervous system development is hierarchical and subject to some plasticity. The focus of NDT is on gait training and motor development, including daily living skills; perceptual abilities, such as eye-hand coordination; and spatial relationships. *Sensory integration therapy* is also used by occupational therapists to structure sensory experience from the tactile, proprioceptive, and vestibular systems to allow for adaptive motor responses.

**Speech-language intervention** by a speech therapist (oral-motor therapist) is usually part of the overall educational program and is based on the tested language strengths and weaknesses of the child. Children needing this type of intervention may show difficulties in reading and other academic areas and develop social and behavioral problems because of their difficulties in being understood and in understanding others. **Hearing intervention**, performed by an audiologist (or an otolaryngologist), includes monitoring hearing acuity and providing amplification when necessary via hearing aids.

**Social and environmental intervention** generally takes the form of nursing or social work involvement with the family. Frequently the task of coordinating the services of other disciplines falls to these specialists. These case managers may be in the private sector, from the child's insurance or Medicaid plan or part of a child protection agency.

**Medical intervention** for a child with a developmental disability involves providing primary care as well as specific treatment of conditions associated with disability. Although curative treatment often is not possible because of the irreversible nature of many disabling conditions, functional impairment can be minimized through thoughtful medical management. Certain general medical problems are found more frequently in delayed and developmentally disabled people (Table 10-5). Many of these children have associated medical conditions, especially if the delay is part of a known syndrome (Down syndrome or vertebral defects, imperforate anus, tracheoesophageal fistula, and radial and renal dysplasia [VATER association]). Some children may have a limited life expectancy. Supporting the family through palliative care, hospice, and bereavement is another important role of the primary care pediatrician.

## SELECTED CLINICAL PROBLEMS: THE SPECIAL NEEDS CHILD

### Mental Retardation

Mental retardation (MR) is defined as significantly subnormal intellectual functioning for a child's developmental stage, existing concurrently with deficits in adaptive

---

**TABLE 10-5 Recurring Medical Issues in Children with Developmental Disabilities**

| Problem | Ask About or Check |
|---|---|
| Motor | Range of motion examination; scoliosis check; assessment of mobility; interaction with orthopedist, physiatrist, and physical therapist/occupational therapist as needed |
| Diet | Dietary history, feeding observation, growth parameter measurement and charting, supplementation as indicated by observations |
| Sensory impairments | Functional vision and hearing screening; interaction as needed with ophthalmologist, audiologist |
| Dermatology | Examination of *all* skin areas for decubitus ulcers or infection |
| Dentistry | Examination of teeth and gums; confirmation of access to dental care |
| Behavioral problems | Aggression, self-injury, pica; sleep problems; psychotropic drug levels and side effects |
| Advocacy | Educational program, family supports, financial supports |
| Seizures | Major motor, absence, other suspicious symptoms; monitoring of anticonvulsant levels and side effects |
| Infectious diseases | Ear infections, diarrhea, respiratory symptoms, aspiration pneumonia, immunizations (especially hepatitis B and influenza) |
| Gastrointestinal problems | Constipation, gastroesophageal reflux, gastrointestinal bleeding (stool for occult blood) |
| Sexuality | Sexuality education, hygiene, contraception (when appropriate), genetic counseling |
| Other syndrome-specific problems | Ongoing evaluation of other "physical" problems as indicated by known mental retardation/developmental disability etiology |

**TABLE 10-6 Levels of Mental Retardation**

| Level of Retardation | ICD-10 IQ Score | WISC-IV IQ Score | Educational Label |
|---|---|---|---|
| Mild | 50–69 | 50–55 to 70 | "Educable (EMR)" |
| Moderate | 35–49 | 35–40 to 50–55 | "Trainable (TMR)" |
| Severe | 20–34 | 20–25 to 35–50 | |
| Profound | <20 | <20–25 | |

ICD-10, International Classification of Diseases (WHO), ed 10; WISC-IV, Wechsler Intelligence Scale for children, ed 4.

behaviors (self-care, home living, communication, and social interactions). MR is defined statistically as cognitive performance that is two standard deviations below the mean (roughly below the third percentile) of the general population as measured on standardized intelligence testing. There have been no longitudinal studies of the prevalence of MR in the United States, and cross-sectional estimates have varied immensely. The last known estimates were about 20,000 per million, or 2%. Levels of MR from IQ scores derived from two typical tests are shown in Table 10-6. Caution must be exercised in interpretation because these categories do not reflect actual functional level of the tested individual.

The etiology of the central nervous system insult resulting in MR may involve genetic disorders, teratogenic influences, perinatal insults, acquired childhood disease, and environmental and social factors (Table 10-7). Mild MR correlates with socioeconomic status, although profound MR does not. Although a single organic cause may be found, each individual's performance should be considered a function of the interaction of environmental influences with the individual's organic substrate. It is common for a child with MR to have behavioral difficulties resulting from the MR itself and from the family's reaction to the child and the condition. More severe forms of MR can be traced to biologic factors. The earlier the cognitive slowing is recognized, the more severe the deviation from normal is likely to be.

The first step in the diagnosis and management of a child with MR is to identify functional strengths and weaknesses for purposes of medical and habilitative therapies. When the developmental delays have been identified, the history and physical examination may suggest a diagnostic approach that, then, may be confirmed by laboratory testing and/or imaging. Frequently used laboratory tests include chromosomal analysis and magnetic resonance imaging of the brain. Almost one third of individuals with MR do not have readily identifiable reasons for their disability.

## Vision Impairment

Significant visual impairment is a problem in many children. **Partial vision** (defined as visual acuity between 20/70 and 20/200) occurs in 1 in 500 school-age children

**TABLE 10-7 Differential Diagnosis of Mental Retardation***

### EARLY ALTERATIONS OF EMBRYONIC DEVELOPMENT

Sporadic events affecting embryogenesis, usually a stable developmental challenge
  Chromosomal changes (e.g., trisomy 21)
  Prenatal influences (e.g., substance abuse, teratogenic medications, intrauterine TORCH infections)[†]

### UNKNOWN CAUSES

No definite issue is identified, or multiple elements present, none of which is diagnostic (may be multifactorial)

### ENVIRONMENTAL AND SOCIAL PROBLEMS

Dynamic influences, commonly associated with other challenges
  Deprivation (neglect)
  Parental mental illness
  Environmental intoxications (e.g., significant lead intoxication)[*]

### PREGNANCY PROBLEMS AND PERINATAL MORBIDITY

Impingement on normal intrauterine development or delivery; neurologic abnormalities frequent, challenges are stable or occasionally worsening
  Fetal malnutrition and placental insufficiency
  Perinatal complications (e.g., prematurity, birth asphyxia, birth trauma)

### HEREDITARY DISORDERS

Preconceptual origin, variable expression in the individual infant, multiple somatic effects, frequently a progressive or degenerative course
  Inborn errors of metabolism (e.g., Tay-Sachs disease, Hunter disease, phenylketonuria)
  Single-gene abnormalities (e.g., neurofibromatosis or tuberous sclerosis)
  Other chromosomal aberrations (e.g., fragile X syndrome, deletion mutations such as Prader-Willi syndrome)
  Polygenic familial syndromes (pervasive developmental disorders)

### ACQUIRED CHILDHOOD ILLNESS

Acute modification of developmental status, variable potential for functional recovery
  Infections (all can ultimately lead to brain damage, but most significant are encephalitis and meningitis)
  Cranial trauma (accidental and child abuse)
  Accidents (e.g., near-drowning, electrocution)
  Environmental intoxications (prototype is lead poisoning)

*Some health problems fit in several categories (e.g., lead intoxication may be involved in several areas).
†This also may be considered as an acquired childhood disease. TORCH, toxoplasmosis, other (congenital syphilis and viruses), rubella, cytomegalovirus, and herpes simplex virus.

in the United States, with about 35,000 children having visual acuity between 20/200 and total blindness. **Legal blindness** is defined as distant visual acuity of 20/200 or worse. Although this definition allows for considerable residual vision, such impairment can be a major barrier to optimal educational development.

The most common cause of **severe visual impairment** in children is retinopathy of prematurity (see Chapter 61). Congenital cataracts may lead to significant amblyopia. Cataracts also are associated with other ocular abnormalities and developmental disabilities. **Amblyopia** is defined as a pathologic alteration of the visual system characterized by a reduction in visual acuity in one or both eyes with no clinically apparent organic abnormality that can completely account for the visual loss. Amblyopia is due to a distortion of the normal clearly formed retinal image (from congenital cataracts or severe refractive errors); abnormal binocular interaction between the eyes with one eye competitively inhibiting the other (strabismus); or a combination of both mechanisms. Albinism, hydrocephalus, congenital cytomegalovirus infection, and birth asphyxia are other significant contributors to blindness in children.

Children with **mild to moderate visual impairment** usually are discovered to have an uncorrected refractive error. The most common presentation is myopia or nearsightedness. Other causes are hyperopia (farsightedness) and astigmatism (alteration in the shape of the cornea leading to visual distortion). In children younger than 6 years of age, high refractive errors in one or both eyes also may cause amblyopia, which aggravates the vision impairment.

The diagnosis of severe visual impairment commonly is made when an infant is 4 to 8 months of age. Clinical suspicion is based on parental concerns aroused by unusual behavior, such as lack of smiling in response to appropriate stimuli, the presence of nystagmus, other wandering eye movements, or motor delays in beginning to reach for objects. Fixation and visual tracking behavior can be seen in most infants by 6 weeks of age. This behavior can be assessed by moving a brightly colored object (or the examiner's face) across the visual field of a quiet but alert infant at a distance of 1 foot. The eyes also should be examined for red reflexes and pupillary reactions to light, although optical alignment (binocular vision with both eyes consistently focusing on the same spot) should not be expected until the infant is beyond the newborn period. Persistent nystagmus is abnormal at any age. If ocular abnormalities are identified, referral to a pediatric ophthalmologist is indicated.

During the newborn period, vision may be assessed by physical examination and by **visual evoked response (VER)**. This test evaluates the conduction of electrical impulses from the optic nerve to the occipital cortex of the brain. The eye is stimulated by a bright flash of light or with an alternating checkerboard of black-and-white squares and the resulting electrical response is recorded from electrodes strategically placed on the scalp, similar to an electroencephalogram.

There are many developmental implications of visual impairment. Perception of body image is abnormal, and imitative behavior, such as smiling, is delayed. Delays in mobility may occur in children who are visually impaired from birth, although their postural milestones (ability to sit) usually are achieved appropriately. Social bonding with the parents also is affected.

Visually impaired children can be helped in various ways. Classroom settings may be augmented with resource-room assistance to present material in a nonvisual format; some schools consult with an experienced teacher of the blind. Fine motor activity development, listening skills, and Braille reading and writing are intrinsic to successful educational intervention with the child who has severe visual impairment.

## Hearing Impairment

The clinical significance of hearing loss varies with its type (conductive vs. sensorineural), its frequency, and its severity as measured in number of decibels heard or the number of decibels of hearing lost. The most common cause of mild to moderate hearing loss in children is a conduction abnormality caused by acquired middle ear disease. This abnormality may have a significant effect on the development of speech and other aspects of language development, particularly if there is chronic fluctuating middle ear fluid. When hearing impairment is more severe, sensorineural hearing loss is more common. Causes of sensorineural deafness include congenital infections (e.g., rubella or cytomegalovirus), meningitis, birth asphyxia, kernicterus, ototoxic drugs (especially aminoglycoside antibiotics), and tumors and their treatments. Genetic deafness may be either dominant or recessive in inheritance; this is the main cause of hearing impairment in schools for the deaf. In Down syndrome, there is a predisposition to conductive loss caused by middle ear infection and sensorineural loss caused by cochlear disease. Any hearing loss may have a significant effect on the child's developing communication skills. These skills then affect all areas of the child's cognitive and skills development (Table 10-8).

It is sometimes quite difficult to determine accurately the presence of hearing in infants and young children. Using developmental surveillance to inquire about a newborn's or infant's response to parental sounds or even observing the response to sounds in the office is unreliable for identifying hearing-impaired children. Universal screening of newborns is required prior to nursery discharge and includes:

- **Auditory brainstem response (ABR)**, which measures how the brain responds to sound. Clicks or tones are played through soft earphones into the infant's ears. Three electrodes placed on the infant's head measure the brain's response.
- **Otoacoustic emissions (OAE)**, which measures sound waves produced in the inner ear. A tiny probe is placed just inside the infant's ear canal. It measures the response (echo) when clicks or tones are played into the infant's ears.

Both of these tests are quick (5 to 10 minutes), painless, and may be performed while the infant is sleeping or lying still. The tests are sensitive but not as specific as more definitive tests. Infants who fail these tests are referred for more comprehensive testing. Many of these infants have normal hearing on definitive testing. Infants who do not having normal hearing are immediately referred for etiologic diagnosis and early intervention.

**TABLE 10-8 Neurodevelopmental-Behavioral Complications of Hearing Loss**

| Severity of Hearing Loss | Possible Etiologic Origins | Complications | | | Types of Therapy |
|---|---|---|---|---|---|
| | | Speech-Language | Educational | Behavioral | |
| *Slight* 15–25 dB (ASA) | Serous otitis media | Difficulty with distant or faint speech | Possible auditory learning dysfunction | Usually none | May require favorable class setting, speech therapy, or auditory training |
| | Perforation of tympanic membrane Sensorineural loss Tympanosclerosis | | May reveal a slight verbal deficit | | Possible value in hearing aid |
| *Mild* 25–40 dB (ASA) | Serous otitis media | Difficulty with conversational speech over 3–5 ft | May miss 50% of class discussions | Psychological problems | Special education resource help |
| | Perforation of tympanic membrane | May have limited vocabulary and speech disorders | Auditory learning dysfunction | May act inappropriately if directions are not heard well | Hearing aid |
| | Sensorineural loss Tympanosclerosis | | | Acting out behavior Poor self-concept | Favorable class setting Lip reading instruction Speech therapy |
| *Moderate* 40–65 dB (ASA) | Chronic otitis media | Conversation must be loud to be understood | Learning disability | Emotional and social problems | Special education resource or special class |
| | Middle ear anomaly | Defective speech | Difficulty with group learning or discussion | Behavioral reactions of childhood | Special help in speech-language development |
| | Sensorineural loss | Deficient language use and comprehension | Auditory processing dysfunction | Acting out | Hearing aid and lip reading |
| | | | Limited vocabulary | Poor self-concept | Speech therapy |
| *Severe* 65–95 dB (ASA) | Sensorineural loss | Loud voices may be heard 2 ft from ear | Marked educational retardation | Emotional and social problems that are associated with handicap | Full-time special education for deaf children |
| | Middle ear disease | Defective speech and language | Marked learning disability | Poor self-concept | Hearing aid, lip reading, speech therapy |
| | | No spontaneous speech development if loss present before 1 yr | Limited vocabulary | | Auditory training |
| | | | | | Counseling Cochlear implant |
| *Profound* ≥95 dB (ASA) | Sensorineural or mixed loss | Relies on vision rather than hearing | Marked learning disability because of lack of understanding of speech | Congenital and prelingually deaf may show severe emotional problems | As above |
| | | Defective speech and language Speech and language will not develop spontaneously if loss present before 1 yr | | | Oral and manual communication Counseling |

ASA, Acoustical Society of America.
From Gottleib MI: Otitis media. In Levine MD, Carey WB, Crocker AC, et al, editors: Developmental-Behavioral Pediatrics, Philadelphia, 1983, WB Saunders.

For children not screened at birth or children with suspected acquired hearing loss, later testing may allow early appropriate intervention. Hearing can be screened by means of an office audiogram, but other techniques are needed (ABR, behavior audiology) for young, neurologically immature or impaired, and behaviorally difficult children. The typical audiologic assessment includes pure-tone audiometry over a variety of sound frequencies (pitches), especially over the range of frequencies in which most speech occurs. Tympanometry is used in the assessment of middle ear function and the evaluation of tympanic membrane compliance for pathology in the middle ear, such as fluid, ossicular dysfunction, and eustachian tube dysfunction (see Chapter 9).

The treatment of conductive hearing loss (largely due to otitis media and middle ear effusions) is discussed in Chapter 105. Treatment of sensorineural hearing impairment may be medical or surgical. The audiologist may believe that amplification is indicated, in which case hearing aids can be tuned preferentially to amplify the frequency ranges in which the patient has decreased acuity. Educational intervention typically includes speech-language therapy and teaching American Sign Language. Even with amplification, many hearing-impaired children show deficits in processing information presented through the auditory pathway, requiring special educational services for helping to read and for other academic skills. Cochlear implants may benefit some children. A cochlear implant is a surgically implantable device that provides hearing sensation to individuals with severe to profound hearing loss who do not benefit from hearing aids. The implants are designed to substitute for the function of the middle ear, cochlear mechanical motion, and sensory cells, transforming sound energy into electrical energy that initiates impulses in the auditory nerve. Cochlear implants are indicated for children between 12 months and 17 years of age with profound bilateral sensorineural hearing loss who have limited benefit from hearing aids. In addition, they have failed to progress in auditory skill development and have no radiologic or medical contraindications. Implanting children as young as possible gives them the most advantageous auditory environment for speech-language learning.

## Speech-Language Impairment

Parents often bring the concern of speech delay to the physician's attention when they compare their young child with others of the same age (Table 10-9). The most common causes of the speech delay are MR, hearing impairment, social deprivation, autism, and oral-motor abnormalities. If a problem is suspected based on screening with tests such as the Denver II or other standard screening test (Early Language Milestone Scale), a referral to a specialized hearing and speech center is indicated. While awaiting the results of testing or initiation of speech-language therapy, parents should be advised to speak slowly and clearly to the child (and avoid *baby talk*). Parents and older siblings should read to the speech-delayed child frequently.

Speech disorders include **articulation, fluency**, and **resonance disorders**. Articulation disorders include

difficulties producing sounds in syllables or saying words incorrectly to the point that other people cannot understand what is being said. Fluency disorders include problems such as **stuttering**, the condition in which the flow of speech is interrupted by abnormal stoppages, repetitions (*st-st-stuttering*), or prolonging sounds and syllables (*sssstuttering*). Resonance or voice disorders include

**TABLE 10-9 Clues to When a Child with a Communication Disorder Needs Help**

**0–11 MONTHS**

Before 6 months, the child does not startle, blink, or change immediate activity in response to sudden, loud sounds
Before 6 months, the child does not attend to the human voice and is not soothed by his or her mother's voice
By 6 months, the child does not babble strings of consonant and vowel syllables or imitate gurgling or cooing sounds
By 10 months, the child does not respond to his or her name
At 10 months, the child's sound-making is limited to shrieks, grunts, or sustained vowel production

**12–23 MONTHS**

At 12 months, the child's babbling or speech is limited to vowel sounds
By 15 months, the child does not respond to "no," "bye-bye," or "bottle"
By 15 months, the child does not imitate sounds or words
By 18 months, the child is not consistently using at least six words with appropriate meaning
By 21 months, the child does not respond correctly to "Give me...," "Sit down," or "Come here" when spoken without gestural cues
By 23 months, two-word phrases that are spoken as single units (e.g., "whatszit," "thank you," "allgone") have not emerged

**24–36 MONTHS**

By 24 months, at least 50% of the child's speech is not understood by familiar listeners
By 24 months, the child does not point to body parts without gestural cues
By 24 months, the child is not combining words into phrases (e.g., "go bye-bye," "go car," "want cookie")
By 30 months, the child does not show understanding of on, in, under, front, and back
By 30 months, the child is not using short sentences (e.g., "Daddy went bye-bye")
By 30 months, the child has not begun to ask questions (using where, what, why)
By 36 months, the child's speech is not understood by unfamiliar listeners

**ALL AGES**

At any age, the child is consistently dysfluent with repetitions, hesitations; blocks or struggles to say words. Struggle may be accompanied by grimaces, eye blinks, or hand gestures

Adapted from Weiss CE, Lillywhite HE: Communication Disorders: A Handbook for Prevention and Early Detection, St Louis, 1976, *Mosby.*

problems with the pitch, volume, or quality of a child's voice that distract listeners from what is being said.

Language disorders can be either receptive or expressive. Receptive disorders refer to difficulties understanding or processing language. Expressive disorders include difficulty putting words together, limited vocabulary, or inability to use language in a socially appropriate way.

Speech-language pathologists (speech or oral-motor therapists) assess the speech, language, cognitive-communication, and swallowing skills of children; determine what types of communication problems exist; and the best way to treat these challenges. Speech-language pathologists skilled at working with infants and young children are also vital in training parents and infants in other oral-motor skills, such as teaching the parent of an infant born with cleft lip and palate how to feed the infant appropriately.

Speech-language therapy involves having a speech-language specialist work with a child on a one-on-one basis, in a small group, or directly in a classroom to overcome a specific disorder using a variety of therapeutic strategies. Language intervention activities involve having a speech-language specialist interact with a child by playing and talking to him or her. The therapist may use pictures, books, objects, or ongoing events to stimulate language development. The therapist also may model correct pronunciation and use repetition exercises to build speech and language skills. Articulation therapy involves having the therapist model correct sounds and syllables for a child, often during play activities.

Children enrolled in therapy early in their development (<3 years of age) tend to have better outcomes than children who begin therapy later. Older children can make progress in therapy, but progress may occur more slowly because these children often have learned patterns that need to be modified or changed. Parental involvement is crucial to the success of a child's progress in speech-language therapy.

## Cerebral Palsy

Cerebral palsy (CP) refers to a group of nonprogressive, but often changing, motor impairment syndromes secondary to anomalies or lesions of the brain usually arising before or after birth. A total of 2 to 2.5 of every 1000 live-born children in developed countries have CP; incidence is higher in premature and twin births. Prematurity and low birth weight infants (leading to perinatal asphyxia), congenital malformations, and kernicterus are causes of CP noted at birth. Ten percent of children with CP have acquired CP that occurs at later ages. Meningitis and head injury (accidental and nonaccidental) are the most common causes of acquired CP (Table 10-10). Nearly 50% of children with CP have no identifiable risk factors.

Most children with CP, except in its mildest forms, are diagnosed in the first 18 months of life when they fail to attain motor milestones or when they show abnormalities such as asymmetric gross motor function, hypertonia, or hypotonia. CP can be characterized further by the affected parts of the body (Table 10-11) and descriptions of the predominant type of motor disorder (Table 10-12). Comorbidities in these children often include epilepsy,

learning difficulties, behavioral challenges, and sensory impairments. Many of these children have an isolated motor defect. Some affected children may be intellectually gifted.

Treatment depends on the pattern of dysfunction. Physical and occupational therapy can facilitate optimal positioning and movement patterns, increasing function of the affected parts. Spasticity management also may include oral medications, botulinum toxin injections, and implantation of intrathecal baclofen pumps. Management of seizures, spasticity, orthopedic impairments, and sensory impairments all may help improve educational attainment. CP cannot be cured, but a host of interventions can improve functional abilities, participation in society, and quality of life.

---

**TABLE 10-10 Risk Factors for Cerebral Palsy**

### PREGNANCY AND BIRTH

Low socioeconomic status
Prematurity
Low birth weight/fetal growth retardation (<1500 g at birth)
Maternal seizures/seizure disorder
Treatment with thyroid hormone, estrogen, or progesterone
Pregnancy complications
    Polyhydramnios
    Eclampsia
    Third-trimester bleeding (including threatened abortion and placenta previa)
    Multiple births
    Abnormal fetal presentation
    Maternal fever
Congenital malformations/syndromes
Newborn hypoxic-ischemic encephalopathy
Bilirubin (kernicterus)

### ACQUIRED AFTER THE NEWBORN PERIOD

Meningitis
Head Injury
    Car crashes
    Child abuse
Stroke

---

**TABLE 10-11 Descriptions of Cerebral Palsy by Site of Involvement**

Hemiparesis (hemiplegia)—predominantly unilateral impairment of the arm and leg on the same (e.g., right or left) side
Diplegia—motor impairment primarily of the legs (often with some limited involvement of the arms; some authors challenge this specific type as not being different from quadriplegia)
Quadriplegia—all four limbs (whole body) are functionally compromised

| **TABLE 10-12 Classification of Cerebral Palsy by Type of Motor Disorder** |
| --- |

**Spastic cerebral palsy:** the most common form of cerebral palsy, it accounts for 70%–80% of cases. It results from injury to the upper motor neurons of the pyramidal tract. It may occasionally be bilateral. It is characterized by at least two of the following:
  Abnormal movement pattern
  Increased tone
  Pathologic reflexes (e.g., Babinski response, hyperreflexia)
**Dyskinetic cerebral palsy:** occurs in 10%–15% of cases. It is dominated by abnormal patterns of movement and involuntary, uncontrolled, recurring movements.
**Ataxic cerebral palsy:** accounts for <5% of cases. This form of the disease results from cerebellar injury and features abnormal posture or movement and loss of orderly muscle coordination or both.
**Dystonic cerebral palsy:** also uncommon. It is characterized by reduced activity and stiff movement (hypokinesia) and hypotonia.
**Choreoathetotic cerebral palsy:** rare now that excessive hyperbilirubinemia is aggressively prevented and treated. This form is dominated by increased and stormy movements (hyperkinesia) and hypotonia.
**Mixed cerebral palsy:** accounts for 10%–15% of cases. This term is used when more than one type of motor pattern is present and when one pattern does not clearly dominate another. It typically is associated with more complications, including sensory deficits, seizures, and cognitive-perceptual impairments.

# SUGGESTED READING

Brosco J, Mattingly M, Sanders L: Impact of specific medical interventions on reducing the prevalence of mental retardation, *Arch Pediatr Adolesc Med* 160:302–309, 2006.

Council on Children With Disabilities: Section on Developmental Behavioral Pediatrics. Bright Futures Steering Committee. Medical Home Initiatives for Children With Special Needs Project Advisory Committee, *Pediatrics* 118(1): 405–420, 2006.

Daniels S, Greer F: Committee on Nutrition: Lipid screening and cardiovascular health in childhood, *Pediatrics* 122:198–208, 2008.

Gardner HG: American Academy of Pediatrics Committee on Injury, Violence, and Poison Prevention. Office-based counseling for unintentional injury prevention, *Pediatrics* 119(1):202–206, 2007.

Hagan J, Shaw J, Duncan P: Bright futures: Guidelines for health supervision of infants, children, and adolescents, 3rd ed, Elk Grove Village Ill, 2008, *American Academy of Pediatrics.*

Kliegman R, Behrman R, Jenson H, et al: Nelson textbook of pediatrics, 18th ed, Philadelphia, 2007, *Elsevier.*

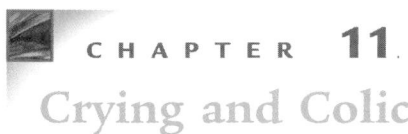

CHAPTER 11

# Crying and Colic

Crying can be a sign of pain, distress, hunger, or tiredness. Humans interpret their infants' cries according to the context of the crying. The cry of a newborn at the time of delivery heralds the health and vigor of the infant. The screams of the same infant at 6 weeks of age after feeding, changing, and soothing may be interpreted as a sign of illness, difficult temperament, or poor parenting. Crying is a manifestation of infant arousal influenced by the environment and interpreted through the lens of the family, social, and cultural context.

## NORMAL DEVELOPMENT

Understanding crying includes attention to the characteristics of timing, duration, frequency, intensity, and modifiability of the cry (Fig. 11-1). Most infants cry little

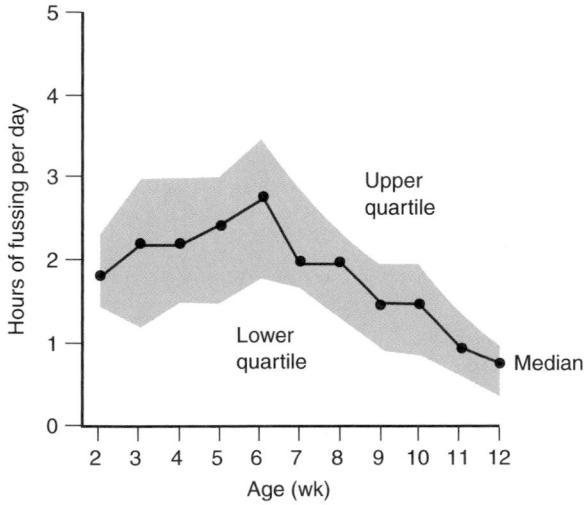

**FIGURE 11-1**

Distribution of total crying time among 80 infants studied from 2 to 12 weeks of age. Data derived from daily crying diaries recorded by mothers. (From Brazelton TB: Crying in infancy, *Pediatrics* 29:582, 1962.)

during the first 2 weeks of life. Between 2 and 6 weeks, total daily crying duration increases from an average of 2 hours per day to 3 hours per day. By 12 weeks of age, the average daily duration of crying is 1 hour.

Cry duration differs by culture and infant care practices; the duration of crying is 50% lower in the !Kung San hunter gatherers, who continuously carry their infants and feed them four times per hour, compared with infants in the United States. Crying may also relate to health status. Premature infants cry little before 40 weeks gestational age and tend to cry more than term infants at 6 weeks' corrected age. Crying behavior in former premature infants also may be influenced by ongoing medical conditions, such as bronchopulmonary dysplasia, visual impairments, and feeding disorders. The duration of crying is modifiable by caregiving strategies.

**Frequency** of crying has less variability than duration of crying. At 6 weeks of age, the mean frequency of combined crying and fussing is 10 episodes in 24 hours (assessed by parental diary and voice-activated radiotelemetric tape recordings). Diurnal variation in crying is the norm, with crying concentrated in the late afternoon and evening.

The **intensity** of infant crying varies, with descriptions ranging from fussing to screaming. An intense infant cry (pitch and loudness) is more likely to elicit concern or even alarm from parents and caregivers than an infant who frets more quietly. Pain cries of newborns are remarkably loud: 80 dB at a distance of 30.5 cm from the infant's mouth. Although pain cries have a higher frequency than hunger cries, when not attended to for a protracted period, hunger cries become acoustically similar to pain cries. Fortunately, most infant crying is of a lesser intensity, consistent with fussing.

## COLIC

Colic often is diagnosed using the **rule of threes**—crying for more than 3 hours per day, for more than 3 days per week, for more than 3 weeks. The limitations of this definition include the lack of definition of crying (does this include fussing?) and the necessity to wait 3 weeks to make a diagnosis in an infant who has excessive crying. The crying of colic is often described as paroxysmal and may be characterized by facial grimacing, drawing up of the legs, and passing flatus.

## Etiology

Fewer than 5% of infants evaluated for excessive crying have an organic etiology. Because the etiology of colic is unknown, this syndrome may represent the extreme of the normal phenomenon of infant crying. Nonetheless, evaluation of infants with excessive crying is warranted.

## Epidemiology

Cumulative incidence rates of colic vary from 5% to 19% in different studies. Girls and boys are affected equally. Studies vary by how colic is defined and by data collection methodology, such as maintaining a cry diary or actual recording of infant vocalizations. Concern about infant crying also varies by culture, and this may influence what is recorded as crying or fussing.

## Clinical Manifestations

The clinician who evaluates a crying infant must differentiate serious disease from colic, which has no identifiable etiology. The history includes a description of the crying, including duration, frequency, intensity, and modifiability. Does the infant have associated symptoms, such as pulling up of the legs, facial grimacing, vomiting, or back arching? When did the crying first begin? Has the crying changed? Does anything relieve or exacerbate the crying? Is there a diurnal pattern to the crying? A review of systems is essential because crying in an infant is a systemic symptom that can herald serious illness. Past medical history also is important, because infants with perinatal problems are at increased risk for neurologic causes of crying. Attention to the feeding history is crucial because some causes of crying are related to feeding problems, including hunger, air swallowing (worsened by crying), gastroesophageal reflux, and food intolerance. Questions concerning the family's ability to handle the stress of the infant's crying and their knowledge of infant soothing strategies assist the clinician in assessing risk for parental mental health comorbidities and developing an intervention plan suitable for the family.

The **physical examination** is an essential component of the evaluation of an infant with colic. The diagnosis of colic is made only when the physical examination reveals no organic cause for the infant's excessive crying. The examination begins with vital signs, weight, length, and head circumference, looking for effects of systemic illness on growth, such as occur with infection or malnutrition. A thorough inspection of the infant is important to identify possible sources of pain, including skin lesions, **corneal abrasions**, **hair tourniquets**, **skeletal infections**, or signs of child abuse such as **fractures** (see Chapters 22 and 198). Infants with common conditions such as otitis media, urinary tract infections, mouth ulcerations, and insect bites may present with crying. A neurologic examination may reveal previously undiagnosed neurologic conditions, such as perinatal brain injuries, as the cause of irritability and crying. Observation of the infant during a crying episode is invaluable to assess the infant's potential for calming and the parents' skills in soothing the infant.

**FIGURE 11-2**

Algorithm for medical evaluation of infants with acute excessive crying. (From Barr RG, et al: Crying complaints in the emergency department. In Crying as a Sign, a Symptom, and a Signal, London, 2000, *MacKeith Press*.)

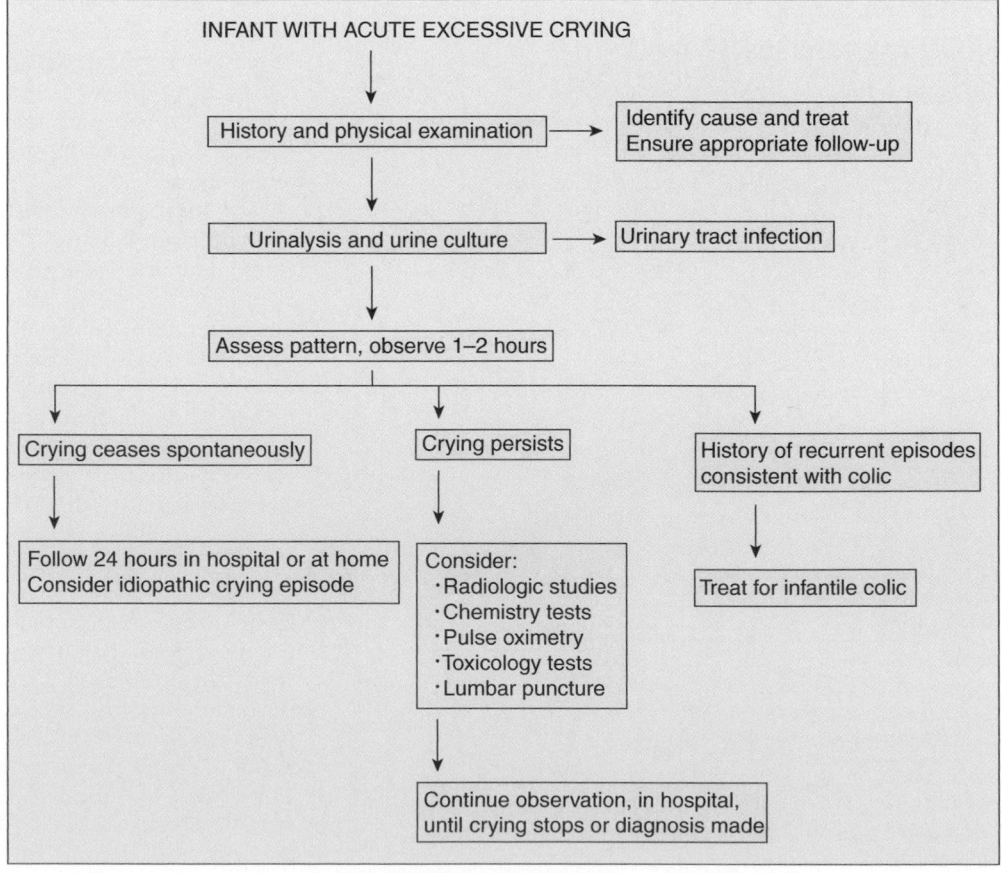

Laboratory and imaging studies are reserved for infants in whom there are history or physical examination findings suggesting an organic cause for excessive crying. An algorithm for the medical evaluation of an infant with excessive crying inconsistent with colic is presented in Figure 11-2.

## Differential Diagnosis

The differential diagnosis for colic is broad and includes any condition that can cause pain or discomfort in the infant and conditions associated with *nonpainful* distress, such as fatigue or sensory overload (Table 11-1). Cow's milk protein intolerance, maternal drug effects (including fluoxetine hydrochloride via breastfeeding), and anomalous left coronary artery all have been reported as causes of persistent crying. In addition, situations associated with poor infant regulation, including fatigue, hunger, parental anxiety, and chaotic environmental conditions, may increase the risk of excessive crying. In most cases, the cause of crying in infants is unexplained. If the condition began before 3 weeks' corrected age, the crying has a diurnal pattern consistent with colic (afternoon and evening clustering), the infant is otherwise developing and thriving, and no organic cause is found, a diagnosis of colic is indicated.

## Treatment

The management of colic begins with education and demystification. When the family and the physician are reassured that the infant is healthy, and no infection, trauma, or underlying disease is present, education about the normal pattern of infant crying is appropriate. Learning about the temporal pattern of colic can be reassuring; the mean crying duration begins to decrease at 6 weeks of age and decreases by half by 12 weeks of age. Parents should not be told that colic resolves by 3 months of age; at that point the mean duration of crying is 1 hour per day. Approximately 15% of infants with colic continue to have excessive crying after 3 months of age.

Helping families develop caregiving schedules that accommodate the infant's fussy period is useful. Techniques for calming infants include soothing vocalizations or singing, swaddling, slow rhythmic rocking, walking, white noise, and gentle vibration (e.g., a ride in a car). Giving caretakers permission to allow the infant to rest when soothing strategies are not working may alleviate overstimulation in some infants; this also relieves families of guilt and allows them a wider range of responses to infant crying. **Avoidance** of dangerous soothing techniques, such as **shaking the infant** or placing the infant on a vibrating clothes dryer (which has resulted in injury from falls), should be stressed.

**Medications**, including phenobarbital, diphenhydramine, alcohol, simethicone, dicyclomine, and lactase, are of no benefit in reducing colic and should be avoided. Parents, especially from Mexico and Eastern Europe, often use chamomile, fennel, vervain, licorice, and balm-mint teas. These teas have not been studied scientifically as remedies for colic. Families should be counseled to limit the volume of tea given because it displaces milk from the infant's diet and may limit caloric intake.

**TABLE 11-1 Diagnoses in 56 Infants Presenting to the Denver Children's Hospital Emergency Department with an Episode of Unexplained, Excessive Crying**

| Diagnosis | No. with Diagnosis |
|---|---|
| **Idiopathic** | 10 |
| **INFECTIOUS** | |
| Otitis media* | 10 |
| Viral illness with anorexia, dehydration* | 2 |
| Urinary tract infection* | 1 |
| Mild prodrome of gastroenteritis | 1 |
| Herpangina* | 1 |
| Herpes stomatitis* | 1 |
| **TRAUMA** | |
| Corneal abrasion* | 3 |
| Foreign body in eye* | 1 |
| Foreign body in oropharynx* | 1 |
| Tibial fracture (from child abuse)* | 1 |
| Clavicular fracture (accidental)* | 1 |
| Brown recluse spider bite* | 1 |
| Hair tourniquet syndrome (hair wrapped tightly around digit) | 1 |
| **GASTROINTESTINAL** | |
| Constipation | 3 |
| Intussusception* | 1 |
| Gastroesophageal reflux* | 1 |
| **CENTRAL NERVOUS SYSTEM** | |
| Subdural hematoma (bleeding around the brain from child abuse)* | 1 |
| Encephalitis* | 1 |
| Pseudotumor cerebri* | 1 |
| **DRUG REACTION/OVERDOSE** | |
| DTP reaction[†] | 1 |
| Inadvertent pseudoephedrine (cold medication) overdose | 1 |
| **BEHAVIORAL** | |
| Night terrors | 1 |
| Overstimulation | 1 |
| **CARDIOVASCULAR** | |
| Supraventricular tachycardia* | 2 |
| **METABOLIC** | |
| Glutaric aciduria type 1* | 1 |
| *Total* | 56 |

*Indicates conditions considered serious.
[†]From diphtheria/tetanus/pertussis (DTP) vaccine.
From Barr RG, et al: Crying complaints in the emergency department. In Crying as a Sign, a Symptom, and a Signal, London, 2000, *MacKeith Press*; with permission.

**Dietary changes** should be considered in certain specific circumstances. There is rationale for change to a non–cow's milk formula if the infant has signs of cow's milk protein colitis. If the infant is breastfeeding, the mother can eliminate dairy products from her diet. In most circumstances, dietary changes are not effective in reducing colic, but they may appear to help because their use coincides with the natural reduction in crying between 6 and 12 weeks of age.

## Prognosis

Infants with colic have not been shown to have adverse long-term outcomes in health or temperament after the neonatal period. Similarly, infantile colic does not have untoward long-term effects on maternal mental health. When colic subsides, the maternal distress resolves. Rarely, cases of child abuse have been associated with inconsolable infant crying.

## Prevention

Much can be done to prevent colic, beginning with education of all prospective parents about the normal pattern of infant crying. Prospective parents often imagine that their infant will cry only briefly for hunger, not realizing that this may be beyond their control. Increased contact and carrying of the infant in the weeks before the onset of colic may decrease the duration of crying episodes. Similarly, other soothing strategies may be more effective if the infant has experienced them before the onset of excessive crying. Infants who have been tightly swaddled for sleep and rest during the first weeks of life often calm to swaddling during a crying episode; this is not true for infants who have not experienced swaddling before a crying episode. Parents also can be coached to learn to read their infant's cues and ask themselves if the infant is hungry, uncomfortable, bored, or overstimulated. Parents also should be counseled that there are times when the infant's cry is not interpretable, and caregivers can only do their best.

CHAPTER **12**

# Temper Tantrums

A temper tantrum is defined as out-of-control behavior, including screaming, stomping, hitting, head banging, falling down, and other violent displays of frustration. In the extreme, tantrums can include breath-holding, vomiting, and serious aggression, including biting. Such behavior is seen most often when the young child experiences frustration, anger, or simple inability to cope with a situation. Temper tantrums can be considered normal behavior in 1- to 3-year-old children, when the temper tantrum period is of short duration and the tantrums are not manipulative in nature.

## ETIOLOGY

Temper tantrums are believed to be a normal human developmental stage. Child temperament may be a determinant of tantrum behavior.

## EPIDEMIOLOGY

This behavior is common in children 18 months to 4 years of age. In U.S. studies, 50% to 80% of 2- to 3-year-old children have had regular tantrums, and 20% are reported to have daily tantrums. The behavior appears to peak late in the third year of life. Approximately 20% of 4-year-olds are still having regular temper tantrums, and explosive temper occurs in approximately 5% of school-age children. Tantrums occur equally in boys and girls during the preschool period.

## CLINICAL MANIFESTATIONS

Temper tantrums are the most commonly reported behavioral problem in 2- and 3-year-old children. The typical frequency of tantrums is approximately one per week, with a great deal of variability (Fig. 12-1). The duration of each tantrum is 2 to 5 minutes, and duration increases with age (Fig. 12-2). Helping the family identify the typical antecedents of the child's tantrums is essential to evaluation and intervention. A child who has tantrums only when he or she misses a routine nap can be treated differently than a child who has frequent tantrums related to minor difficulties or disappointments.

The **evaluation** of a child who is having temper tantrums requires a complete history, including perinatal and developmental information. Careful attention to the child's daily routines may reveal problems associated with hunger, fatigue, inadequate physical activity, or overstimulation. A social history is important, because family stress can exacerbate or prolong what begins as a normal developmental phase. Some children may be exposed to violence in the home and may be exhibiting learned behavior. The coexistence of other behavioral problems, such as sleep problems, learning problems, and social problems, suggests the possibility of a more serious mental health disorder.

The physical examination focuses on discovering underlying illness that could decrease the child's ability to self-regulate. Thorough examination of the skin to identify child abuse is recommended (see Chapter 22). The neurologic examination identifies underlying brain disorders. Dysmorphic features may reveal a genetic syndrome. Behavioral observations reveal a child's ability to follow instructions, play with age-appropriate toys, and interact with parents and clinician.

Laboratory studies screening for iron deficiency anemia and lead exposure are important. Other laboratory and imaging studies are performed only when the history and physical examination suggest a possible underlying etiology. Some children with excessive tantrums should have a formal developmental evaluation.

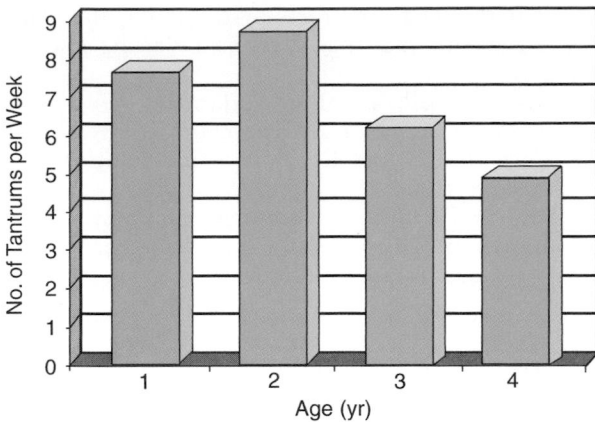

**FIGURE 12-1**

**Mean tantrum frequency per week.** Children 1 to 4 years of age who have tantrums typically have four to nine tantrums per week.

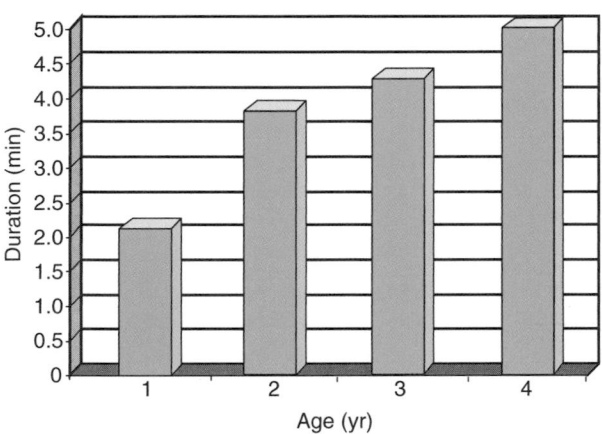

**FIGURE 12-2**

**Mean duration of tantrums.** The typical duration of a tantrum increases with the age of the child.

## DIFFERENTIAL DIAGNOSIS

Most children who have temper tantrums have no underlying medical problem. In rare instances, seizures may mimic a tantrum. Hearing loss and language delay may be associated with temper tantrums. Children with brain injury and other brain disorders are at increased risk for prolonged temper tantrum behavior (in terms of actual tantrum duration and continued manifestation after the normal tantrum age). These children include former premature infants and children with autism, traumatic brain injury, cognitive impairment, and Prader-Willi and Smith-Magenis syndromes. Children with rare conditions, such as congenital adrenal hyperplasia and precocious puberty, also may present with severe and persistent tantrums.

## TREATMENT

Intervention begins with parental education about temper tantrums, stressing that tantrums are a normal developmental phase. Parents may have unwarranted concerns about their child's mental health. The clinician can help parents understand their role in helping the child move toward self-regulation of frustration and anger. The environment can be structured to limit toddler frustration; age-inappropriate demands on the child; and hunger, fatigue, loneliness, or hyperstimulation. It is important to review the child's daily routine to understand if the child's behavior is communicating an essential unmet need. Children who behave well all day at day care and exhibit temper tantrums at home in the evening may be signaling fatigue or need for parental attention. Identification of underlying stress is the cornerstone of treatment because many stressors can be eliminated. If the child is required to put away toys before a snack and always has a tantrum, the parent could consider switching the order of the activities. It is possible that the child is hungry at that moment and cannot handle the delay in nourishment. Parents may consider some changes in the home environment so that they do not have to say "No" to the child as frequently. At the moment of a tantrum, the parent can consider how to move the child quickly back into a state of control without reinforcing an unreasonable demand.

In some cases, parents inadvertently reinforce tantrum behavior by complying with the child's demands. A 2-year-old who has learned that her mother will give her soda pop when she screams may repeat this behavior to get what she wants. The child's behavior can be seen as manipulative or simply as learned behavior from a prior successful experience. Parental ambivalence about acceptable toddler behavior also may lead to inconsistent expectations and restrictions. Helping parents clarify what behavior is allowed and what is off limits can avert the temptation to give in when the child screams loudly or publicly.

Distraction from the frustrating object or event is an effective means of short-circuiting impending tantrums. Physically removing the child from an environment that is associated with the child's difficulty is sometimes helpful. Children who have difficulty with noisy or visually stimulating environments can be protected from that type of overstimulation until they are more mature.

Further behavioral interventions are recommended only after strategies to help the child gain control by meeting basic needs, altering the environment, and anticipating meltdowns are in place. Recommended behavioral strategies include behavior modification with positive and negative reinforcement and extinction. During the first week of any behavioral intervention, a child may increase tantrum behavior. Parents must be warned that it will probably get worse before it gets better. At the same time that parents are working to extinguish or decrease the tantrums, it is important that they provide positive reinforcement for good behavior. It also is advisable to spend time with the child when his or her behavior is desirable, reinforcing behavior that the parents enjoy.

## PREVENTION

Providing parents with knowledge about the temper tantrum stage and strategies for assisting the child with emotional regulation is recommended at a health care maintenance visit between 12 and 18 months of age. Regular routines for sleeping, eating, and physical activity in a childproofed home (or day care center) provided by well-rested and psychologically healthy parents (or caregivers) usually result in a quick transition through this challenging period.

CHAPTER **13**

# Attention-Deficit/ Hyperactivity Disorder

Attention-deficit/hyperactivity disorder (ADHD) is a neurobehavioral disorder defined by symptoms of inattention, hyperactivity, and impulsivity. Clinical guidelines emphasize the use of the *Diagnostic and Statistical Manual of Mental Health Disorders, Fourth Edition,* criteria to diagnose ADHD (Table 13-1). These criteria require that the child have symptoms in at least two environments and functional impairment in addition to the symptoms of the disorder for diagnosis.

## ETIOLOGY

ADHD is a complex of symptoms with diverse etiology. There is evidence that ADHD runs in some families, but there is no evidence of any single gene that determines ADHD type. Although most cases of ADHD occur in typically developing children, ADHD can be seen in children who have developmental disorders, including fetal alcohol syndrome and Down syndrome, as well as in children who have had varying levels of brain injury, including perinatal brain damage. Most commonly, there is no identified cause of ADHD. It is likely that the symptoms of ADHD represent a final common pathway of diverse causes, including genetic, organic, and environmental etiologies (perhaps in combination).

## EPIDEMIOLOGY

The estimated prevalence of ADHD in U.S. school-age community populations is 8% to 10%. There is a twofold to threefold higher prevalence in boys than in girls. Girls are more likely to be diagnosed with inattentive-type ADHD. Symptoms of ADHD persist into adolescence in 60% to 80% of patients. Many continue to have symptoms into adulthood.

## CLINICAL MANIFESTATIONS

The diagnosis of ADHD is made by **history**. The clinician should elicit the history by interview using open-ended questions focused on specific behaviors and by using ADHD-specific rating scales. ADHD rating scales are sensitive and specific for diagnosing ADHD. The Conners Questionnaires and the Vanderbilt forms are two commonly used parent and teacher questionnaires.

A **physical examination** is essential to rule out underlying medical or developmental problems. The examination should include the observation of the child and the parents and their relationship. It is a mistake to interpret absence of hyperactivity in the office as a sign that the child does not have ADHD. It is common for children with ADHD to focus without hyperactivity in an environment that has low stimulation and little distraction.

**Laboratory and imaging** studies are not routinely recommended. The clinician may consider thyroid function studies, blood lead levels, genetic karyotyping, and brain imaging studies if any of these studies are indicated by past medical history, environmental history, or physical examination. These studies do not confirm ADHD, but they are useful in excluding other conditions.

## DIFFERENTIAL DIAGNOSIS

The differential diagnosis includes the possibility that the child's behavior is within the range of normal. Other possibilities include hyperactivity and distractibility secondary to hyperthyroidism or lead intoxication. Chaotic living situations also can lead to symptoms of hyperactivity, distractibility, and inattention. Children who have symptoms of ADHD in only one setting may be having problems secondary to cognitive level, level of emotional maturity, or feelings of well-being in that setting.

Speech-language delay and learning disabilities can occur with ADHD (see Chapter 8). Psychiatric conditions, such as conduct disorder, depression, and anxiety disorder, also are more common in children with ADHD than in the general population (see Section 4).

## TREATMENT

Management begins with recognizing ADHD as a chronic condition and educating affected children and their parents about the symptoms of ADHD and strategies to control adverse effects on learning, school functioning, social relationships, and family life. Children with ADHD benefit from **behavioral approaches** to accommodate their condition. It is helpful to provide structure, routine, and appropriate behavioral goals. Some children benefit from social skills counseling or mental health treatment to assist behavior change or to preserve self-esteem.

**Stimulant medication** is effective for managing the symptoms of inattention, hyperactivity, and distractibility in most children with ADHD. Stimulant medications do not treat the comorbid conditions and do not improve intelligence. Short-acting, intermediate-acting, and long-acting methylphenidate and long-acting dextroamphetamine are widely used stimulant medications. Nonstimulant medications, including atomoxetine, may be helpful for children who have not responded to stimulant medications. Alpha agonists such as clonidine and guanfacine hydrochloride also can be helpful for children with ADHD, especially for children with sleep disorders. Dosing for ADHD medications is listed in Table 13-2. Common side effects of stimulant medication include appetite suppression and sleep disturbance. These side effects usually can be managed by careful adjustment of dosage and timing of the medication.

Many parents worry that their child may develop illicit drug use and even addiction because of taking stimulant

| TABLE 13-1 Diagnostic Criteria for Attention-Deficit/Hyperactivity Disorder |
|---|

A. Either 1 or 2
  1. Six (or more) of the following symptoms of **inattention** have persisted for at least 6 mo to a degree that is maladaptive and inconsistent with developmental level
  *Inattention*
    a. Often fails to give close attention to details or makes careless mistakes in schoolwork, work, or other activities
    b. Often has difficulty sustaining attention in tasks or play activities
    c. Often does not seem to listen when spoken to directly
    d. Often does not follow through on instructions and fails to finish schoolwork, chores, or duties in the workplace (not due to oppositional behavior or failure to understand instructions)
    e. Often has difficulty organizing tasks and activities
    f. Often avoids, dislikes, or is reluctant to engage in tasks that require sustained mental effort (e.g., schoolwork or homework)
    g. Often loses things necessary for tasks or activities (e.g., toys, school assignments, pencils, books, or tools)
    h. Is often easily distracted by extraneous stimuli
    i. Is often forgetful in daily activities
  2. Six (or more) of the following symptoms of **hyperactivity-impulsivity** have persisted for at least 6 mo to a degree that is maladaptive and inconsistent with developmental level
  *Hyperactivity*
    a. Often fidgets with hands or feet or squirms in seat
    b. Often leaves seat in classroom or in other situations in which remaining seated is expected
    c. Often runs about or climbs excessively in situations in which it is inappropriate (in adolescents or adults, may be limited to subjective feelings of restlessness)
    d. Often has difficulty playing or engaging in leisure activities quietly
    e. Is often "on the go" or often acts as if "driven by a motor"
    f. Often talks excessively
  *Impulsivity*
    g. Often blurts out answers before questions have been completed
    h. Often has difficulty awaiting turn
    i. Often interrupts or intrudes on others (e.g., butts into conversations or games)
B. Some hyperactive-impulsive or inattentive symptoms that caused impairment were present <7 yr of age
C. Some impairment from the symptoms is present in two or more settings (e.g., at school [or work] and at home)
D. There must be clear evidence of clinically significant impairment in social, academic, or occupational functioning
E. The symptoms do not occur exclusively during the course of a pervasive developmental disorder, schizophrenia, or other psychotic disorder and are not better accounted for by another mental disorder (e.g., mood disorder, anxiety disorder, dissociative disorder, or personality disorder)

Code based on type:
**314.01 Attention-Deficit/Hyperactivity Disorder, Combined Type:** if both criteria A1 and A2 are met for the past 6 mo
**314.00 Attention-Deficit/Hyperactivity Disorder, Predominantly Inattentive Type:** if criterion A1 is met but criterion A2 is not met for the past 6 mo
**314.01 Attention-Deficit/Hyperactivity Disorder, Predominantly Hyperactive, Impulsive Type:** if criterion A2 is met but criterion A1 is not met for the past 6 mo
**314.9 Attention-Deficit/Hyperactivity Disorder Not Otherwise Specified**

From the American Psychiatric Association: *Diagnostic and Statistical Manual of Mental Disorders*, 4th ed (DSM-IV), Arlington, Va, 1994, American Psychiatric Association.

medication. Children with ADHD may be at increased risk for drug use during adolescence because of their impulsivity. Nonetheless, there is a decreased risk of drug abuse in children with ADHD who are well managed medically.

## COMPLICATIONS

ADHD may be associated with academic underachievement, difficulties in interpersonal relationships, and poor self-esteem.

## PREVENTION

Child-rearing practices that include promoting calm environments and opportunities for increasing length of focus on age-appropriate activities may be helpful. Limiting time spent watching television and playing rapid-response video games also may be prudent because these activities reinforce short attention span. Prevention of secondary disabilities can be achieved by education of medical professionals and educators about the signs and symptoms of ADHD and the most appropriate behavioral and pharmaceutical interventions.

**TABLE 13-2  Medications Used in Attention-Deficit/Hyperactivity Disorder**

| Generic Medication | Brand Name | Daily Dose (mg/kg)* | Common Adverse Effects |
|---|---|---|---|
| **Stimulants** | | | All age groups: |
| Methylphenidate | Ritalin (LA†) | 1.0–2.0 | ● Insomnia, decreased appetite, weight loss, dysphoria |
| | Concerta† | 0.5–1.0 | |
| | Metadate (CD†) | 0.3–1.5 | |
| | MTS (patch)†,‡ | 1.0 | |
| D-Methylphenidate | Focalin (XR†) | 1.0 | ● Possible reduction in growth velocity with chronic use |
| Amphetamines | | | |
| Dextroamphetamine | Dexedrine | 1.0 | ● Rebound phenomena with immediate release |
| Lisdexamfetamine | Vyvanse | 1.0 | |
| Amphetamine compound | Adderall (XR†) | 1.0 | |
| Noradrenergic agents | | | |
| Atomoxetine | Strattera | 0.5–1.8 | ● GI upset |
| | | | ● Hypersomnia and insomnia |
| | | | ● Irritability/activation |
| Arousal Agents | | | |
| Modafinil§ | Provigil | 200–400 mg/day | ● Insomnia |
| | | | ● Appetite suppression |
| | | | ● Headache |
| **Antidepressants** | | | All age groups |
| Bupropion§ | Wellbutrin (SR, XL) | 3.0–6.0 | ● Irritability, insomnia, seizure risk |
| | | | ● Contraindicated in bulimics |
| Tricyclics (TCAs)§ | | | ● Dry mouth, constipation |
| Imipramine, desipramine | Tofranil, Norpramin | 2.0–5.0 | ● Weight loss |
| Nortriptyline | Pamelor | 1.0–3.0 | ● Vital sign and ECG changes |
| | | | ● Nausea |
| | | | ● Sedation |
| Antihypertensives | | | Juveniles only: |
| Clonidine§ | Catapres | 3–10 μg/kg | ● Sedation, depression, confusion |
| | | | ● Rebound hypertension |
| | | | ● Dermatitis with patch |
| Guanfacine§ | Tenex | 30–100 μg/kg | Similar to clonidine but less sedation |

*Exceeds dosage recommended by the manufacturer.
†Denotes extended-release preparation of stimulant.
‡Not yet approved for use in the United States.
§Not approved by the Food and Drug Administration for this indication.
ECG, electrocardiographic.
From Wilens T, Spencer T, Biederman J: Attention deficit hyperactivity disorder. In Rakel RE, Bope ER, editors: Conn's Current Therapy, 60th ed, Philadelphia, *Saunders*, 2008.

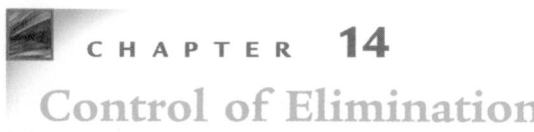

CHAPTER **14**

# Control of Elimination

## NORMAL DEVELOPMENT OF ELIMINATION

Development of control of urination and defecation involves physical and cognitive maturation and is strongly influenced by cultural norms and practices. Toilet training practices differ in various cultural and economic groups in the United States. There is even greater diversity of toilet training practices and age of acquisition of toilet mastery throughout the world. In the first half of the 20th century,

toilet mastery by 18 months of age was the norm in the United States. Concern about harsh toilet training and possible later psychological distress led to professional endorsement of later toilet training. In 1962, Brazelton introduced the *child-centered approach,* which respects the child's autonomy and pride in mastery. The invention of disposable diapers also facilitated later toilet training. Social changes, including increased maternal work outside the home and group child care, also have influenced this trend. Some families choose to wait until the child is older because the duration of the training period is usually shorter. Toilet training usually begins after the second birthday and is achieved at about 3 years of age in middle-class white U.S. populations. Toilet training between 12 and 18 months of age continues to be accepted in lower-income families.

Prerequisites for achieving elimination in the toilet include the child's ability to recognize the urge for urination and defecation; get to the toilet; understand the sequence of tasks required; avoid oppositional behavior; and take pride in achievement. The entire process of toilet training can take 6 months and need not be hurried. Successful parent-child interaction around the goal of toilet mastery can set the stage for future active parental teaching and training (e.g., manners, kindness, rules and laws, and limit setting).

## ENURESIS

Enuresis is urinary incontinence in a child who is considered adequately mature to have achieved continence. Enuresis is classified as diurnal (daytime) or nocturnal (nighttime). Daytime dryness is expected in the United States by 4 years of age. Nighttime dryness is expected by 6 years of age. Another useful classification of enuresis is **primary** (incontinence in a child who has never achieved dryness) and **secondary** (incontinence in a child who has been dry for at least 6 months).

### Etiology

Enuresis is a symptom with multiple possible etiologic factors, including developmental difference, organic illness, or psychological distress. Primary enuresis often is associated with a family history of delayed acquisition of bladder control. A genetic etiology has been hypothesized, and familial groups with autosomal dominant phenotypic patterns for nocturnal enuresis have been identified. Although most children with enuresis do not have a psychiatric disorder, stressful life events can trigger loss of bladder control. Sleep physiology may play a role in the etiology of nocturnal enuresis, with a high arousal threshold commonly noted. In a subgroup of enuretic children, nocturnal polyuria relates to a lack of a nocturnal vasopressin peak. Another possible etiology is malfunction of the detrusor muscle such that it has a tendency for involuntary contractions even when the bladder contains small amounts of urine. Reduced bladder capacity can be associated with enuresis and is commonly seen in children who have chronic constipation with a large dilated distal colon, which impinges on the bladder.

### Epidemiology

Enuresis is the most common urologic condition in children. Nocturnal enuresis has a reported prevalence of 7% in 8-year-olds and 1% in 15-year-olds. The spontaneous remission rate is reported to be 15% per year. The odds ratio of nocturnal enuresis in boys compared with girls is 1.4:1. The prevalence of daytime enuresis is lower than nocturnal enuresis but has a female predominance. Estimates of prevalence are 2% in boys and 3% in girls at 7 years of age. Of children with enuresis, 22% wet only during the day, 17% wet during the day and at night, and 61% wet at night only. Large family size and father absence have been independently associated with enuresis.

### Clinical Manifestations

The history focuses on elucidating the pattern of voiding: How often does wetting occur? Does it occur during the day, night, or both? Are there any associated conditions with wetting episodes (e.g., bad dreams, consumption of caffeinated beverages, or exhausting days)? Has the child had a period of dryness in the past? Was a change in wetting pattern preceded by a stressful event? A review of systems should include a developmental history and detailed information about the neurologic, urinary, and gastrointestinal systems (including patterns of defecation). A history of sleep patterns also is important, including snoring, parasomnias, and timing of nighttime urination. A family history often reveals that one or both parents had enuresis as children. Although enuresis is rarely associated with child abuse, physical and sexual abuse history should be included as part of the psychosocial history. Many families have tried numerous interventions before seeking a physician's help. Identifying these interventions and how they were carried out aids the understanding of the child's condition and its role within the family.

The **physical examination** begins with observation of the child and the parent for clues about child developmental and parent-child interaction patterns. Special attention is paid to the abdominal, neurologic, and genital examination. A rectal examination is recommended if the child has constipation. Observation of voiding is recommended if a history of voiding problems, such as hesitancy or dribbling, is elicited. The lumbosacral spine should be examined for signs of spinal dysraphism or a tethered cord.

For most children with enuresis, the only laboratory test recommended is a clean catch urinalysis to look for chronic urinary tract infection (UTI), renal disease, and diabetes mellitus. Further testing, such as urine culture, is based on the urinalysis. Children with complicated enuresis, including children with previous or current UTI, severe voiding dysfunction, or a neurologic finding, are evaluated with a renal sonogram and a voiding cystourethrogram. If vesicoureteral reflux, hydronephrosis, or posterior urethral valves are found, the child is referred to a urologist for further evaluation and treatment.

### Differential Diagnosis

Commonly, there is no identified cause of enuresis and in most cases, enuresis resolves by adolescence without treatment. Children with primary nocturnal enuresis are most likely to have a family history and are least likely to have an identified etiology. Children with secondary diurnal and nocturnal enuresis are more likely to have an organic etiology, such as UTI, diabetes mellitus, or diabetes insipidus, to explain their symptoms. Children with primary diurnal and nocturnal enuresis may have a neurodevelopmental condition or a problem with bladder function. Children with secondary nocturnal enuresis may have a psychosocial stressor or a sleep disturbance as a predisposing condition for enuresis.

### Treatment

Treatment begins with treating any diagnosed underlying organic causes of enuresis, including UTIs, diabetes mellitus, sleep disorders, and urologic abnormalities. Elimination of underlying chronic constipation is often curative. For a child whose enuresis is not associated with an identifiable disorder, all therapies must be considered in terms of cost in time, money, disruption to the family, the treatment's known success rate, and the child's likelihood to recover from the condition without treatment. Treatment options include **conditioning therapy**, **pharmacotherapy**, and **hypnotherapy**. The clinician can also assist the family in making a plan to help the child cope with this problem until it is resolved. Many children have to live with enuresis for months to years before a cure is achieved, and a few children have symptoms into adulthood. A plan for handling wet garments and linens in a nonhumiliating and hygienic manner preserves the child's self-esteem. The child should take as much responsibility as he or she is able, depending on age, development, and family culture.

The most widely used **conditioning therapy** for nocturnal enuresis is the **enuresis alarm**. Enuresis alarms have an initial success rate of 70% with a relapse rate of 10%. The use of an alarm requires commitment from the parent and the child. The alarm is worn on the wrist or clipped onto a layer of clothing and has a probe that is placed in the underpants or pajamas in front of the urethra. The alarm sounds when the first drop of urine contacts the probe. The child is instructed to get up and finish voiding in the bathroom when the alarm sounds. After 3 to 5 months, 70% of children are dry through the night, either because they become conditioned to awaken to a full bladder or because they become able to complete a night without urination.

**Pharmacotherapy** for nighttime enuresis includes tricyclic antidepressants and desmopressin acetate. **Imipramine** reduces the frequency of nighttime wetting. The initial dose for children 6 years of age and older is 25 mg 1 hour before bedtime. The dose may be increased to 50 mg after 1 week. The maximum dose for children younger than 12 years of age is 50 mg, and it is 75 mg for those 12 years of age and older. The initial success rate is 50%. Imipramine is effective only during treatment, with a relapse rate of 90% on discontinuation of the medication. The most important contraindication is risk of overdose (associated with fatal cardiac arrhythmia). **Desmopressin** is also used to treat enuresis and has proved to be safe. It is available in an oral form, which is more acceptable than the nasal spray formulation. The oral medication is started at 0.2 mg per dose (one dose at bedtime) and on subsequent nights is increased to 0.4 mg and then to 0.6 mg if needed. Desmopressin decreases the number of wet nights per week. This treatment must be considered symptomatic, not curative, and has a relapse rate of 90% when the medication is discontinued.

**Hypnotherapy** has a reported 44% success rate without relapse, with significant improvement in the number of dry nights in an additional 31% of patients. Hypnotherapy for enuresis should be offered by health or mental health professionals who are qualified to evaluate and treat enuresis by other modalities and who have training in pediatric hypnotherapy.

## Complications

The psychological consequences can be severe. Families can minimize the impact on the child's self-esteem by avoiding punitive approaches and ensuring that the child is competent to handle issues of their own comfort, hygiene, and aesthetics.

## Prevention

Early identification of chronic constipation can eliminate one common cause of enuresis. Early diagnosis and treatment of sleep disorders can eliminate another cause of nocturnal enuresis. Appropriate anticipatory guidance concerning toilet training to educate parents that 15% of 5-year-olds and 7% of 8-year-olds regularly wet the bed helps alleviate considerable anxiety about children who do not achieve nighttime dryness early in childhood.

# FUNCTIONAL CONSTIPATION AND SOILING

**Constipation** is decreased frequency of bowel movements usually associated with a hard stool consistency. The occurrence of pain at defecation frequently accompanies constipation. Although underlying gastrointestinal, endocrinologic, or neurologic disorders can cause constipation, *functional constipation* implies that there is no identifiable causative organic condition. **Encopresis** is the regular, voluntary or involuntary passage of feces into a place other than the toilet after 4 years of age. Encopresis without constipation is uncommon and may be a symptom of oppositional defiant disorder or other psychiatric illness. *Soiling* is the involuntary passage of stool and often is associated with fecal impaction. The normal frequency of bowel movements declines between birth and 4 years of age, beginning with greater than four stools per day to approximately one per day.

## Etiology

The etiology of functional constipation and soiling includes a low-fiber diet, slow gastrointestinal transit time for neurologic or genetic reasons, and chronic withholding of bowel movements usually because of past painful defecation experiences. Approximately 95% of children referred to a subspecialist for encopresis have no other underlying pathologic condition.

## Epidemiology

In U.S. studies, 16% to 37% of children experience constipation between 5 and 12 years of age. Constipation with overflow soiling occurs in 1% to 2% of preschool children and 4% of school-age children. The incidence of constipation and soiling is equal in preschool girls and boys, whereas there is a male predominance during school age.

## Clinical Manifestations

The presenting complaint for constipation with soiling is typically a complaint of uncontrolled defecation in the underwear. Parents may report that the child has diarrhea because of soiling of liquid stool. Soiling may be frequent or continuous. On further questioning, the clinician learns that the child is passing large-caliber bowel movements that occasionally block the toilet. Children younger than 3 years of age often present with painful defecation, impaction, and withholding. The history should include a complete review of systems for gastrointestinal, endocrine, and neurologic disorders and a developmental and psychosocial history.

**Stool impaction** can be felt on abdominal examination in about 50% of patients at presentation. Firm packed stool in the rectum is highly predictive of fecal impaction. A rectal examination allows assessment of sphincter tone and size of the rectal vault. Evaluation of anal placement and existence of anal fissures also is helpful in considering etiology and severity. A neurologic examination, including lower extremity reflexes, anal wink, and cremasteric reflexes, may reveal underlying spinal cord abnormalities.

Abdominal x-ray is not required. It can be helpful to show to the family the degree of colonic distention and fecal impaction. In obese children or children who cannot cooperate with a physical examination, a flat plate provides the evidence needed to make the diagnosis. In general, further studies, such as barium enema and rectal biopsy, are indicated only if an organic cause for the constipation is indicated by history or physical examination (see Chapter 129). Similarly, although endocrinologic conditions such as hypothyroidism can cause chronic constipation, laboratory studies are not indicated without history or physical examination suggesting such a disorder.

## Differential Diagnosis

The differential diagnosis for functional constipation and soiling includes organic causes of constipation (e.g., neurogenic, anatomic, endocrinologic, gastrointestinal, and pharmacologic). A child with chronic constipation and soiling who had delayed passage of meconium and has an empty rectum and a tight sphincter may have Hirschsprung disease (see Chapter 129). Chronic constipation may be a presenting sign of spinal cord abnormalities, such as a spinal cord tumor or a tethered cord. Physical examination findings of altered lower extremity reflexes, absent anal wink, or a sacral hairy tuft or sacral sinus may be a clue to these anomalies. Hypothyroidism can present with chronic constipation and typically is accompanied by poor linear growth and bradycardia. Anal stenosis may lead to chronic constipation. The use of opiates, phenothiazine, antidepressants, and anticholinergics also may lead to chronic constipation. Developmental problems, including mental retardation and autism, may be associated with chronic constipation.

## Treatment

Treatment begins with education and demystification for the child and family about chronic constipation and soiling, emphasizing the chronic nature of this condition and the good prognosis with optimal management. Explaining the physiologic basis of constipation and soiling to the child and the family alleviates blame and enlists cooperation. Education may improve adherence to the long-term treatment plan (Table 14-1). One half to two thirds of children with functional constipation recover completely and no longer require medication. The younger the child is when diagnosis and treatment begin, the higher the success rate. Treatment involves a combination of behavioral training and laxative therapy. Successful treatment requires 6 to 24 months. The next step is adequate colonic cleanout or disimpaction. Clean-out methods include enemas alone or combinations of enema, suppository, and oral laxatives. High-dose oral mineral oil is a slower approach to cleanout.

| TABLE 14-1 Education About Chronic Constipation and Soiling |
| --- |

Constipation affects 16%–37% of children, and 1%–4% of children have functional constipation and soiling.

Functional constipation with or without soiling begins early in life for most children owing to a combination of common factors:

- Uncomfortable/painful stool passage
- Withholding of stool to avoid discomfort
- Diets higher in constipating foods and lower in fiber and fluid intake*
- Use of medications that are constipating
- Developmental features—increasing autonomy and perhaps toilet avoidance
- Perhaps family genetic factors—slower colonic transit

When chronic impaction of stool has occurred, physiologic changes at the rectum reduce a child's ability to control his or her bowel movements.

- Rectal vault is dilated resulting in reduced sensation to standard fecal volume.
- Rehabilitation of rectal musculature and strength requires several months. Until then, the dilated rectal musculature may be less able to expel stool effectively.
- Some children have paradoxical anal sphincter contraction when the urge to defecate is felt; this can lead to incomplete emptying of stool at defecation attempt.

Many children do not recognize their soiling accidents owing to olfactory accommodation.

Although children frequently present with low self-esteem or other behavioral concerns, these symptoms are improved for most with education and management for the constipation and soiling.

Effective management of functional constipation requires a substantial commitment of the child and family, usually for 6–24 mo.

Degree of child and family adherence is likely a predictor of the child's success.

---

*The common features of the transition to the toddler diet (decreased fluid intake, continued high dairy intake, and *finicky* eating patterns) make this a high-risk time during development for constipation problems

Choice of disimpaction method depends on the age of the child, family choice, and the clinician's experience with a particular method. Methods and side effects are summarized in Table 14-2. The child and family should be included in the process of choosing the clean-out method. Because enemas may be invasive and oral medication may be unpleasant, allowing points of choice and control for the child and praising all signs of cooperation are important.

**Behavioral training** is essential to the treatment of chronic constipation and soiling. The child and family are asked to monitor and document stool output. Routine toilet sitting is instituted for 5 to 10 minutes three to four times per day. The child is asked to demonstrate proper toilet sitting position with the upper body flexed forward slightly and feet on the floor or foot support. The child should be praised for all components of cooperation with this program, and punishment and embarrassment

| TABLE 14-2 Clean-Out Disimpaction | |
|---|---|
| **Medication** | **Side Effects/Comments** |
| **INFANTS** | |
| Glycerin suppositories | No side effects |
| Enema—6 mL/kg up to 4.5 oz (135 mL) | If enemas are considered, administer first in physician's office |
| **CHILDREN** | |
| *Rapid Cleanout* | |
| Enema—6 mL/kg up to 4.5 oz (135 mL) every 12–24 hr × 1–3 | Invasive; risk of mechanical trauma |
| | Large impaction: mineral oil enema followed 1–3 hr later by normal saline or phosphate enema |
| | Small impaction: normal saline or phosphate enema |
| Mineral oil | Lubricates hard impaction; may not see return after administration |
| Normal saline | Abdominal cramping; may not be as effective as hypertonic phosphate |
| Hypertonic phosphate | Abdominal cramping; risk of hyperphosphatemia, hypokalemia, and hypocalcemia especially with Hirschsprung or renal insufficiency or if retained. Some experts do not recommend phosphate enema for children <4 yr, others for children <2 yr |
| Milk of molasses: 1:1 milk:molasses | For difficult to clear impaction |
| Combination: enema, suppository, oral laxative | |
| Day 1: Enema q12–24 h | See enemas above |
| Day 2: Bisacodyl suppository (10 mg) q12–24 h | Abdominal cramping, diarrhea, hypokalemia |
| Day 3: Bisacodyl tablet (5 mg) q12–24 h | Abdominal cramping, diarrhea, hypokalemia |
| Repeat 3-day cycle if needed × 1–2 | |
| Oral/nasogastric tube: Polyethylene glycol electrolyte solution (GoLYTELY or NuLYTELY)—25 mL/kg/hr up to 1000 mL/hr × 4 hr/day | Nausea, cramping, vomiting, bloating, aspiration. Large volume. Usually requires nasogastric tube and hospitalization to administer |
| *Slower Cleanout* | |
| Oral high-dose mineral oil—15–30 mL per year of age per day up to 8 oz × 3–4 days | Aspiration—lipoid pneumonia. Give chilled |
| X-Prep (senna): 15 mL q12h × 3 | Abdominal cramping. May not see output until dose 2 or 3 |
| Magnesium citrate: 1 oz/yr of age to maximum of 10 oz per day for 2–3 days | Hypermagnesemia |
| Maintenance medications—also may be used for cleanout | |

should be avoided. As symptoms resolve, toilet sitting is decreased to twice daily and finally to once a day.

When disimpaction is achieved, the child begins the maintenance phase of treatment. This phase promotes regular stool production and prevents reimpaction. It involves attention to diet, medications to promote stool regularity, and behavioral training. Increasing dietary fiber and fluid are recommended. The recommended daily dose of fiber in grams is calculated as 5 plus the child's age in years (e.g., a 10-year-old should take 15 g of fiber per day). For children with chronic constipation, the recommended dose is 10 grams plus the child's age in years. Families need to learn to read food labels and to plan for their child's daily intake of fiber. At least 2 oz of nondairy fluid intake per gram of fiber intake is recommended. Sorbitol-based juices, including prune, pear, and apple juice, increase the water content of bowel movements. Lubricants or osmotic laxatives are used to promote regular soft bowel movements. The use of medication during the maintenance phase is more effective than behavioral therapy alone. Maintenance medications, including side effects, are listed in Table 14-3. Polyethylene glycol powder is well tolerated because the taste and texture are palatable. Some children may require the use of a lubricant in addition to an osmotic laxative, and children with severe constipation may require a stimulant laxative. Treatment failure occurs in approximately one in five children secondary to problems with adherence or poor recognition of inadequate treatment resulting in reimpaction.

## Complications

Chronic constipation and soiling interfere with social functioning and self-esteem. Discomfort and fear of accidents may distract children from their schoolwork and other important tasks. Children also may develop unusual eating habits in response to chronic constipation and their beliefs about this condition. Case reports of child abuse related to soiling have been published.

## Prevention

The primary care physician can recommend adequate fiber intake in all children and encourage families to help their children institute regular toileting habits at an early age as preventive measures. Earlier diagnosis of chronic constipation can prevent much secondary disability and shorten the length of treatment required.

## TABLE 14-3 Maintenance Medications*

| Medication | Side Effects/Comments |
|---|---|
| **INFANTS** | |
| *Oral Medications/Other* | |
| Juices containing sorbitol | Pear, prune, apple |
| Lactulose or sorbitol: 1–3 mL/kg/day ÷ doses bid | See below |
| Corn syrup (light or dark): 1–3 mL/kg/day ÷ doses bid | Not considered risk for *Clostridium botulinum* spores |
| *Per Rectum* | |
| Glycerin suppository | No side effects |
| **CHILDREN** | |
| *Oral Medications* | |
| Lubricant | Softens stool and eases passage |
|    Mineral oil: 1–3 mL/kg day as one dose or ÷ bid | Aspiration—lipoid pneumonia |
| | Chill or give with juice. |
| | Adherence problems |
| | Leakage: dose too high or impaction |
| Osmotics | Retain water in stool, aiding bulk and softness |
|    Lactulose: 10 g/15 mL, 1–3 cc/kg/day ÷ doses bid | Synthetic disaccharide: abdominal cramping, flatus |
|    Magnesium hydroxide (milk of magnesia): | Risk of hypermagnesemia, hypophosphatemia, secondary |
|       400 mg/5 mL, 1–3 mL/kg/day ÷ bid |   hypocalcemia with overdose or renal insufficiency |
|       800 mg/5 mL, 0.5 mL/kg ÷ bid | |
|    MiraLAX (polyethylene glycol powder): | Titrate dose at 3-day intervals to achieve mushy stool consistency |
|       17 g/240 cc water or juice stock, 1.0 g/kg/day ÷ doses | May make stock solutions to administer over 1–2 days |
|       bid (approximately 15 cc/kg/day) | Excellent adherence |
|    Sorbitol: 1–3 mL/kg/day ÷ doses bid | Less costly than lactulose |
| Stimulants† | Improve effectiveness of colonic and rectal muscle contractions |
|    Senna: syrup—8.8 g sennoside/5 mL | Idiosyncratic hepatitis, melanosis coli, hypertrophic |
|       2–6 yr: 2.5–7.5 cc/day ÷ doses bid |   osteoarthropathy, analgesic nephropathy; abdominal |
|       6–12 yr: 5–15 cc/day ÷ doses bid |   cramping. Improvement of melanosis coli after medication |
|       (Tablets and granules available) |   stopped |
|    Bisacodyl: 5-mg tablets, 1–3 tablets/dose 1-2 × daily | Abdominal cramping, diarrhea, hypokalemia |
| *Per Rectum* | |
|    Glycerin suppository | No side effects |
|    Bisacodyl: 10-mg suppositories, 0.5–1 suppository, 1–2 × daily | Abdominal cramping, diarrhea, hypokalemia |

*Single agent may suffice to achieve daily, comfortable stools.
†Stimulants should be reserved for short-term use.

# CHAPTER 15

# Normal Sleep and Pediatric Sleep Disorders

Sleep is a complex physiologic and behavioral process in which the person achieves a reversible state of disengagement from the environment and partial unresponsiveness. Sleep physiology rapidly changes from fetal life through infancy and childhood. Polysomnographic recordings show two broad categories of sleep: rapid eye movement (REM) sleep and non–rapid eye movement (NREM) sleep. NREM sleep is divided into four stages—from stage 1, which has relatively low voltage with mixed frequency activity, to stage 4, which has greater than 50% high-amplitude waves with slow frequency activity. In the fetus and neonate, sleep is categorized into active sleep and quiet sleep. Active sleep becomes REM sleep in the child and adult. There is significant motor activity during active sleep. Periodic breathing and rapid eye movements accompany active sleep. Quiet sleep matures into NREM sleep.

Full-term infants sleep two thirds of the day. The longest sleep period at 6 weeks of age is variable, with two standard deviations ranging between 3 and 11 hours. It is typical of neonates to start their sleep cycle in active sleep, whereas older children and adults begin sleep in NREM sleep. Sleep cycles typically last 60 minutes in newborns compared with 90 minutes in children and adults. Slow-wave sleep (stages 3 and 4) is not seen before 3 to 6 months of age. Between 6 and 12 months, active sleep shifts toward the last third of the night and continues this pattern into adulthood.

One-year-old children sleep on average 15 hours a day. At this age, most U.S. children sleep 2 to 3 hours during the day and the remainder at night. By 12 years of age, the average child sleeps 9 hours a day. During adolescence, sleep physiology changes, with decreased stages 3 and 4 NREM sleep and decreased REM sleep. Adolescents continue to need on average 9 hours of sleep per day. Cultural influences strongly determine whether children sleep independently (the norm in the United States) or with parents, other siblings, or grandparents (the norm in other cultures).

## ETIOLOGY

Numerous sleep disorders exist, including sleep-onset association disorders (infancy), parasomnias, or circadian rhythm disorders (adolescence) (Table 15-1). Sudden infant death syndrome (SIDS), obstructive sleep apnea (OSA), and sleep disorders associated with mental and physical illness are included in the discussion of the differential diagnosis.

## EPIDEMIOLOGY

Almost half of mothers of infants complain to the pediatrician about their infants' sleep rhythms. OSA is reported in 2% of children. Adolescent insomnia is much more common. Night talking is the most common parasomnia experienced by almost all people at one time in their life. Sleepwalking occurs in approximately 15% of children between 5 and 12 years of age at least once. Night terrors also are common.

## CLINICAL MANIFESTATIONS

Because sleep problems in children are common, screening is recommended as part of primary care. Five sleep domains can be addressed as part of a standard sleep history. These domains include bedtime problems, excessive daytime sleepiness, awakenings during the night, regularity and duration of sleep, and presence or absence of sleep-disordered breathing. Examples of screening questions include "Do you feel tired during the day?," "Do you wake up during the night?," and "Does your child snore?" Parents provide sleep history for preschool and school-aged children and adolescents report on their own sleep patterns.

The assessment of sleep complaints begins with a detailed **history** of sleep habits, including bedtime, times of achieving sleep, and waking. A detailed description of the sleep environment, including the type of bed, who shares it, the ambient light, noise, and temperature, and the bedtime routine, can lead to a dynamic understanding of the challenges to and resources for achieving normal sleep. Parental work patterns may be important because some children resist sleep until a parent is at home, and infants have been known to reverse their day-night cycle to breastfeed during the night when the mother is at home. Dietary practices, including timing of meals, undernutrition and overnutrition, and caffeine intake, influence sleep patterns. Documentation of snoring and breathing pauses during sleep can lead to a diagnosis related to

OSA. New-onset sleep disorders may be associated with a psychological trauma. When the history does not reveal the cause of the sleep disorder, a sleep diary can be helpful.

A complete **physical examination** is important to rule out medical causes of sleep disturbance, such as conditions that cause pain, neurologic conditions that could be associated with seizure disorder, and other central nervous system disorders. Children with genetic syndromes associated with developmental delay may have sleep disorder. Similarly, children with attention-deficit/hyperactivity disorder and fetal alcohol syndrome are at higher risk for sleep disorder than children without these conditions. Careful attention to the upper airway and pulmonary examination may reveal enlarged tonsils or adenoids or other signs of obstruction.

A **polysomnogram** is used to detect obstructive and central apnea, excessive limb movements, and seizure disorder. Children can be admitted for an overnight polysomnogram, and 24-hour ambulatory recordings are available. Children who have a history consistent with a behavioral sleep disorder, such as sleep-onset association disorder and difficulty falling asleep, do not need a polysomnogram, unless they do not improve with intervention.

## DIFFERENTIAL DIAGNOSIS

### Infancy

The incidence of **SIDS** has decreased by 60% as a result of placing infants on their backs to sleep and reducing overbundling and cigarette smoke exposure (see Chapter 134). Although SIDS is probably a final common pathway for a variety of different etiologies, decreased arousal to hypoxia or hypercapnia may be a mechanism in some cases.

**Sleep-onset association disorders** are common in the United States, where a high degree of independence is expected for infant sleep. Infants experience arousal during each sleep cycle as they go back into light sleep (stage 1). Infants who wake under conditions different from those they experienced as they fell asleep are likely to become more aroused.

### Childhood

Difficulty falling asleep includes bedtime resistance, delayed sleep onset, sleep anxiety, and fears. Bedtime resistance is most common in preschool children. Psychologically, bedtime is experienced as separation from parents, with morning being a reunion experience. Children with insecure attachment may be more prone to distress at bedtime. Bedtime resistance does not rule out other sleep pathology and is more common in children with sleep-disordered breathing.

**OSA** in childhood is not always obvious or easy to diagnose. OSA is commonly caused by tonsillar or adenoidal hypertrophy. Some prefer the term *sleep-disordered breathing* because obstruction is often partial. These children typically present with a history of snoring, and some may have excessive daytime sleepiness. Obese children are at increased risk for OSA. In toddlers, OSA often is

**TABLE 15-1 Childhood Sleep Disruption Disorders**

| Type | Cause | Symptoms | Treatment |
|------|-------|----------|-----------|
| **ORGANIC** | | | |
| Colic | Unknown | Crying, irritability | Rocking, pacifier, nursing Support until resolution |
| Medications | Stimulants Bronchodilators Anticonvulsants | Failure to fall asleep; restless sleep | Adjust dosage/timing; change medication |
| Illness | Any chronically irritating disorder (e.g., otitis, dermatitis, asthma, or esophageal reflux) | Painful crying out | Treat disease symptomatically |
| Central nervous system disorders | Variable; rule out seizures | Decreased sleep | Evaluate environment Sedatives as last resort |
| **PARASOMNIAS** | | | |
| Sleepwalking, sleep terrors | Stage 4 (deep) sleep instability | Awakening 1–3 hr after falling asleep | Reassurance; protective environment |
| Confusional arousals | | Intense crying, walking, disorientation, talking | |
| Enuresis | ? Stage 4 instability Metabolic disease (e.g., diabetes) Urinary tract infection Urinary anatomic anomaly | Bed-wetting | Rule out medical conditions Fluid limitation Prebed voiding Behavioral approaches (bell and pad) Emotional support Medication (e.g., imipramine, DDAVP) Reassurance |
| **SLEEP-WAKE SCHEDULE DISORDERS** | | | |
| Irregular sleep-wake pattern | No defined schedule | Variable waking and sleeping | Regularize schedule |
| Regular but inappropriate sleep-wake schedule | Napping at wrong times Prematurely eliminated nap | Morning sleepiness Night wakings | Rework schedule |
| Delayed sleep phase | Late sleep onset with resetting of circadian rhythm | Late sleep onset Morning sleepiness Not sleepy at bedtime | Enforce wake-up time Gradually move bedtime earlier or keep awake overnight to create drowsy state |
| **ENVIRONMENTAL AND PSYCHOSOCIAL FACTORS** | | | |
| Inappropriate sleep-onset associations | No defined bedtime routine Child falls asleep in conditions different from those of the rest of the night | Night wakenings requiring intervention | Regularize routine Minimize nocturnal parental response |
| Excessive nocturnal fluid | Child gets food/drink with each awakening | Night wakening or wanting drink | Gradually decrease nocturnal fluid |
| Inconsistent limit setting | Parental anxiety | Delayed bedtime Excessive expression of "needs" by child | Modify parental behavior to improve limit setting Gradually increase limits |
| Anxieties; fears | Separation anxieties | Night waking Refusal to sleep | Reassurance when appropriate Counseling in severe cases |
| Social disruptions | Family stressors | Night waking Refusal to sleep | Family counseling Regularize routines |

DDAVP, 1-desamino-8-D-arginine vasopressin

associated with poor growth, which improves when the obstruction is relieved by tonsillectomy or adenoidectomy. Many children with OSA experience cognitive difficulties and school problems. Hyperactivity also is more common in these children than in age-matched controls.

**Parasomnias** include night terrors, sleepwalking, and sleep talk and involve movement from stage 3 or 4 sleep into REM. Night terrors are common, occur in preschool children, and are likely to resolve with time and developmental maturation. Night terrors are differentiated from nightmares, which occur later in the night and result from arousal from REM or dreaming sleep. Children typically remember their nightmares but have no recollection of night terrors. Parents often report distress at their child's night terrors because the child may scream and not recognize them during the episode.

### Adolescence

Circadian rhythm disorder in adolescence is caused by irregularities in sleep hygiene, leading to delayed sleep phase syndrome. Many adolescents stay up late and sleep 7 hours or less a night during the week with attempts to recoup lost sleep on the weekend. This schedule disrupts the biologic clock and can lead to bedtime insomnia, difficulty maintaining sleep during the night, or inability to arouse in the morning. Resulting sleep deprivation leads to cognitive problems and problems of emotional regulation.

Primary sleep disorders must be differentiated from sleep disorders associated with psychiatric and medical disorders. Psychoses, anxiety disorders, and substance abuse can present with disordered sleep. The clinician also should consider sleep-related epilepsy, sleep-related headaches, and degenerative and developmental disorders. Asthma and gastroesophageal reflux also can disrupt sleep.

## TREATMENT

The management of sleep-onset association disorder, difficulty falling asleep, and circadian rhythm disorder is challenging. Treatment involves the following behavioral management principles:

1. Education and demystification
2. Setting objectives and a timetable
3. Positive reinforcement and rewards
4. Negative reinforcement and withdrawal of attention or privileges

It is recommended that infants be put in bed slightly awake after they have had a diaper change, food, and comfort. A safe sleep environment is essential. Some toleration of infant crying is required for the infant to achieve self-regulation of sleep. Children younger than 4 months of age need nighttime feeding. Difficulty falling asleep and bedtime resistance are treated by meticulous attention to sleep hygiene of the youngster. Children who are experiencing separation anxiety can benefit from behavioral therapy aimed at reinforcing feelings of safety and parental presence. Objects of attachment, such as a favorite blanket or stuffed animal, are helpful. Removing televisions and

VCRs from the bedroom is advised because television at bedtime also may delay sleep onset and increase arousal during the night.

Rarely, children with insomnia are treated pharmacologically. Melatonin (dose, 2.5 to 10 mg) has soporific properties useful in treating delayed sleep phase syndrome. Developmentally normal and developmentally delayed children have been treated successfully with melatonin for difficulty falling asleep. Melatonin is available without prescription in stores that sell dietary supplements. The α-agonist clonidine acts preferentially on presynaptic $\alpha_2$ neurons to inhibit noradrenergic activity. Somnolence is a side effect of clonidine, which can be put to use in cases of refractory sleep difficulties. Clonidine usually is started in a dose of 0.05 mg at bedtime and increased to 0.1 mg at bedtime if needed. There are data on treating children as young as 4 years of age with clonidine; this is an *off-label* use in children. Weaning off clonidine is recommended at the end of treatment.

Night terrors are best managed by minimal intervention. Conversation with the child is not possible at the time of the night terror. Children who have frequent or prolonged night terrors have been treated successfully with soporific medications and with clinical hypnosis. Children with atypical night terrors may need a sleep study to evaluate possible coexisting sleep disorders.

Circadian rhythm disorder in adolescents can be treated by meticulous attention to sleep hygiene and gradual resetting of the biologic clock. Advancing the bedtime forward is one treatment. This therapy requires the adolescent to stay awake for 1 night followed by going to bed at the desired time the next day. He or she then is required to maintain a consistent bedtime (including weekend nights) for the duration of treatment and maintenance. The adolescent also is required to arise at a consistent time on the weekends, not more than several hours after their weekday wake-up time. Another method of resetting the biologic clock involves gradually shifting the bedtime and waking times earlier over the course of several weeks. Both therapies are supplemented by attention to regular mealtimes, avoidance of caffeine, exclusion of the television from the bedroom, and use of soporific medications if needed. Families require a great deal of support and counseling during this intervention.

## COMPLICATIONS

The most obvious and serious complication associated with childhood sleep disorders is impairment of cognitive ability and emotional regulation. This impairment puts children at risk for school failure, family difficulties, and social problems. It is likely that sleep-deprived children are at increased risk for acute illness and psychiatric disorders.

## PREVENTION

The principles of prevention for pediatric behavioral sleep disorders are outlined in Table 15-2. Sleep-onset association disorder in infancy usually can be prevented by parental understanding of infant sleep physiology, developmentally appropriate expectations, and planning the

| TABLE 15-2 Prevention of Pediatric Behavioral Sleep Disorders |
|---|
| Consistent ambient noise, light, temperature in bedroom |
| Adequate food, liquid, socialization, and physical activity during the day |
| Caffeine avoidance |
| Regular bedtime |
| Regular wake-up time |
| Consistent bedtime routine (15–30 min) to cue sleep |
| No television in bedroom |
| Child feels safe and protected |
| Child allowed to develop self-soothing strategies |
| Parents are comfortable setting limits/boundaries |

infant sleep environment to coincide with family needs. It is important for parents to understand that it is normal for their infant to wake frequently for the first 6 weeks before settling into a routine of waking every 3 to 4 hours for feeding. Infants typically do not sleep through the night before 6 months of age, and many do not sleep through the night before 18 months of age. Even though cosleeping (mother and infant sleeping together) is common, it is not recommended because of increased risk of SIDS.

Difficulty falling asleep in toddlers and preschool children can be largely prevented by a structured daily routine, including good sleep hygiene at a bedtime that takes into account the child's needs for sleep and for time with the parents. A consistent bedtime ensures that the child's circadian rhythm matches the parental expectation. Designating special parent-child time can alleviate the child's need to delay bedtime. Bedtime routines should last no more than 30 minutes and include a set combination of activities that might include bath, teeth brushing, story, and cuddle. Including physical activity in the daily routine is advised so that the child is physically and mentally tired at bedtime. During times of illness or stress in the family, young children may begin to sleep in their parent's bed. Proactively considering the desirability of bed sharing allows parents to be in control rather than ceding control to the young child.

Requiring a consistent bedtime during the week can prevent circadian rhythm disorders in adolescence; this may require limiting extracurricular activities, television, and video games. Similarly, setting a weekend wake-up time can prevent significant shifting of the biologic clock. Setting limits with adolescents is challenging. Beginning to lay the groundwork for these expectations earlier in the adolescent years is often helpful. Some professionals believe that adolescents would be less likely to have sleep disorders if high schools started at 9:00 AM instead of 7:30 AM. This is not the norm in the United States because many adolescents are employed, and many participate in athletic and other extracurricular activities after school.

 **SUGGESTED   READING**

Blass EM, Camp CA: Changing determinants of crying termination in 6- to 12-week-old human infants, *Dev Psychobiol* 42:312–316, 2003.

Brown RT, Amler RW, Freeman WS, et al: American Academy of Pediatrics committee on quality improvement. American Academy of Pediatrics subcommittee on attention-deficit/hyperactivity disorder. Treatment of attention-deficit/hyperactivity disorder: overview of the evidence, *Pediatrics* 115(6):e749–e757, 2005.

Glazener CM, Evans JH, Peto RE: Alarm interventions for nocturnal enuresis in children, *Cochrane Database of Syst Rev* (2): CD002911, 2005.

Meltzer LJ, Mindell JA: Sleep and sleep disorders in children and adolescents, *Psychiatr Clin North Am* 29:1059–1076, 2006.

Owens JA, Dalzell V: Use of the "BEARS" sleep screening tool in a pediatric residents' continuity clinic: a pilot study, *Sleep Med* 6:63–69, 2005.

Potegal M, Davidson RJ: Temper tantrums in young children: 1. Behavioral composition. *J Dev, Behav Pediatr* 24:140–147, 2003.

Rubin G, Dale A: Chronic constipation in children, *BMJ* 333:1051–1055, 2006.

CHAPTER 16

# Somatoform Disorders

The somatoform disorders involve a complaint of physical symptoms (pain or loss of function) that suggest a medical condition but are not fully explained by either a medical condition, a pharmacologic effect, or another psychiatric condition (Table 16-1). The symptoms are usually recurrent and involve multiple clinically significant complaints (Table 16-2). In evaluating somatic complaints, the evidence for medical disorders and for psychological symptoms should be sought simultaneously. The physical complaints are commonly *signals of distress,* not indication of a serious psychiatric illness.

Affected children are more likely to come from families with a history of marital conflict. Other members of the child's family may also have unexplained symptoms. Lifetime prevalence of somatoform disorders is 3% and subclinical somatoform illness as high as 10%. Somatoform illness is relatively stable and persistent, but with time, the overall symptom profile changes. Polysymptomatic presentations, including somatization disorders, hypochondriasis, conversion disorder, and body dysmorphic disorder, are more common with increasing age. Somatoform illness is more common in females, and children with lower socioeconomic status, history of sexual trauma or physical threats, parental neglect, substance abuse, depression, and premorbid anxiety.

Youths with somatoform disorders have high rates of anxiety and depressive symptoms. Cough and dyspnea are highly associated with anxiety, depression, attention-deficit/hyperactivity disorder (ADHD), and substance abuse. Vocal cord dysfunction is suspected in 10% of dyspneic people who are being evaluated for unresponsive asthma. In vocal cord dysfunction, vocal cord spasm mimics acute asthma. Vocal cord dysfunction is differentiated from asthma by lack of improvement despite aggressive asthma management, the absence of nocturnal symptoms, normal blood gases despite severe symptoms, and significant adduction of the vocal cords on laryngoscopy.

**Treatment** approaches for somatoform problems are complex. The patient must believe that the physician, in finding no evidence of disease, will not judge the symptoms to be feigned or imagined. Reassurance that a life-threatening or serious physical disease is not present helps decrease anxiety. Avoiding unnecessary medical procedures after the diagnosis is made decreases morbidity.

Antidepressant medications (fluoxetine, citalopram, clomipramine) may be of benefit in the treatment of unexplained headaches, fibromyalgia, body dysmorphic disorder, somatoform pain, irritable bowel syndrome, and functional gastrointestinal disorders. Tricyclic antidepressants should be avoided in youth with **functional abdominal pain (FAP)** because they have no proven efficacy in either pain management or mood disorders. In **chronic fatigue syndrome (CFS)** with comorbid depression and anxiety, a more activating antidepressant, bupropion, is useful. Stimulants may also be helpful in CFS. **Cognitive-behavioral methods,** which reward health-promoting behaviors and discourage disability and illness behaviors, help in the treatment of recurrent pain, CFS, fibromyalgia, and FAP. Interpersonal and expressive psychotherapies in the presence of psychological trauma are particularly useful. Self-management strategies, such as self-monitoring, relaxation, hypnosis, and biofeedback, provide some degree of symptomatic relief and encourage more active coping strategies. Family therapy and family-based interventions are very useful in some cases. Home schooling should be avoided, and school attendance and performance should be emphasized as important indicators of appropriate functioning.

**Somatization disorder** involves multiple unexplained physical complaints, including pain, gastrointestinal, sexual, and pseudoneurologic symptoms. These physical symptoms are not caused by known mechanisms and may be related to the patient's need to maintain a sick role. The patient is frequently convinced that the symptoms are unrelated to psychological factors. The criteria used to diagnose this disorder are listed in Table 16-2. Given the requirement for at least one sexual or reproductive symptom, the diagnosis is somewhat unusual in children.

The onset of the condition is common during adolescence. Prevalence estimates range from 0.2% to 2% in females and less than 0.2% in males. The symptoms tend to persist or vary in intensity and character despite ongoing treatment. There is an increased risk of the disorder in first-degree relatives, especially female relatives (10% to 20%).

## TABLE 16-1 Features of Somatoform Disorders of Children and Adolescents

### PSYCHOPHYSIOLOGIC DISORDER

Presenting complaint is a physical symptom

Physical symptom caused by a known physiologic mechanism

Physical symptom is stress induced

Patient may recognize association between symptom and stress

Frequently responds to medication, biofeedback, and stress reduction

### CONVERSION REACTION

Presenting complaint is physical (loss of function, pain, or both)

Physical symptom not caused by a known physiologic mechanism

Physical symptom related to unconscious idea, fantasy, or conflict

Patient does not recognize association between symptom and the unconscious

Symptom responds slowly to resolution of unconscious factors

### SOMATIZATION DISORDER

Requires more than 13 physical symptoms in girls, more than 11 in boys (see Table 16-2)

Physical symptoms not caused by a known physiologic or pathologic mechanism

Physical symptoms related to need to maintain the sick role

Patient convinced that symptoms unrelated to psychological factors

Symptoms tend to persist or change character despite treatment

### HYPOCHONDRIASIS

Presenting complaint is a physical sign or symptom

Patient interprets physical symptom to indicate disease

Conviction regarding illness may be related to depression or anxiety

Symptom does not respond to reassurance

Medication directed at underlying psychological problems often helps

### MALINGERING

Presenting complaint is a physical symptom

Physical symptom is under voluntary control

Physical symptom is used to gain reward (e.g., money, avoidance of military service)

Patient consciously recognizes symptom as factitious

Symptom may not lessen when reward is attained (need to retain reward)

### FACTITIOUS DISORDER (E.G., MUNCHAUSEN SYNDROME)

Presenting complaint is symptom complex mimicking known syndrome

Symptom complex is under voluntary control

Symptom complex is used to attain medical treatment (including surgery)

Patient consciously recognizes symptom complex as factitious, but is often psychologically disturbed so that unconscious factors also are operating

Symptom complex often results in multiple diagnoses and multiple operations

## TABLE 16-2 Criteria for Diagnosis of Somatization Disorder

Each of the following criteria must be met. Individual symptoms may occur at any time during the course of disturbance.

1. **Four pain symptoms**: pain related to at least four different sites or functions (e.g., head, abdomen, back, joints, extremities, chest, rectum; during menstruation, sexual intercourse, or urination)
2. **Two gastrointestinal symptoms**: at least two gastrointestinal symptoms other than pain (e.g., nausea, bloating, vomiting, diarrhea, or intolerance of several foods)
3. **One sexual symptom**: at least one sexual or reproductive symptom other than pain (e.g., sexual indifference, erectile or ejaculatory dysfunction, irregular menses, excessive menstrual bleeding, vomiting throughout pregnancy)
4. **One pseudoneurologic symptom**: at least one symptom or deficit suggesting a neurologic condition not limited to pain (conversion symptoms such as impaired coordination or balance, paralysis or localized weakness, difficulty swallowing or lump in throat, aphonia, urinary retention, hallucinations, loss of touch or pain sensation, double vision, blindness, deafness, seizures; dissociative symptoms such as amnesia; or loss of consciousness other than fainting)

Either (1) or (2)

1. After appropriate investigation, each of the symptoms is not fully explained by a known general medical condition or the direct effects of a substance (e.g., drug, medication)
2. When there is a related general medical condition, the physical complaints, social or occupational impairment are in excess of what is expected from the history, physical examination, or laboratory findings.

Patients with somatization disorder and their family members experience higher rates of major depression, anxiety, personality disorders (antisocial, histrionic, borderline), and substance abuse and dependence. Medical conditions with multiple systemic symptoms need to be ruled out. Factitious disorder or malingering may coexist with somatization disorder. Extensive workup is often performed, so once a diagnosis is made, the major goal is to limit morbidity from unnecessary medical procedures and tests. Early onset of somatization disorder is associated with poor prognosis.

**Undifferentiated somatoform disorder** includes one or more unexplained physical complaints that last for at least 6 months. The number of physical complaints is less than that required for a diagnosis of somatization disorder (Table 16-3). These symptoms are not explained by medical conditions or drugs. Patients may recognize an association between their symptoms and stress.

**Conversion disorder** symptoms, suggestive of a neurologic illness in the absence of disease, include nonepileptic seizures, unresponsiveness, faints, falls, and abnormalities of gait or sensation (Table 16-4).

**Falling out syndrome** (falling down with altered consciousness) is common in several cultures throughout the

**TABLE 16-3 Criteria for Diagnosis of Undifferentiated Somatoform Disorder**

A. One or more physical complaints (e.g., fatigue, loss of appetite, gastrointestinal complaints)
B. Either (1) or (2)
1. After appropriate investigation, the symptoms cannot be fully explained by a known general medical condition or the direct effects of a substance (e.g., drug or medication)
2. When there is a related general medical condition, the physical complaints, social or occupational impairment is in excess of what is expected from the history, physical examination, or laboratory findings
C. The symptoms cause clinically significant distress or impairment in social, occupational, or other important areas of functioning
D. At least 6 months of disturbance
E. The disturbance is not better accounted for by another mental disorder (e.g., another somatoform disorder, sexual dysfunction, mood disorder, anxiety disorder, sleep disorder, or psychotic disorder)
F. The symptom is not intentionally produced or feigned (factitious disorder, malingering)

world. Stocking glove (nonanatomic) anesthesia is another common finding. Symptoms are often inconstant; patients may move a *paralyzed* extremity when they think that no one is watching. Presenting symptoms follow the psychological stressor by hours to weeks and may cause more distress for others than for the patient (*la belle indifference*). Symptoms are usually self-limited but may be associated with chronic sequelae, such as

**TABLE 16-4 Criteria for Diagnosis of Conversion Disorder**

A. One or more symptoms affecting voluntary motor or sensory function that suggest a neurologic or other general medical condition
B. Psychological factors are judged to be associated with the symptom or deficit because the initiation or exacerbation is preceded by conflicts or other stressors
C. The symptom is not intentionally produced or feigned (factitious disorder, malingering)
D. After appropriate investigation, the symptom cannot be fully explained by a general medical condition, by the direct effects of a substance, or as a culturally sanctioned behavior or experience
E. The symptom causes clinically significant distress or impairment in social, occupational, or other function or warrants medical evaluation
F. The symptom is not limited to pain or sexual dysfunction, does not occur exclusively during the course of somatization disorder, and is not better accounted for by another mental disorder

contractures or iatrogenic injury. There are four subtypes of conversion disorder based on whether the symptoms presented are primarily motor, sensory, nonepileptic (seizures), or mixed.

**Nonepileptic seizures**, sometimes described as *pseudoseizures*, resemble epileptic seizures but are not associated with the electroencephalographic abnormalities or a clinical course characteristic of true epilepsy. Affected individuals may also suffer from concomitant epilepsy. Most cases resolve within 3 months of diagnosis.

The cause of conversion symptoms may be related to an unconscious idea, fantasy, or conflict. The patient does not recognize an association between the symptoms and the conflict. The rate of misdiagnosis of conversion symptoms averages 4%. Myasthenia gravis, multiple sclerosis, dystonias, and dyskinesias (abnormal movements) are conditions commonly mistaken for conversion disorder.

Conversion disorders are uncommon in children and adolescents, with a lifetime prevalence of 0.3%. They are practically nonexistent in children older than 6 years of age. The prevalence increases in psychiatric (1% to 3%) and surgical (1% to 14%) patients. Conversion symptoms are more commonly seen in first-degree relatives of affected people, in patients with family history of unexplainable medical problems, in people living in rural areas, and in people of low socioeconomic status.

**Treatment** is best accomplished by reassuring patients that the symptoms usually go away. Multiple medical treatments and diagnostic interventions can solidify the symptoms, delay recovery, and increase morbidity. The course of the condition is often benign, although 20% to 25% of patients experience a recurrence. Good prognostic characteristics include symptoms of paralysis, aphonia, blindness; acute onset, above-average intelligence, presence of an identifiable stressor, and early diagnosis and psychiatric treatment. Poor prognostic characteristics include tremor and pseudoseizures.

**Pain disorder** is characterized by pain as the predominant complaint. Psychological factors are important in the onset, severity, and maintenance of this disorder (Table 16-5). The diagnosis is considered acute if the condition lasts less than 6 months and chronic when it lasts 6 months or more. Chronic, recurrent pain disorders in childhood most commonly involve abdominal pain, headache, limb pain, or chest pain. It is unusual for children to exhibit more than one pain syndrome at the same time, although chronic, recurrent pain in a different location in the past is not uncommon. Most chronic, recurrent pain disorders have no clear organic or emotional origin; organic etiology is found in only about 10% of children.

Pain disorder is the most common pain-related diagnosis. FAP appears to be the most common pain complaint in preschoolers (responsible for up to 4% of pediatric visits in this age group) followed by headache (responsible for up to 2% of pediatric ambulatory visits), which peaks at approximately 12 years of age. FAP may present with nausea, vomiting, and bowel-related complaints. Most cases of pediatric abdominal pain are considered functional in the absence of weight loss, intestinal bleeding, fever, other systemic symptoms, or laboratory abnormalities. Seventy-five percent of children with FAP have an anxiety disorder. Common types of headaches are

---

**TABLE 16-5  Criteria for Diagnosis of Pain Disorder**

A. Pain in one or more anatomic sites is the predominant focus and is of sufficient severity to warrant clinical attention

B. The pain causes clinically significant distress or impairment in social, occupational, or other important functions

C. Psychological factors have an important role in the onset, severity, exacerbation, or maintenance of the pain

D. The symptom or deficit is not intentionally produced or feigned (factitious disorder, malingering)

E. The pain is not better accounted for by a mood, anxiety, or psychotic disorder and does not meet criteria for dyspareunia

Specify if:
● Acute: duration <6 months
● Chronic: duration ≥6 months

---

migraine and tension-type headache. Migraine may be associated with dizziness, gastrointestinal symptoms, and cyclical vomiting syndrome, characterized by recurrent and stereotypical episodes of intense, unexplained vomiting. Patients with functional chest pain, a condition that is seen in 10% of school-aged children and adolescents, may present to the emergency department. Other common pain disorders are musculoskeletal pains (limb pain and back pain), fibromyalgia, and complex regional pain syndrome type I (previously known as reflex sympathetic dystrophy).

Diagnostic studies should be undertaken in response to specific findings that suggest an organic etiology. Evidence of psychological stress usually is found by the time the child exhibits a chronic problem. The nurturing responses of the family may provide secondary gain that prolongs the pain. Complaints or frustration with failure to find a specific cause may lead to accusations of malingering and to increased stress on the child, exacerbating the problem.

Reassurance is the primary treatment of pain disorder. Symptom diaries, including the events that precede and follow the pain episode, aid in initial assessment and ongoing management of the problem. Minimizing secondary psychological consequences of recurrent pain syndromes is important.

**Hypochondriasis** is the preoccupation with the fear of having a serious disease based on misinterpretation of bodily symptoms and functions. This fear should be present for 6 months. The presenting complaint is a physical sign or symptom, which is normal but is interpreted by the patient to indicate disease despite reassurance of a physician (e.g., a tension headache perceived as a brain tumor). Symptoms typically do not respond to reassurance. An underlying depression or anxiety disorder may be related to the symptoms. Hypochondriasis may overlap with obsessive-compulsive disorder and can be considered a health anxiety disorder or phobia. When the belief or preoccupation is limited to an imagined defect in appearance, the diagnosis is body dysmorphic disorder, not hypochondriasis.

Psychotropic medications directed at underlying psychiatric problems can be helpful. Limiting medical procedures can help decrease morbidity.

**Body dysmorphic disorder (BDD)** is a preoccupation with an imagined or slight defect in physical appearance that causes clinically significant distress or impairment in functioning. It is usually seen in adolescents and is distinguished from common developmental preoccupations with appearance by the presence of clinically significant distress and/or impairment in functioning. Any body area can be a focus, but excessive concerns about the skin (scars and acne) and body shape are common. Patients may cause self-injury as a consequence of attempts to fix the perceived flaw. Insight is often poor, and patients often seek costly and potentially dangerous treatments. Because BDD can be associated with shame and the need for secrecy, the diagnosis may be missed unless clinicians ask directly about symptoms. Parents of children with BDD report excessive mirror checking, grooming, attempts to *camouflage* a particular body area, and reassurance-seeking. BDD is considered to be related to obsessive-compulsive disorder. The prevalence of BDD has been reported to be 0.7% in children, 2% in adolescents, and up to 5% in patients seeking cosmetic surgery.

**Psychological factors affecting physical condition** is a diagnosis in which physical illness is exacerbated by psychological or behavioral factors, often in patients with chronic medical conditions. These factors can worsen the underlying illness or affect its treatment (e.g., a child with type 1 diabetes mellitus whose stressors and maladaptive behaviors interfere with the ability to effectively monitor blood glucose levels).

**Fatigue** is a common physical complaint, affecting up to 50% of adolescents. **CFS** specifically refers to a condition characterized by severe, disabling fatigue of at least 6 months' duration that is associated with self-reported limitations in concentration and short-term memory, sleep disturbance, and musculoskeletal aches and pains, where alternative medical and psychiatric explanations (e.g., hypothyroidism, malignancy, hepatitis, narcolepsy, obstructive sleep apnea, medication side effects, major mood disorder, schizophrenia, or eating disorder) have been excluded. CFS is rare in childhood and uncommon in adolescence, with prevalence below 1%. Onset typically follows an acute febrile illness (postviral) in approximately two thirds of cases. It is often associated with depression and can be incapacitating. Treatment is nonspecific, unless a psychological or general medical cause is uncovered.

**Malingering** is a condition in which a physical symptom that is under voluntary control is used to gain reward (money or avoidance of school, jail, or military service). The motivation is usually not readily apparent, but the patient consciously recognizes the symptom as factitious. Malingering is difficult to prove unless the patient is directly observed or confesses. Symptoms may not lessen when the reward is attained.

**Factitious disorder** is a condition in which physical or psychological symptoms are produced intentionally to assume the sick role. This diagnosis is made either by direct observation or by eliminating other possible causes. The presenting complaint, often a symptom complex that mimics a known syndrome, can include subjective complaints (abdominal pain), falsified objective signs (blood in urine), or self-inflicted injury. It can also be an exaggeration of symptoms of existing conditions (e.g., pseudoseizures in patients with epilepsy). This condition often leads to unnecessary medical tests, procedures, and treatments, including surgeries. The patient, usually female, may not know the motivation for feigning symptoms. Approximately 1% of patients who receive psychiatric consultation have factitious disorder. The most common comorbid condition is substance abuse.

The evaluation of factitious disorder must include a thorough medical evaluation or a psychiatric evaluation if the symptoms are psychiatric. Approximate answers reported during a mental status examination are most commonly found in factitious disorders. This term is applied when patients give close answers (e.g., $20 - 3 = 18$).

**Munchausen syndrome by proxy (MBP)** is a form of factitious disorder by proxy, where a parent mimics symptoms in his or her child. The motivation is believed to be a psychological need to assume a sick role through the child. MBP is a type of child abuse. Boys are more commonly abused in this way, and neonates and preschoolers are the most common victims. The overwhelming majority of MBP perpetrators are women, usually the child's mothers. Of these mothers, more than 72% have a history of factitious disorder or a somatoform disorder. Up to 80% of involved parents have some health care background.

Both *factitious disorder by proxy* and *pediatric condition falsification* are needed for diagnosis. Pediatric condition falsification occurs through simulation (i.e., false reporting of symptoms or contaminating laboratory samples) and/or production of symptoms. The estimated incidence of MBP is 2 to 2.8 per 100,000 in children younger than 1 year of age and 0.4 per 100,000 in children younger than 16 years of age. The mean age of children with MBP is 1 to 2 years.

Differentiating MBP from other cases of factitious illness is crucial, because children with MBP are in much greater danger. Mortality may be as high as 33% when suffocation or poisoning is involved. Siblings of these children are also at risk; 61% have symptoms similar to the victims, and 25% die. Virtually all children suffer serious psychological sequelae from this form of abuse, and 8% of victims of MBP suffer long-term morbidity. It is likely that as many as 5% of patients in allergy clinics and 1% of those in asthma clinics have MBP.

Common presenting symptoms include vomiting, diarrhea, respiratory arrest, asthma, seizures, incoordination, fever, bleeding, failure to thrive, rash, hypoglycemia, and loss of consciousness. Simulation of psychiatric disorders is rare.

Nearly 75% of the morbidity to the child occurs in hospitals from invasive procedures. Once confronted with negative test results or discharge planning, the perpetrators may become intensely enraged and acutely suicidal. They may initiate legal action. The treatment team should take appropriate precautions. Treatment involves protecting the child from further abuse and reporting to child protective services.

## CHAPTER 17
# Anxiety and Phobias

## ANXIETY DISORDERS

Anxiety disorders tend to be chronic, recurring conditions that vary in intensity over time. They affect 5% to 10% of children and adolescents.

**Panic disorder** is the presence of recurrent, unexpected panic attacks. At least 1 month of persistent worrying about having another panic attack is required to make the diagnosis (Table 17-1). Panic disorder most often begins in adolescence or early adulthood; onset before puberty is significantly less common. The course of illness tends to be chronic with waxing and waning of symptom severity over time.

A **panic attack** is a sudden onset of intense fear associated with a feeling of impending doom in the absence of real danger. These attacks occur unexpectedly. Characteristic symptoms include shortness of breath, palpitations, chest pain, a choking or smothering sensation, and a fear of losing control or going *crazy* (Table 17-2). Panic attacks are classified as spontaneous, bound to situations (occur immediately on exposure), and predisposed to situations (attacks occur while at school, but not every time). Triggers can be external (life-threatening situation) or internal (worries about a situation). Situational attacks are common and occur in many patients with other anxiety disorders.

Panic attacks are time-limited and are accompanied by physical symptoms of anxiety. It is common for patients to think that they are about to die of a heart attack. Patients with asthma have a high incidence of panic attacks.

---

**TABLE 17-1 Criteria for Diagnosis of Panic Disorder**

A. Both (1) and (2)
 1. Recurrent unexpected panic attacks
 2. At least one attack is followed by ≥1 month of one or more of the following:
  a. Persistent concern about having additional attacks
  b. Worry about the implications of the attack or its consequences (e.g., losing control, having a heart attack, "going crazy")
  c. A significant change in behavior related to the attacks
B. The presence of agoraphobia
C. The panic attacks are not due to direct physiologic effects of drugs of abuse or medication or a general medical condition (e.g., hyperthyroidism)
D. The panic attacks are not better accounted for by another mental disorder, such as social phobia, specific phobia, obsessive-compulsive disorder, post-traumatic stress disorder, or separation anxiety disorder

---

**TABLE 17-2 Criteria for Diagnosis of a Panic Attack**

A discrete period of intense fear or discomfort, in which four or more of the following symptoms developed abruptly and reached a peak within 10 minutes:

   Palpitations, pounding heart, or accelerated heart rate
   Sweating
   Trembling or shaking
   Sensations of shortness of breath or smothering
   Feeling of choking
   Chest pain or discomfort
   Nausea or abdominal distress
   Feeling dizzy, unsteady, lightheaded, or faint
   Derealization (feelings of unreality) or depersonalization
    (being detached from oneself)
Fear of losing control or going crazy
Paresthesias (numbness or tingling sensations)
Chills or hot flashes

---

Prevalence rates for panic disorder in pediatric psychiatric clinics range from 0.2% to 10%; rates are similar in all racial groups. The condition is eight times more common in family members of affected individuals than in the general population. This family association increases the likelihood of an early onset. Twin studies suggest a genetic component. Children with separation anxiety disorder seem to be at particular risk for subsequent development of panic disorder. Agoraphobia is present in approximately half of patients with panic disorder.

There are no diagnostic laboratory or neuroimaging studies for panic disorder or any other anxiety disorder, although infusions of sodium lactate and breathing into a paper bag have been used as provocative tests in laboratory settings. Patients experiencing a panic attack may present with respiratory alkalosis (due to hyperventilation). The differential diagnosis for panic disorder includes the other anxiety disorders, especially those secondary to general medical conditions and substance-induced anxiety disorders.

**Anxiety disorder due to a general medical condition** is characterized by impairing symptoms of anxiety that are judged to be the direct consequence of another medical illness. Medical illnesses that can mimic panic disorder and other anxiety disorders include cardiovascular disease (dysrhythmias, mitral valve prolapse), hyperthyroidism, asthma, irritable bowel syndrome, chronic obstructive pulmonary disease, and pheochromocytoma. **Substance-induced anxiety disorder** is characterized by symptoms of anxiety that are judged to be the direct consequence of a drug (caffeine or other stimulants). A variety of psychiatric illnesses may occur concurrently with panic disorder, including major depression, obsessive-compulsive disorder (OCD), and other anxiety disorders. Patients with anxiety disorders abuse substances at higher rates than the general population.

**Agoraphobia** literally means *fear of the marketplace*. In common usage, the term is applied to a pathologic condition describing fear of situations where escape is difficult or would draw unwanted attention to the person.

Agoraphobia is often persistent and can leave people homebound. It can occur independently or in relationship to panic disorder; 95% of patients with agoraphobia also have panic disorder. The condition is more common in females. Consider the diagnosis of a specific phobia (as opposed to agoraphobia) if the avoidance is limited to one or a few specific situations or social phobia if avoidance is limited to social situations in general.

**Generalized anxiety disorder (GAD)** is characterized by 6 or more months of persistent and excessive anxiety and worry and includes a historical diagnosis of overanxious disorder of childhood. It is common in patients referred to a psychiatrist. The anxiety must be accompanied by at least three of the following symptoms: restlessness, easy fatigability, difficulty concentrating, irritability, muscle tension, and disturbed sleep. The fear or anxiety must be out of proportion to what is realistic. The worries should be multiple, not paroxysmal, and not focused on a single theme, as in separation anxiety disorder (Table 17-3).

The etiology of GAD is unknown. The lifetime prevalence rate is 5%. Biologic relatives have an increased risk of developing GAD and an increased risk of major depression. Physical signs of anxiety are often present, including shakiness, trembling, and myalgias. Gastrointestinal symptoms (nausea, vomiting, diarrhea) and

---

**TABLE 17-3 Criteria for Diagnosis of Generalized Anxiety Disorder**

A. Excessive anxiety and worry (apprehensive expectation), occurring more days than not for at least 6 months, about numerous events or activities
B. The person finds it difficult to control the worry
C. The anxiety and worry are associated with three or more of the following six symptoms (with at least some symptoms present for more days than not for the past 6 months). Note: Only one symptom is required in children.
  1. Restlessness or feeling keyed up or on edge
  2. Being easily fatigued
  3. Difficulty concentrating or mind going blank
  4. Irritability
  5. Muscle tension
  6. Sleep disturbance (difficulty falling or staying asleep or restless, unsatisfying sleep)
D. The focus of the anxiety and worry is not confined to features of a disorder (e.g., panic disorder, social phobia, obsessive-compulsive disorder, separation anxiety disorder, anorexia nervosa, somatization disorder, hypochondriasis), and the anxiety and worry do not occur exclusively during post-traumatic stress disorder
E. The anxiety, worry, or physical symptoms cause clinically significant distress or impairment in social, occupational, or other important areas of functioning
F. The disturbance is not due to the direct physiologic effects of a drug or a general medical condition (e.g., hyperthyroidism) and does not occur exclusively during a mood disorder, a psychotic disorder, or a pervasive developmental disorder

---

autonomic symptoms (tachycardia, shortness of breath) commonly coexist. In children and adolescents, the specific symptoms of autonomic arousal are less prominent. Symptoms are often related to school performance or sports. Children with GAD are often perfectionists and overly concerned about the approval of others. Patients with GAD describe having been anxious all their lives and have more sleep disturbance than patients with any other kind of anxiety disorder.

There are no laboratory or imaging studies diagnostic for GAD. The differential diagnosis for GAD includes normal anxiety, other anxiety disorders (OCD, separation anxiety disorder, social phobia), anorexia nervosa, somatoform disorders, and major depression. Substance-induced anxiety disorder must also be considered (caffeine, sedative-hypnotic withdrawal). Care must be taken to elicit internalizing symptoms of negative cognitions about the self (hopelessness, helplessness, worthlessness, suicidal ideation),

as well as those concerning relationships (embarrassment, self-consciousness) and associated with anxieties. Enquiry about eating, weight, and energy, and interests should also be carried out to eliminate a mood disorder.

**Post-traumatic stress disorder (PTSD)** is characterized by re-experiencing a traumatic event in which actual or threatened death or serious injury was possible. The re-experiencing is accompanied by avoidance of stimuli that remind the person of the trauma and by autonomic hyperarousal (Table 17-4). Stressors including rape and torture are particularly traumatic. PTSD can result from one dramatic incident (e.g., a motor vehicle accident), but in children it is often the result of repeated trauma and may be more difficult to treat.

Severity, duration, and proximity of the traumatic event are the most likely predictors of PTSD. Dissociative states lasting a few seconds to many hours, in which the person relives the traumatic event, are referred to as

---

**TABLE 17-4 Criteria for Diagnosis of Post-Traumatic Stress Disorder**

A. The person has been exposed to a traumatic event in which both of the following were present:
   1. The person experienced, witnessed, or was confronted with an event or events that involved actual or threatened death or serious injury or a threat to the physical integrity of self or others
   2. The person's response involved intense fear, helplessness, or horror. Note: In children, this may be expressed instead by disorganized or agitated behavior
B. The traumatic event is persistently re-experienced in one or more of the following ways:
   1. Recurrent and intrusive distressing recollections of the event, including images, thoughts, or perceptions. Note: In young children, repetitive play may occur in which themes or aspects of the trauma are expressed
   2. Recurrent distressing dreams of the event. Note: In children, there may be frightening dreams without recognizable content
   3. Acting or feeling as if the traumatic event were recurring (includes a sense of reliving the experience, illusions, hallucinations, and dissociative flashback episodes, including flashbacks that occur on awakening or when intoxicated). Note: In young children, trauma-specific re-enactment may occur
   4. Intense psychological distress at exposure to internal or external cues that symbolize or resemble an aspect of the traumatic event
   5. Physiologic reactivity on exposure to internal or external cues that symbolize or resemble an aspect of the traumatic event
C. Persistent avoidance of stimuli associated with the trauma and numbing of general responsiveness (not present before the trauma), as indicated by three or more of the following:
   1. Efforts to avoid thoughts, feelings, or conversations associated with the trauma
   2. Efforts to avoid activities, places, or people that arouse recollections of the trauma
   3. Inability to recall an important aspect of the trauma
   4. Markedly diminished interest or participation in significant activities
   5. Feeling of detachment or estrangement from others
   6. Restricted range of affect (e.g., unable to have loving feelings)
   7. Sense of a foreshortened future (e.g., does not expect to have a career, marriage, children, or a normal life span)
D. Persistent symptoms of increased arousal (not present before the trauma), as indicated by two or more of the following:
   1. Difficulty falling or staying asleep
   2. Irritability or outbursts of anger
   3. Difficulty concentrating
   4. Hypervigilance
   5. Exaggerated startle response
E. Duration of the disturbance (symptoms in criteria B, C, and D) is >1 month
F. The disturbance causes clinically significant distress or impairment in social, occupational, or other important areas of functioning

Specify if:
● Acute: if duration of symptoms is <3 months
● Chronic: if duration of symptoms is ≥3 months
● With delayed onset: if onset of symptoms is at least 6 mo after the stressor

*flashbacks.* Re-experiencing trauma in children may be nonspecific to the trauma (e.g., dreams of monsters). In children, play may revolve repetitively around the circumstances of the trauma. In adolescents, anticipation of unwanted visual imagery increases the risk of irritable mood, anger, and sleep deprivation (sleep is associated with nightmares and undesirable visual experiences). When faced with reminders of the original trauma, physical signs of anxiety or increased arousal, including difficulty falling or staying asleep, hypervigilance, exaggerated startle response, irritability, angry outbursts, and difficulty concentrating, occur.

Most PSTD symptoms are adaptive until they interfere with the person's functioning. PTSD usually begins within 3 months of the trauma, although delay in symptom expression can occur. Typically, an acute stress disorder is present immediately after the trauma. The risk of chronic PTSD increases when symptoms are unresolved by 6 weeks and there are higher premorbid levels of anxiety or depression. Rates of suicide attempts are threefold higher than unaffected controls. There is an increased risk of PTSD in girls and less able children, especially when there is concurrent experience of death or severe injury to a member of close family. There is an increased risk of developing PTSD in family members of patients with PTSD. The lifetime prevalence estimates of PTSD vary, but 8% is most commonly cited (11.5% in children from war zones).

The differential diagnosis of PTSD includes other anxiety disorders, adjustment disorders, acute stress disorder, OCD, psychotic disorders, substance-induced disorders, and psychotic disorders secondary to general medical conditions. Although rare, if financial compensation is at issue, malingering should be ruled out.

The prognosis for people with PTSD varies. Some patients have excellent recovery, and others have significant functional decline. Early intervention to decrease morbidity is important. There is no proven primary prevention for PTSD.

For PTSD, antidepressants may be augmented by clonidine (also useful in hyperarousal and impulsivity) in the presence of severe affective dyscontrol. Atypical antipsychotics are used if self-injurious behavior, dissociation, psychosis, and aggression are present. Atomoxetine is useful in PTSD with concurrent ADHD. Asking children to draw on their experience often assists recall of both the event and the associated emotion. It is important to ensure that re-experiencing the event results in mastery of the associated distress and diminishes personal impairment, rather than increasing it by magnifying the impact of the original trauma. Critical-incident stress debriefing soon after the event greatly reduces distress and involves discussing the nature and impact of the trauma event in a group format.

**Acute stress disorder** is characterized by the same signs and symptoms as PTSD but occurs immediately after a traumatic event. These symptoms do not always progress to PTSD. If impaired function persists after 1 month, the diagnosis is PTSD.

**Anxiety disorder not otherwise specified** is a common condition in clinical practice. This diagnosis is used when there is impairing anxiety or phobic symptoms that do not meet full criteria for another anxiety disorder.

**School phobia** and **separation anxiety disorder** (SAD) are often intertwined. Children and adolescents who avoid or refuse to go to school may have histories of separation anxiety and vague somatic complaints (e.g., headaches, abdominal pain, fatigue). They often have been seen by numerous specialists and have undergone elaborate medical evaluations. Their absence from school often is mistakenly seen as a consequence of their symptoms.

SAD occurs in 2% to 4% of children and adolescents. It is most often seen in prepubertal children, with proximity-seeking clinging behavior as a common presenting complaint. There is no marked sex difference. The expression of the somatic symptoms is a means to avoid school and gain parental attention. Patients may have a valid or an irrational concern about a parent or have had an unpleasant experience in school. The prospect of returning to school provokes extreme anxiety and escalating symptoms. True phobia related to schoolwork is rare. School phobia that first presents during adolescence may be an expression of a severe underlying psychopathologic condition, and psychiatric consultation is needed. SAD is a strong (78%) risk factor for developing problems in adulthood, such as panic disorder, agoraphobia, and depression. The most effective treatment is for the child to return to school (or the exposure).

In the **management of anxiety disorders,** likely medical conditions, including hyperthyroidism, medication side effects, substance abuse, or other medical conditions, should be ruled out. The patient should be screened for comorbid psychiatric disorders, such as mood disorders, psychosis, eating disorders, tic disorders, and disruptive behavior disorders. A history from multiple sources is important, because the child may be unable to effectively communicate symptoms. A detailed history that includes the nature of the anxiety triggers; psychosocial history; and family history of tics, anxiety disorders, depression, and other mood disorders should be taken. The younger child may communicate his or her anxieties better through drawings or play.

Combined pharmacologic and psychotherapy is better than either alone for the **treatment** for all anxiety disorders. Selective serotonin reuptake inhibitors (SSRIs) are the medication of choice. The SSRIs approved for children by the U.S. Food and Drug Administration are fluoxetine, sertraline, and fluvoxamine. They can initially exacerbate anxiety or even panic symptoms. Clomipramine requires electrocardiographic and blood level monitoring but may be effective, and it is approved by the U.S. Food and Drug Administration for OCD. Benzodiazepines include a risk of causing disinhibition in children. Alpha-2a-agonists (guanfacine and clonidine) may be useful if autonomic symptoms are present. Anticonvulsant agents (gabapentin, topiramate, and oxcarbazepine) are used when other agents are ineffective. Co-occurrence of the inattentive type of ADHD and an anxiety disorder is common. When using a stimulant, it is advisable to start at a low dose, increasing slowly to minimize the risk of increasing anxiety. Patients with anxiety disorders are often less tolerant of medication side effects. Extra support helps them maintain treatment regimens.

Cognitive and behavioral therapy can be beneficial in a variety of anxiety disorders. For mild to moderate anxiety, evidence-based psychotherapies and psychoeducation should be used first. Reassurance that the patient does not have a life-threatening illness is important. Other psychosocial treatments include stress management, supportive therapies, and biofeedback. Panic disorder tends to be chronic but usually is responsive to treatment. Emphasis is placed on decreasing morbidity through proper treatment. There are no proven primary prevention techniques.

## SPECIFIC PHOBIAS

Specific phobias are marked persistent fears of things or situations, which often lead to avoidance behaviors (Table 17-5). The associated anxiety is almost always felt immediately when the person is confronted with the feared object or situation. The greater the proximity or the more difficult it is to escape, the higher the anxiety. Many patients have had actual fearful experiences with the object or situation (traumatic event). The response to the fear can range from limited symptoms of anxiety to full panic attacks. Although adults and adolescents usually can recognize that their fears are out of proportion to the circumstances, children may not. Children may express their anxiety as crying, tantrums, freezing, or clinging.

Phobia prevalence rates in children and adolescents are estimated at about 2%. The ratio of females to males is 2:1. There is an increased risk of specific phobias in first-degree relatives of patients with specific phobias. Comorbidity with other anxiety disorders is high. Adults with panic and agoraphobia usually have a childhood history of simple phobias, suggesting that some childhood phobias persist over time.

**School phobia** is one of a range of reasons for school nonattendance. In severely worried children, defensive aggression may be used to prevent attendance. Otherwise, these patients do not have antisocial tendencies. Boys and girls are equally affected and there is no association with social class, intelligence, or academic ability. The youngest in a family of several children is more likely to be affected as well as children of older parents. Truancy is generally associated with older adolescents with lower levels of fear. Unlike anxious school refusers, truants hide their school nonattendance from their parents.

**Social phobia** is a common (3% to 13% prevalence) type of phobia characterized by a marked and persistent fear of social or performance situations in which embarrassment might occur (Table 17-6). In other ways, social phobia is similar to specific phobias. There is a wariness of strangers and social apprehension or anxiety when encountering new, strange, or socially threatening situations. Children appear to have a lower rate of negative cognitions (e.g., embarrassment, overconcern, self-consciousness) than adults. Children with simple avoidant disorders are younger than those with more socialized phobic conditions. Left untreated or poorly treated, phobias can become immobilizing and result in significant morbidity. People with specific phobias often significantly restrict their lives. A vasovagal fainting response is common in blood/injection/injury-type phobias. In addition, blood/injection/injury-type phobias may lead patients to avoid needed medical care.

No laboratory or imaging studies can diagnose a specific phobia. Specific phobias share many symptoms with other anxiety disorders. Concurrent illnesses often include major depression and substance-related disorders; 60% of patients with a specific phobia meet diagnostic criteria for another psychiatric disorder. The diagnosis requires that anticipation of fear or actual fear must interfere with the child's daily living.

Cognitive and behavioral techniques are frequently successful in the **treatment** of phobias. Common

---

### TABLE 17-5 Criteria for Diagnosis of Specific Phobia

A. Marked and persistent fear that is excessive or unreasonable, cued by the presence or anticipation of a specific object or situation (e.g., flying, heights, animals, receiving an injection, seeing blood)

B. Exposure to the phobic stimulus almost invariably provokes an immediate anxiety response, which may take the form of a situationally bound or situationally predisposed panic attack. Note: In children, the anxiety may be expressed by crying, tantrums, freezing, or clinging

C. The person recognizes that the fear is excessive or unreasonable. Note: In children, this feature may be absent

D. The phobic situation is avoided or else is endured with intense anxiety or distress

E. The avoidance, anxious anticipation, or distress in the feared situation interferes significantly with the person's normal routine, occupational (or academic) functioning, or social activities or relationships, or there is marked distress about having the phobia

F. In children <18 years, the duration is at least 6 months

G. The anxiety, panic attacks, or phobic avoidance associated with the specific object or situation are not better accounted for by another mental disorder, such as obsessive-compulsive disorder, post-traumatic stress disorder, separation anxiety disorder, social phobia, panic disorder with agoraphobia, or agoraphobia without history of panic disorder

Specify type:
● Animal type is fear elicited by animals or insects
● Natural environment type (e.g., heights, storms, water)
● Blood/injection/injury type is fear related to seeing blood, injuries, injections, or having an invasive medical procedure
● Situational type is fear caused by specific situations (e.g., airplanes, elevators, enclosed places)
● Other type (e.g., fear of choking, vomiting, or contracting an illness; in children, fear of loud sounds or costumed characters)

**TABLE 17-6 Criteria for Diagnosis of Social Phobia**

A. A marked and persistent fear of one or more social or performance situations in which the person is exposed to unfamiliar people or to possible scrutiny by others. The individual fears that he or she will act in a way (or show anxiety symptoms) that will be humiliating or embarrassing. Note: In children, there must be evidence of the capacity for age-appropriate social relationships with familiar people, and the anxiety must occur in peer settings, not just in interactions with adults

B. Exposure to the feared social situation almost invariably provokes anxiety, which may take the form of a situationally bound or situationally predisposed panic attack. Note: In children, the anxiety may be expressed by crying, tantrums, freezing, or shrinking from social situations or unfamiliar people

C. The person recognizes that the fear is excessive or unreasonable. Note: In children, this feature may be absent

D. The feared social or performance situations are avoided or else are endured with intense anxiety or distress

E. The avoidance, anxious anticipation, or distress in the feared social or performance situation interferes significantly with the person's normal routine, occupational (academic) functioning, or social activities or relationships, or there is marked distress about having the phobia

F. In children <18 years, the duration is at least 6 months

G. The fear or avoidance is not due to the direct physiologic effects of a drug of abuse, a medication, or a general medical condition and is not better accounted for by another mental disorder (e.g., panic disorder with or without agoraphobia, separation anxiety disorder, body dysmorphic disorder, pervasive developmental disorder, or schizoid personality disorder)

H. If a general medical condition or another mental disorder is present, the fear in criterion A is unrelated to it (e.g., the fear is not of stuttering, or exhibiting abnormal eating behavior in anorexia nervosa or bulimia nervosa)

Specify if:

Generalized: if the fears include most social situations (e.g., initiating or maintaining conversations, participating in small groups, dating, speaking to authority figures, attending parties). Note: Also consider the additional diagnosis of avoidant personality disorder.

techniques include rapid exposure (flooding) or systematic desensitization (slowly getting closer to the feared object). SSRIs or buspirone are used in more extreme or urgent cases. The psychotherapeutic techniques are more likely to have persistent effects than medications. If a phobia persists into adulthood, there is only a 20% chance of full remission. There are no well-studied primary prevention techniques. Preventing a cycle of exposure and escape (which reinforces the phobic response) can decrease the likelihood of prolonged impairment.

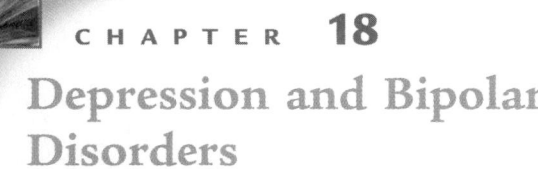

# CHAPTER 18

# Depression and Bipolar Disorders

## DEPRESSION

**Major depression** is a diagnosis that requires a minimum of 2 weeks of symptoms, including either a depressed mood or loss of interest or pleasure in nearly all activities. Four additional symptoms also must be present (Table 18-1).

The signs and symptoms of major depression can be remembered using the mnemonic SIGECAPS:

S: Sleep disturbance (usually decreased, can be increased)
I: Interests (decreased, for usual activities)
G: Guilt (excessive or inappropriate)
E: Energy (decreased)
C: Concentration problems

A: Appetite change (usually decreased, can be increased)
P: Pleasure (decreased)
S: Suicidal thoughts or actions

Patients usually present with *boredom*, restlessness, and somatic complaints (fatigue or vague or localized pains). Depressed children and adolescents may not be able to identify their affective state. Instead of depressed mood, they may present with a new onset of irritability or failure to gain weight. Sudden drops in grades may be a clue. Patients with depression have disturbed sleep (decreased rapid eye movement latency, middle and terminal insomnia) and decreased appetite (weight loss or failure to gain appropriate weight). Discussion of suicidal thoughts is important when evaluating depressed patients because suicidal thoughts and attempts are common. There is no evidence that discussing suicide leads to increased suicidal thoughts.

Depression occurs in approximately 2% (0.4% to 2.50%) of prepubertal children, with equal prevalence in boys and girls. The prevalence is approximately 6% (1.6% to 8.0%) in adolescents, with a female-to-male ratio of 2:1, similar to adults. The average duration of an untreated major depressive episode in a child or adolescent is 7 to 9 months. Fifty percent of youth relapse; 10% have a chronic course that continues into adulthood.

The etiology of depression is not completely understood. There is a genetic predisposition. Potential factors include genetic heritability, dysregulation of central serotonergic or noradrenergic systems, hypothalamic-pituitary-adrenal axis dysfunction, and the influence of pubertal sex hormones. Personality factors, such as a negative cognitive style (pessimistic approach), have been implicated. The stress-diathesis model suggests that a negative cognitive style combined with negative life events and environmental adversity contributes to depression.

## TABLE 18-1  Criteria for Diagnosis of Major Depressive Episode

A. Five or more of the following symptoms have been present during the same 2-week period and represent a change from previous functioning; at least one of the symptoms is either (1) depressed mood or (2) loss of interest or pleasure. Note: Do not include symptoms that are clearly due to a general medical condition or mood-incongruent delusions or hallucinations
   1. Depressed mood most of the day, nearly every day, as indicated by either subjective report (e.g., feels sad or empty) or observation made by others (e.g., appears tearful). Note: In children and adolescents, mood can be irritable
   2. Markedly diminished interest or pleasure in all, or almost all, activities most of the day, nearly every day (as indicated subjective account or observation by others)
   3. Significant weight loss when not dieting or weight gain or decrease or increase in appetite nearly every day. Note: In children, consider failure to make expected weight gains
   4. Insomnia or hypersomnia nearly every day
   5. Psychomotor agitation or retardation nearly every day (observable by others)
   6. Fatigue or loss of energy nearly every day
   7. Feelings of worthlessness or excessive or inappropriate guilt (which may be delusional) nearly every day (not self-reproach or guilt about being sick)
   8. Diminished ability to think, concentrate, or be decisive nearly every day (either by subjective account or as observed by others)
   9. Recurrent thoughts of death (not just fear of dying), recurrent suicidal ideation without a specific plan, a suicide attempt or a specific plan for committing suicide
B. The symptoms do not meet criteria for a mixed manic episode
C. The symptoms cause clinically significant distress or impairment in social, occupational, or other important areas of functioning
D. The symptoms are not due to the direct physiologic effects of a drug of abuse, a medication, or a general medical condition (e.g., hypothyroidism)
E. The symptoms are not better accounted for by bereavement, and the symptoms persist >2 mo or are characterized by marked functional impairment, morbid preoccupation with worthlessness, suicidal ideation, psychotic symptoms, or psychomotor retardation.

One comorbid psychiatric disorder is seen in 40% to 70% of depressed children and adolescents, and 20% to 50% have more than one such condition. The most frequent comorbid diagnoses are dysthymic disorder and anxiety disorders (30% to 80 for both), substance abuse (20% to 30%), and disruptive behavior disorders (10% to 20%). Comorbid conditions appear to influence the risk of recurrent depression, duration of the episode, suicide attempt or behaviors, functional outcome, and response to treatment. Depressed patients with comorbid disruptive behavior have poorer short-term outcomes, fewer melancholic symptoms, fewer recurrences, a lower familial aggregation of mood disorders, a higher incidence of adult criminality, more suicide attempts, and a better response to placebo.

Symptoms of depression overlap with other disorders. One should also be alert to the possibility of mania, because juvenile bipolar disorder frequently presents with a mixed state of depressive and manic symptoms.

No laboratory or imaging studies can diagnose major depression. Dysthymia and other affective disorders are the primary psychiatric disorders in the differential diagnosis for major depression. Adjustment disorders are common and respond to psychosocial interventions, including brief hospitalizations and supportive therapy. In addition, mood disorder, due to a general medical condition (e.g., hypothyroidism), and substance-induced mood disorders should be considered.

**Dysthymic disorder** (prevalence rate 0.6% to 1.7%) is a chronic, milder form of depression characterized by a depressed or irritable mood (indicated subjectively or described by others) present for at least 1 year. Two of the following also are required: changes in appetite; sleep difficulty, fatigue, low self-esteem, poor concentration or difficulty with making decisions, and feelings of hopelessness. About 70% of children and adolescents with dysthymic disorder eventually develop major depression.

**Atypical depression** is characterized by hypersomnia, increased appetite with carbohydrate craving, weight gain, interpersonal rejection sensitivity, and mood reactivity.

**Adjustment disorder with depressed mood** is the most common depressive mood disorder in children and adolescents. Symptoms start within 3 months of an identifiable stressor (e.g., loss of a relationship), with distress in excess of what would be expected and interference with social, occupational, or school functioning. Symptoms should not meet criteria for another psychiatric disorder, should not be caused by bereavement, and should not last longer than 6 months after the stressor has stopped.

**Seasonal affective disorder** is a condition in which depressive symptoms occur in the late fall and early winter when the hours of daylight are shortening. It is most common in northern latitudes.

**Depressive disorder not otherwise specified** is a diagnosis used when patients have functionally impairing depressive symptoms that do not meet criteria for another condition.

Suicide is a complication of major depression and is the third leading cause of death in adolescents. Fifteen to 20% of high school students contemplate suicide and 8% attempt it. The risk of suicide may increase as a patient begins to recover from depression as his or her energy and motivation increase, leading to suicide attempts. There are no known primary prevention interventions. **Treatment** is targeted toward decreasing morbidity and suicide. To ensure safety, modalities such as hospitalization, partial hospital and therapeutic after-school programs, or psycho-education may be needed.

In the 1990s, there was a 28% decrease in suicides in adolescents because of improved detection of depression, along with the proper use of antidepressants. Since 2004, a 14% increase in suicides has coincided with the U.S. Food and Drug Administration (FDA) black box warning about increased risk of suicidal thoughts and behavior about children and youth receiving selective serotonin reuptake inhibitors (SSRIs), along with the resultant decrease in SSRI prescriptions. Substance use, concomitant conduct problems, and impulsivity increase the risk of suicide.

Fluoxetine is the only agent approved by the FDA for treatment of youth. Citalopram and escitalopram have positive clinical trial results as well. The data suggest that antidepressants (notably paroxetine and venlafaxine) pose a 4% risk, versus a 2% risk in placebo, of suicidal thinking or behavior. The FDA has issued a black box warning for suicidality for all antidepressants, not just the SSRIs. The risk of using antidepressants is much less than the high rate of suicide in children and adolescents with untreated depression. Clinicians are not able to determine in advance which medication might work. Medications should be chosen according to side effect profile and drug interactions.

An antidepressant should be given an adequate trial (6 weeks at *therapeutic* doses) before switching or discontinuing unless there are serious side effects. For a first episode of depression in children and adolescents, treatment for 6 to 9 months after remission of symptoms is recommended. Patients with recurrent or chronic depression may need to take antidepressants for extended periods (years or even a lifetime). If a patient does not respond to adequate trials of two or more antidepressants, a child psychiatrist should be consulted. The psychiatrist's evaluation should focus on diagnostic clarity and psychosocial issues that might be preventing full response. An initial evaluation by a child psychiatrist to confirm diagnosis is also helpful. Usually, starting an SSRI and subsequently referring to a child psychiatrist can decrease the time it takes for the child to receive adequate treatment. For acute depression, weekly visits for the first month, then twice monthly for a month, and at least once monthly thereafter are indicated. Telephone calls may substitute for face-to-face visits. The risks of medication (including suicidal and self-destructive behavior) should be discussed with parents, guardians, and patients. They should also be educated about what symptoms (increased agitation, thoughts of suicide, or anxiety and restlessness) to watch for and to call right away if these new symptoms occur. The family should be engaged in treatment.

Psychotherapy is another potential treatment for depression. Cognitive-behavioral therapy, interpersonal therapy, and dialectic behavioral therapy all show promise in the treatment of children and adolescents.

Comorbid psychiatric disorders (especially conduct disorder), exposure to negative life events, family history of major depressive disorder, and conflict within the family all lead to a worse prognosis. Additionally, 20% to 40% of those with childhood-onset depression with psychotic features, family history of bipolar disorder, or a hypomanic episode as a result of antidepressant medications, will develop bipolar disorder.

# BIPOLAR DISORDERS

**Bipolar disorder** (BD), previously called manic-depressive disorder, often has its onset during childhood or adolescence. Mania consists of distinct periods of elevated, expansive, or irritable moods associated with hyperactivity and distractibility that may alternate with periods of severe depression lasting several days or weeks (Table 18-2).

To diagnose mania associated with BD, euphoria (elevated or expansive mood) and three additional symptoms, or irritability and four additional manic symptoms are required. Children and adolescents with euphoric mood are bubbly, giggly, *over-the-top* happy, to a degree that it is socially unacceptable and irritating to others. Grandiosity in children is often dramatic. Children act as if they are superior even in situations in which it is obvious that this is not true and behave as if the laws of nature do not apply to them; they may tell adults what to do and how to do it. Racing thoughts are common in bipolar disorder and occur when thoughts are generated too quickly for a person to keep up. Periods of extreme rage also are common. These rages or tantrums are not a diagnostic criterion, because many children with BD do not exhibit them.

A decreased need for sleep is a hallmark of mania. Although decreased sleep is not absolutely required to make the diagnosis, there are no other diagnoses where a child has a greatly decreased amount of total sleep

---

**TABLE 18-2  Mania Symptoms**

A. A distinct period of abnormally and persistently elevated, expansive, or irritable mood, lasting at least 1 week (or any duration if hospitalization is necessary)

B. During the period of mood disturbance, three or more of the following symptoms have persisted (four if the mood is only irritability) and are present to a significant degree
 1. Inflated self-esteem or grandiosity
 2. Decreased need for sleep (e.g., feels rested after only 3 hours of sleep)
 3. More talkative than usual or pressure to keep talking
 4. Flight of ideas or subjective experience that thoughts are racing
 5. Distractibility (i.e., easily drawn to unimportant or irrelevant external stimuli)
 6. Increased goal-directed activity (socially, at work or school, or sexually) or psychomotor agitation

C. Excessive involvement in pleasurable activities that have a high potential for painful consequences (e.g., unrestrained buying sprees, sexual indiscretions, or foolish investments)

D. The symptoms do not meet criteria for a mixed episode

E. The mood disturbance is sufficiently severe to cause marked impairment in occupational functioning, usual social activities or relationships with others or to necessitate hospitalization to prevent harm to self or others, or with psychotic features

F. The symptoms are not due to the direct physiologic effects of a substance or a general medical condition. Note: Manic-like episodes that are clearly caused by somatic antidepressant treatment (e.g., medication, electroconvulsive therapy, light therapy) should not count toward a diagnosis of bipolar I disorder.

(compared with age-appropriate norms) and is not fatigued. Sleep deprivation, substance abuse, and antidepressants may trigger mania. Children with BD often present with rapid or ultra-rapid cycling with multiple shifts between euthymia, mania, and depression within a single day. Early-onset BD has a highly variable, chronic, nonepisodic presentation. Irritability as well as labile mood and psychotic features may be more common in young people with BD. BD often begins with an episode of depression. It is estimated that 20% to 40% of youth will develop BD within 5 years of a depression. Features associated with switching include early-onset depression, psychomotor retardation, psychosis, mood lability, seasonal pattern, family history of BD or mood disorders, and antidepressant-induced hypomania. A mixed episode requires 1 week of symptoms from both a manic and major depressive episode. *Dysphoric mania* is another term used to describe periods of mania that are accompanied by *bad feelings*. *Hypomania* is used to describe a period of more than 4 but less than 7 days of manic symptoms. It also is used to describe less intense mania.

**Bipolar II disorder** includes at least one full major depressive episode and at least one period of hypomania (4 days). This is in contrast to bipolar I disorder, in which impairing symptoms of mania have to be present for at least 7 days. **Bipolar disorder not otherwise specified** is used to describe prominent symptoms of BD that do not meet full diagnostic criteria. It also is used when historical information is unclear or contradictory.

**Cyclothymic disorder** is characterized by 2 years or more (1 year in children) of numerous periods of hypomania and depression that do not meet full criteria for either a manic or a major depressive episode.

BD is an even higher risk factor for suicide than depression. Twenty-five to 33% of children and 50% of adolescents with BD attempt suicide. High levels of irritability, impulsivity, and poor ability to consider consequences increase the risk of completed suicide. Attempters are usually older, more likely to have mixed episodes and psychotic features, comorbid substance use, panic disorder, nonsuicidal self-injurious behaviors, a family history of suicide attempts, history of hospitalizations, and history of physical or sexual abuse. Ensuring safety is the first consideration. Hospitalization, partial hospitalization, intensive outpatient treatment, and intensive in-home services are used as needed for stabilization and safety.

BD occurs in about 4% of the general population. It is estimated that 1% of children and adolescents meet diagnostic criteria for bipolar disorder. Although BD in adults tends to be gender neutral, it is estimated that prepubertal BD is almost four times more frequently diagnosed in boys.

The etiology of BD is multifactorial. The family history of children with BD is often positive for mental illness, such as major depression, bipolar disorder, schizophrenia, or attention-deficit/hyperactivity disorder (ADHD). An earlier onset of BD in adults increases the risk of BD in offspring during childhood or adolescence and often has a more chronic and debilitating course. A first-degree relative with BD leads to a 10-fold increase in a child's chance of developing BD. Compared with adults, children and adolescents with BD may have a more prolonged early course and are less responsive to treatment.

Patients with BD often have concurrent conditions that warrant treatment. ADHD occurs in approximately 60% to 90% of children with BD. Patients with untreated ADHD are often demoralized, are not grandiose, and do not have decreased need for sleep. Anxiety disorders also commonly occur with BD and do not respond to antimanic agents. Substance abuse can precipitate and perpetuate mania and depression. Many patients with BD are aggressive; they damage property and impulsively commit other crimes. They may meet criteria for conduct disorder. Prominent symptoms of mania assist in differentiating between conduct disorder and BD.

The differential diagnosis for bipolar disorder includes ADHD, major depression, conduct disorder, mood disorder due to a general medical condition, substance-induced mood disorder, and schizophrenia. No laboratory or imaging studies can diagnose BD. Physical examination, careful history, review of systems, and laboratory testing are done to rule out suspected medical etiologies, including neurologic, systemic, and substance-induced disorders.

**Treatment** of BD includes decreasing acute symptoms. The FDA has approved lithium, divalproex sodium, carbamazepine, olanzapine, risperidone, quetiapine, ziprasidone, and aripiprazole for adults with BD. Lithium is the oldest proven treatment for mania and has been used effectively in children and adolescents for years. Common side effects of lithium include hypothyroidism, polyuria, and acne. Divalproex is also a first-line agent (preferable for mixed or rapid cycling cases). Periodic monitoring of blood levels for select medications (lithium and divalproex sodium) can help ensure both the treatment safety and the receipt of therapeutic amounts of the medication. Antipsychotics (risperidone, olanzepine, quetiapine, aripiprazole, and ziprasidone) have had positive results in youth with BD.

Treating comorbid psychiatric disorders must be done carefully. Stimulants may be used to treat ADHD once the patient has been stabilized on a mood stabilizer. Antidepressants should be avoided; if the youth is depressed or has significant anxiety and is not responsive to other pharmacotherapy, cautious use of antidepressants may be necessary. Careful monitoring for manic reactivation, cycling, and suicidality is needed.

Cognitive and behavioral therapies are aimed at improving adherence to medication treatments and ameliorating anxiety and depressive symptoms. These therapies may be the treatment of choice for concurrent anxiety and depressive symptoms. Psychoeducation and family therapy are needed to stabilize the patient's environment and improve prognosis. Cognitive-behavioral therapy, anger management, or insight-oriented work may be helpful. There should be continuous ongoing safety assessment. Collaboration with school regarding behavioral management, special educational needs, and appropriate individualized educational plan is also needed.

Long episode duration, high prevalence of mixed mania, psychosis, and rapid cycling are risk factors for poor outcome. Suicide, school and occupational failures, social difficulties, and criminal activity are common in patients who do not obtain or adhere to thoughtful treatment regimens. Developmental delays are also common in young children with bipolar disorder due to poor learning while symptomatic.

CHAPTER 19

# Obsessive-Compulsive Disorder

Obsessive-compulsive disorder (OCD) is characterized by obsessions, compulsions, or both (Table 19-1). The most common obsessions are fears of contamination, repeated doubts, need for orderliness, aggressive or horrific impulses, and sexual imagery. The most common compulsions are handwashing, ordering, checking, requesting or demanding reassurance, praying, counting, repeating words silently, and hoarding. Compulsions predominate in children, who often do not complain about the symptoms because they frequently have less insight than adults. In some cases, children show some voluntary control or may hide the symptoms, which may shift over time.

Prevalence of OCD in children and adolescents ranges from 1% to 4%, increasing with age. Nearly 80% of adults with OCD had symptoms in childhood. OCD is more common in boys at a younger age and in girls during adolescence. Family studies reflect a genetic component in OCD, with monozygotic twins affected more commonly than dizygotic twins. OCD may be related to group A streptococcal infection and is referred to as **pediatric autoimmune neuropsychiatric disorder associated with streptococcal infections (PANDAS)**. The onset of PANDAS is often before puberty. It is frequently associated with neurologic abnormalities.

The overall lifetime psychiatric comorbidity, including tic, mood and anxiety disorders, disruptive behavior (attention-deficit/hyperactivity disorder [ADHD] and oppositional defiant disorder), and specific developmental disorders, is as high as 75% (8% to 73% for mood disorders, and 13% to 70% for anxiety disorders). There are strong relationships between OCD, Tourette's disorder, body dysmorphic disorder, hypochondriasis, obsessive-compulsive personality disorder, and PANDAS.

No laboratory or imaging studies confirm or disprove the diagnosis. Physical examination may reveal rough, cracked skin as evidence of excessive handwashing.

The differential diagnosis for OCD includes psychotic disorders, other anxiety disorders, and obsessive-compulsive personality disorder. **Obsessive-compulsive personality disorder** is a character style involving preoccupation with orderliness, perfectionism, and control. No obsessions or compulsions are present. **Body dysmorphic disorder**, a delusional fixation on appearance, can be confused with OCD. **Trichotillomania** or hair pulling to relieve anxiety or tension also can be confused with OCD. Schizophrenia can be concurrent with OCD. Intrusive thoughts of OCD can be confused with hallucinations. Complex tics may be confused with simple compulsions such as touching oneself. Of particular importance in pediatric OCD is the high rate of comorbid tic disorders (13% to 23%), including Tourette's syndrome (50%). Major depression, other anxiety disorders, eating disorders, and obsessive-compulsive personality disorder commonly coexist with OCD. Learning disorders and disruptive behavior disorders are also common.

Cognitive-behavioral therapy (CBT) alone is the initial **treatment** of choice in milder cases. High severity of

---

### TABLE 19-1 Criteria for Diagnosis of Obsessive-Compulsive Disorder

A. Either obsessions or compulsions

Obsessions are defined by (1), (2), (3), and (4)

1. Recurrent and persistent thoughts, impulses, or images experienced, at some time during the disturbance, as intrusive and inappropriate and causing marked anxiety or distress
2. Thoughts, impulses, or images are not simply excessive worries about real life problems
3. The person attempts to ignore or suppress such thoughts, impulses, or images or to neutralize them with some other thought or action
4. The person recognizes that the obsessional thoughts, impulses, or images are a product of his or her own mind (not imposed from without as in thought insertion)

Compulsions are defined by (1) and (2)

1. Repetitive behaviors (e.g., handwashing, ordering, checking) or mental acts (e.g., praying, counting, repeating words silently) that the person feels driven to perform in response to an obsession or according to rigidly applied rules
2. The behaviors or mental acts are aimed at preventing or reducing distress or preventing some dreaded event or situation; however, these behaviors or mental acts are not realistically connected with what they are designed to neutralize/prevent or are clearly excessive

B. At some point, the person recognizes that the obsessions or compulsions are excessive or unreasonable. Note: This is not required for children

C. The obsessions or compulsions cause marked distress; are time-consuming (taking >1 hour a day); or significantly interfere with a normal routine, occupational (or academic) functioning, or usual social activities or relationships

D. If another Axis I disorder is present, the content of the obsessions or compulsions is not restricted to it (e.g., preoccupation with food in the presence of an eating disorder)

E. The disturbance is not due to the direct physiologic effects of a drug of abuse, a medication, or a general medical condition

Specify if:

With poor insight: if, for most of the time during the current episode, the person does not recognize that the obsessions and compulsions are excessive or unreasonable

symptoms and complication with comorbidities or insufficient cognitive or emotional ability to cooperate in CBT are indications for selective serotonin reuptake inhibitor (SSRI) treatment. Benefits of using CBT include the apparent durability of symptom relief and avoidance of potential pharmacotherapy-associated side effects. However, the combination of CBT and SSRI may be more efficient than either one alone.

SSRI treatment is generally thought to show a favorable risk-to-benefit ratio in OCD. Behavioral side effects such as activation, akathisia, disinhibition, impulsivity, and hyperactivity may be seen. Monitoring of height may be advisable due to possible growth suppression associated with the SSRIs. In the case of nonresponse, a second SSRI is recommended. (SSRI switching can be done quickly without a cross titration.) Failing this, a clomipramine trial can be attempted. Combinations are considered if single drug therapy fails. Antipsychotics may be needed in severe or treatment refractory cases. Tapering medication should occur during times of low stress (e.g., summer vacation). The response rate to SSRI is lower in the presence of comorbidities. These patients may also be more vulnerable to relapse with SSRI discontinuation. CBT may counter this.

For children and adolescents with OCD and comorbid tic disorder, improvement in tic severity is frequently seen with the improvement of mood and anxiety symptoms. A low dose of risperidone or another atypical antipsychotic medication may be helpful. In OCD comorbid with ADHD, it is common to combine SSRIs (or clomipramine) with a psychostimulant, even though there is theoretical risk that stimulants may increase obsessional symptoms. Intravenous immunoglobulin and other techniques aimed at the streptococcal cases (PANDAS) show promise. One should suspect PANDAS in children with an abrupt onset or exacerbation of OCD and/or tic after an upper respiratory tract infection. Antistreptolysin O, antistreptococcal DNAase B titers, and a throat culture assist in diagnosing a group A beta-hemolytic streptococcal infection.

As many as one third of young people with OCD are refractory to treatment. Many *responders* exhibit only partial response. Poor prognostic factors include comorbid psychiatric illness and a poor initial treatment response.

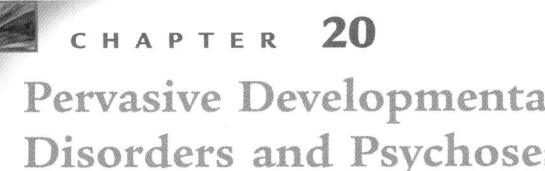

## CHAPTER **20**

# Pervasive Developmental Disorders and Psychoses

## AUTISM

Pervasive developmental disorders, also known as **autism spectrum disorders** (ASDs) consist of five disorders: autism, Asperger's disorder, childhood disintegrative disorder, Rett disorder, and pervasive developmental disorder not otherwise specified. These disorders are marked by their onset in infancy and preschool years. Hallmarks of these disorders include impaired communication and impaired social interaction as well as stereotypic behaviors, interests, and activities. Mental retardation is common. Some children with ASDs show remarkable isolated abilities (savant or splinter skills). ASDs are seen in less than 1% of the population, although the number diagnosed has increased rapidly in the last decade. The prevalence is greater in boys (except for Rett disorder), but girls with the disorders tend to be more severely affected. ASDs are present in equal prevalence among all racial and ethnic groups.

**Autism** is characterized by lifelong marked impairment in reciprocal social interaction, communication, and a restricted range of activities and interests (Table 20-1). Clinical manifestations of the disorder should be present by 3 years of age. Otherwise, Rett disorder or childhood disintegrative disorder should be considered. Approximately 20% of parents report relatively normal development until 1 or 2 years of age, followed by a steady or sudden decline. As an infant, there is delayed or absent social smiling. The young child may spend hours in solitary play and be socially withdrawn with indifference to attempts at communication. Patients with autism often are not able to understand nonverbal communication (eye contact) and do not interact with people as significantly different from objects. Intense absorbing interests, ritualistic behavior, and compulsive routines are characteristic, and their disruption invokes tantrum or rage reactions. Head banging, teeth grinding, rocking, diminished responsiveness to pain and external stimuli, and self-mutilation may be noted. Speech often is delayed and, when present, it is frequently dominated by echolalia (can be mistaken as a sign of obsessive-compulsive disorder [OCD]), perseveration (confused with psychosis or OCD), pronoun reversal, nonsense rhyming, and other abnormalities.

Although the etiology of autistic disorder is unknown, there is an increased risk of autistic disorder in siblings compared with the general population. The prevalence rate is approximately 10 cases per 10,000. Males are affected four to five times more frequently than females. Affected females often have severe mental retardation.

Common comorbidities are mental retardation (in up to 80%), seizure disorder (in 25% and usually beginning in adolescence), anxiety disorders, OCD, and attention-deficit/hyperactivity disorder. Higher IQ and better language skills are related to improved prognosis. Good communication predicts the likelihood of living in less structured group living situations or even independently.

There are no definitive laboratory studies for autistic disorder, but they can help in identifying medical causes that may mimic autism. Hearing should be tested to determine if a deficit may account for the language problems. Chromosomal abnormalities (fragile X syndrome), genetic polymorphisms, congenital viral infections, metabolic disorders (phenylketonuria), and structural brain abnormalities (tuberous sclerosis) should be evaluated as possible etiologic causes of the autistic symptoms. Expressive and mixed receptive and expressive language disorders should be considered. Speech pathology consultation can be helpful in evaluating the communication difficulties. Nonspecific electroencephalographic abnormalities are common even without seizures.

---

**TABLE 20-1  Criteria for Diagnosis of Autistic Disorder**

A. Six or more items from (1), (2), and (3), with at least two from (1) and one each from (2) and (3)
　1. Qualitative impairment in social interaction, as manifested by at least two of the following:
　　a. Marked impairment in the use of multiple nonverbal behaviors, such as eye-to-eye gaze, facial expression, body postures, and gestures to regulate social interaction
　　b. Failure to develop peer relationships appropriate to developmental level
　　c. A lack of spontaneously seeking to share enjoyment, interests, or achievements with other people (e.g., by a lack of showing, bringing, or pointing out objects of interest)
　　d. Lack of social or emotional reciprocity
　2. Qualitative impairments in communication as manifested by at least one of the following:
　　a. Delay in, or total lack of, the development of spoken language (not accompanied by attempts to compensate through alternative modes of communication, such as gesture or mime)
　　b. In individuals with adequate speech, marked impairment in the ability to initiate or sustain a conversation with others
　　c. Stereotyped and repetitive use of language or idiosyncratic language
　　d. Lack of varied, spontaneous make-believe play or social imitative play appropriate to developmental level
　3. Restricted repetitive and stereotyped patterns of behavior, interests, and activities, as manifested by at least one of the following:
　　a. Encompassing preoccupation with stereotyped and restricted patterns of interest that is abnormal either in intensity or focus
　　b. Apparently inflexible adherence to specific, nonfunctional routines or rituals
　　c. Stereotyped and repetitive motor mannerisms (e.g., hand- or finger-flapping or twisting or complex whole body movements)
　　d. Persistent preoccupation with parts of objects
B. Delays or abnormal functioning in at least one of the following areas, with onset before age 3 yr
　1. Social interaction
　2. Language as used in social communication
　3. Symbolic or imaginative play
C. The disturbance is not better accounted for by Rett syndrome or childhood disintegrative disorder

---

The American Academy of Pediatrics recommends screening for autism at 18 and 24 months of age. Comprehensive testing should be done if there is an affected sibling or parental, other caregiver, or pediatrician concern.

Other pervasive developmental disorders can also be confused with autism:

**Asperger's disorder** (2.5 per 10,000 and 5:1 male-to-female ratio) can be distinguished from autistic disorder by a preservation of language development. **Childhood disintegrative disorder** (0.11 per 10,000) has a distinctive pattern of severe developmental regression. This regression occurs after developmental milestones are achieved relatively normally in the first 2 years of life. A rapid deterioration in multiple functional areas is the hallmark of the disorder.

**Rett disorder** (0.44 to 2.1 per 10,000) has been diagnosed only in girls and is associated with mutations in the *MECP2* gene. The characteristic pattern of developmental regression occurs after relatively normal development in the first few months of life. Head circumference growth dramatically decelerates. A characteristic hand-wringing stereotypical movement exists. Motor coordination problems are prominent.

Pervasive developmental disorder not otherwise specified (2 to 16 per 10,000) is a diagnosis made when significant impairment exists in the developmental trajectory but the patient does not meet full criteria for one of the aforementioned disorders.

Many types of medications are used to treat symptoms commonly found in patients with ASD. Antipsychotics (risperidone, olanzapine, quetiapine, aripiprazole, ziprasidone, paliperidone, haloperidol, thioridazine) are used for aggression, agitation, irritability, hyperactivity, and self-injurious behavior. Anticonvulsants and lithium can be used for aggression. Naltrexone has been used to decrease self-injurious behavior. Selective serotonin reuptake inhibitors are given for anxiety, perseveration, compulsions, depression, and social isolation. Stimulants are useful for hyperactivity and inattention (better response with Asperger's disorder). Alpha-2 agonists (guanfacine, clonidine) are used for hyperactivity, aggression, and sleep dysregulation, although melatonin is first-line medication for the common sleep dysregulation. Parent behavioral management training is useful to teach the parents protocols to help their child learn appropriate behavior. Special educational services need to be individualized for the child. Occupational, speech, and physical therapy are required. Also important is the referral for disability services and support. Potentially useful therapies tailored to the individual include applied behavioral analysis, discrete trial training, and structured teaching. There is need for family support groups and individual supportive counseling for parents. The prognosis for autism is guarded. There are no known methods of primary prevention. Treatment and educational interventions are aimed at decreasing morbidity and maximizing function.

## SCHIZOPHRENIA

Schizophrenia generally presents in adolescence or early adulthood; the onset resembles that in adults. To diagnose schizophrenia in children, the same diagnostic criteria are applied as in adults but must be interpreted in terms of the developmental stage of the child because symptoms at an early age are less specific and overlap with a number of developmental disorders (Table 20-2).

Childhood-onset schizophrenia is a rare disorder (<1 in 10,000 children). The frequency increases between 13 and 18 years of age. Boys tend to be affected about twice as often as girls, regardless of ethnic or other cultural factors. The etiology of schizophrenia is unknown. Numerous studies have shown genetic predisposition and linkages for the disorder. In addition, family studies consistently have shown a higher risk in monozygotic twins compared with dizygotic twins and siblings. First-degree relatives of patients with schizophrenia have a 10-fold higher risk.

Schizophrenia is characterized by hallucinations; delusions; disorganization; loosening of associations; inappropriate affect; ambivalent emotional state; and marked withdrawal from family, school, and peers. The symptoms of schizophrenia typically fall into four broad categories:

- **Positive symptoms** include hallucinations and delusions. Hallucinations are auditory or visual misperceptions that occur without external stimuli. Delusions are fixed false beliefs and can be bizarre or nonbizarre, depending on cultural norms.
- **Negative symptoms** include a lack of motivation and social interactions, and flat effect. Negative symptoms are most frequent in early childhood and later adolescence. Children with high IQs showed more positive and fewer negative symptoms than children with low IQs.
- **Disorganization of thoughts and behavior** is another category of symptoms that cause significant impairment.
- **Cognitive impairment** is common and is perhaps the most disabling feature of schizophrenia, causing marked social and functional impairment.

There are five subtypes of schizophrenia: paranoid, disorganized, catatonic, undifferentiated, and residual.

- **Paranoid type**: prominent hallucinations and delusions with relatively normal cognition. The delusions are often persecutory, but other types also may occur.
- **Disorganized type**: disorganized speech, disorganized behavior, and flat or inappropriate affect

---

**TABLE 20-2  Criteria for Diagnosis of Schizophrenia**

A. Characteristic symptoms: two of the following, each present for a significant portion of time during a 1-month period (or less if successfully treated)
  1. Delusions
  2. Hallucinations
  3. Disorganized speech (e.g., frequent derailment or incoherence)
  4. Grossly disorganized or catatonic behavior
  5. Negative symptoms (i.e., affective flattening, alogia, or avolition)
  Note: Only one criterion A symptom is required if delusions are bizarre or hallucinations consist of a voice keeping up a running commentary on the person's behavior or thoughts or two or more voices conversing with each other
B. Social/occupational dysfunction: For a significant portion of the time since the onset of the disturbance, major areas of functioning, such as work, interpersonal relations, or self-care, are markedly below the level achieved before the onset (or when the onset is in childhood or adolescence, failure to achieve expected level of interpersonal, academic, or occupational achievement)
C. Duration: Continuous signs of the disturbance persist for at least 6 months. This 6-month period must include at least 1 month of symptoms (or less if successfully treated) that meet criterion A (i.e., active-phase symptoms) and may include periods of prodromal or residual symptoms. During prodromal or residual periods, signs of disturbance may be manifested by only negative symptoms or symptoms listed in criterion A present in an attenuated form (e.g., odd beliefs, unusual perceptual experiences)
D. Schizoaffective and mood disorder exclusion: Schizoaffective disorder and mood disorder with psychotic features have been ruled out because either (1) no major depressive, manic, or mixed episodes have occurred concurrently with the active-phase symptoms or (2) if mood episodes have occurred during active-phase symptoms, their total duration has been brief relative to the duration of the active and residual periods
E. The disturbance is not due to the direct physiologic effects of a drug of abuse, a medication, or a general medical condition
F. If there is a history of autistic disorder or another pervasive developmental disorder, the additional diagnosis of schizophrenia is made only if prominent delusions or hallucinations also are present for at least 1 month (or less if successfully treated)

Classification of longitudinal course (can be applied only after at least 1 year has elapsed since the initial onset of active-phase symptoms):
  Episodic with interepisode residual symptoms (episodes are defined by the re-emergence of prominent psychotic symptoms); also specify if: with prominent negative symptoms.
  Episodic with no interepisode residual symptoms
  Continuous (prominent psychotic symptoms are present throughout the period of observation); also specify if with prominent negative symptoms

- **Catatonic type**: prominent psychomotor abnormalities that may include extreme inactivity or excessive motor activity. **Cataplexy** (waxy flexibility) is rare in children and adolescents.
- **Undifferentiated type**: case in which a patient meets the diagnostic criteria for schizophrenia but not paranoid, disorganized, or catatonic type.
- **Residual type**: clinical situation in which full diagnostic criteria have been met previously but no current, prominent positive symptoms.

To meet criteria for diagnosing schizophrenia, clinical symptoms should be present for at least 6 months. If symptoms are present for less than 1 month, the condition is called a **brief psychotic disorder**. If symptoms are present for more than 1 month but less than 6 months, a diagnosis of **schizophreniform disorder** is made. Psychotic symptoms that do not meet full diagnostic criteria for schizophrenia but are clinically significant are diagnosed as **psychotic disorder not otherwise specified**. There are several disorders that have to be distinguished from schizophrenia.

**Schizoaffective disorder** is diagnosed when a person has clear symptoms of schizophrenia for at least 2 weeks without active symptoms of depression or mania. These affective syndromes occur at other times, even when psychotic symptoms are present.

**Major depression with psychotic features** and **bipolar disorder with psychotic features** are diagnoses made when psychotic symptoms occur only during the course of depression or mania. Psychotic disorder due to a general medical condition describes psychotic symptoms that are judged to be the direct result of a general medical condition.

**Substance-induced psychotic disorders** have psychotic symptoms that are related to drug or alcohol ingestion.

**Shared psychotic disorder, folie à deux,** occurs when delusional symptoms from one person influence delusions, with similar content, in another person.

Other disorders in the differential diagnoses are autism, childhood disintegrative disorder (Heller's syndrome), Asperger's disorder, drug-induced psychosis, and organic brain disorders. No diagnostic tests or imaging studies are specific for schizophrenia. It is a diagnosis of exclusion. Structural brain imaging studies typically reveal large cerebral ventricles and an increased ventricle-to-brain ratio (less cortex, more cerebrospinal fluid). Numerous neurochemical and neuropsychological abnormalities are reported in patients with schizophrenia. None of these studies are clinically useful. Magnetic resonance imaging of the brain should be performed for new-onset psychosis to evaluate for intracranial lesions that could mimic schizophrenia. Temporal lobe epilepsy is a condition that mimics symptoms of schizophrenia but is etiologically related to a seizure disorder. Special electroencephalogram lead placement may be necessary to diagnose this condition.

**Treatment** is based on a multimodal approach including antipsychotic medications. First-line drugs are atypical antipsychotics (risperidone, olanzapine, quetiapine, aripiprazole, ziprasidone, paliperidone). Second-line medications are typical antipsychotics (haloperidol, thiothixene, chlorpromazine, trifluoperazine, loxapine, and molindone). These medications can be augmented with lithium or another mood stabilizer. Clozapine or electroconvulsive therapy is generally reserved for resistant cases.

Psychosocial treatments, including skills training, supportive psychotherapy, behavior modification, and cognitive-behavioral therapy are all appropriate and should be considered as needed for individual patients. Attention should be paid to psychoeducation for parents and the child about the disease and the treatment. School interventions are done to ensure that any special learning needs are addressed.

The course of illness for schizophrenia varies. Rarely, a patient may respond well initially and have no additional psychotic episodes. Others respond but have intermittent episodes throughout their lives. Still others have a chronic deteriorating course. The poorest prognosis is seen if the onset is at an age younger than 14 years, with poor premorbid function, when negative symptoms are present, and a family history of schizophrenia exists.

 **SUGGESTED READING**

Dyl J, Kittler J, Phillips KA, et al: Body dysmorphic disorder and other clinically significant body image concerns in adolescent psychiatric inpatients: prevalence and clinical characteristics, *Child Psychiatry Hum Dev* 36:369–382, 2006.

Fisher PL, Wells A: How effective are cognitive and behavioral treatments for obsessive-compulsive disorder? A clinical significance analysis, *Behav Res Ther* 43(12):1543–1558, 2005.

Johnson CP, Myers SM: Council on Children with Disabilities: Identification and evaluation of children with autism spectrum disorders, *Pediatrics* 120: 1183–1215, 2007.

Kliegman RM, Behrman RE, Jenson HB, et al: Nelson Textbook of Pediatrics, 18th ed, Philadelphia, 2007, *Saunders*.

Mancini C, Van Ameringen M, Bennett M, et al: Emerging treatments for child and adolescent social phobia: a review, *J Child Adolesc Psychopharmacol* 15:589–607, 2005.

Pavuluri MN, Birmaher B, Naylor MW: Pediatric bipolar disorder: a review of the past 10 years, *J Am Acad Child Adolesc Psychiatry* 44(9):846–871, 2005.

Post Traumatic Stress Disorder (PTSD): The Management of PTSD in Adults and Children in Primary and Secondary Care (2005), *National Institute of Clinical Excellence*. www.nice.org.uk.

Rappaport N, Bostic JQ, Prince JB, et al: Treating pediatric depression in primary care: coping with the patients' blue mood and the FDA's black box, *J Pediatr* 148:567–568, 2006.

# PSYCHOSOCIAL ISSUES

Cindy W. Christian and Nathan J. Blum

---

## CHAPTER 21

## Failure to Thrive

**Failure to thrive (FTT)** is a term given to malnourished infants and young children who fail to meet expected standards of growth. The term FTT is most often used to describe malnutrition that is related to environmental or psychosocial causes, although in many children with inadequate growth, organic, and environmental contributors coexist. It is important to assess the potential medical, nutritional, developmental, psychosocial, and environmental contributors to FTT.

FTT is diagnosed by weight that falls or remains below the third percentile for age; that decreases, crossing two major percentile lines on the growth chart over time; or that is less than 80% of the median weight for the height of the child. Caveats to these definitions exist. According to growth chart standards, 3% of the population naturally falls below the third percentile. These children, who typically have short stature or constitutional delay of growth, usually are proportional (normal weight for height). Additionally, in the first few years of life, large fluctuations in percentile position can occur in normal children. Changes in weight should be assessed in relation to height (length) and head circumference.

Weight that decreases from a disproportionately high percentile to one that is proportional causes no concern, but weight that decreases to a percentile that is disproportionately low is of concern. Allowances must be made for prematurity; weight corrections are needed until 24 months of age, height corrections until 40 months of age, and head circumference corrections until 18 months of age. Although some growth variants can be difficult to distinguish from FTT, growth velocity and height-for-weight determinations can be useful in distinguishing the cause of growth failure. In children with FTT, malnutrition initially results in wasting (deficiency in weight gain). Stunting (deficiency in linear growth) generally occurs after months of malnutrition, and head circumference is spared except with chronic, severe malnutrition. FTT that is *symmetric* (weight, height/length, and head circumference are proportional) suggests long-standing malnutrition, chromosomal

abnormalities, congenital infection, or teratogenic exposures. FTT is a common problem in pediatrics, affecting 5% to 10% of young children, 3% to 5% of children admitted to teaching hospitals, and 15% of children living in poverty and foster care.

## ETIOLOGY

Diseases of any organ system can cause malnutrition. Because possible causes of growth failure are so diverse and often multifactorial, the management of FTT begins with a careful search for its etiology (Table 21-1). The common causes of FTT vary by age, which should be reflected in the evaluation (Table 21-2). In most cases, a comprehensive history and physical examination are sufficient to suggest or eliminate medical disease as the primary cause of FTT. Medical diseases are diagnosed in fewer than 50% of children hospitalized for growth failure and even less frequently in children managed in the outpatient setting. Growth failure is often a manifestation of more extensive family problems.

## DIAGNOSIS AND CLINICAL MANIFESTATIONS

A medical history should include the history of prenatal care, maternal illnesses during pregnancy, identified fetal growth problems, prematurity, and birth size (weight, length, and head circumference). Indicators of medical diseases, such as vomiting, diarrhea, fever, respiratory symptoms, and fatigue, should be noted. A careful diet history is essential to the evaluation. Lactation problems in breastfed infants and improper formula preparation are frequent causes of growth failure early in infancy; the adequacy of the maternal milk supply or the precise preparation of formula should be evaluated. For older infants and young children, a detailed diet history is helpful, although it may be difficult to obtain. It is essential to evaluate intake of solid foods and liquids. Because of parental dietary beliefs, some children have inappropriately restricted diets. Others drink excessive amounts of fruit juice, leading to malabsorption or anorexia. The child's daily schedule, including the timing, frequency, and location of meals, is important. Mealtime practices,

## TABLE 21-1  Causes of Failure to Thrive

### ENVIRONMENTAL (COMMON)

Emotional deprivation
Rumination
Child maltreatment
Maternal depression
Poverty
Poor feeding techniques
Improper formula preparation
Improper mealtime environment
Unusual parental nutritional beliefs

### GASTROINTESTINAL

Cystic fibrosis and other causes of pancreatic insufficiency
Celiac disease
Other malabsorption syndromes
Gastrointestinal reflux

### CONGENITAL/ANATOMIC

Chromosomal abnormalities, genetic syndromes
Congenital heart disease
Gastrointestinal abnormalities (e.g., pyloric stenosis,
  malrotation)
Vascular rings
Upper airway obstruction
Dental caries
Congenital immunodeficiency syndromes

### INFECTIONS

Human immunodeficiency virus
Tuberculosis
Hepatitis
Urinary tract infection
Chronic sinusitis
Parasitic infection

### METABOLIC

Thyroid disease
Adrenal or pituitary disease
Aminoaciduria, organic aciduria
Galactosemia

### NEUROLOGIC

Cerebral palsy
Hypothalamic and other central nervous system tumors
Hypotonia syndromes
Neuromuscular diseases
Degenerative and storage diseases

### RENAL

Chronic renal failure
Renal tubular acidosis
Urinary tract infection

### HEMATOLOGIC

Sickle cell disease
Iron deficiency anemia

## TABLE 21-2  Common Causes of Malnutrition in Early Life

### NEONATE

Failed breastfeeding
Improper formula preparation
Congenital syndromes
Prenatal infections
Teratogenic exposures

### EARLY INFANCY

Maternal depression
Improper formula preparation
Gastroesophageal reflux
Poverty
Congenital heart disease
Cystic fibrosis
Neurologic abnormalities
Child neglect

### LATER INFANCY

Celiac disease
Food intolerance
Child neglect
Delayed introduction of age-appropriate foods
Juice consumption

### AFTER INFANCY

Acquired diseases
Highly distractible child
Juice consumption
Autonomy struggles
Inappropriate mealtime environment
Inappropriate diet

especially distractions that interfere with completing meals, can influence growth. A complete psychosocial assessment of the child and family is required. Child factors (temperament, development), parental factors (depression, domestic violence, social isolation, mental retardation, substance abuse), and environmental and societal factors (poverty, unemployment, illiteracy, lead toxicity) all may contribute to growth failure. In some cases, the history provided by parents is inaccurate, which complicates the evaluation and management of the problem.

A complete physical examination and developmental screening should assess signs of inflicted injury; oral or dental problems; indicators of pulmonary, cardiac, or gastrointestinal disease; and dysmorphic features that may suggest a genetic or teratogenic cause for growth failure. A complete neurologic examination may reveal spasticity or hypotonia, both of which can have untoward effects on feeding and growth. Physical findings related to malnutrition include dermatitis, hepatomegaly, cheilosis, or edema (see Chapter 30). Additionally, children with FTT have more otitis media as well as respiratory and gastrointestinal infections than age-matched controls; severely malnourished children are at risk for a variety of serious infections.

The history and physical examination findings guide the laboratory evaluation, but an extensive search has no merit. Simple screening tests are recommended to identify common illnesses that cause growth failure and to search for medical problems that result from malnutrition. Recommended laboratory tests include screening for iron deficiency anemia and lead toxicity; urinalysis, urine culture, and serum electrolytes to assess renal infection or dysfunction; and a protein purified derivative test to screen for tuberculosis. Human immunodeficiency virus testing may be indicated for selected children. For children with diarrhea, abdominal pain, or malodorous stools, a stool sample for culture and ova and parasites may be indicated. Observation during feeding and home visitation, if possible, are of great diagnostic value in assessing feeding problems, food preferences, mealtime distractions, unusual or disruptive parent-child interactions, and the home environment.

## TREATMENT

Treatment must address the nutritional requirements of the child and the social issues of the family. Initial treatment should focus on the nutritional and medical management of the child while engaging the family in the treatment plan. Parents of malnourished children may feel personally responsible and threatened by the diagnosis of FTT. Parents may be so depressed or dysfunctional that they cannot focus on their child's needs; they may not recognize the psychosocial and family contributors to the malnutrition. These issues can have a profound effect on the success of treatment, and, in the course of therapy, they need to be addressed.

Children with mild malnutrition whose cause is easily identified can be managed by the primary care physician and family. In more challenging cases, a multidisciplinary team, including pediatricians, nutritionists, developmental specialists, nurses, and social workers, improves nutritional outcome in children with FTT. Most children with FTT can be treated in the outpatient setting. Children with severe malnutrition, underlying diagnoses that require hospitalization for evaluation or treatment, or whose safety is in jeopardy because of maltreatment require hospitalization. Admitting children to the hospital to induce and document weight gain is not recommended unless intensive outpatient evaluation and intervention has failed or the social circumstances are a contraindication for attempting outpatient management.

Nutritional management is the cornerstone of treatment, regardless of the etiology. Children with FTT may require more than 1.5 times the expected calorie and protein intake for their age for catch-up growth. Children with FTT who are anorexic and picky eaters may not be able to consume this amount in volume and require calorically dense foods. For formula-fed infants, the concentration of formula can be changed from 20 cal/oz to 24 or 27 cal/oz (Table 21-3). For toddlers, dietary changes should include increasing the caloric density of favorite foods by adding butter, oil, sour cream, peanut butter, or other high-calorie foods. High-calorie oral supplements that provide 30 cal/oz are often well tolerated by toddlers. In some cases, specific carbohydrate, fat, or protein additives are used to boost calories by increasing calories without increasing volume requirements. They can be used to supplement formulas for infants and older children. In addition, vitamin and mineral supplementation is needed, especially during catch-up growth. In general, the simplest and least costly approach to dietary change is warranted.

Depending on the severity of the malnutrition, initiation of catch-up growth may take 2 weeks. Initial weight gain of more than double normal growth can be seen. Weight improvement precedes improvement in stature. For children with chronic, severe malnutrition, many months are needed to reverse all trends in growth. Although many children with FTT eventually reach normal size, they continue to be at risk for developmental, learning, and behavioral problems.

## COMPLICATIONS

Malnutrition causes defects in host defenses. Conversely, infection increases the metabolic needs of the patient and often is associated with anorexia. Children with FTT

---

**TABLE 21-3 Infant Formula Preparation***

| Amount of Powder/Liquid | Amount of Water (oz) | Final Concentration |
| --- | --- | --- |
| 1 cup powdered formula | 29 | 20 kcal/oz |
| 4 scoops powdered formula | 8 | 20 kcal/oz |
| 13 oz liquid concentrate | 13 | 20 kcal/oz |
| 1 cup powdered formula | 24 | 24 kcal/oz |
| 5 scoops powdered formula | 8 | 24 kcal/oz |
| 13 oz liquid concentrate | 9 | 24 kcal/oz |
| 1 cup powdered formula | 21 | 27 kcal/oz |
| 5.5 scoops powdered formula | 8 | 27 kcal/oz |
| 13 oz liquid concentrate | 6 | 27 kcal/oz |

*Final concentrations are reached by adding formula to water. One scoop of powdered formula = one measuring tablespoon. For healthy infants, formulas are prepared to provide 20 kcal/oz.

From Jew R, editor: Department of Pharmacy Services Pharmacy Handbook and Formulary, 2000-2001. Hudson, Ohio, 2000, *Department of Pharmacy Services*, p 422.

may suffer from a **malnutrition-infection cycle**, in which recurrent infections exacerbate malnutrition, which leads to greater susceptibility to infection. Children with FTT must be evaluated and treated promptly for infection and followed closely.

During starvation, the body slows metabolic processes and growth to minimize the need for nutrients and uses its stores of glycogen, fat, and protein to maintain normal metabolic requirements. During starvation, the body also generally maintains homeostasis and normal serum concentrations of electrolytes. With the rapid reinstitution of feeding after starvation, fluid and electrolyte homeostasis may be lost. Changes in serum electrolyte concentrations and the associated complications are collectively termed the **refeeding syndrome**. These changes typically affect phosphorus, potassium, calcium, and magnesium and can result in life-threatening cardiac, pulmonary, or neurologic problems. Infants and children with marasmus, kwashiorkor, and anorexia nervosa and who have had prolonged fasting are at risk for refeeding syndrome. Refeeding syndrome can be avoided by slow institution of nutrition, close monitoring of serum electrolytes during the initial days of feeding, and prompt replacement of depleted electrolytes.

Occasionally, children who live in psychological deprivation develop short stature with or without concomitant FTT or delayed puberty, a syndrome called **psychosocial short stature**. The signs and symptoms found in children with psychosocial short stature include polyphagia, polydipsia, hoarding and stealing of food, gorging and vomiting, drinking from toilet bowls, and other notable behaviors. Affected children are often shy and passive and are typically depressed and socially withdrawn. Endocrine dysfunction is often identified in affected children, who may have decreased growth hormone secretion and a muted response to exogenous growth hormone. Removal of the child from the adverse environment typically results in rapid improvement in endocrine function and subsequent rapid somatic and pubertal growth of the child. The prognosis for children with psychosocial short stature depends on the age at diagnosis and the degree of psychological trauma. Early identification and removal from the environment portends a healthy prognosis. Children who are diagnosed in later childhood or adolescence may not reach their genetic potential for growth and have a poorer psychosocial prognosis.

CHAPTER **22**

# Child Abuse and Neglect

Few social problems have as profound an impact on the well-being of children as child abuse and neglect. Each year in the United States, 3 million reports of suspected maltreatment are made to child welfare agencies. Approximately 1 million of these reports are substantiated after investigation by Child Protective Services (CPS). These reports represent only a small portion of the children who suffer from maltreatment. Parental surveys indicate that several million adults admit to physical violence against their children each year, and many more adults report abusive experiences as children. Federal and state laws define child abuse and neglect. Each state determines the process of investigating abuse, protecting children, and punishing perpetrators for their crimes. Much of the abuse that is recognized by mandated reporters does not get reported to CPS for investigation. Adverse childhood events, such as child abuse and neglect, increase the risk of the individual's developing behaviors in adolescence and adulthood that predict adult morbidity and early mortality. The ability to recognize child maltreatment and effectively advocate for the protection and safety of a child is a great challenge in pediatric practice that can have a profound influence on the health and future well-being of a child.

Child abuse is parental behavior destructive to the normal physical or emotional development of a child. Because personal definitions of abuse vary according to religious and cultural beliefs, individual experiences, and family upbringing, various physicians have different thresholds for reporting suspected abuse to CPS. In every state, physicians are mandated by law to identify and report all cases of *suspected* child abuse and neglect. It is the responsibility of CPS to investigate reports of suspected abuse to determine whether abuse has occurred and to ensure the ongoing safety of the child. State laws also define intentional or reckless acts that cause harm to a child as crimes. Law enforcement investigates crimes such as sexual abuse and serious physical abuse or neglect for possible prosecution of the perpetrator.

Child abuse and neglect are often considered in broad categories that include physical abuse, sexual abuse, emotional abuse, and neglect. Neglect is the most common, accounting for approximately half of the reports made to child welfare agencies. **Child neglect** is defined by omissions that prevent a child's basic needs from being met. These needs include adequate food, clothing, supervision, housing, health care, education, and nurturance. Child abuse and neglect result from a complex interaction of individual, family, and societal risk factors. Although some risk factors, such as parental substance abuse, maternal depression, and domestic violence are strong risk factors for maltreatment, these and other risk factors are better considered as broadly defined markers to alert a physician to a potential risk, rather than determinants of specific abuse and neglect. These risk factors, although important for developing public policies and prevention strategies for maltreatment, should not be used to determine whether a specific patient is a victim of child maltreatment.

The ability to identify victims of child abuse varies by the age of the patient and the type of maltreatment sustained. Children who are victims of sexual abuse are often brought for medical care after the child makes a disclosure, and the diagnosis is obvious. Physically abused infants may be brought for medical evaluation of irritability or lethargy, without a disclosure of trauma. If the infant's injuries are not severe or visible, the diagnosis may be missed. Approximately one third of infants with abusive head trauma initially are misdiagnosed by unsuspecting physicians, only to be identified after sustaining further injury. Although physicians are inherently trusting of parents, a constant awareness of the possibility of abuse is needed.

## PHYSICAL ABUSE

The physical abuse of children by parents affects children of all ages. It is estimated that 1% to 2% of children are physically abused during childhood and that approximately 2000 children are fatally injured each year. Although mothers are most frequently reported as the perpetrators of physical abuse, serious injuries, such as head or abdominal trauma, are more likely to be inflicted by fathers or maternal boyfriends. The diagnosis of physical abuse can be made easily if the child is battered, has obvious external injuries, or is capable of providing a history of the abuse. In many cases, the diagnosis is not obvious. The history provided by the parent is often inaccurate because the parent is unwilling to provide the correct history or is a nonoffending parent who is unaware of the abuse. The child may be too young or ill to provide a history of the assault. An older child may be too scared to do so or may have a strong sense of loyalty to the perpetrator.

A **diagnosis** of physical abuse initially is suggested by a history that seems incongruent with the clinical presentation of the child (Table 22-1). Although injury to any organ system can occur from physical abuse, some injuries are more common. Bruises are universal findings in nonabused ambulatory children but also are among the most common injury identified in abused children. Bruises suggestive of abuse include those that are patterned, such as a slap mark on the face or looped extension cord marks on the body (Fig. 22-1). Bruises in healthy children generally are distributed over bony prominences; bruises that occur

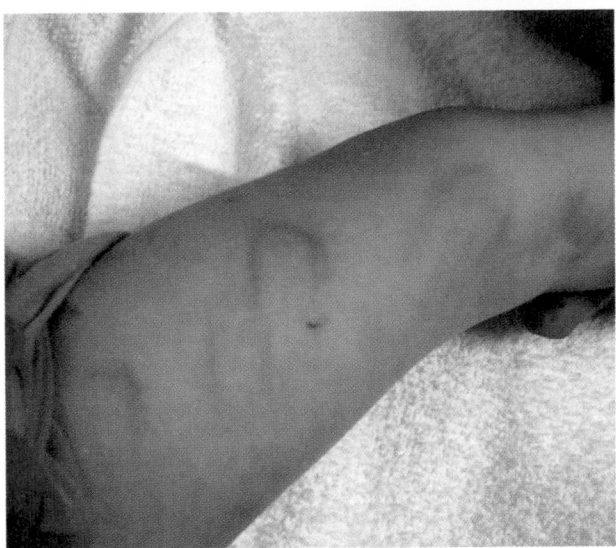

**FIGURE 22-1**

Multiple looped cord marks on a 2-year-old abused child who presented to the hospital with multiple untreated burns to the back, arms, and feet.

in an unusual distribution, such as isolated to the trunk or neck, should raise concern. Bruises in nonambulatory infants are unusual, occurring in less than 2% of healthy infants seen for routine medical care. Occasionally, a subtle bruise may be the only external clue to abuse and can be associated with significant internal injury.

Burns are common pediatric injuries and usually represent preventable unintentional trauma (see Chapter 44). Approximately 10% of children hospitalized with burns are victims of abuse. Inflicted burns can be the result of contact with hot objects (irons, radiators, or cigarettes) but more commonly result from scalding injuries (Fig. 22-2).

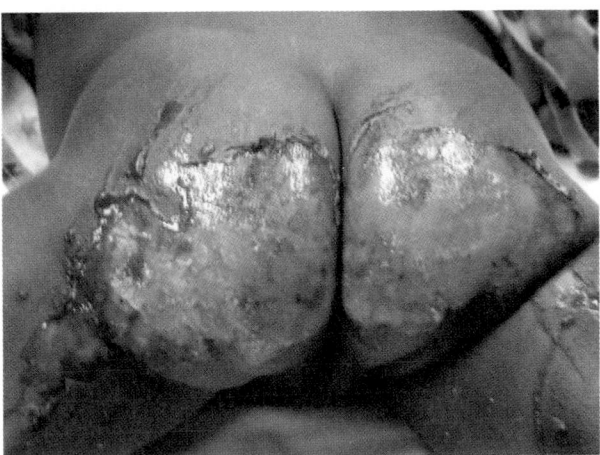

**FIGURE 22-2**

A 1-year-old child brought to the hospital with a history that she sat on a hot radiator. Suspicious injuries such as this require a full medical and social investigation, including a skeletal survey to look for occult skeletal injuries and a child welfare evaluation.

| TABLE 22-1 Clues to the Diagnosis of Physical Abuse |
|---|
| A child presents for medical care with significant injuries, and a history of trauma is denied, especially if the child is an infant or toddler |
| The history provided by the caregiver does not explain the injuries identified |
| The history of the injury changes significantly over time |
| A history of self-inflicted trauma does not correlate with the child's developmental abilities |
| There is an unexpected or unexplained delay in seeking medical care |
| Multiple organ systems are injured, including injuries of various ages |
| The injuries are pathognomonic for child abuse |

Hot tap water burns in infants and toddlers are sometimes the result of intentional immersion injuries, which often occur around toilet training issues. These burns have clear lines of demarcation, uniformity of burn depth, and characteristic pattern.

Inflicted fractures occur more commonly in infants and young children. Although diaphyseal fractures are most common in abuse, they are nonspecific for inflicted injury. Fractures that should raise suspicion for abuse include fractures that are unexplained; occur in young, non-ambulatory children; or involve multiple bones. Certain fractures have a high specificity for abuse, such as rib, metaphyseal, scapular, vertebral, or other unusual fractures (Fig. 22-3).

Abdominal injury is an uncommon but serious form of physical abuse. Blunt trauma to the abdomen is the primary mechanism of injury, and infants and toddlers are the most common victims. Injuries to solid organs, such as the liver or pancreas, predominate. Hollow viscus injury occurs more commonly with inflicted trauma than accidental, and injury to solid and hollow organs occurs almost exclusively with abuse. Even in severe cases of trauma, there may be no bruising to the abdominal wall. The lack of external trauma, along with the usual inaccurate history, can cause delay in diagnosis. A careful evaluation often reveals additional injuries. Abdominal trauma is the second leading cause of mortality from physical abuse, although the prognosis is generally good for children who survive the acute assault.

Abusive head trauma is the leading cause of mortality and morbidity from physical abuse. Most victims are young; infants predominate. Shaking and blunt impact trauma cause injuries. The perpetrators are most commonly fathers and boyfriends, and the trauma typically is precipitated by the perpetrator's intolerance to a crying, fussy infant. Victims present with neurologic symptoms ranging from lethargy and irritability to seizures, apnea, and coma. Unsuspecting physicians misdiagnose approximately one third of infants, and of these, more than 25% are reinjured before diagnosis. Infants most likely to be misdiagnosed include infants with mild injuries, infants who are younger than 6 months of age, and white infants who live in two-parent households. A common finding on presentation is subdural hemorrhage, often associated with progressive cerebral edema (Fig. 22-4). Secondary hypoxic injury is a significant contributor to the pathophysiology of the brain injury. Associated findings include retinal hemorrhages (seen in many, but not all, victims) and skeletal trauma, including rib and metaphyseal fractures. At the time of diagnosis, many head-injured infants have evidence of previous injury. Survivors are at high risk for permanent neurologic sequelae.

The extensive **differential diagnosis** of physical abuse depends on the type of injury (Table 22-2). For children who present with pathognomonic injuries to multiple organ systems, an exhaustive search for medical diagnoses is unwarranted. Children with unusual medical diseases have been incorrectly diagnosed as victims of abuse, emphasizing the need for careful, objective assessments of all children. All infants and young toddlers who present with suspicious injuries should undergo a skeletal survey looking for occult or healing fractures. One third of young infants with multiple fractures, facial injuries, or rib fractures may have occult head trauma. Brain imaging may be indicated for these infants.

## SEXUAL ABUSE

Child sexual abuse is the involvement of children in sexual activities that they cannot understand, for which they are developmentally unprepared and cannot give consent to, and that violates societal taboos. Sexual abuse can be a single event, but more commonly it is chronic. Most perpetrators are adults or adolescents who are known to the child and who have real or perceived power over the child. Most sexual abuse involves manipulation and coercion and is typically a physically nonviolent assault. Although assaults by strangers occur, they are infrequent. Perpetrators are more often male than female and include parents, relatives, teachers, family friends, members of the clergy, and other individuals who have access to children. All perpetrators strive to keep the child from disclosing the abuse and often do so with coercion or threats.

Each year, more than 150,000 cases of sexual abuse are substantiated by CPS, which is likely to be a significant underestimation of the incidence. Approximately 80% of victims are girls, although the sexual abuse of boys is under-recognized and under-reported. Children generally come to attention after they have made a disclosure of their abuse. They may disclose to a nonoffending parent, sibling, relative, friend, or teacher. Children seldom disclose their abuse after a single event, and it is common for children to delay disclosure for many weeks, months, or years, especially if the perpetrator has ongoing access to the child. Sexual abuse also should be considered in children who have behavioral problems, although no behavior is pathognomonic. Hypersexual behaviors should raise the possibility of abuse, although some children with these behaviors are exposed to inappropriate sexual behaviors on television or videos or by witnessing adult sexual activity. Sexual abuse occasionally is recognized by the discovery of an unexplained vaginal, penile, or anal injury or by the discovery of a sexually transmitted infection.

In most cases, the diagnosis of sexual abuse is made by the history obtained from the child. In cases in which the sexual abuse has been reported to CPS or the police (or both), and the child has been interviewed before the medical visit, a complete, forensic interview at the physician's office is not needed. Many communities have systems in place to ensure quality investigative interviews of sexually abused children, and repetitive interviewing of the child should be avoided. If no other professional has spoken to the child about the abuse, or the child makes a spontaneous disclosure to the physician, the child should be interviewed with questions that are open-ended and nonleading. In all cases, the child should be questioned about medical issues related to the abuse, such as timing of the assault and symptoms (bleeding, discharge, or genital pain).

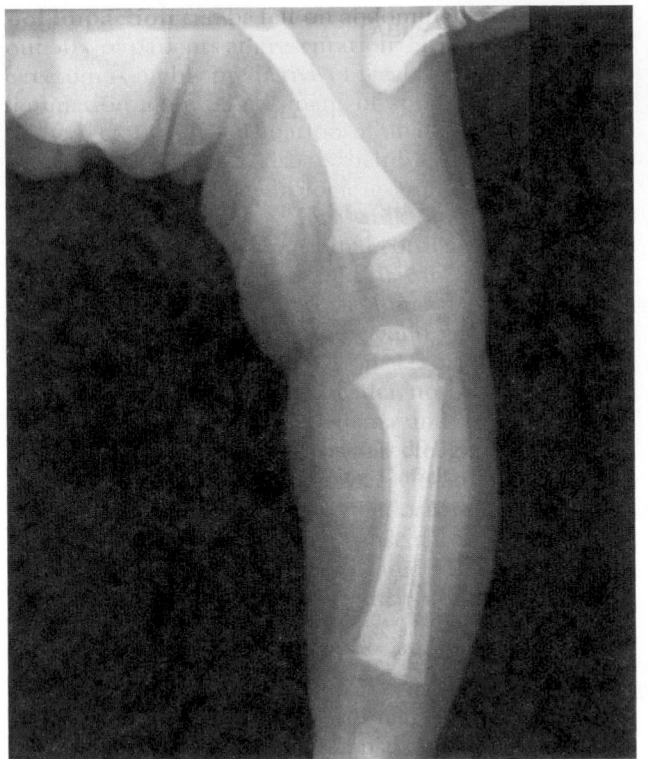

A

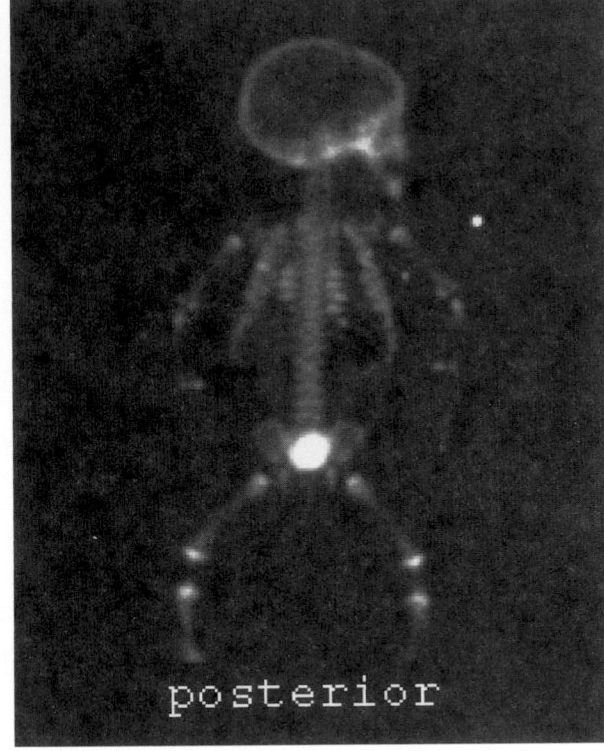

B

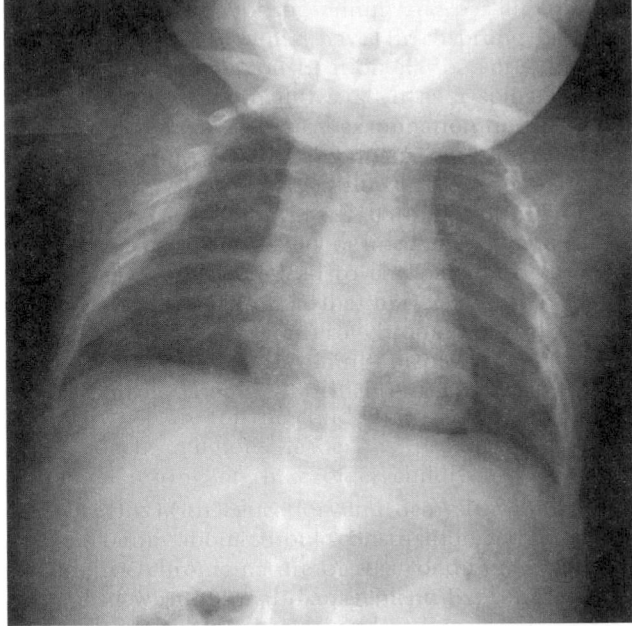

C

**FIGURE 22-3**

**A,** Metaphyseal fracture of the distal tibia in a 3-month-old infant admitted to the hospital with severe head injury. There also is periosteal new bone formation of that tibia, perhaps from a previous injury. **B,** Bone scan of same infant. Initial chest x-ray showed a single fracture of the right posterior fourth rib. A radionuclide bone scan performed 2 days later revealed multiple previously unrecognized fractures of the posterior and lateral ribs. **C,** Follow-up radiographs 2 weeks later showed multiple healing rib fractures. This pattern of fracture is highly specific for child abuse. The mechanism of these injuries is usually violent squeezing of the chest.

The **physical examination** should be complete, with careful inspection of the genitals and anus. Most sexually abused children have a normal genital examination at the time of the medical evaluation. Genital injuries are seen more commonly in children who present for medical care within 72 hours of their most recent assault and in children who report genital bleeding, but they are diagnosed in only 5% to 10% of sexually abused children. Many types of sexual abuse (fondling, vulvar coitus, oral-genital contact) do not injure genital tissue, and genital mucosa heals so rapidly and completely that injuries often heal by the time of the medical examination. For children

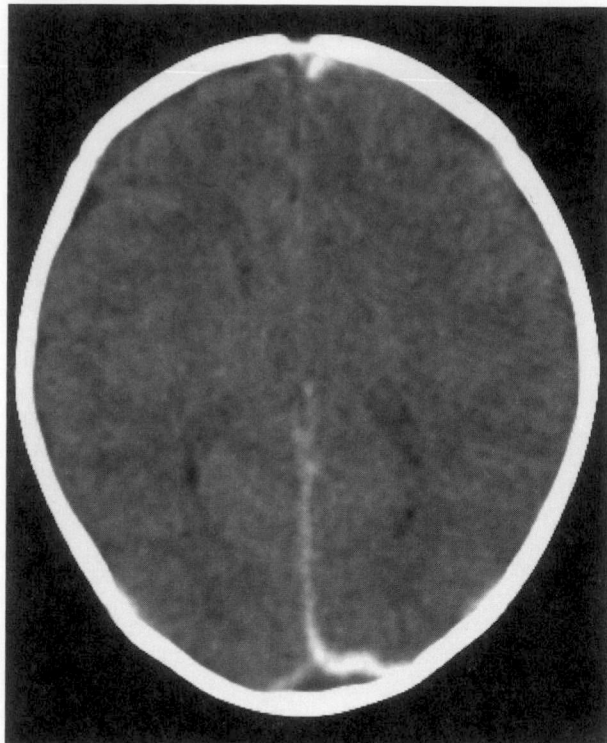

**FIGURE 22-4**

Acute subdural hemorrhage in the posterior interhemispheric fissure in an abused infant.

who present within 72 hours of the most recent assault, special attention should be given to identifying acute injury and the presence of blood or semen on the child. Injuries to the oral mucosa, breasts, or thighs should not be overlooked. Forensic evidence collection is needed in a few cases and has the greatest yield when collected in the first 24 hours after an acute assault. Highest yields come from the child's clothing or bed linens, and efforts should be made to secure these items. Few findings are diagnostic of sexual assault, but findings with the most specificity include acute, unexplained lacerations or ecchymoses of the hymen, posterior fourchette or anus, complete transection of the hymen, unexplained anogenital scarring, or pregnancy in an adolescent with no other history of sexual activity.

The **laboratory evaluation** of a sexually abused child is dictated by the child's age, history, and symptoms. Universal screening for sexually transmitted infections for prepubertal children is unnecessary because the risk of infection is low in asymptomatic young children. The type of assault, identity and known medical history of the perpetrator, and the epidemiology of sexually transmitted infections in the community also are considered. Because of the medicolegal implications of the diagnosis, proper methods must be used for testing. In prepubertal children, culture diagnosis remains the gold standard; non-culture diagnosis of *Neisseria gonorrhoeae* and *Chlamydia trachomatis* do not meet medical or legal standards at this time, although these standards may change in the future, with further experience with nucleic acid amplification

## TABLE 22-2  Differential Diagnosis of Physical Abuse*

### BRUISES

**Accidental injury** (common)
**Dermatologic disorders**
  Mongolian spots
  Erythema multiforme
  Phytophotodermatitis
**Hematologic disorders**
  Idiopathic thrombocytopenic purpura
  Leukemia
  Hemophilia
  Vitamin K deficiency
  Disseminated intravascular coagulopathy
**Cultural practices**
  Cao gio (coining)
  Quat sha (spoon rubbing)
**Infection**
  Sepsis
  Purpura fulminans (meningococcemia)
**Genetic diseases**
  Ehlers-Danlos syndrome
  Familial dysautonomia (with congenital indifference to pain)
  Vasculitis
  Henoch-Schönlein purpura

### BURNS

**Accidental burns** (common)
**Infection**
  Staphylococcal scalded skin syndrome
  Impetigo
**Dermatologic**
  Phytophotodermatitis
  Stevens-Johnson syndrome
  Fixed drug eruption
  Epidermolysis bullosa
  Severe diaper dermatitis, including Ex-Lax ingestion
**Cultural practices**
  Cupping
  Moxibustion

### FRACTURES

**Accidental injury**
**Birth trauma**
**Metabolic bone disease**
  Osteogenesis imperfecta
  Copper deficiency
**Rickets**
**Infection**
  Congenital syphilis
  Osteomyelitis

### HEAD TRAUMA

**Accidental head injury**
**Hematologic disorders**
  Vitamin K deficiency (hemorrhagic disease of the newborn)
  Hemophilia
**Intracranial vascular abnormalities**
**Infection**
**Metabolic diseases**
  Glutaric aciduria type I

*The differential diagnosis of physical abuse varies by the type of injury and organ system involved.
Data from Christian CW: Child abuse physical. In Schwartz MW, editor: The 5-minute pediatric consult, 3rd ed. Philadelphia, 2003, *Lippincott Williams & Wilkins.*

**TABLE 22-3 Proper Testing Methods for Sexually Transmitted Infections in Children and Adolescents**

| Organism | Infants and Prepubertal Children | Adolescents |
|---|---|---|
| *Neisseria gonorrhoeae* | Culture* | Culture, NAAT[†] |
| *Chlamydia trachomatis* | Culture[‡] | Culture, NAAT[†] |
| *Trichomonas vaginalis* | Vaginal wet mount and culture | Vaginal wet mount and culture |
| Syphilis, HIV, hepatitis B and C | Serum tests | Serum tests |
| Herpes simplex virus | Culture | Culture |

*Culture from pharynx, anus, vagina, or urethra (boys) is positive for gram-negative, oxidase-positive diplococcus, with two of three confirmatory tests positive (e.g., carbohydrate utilization, direct fluorescent antibody testing, enzyme substrate testing).
[†]NAAT can be substituted, with positive test confirmed by second NAAT test. Non-NAAT, direct fluorescent antibody, and enzyme immunoassay are *not* recommended. NAAT, nucleic acid amplification test.
[‡]Data are insufficient to adequately assess the utility of nucleic acid amplification tests, but these tests might be an alternative if confirmation is available and culture systems for *C. trachomatis* are unavailable. Confirmation tests should consist of a second FDA-cleared nucleic acid amplification test that targets a different sequence from the initial test.
FDA, U.S. Food and Drug Administration; HIV, human immunodeficiency virus; NAAT, nucleic acid amplification test.

**TABLE 22-4 Implications of Commonly Encountered or Sexually Associated Infections for Diagnosis and Reporting of Sexual Abuse among Infants and Prepubertal Children**

| Sexually Transmitted or Sexually Associated Infections Confirmed | Evidence of Sexual Abuse | Suggested Action |
|---|---|---|
| Gonorrhea | Diagnostic | Report |
| Syphilis | Diagnostic | Report |
| Human immunodeficiency virus | Diagnostic | Report |
| *Chlamydia trachomatis* | Diagnostic | Report |
| *Trichomonas vaginalis* | Highly suspicious | Report |
| Condylomata acuminata (anogenital warts) | Suspicious | Report |
| Genital herpes | Suspicious | Report |
| Bacterial vaginosis | Inconclusive | Medical follow-up |

Adapted from the American Academy of Pediatrics Committee on Child Abuse and Neglect. Guidelines for the evaluation of sexual abuse of children. *Pediatrics* 103:186–191, 1999. [Published correction *Pediatrics* 103:149, 1999.] www.cdc.gov/std/treatment/8-2002TG.htm.

testing in young children (Table 22-3). The diagnosis of most sexually transmitted infections in young children requires an investigation for sexual abuse (Table 22-4) (see Chapter 116).

## MANAGEMENT

The management of child abuse includes medical treatment for injuries and infections, careful medical documentation of verbal statements and findings, and ongoing advocacy for the safety and health of the child (Fig. 22-5). Parents always should be informed of the suspicion of abuse and the need to report to CPS, focusing on the need to ensure the safety and well-being of the child. Crimes that are committed against children also are investigated by law enforcement, so the police become involved in some, but not all, cases of suspected abuse. Physicians occasionally are called to testify in court hearings regarding civil issues, such as dependency and custody, or criminal issues. Careful review of the medical records and preparation for court are needed to provide an educated, unbiased account of the child's medical condition and diagnoses.

The need to prevent child abuse is obvious, yet it is premature to consider the primary prevention of maltreatment an attainable goal. Much of what we consider prevention is in reality reactive: High-risk families are identified and monitored, counseling and therapy are provided when available, and the criminal justice system assists in protecting children and attempting to modify behavior. There are a few partially successful primary prevention programs. Visiting home nursing programs that begin during pregnancy and continue through early childhood may reduce the risk of abuse and neglect. A number of states have mandated educational programs in newborn nurseries for reducing abusive head trauma, and evaluation of the effectiveness of these programs is under way. Physicians always need to remain cognizant of the diagnosis, aware of their professional mandates, and willing to advocate on behalf of these vulnerable patients.

**FIGURE 22-5**

A, Approach to initiating the civil and criminal investigation of suspected abuse. B, Reporting to Child Protective Services (CPS) or law enforcement or both in child abuse cases. CPS reports are required when a child is injured by a parent, by an adult acting as a parent, or by a caregiver of the child. The police investigate crimes against children committed by any person, including parents or other caregivers. (From Christian CW: Child abuse. In Schwartz MW, editor: Clinical handbook of pediatrics, ed 3. Baltimore, 2003, *Lippincott Williams & Wilkins,* pp 192-193.)

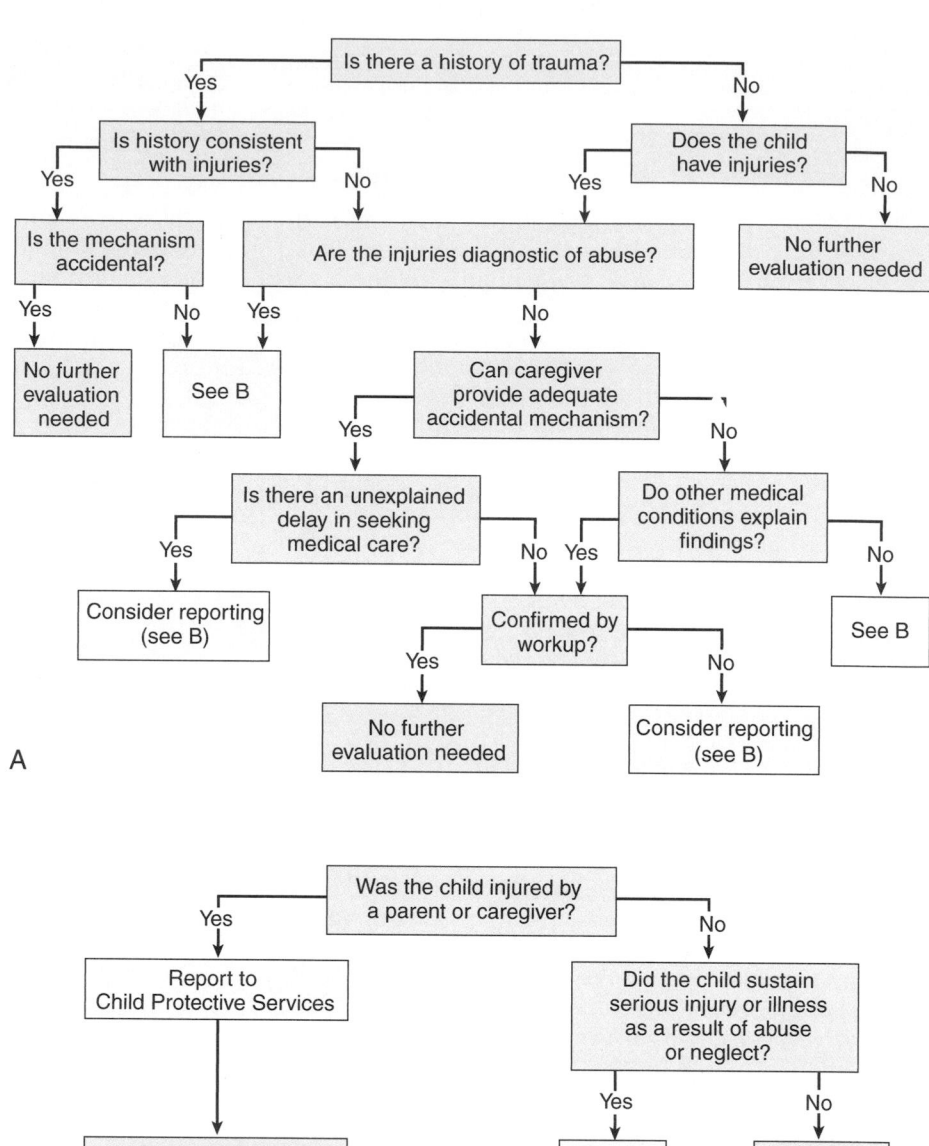

A

B

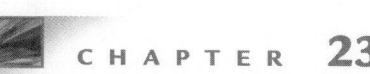

CHAPTER **23**

# Homosexuality and Gender Identity

The development of sexuality occurs throughout a child's life. Sexuality includes gender roles, gender identity, sexual orientation, and sexual behaviors. It is influenced by biologic and social factors and individual experience. Pediatricians are likely to be consulted if parents have a concern about their child's sexual development. A pediatrician who provides an open and nonjudgmental environment may be a valuable resource for an adolescent with questions about heterosexual behaviors, homosexuality, or gender identity (Table 23-1).

## DEVELOPMENT OF SEXUAL IDENTITY

Sexual behaviors occur throughout childhood. In the first few days of life male infants can have erections and female infants are capable of vaginal lubrication. During the preschool period, masturbation occurs in both sexes but is more common in boys. Between 2 and 3 years of age,

---

**TABLE 23-1 Terminology**

**Gender identity**
Perception of oneself as male or female

**Gender Role**
Behaviors and appearance that signal to others being male or female

**Heterosexual**
Sexual attraction to members of the opposite sex with weak attraction to members of the same sex

**Homosexual**
Sexual attraction to members of the same sex with weak attraction to members of the opposite sex

---

children identify themselves as a boy or a girl, but the understanding that one is always a male or always a female may not develop until 4 to 5 years of age. Stating that one wants to be a member of the opposite sex and pretending to be a member of the opposite sex are not unusual behaviors in this age group. Preschool children need to begin to learn that genitals and sexual behaviors are private; it is common for preschool children to touch their genitals in public, show their genitals to others, or undress in public. It would be highly unusual for a preschool child to imitate intercourse or other adult sexual behaviors. If this behavior is occurring, the child should be evaluated for exposure to inappropriate sexual material and possible sexual abuse (see Chapter 22).

Most elementary school–age children show a strong and consistent **gender identity**, and their behaviors (**gender roles**) reflect this. If a child this age is engaging in gender role behaviors typical of the opposite sex, parents may be concerned about teasing and the possibility of their child having a homosexual sexual orientation. This concern is particularly true if a boy is engaged in effeminate behaviors that are generally viewed as less socially acceptable than a girl acting as a *tomboy*. By this age, dressing as a member of the opposite sex and, particularly, stating a desire to be the opposite sex are uncommon, but playing with toys *designed* for the opposite sex remains common. In assessing parental concerns about atypical gender role behaviors, the type of behavior exhibited and the consistency of these behaviors should be considered. Reassurance that the behavior is consistent with typical child development is appropriate when these behaviors are part of a flexible repertoire of male and female gender role behaviors. Reassurance is appropriate if the behaviors occur in response to a stress, such as the birth of an infant of the opposite sex from the child or divorce of the parents. In contrast, if these behaviors occur as a consistent and persistent pattern of nearly exclusive interest in behaviors typical of the gender role opposite that of the child's anatomic sex, referral for evaluation for **gender identity disorder** (GID) would be appropriate.

The biologic, social, and cognitive changes during adolescence place a focus on sexuality. Becoming comfortable with one's sexuality is one of the principal developmental tasks of this period and is likely to include questioning and experimentation. Almost half of high school students report that they have had sexual intercourse. Ten to 25% have at least one homosexual experience, with this behavior being reported more commonly by boys than girls. Although many adolescents have sexual experiences with a same-sex partner, only a few have a homosexual sexual orientation by late adolescence. When adolescents develop a consistent sexual orientation is probably affected by many different factors (societal, family, individual). Some adolescents report that they are certain of their sexual orientation in the early teenage years, whereas for others this does not develop until later. By 18 years of age, only a small proportion of individuals report being uncertain of their sexual orientation.

## GENDER IDENTITY DISORDER

GID is characterized by intense and persistent cross-gender identification and discomfort with one's own sex. In children, these feelings may be manifested by behaviors such as cross-dressing, stating that one wants to be or is the opposite sex, and a strong and almost exclusive preference for cross-sex roles, games, and playmates. The onset of these behaviors often can be traced back to the preschool period. However, referral for evaluation often occurs at school age, when it becomes clear that the behaviors do not represent a transient phase, and the behaviors may begin to interfere with social relationships.

In adults, GID may be characterized by a belief that one was born the wrong sex and by a persistent desire to live and be treated as the opposite sex. Adults may request hormones or surgical procedures to alter sexual characteristics to simulate the other sex. Long-term follow-up studies of children with GID suggest that only 2% to 20% have GID as adults, but persistence is more likely in adolescents with GID. Forty to 80% of children with GID have a bisexual or homosexual sexual orientation as adults. Although one must acknowledge that these children are significantly more likely to have a homosexual orientation than the general population, there is no reliable way to predict the sexual orientation of any one particular child. There is no evidence that parental behavior would alter the developmental pathway toward homosexual or heterosexual behavior (see Chapter 24).

## HOMOSEXUALITY

Identical twins (even twins raised in separate families) show a higher concordance rate for sexual orientation than would be expected by chance alone, but nowhere near 100%, as would be expected if genetics alone determined sexual orientation. Some studies have found differences in the size of certain brain regions in homosexual individuals, but the findings are inconsistent. The levels of androgens and estrogens have not been found to differ in homosexual and heterosexual adults. Although it is well documented that parents tend to treat boys and girls differently, if, or how, these interactions affect sexual orientation is unknown.

It is currently estimated that about 1% to 4% of adults identify themselves as homosexual. Given the prevalent negative societal attitudes toward homosexuality, these children are at high risk for having a negative self-esteem, being isolated, being verbally harassed, and often being physically assaulted. Although sexual behaviors, not sexual orientation, determine risk of sexually transmitted infections, homosexual male adolescents engage in high-risk behaviors despite the threat of infection from human immunodeficiency virus (HIV). For medical and psychosocial reasons, health care providers need to provide an environment in which adolescents feel comfortable discussing their sexual orientation (Table 23-2).

Acknowledging that one is homosexual and disclosing it to one's parents is often extremely stressful. Although many parents come to accept their child's homosexuality, some parents, particularly those who view this behavior as immoral, may reject their child. Homosexual youth are at a high risk for homelessness. Adolescents need to be made aware that even parents who eventually come to accept their child's homosexuality initially may be shocked, fearful about their child's well-being, or upset about the loss of the adulthood they had expected for their child. Parents may need to be reassured that they did not cause their child to have a homosexual orientation. Likewise, they may need to be informed that therapies designed to change sexual orientation not only are unsuccessful, but often lead to the child having more feelings of guilt and a lower self-esteem. The health care provider should have knowledge of support groups and counselors who can discuss these issues with the adolescent or his or her parents when the information the health care provider offers is not sufficient.

The homosexual youth is affected by how homosexuality is addressed in schools, by peers, and by other community groups. Unbiased information about homosexuality is often not available in these settings, and homophobic jokes, teasing, and violence are common. It is not surprising that homosexual youth and adults have higher rates of anxiety and mood disorders than are found in the general population. Increased rates of substance abuse and suicide are reported. Health care providers have an important role in detecting these problems.

Although education about safe sexual practices should be part of all adolescent well-child visits, health care providers should be aware that certain sexual behaviors of homosexual males increase the risk of certain types of sexually transmitted infections. Anal intercourse is an efficient route for infection by hepatitis B virus, cytomegalovirus, and HIV. Proctitis caused by gonorrhea, chlamydia, herpes simplex virus, syphilis, or human papillomavirus may occur (see Chapter 116).

---

**TABLE 23-2 Providing Supportive Health Care Environments for Homosexual Youth**

Ensure confidentiality
Implement policies against homophobic jokes and remarks
Ensure information-gathering forms use gender-neutral
  language (e.g., *partner* as opposed to *husband/wife*)
Ensure that one uses gender-neutral questions when asking
  about dating or sexual behaviors
Display posters, brochures, and information that show concern
  for issues important to homosexual youth and their families
Provide information about support groups and other
  resources for homosexual youth and their families

Adapted from Perrin EC: Sexual orientation in child and adolescent health care. New York, 2002, *Kluwer Academic/Plenum Publishers*.

---

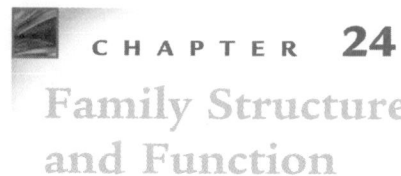

CHAPTER **24**

# Family Structure and Function

A family is a dynamic system of interactions among biologically, socially, or legally related individuals; families have a unique power to promote or interfere with health and development. When a family functions well, interactions support the physical and emotional needs of all family members, and the family serves as a resource for an individual member who is having difficulty. Alternatively, the problems of an individual member or the interactions among members may prevent the family from meeting the physical or emotional needs of one or more family members or, in the worst-case scenario, may cause physical or emotional harm to a member of the family. These situations are often referred to as **family dysfunction**.

## FAMILY FUNCTIONS

The functions that families carry out in support of their children can be categorized broadly as providing for physical needs, emotional support, education, and socialization (Table 24-1). Within these categories, all families have strengths and weaknesses. The amount of support that an individual child needs in these categories varies with the child's development, personality, temperament, health status, experiences, and stressors. Too much and too little support can interfere with optimal child health and development. Most cases of child abuse involve the failure of the family to provide a safe environment for the child and, in cases of neglect, inappropriate support for the child's physical, emotional, or social development. At the other extreme, overprotective parents may limit

---

**TABLE 24-1 Important Roles Families Play in Supporting Children**

**PHYSICAL NEEDS**

Safety
Food
Shelter
Health and health care

**EMOTIONAL SUPPORT**

Affection
Stimulation
Communication
Guidance/discipline

**EDUCATION AND SOCIALIZATION**

Values
Relationships
Community
Formal schooling

friendships and other growth-promoting experiences or seek excessive health care, as may occur in the vulnerable child syndrome. Parental perfectionism may create intense pressure on children related to achievement that may contribute to problems such as anxiety disorders.

## FAMILY STRUCTURE

The traditional family consists of a married mother and father and their biologic children. The diversity in the structure of the family in the United States has increased dramatically; less than half of children now live in the traditional nuclear family. Today, children may live with unmarried parents, single parents of either gender, a parent and a stepparent, grandparents, parents living as a same-sex couple, or foster care families. There is little evidence that family structure alone is a significant predictor of child health or development. Regardless of family structure, the presence of a loving adult or adults serving as a parent or parents committed to the fulfilling of a child's physical, emotional, and socialization needs is the best predictor of a child's optimal health and development. Different family structures create different types of family stresses.

### Single-Parent Families

Some children live in single-parent families because of divorce or the death of a parent (see Chapter 26). More than 20% of children are born to unmarried mothers. Many of these children live in single-parent families for some, if not all, of their childhood. Although some women elect to have children without getting married, in many situations the single parent is a young mother who had an unplanned pregnancy.

Single parents often have fewer financial resources and social supports. The mean income of households headed by single mothers is only 40% of that of two-parent families. More than half of these households live in poverty. Single parents also must rely to a greater extent on other adults for child care. Although these adults may be sources of support for the single parent, they also may criticize the parent, decreasing confidence in parenting skills. This decreased confidence, in combination with the fatigue associated with working and raising a child, makes consistent discipline more difficult to maintain, which may exacerbate behavioral problems. These parents are likely to have less time for a social life or other activities, which may increase their isolation. When the increased burdens of being a single parent are associated with exhaustion, isolation, and depression, optimal child development is less likely.

When the parent is a teenage mother, problems of parenting may be exacerbated further (see Section 12). Being a teenage parent is associated with lower educational attainment, lower paying jobs without much opportunity for autonomy or advancement, and lower self-esteem. They are even less likely than other single mothers to have any support from the child's father. Children of adolescent mothers are at high risk for cognitive delays, behavioral problems, and difficulties in school. Referral to

early intervention services or Head Start programs is important in these situations.

When a single parent has good social supports, is able to collaborate well with other care providers, and has sufficient financial resources, he or she is likely to be successful in raising a child. Pediatricians can improve parental confidence through education about child development and behavior and validation of parenting behaviors. Empathetic understanding of the difficulties of being a single parent can have a healing effect or help a parent to discuss difficulties that may suggest the need for a referral to other professionals.

### Children Living with Homosexual Parents

Many children with a gay or lesbian parent were conceived in the context of a heterosexual relationship. Some parents were unaware of their homosexuality at the time that they married, whereas others may view themselves as bisexual or marry despite the recognition that they are homosexual. Gay men and lesbian women also become parents on their own or in the context of an already established relationship with a same-sex partner through adoption, insemination, or surrogacy. Children living with homosexual parents may encompass many possible family structures.

Parents in these families are likely to have concerns about how disclosure of the homosexuality and the associated social stigma will affect the child. In general, earlier disclosure of a parent's homosexuality to children, especially before adolescence, is associated with better acceptance. Most children of homosexual parents experience some social stigma associated with having a gay or lesbian parent; this may occur in the form of teasing by peers, disapproval from adults, and stress or isolation related to keeping the parent's homosexuality a secret.

Evidence suggests that having a homosexual parent does not cause increased problems in the parent-child relationship or the child's social-emotional development. Gender and gender role behaviors are typical for the child's age. Nonetheless, distress related to teasing or maintaining the parent's secret may be great for some children, especially in early adolescence when issues of peer acceptance, sexual identity, and separation from one's parents are especially strong.

### Adoption

Adoption is a legal and social process that provides full family membership to a child not born to the adoptive parents. Approximately 2% of children in the United States are adopted. A significant proportion of legal and informal adoptions are by stepparents or relatives of the child. Most adoptions in the United States involve U.S. parents adopting U.S. children, but shifting cultural trends and a shortage of healthy U.S. children available for adoption have increased the diversity in the ways in which adoptions occur (e.g., international adoptions, privately arranged adoptions, and the use of a surrogate parent). These types of adoption each raise unique issues for families and health care providers. *Open adoptions* in which the biologic parents and birth parents agree to interact are occurring with increased frequency and create new issues for the adoption triad (biologic parent, adoptive parent, and child). Adoptions by single parents create another set of issues.

Pediatricians are in an ideal position to help adoptive parents. Pediatricians can help parents obtain and evaluate medical information, consider the unique medical needs of the adopted child, and provide a source of advice and counseling from the preadoption period through the issues that may arise when the child is an adolescent. A *preadoption visit* may allow parents to address the medical information they have received about the child and identify important pieces of the medical history that may be missing, such as the medical history of the biologic family and the educational and social history of the biologic parents. The preadoption period is the time that families are most likely to be able to obtain this information. When children are adopted from another country, there may be risks of infections, in utero substance exposure, poor nutrition, or inadequate infant care that are specific to individual countries and should be discussed with adoptive parents.

When the adopted child is first seen, screening for medical disorders beyond the typical age-appropriate screening tests should be considered. If the child has not had the standard newborn screening tests, the pediatrician may need to obtain these tests. Documented immunizations should be reviewed, and, if needed, a plan developed to complete the needed immunizations (see Chapter 94). Children may be at high risk for infection based on the biologic mother's social history or the country from which the child was adopted including infection with human immunodeficiency virus, hepatitis B, cytomegalovirus, tuberculosis, syphilis, and parasites. A complete blood count may be needed to screen for iron deficiency.

A knowledgeable pediatrician also can be a valuable source of support and advice about psychosocial issues. The pediatrician should help the adoptive parents think about how they will raise the child while helping the child to understand the fact that he or she is adopted. Neither denial of nor intense focus on the adoption is healthy. Parents should use the term *adoption* around their children during the toddler years and explain the simplest facts first. Children's questions should be answered honestly. Parents should expect the same or similar questions repeatedly, and that during the preschool period the child's cognitive limitations make it likely the child will not fully understand the meaning of adoption. As children get older, they may have fantasies of being reunited with their biologic parents, and there may be new challenges as the child begins to interact more with individuals outside the family. Families may want advice about difficulties created by school assignments such as creating a genealogic chart or teasing by peers. During the teenage years, the child may have questions about his or her identity and a desire to find his or her biologic parents. Adoptive parents may need reassurance that these desires do not represent rejection of the adoptive family, but the child's desire to understand more about his or her life. In general, adopted adolescents should be supported in efforts to learn about their past, but most experts recommend encouraging children to wait until late adolescence before deciding to search actively for the biologic parents.

Although adopted children have a higher rate of school, learning, and behavioral problems, much of this increase is likely to be related to biologic and social influences before the adoption. The pediatrician can play an important role in helping families distinguish developmental and behavioral variations from problems that may require recommendations for early intervention, counseling, or other services.

## Foster Care

Foster care is a means of providing protection for children who require out-of-home placement, most commonly because of homelessness, parental inability to care for the child, parental substance abuse, or child neglect or abuse. The number of children in foster care doubled between 1987 and 2001, and currently more than 0.5 million children live in foster care. For these children, reunification with the biologic family is the goal for approximately 40%, and adoption or placement with relatives is the goal for 25% to 35%. Ten percent of children are in long-term foster care. For the remaining 20%, no long-term goal has been established.

Children in foster care are at extremely high risk for medical, nutritional, developmental, behavioral, and mental health problems. At the time of placement in foster care, most of these children have received incomplete medical care and have had multiple detrimental life experiences. Comprehensive assessments at the time of placement reveal many untreated acute medical problems; 40% to 70% of foster children have chronic illnesses. More than half have significant developmental delays, and behavioral disorders are common. Ideally, foster care provides a healing service for these children and families, leading to reunification or adoption. Too often, inadequate programs contribute to the ongoing difficulties of the children.

Consistent, multidisciplinary, and coordinated care is needed to address the complex needs of children entering foster care. For children in foster care for more than 1 year, more than 40% experience three or more home placements, and for children in foster care for more than 4 years, this figure is approximately 60%. Poor case coordination in conjunction with these multiple placements leads to frequent changes in schools and medical providers, further fragmenting the health care and education these children receive. In some locations, one third of children received no immunizations while in foster care. Frequent changes in placement exacerbate the problems foster children often have in forming a secure relationship with adult caregivers. Children may manifest this difficulty by resisting foster parents' attempts to develop a close relationship. This detachment from the foster parent may be difficult for the foster parent to endure, which may perpetuate a cycle of placement failures. Although the *protections* of the foster care system end at 18 years of age, these adolescents rarely have the skills and maturity that allow them to live independently. In the first 2 years following discharge from the foster care system when they become 18, approximately 25% of males and 10% of females are incarcerated at least once.

When health care providers see a child in foster care, it is crucial that they perform a comprehensive health assessment for acute and chronic medical problems and developmental and behavioral disorders. When children are placed with competent and nurturing foster parents and provided coordinated care from skilled professionals, significant improvements in a child's health status, development, and academic achievement usually occur.

## FAMILY DYSFUNCTION

### Physical Needs

Failure to meet a child's physical needs for protection or nutrition results in some of the most severe forms of family dysfunction (see Chapters 21 and 22). There are many other ways in which parental behaviors can interfere with a child having a healthy and safe environment, such as prenatal and postnatal substance abuse. Prenatal use of alcohol exposes children to potentially devastating consequences of this teratogen. Children with **fetal alcohol syndrome** have in utero and postnatal growth retardation, microcephaly, mental retardation, and a characteristic dysmorphic facial appearance. Even in the absence of growth retardation and a dysmorphic appearance, some children exposed to alcohol in utero develop problems with coordination, attention, hyperactivity, impulsivity, and other learning or behavioral problems related to the alcohol exposure. In the past, these children have been described as having fetal alcohol effects, but the currently recommended terminology is *alcohol-related neurodevelopmental disorder*.

Other substances also may affect the fetus, but investigation of these effects is complicated by the fact that often more than one substance is used, and nutrition and prenatal care are not optimal. Cigarette smoking during pregnancy is associated with lower birth weight and increased child behavioral problems. Use of cocaine in the perinatal period has been associated with intracranial hemorrhages and abruptio placentae. Similarly, although exposure to opiates in utero can result in a neonatal withdrawal syndrome, significant cognitive deficits do not seem to be associated with the use of opiates alone. Cocaine- and opiate-exposed infants often have coexisting high risk factors for cognitive deficits, such as low birth weight.

Parental substance abuse after the child's birth is associated with increased family conflict, decreased organization, increased isolation, and increased family stress related to marital and work problems. Family violence may be more frequent. Despite the fact that these parents often have difficulty providing discipline and structure, they may expect their children to be competent at a variety of tasks at a younger age than non–substance-abusing parents. This sets the children up for failure and contributes to increased rates of depression, anxiety, and low self-esteem. The parents' more accepting attitude toward alcohol and drugs seems to increase the chance that their children will use substances during adolescence.

Parents also may expose children directly to the harmful effects of other substances, such as exposure to *secondhand cigarette smoke*, which is consistently associated with increased rates of childhood respiratory illnesses, otitis media, and sudden infant death syndrome. Despite these effects, only a few parents restrict smoking in their homes. There are many other ways in which parents may not physically protect their children. Failing to immunize children, to childproof the home adequately, and to provide adequate supervision are other examples.

Parents' attempts to provide too much protection for their child also can cause problems. One example of this is the **vulnerable child syndrome**. A child who is ill early in life continues to be viewed as vulnerable by the parents despite the fact that the child has fully recovered. Behavioral difficulties may result if parents are overindulgent and fail to set limits. Parental reluctance to leave the child may contribute to the child having separation anxiety. Parents may be particularly attentive to minor variations in bodily functions, leading them to seek excess medical care. If the physician does not recognize this situation, the child may be exposed to unnecessary medical procedures.

### Emotional Support, Education, and Socialization

Failure to meet a child's emotional or educational needs can have a severe and enduring negative impact on child development and behavior. Infants need a consistent adult who learns to understand their signals and meets the infant's needs for attention as well as food. As the adult caregiver learns these signals, he or she responds more rapidly and appropriately to the infant's attempts at communication. Through this process, often referred to as **attachment**, the special relationship between parent and child develops. When affectionate and responsive adults are not consistently available, infants often are less willing to explore the environment and may become unusually clingy, angry, or difficult to comfort.

Appropriate stimulation also is vital for a child's cognitive development. Children whose parents do not read to them and do not play developmentally appropriate games with them have lower scores on intelligence tests and more school problems. In these situations, early intervention has been shown to be particularly effective in improving skill development and subsequent school performance. At the other extreme, there are increasing concerns that some parents may provide too much stimulation and scheduling of the child's day. There may be such emphasis on achievement that children come to feel that parental love is contingent on achievement. There are concerns that this narrow definition of success may contribute to problems with anxiety and self-esteem for some children.

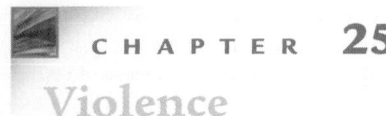

CHAPTER **25**

Violence

## DOMESTIC VIOLENCE AND CHILDREN

Intimate partner violence between adults affects the lives of millions of children each year. Children experience domestic violence by seeing or hearing the violence or seeing its aftermath. Children who live in households with domestic violence often develop psychological and behavioral problems that interfere with their ability to function normally in school, at home, and with peers. They may be injured during violent outbursts, sometimes while attempting to intervene on behalf of a parent. Many children are victims of abuse themselves. It is estimated that there is at least a 50% concurrence rate between domestic violence and child abuse. Children who grow up in violent households learn that violence is appropriate in intimate relationships. A history of having witnessed domestic violence as a child is a strong predictor for becoming a batterer in adulthood. Children who live with domestic violence have experienced more than sporadic outbursts of violence. They live in households in which one partner, usually the mother, is isolated, belittled, made to feel worthless, and the victim of physical violence. This type of environment is filled with disruptive events that can overtly or subtly affect the child's normal development. Most domestic violence is perpetrated by men against women. Levels of physical violence against women are high during pregnancy and in the postpartum period.

There is no particular behavioral consequence or disturbance that is specific to children who witness domestic violence. Some children are traumatized by fear for their mother's safety and feel helpless to protect her. Others may blame themselves for the violence. Children may have symptoms of **post-traumatic stress disorder**, depression, anxiety, aggression, or hypervigilance. Older children may have conduct disorders, poor school performance, low self-esteem, or other nonspecific behaviors. Infants and young toddlers are at risk for disrupted attachment and routines around eating and sleeping. Preschoolers may show signs of regression, irritable behavior, or temper tantrums. During school-age years, gender differences begin to emerge, although any given child may not follow these patterns. Boys who have witnessed violence tend to be more aggressive or disruptive, whereas girls become more withdrawn and passive. Boys and girls may have loss of confidence or academic problems. Because of family isolation, some children have no opportunity to participate in extracurricular activities at school and do not form friendships outside of the family. Adolescent girls who have lived with domestic violence are at risk for becoming victims of physical violence by their boyfriends; adolescent boys may become victimizers. Although some adolescents learn to assume the parent role, others turn on the victimized parent and identify themselves with the abusive parent.

Because of the high concurrence of domestic violence and child abuse, asking about domestic violence is part of the screening for violence against children. Many women's advocates suggest that intervening on behalf of battered women is an active form of child abuse prevention. Recognizing the importance of domestic violence screening in pediatric practice, the American Academy of Pediatrics has endorsed universal domestic violence screening in this setting. Without standardized screening, pediatricians may underestimate the prevalence of domestic violence in their practices. Screening is recommended for all families intermittently, especially in the first few years of the child's life. Parents should not be screened together. Questions about family violence should be direct, nonjudgmental, and done in the context of child safety and anticipatory guidance (Table 25-1).

Intervention is needed for women who disclose domestic violence. It is appropriate to show concern and to inform the woman of available community resources. It is important to assess her safety and inquire about whether the children are in physical danger. In some states, physicians are mandated to report domestic violence. Information for women that provides details about community resources and state laws is helpful.

### TABLE 25-1  Questions for Adults and Children Related to Family Violence

#### FOR THE CHILD

How are things at home, at school?
Who lives with you?
How do you get along with your family members?
What do you like to do with them?
What do you do if something is bothering you?
Do you feel safe at home?
Do people fight at home? What do they fight about? How do they fight?

#### ADDITIONAL QUESTIONS FOR THE ADOLESCENT

Do your friends get into fights often? How about you?
When was your last physical fight?
Have you ever been injured during a fight?
Has anyone you know been injured or killed?
Have you ever been forced to have sex against your will?
Have you ever been threatened with a gun? A knife?
How do you avoid getting in fights?
Do you carry a weapon for self-defense?

#### FOR THE PARENT

Do you have any concerns about your child?
Who helps with your children?
How do you feel about your neighborhood?
Do you feel safe at home?
Is there any fighting or violence at home?
Does anyone at home use drugs?
Have you been frightened by your partner?
Does your partner ever threaten you? Hurt you?

## YOUTH VIOLENCE

Youth violence is a leading cause of pediatric mortality in the United States. Each year, more than 2500 children, primarily adolescents, are victims of homicide, and almost 2000 more commit suicide. Youth violence is a problem in urban, suburban, and rural communities and affects children of all races and both genders. Surveys of adolescents show that 30% to 40% of boys and 15% to 30% of girls report having committed a serious violent offense during childhood, including robbery, rape, aggravated assault, or homicide. Most of these crimes are not reported to the police, and the perpetrator is arrested in only a few cases. Although boys commit more crimes than girls, this gap has narrowed. Boys are much more likely to be arrested for their crimes. Self-reported violent events do not differ much between white and minority adolescents; the latter are more likely to be arrested for their crimes.

Most violent youth begin to exhibit their violent behaviors during early adolescence. More mild forms of aggression, such as **bullying**, which can involve verbal and physical aggression, peak during middle school years. Children who bully others are more likely to be involved with other problem behaviors, such as smoking and alcohol use. Although most bullies do not progress into serious violent offenders, violent behavior that continues into high school years indicates the potential for severe violent behavior in adulthood. Another subset of violent youth begins at a very young age. These children tend to be more serious offenders, perpetrate more crimes, and more often continue their violence into adulthood. The peak age of onset for serious violence is 15 to 16 years for boys and a few years earlier for girls. Most adolescent violence ends by young adulthood. Most violent youth are only intermittently violent. Frequent acts of violence are committed more commonly by youth who start their violence before the onset of puberty. These violent youth need to be evaluated for cognitive impairments or mental illness.

Serious youth violence is not an isolated problem but usually coexists with other adolescent risk-taking behaviors, such as drug use, truancy and school dropout, early sexual activity, and gun ownership. Risk factors for youth violence are slightly different for children who begin their violence early in life compared with youth who begin during adolescence. Often, these risk factors exist in clusters, and they tend to be additive. Although understanding risk factors for violence is crucial for developing prevention strategies, the risk factors do not predict whether a particular individual will become violent. For children who begin their violence early in life, the strongest risk factors are early substance abuse (<12 years of age) and perpetration of nonviolent, serious crimes during childhood. Additional risk factors include poverty, male gender, and antisocial behavior. For children who begin their violence during adolescence, individual risk factors are less important, whereas factors related to peer groups are most important. Membership in a gang, associating with antisocial or delinquent friends, being unpopular in school, and having weak ties to conventional peer groups are important risk factors for adolescent-onset violence (Table 25-2). The strength of the listed risk factors is not uniform, and some factors show only a small effect. Table 25-2 also lists protective factors that seem to buffer the effects of risk factors. One important protective factor is the child's level of school connectedness, such as involvement in class and extracurricular activities, and how positively the child regards the school's personnel. Another protective factor is the support of nonviolent family members and close friends.

Violence prevention efforts that target risk and protective factors need to be developmentally appropriate. Education about the dangers of substance abuse should begin before the onset of puberty, whereas adolescent programs must consider the importance of peer group identification. Many violence prevention programs fail to show long-term effects. Effective violence prevention programs must address simultaneously individual, family, and environmental (school, peer group, social) risk factors; capitalize on the child's strengths; involve family and other supports; and be implemented over an extended period.

## DATING VIOLENCE AND DATE RAPE

Dating violence and date rape are relatively common problems. It is estimated that 15% to 40% of adolescents have experienced violence in a dating relationship. Adolescent and young adult women experience higher rates of sexual assault than any other age group. An acquaintance or partner of the victim perpetrates most adolescent sexual assaults; assaults by strangers are the exception. Risk factors for date rape include initiating dating at a young age, initiating early sexual activity, and having a history of past sexual abuse or victimization. A history of child abuse or sexual abuse by parents or siblings increases the risk of being a perpetrator or a victim of dating violence. Adolescent boys who hold opinions that are accepting of dating violence are at risk for becoming perpetrators. These opinions include believing that it is appropriate to strike a girl if she insulted or embarrassed him or intentionally tried to make him jealous. Date-specific factors put some teens at risk for date rape, including who initiated the date, the activities of the date, which person drove, and who paid for the date.

Alcohol use is extremely common in episodes of adolescent sexual assault, occurring in approximately 50% of cases. Drugs such as benzodiazepines, cocaine, and marijuana may also contribute. Flunitrazepam (Rohypnol) and gamma hydroxybutyrate are two commonly implicated drugs that cause sedation and amnesia, especially when used in conjunction with alcohol.

Relatively few victims of date rape report the assault to law enforcement. Reporting rates are even lower when the victim knows the perpetrator rather than when the perpetrator is a stranger. Women who report assaults to the police are more likely to receive timely medical care; it is likely that many sexually assaulted adolescents do not receive medical attention, putting them at risk for physical and mental health consequences. Routine adolescent health care should screen for adolescent dating violence and sexual assault, provide routine sexually transmitted infection evaluation, and be able to identify counseling resources for teens who are victims or perpetrators of dating violence (see Chapter 116).

**TABLE 25-2  Risk and Protective Factors for Serious Youth Violence by Age of Onset**

| Factors | Early Onset (<12 yr) | Later Onset (>12 yr) | Protective Factors |
|---|---|---|---|
| Individual | **Substance use*** | General offenses | Intolerance toward deviance |
| | **General offenses** | Aggression[†] | High IQ |
| | Being male | Being male | Being female |
| | Antisocial behavior | Physical violence | Positive social orientation |
| | Aggression[†] | Antisocial attitudes | Perceived sanctions for transgressions |
| | Hyperactivity | Crimes against persons | |
| | Exposure to TV violence | Low IQ | |
| | Low IQ | Substance abuse | |
| | Antisocial attitudes | Risk-taking behaviors | |
| | Dishonesty[†] | | |
| Family | Low SES/poverty | Poor parent-child relations | Supportive parents or other adults |
| | Antisocial parents | Low parent involvement | Parental monitoring |
| | Poor parent-child relations | Antisocial parents | Parents' positive evaluation of peers |
| | Broken home | Broken home | |
| | Abusive, neglectful parents | Low SES/poverty | |
| | | Abusive parents | |
| School | Poor attitude | Poor attitude | Commitment to school |
| | Poor performance | Poor performance | Recognition for involvement in school activities |
| | | Academic failure | |
| Peer | Weak social ties | **Weak social ties** | Friends who engage in conventional behavior |
| | Antisocial peers | **Antisocial delinquent peers** | |
| | | **Gang membership** | |
| Community | | Neighborhood crime | |
| | | Neighborhood drugs | |
| | | Neighborhood disorganization | |

*__Bold__ = factors with strongest effect.
[†]Males only.
SES, socioeconomic status.
From National Center for Injury Prevention and Control, Substance Abuse and Mental Health Services Administration: Youth violence: a report of the surgeon general. Rockville, Md, 2001, *U.S. Department of Health and Human Services.*

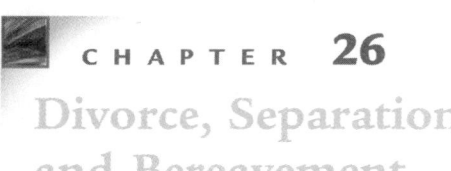

CHAPTER **26**

# Divorce, Separation, and Bereavement

The family is the child's principal resource for meeting his or her needs for protection, emotional support, education, and socialization. A variety of different events can result in disruptions that cause the child to be separated from his or her parents. At times, these separations may be relatively brief but unexpected (e.g., a parent's acute illness or injury). The separation may occur in the context of significant parental discord, as often occurs with a divorce. The death of a parent results in a permanent separation that may be anticipated or unanticipated. All of these disruptions cause significant stress for the child, with the potential for long-term adverse consequences. The child's adaptation to these stresses is affected by the reasons for the separation and the child's age, temperament, and available support systems.

## DIVORCE

Approximately 40% of first marriages end in divorce. About half of these divorces occur in the first 10 years of marriage, so there are often young children in the family when the parents divorce. At least 25% of children experience the divorce or separation of their parents. Few events in childhood are as dramatic and challenging for the child as divorce.

Divorce is likely to be accompanied by changes in behavioral and emotional adjustment. In the immediate postdivorce period, many children exhibit anger, noncompliance, anxiety, and depression. Children from divorced families require psychological help two to three times more frequently than children with married parents. Long-term studies suggest that in the absence of ongoing stressors, most children demonstrate good adjustment a few years after the divorce, but some have enduring difficulties. Overall, when groups of children from divorced families are compared with groups of children from married families on standardized measures of psychological adjustment, the children from divorced families have only a relatively small increase in problems.

Divorce is not a single event, but a process that occurs over time. In most cases, marital conflict begins long before the physical or legal separation, and the divorce brings about permanent changes in the family structure. Multiple potential stressors for the child are associated with divorce, including parental discord before and after the divorce, changes in living arrangements and sometimes location, and changes in the child's relationship with both parents.

The child's relationship with each parent is changed by the divorce. In the short-term, the parent is likely to experience new burdens and feelings of guilt, anger, or disappointment that may disrupt parenting skills and family routines. Contact with the noncustodial parent may decline greatly. Parents may be perceived by their children as being unaware of the child's distress around the time of the divorce. Pediatricians can help parents understand things they can do that will be reassuring to the child. Maintaining contact with both parents, seeing where the noncustodial parent is living, and in particular, maintaining familiar routines are comforting to the child in the midst of the turmoil of a separation and divorce. The child should attend school and continue to have opportunities to interact with friends. Given the parents' distress, assistance from the extended family can be helpful, but these family members may not offer to help for fear of "interfering." It may be helpful for pediatricians to encourage parents to ask for this assistance. Pediatricians should look for maladaptive coping responses. Some parents may respond to their increased burdens and distress by treating their children as friends with whom they share their distress. Alternatively, they may place excessive responsibilities on the child or leave the child unsupervised for longer periods of time. Responses such as these increase the burdens on the child and increase the chance that the child will develop behavioral or emotional problems.

## Reaction to Divorce at Different Ages

The child's reaction to the divorce is influenced by the child's age and developmental level. Infants do not react directly to the divorce, but if the divorce results in prolonged or more frequent separations from a primary caregiver, developing a secure relationship with this individual may be more difficult. Infants require special consideration in relation to custody and visitation. Separations from a primary caregiver should be brief. **Preschool children** are characterized by having magical beliefs about cause and effects and an egocentric view of the world. They may believe that something they did caused the divorce, leading them to be particularly upset. They may engage in unusual behaviors that they believe will bring the parents back together again. At this age, parents need to deliver a clear message that the divorce was related to disagreements between the parents, that nothing the child did caused the divorce, and that nothing the child could do would bring the parents back together again. Preschool children may reason that if the parents left each other they also might leave the child. To counteract this fear of abandonment, children may need to be reassured that although parents separated, they will not abandon the child and that the child's relationship with both parents will endure.

**School-age children** have a concrete understanding of cause and effect; if something bad happened, they understand that something caused it to happen. However, they are not likely to understand fully the subtleties of parental conflict or the idea that multiple factors contribute to a conflict. Children at this age may express more anger than younger children and often feel rejected. Many young school-age children worry about what will happen to one or both parents. School performance often deteriorates. Older elementary school–age children may believe that one parent was wronged by the other, further contributing to their anger. This belief, in conjunction with their concrete understanding of cause and effect, allows children to be easily co-opted by one parent to take sides against the other. Parents need to understand this vulnerability and resist the temptation to support their child in taking sides.

**Adolescents** may respond to the divorce by acting out, becoming depressed, or experiencing somatic symptoms. Adolescents are developing a sense of autonomy, a sense of morality, and the capacity for intimacy, and divorce may lead them to question previously held beliefs. They may be concerned about what the divorce means for their future and whether they, too, will experience marital failure. Questioning of previous beliefs in conjunction with decreased supervision may set the stage for risk-taking behaviors, such as truancy, sexual behaviors, and alcohol or drug use.

## Outcome of Divorce

One of the best predictors of children's adaptation to divorce is whether the physical separation is associated with a decrease in the child's exposure to parental discord. In most cases, divorced parents still must interact with each other around the child's schedule, child custody and support, and other parenting issues. These types of issues create the potential for the child to have ongoing exposure to significant discord between the parents. For example, if one parent tends to keep the child up much later than the bedtime at the other parent's house, sleep problems may develop. When children feel caught in the middle of ongoing conflicts between their divorced parents, behavior or emotional problems are much more likely. Regardless of how angry parents are with each other, the parents should be counseled that they must shield their child from this animosity. Clear rules about schedules, discipline, and other parenting roles often are helpful in minimizing conflicts. When parents have trouble resolving these issues, mediation may be helpful. Pediatricians need to be wary of parents' attempts to recruit them into custody battles to substantiate claims of poor parenting, unless the pediatrician has first-hand knowledge that the concerns are valid.

Although the primary physical residence for most children is still with the mother, the court's bias toward preferring mothers in custody decisions has decreased, and there is more emphasis on including both parents in the child's life. In the early 1980s, 50% of children had no contact with their fathers 2 or 3 years after a divorce, whereas today only 20% to 25% of children have no contact with their father. Most states now allow joint physical or legal custody. In joint physical custody, the child spends an approximately equal amount of time with both parents, and in joint legal custody, parents share authority in decision making. Although joint custody arrangements may promote the involvement of both parents in the child's life, they also can be a vehicle through which parents continue to express their anger at each other. When parents have severe difficulty working together, joint custody is an inappropriate arrangement and has been associated with deterioration in the child's psychological and social adjustment.

Divorce often creates financial difficulties for the mother and child. The mother's family income often declines by 30% or more in the first year after the divorce. Only about half of mothers who have child support awards receive the full amount, and one fourth receive no money at all. These financial changes may have multiple adverse affects on the child. The family may have to move to a new house and the child may have to attend a new school, disrupting peer and family relationships. The child may spend more time in child care if the mother has to return to work or increase her work hours.

## Role of the Pediatrician

Pediatricians may be confronted with issues related to marital discord before the divorce, may be consulted around the time of the divorce, or may be involved in helping the family to manage issues in the years after the divorce. The pediatrician can be an important voice in helping the parents understand and meet the child's needs (Table 26-1). Before the divorce, parents may wonder what they should tell their children. Children should

---

**TABLE 26-1 General Recommendations for Pediatricians to Help Children During Separation, Divorce, or Death of a Close Relative**

Acknowledge and provide support for grief the parent/ caregiver is experiencing

Help parent/caregiver to consider child's needs

Encourage parent/caregiver to maintain routines familiar to the child

Encourage continued contact between child and his or her friends

If primary residence changes, the child should take transitional objects, familiar toys, and other important objects to the new residence

Minimize frequent changes in caregivers, and for infants keep times away from primary caregiver brief

Have parent/caregiver reassure the child that he or she will continue to be cared for

Have parent/caregiver reassure the child that he or she did not cause the separation, divorce, or death (especially important in preschool children)

Encourage parent/caregiver to create times or rituals that allow the child to discuss questions and feelings if the child wishes

---

be told of the parents' decision before the physical separation. The separation should be presented as a rational step in managing marital conflict and should prepare the child for the changes that will occur. Parents should be prepared to answer children's questions, and they should expect that the questions will be repeated over the next months. Once parents have told children of the separation, it may be confusing to the child if the parents continue to appear to live together and may raise false hopes that the parents will not divorce.

Many parents report not feeling like their life had stabilized until 2 to 3 years or more after the divorce, and for some the divorce remains a painful issue 10 years later. Children's understanding of the divorce changes at different developmental stages, and their questions may change as they try to understand their family's history. Although most children ultimately show good adjustment to the divorce, some have significant acting-out behaviors or depression that requires referral to a mental health professional. Some parents need the assistance of a mediator or family therapist to help them stay focused on their child's needs. In the most contentious situations, a guardian ad litem may need to be appointed by the court. This individual is usually a lawyer or mental health professional with the power to investigate the child and family's background and relationships to make a recommendation to the court as to what would be in the best interests of the child.

## SEPARATIONS FROM PARENTS

Children experience separations from their primary caregiver for a variety of reasons. Brief separations, such as those to attend school, camp, or other activities, are nearly a universal experience. Many children experience longer separations for a variety of reasons, including parental business trips, military service, or hospitalization. Child adjustment to separation is affected by child factors, such as the age of the child and the child's temperament; factors related to the separation, such as the length of and reason for the separation, whether the separation was planned or unplanned, and factors related to the caregiving environment during the separation, such as how familiar the child is with the caregiver and whether the child has access to friends and familiar toys and routines.

Children between 6 months and 3 to 4 years of age often have the most difficulty adjusting to a separation from their primary caregiver. Older children have cognitive and emotional skills that help them adjust. They may be better able to understand the reason for the separation, communicate their feelings, and comprehend the passage of time, allowing them to anticipate the parent's return. For older children, the period immediately before a planned separation may be particularly difficult if the reason for the separation causes significant family tension, as it may in the case of hospitalization or military service.

If parents anticipate a separation, they should explain the reason for the separation and, to the extent possible, give concrete information about when they will be in contact with the child and when they will return home. If the child can remain at home with a familiar and responsive caregiver, this is likely to help adjustment. If children cannot remain at home, they should be encouraged to take with them transitional objects, such as a favorite pillow, blanket, or stuffed animal. Familiar toys and important objects such as a picture of the parent should be taken to the new environment. Maintenance of familiar family routines and relationships with friends should be encouraged.

## DEATH OF A PARENT OR FAMILY MEMBER AND BEREAVEMENT

Death of a close family member is a sad and difficult experience. When a child loses a parent, it is a devastating experience. This experience is not rare. By 15 years of age, 4% of children in the United States experience the death of a parent. This experience is likely to alter forever the child's view of the world as a secure and safe place. Similar to the other separations, a child's cognitive development and temperament along with the available support systems affect the child's adjustment after the death of a parent. Many of the recommendations in Table 26-1 are helpful. The death of a parent or close family member also brings up some unique issues.

### Explaining Death to a Child

Children's understanding of death changes with their cognitive development and experiences (see Chapter 4). Preschool children often do not view death as permanent and may have magical beliefs about what caused death. As children become older, they understand death as permanent and inevitable, but the concept that death represents the cessation of all bodily functions and has a biologic cause may not be fully appreciated until adolescence.

Death should not be hidden from the child. It should be explained in simple and honest terms that are consistent with the family's beliefs. The explanation should help the child to understand that the dead person's body stopped functioning and that the dead person will not return. Preschool children should be reassured that nothing they did caused the individual to die. One should be prepared to answer questions about where the body is and let the child's questions help determine what information the child is prepared to hear. False or misleading information should be avoided. Comparisons of death to sleep may contribute to sleep problems in the child.

There are many possible reactions of children to the death of a parent or close relative. Sadness and a yearning to be with the dead relative are common. Sometimes a child might express a wish to die so that he or she can visit the dead relative, but a plan or desire to commit suicide is uncommon and would need immediate evaluation. A decrease in academic functioning, lack of enjoyment with activities, and changes in appetite and sleep can occur. About half of children have their most severe symptoms about 1 month after the death, but for many the most severe symptoms in reaction to the death do not occur until 6 to 12 months after the death.

### Should the Child Attend the Funeral?

Children often find it helpful to attend the funeral. It may help the child to understand that the death occurred and provide an opportunity to say good-bye. Seeing others express their grief and sadness may help the child to express these feelings. Going to the funeral helps prevent the child from having fears or fantasies about what happened at the funeral. If the child is going to attend the funeral, he or she should be informed of what will happen. If a preschool-age child expresses a desire not to attend the funeral, he or she should not be encouraged to attend. For older children, it may be appropriate to encourage attendance, but a child who feels strongly about not wanting to go to the funeral should not be required to attend.

 **S U G G E S T E D    R E A D I N G**

American Academy of Pediatrics Committee on Early Childhood: Adoption, and Dependent Care: Health care of young children in foster care, *Pediatrics* 109:536–541, 2002.

Hetherington EM: Divorce and the adjustment of children, *Pediatr Rev* 26:163–169, 2005.

Jenista JA: The immigrant, refugee, or internationally adopted child, *Pediatr Rev* 22:419–429, 2001.

Keane V, Feigelman S: Failure to thrive and malnutrition. In Kliegman RM, Greenbaum PS, Lye PS, editors: Practical strategies in pediatric diagnosis and therapy, 2nd ed, Philadelphia, 2004, *WB Saunders*, pp 233–248.

Kellogg ND and the Committee on child abuse and neglect: The evaluation of sexual abuse in children, *Pediatrics* 116:506–512, 2005.

Kellogg ND and the Committee on child abuse and neglect: Evaluation of suspected child physical abuse, *Pediatrics* 119:1232–1241, 2007.

Kliegman RE, Behrman RE, Jenson HB, et al: Children with special needs. In Nelson textbook of pediatrics, 18th ed, Philadelphia, 2007, *WB Saunders*, pp 163–206.

Reece RM, Christian CW, editors: Child abuse: medical diagnosis and management, 3rd ed, Elk Grove Village, Ill, 2009, *American Academy of Pediatrics*.

Silovsky JF, Swisher LM, Zucker K, et al: Sexuality. In Wolraich ML, Drotar DD, Dworkin PH, et al, editors: Developmental-behavioral pediatrics: evidence and practice, Philadelphia, 2008, *Mosby*.

# PEDIATRIC NUTRITION AND NUTRITIONAL DISORDERS

**Nancy F. Krebs and Laura E. Primak**

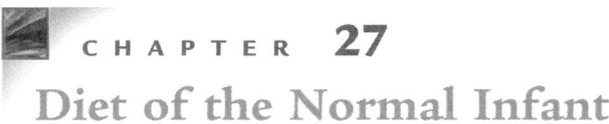

## CHAPTER 27

## Diet of the Normal Infant

Infancy, especially the first 6 months, is a period of exceptionally rapid growth and high nutrient requirements relative to body weight (see Chapter 5). If inadequate total intake or inappropriate choice of food occurs, there is risk of rapid deterioration in growth and nutritional status, with potential for adverse consequences on neurocognitive development.

## BREASTFEEDING

Human milk is the ideal and uniquely superior food for infants. The American Academy of Pediatrics recommends human milk as the sole source of nutrition for the first 6 months of life, with continued intake for the first year and as long as desired thereafter. Breastfeeding offers infants, mothers, and society compelling advantages. Human milk feeding decreases the incidence or severity of diarrhea, respiratory illnesses, otitis media, bacteremia, bacterial meningitis, and necrotizing enterocolitis. Mothers who breastfeed experience a decreased risk of postpartum hemorrhage, longer period of amenorrhea, reduced risk of ovarian and premenopausal breast cancers, and, possibly a reduced risk of osteoporosis. Advantages to society include reduced health care costs because of lower incidence of illness in breastfed infants and reduced employee absenteeism for care attributable to infant illness. Human milk may reduce the incidence of food allergies and eczema. It also contains protective bacterial and viral antibodies (secretory IgA) and nonspecific immune factors, including macrophages and nucleotides, which also help limit infections.

Breastfeeding initiation rates in 2005 were at an all-time high of approximately 74%. However, the number of infants still breastfeeding by 6 months decreased to 43% and was even lower by 1 year (approximately 21%). Breastfeeding rates are lower in several subpopulations of women, especially low-income, minority, and young mothers. Many mothers face obstacles in maintaining lactation because of lack of support from health care professionals and family as well as the need to return to work. Skilled use of a breast pump may help maintain lactation in many circumstances. Primary lactation failure is rare; most women can succeed at breastfeeding if given adequate information and support, especially in the early postpartum period. Multiple excellent resources are readily available at maternity or children's hospitals, in print, and on the Internet, with guidelines on breastfeeding initiation, positioning, and troubleshooting.

Human milk has several nutritional and non-nutritional advantages over infant formula. The nutrient composition of human milk is summarized and compared with infant formulas in Table 27-1. Outstanding characteristics include the relatively low but highly bioavailable protein content; a generous quantity of essential fatty acids; the presence of long-chain unsaturated fatty acids of the $\omega$-3 series (docosahexaenoic acid is thought to be especially important); a relatively low sodium and solute load; and low but highly bioavailable concentrations of calcium, iron, and zinc, which provide adequate quantities of these nutrients to a normal breastfed infant for approximately 6 months. Breast milk does not need to be warmed, does not require a clean water supply, and is generally free of microorganisms.

### Exclusive Breastfeeding

Colostrum, a high-protein, low-fat fluid, is produced in small amounts during the first few postpartum days. It has some nutritional value but primarily has important immunologic and maturational properties. Primiparous women often experience breast **engorgement** before the milk comes in around the third postpartum day; the breasts become hard and are painful, the nipples become nonprotractile, and the mother's temperature may increase slightly. Enhancement of milk flow is the best management. If severe engorgement occurs, areolar rigidity may prevent the infant from grasping the nipple and areola. Attention to proper latch-on and hand expression of milk assists in drainage.

**TABLE 27-1 Composition of Breast Milk and Representative Infant Formulas**

| | Breast Milk (per dL) | Standard Formula (per dL) | Premature Formula (per dL) | Soy Formula (per dL) | Nutramigen (per dL) | Pregestimil (per dL) |
|---|---|---|---|---|---|---|
| Calories (kcal) | 67 | 67 | 67-81 | 67 | 67 | 67 |
| **Protein** (g) | 1.1 | 1.5 | 2.0-2.4 | 1.7 | 1.9 | 1.9 |
| (% calories) | (6%) | (9%) | (12%) | (10%) | (11%) | (11%) |
| Whey-to-casein protein ratio | 80:20 | 60:40, 18:82 | 60:40 | Soy protein, methionine | Casein hydrolysate plus L-cystine, L-tyrosine, and L-tryptophan | Casein hydrolysate plus L-cystine, L-tyrosine, and L-tryptophan |
| **Fat** (g) | 4.0 | 3.6 | 3.4-4.4 | 3.6 | 3.3 | 3.8 |
| (% calories) | (55%) | (50%) | (45%) | (48%) | (45%) | (48%) |
| MCT (%) | 0 | 0 | 40-50 | 0 | 0 | 55 |
| **Carbohydrate** (g) | 7.2 | 6.9-7.2 | 8.5-8.9 | 6.8 | 7.3 | 6.9 |
| (% calories) | (40%) | (41%) | (42%) | (40%) | (44%) | (41%) |
| Source | Lactose | Lactose | Lactose, corn syrup | Corn syrup, sucrose | Corn syrup solids, cornstarch | Corn syrup solids, cornstarch, dextrose |
| **Minerals** | | | | | | |
| Calcium (mg/L) | 290 | 420-550 | 1115-1452 | 700 | 635 | 777 |
| Phosphorus (mg/L) | 140 | 280-390 | 561-806 | 500 | 420 | 500 |
| Sodium (mEq/L) | 8.0 | 6.5-8.3 | 11-15 | 13 | 14 | 14 |
| Vitamin D | Variable | 400 | 1000-1800 | 400 | 400 | 400 |
| Osmolality (mOsm/L) | 253 | 270 | 230-270 | 200-220 | 290 | 290 |
| Renal solute load (mOsm/L) | 75 | 100-126 | 175-213 | 126-150 | 175 | 125 |
| **Comments** | Reference standard, deficient in vitamin K; may be deficient in Na, $Ca^{2+}$, protein, vitamin D for VLBW infants | Risk of milk protein intolerance—gastrointestinal bleeding, anemia, wheezing, eczema | Specifically fortified with additional protein, $Ca^{2+}$, P, Na, vitamin D, and MCT oil | Useful for milk protein intolerance; may lead to soy protein intolerance; rickets develops in VLBW infants | Useful for milk protein intolerance (allergy) | Useful for malabsorption states, lactose and milk protein intolerance (allergy) |

MCT, medium-chain triglyceride; VLBW, very low birth weight.

**Adequacy of milk intake** can be assessed by voiding and stooling patterns of the infant. A well-hydrated infant voids six to eight times a day. Each voiding should soak, not merely moisten, a diaper, and urine should be colorless. By 5 to 7 days, loose yellow stools should be passed at least four times a day. Rate of weight gain provides the most objective indicator of adequate milk intake. Total weight loss after birth should not exceed 7%, and birth weight should be regained by 10 days. An infant may be adequately hydrated while not receiving enough milk to achieve adequate energy and nutrient intake. Telephone follow-up is valuable during the interim between discharge and the first physician visit to monitor the progress of lactation. A follow-up visit should be scheduled by 3 to 5 days of age, and again by 2 weeks of age. The mean feeding frequency during the early weeks postpartum is 8 to 12 times per day.

The characteristics of the stools of breastfed infants may alarm parents. Stools are unformed, yellow, and seedy in appearance. Parents commonly think their breastfed infant has diarrhea. Stool frequencies vary; during the first 4 to 6 weeks, breastfed infants tend to produce stool more frequently than formula-fed infants. After 6 to 8 weeks, breastfed infants may go several days without passing a stool.

In the newborn period, elevated concentrations of serum bilirubin are present more often in breastfed infants than in formula-fed infants (see Chapter 62). Feeding frequency during the first 3 days of life of breastfed infants is inversely related to the level of bilirubin; frequent feedings stimulate meconium passage and excretion of bilirubin in the stool. Infants who have insufficient milk intake and poor weight gain in the first week of life may have an increase in unconjugated bilirubin secondary to an exaggerated enterohepatic circulation of bilirubin. This is known as **breastfeeding jaundice**. Attention should be directed toward improved milk production and intake. The use of water supplements in breastfed infants has no effect on bilirubin levels and is not recommended. After the first week of life in a breastfed infant, prolonged elevated serum bilirubin may be due to presence of an unknown factor in milk that enhances intestinal absorption of bilirubin. This is termed **breast milk jaundice**, which is a diagnosis of exclusion and should be made only if an infant is otherwise thriving, with normal growth and no evidence of hemolysis, infection, biliary atresia, or metabolic disease (see Chapter 62). Breast milk jaundice usually lasts no more than 1 to 2 weeks. The American Academy of Pediatrics recommends vitamin D supplementation (400 IU/day starting soon after birth), and, when needed, fluoride after 6 months for breastfed infants.

## Common Breastfeeding Problems

Breast tenderness, engorgement, and cracked nipples are the most common problems encountered by breastfeeding mothers. Engorgement, one of the most common causes of lactation failure, should receive prompt attention because milk supply can decrease quickly if the breasts are not adequately emptied. Applying warm or cold compresses to the breasts before nursing and hand expression or pumping of some milk can provide relief to the mother and make the areola easier to grasp by the infant. Nipple tenderness requires attention to proper latch-on and positioning of the infant. Supportive measures include nursing for shorter periods, beginning feedings on the less sore side, air drying the nipples well after nursing, and applying lanolin cream after each nursing session. Severe nipple pain and cracking usually indicate improper latch-on. Temporary pumping, which is well tolerated, may be needed. Meeting with a lactation consultant may help minimize these problems and allow the successful continuation of breastfeeding.

If a lactating woman reports fever, chills, and malaise, **mastitis** should be considered. Treatment includes frequent and complete emptying of the breast and antibiotics. Breastfeeding usually should not be stopped, because the mother's mastitis commonly has no adverse effects on the breastfed infant. Untreated mastitis may also progress to a **breast abscess**. If an abscess is diagnosed, treatment includes incision and drainage, antibiotics, and regular emptying of the breast. Nursing from the contralateral breast can be continued with a healthy infant. If maternal comfort allows, nursing can continue on the affected side.

Maternal infection with human immunodeficiency virus is considered a contraindication for breastfeeding in developed countries. When the mother has active tuberculosis, syphilis, or varicella, restarting breastfeeding may be considered after therapy is initiated. If a woman has herpetic lesions on her breast, nursing and contact with the infant on that breast should be avoided. Women with genital herpes can breastfeed. Proper handwashing procedures should be stressed. Galactosemia in the infant also is a contraindication to breastfeeding.

## Maternal Drug Use

Any drug prescribed therapeutically to newborns usually can be consumed via breast milk without ill effect. The factors that determine the effects of maternal drug therapy on the nursing infant include the route of administration, dosage, molecular weight, pH, and protein binding. Few therapeutic drugs are absolutely contraindicated; these include radioactive compounds, antimetabolites, lithium, and certain antithyroid drugs. The mother should be advised against the use of unprescribed drugs, including alcohol, nicotine, caffeine, or *street drugs*.

Maternal use of illicit or recreational drugs is a contraindication to breastfeeding. If a woman is unable to discontinue drug use, she should not breastfeed. Expression of milk for a feeding or two after use of a drug is not acceptable. Breastfed infants of mothers taking methadone (but no alcohol or other drugs) as part of a treatment program generally have not experienced ill effects.

# FORMULA FEEDING

## Cow's Milk–Based Formulas

The alternative to human milk is iron-fortified formula, which permits adequate growth of most infants and is formulated to mimic human milk. No vitamin or mineral supplements (other than possibly fluoride after 6 months) are needed with such formulas. Cow's milk formulas

**TABLE 27-2 Infant Feedings and Standard and Specialized Formulas**

| Formula Category | Example Formulas | Features and Typical Uses |
|---|---|---|
| Human milk | | *Gold standard* |
| | | Expressed milk can be delivered by gavage or nasogastric tube |
| Cow's milk–based (with lactose) | Enfamil | Standard substitute for breast milk |
| | Similac | |
| | Carnation Good Start | |
| Cow's milk–based (without lactose) | LactoFree | Useful for transient lactase deficiency or lactose intolerance |
| | Similac Lactose Free | |
| Soy protein–based/lactose-free | ProSobee | Alternative to milk protein-based formulas |
| | Isomil | Not recommended for premature infants |
| Premature formula: cow's milk (reduced lactose) | Similac Special Care | Indicated for premature and LBW infants |
| | Enfamil Premature | Fat is 50% MCT, higher in many micronutrients |
| Predigested | Pregestimil (50% fat MCT) | Casein hydrolysate, useful for protein allergies and malabsorptive disorders |
| | Nutramigen (no MCT) | |
| | Alimentum (50% fat MCT) | |
| Elemental | Neocate | Free amino acids for severe protein allergy; malabsorption |
| | EleCare (high MCT) | |
| Premature transitional | EnfaCare | Standard at 22 kcal/oz, intermediate in protein and micronutrients to promote growth postdischarge |
| | NeoSure | |
| Fat modified | Lipisorb | High MCT, useful for chylous effusions and for some malabsorptive disorders |
| | Portagen | |
| Prethickened | Enfamil AR | May be useful for dysphagia, mild GER |
| Carbohydrate intolerance | 3232A | All monosaccharides and disaccharides removed; can titrate dextrose or fructose additives to tolerance |
| | Ross Carbohydrate Free | |

GER, gastroesophageal reflux; LBW, low birth weight; MCT, medium-chain triglyceride.

(see Table 27-1; Table 27-2) are composed of reconstituted, skimmed cow's milk or a mixture of skimmed cow's milk and electrolyte-depleted cow's milk whey or casein proteins. The fat used in infant formulas is a mixture of vegetable oils, commonly including soy, palm, coconut, corn, oleo, or safflower oils. The carbohydrate is generally lactose, although lactose-free cow's milk–based formulas are available. The caloric density of formulas is 20 kcal/oz (0.67 kcal/mL), similar to that of human milk. Formula-fed infants often gain weight more rapidly than breastfed infants, especially after the first 3 to 4 months of life. Formula-fed infants are at higher risk for obesity later in childhood; this may be related to differences in feeding practices for formula-fed infants compared with breastfed infants. Cow's milk–based infant formulas are used as substitutes for breast milk for infants whose mothers choose not to or cannot breastfeed or as supplements for breastfeeding. Nondairy milk substitutes such as rice or nut milks are inappropriate to feed to infants and can result in severe nutritional deficiencies. Human milk fortifiers, which when mixed with breast milk boost the caloric (24 kcal/oz) and nutrient content, also are available for use with premature infants when adequate growth cannot be achieved with human milk alone.

## Soy Formulas

Soy protein–based formulas provide a nutritionally safe alternative to cow's milk–based formulas when intolerance occurs from immune reactions to cow's milk proteins.

However, a proportion of infants allergic to cow's milk protein also are allergic to soy protein. The soy protein is supplemented with methionine to improve its nutritional qualities. The carbohydrates in soy formulas are glucose oligomers (smaller molecular weight corn starches) and, sometimes, sucrose. The fat mixture is similar to that used in cow's milk formulas. Caloric density is the same as for cow's milk formulas.

Soy protein formulas do not prevent the development of allergic disorders in later life. Clinical intolerance to soy protein or cow's milk protein occurs with similar frequency. Soy protein formulas can be recommended for use by vegetarian families and in the management of galactosemia and primary and secondary lactose intolerance. Soy formulas should not be used indiscriminately to "treat" poorly evaluated patients with colic, formula intolerance, or more serious diseases. Soy protein–based formulas are not recommended for premature infants with birth weights less than 1800 g.

## Therapeutic Formulas

The composition of specialized infant and pediatric formulas is modified to meet specific therapeutic requirements (see Table 27-2; Table 27-3). Therapeutic formulas are designed to treat **digestive** and **absorptive insufficiency** or protein hypersensitivity. Semi-elemental formulas include protein hydrolysate formulas, the major nitrogen source of which is a casein or whey hydrolysate, supplemented with selected amino acids. These formulas contain

**TABLE 27-3 Pediatric Enteral Formulas**

| Formula Category | Formula Examples | Typical Uses |
|---|---|---|
| Standard, milk protein–based | Nutren Junior<br>PediaSure (with/without fiber)<br>Kindercal (with/without fiber) | Nutritionally complete for ages 1 to 10. Can be used for tube feeds or oral supplements |
| Food-based | Compleat Pediatric | Made with beef protein, fruits, and vegetables—contains lactose. Fortified with vitamins/minerals |
| Semi-elemental | Peptamen Jr. | Indicated for impaired gut function with peptides as protein source, high MCT content with lower total fat percentage than standard pediatric formulas |
| Elemental | Pediatric Vivonex (24 kcal/oz)<br>EleCare<br>Neocate One Plus | Indicated for impaired gut function or protein allergy, contains free amino acids. Lower fat, with most as MCT |

MCT, medium-chain triglyceride.

an abundance of essential fatty acids from vegetable oil. Certain brands also provide substantial amounts (25% to 50% of total fat) of medium-chain triglycerides, which are water soluble and are more easily absorbed than long-chain fatty acids; this is a useful feature for patients with malabsorption resulting from such conditions as short gut syndrome, intestinal mucosal atrophy or injury, chronic diarrhea, or cholestasis. Elemental formulas also are available that contain synthetic free amino acids and varying quantities and types of fat components. These are especially designed for patients with protein allergy or sensitivity. The carbohydrate content of these specialized formulas varies, but all are lactose free; some contain glucose oligomers and soluble starches.

## COMPLEMENTARY FOODS AND WEANING

By approximately 6 months, complementary feeding of semisolid foods is suggested. By this age, an exclusively breastfed infant requires additional sources of several nutrients, including protein, iron, and zinc. If the introduction of solid foods is delayed, nutritional deficiencies can develop, and oral sensory issues (texture and oral aversion) may occur. General signs of **readiness** include the ability to hold the head up and sit unassisted, bringing objects to the mouth, showing interest in foods, and the ability to track a spoon and open the mouth. Although the growth rate of the infant is decreasing, energy needs for activity increase (Fig. 27-1). A relatively high-fat and calorically dense diet (human milk or formula) is needed to deliver adequate calories. The choice of foods to meet micronutrient needs is less critical for formula-fed infants because of the nutrient fortification of formula. The exposure to different textures and the process of self-feeding are important developmental experiences for formula-fed infants.

Commercially prepared or homemade foods help meet the nutritional needs of the infant. Because infant foods are usually less energy dense than human milk and formula, they generally should not be used in young infants to compensate for inadequate intake from breastfeeding or formula. Oropharyngeal coordination is immature

before 3 months, making feeding with solid foods difficult. Vitamin-fortified and iron-fortified dry cereals are often used as a source of calories and micronutrients (particularly iron) to supplement the diet of infants whose needs for these nutrients are not met by human milk after about 6 months of age. Cereals commonly are mixed with breast milk, formula, or water and later with fruits. To help identify possible allergies or food intolerances that may arise when new foods are added to the diet, single-grain cereals (rice, oatmeal, barley) are recommended as starting cereals. New single-ingredient foods generally can be offered approximately every week. Mixed cereal (oat, corn, wheat, and soy) provides greater variety to older infants.

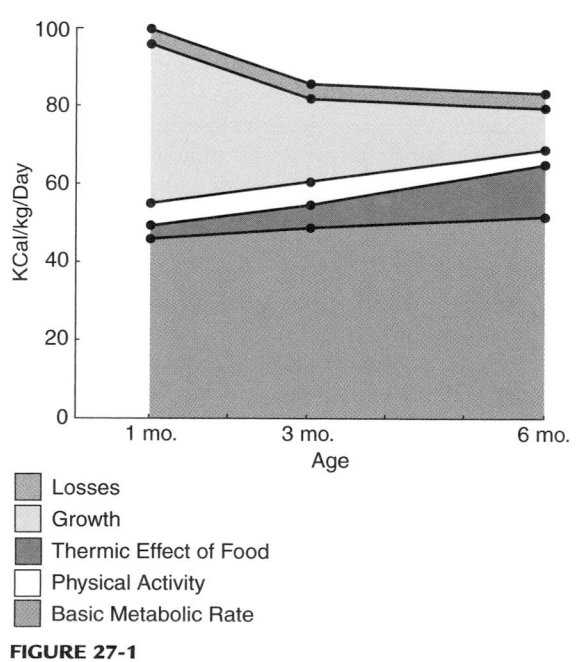

**FIGURE 27-1**

Energy requirements of infants. (From Waterlow JC: Basic concepts in the determination of nutritional requirements of normal infants. In Tsang RC, Nichols BL, editors: Nutrition during infancy. Philadelphia, 1988, *Hanley & Belfus*.)

Puréed fruits, vegetables, and meats are available in containers that provide an appropriate serving size for infants. By approximately 6 months, the infant's gastro-intestinal tract is mature, and the order of introducing complementary foods is not critical. Introduction of sin-gle-ingredient meats (versus combination dinners) as an early complementary food provides an excellent source of bioavailable iron and zinc, both of which are important for the older breastfed infant. Parents who prefer to make homemade infant foods using a food processor or food mill should be encouraged to practice safe food handling techniques and avoid flavor additives such as salt. If juice is given, it should be started only after 6 months of age, be given in a cup (as opposed to a bottle), and limited to 4 oz daily. An infant should never be put to sleep with a bottle or sippy cup filled with milk, formula, or juice, because this can result in **infant bottle tooth decay** (see Chapter 127). Foods with high allergic potential that should be avoided during infancy, especially for infants with a strong family history of **food allergy**, include fish, peanuts, tree nuts, dairy products, and eggs. Hot dogs, grapes, popcorn, and nuts present a risk of aspira-tion and airway obstruction. All foods with the potential to obstruct the young infant's airway should be cut into sizes smaller than an infant's main airway. In general, such foods should be avoided until 4 years of age or older. Honey (risk of infant botulism) should not be given before 1 year of age.

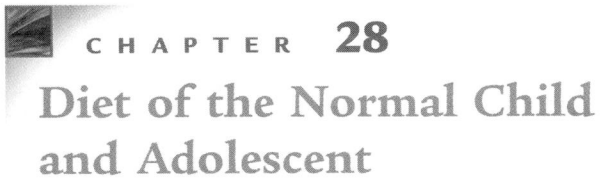

# CHAPTER 28
# Diet of the Normal Child and Adolescent

For a discussion of nutrient needs for children and adoles-cents, go to http://www.health.gov/dietaryguidelines.

## NUTRITION ISSUES FOR TODDLERS AND OLDER CHILDREN

Cow's milk ideally is not introduced until approximately 1 year of age to avoid occult intestinal blood loss. Low fat (2%) or whole milk is recommended until 2 years of age, after which fat free milk is recommended. Excessive milk (>24 oz/day) intake should be avoided in toddlers because larger intakes may reduce the intake of a good variety of nutritionally important solid foods and result in iron deficiency anemia; large intakes also may contrib-ute to excessive caloric intake. Juice intake for toddlers and young children should be limited to 4 to 6 oz/day, and juice intake for children 7 to 18 years of age should be limited to 8 to 12 oz/day. By 1 year of age, infants should be eating meals with the family, have a regular schedule of meals and snacks, and be encouraged to self-feed with appropriate finger foods. The Food Guide Pyramid developed by the U.S. Department of Agriculture can provide parents with a general guideline for the types of foods to be offered on a regular basis. A general rule for the quantity of food to offer is 1 tablespoon of each food provided per meal, with more given if the toddler requests. Power struggles over eating are common between parents and toddlers. The **parent's role** is to decide the what, when, and where of the meals. The **child's role** is to decide if, what, and how much to eat. Breastfeeding of the older infant can continue as long as mutually desired, with care taken to ensure the infant is consuming a variety of other foods and is not depending excessively on breastfeeding for nutritional or comfort needs.

Iron intake may be inadequate in some children between 1 and 3 years of age in the United States. The incidence of iron deficiency anemia has decreased in young children in the United States. Significant iron deficiency and iron deficiency anemia exist in some high-risk minority or poor populations of young children. Toddlers with excessive milk intakes (> 32 oz/day) and/or those who consume little meat are at risk for iron deficiency.

Ten percent of 2- to 5-year-old children have weight-for-length or body mass index percentiles at or above the 95th percentile for age. The relatively high prevalence of **underweight** and **overweight** emphasizes the importance of surveillance of growth velocity in all young children to allow early detection of abnormal rates of weight gain rel-ative to linear growth.

Learning healthy eating behaviors at an early age is an important preventive measure because of the association of diet with several chronic adult diseases, such as obesity, diabetes, and cardiovascular disease. Table 28-1 provides guidelines for a **prudent diet** appropriate for most chil-dren older than 2 years of age. After 2 years, it is recom-mended that the fat intake gradually be reduced to approximately 30% and not less than 20% of calories.

## NUTRITION ISSUES FOR ADOLESCENTS

Adolescence can be a time when poor eating habits develop. Skipped meals (especially breakfast), binge eating with friends or alone, dieting, and consumption of nutri-ent-poor, calorically dense foods are common problems. Excessive consumption of sugar from soda, fruit drinks, and specialty coffee and tea drinks may contribute to excess weight gain and tooth decay and may displace other needed nutrients. Poor calcium intake during ado-lescence may predispose adults to osteoporotic hip frac-tures in later life. **Osteoporosis** (osteopenia) caused by poor dietary calcium or vitamin intake or poor absorp-tion of ingested calcium in children and adolescents is becoming more clinically recognized and treated. Inad-equate iron intake may result in symptoms of fatigue and iron deficiency anemia. Student athletes may be espe-cially vulnerable to inadequate iron intakes, severely restrictive eating patterns, and use of inappropriate nutri-tional and vitamin supplements. Adolescents should be counseled on appropriate dietary recommendations (see Chapter 70).

**TABLE 28-1 Prudent Diet Guidelines for Children Older than 2 Years**

### GENERAL RECOMMENDATIONS

Consume 3 regular meals daily with healthful snacks (2–3/day) according to appetite, activity, and growth needs

Include a variety of foods with abundant vegetables and fruits

### KEY NUTRIENTS

**Carbohydrates**

Complex carbohydrates should provide ≥55%–60% of daily calories; half of all grains should be whole-grain, high-fiber foods

Simple sugars should be limited to <10% daily calories

**Fat**

<30% of total calories should come from dietary fat

Saturated and polyunsaturated fats should make up <10% total calories each

Monounsaturated fats should provide at least 10% total calories

Encourage lean cuts of meat, fish, low-fat dairy products, vegetable oils

Cholesterol intake should approximate 100 mg/1000 kcal/day (maximum of 300 mg/day)

Severe fat restriction (≤15%–20% total calories) should be avoided because it may result in growth failure

**Sodium**

Limit sodium intake by choosing fresh over highly processed foods

### BEHAVIORAL

Limit grazing behavior, eating while watching television, and regular consumption of high-calorie, low-nutrient foods

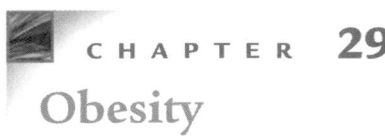

CHAPTER **29**

# Obesity

## EPIDEMIOLOGY AND DEFINITIONS

The prevalence of obesity in children has increased dramatically. Data from 2004 to 2006 indicate that 16.3% of American children 2 to 19 years of age are considered **obese** (body mass index [BMI] ≥95th percentile). The largest increases in the prevalence of obesity are seen in the most overweight classifications and in certain ethnic groups, such as African-American and Mexican-American children, of whom more than 30% are overweight.

Many obese children become obese adults. The risk of remaining obese increases with age and degree of obesity. Eleven-year-old children who are overweight are more than twice as likely to remain overweight at 15 years of age than are 7-year-old overweight children. The risk of becoming obese as a child and remaining obese as an adult is also influenced by family history. If one parent is obese, the odds ratio for the child to be obese in adulthood is 3, but if both parents are obese, the ratio increases to 10.

Obesity runs in families; this could be related to genetic influences or the influence of a common, shared environment. Eighty percent of the variance in weight for height or skin-fold thickness in adopted twin pairs may be explained on the basis of genetics. A strong relationship exists between the BMI of adoptees and that of their biologic parents; a weaker relationship exists between the BMI of adoptees and that of their adoptive parents. The association between obesity and television watching and dietary intake, the different rates of obesity observed in urban versus rural areas, and changes in obesity with seasons support the important influence of environment.

## CLINICAL MANIFESTATIONS

**Complications** of obesity in children and adolescents can affect virtually every major organ system. The history and physical examination should screen for many potential complications noted among obese patients (Table 29-1) in addition to specific diseases associated with obesity (Table 29-2). Medical complications usually are related to the degree of obesity and usually decrease in severity or resolve with weight reduction.

The **diagnosis** of obesity depends on the measurement of excess body fat. Actual measurement of body composition is not practical in most clinical situations. **BMI** is a convenient screening tool that correlates fairly strongly with body fatness in children and adults. **BMI age-specific and gender-specific percentile curves** (for 2- to 20-year-olds) allow an assessment of BMI percentile (available online at http://www.cdc.gov/growthcharts). Table 29-3 provides BMI interpretation guidelines. For children younger than 2 years of age, weight-for-length measurements greater than 95th percentile may indicate overweight and warrant further assessment. A BMI for age and gender above the 99th percentile is strongly associated with excessive body fat and is associated with multiple cardiovascular disease risk factors.

**TABLE 29-1 Complications of Obesity**

| Complication | Effects |
|---|---|
| Psychosocial | Peer discrimination, teasing, reduced college acceptance, isolation, reduced job promotion* |
| Growth | Advance bone age, increased height, early menarche |
| Central nervous system | Pseudotumor cerebri |
| Respiratory | Sleep apnea, pickwickian syndrome |
| Cardiovascular | Hypertension, cardiac hypertrophy, ischemic heart disease,* sudden death* |
| Orthopedic | Slipped capital femoral epiphysis, Blount disease |
| Metabolic | Insulin resistance, type 2 diabetes mellitus, hypertriglyceridemia, hypercholesterolemia, gout,* hepatic steatosis, polycystic ovary disease, cholelithiasis |

*Complications unusual until adulthood.

**TABLE 29-2  Diseases Associated with Childhood Obesity***

| Syndrome | Manifestations |
| --- | --- |
| Alström syndrome | Hypogonadism, retinal degeneration, deafness, diabetes mellitus |
| Carpenter syndrome | Polydactyly, syndactyly, cranial synostosis, mental retardation |
| Cushing syndrome | Adrenal hyperplasia or pituitary tumor |
| Fröhlich syndrome | Hypothalamic tumor |
| Hyperinsulinism | Nesidioblastosis, pancreatic adenoma, hypoglycemia, Mauriac syndrome |
| Laurence-Moon-Bardet-Biedl syndrome | Retinal degeneration, syndactyly, hypogonadism, mental retardation; autosomal recessive |
| Muscular dystrophy | Late onset of obesity |
| Myelodysplasia | Spina bifida |
| Prader-Willi syndrome | Neonatal hypotonia, normal growth immediately after birth, small hands and feet, mental retardation, hypogonadism; some have partial deletion of chromosome 15 |
| Pseudohypoparathyroidism | Variable hypocalcemia, cutaneous calcifications |
| Turner syndrome | Ovarian dysgenesis, lymphedema, web neck; XO chromosome |

*These diseases represent <5% of cases of childhood obesity.

**TABLE 29-3  Body Mass Index (BMI) Interpretation**

| BMI/Age percentile | Interpretation |
| --- | --- |
| <5th | Underweight |
| 5–85th | Normal |
| 85–95th | Overweight |
| ≥95th | Obese |
| >99th | Severely obese |

**TABLE 29-4  Eating and Activity Habits for Overweight/Obesity Prevention and Treatment**

| DIET |
| --- |
| Consume five or more servings of fruits and vegetables per day |
| Minimize consumption of sugar-sweetened beverages |
| Prepare more meals at home rather than purchasing restaurant food |
| Eat at table, as a family, at least five to six times per week |
| Consume a healthy breakfast every day |
| Allow child to self-regulate his or her meals and avoid overly restrictive feeding behaviors |

| ACTIVITY |
| --- |
| Limit screen time (television, computer games/Internet, video games) to ≤2 hours per day (no TV for child <2 yr of age) |
| Be physically active ≥1 hour per day; engage in both unstructured and structured activities |

## ASSESSMENT

Early recognition of excessive rates of weight gain, overweight, or obesity in children is essential because family counseling and treatment interventions are more likely to be successful before obesity becomes severe. Routine evaluation at well-child visits should include the following:

1. **Anthropometric data**, including weight, height, and calculation of BMI. Data should be plotted on age-appropriate and gender-appropriate growth charts and assessed for weight gain trends and upward crossing of percentiles.
2. **Dietary and physical activity history** (Table 29-4). Assess patterns and potential targets for behavioral change.
3. **Physical examination.** Assess blood pressure, adiposity distribution (central versus generalized), markers of comorbidities (acanthosis nigricans, hirsutism, hepatomegaly, orthopedic abnormalities), and physical stigmata of genetic syndrome (Prader-Willi syndrome).
4. **Laboratory studies.** These are generally reserved for children who are obese (BMI >95th percentile), who have evidence of comorbidities or both. Useful laboratory tests may include a fasting lipid profile, fasting glucose levels, liver function tests, and thyroid function tests (if evidence of plateau in linear growth). Other studies should be guided by findings in the history and physical examination.

## TREATMENT

The approach to therapy and aggressiveness of treatment should be based on risk factors, including age, severity of overweight and obesity and comorbidities, and family history and support. The primary goal for all children with uncomplicated overweight is to achieve **healthy eating and activity patterns**. For children with a secondary complication, improvement of the complication is an important goal. Childhood and adolescent obesity treatment programs can lead to sustained weight loss and decreases in BMI when treatment focuses on behavioral changes and is family-centered. Concurrent changes in dietary and physical activity patterns are most likely to provide success.

Treatment recommendations by an Expert Committee include a systematic approach that promotes brief, office-based interventions for the greatest number of overweight and obese children, as well as a systematic intensification of efforts, tailored to the capacity of the clinical office, the motivation of the family, and the degree of obesity. The most aggressive therapy is considered only for those who have not responded to other interventions. The four levels or stages of treatment are described below.

1. **Prevention plus**: The goal is improved BMI status. Problem areas identified by dietary and physical activity history should be provided (see Table 29-4), and emphasis should be placed on healthy eating and physical activity patterns. This is especially appropriate for preventing further weight gain and for overweight and mildly obese children. This stage of treatment can take place in the office setting.

2. **Structured weight management**: The approach may include planned diet, structured daily meals, and planned snacks; additional reduction in screen (computer/video game/television) time; planned, supervised activity; self-monitoring of behaviors, including logs; and planned reinforcement for achievement of targeted behavior change. This may be done in the primary care setting but generally requires a registered dietitian or a clinician who has specialized training. Monthly follow-up visits are recommended.

3. **Comprehensive multidisciplinary intervention**: This level of treatment increases the intensity of behavior change, frequency of visits, and the specialists involved. Programs at this level are presumed to be beyond the capacity of most primary care office settings. Typical components of a program include structured behavior modification, food monitoring, diet and physical activity goal setting, and contingency management. A multidisciplinary team with expertise in childhood obesity typically includes a behavior counselor, registered dietitian, exercise specialist, and primary care provider to monitor ongoing medical issues. Frequency of visits is typically weekly for 8 to 10 weeks, with subsequent monthly visits. Group visits and treatment programs, including commercial weight management programs, should be considered. The Weight Information Network, a service available through the National Institutes of Health, disseminates information on weight control programs (http://www.niddk.nih.gov//NutritionDocs.html).

4. **Tertiary care intervention**: This more intensive approach should be considered for severely obese children. Approaches include medications, very low calorie diets, and weight control surgery, in addition to the attainment of behavior changes to improve diet and activity patterns. This level of intervention also includes a multidisciplinary team with expertise in obesity and its comorbidities and takes place in a pediatric weight management center.

## PREVENTION

Obesity is challenging to treat and can cause significant medical and psychosocial issues for young children and adolescents. Families need to be counseled on age-appropriate and healthy eating patterns beginning with the promotion of **breastfeeding**. For infants, transition to complementary and table foods and the importance of regularly scheduled meals and snacks, versus grazing behavior, should be emphasized. Age-appropriate **portion sizes** for meals and snacks should be encouraged. Children should be taught to recognize hunger and satiety cues, guided by reasonable portions and healthy food choices by parents. Children should never be forced to eat when they are not willing, and overemphasis of food as a reward should be avoided. The U.S. Department of Agriculture MyPyramid (http://www.mypyramid.gov) provides a good framework for a healthy diet, with an emphasis on whole grains, fruits, and vegetables and with age-appropriate portion sizes. After 2 years of age, most children should change from whole or 2% milk to skim milk, because other food sources provide adequate fat for growth and development.

The importance of physical activity should be emphasized. For some children, organized sports and school-based activities provide opportunities for vigorous activity and fun, whereas for others a focus on activities of daily living, such as increased walking, using stairs, and more active play may be better received. Time spent in **sedentary behavior**, such as television viewing and video/computer games, should be limited. Television in children's rooms is associated with more television time and with higher rates of overweight, and the risks of this practice should be discussed with parents. Clinicians may need to help families identify alternatives to sedentary activities, especially for families with deterrents to activity, such as unsafe neighborhoods or lack of supervision after school.

# CHAPTER 30
# Pediatric Undernutrition

Worldwide, protein-energy malnutrition (PEM) is a leading cause of death in children younger than 5 years of age. PEM is a spectrum of conditions caused by varying levels of protein and calorie deficiencies. Primary PEM is caused by social or economic factors that result in a lack of food. Secondary PEM occurs in children with various conditions associated with increased caloric requirements (infection, trauma, cancer) (Fig. 30-1), increased caloric loss (malabsorption), reduced caloric intake (anorexia, cancer, oral intake restriction, social factors), or a combination of these three variables. See Table 30-1 for guidelines on the classification of pediatric undernutrition. Protein and calorie malnutrition may be associated with other nutrient deficiencies, which may be evident on the physical examination (Table 30-2).

## FAILURE TO THRIVE

The most common diagnosis of pediatric **undernutrition** in the United States is often termed **failure to thrive** and is estimated to have a prevalence of 5% to 10% in young children (see Chapter 21). Psychosocial risk factors may develop as a result of medical problems or may be a primary cause of undernutrition. In the United States, most factors that contribute to poor growth are likely to be due to behavioral and psychosocial factors. The terms **organic** and **nonorganic** failure to thrive have lost favor

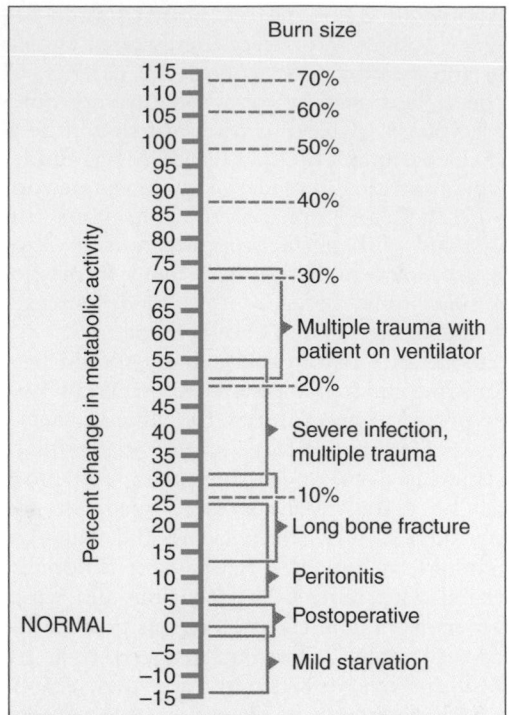

**FIGURE 30-1**

Increased energy needs with stress. (Adapted from Wilmore D: The metabolic management of the critically ill, New York, 1977, Plenum Publishing. Revised in Walker W, Watkins J, editors: Nutrition in pediatrics: basic science and clinical application. Boston, 1985, *Little, Brown*.)

in recognition of the frequent interplay between underlying medical conditions that may cause maladaptive behaviors. Similarly, social and behavioral factors that initially may have been associated with feeding problems and poor growth also may be associated with medical problems, including frequent minor acute illnesses.

## MARASMUS

*Marasmus* is the term used for **severe PEM** and wasting (low wt/ht). Many secondary forms of marasmic PEM are associated with chronic diseases (cystic fibrosis, tuberculosis, cancer, acquired immunodeficiency virus, celiac disease). The principal clinical manifestation in a child with severe malnutrition is **emaciation** with a body weight less than 60% of the median (50th percentile) for age or less than 70% of the ideal weight for height and depleted body fat stores. Loss of muscle mass and subcutaneous fat stores are confirmed by inspection or palpation and quantified by anthropometric measurements. The head may appear large but generally is proportional to the body length. Edema usually is absent. The skin is dry and thin, and the hair may be thin, sparse, and easily pulled out. Marasmic children may be apathetic and weak. Bradycardia and hypothermia signify severe and life-threatening malnutrition. Atrophy of the filiform papillae of the tongue is common, and monilial stomatitis is frequent. Inappropriate or inadequate weaning practices and chronic diarrhea are common findings in developing countries. Stunting (impaired linear growth (Table 30-1)) results from a combination of malnutrition, especially micronutrients, and recurrent infections. Stunting is more prevalent than wasting.

## KWASHIORKOR

Kwashiorkor is **hypoalbuminemic, edematous malnutrition** and presents with pitting edema that starts in the lower extremities and ascends with increasing severity. It is classically described as being caused by inadequate protein intake in the presence of fair to good caloric intake. Other factors, such as acute infection, toxins, and possibly specific micronutrient or amino acid imbalances, are likely to contribute to the etiology. The major **clinical manifestation** of kwashiorkor is that the body weight of the child ranges from 60% to 80% of the expected weight for age; weight alone may not accurately reflect the nutritional status because of edema. **Physical examination** reveals a relative maintenance of subcutaneous adipose tissue and a marked atrophy of muscle mass. Edema varies from a minor pitting of the dorsum of the foot to generalized edema with involvement of the eyelids and scrotum. The hair is sparse; is easily plucked; and appears dull brown, red, or yellow-white. Nutritional repletion restores hair color, leaving a band of hair with altered pigmentation followed by a band with normal pigmentation (flag sign). Skin changes are common and range from hyperpigmented hyperkeratosis to an erythematous macular rash (pellagroid) on the trunk and extremities. In the most severe form of kwashiorkor, a superficial desquamation occurs over pressure surfaces ("flaky paint" rash). Angular cheilosis, atrophy of the filiform papillae of the tongue, and monilial stomatitis are common. Enlarged parotid glands and facial edema result in moon facies;

| TABLE 30-1  Classification Guidelines for Pediatric Undernutrition | | | | |
|---|---|---|---|---|
| Nutrition Status | Weight/Age | Height/Age | Weight/Height | % IBW |
| Wasting | Normal or low | Normal | <5th percentile | <85%–90% |
| Stunting | <5th percentile | <5th percentile | Normal | Normal |
| Mild malnutrition | Normal or low | Normal | <5th percentile | 81%–90% |
| Moderate malnutrition | Normal or low | Normal | <5th percentile | 70%–80% |
| Kwashiorkor | Normal or low | Normal or low | Normal (edema) | Normal |
| Marasmus (severe wasting) | Low | Normal or low | <5th percentile | <70% |

IBW, ideal body weight.

**TABLE 30-2 Physical Signs of Nutritional Deficiency Disorders**

| System | Sign | Deficiency |
|---|---|---|
| General appearance | Reduced weight for height | Calories |
| Skin and hair | Pallor | Anemias (iron, vitamin $B_{12}$, vitamin E, folate, and copper) |
| | Edema | Protein, thiamine |
| | Nasolabial seborrhea | Calories, protein, vitamin $B_6$, niacin, riboflavin |
| | Dermatitis | Riboflavin, essential fatty acids, biotin |
| | Photosensitivity dermatitis | Niacin |
| | Acrodermatitis | Zinc |
| | Follicular hyperkeratosis (sandpaper-like) | Vitamin A |
| | Depigmented skin | Calories, protein |
| | Purpura | Vitamins C, K |
| | Scrotal, vulval dermatitis | Riboflavin |
| | Alopecia | Zinc, biotin, protein |
| | Depigmented, dull hair, easily pluckable | Protein, calories, copper |
| Subcutaneous tissue | Decreased | Calories |
| Eye (vision) | Adaptation to dark | Vitamins A, E, zinc |
| | Color discrimination | Vitamin A |
| | Bitot spots, xerophthalmia, keratomalacia | Vitamin A |
| | Conjunctival pallor | Nutritional anemias |
| | Fundal capillary microaneurysms | Vitamin C |
| Face, mouth, and neck | Angular stomatitis | Riboflavin, iron |
| | Cheilosis | Vitamins $B_6$, niacin, riboflavin |
| | Bleeding gums | Vitamins C, K |
| | Atrophic papillae | Riboflavin, iron, niacin, folate, vitamin $B_{12}$ |
| | Smooth tongue | Iron |
| | Red tongue (glossitis) | Vitamins $B_6$, $B_{12}$, niacin, riboflavin, folate |
| | Parotid swelling | Protein |
| | Caries | Fluoride |
| | Anosmia | Vitamins A, $B_{12}$, zinc |
| | Hypogeusia | Vitamin A, zinc |
| | Goiter | Iodine |
| Cardiovascular | Heart failure | Thiamine, selenium, nutritional anemias |
| Genital | Hypogonadism | Zinc |
| Skeletal | Costochondral beading | Vitamins D, C |
| | Subperiosteal hemorrhage | Vitamin C, copper |
| | Cranial bossing | Vitamin D |
| | Wide fontanel | Vitamin D |
| | Epiphyseal enlargement | Vitamin D |
| | Craniotabes | Vitamin D, calcium |
| | Tender bones | Vitamin C |
| | Tender calves | Thiamine, selenium, vitamin C |
| | Spoon-shaped nails (koilonychia) | Iron |
| | Transverse nail line | Protein |
| Neurologic | Sensory, motor neuropathy | Thiamine, vitamins E, $B_6$, $B_{12}$ |
| | Ataxia, areflexia | Vitamin E |
| | Ophthalmoplegia | Vitamin E, thiamine |
| | Tetany | Vitamin D, $Ca^2$, $Mg^2$ |
| | Retardation | Iodine, niacin |
| | Dementia, delirium | Vitamin E, niacin, thiamine |
| | Poor position sense, ataxia | Thiamine, vitamin $B_{12}$ |

apathy and disinterest in eating are typical of kwashior-kor. Examination of the abdomen may reveal an enlarged, soft liver with an indefinite edge. Lymphatic tissue commonly is atrophic. Chest examination may reveal basilar rales. The abdomen is distended, and bowel sounds tend to be hypoactive.

## TREATMENT OF MALNUTRITION

The basal metabolic rate and immediate nutrient needs decrease in cases of malnutrition. When nutrients are provided, the metabolic rate increases, stimulating anabolism and increasing nutrient requirements. The body of the malnourished child may have compensated for micronutrient deficiencies with lower metabolic and growth rates; refeeding may unmask these deficiencies. The gastrointestinal tract may not tolerate a rapid increase in intake. Nutritional rehabilitation should be initiated and advanced *slowly* to minimize these complications. Intravenous fluid should be avoided if possible to avoid excessive fluid and solute load and resultant heart or renal failure. If edema develops in the child during refeeding, caloric intake should be kept stable until the edema begins to resolve.

When nutritional rehabilitation is initiated, calories can be safely started at 20% above the child's recent intake. If no estimate of the caloric intake is available, 50% to 75% of the normal energy requirement is safe. Following these guidelines should help avoid the **refeeding syndrome**, which is characterized by fluid retention, hypophosphatemia, hypomagnesemia, and hypokalemia. Careful monitoring of laboratory values and clinical status with severe malnutrition is essential.

When nutritional rehabilitation has begun, caloric intake can be increased 10% to 20% per day, monitoring for electrolyte imbalances, poor cardiac function, edema, or feeding intolerance. If any of these occurs, further caloric increases are not made until the child's status stabilizes. Caloric intake is increased until appropriate regrowth or catch-up growth is initiated. Catch-up growth refers to gaining weight at greater than 50th percentile for age and may require 150% or more of the recommended calories for an age-matched, well-nourished child. A general rule of thumb for infants and children up to 3 years of age is to provide 100 to 120 kcal/kg based on *ideal* weight for height. Protein needs also are increased as anabolism begins and are provided in proportion to the caloric intake. Vitamin and mineral intake in excess of the daily recommended intake is provided to account for the increased requirements; this is frequently accomplished by giving an age-appropriate daily multiple vitamin, with other individual micronutrient supplements as warranted by history, physical examination, or laboratory studies. Iron supplements are not recommended during the acute rehabilitation phase, especially for children with kwashiorkor, for whom ferritin levels are often high. Additional iron may pose an oxidative stress; iron supplementation is associated with higher morbidity and mortality.

In most cases, cow's milk–based formulas are tolerated and provide an appropriate mix of nutrients. Other easily digested foods, appropriate for the age, also may be introduced slowly. If feeding intolerance occurs, lactose-free or semielemental formulas should be considered.

## COMPLICATIONS OF MALNUTRITION

Malnourished children are more susceptible to **infection**, especially sepsis, pneumonia, and gastroenteritis. Hypoglycemia is common after periods of severe fasting but also may be a sign of sepsis. Hypothermia may signify infection or, with bradycardia, may signify a decreased metabolic rate to conserve energy. Bradycardia and poor cardiac output predispose the malnourished child to heart failure, which is exacerbated by acute fluid or solute loads. **Micronutrient deficiencies** also can complicate malnutrition. Vitamin A and zinc deficiencies are common in the developing world and are an important cause of altered immune response and increased morbidity and mortality. Depending on the age at onset and the duration of the malnutrition, malnourished children may have permanent growth stunting (from malnutrition in utero, infancy, or adolescence) and delayed development (from malnutrition in infancy or adolescence). Environmental (social) deprivation may interact with the effects of the malnutrition to impair further development and cognitive function.

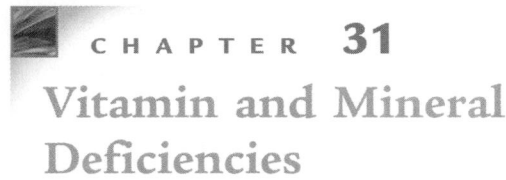

## CHAPTER 31
# Vitamin and Mineral Deficiencies

**Micronutrients** comprise 13 vitamins and 17 essential minerals. In industrialized societies, frank clinical deficiencies are unusual in healthy children, but they can and do occur in certain high-risk circumstances. Risk factors include diets that are consistently limited in variety, especially with the exclusion of entire food groups, malabsorption syndromes, and conditions causing high physiologic requirements. Various common etiologies of vitamin and nutrient deficiency states are highlighted in Table 31-1, and characteristics of vitamin deficiencies are outlined in Table 31-2.

## WATER-SOLUBLE VITAMINS

Water-soluble vitamins are not *stored* in the body except for vitamin $B_{12}$; intake alters tissue levels. Absorption from the diet is usually high, and the compounds exchange readily between intracellular and extracellular fluids; excretion is via the urine. Water-soluble vitamins typically function as coenzymes in energy, protein, amino acid, and nucleic acid metabolism; as cosubstrates in enzymatic reactions; and as structural components.

### Ascorbic Acid

The principal forms of vitamin C are ascorbic acid and the oxidized form, dehydroascorbic acid. Ascorbic acid accelerates hydroxylation reactions in many biosynthetic reactions, including hydroxylation of proline in the formation of collagen. The needs of full-term infants for ascorbic acid and dehydroascorbic acid are calculated by estimating the availability in human milk.

A deficiency of ascorbic acid results in the clinical manifestations of **scurvy**. Infantile scurvy is manifested by irritability, bone tenderness with swelling, and pseudoparalysis of the legs. The disease may occur if infants are fed unsupplemented cow's milk in the first year of life or if the diet is devoid of fruits and vegetables. Subperiosteal hemorrhage, bleeding gums and petechiae, hyperkeratosis of hair follicles, and a succession of mental changes characterize the progression of the illness. Anemia secondary to bleeding, decreased iron absorption, or abnormal folate metabolism is also seen in chronic scurvy. **Treatment** of several vitamin related diseases is presented in Table 31-3.

**TABLE 31-1 Etiology of Vitamin and Nutrient Deficiency States**

| Etiology | Deficiency |
|---|---|
| **DIET** | |
| Vegans (strict) | Protein, vitamins $B_{12}$, D, riboflavin |
| Breastfed infant | Vitamins K, D |
| Cow's milk–fed infant | Iron |
| Bulimia, anorexia nervosa | Electrolytes, other deficiencies |
| Parenteral alimentation | Essential fatty acids, trace elements |
| Alcoholism | Calories, vitamin $B_1$, $B_6$, folate |
| **MEDICAL PROBLEMS** | |
| Malabsorption syndromes | Vitamins A, D, E, K, zinc, essential fatty acids |
| Cholestasis | Vitamins E, D, K, A, zinc, essential fatty acids |
| **MEDICATIONS** | |
| Sulfonamides | Folate |
| Phenytoin, phenobarbital | Vitamins D, K, folate |
| Mineral oil | Vitamins A, D, E, K |
| Antibiotics | Vitamin K |
| Isoniazid | Vitamin $B_6$ |
| Antacids | Iron, phosphate, calcium |
| Digitalis | Magnesium, calcium |
| Penicillamine | Vitamin $B_6$ |
| **SPECIFIC MECHANISMS** | |
| Transcobalamin II or intrinsic factor deficiency | Vitamin $B_{12}$ |
| Other digestive enzyme | Carbohydrate, fat, protein deficiencies |
| Menkes kinky hair syndrome | Copper |
| Acrodermatitis enteropathica | Zinc |
| Reduced exposure to direct sunlight | Vitamin D |

## B Vitamins

The B vitamins thiamine, riboflavin, and niacin are routinely added to enriched grain products; deficiencies in normal hosts are rare in the United States. Levels from human milk reflect maternal intake, and deficiency can develop in breastfed infants of deficient mothers.

### Thiamine

Vitamin $B_1$ functions as a coenzyme in biochemical reactions related to carbohydrate metabolism, decarboxylation of α-ketoacids and pyruvate, and transketolase reactions of the pentose pathway. Thiamine also is involved in the decarboxylation of branched-chain amino acids. Thiamine is lost during milk pasteurization and sterilization.

Thiamine deficiency occurs in alcoholics and has been reported in adolescents who have undergone bariatric surgery for severe obesity. **Infantile beriberi** occurs between 1 and 4 months of age in breastfed infants whose mothers have a thiamine deficiency (alcoholism), in infants with protein-calorie malnutrition, in infants receiving unsupplemented hyperalimentation fluid, and in infants receiving boiled milk. Acute **wet beriberi** with cardiac symptoms and signs predominates in infantile beriberi. Anorexia, apathy, vomiting, restlessness, and pallor progress to dyspnea, cyanosis, and death from heart failure. Infants with beriberi have a characteristic aphonic cry; they appear to be crying, but no sound is uttered. Other signs include peripheral neuropathy and paresthesias.

### Riboflavin

Vitamin $B_2$ is a constituent of two coenzymes, riboflavin 5′-phosphate and flavin-adenine dinucleotide, essential components of glutathione reductase and xanthine oxidase, which are involved in electron transport. A deficiency of riboflavin affects glucose, fatty acid, and amino acid metabolism. Riboflavin and its phosphate are decomposed by exposure to light and by strong alkaline solutions.

**Ariboflavinosis** is characterized by an angular stomatitis; glossitis; cheilosis; seborrheic dermatitis around the nose and mouth; and eye changes that include reduced tearing, photophobia, corneal vascularization, and the formation of cataracts. Subclinical riboflavin deficiencies have been found in diabetic subjects, children in families with low socioeconomic status, children with chronic cardiac disease, and infants undergoing prolonged phototherapy for hyperbilirubinemia.

### Niacin

Niacin consists of the compounds nicotinic acid and nicotinamide (niacinamide). Nicotinamide, the predominant form of the vitamin, functions as a component of the coenzymes nicotinamide adenine dinucleotide (NAD) and nicotinamide adenine dinucleotide phosphate (NADP). Niacin is involved in multiple metabolic processes, including fat synthesis, intracellular respiratory metabolism, and glycolysis.

In determining the needs for niacin, the content of tryptophan in the diet must be considered because tryptophan is converted to niacin. Niacin is stable in foods and withstands heating and prolonged storage. Approximately 70% of the total niacin equivalents in human milk are derived from tryptophan. **Pellagra**, or niacin deficiency disease, is characterized by weakness, lassitude, dermatitis, photosensitivity, inflammation of mucous membranes, diarrhea, vomiting, dysphagia, and, in severe cases, dementia.

### Vitamin $B_6$

Vitamin $B_6$ refers to three naturally occurring pyridines: pyridoxine (pyridoxol), pyridoxal, and pyridoxamine. The phosphates of the latter two pyridines are metabolically and functionally related and are converted in the liver to the coenzyme form, pyridoxal phosphate. The metabolic

## TABLE 31-2  Characteristics of Vitamin Deficiencies

| Vitamin | Purpose | Deficiency | Comments | Source |
|---|---|---|---|---|
| **WATER SOLUBLE** | | | | |
| Thiamine (B₁) | Coenzyme in ketoacid decarboxylation (e.g., pyruvate → acetyl-CoA transketolase reaction) | *Beriberi:* polyneuropathy, calf tenderness, heart failure, edema, ophthalmoplegia | Inborn errors of lactate metabolism; boiling milk destroys B₁ | Liver, meat, milk, cereals, nuts, legumes |
| Riboflavin (B₂) | FAD coenzyme in oxidation-reduction reactions | Anorexia, mucositis, anemia, cheilosis, nasolabial seborrhea | Photosensitizer | Milk, cheese, liver, meat, eggs, whole grains, green leafy vegetables |
| Niacin (B₃) | NAD coenzyme in oxidation-reduction reactions | *Pellagra:* photosensitivity, dermatitis, dementia, diarrhea, death | Tryptophan is a precursor | Meat, fish, live, whole grains, green leafy vegetables |
| Pyridoxine (B₆) | Cofactor in amino acid metabolism | Seizures, hyperacusis, microcytic anemia, nasolabial seborrhea, neuropathy | Dependency state: deficiency secondary to drugs | Meat, liver, whole grains, peanuts, soybeans |
| Pantothenic acid | CoA in Krebs cycle | None reported | | Meat, vegetables |
| Biotin | Cofactor in carboxylase reactions of amino acids | Alopecia, dermatitis, hypotonia, death | Bowel resection, inborn error of metabolism,* and ingestion of raw eggs | Yeast, meats; made by intestinal flora |
| B₁₂ | Coenzyme for 5-methyl-tetrahydrofolate formation; DNA synthesis | Megaloblastic anemia, peripheral neuropathy, posterior lateral spinal column disease, vitiligo | Vegans; fish tapeworm; short gut syndrome; transcobalamin or intrinsic factor deficiencies | Meat, fish, cheese, eggs |
| Folate | DNA synthesis | Megaloblastic anemia; neural tube defects | Goat milk deficient; drug antagonists; heat inactivates | Liver, greens, vegetables, cereals, cheese |
| Ascorbic acid (C) | Reducing agent; collagen metabolism | *Scurvy:* irritability, purpura, bleeding gums, periosteal hemorrhage, aching bones | May improve tyrosine metabolism in preterm infants | Citrus fruits, green vegetables; cooking destroys it |
| **FAT SOLUBLE** | | | | |
| A | Epithelial cell integrity; vision | Night blindness, xerophthalmia, Bitot spots, follicular hyperkeratosis; immune defects | Common with protein-calorie malnutrition; malabsorption | Liver, milk, eggs, green and yellow vegetables, fruits |
| D | Maintain serum calcium, phosphorus levels | *Rickets:* reduced bone mineralization | Prohormone of 25- and 1,25-vitamin D | Fortified milk, cheese, liver; sunlight |
| E | Antioxidant | Hemolysis in preterm infants; areflexia, ataxia, ophthalmoplegia | May benefit patients with G6PD deficiency | Seeds, vegetables, germ oils, grains |
| K | Post-translation carboxylation of clotting factors II, VII, IX, X and proteins C, S | Prolonged prothrombin time; hemorrhage; elevated protein induced in vitamin K absence (PIVKA) | Malabsorption; breastfed infants | Liver, green vegetables; made by intestinal flora |

*Biotinidase deficiency.
CoA, coenzyme A; FAD, flavin adenine dinucleotide; G6PD, glucose-6-phosphate dehydrogenase; NAD, nicotinamide adenine dinucleotide.

**TABLE 31–3 Recommended Daily Dose Ranges for Treatment of Vitamin-Related Diseases**

| Vitamin | Treatment of Vitamin Deficiency | Treatment of Deficiency in Patients with Malabsorption | Treatment of Dependency Syndrome |
|---|---|---|---|
| A (IU) | 5000–10,000 | 10,000–25,000 | — |
| D (IU) | 400–5000 | 4,000–20,000 | 50,000–200,000 |
|   Calcifediol (μg) | — | 20–100 | 50–100 |
|   Calcitriol (1,25-[OH]$_2$-D) (μg) | — | 1–3 | 1–3 |
| E (IU) | — | 100–1000 | — |
| K (mg) | 1* | 5–10* | — |
| Ascorbic acid (C) (mg) | 250–500 | 500 | — |
| Thiamine (mg) | 5–25 | 5–25 | 25–500 |
| Riboflavin (mg) | 5–25 | 5–25 | — |
| Niacin (mg) | 25–50 | 25–50 | 50–250 |
| B$_6$ (mg) | 5–25 | 2–25 | 10–250 |
| Biotin (mg) | 0.15–0.3 | 0.3–1.0 | 10 |
| Folic acid (mg) | 1 | 1 | —† |
| B$_{12}$ (μg) | —* | —* | 1–40 |

*To be used parenterally as needed.
†To be used only in conjunction with multivitamin mixtures.
From AMA Council on Scientific Affairs: Vitamin preparations as dietary supplements and as therapeutic agents. *JAMA* 257:1929–1936, 1987.

functions of vitamin B$_6$ include interconversion reactions of amino acids, conversion of tryptophan to niacin and serotonin, metabolic reactions in the brain, carbohydrate metabolism, immune development, and the biosynthesis of heme and prostaglandins. The pyridoxal and pyridoxamine forms of the vitamin are destroyed by heat; heat treatment was responsible for vitamin B$_6$ deficiency and seizures in infants fed improperly processed formulas. Goat's milk is deficient in vitamin B$_6$.

Dietary deprivation or malabsorption of vitamin B$_6$ in children results in hypochromic microcytic anemia, vomiting, diarrhea, failure to thrive, listlessness, hyperirritability, and seizures. Children receiving isoniazid or penicillamine may require additional vitamin B$_6$ because the drug binds to the vitamin. Vitamin B$_6$ is unusual as a water-soluble vitamin in that very large doses ($\geq 500$ mg/day) have been associated with a sensory neuropathy. Megadoses have been claimed to promote improved neurocognitive development in children with Down syndrome, but data from controlled trials are lacking, and the practice is not currently justified.

## Folate

A variety of chemical forms of folate are nutritionally active. Folate functions in transport of single-carbon fragments in synthesis of nucleic acids and for normal metabolism of certain amino acids and in conversion of homocysteine to methionine. Food sources include green leafy vegetables, oranges, and whole grains; folate fortification of grains is now routine in the United States.

Folate deficiency, characterized by **hypersegmented neutrophils**, **macrocytic anemia**, and glossitis, may result from a low dietary intake, malabsorption, or vitamin-drug interactions. Deficiency can develop within a few weeks of birth because infants require 10 times as

much folate as adults relative to body weight but have scant stores of folate in the newborn period. Folate is particularly heat labile. Heat-sterilizing home-prepared formula can decrease the folate content by half. Evaporated milk and goat's milk are low in folate. Patients with chronic hemolysis (sickle cell anemia, thalassemia) may require extra folate to avoid deficiency because of the relatively high requirement of the vitamin to support erythropoiesis. Other conditions with risk of deficiency include pregnancy, alcoholism, and treatment with anticonvulsants (phenytoin) or antimetabolites (methotrexate). First occurrence and recurrence of **neural tube defects** are reduced significantly by maternal supplementation during embryogenesis. Because closure of the neural tube occurs before usual recognition of pregnancy, all women of reproductive age are recommended to have a folate intake of at least 400 μg/day as prophylaxis.

## Vitamin B$_{12}$

Vitamin B$_{12}$ is one of the most complex of the vitamin molecules, containing an atom of cobalt held in a *corrin ring* (similar to that of iron in hemoglobin). The cobalt ion is at the active center of the ring and serves as the site for attachment of alkyl groups during their transfer. The vitamin functions in single-carbon transfers and is intimately related to folate function and interconversions. Vitamin B$_{12}$ is essential for normal lipid and carbohydrate metabolism in energy production and in protein biosynthesis and nucleic acid synthesis.

In contrast to other water-soluble vitamins, absorption of vitamin B$_{12}$ is complex, involving cleavage of the vitamin from dietary protein and binding to a glycoprotein called *intrinsic factor*, which is secreted by the gastric mucosa (parietal cells). The cobalamin–intrinsic factor complex is efficiently absorbed from the distal ileum.

As vitamin $B_{12}$ is absorbed into the portal circulation, it is transported bound to a specific protein, transcobalamin II. Its large stores in the liver also are unusual as a water-soluble vitamin. Efficient enterohepatic circulation normally protects from deficiency for months to years. Dietary sources of the vitamin are animal products only. Strict vegetarians should take a vitamin $B_{12}$ supplement.

Vitamin $B_{12}$ deficiency is rare. Early diagnosis and treatment of this disorder in childhood are important because of the danger of irreversible neurologic damage. Most cases in childhood result from a specific defect in absorption (see Table 31-2). Such defects include **congenital pernicious anemia** (absent intrinsic factor), **juvenile pernicious anemia** (autoimmune), and deficiency of transcobalamin II transport. Gastric or intestinal resection and small bowel bacterial overgrowth also cause vitamin $B_{12}$ deficiency. Exclusively breastfed infants ingest adequate vitamin $B_{12}$ unless the mother is a strict vegetarian without supplementation.

Depression of serum vitamin $B_{12}$ and the appearance of hypersegmented neutrophils and macrocytosis (indistinguishable from folate deficiency) are early clinical manifestations of deficiency. Vitamin $B_{12}$ deficiency also causes **neurologic manifestations**, including depression, peripheral neuropathy, posterior spinal column signs, dementia, and eventual coma. The neurologic signs do not occur in folate deficiency, but administration of folate may mask the hematologic signs of vitamin $B_{12}$ deficiency, while the neurologic manifestations progress. Patients with vitamin $B_{12}$ deficiency also have increased urine levels of methylmalonic acid. Most cases of vitamin $B_{12}$ deficiency in infants and children are not of dietary origin and require treatment throughout life. Maintenance therapy consists of repeated monthly intramuscular injections, although a form of vitamin $B_{12}$ is administered intranasally.

## FAT-SOLUBLE VITAMINS

Fat-soluble vitamins generally have stores in the body, and dietary deficiencies generally develop more slowly than for water-soluble vitamins. Absorption of fat-soluble vitamins depends on normal fat intake, digestion, and absorption. The complexity of normal fat absorption and the potential for perturbation in many disease states explains the more common occurrence of deficiencies of these vitamins.

## Vitamin A

The basic constituent of the vitamin A group is retinol. Ingested plant carotene or animal tissue retinol esters release retinol after hydrolysis by pancreatic and intestinal enzymes. Chylomicron-transported retinol esters are stored in the liver as retinol palmitate. Retinol is transported from the liver to target tissues by retinol-binding protein, releasing free retinol to the target tissues. The kidney then excretes the retinol-binding protein. Diseases of the kidney diminish excretion of retinol-binding protein, whereas liver parenchymal disease or malnutrition lowers the synthesis of retinol-binding protein. Specific cellular binding proteins facilitate the uptake of retinol by target tissues. In the eye, retinol is metabolized to form **rhodopsin**; the action of light on rhodopsin is the first step of the visual process. Retinol also influences the growth and differentiation of epithelia. The clinical manifestations of vitamin A deficiency in humans appear as a group of ocular signs termed **xerophthalmia**. The earliest symptom is **night blindness**, which is followed by **xerosis** of the conjunctiva and cornea. Untreated, xerophthalmia can result in ulceration, necrosis, keratomalacia, and a permanent corneal scar. Clinical and subclinical vitamin A deficiencies are associated with **immunodeficiency**; increased risk of infection, especially measles; and increased risk of mortality, especially in developing nations. Xerophthalmia and vitamin A deficiency should be urgently treated. Treatment is summarized in Table 31-3. Hypervitaminosis A also has serious sequelae, including headaches, pseudotumor cerebri, hepatotoxicity, and teratogenicity.

## Vitamin E

Eight naturally occurring compounds have vitamin E activity. The most active of these, $\alpha$-tocopherol, accounts for 90% of the vitamin E present in human tissues and is commercially available as an acetate or succinate. Vitamin E acts as a biologic **antioxidant** by inhibiting the peroxidation of polyunsaturated fatty acids present in cell membranes. It scavenges free radicals generated by the reduction of molecular oxygen and by the action of oxidative enzymes.

Vitamin E deficiency occurs in children with fat malabsorption secondary to liver disease, untreated celiac disease, cystic fibrosis, and abetalipoproteinemia. In these children, without vitamin E supplementation, a syndrome of progressive **sensory and motor neuropathy** develops; the first sign of deficiency is loss of deep tendon reflexes. Deficient preterm infants at 1 to 2 months of age have hemolytic anemia characterized by an elevated reticulocyte count, an increased sensitivity of the erythrocytes to hemolysis in hydrogen peroxide, peripheral edema, and thrombocytosis. All the abnormalities are corrected after oral, lipid, or water-soluble vitamin E therapy.

## Vitamin D

Cholecalciferol (vitamin $D_3$) is the mammalian form of vitamin D and is produced by ultraviolet irradiation of inactive precursors in the skin. Ergocalciferol (vitamin $D_2$) is derived from plants. Vitamin $D_2$ and vitamin $D_3$ require further metabolism to become active. They are of equivalent potency. Clothing, lack of sunlight exposure, and skin pigmentation decrease generation of vitamin D in the epidermis and dermis.

Vitamin D ($D_2$ and $D_3$) is metabolized in the liver to calcidiol, or 25-hydroxyvitamin D (25-[OH]-D); this metabolite, which has little intrinsic activity, is transported by a plasma-binding globulin to the kidney, where it is converted to the most active metabolite calcitriol, or 1,25-dihydroxyvitamin D (1,25-[OH]$_2$-D). The action of 1,25-(OH)$_2$-D results in a decrease in the concentration of messenger RNA (mRNA) for collagen in bone and an increase in the concentration of mRNA for vitamin D–dependent calcium-binding protein in the intestine (directly mediating increased intestinal calcium transport). The antirachitic action of vitamin D probably is mediated by provision of appropriate concentrations of calcium and phosphate in the extracellular space of bone and by enhanced intestinal absorption of these minerals. Vitamin D also may have a direct anabolic effect on bone. $1,25\text{-}(OH)_2\text{-}D$ has direct feedback to the parathyroid gland and inhibits secretion of parathyroid hormone.

Vitamin D deficiency appears as **rickets** in children and as **osteomalacia** in postpubertal adolescents. Inadequate direct sun exposure and vitamin D intake are sufficient causes, but other factors, such as various drugs (phenobarbital, phenytoin) and malabsorption, may increase the risk of development of vitamin-deficiency rickets. Breastfed infants, especially those with dark-pigmented skin, are at risk for vitamin D deficiency.

The pathophysiology of rickets results from defective bone growth, especially at the epiphyseal cartilage matrix, which fails to mineralize. The uncalcified osteoid results in a wide, irregular zone of poorly supported tissue, the rachitic metaphysis. This soft, rather than hardened, zone produces many of the skeletal deformities through compression and lateral bulging or flaring of the ends of bones.

The **clinical manifestations** of rickets are most common during the first 2 years of life and may become evident only after several months of a vitamin D–deficient diet. **Craniotabes** is caused by thinning of the outer table of the skull, which when compressed feels like a ping pong ball to the touch. Enlargement of the costochondral junction (**rachitic rosary**) and thickening of the wrists and ankles may be palpated. The anterior fontanelle is enlarged and its closure may be delayed. In advanced rickets, scoliosis and exaggerated lordosis may be present. Bowlegs or knock-knees may be evident in older infants, and greenstick fractures may be observed in long bones.

The **diagnosis** of rickets is based on a history of poor vitamin D intake and little exposure to direct ultraviolet sunlight. The serum calcium usually is normal but may be low; the serum phosphorus level usually is reduced, and serum alkaline phosphatase activity is elevated. When serum calcium levels decline to less than 7.5 mg/dL, tetany may occur. Levels of $24,25\text{-}(OH)_2\text{-}D$ are undetectable, and serum $1,25\text{-}(OH)2\text{-}D$ levels are commonly less than 7 ng/mL, although $1,25\text{-}(OH)_2\text{-}D$ levels also may be normal. The best measure of vitamin D status is the level of $25\text{-}(OH)\text{-}D$. Characteristic **radiographic** changes of the distal ulna and radius include widening; concave cupping; and frayed, poorly demarcated ends. The increased space seen between the distal ends of the radius and ulna and the metacarpal bones is the enlarged, nonossified metaphysis.

The **treatment** of vitamin D–deficiency rickets and osteomalacia is presented in Table 31-3. Breastfed infants born of mothers with adequate vitamin D stores usually maintain adequate serum vitamin D levels for at least 2 months, but rickets may develop subsequently if these infants are not exposed to the sun or do not receive supplementary vitamin D. The American Academy of Pediatrics recommends vitamin D supplementation of all breastfed infants in the amount of 400 IU/day, started soon after birth and given until the infant is taking more than 500 mL/day of formula or vitamin D–fortified milk (for age >1 year). Toxic effects of excessive vitamin D include hypercalcemia, muscle weakness, polyuria, and nephrocalcinosis.

## Vitamin K

The plant form of vitamin K is phylloquinone, or vitamin $K_1$. Another form is menaquinone, or vitamin $K_2$, one of a series of compounds with unsaturated side chains synthesized by intestinal bacteria. Plasma factors II (prothrombin), VII, IX, and X in the cascade of blood coagulation factors depend on vitamin K for synthesis and for post-translational conversion of their precursor proteins. The post-translational conversion of glutamyl residues to carboxyglutamic acid residues of a prothrombin molecule creates effective calcium-binding sites, making the protein active.

Other vitamin K–dependent proteins include proteins C, S, and Z in plasma and γ-carboxyglutamic acid–containing proteins in several tissues. Bone contains a major vitamin K–dependent protein, osteocalcin, and lesser amounts of other glutamic acid–containing proteins.

Phylloquinone is absorbed from the intestine and transported by chylomicrons. The rarity of dietary vitamin K deficiency in humans with normal intestinal function suggests that the absorption of menaquinones is possible. Vitamin K deficiency has been observed in subjects with impaired fat absorption caused by obstructive jaundice, pancreatic insufficiency, and celiac disease; often these problems are combined with the use of antibiotics that change intestinal flora.

**Hemorrhagic disease of the newborn**, a disease more common among breastfed infants, occurs in the first few weeks of life. It is rare in infants who receive prophylactic intramuscular vitamin K on the first day of life. Hemorrhagic disease of the newborn usually is marked by generalized ecchymoses, gastrointestinal hemorrhage, or bleeding from a circumcision or umbilical stump; intracranial hemorrhage can occur, but is uncommon. The American Academy of Pediatrics recommends that parenteral vitamin K (0.5 to 1 mg) be given to all newborns shortly after birth.

# MINERALS

The major minerals are those that require intakes of more than 100 mg/day and contribute at least 0.1% of total body weight. There are seven essential major minerals: calcium, phosphorus, magnesium, sodium, potassium, chloride, and sulfur. Ten trace minerals, which constitute less than 0.1% of body weight, have essential physiologic roles. Characteristics of trace mineral deficiencies are listed in Table 31-4.

## Calcium

Calcium is the most abundant major mineral. Ninety-nine percent of calcium is in the skeleton; the remaining 1% is in extracellular fluids, intracellular compartments, and cell membranes. The nonskeletal calcium has a role in nerve conduction, muscle contraction, blood clotting, and membrane permeability. There are two distinct bone calcium phosphate pools—a large, crystalline form and a

## TABLE 31–4 Characteristics of Trace Mineral Deficiencies

| Mineral | Function | Manifestations of Deficiency | Comments | Sources |
|---|---|---|---|---|
| Iron | Heme-containing macromolecules (e.g., hemoglobin, cytochrome, and myoglobin) | Anemia, spoon nails, reduced muscle and mental performance | History of pica, cow's milk, gastrointestinal bleeding | Meat, liver, grains, legumes |
| Copper | Redox reactions (e.g., cytochrome oxidase) | Hypochromic anemia, neutropenia, osteoporosis, hypotonia, hypoproteinemia | Inborn error, Menkes kinky hair syndrome | Liver, nuts, grains, legumes, chocolate |
| Zinc | Metalloenzymes (e.g., alkaline phosphatase, carbonic anhydrase, DNA polymerase); wound healing | *Acrodermatitis enteropathica:* poor growth, acro-orificial rash, alopecia, delayed sexual development, hypogeusia, infection | Protein-calorie malnutrition; weaning; malabsorption syndromes | Meat, grains, legumes |
| Selenium | Antioxidant; glutathione peroxidase | Keshan cardiomyopathy in China | Endemic areas; long-term TPN without Se | Meat, vegetables |
| Chromium | Insulin cofactor | Poor weight gain, glucose intolerance, neuropathy | Protein-calorie malnutrition, long-term TPN without Cr | Yeast, breads |
| Fluoride | Strengthening of dental enamel | Caries | Supplementation during tooth growth, narrow therapeutic range, fluorosis may cause staining of the teeth | Seafood, fortified water |
| Iodine | Thyroxine, triiodothyronine production | Simple endemic goiter *Myxedematous cretinism:* congenital hypothyroidism *Neurologic cretinism:* mental retardation, deafness, spasticity, normal thyroxine level at birth | Endemic in New Guinea, the Congo; endemic in Great Lakes area before use of iodized salt | Seafood, iodized salt |

TPN, total parenteral nutrition.

smaller, amorphous phase. Bone calcium constantly turns over, with concurrent bone resorption and formation. Approximately half of **bone mineral accretion** occurs during adolescence. Bone mineral density peaks in early adulthood and is influenced by prior and concurrent dietary calcium intake, exercise, and hormone status (testosterone, estrogen).

Calcium intake can come from a variety of sources, with dairy products providing the most common and concentrated source. The calcium equivalent of 1 cup of milk (about 300 mg of calcium) is ¾ cup of plain yogurt, 1.5 oz of cheddar cheese, 2 cups of ice cream, ⅘ cup of almonds, or 2.5 oz of sardines. Other sources of calcium include some leafy green vegetables (broccoli, kale, collards); lime-processed tortillas; calcium-precipitated tofu; and calcium-fortified juices, cereals, and breads.

There is no classic calcium deficiency syndrome because blood and cell levels are closely regulated. The body can mobilize skeletal calcium and increase the absorptive efficiency of dietary calcium. **Osteoporosis** that occurs in childhood is related to protein-calorie malnutrition, vitamin C deficiency, steroid therapy, endocrine disorders, immobilization and disuse, osteogenesis imperfecta, or calcium deficiency (in premature infants). It is believed that the primary method of prevention of **postmenopausal osteoporosis** is to ensure maximum peak bone mass by providing optimal calcium intake during childhood and adolescence. Bone mineral status can be monitored by dual-energy x-ray absorptiometry.

No adverse effects are observed in adults with dietary calcium intakes of 2.5 g/day. There is concern that higher intakes may increase the risk of urinary stone formation, constipation, and decreased renal function and may inhibit intestinal absorption of other minerals (iron, zinc).

## Iron

Iron, the most abundant trace mineral, is used in the synthesis of hemoglobin, myoglobin, and enzyme iron. Body iron content is regulated primarily through modulation of iron absorption, which depends on the state of body iron stores, the form and amount of iron in foods, and the mixture of foods in the diet. There are two categories of iron in food. The first is **heme iron**, present in hemoglobin and myoglobin, which is supplied by meat and rarely accounts for more than one fourth of the iron ingested by infants. The absorption of heme iron is relatively efficient and is not influenced by other constituents of the diet. The second category is **nonheme iron**, which represents the preponderance of iron intake consumed by infants and exists in the form of iron salts. The absorption of nonheme iron is influenced by the composition of consumed foods. Enhancers of nonheme iron absorption are ascorbic acid, meat, fish, and poultry. Inhibitors are bran, polyphenols (including the tannates in tea), and phytic acid, a compound found in legumes and whole grains. The percent intestinal absorption of the small amount of iron in human milk is 10%; 4% is absorbed from iron-fortified cow's milk formula and from iron-fortified infant dry cereals.

In a normal term infant, there is little change in total body iron and little need for exogenous iron before 4 months of age. Iron deficiency is rare in term infants during the first 4 months, unless there has been substantial blood loss (see Chapter 62). After about 4 months of age, iron reserves become marginal, and, unless exogenous sources of iron are provided, the infant becomes progressively at risk for anemia as the iron requirement to support erythropoiesis and growth increases (see Chapter 150). Premature or low birth weight infants have a lower amount of stored iron because significant amounts of iron are transferred from the mother in the third trimester. In addition, their postnatal iron needs are greater because of rapid rates of growth and when frequent phlebotomy occurs. Iron needs can be met by supplementation (ferrous sulfate) or by iron-containing complementary foods. Under normal circumstances, iron-fortified formula should be the only alternative to breast milk in infants younger than 1 year of age. Premature infants fed human milk may develop iron deficiency anemia earlier unless they receive iron supplements. Formula-fed preterm infants should receive iron-fortified formula.

In older children, iron deficiency may result from inadequate iron intake with excessive cow's milk intake or from intake of foods with poor iron bioavailability. Iron deficiency also can result from blood loss from such sources as menses or gastric ulceration. Iron deficiency affects many tissues (muscle and central nervous system) in addition to producing anemia. **Iron deficiency** and **anemia** have been associated with lethargy and decreased work capacity and **impaired neurocognitive development**, the deficits of which may be irreversible when onset is in the first 2 years of life.

The diagnosis of iron deficiency anemia is established by the presence of a microcytic hypochromic anemia, low serum ferritin levels, low serum iron levels, reduced transferrin saturation, normal to elevated red blood cell width distribution, and enhanced iron-binding capacity. The mean corpuscular volume and red blood cell indices are reduced, and the reticulocyte count is low. Iron deficiency may be present without anemia. Clinical manifestations are noted in Table 31-4.

**Treatment** of iron deficiency anemia includes changes in the diet to provide adequate iron and the administration of 2 to 6 mg iron/kg/24 hr (as ferrous sulfate) divided BID or TID. Reticulocytosis is noted within 3 to 7 days of starting treatment. Oral treatment should be continued for 5 months. Rarely, intramuscular or intravenous iron therapy is needed if oral iron cannot be given. Parenteral therapy carries the risk of anaphylaxis and should be administered according to a strict protocol, including a test dose.

### Zinc

Zinc is the second most abundant trace mineral and is important in protein metabolism and synthesis, in nucleic acid metabolism, and in stabilization of cell membranes. Zinc functions as a cofactor for more than 200 enzymes and is essential to numerous cellular metabolic functions. Adequate zinc status is especially crucial during periods of growth and for tissue proliferation (immune system, wound healing, skin and gastrointestinal tract integrity); physiologic functions for which zinc is essential include normal growth, sexual maturation, and immune function.

Dietary zinc is absorbed (20% to 40%) in the duodenum and proximal small intestine. The best dietary sources of zinc are animal products, including human milk, from which it is readily absorbed. Whole grains and legumes also contain moderate amounts of zinc, but phytic acid inhibits absorption from these sources. On a global basis, poor bioavailability secondary to phytic acid is thought to be a more important factor than low intake in the widespread occurrence of zinc deficiency. Excretion of zinc occurs from the gastrointestinal tract. In the presence of ongoing losses, such as in chronic diarrhea, requirements can drastically increase.

**Zinc deficiency dwarfism** syndrome was first described in a group of children in the Middle East with low levels of zinc in their hair, poor appetite, diminished taste acuity, hypogonadism, and short stature. Zinc supplementation reduces morbidity and mortality from **diarrhea** and **pneumonia** and enhances growth in developing countries. Mild to moderate zinc deficiency is considered to be highly prevalent in developing countries, particularly in populations with high rates of **stunting**. Mild zinc deficiency occurs in older breastfed infants without adequate zinc intake from complementary foods or in young children with poor total or bioavailable zinc intake in the general diet. A high infectious burden also may increase the risk of zinc deficiency in developing countries. Acute, acquired severe zinc deficiency occurs in patients receiving total parenteral nutrition without zinc supplementation and in premature infants fed human milk without fortification. **Clinical manifestations** of mild zinc deficiency include anorexia, growth faltering, and immune impairment. Moderately severe manifestations include delayed sexual maturation, rough skin, and hepatosplenomegaly. The signs of severe deficiency include acral and periorificial erythematous, scaling dermatitis; growth and immune impairment; diarrhea; mood changes; alopecia; night blindness; and photophobia.

**Diagnosis** of zinc deficiency is challenging. Plasma zinc concentration is most commonly used, but levels are frequently normal in conditions of mild deficiency; levels in moderate to severe deficiency are typically less than 60 µg/dL. Acute infection also can result in depression of circulating zinc levels. The standard for the diagnosis of deficiency is response to a trial of supplementation, with outcomes such as improved linear growth or weight gain, improved appetite, and improved immune function. Because there is no pharmacologic effect of zinc on these functions, a positive response to supplementation is considered evidence of a preexisting deficiency. Clinically an empirical trial of zinc supplementation (1 mg/kg/day) is a safe and reasonable approach in situations in which deficiency is considered possible.

**Acrodermatitis enteropathica** is an autosomal recessive disorder that begins within 2 to 4 weeks after infants have been weaned from breast milk. It is characterized by an acute perioral and perianal dermatitis, alopecia, and failure to thrive. The disease is caused by severe zinc deficiency from a specific defect of intestinal zinc absorption. Plasma zinc levels are markedly reduced, and serum alkaline phosphatase activity is low. **Treatment** is with high-dose oral zinc supplements. A relatively uncommon condition associated with presentation of severe zinc deficiency is due to a defect in the secretion of zinc from the mammary gland, resulting in abnormally low milk zinc concentrations. Breastfed infants, especially those born prematurely, present with classic signs of zinc deficiency: growth failure, diarrhea, and dermatitis. Because there is no defect in the infant's ability to absorb zinc, treatment consists of supplementing the infant with zinc for the duration of breastfeeding, which can be successfully continued. Subsequent infants born to the mother will also need zinc supplementation if breastfed. Zinc is relatively nontoxic. Excess intake produces nausea, emesis, abdominal pain, headache, vertigo, and seizures.

## Fluoride

Dental enamel is strengthened when fluoride is substituted for hydroxyl ions in the hydroxyapatite crystalline mineral matrix of the enamel. The resulting fluoroapatite is more resistant to chemical and physical damage. Fluoride is incorporated into the enamel during the mineralization stages of tooth formation and by surface interaction after the tooth has erupted. Fluoride is similarly incorporated into bone mineral and may protect against osteoporosis later in life.

Because of concern about the risk of **fluorosis**, infants should not receive fluoride supplements before 6 months of age. Commercial formulas are made with defluoridated water and contain small amounts of fluoride. An infant older than 6 months of age who receives only ready-feed formula or is exclusively breastfed may benefit from supplemental fluoride. The fluoride content of human milk is low and is not influenced significantly by maternal intake. Fluoride levels of the water supply to which the child is exposed should be determined before fluoride supplements are prescribed. If the concentration of fluoride in the drinking water is less than 0.3 ppm, a supplement of 0.25 mg/day is recommended for infants and children 6 months to 3 years of age.

## SUGGESTED READING

Barlow SE: Expert Committee recommendations regarding the prevention, assessment, and treatment of child and adolescent overweight and obesity: summary report, *Pediatrics* 120:S165, 2007.

Centers for Disease Control: Provisional rates of any and exclusive breastfeeding by age among children born in 2005. http://www.cdc.gov/breastfeeding/data/NIS_data/2005/age.htm.

Daniels SR, Greer FR: the AAP Committee on Nutrition: Lipid screening and cardiovascular health in childhood, *Pediatrics* 122:198–208, 2008.

Gidding SS, Dennison BA, Birch LL, et al: Dietary recommendations for children and adolescents: a guide for practitioners: consensus statement form the American Heart Association, *Circulation* 112:2061–2075, 2005.

Kleinman RE, editor: Pediatric Nutrition Handbook, 6th ed, Washington, DC, 2008, *American Academy of Pediatrics*.

Kliegman RM, Behrman RE, Jenson HB, et al: Nelson Textbook of Pediatrics, 18th ed, Chap. 40–44, Philadelphia, 2007, *Saunders*.

Kramer MS, Guo T, Platt RW, et al: Infant growth and health outcomes associated with 3 compared with 6 mo of exclusive breastfeeding, *Am J Clin Nutr* 78:291–295, 2003.

Krebs NF: Food choices to meet nutritional needs of breast fed infants and toddlers on mixed diets, *J Nutr* 137(2):511S–517S, 2007.

Krebs NF, Hambidge KM, Trace elements. In Duggan C, Watkins JB, Walker WA, editors: Nutrition in Pediatrics: Basic Science and Clinical Applications, 4th ed, Hamilton, Ontario, 2008, *BC Decker*, pp 67–82.

Penny ME, Protein-energy malnutrition: pathophysiology, clinical consequences, and treatment. In Duggan C, Watkins JB, Walker WA, editors: Nutrition in Pediatrics: Basic Science and Clinical Applications, 4th ed, Hamilton, Ontario, 2008, *BC Decker*, pp 127–142.

Wagner CL, Greer FR: Section on Breastfeeding and Committee on Nutrition, American Academy of Pediatrics: Prevention of rickets and vitamin D deficiency: new guidelines for vitamin D intake, *Pediatrics* 122:1142–1152, 2008.

# FLUIDS AND ELECTROLYTES

Larry A. Greenbaum

CHAPTER **32**

# Maintenance Fluid Therapy

## BODY COMPOSITION

Water is the most plentiful constituent of the human body. **Total body water** (TBW) as a percentage of body weight varies with age. The fetus has a high TBW, which gradually decreases to about 75% of birth weight for a term infant. Premature infants have a higher TBW content than term infants. During the first year of life, TBW decreases to about 60% of body weight and basically remains at this level until puberty. At puberty, the fat content of females increases more than males, who acquire more muscle mass than females. Because fat has low water content, and muscle has high water content, by the end of puberty TBW in males remains at 60%, but it decreases to 50% of body weight in females. During dehydration, TBW decreases and is a smaller percentage of body weight.

TBW has two main compartments: **intracellular fluid (ICF)** and **extracellular fluid (ECF)**. In the fetus and newborn, the ECF volume is larger than the ICF volume. The normal postnatal diuresis causes an immediate decrease in the ECF volume. This decrease in ECF volume is followed by continued expansion of the ICF volume because of cellular growth. By 1 year of age, the ratio of the ICF volume to the ECF volume approaches adult levels. The ECF volume is 20% to 25% of body weight, and the ICF volume is 30% to 40% of body weight (Fig. 32-1). With puberty, the increased muscle mass of males results in a higher ICF volume than females.

The ECF is divided further into **plasma water** and **interstitial fluid** (see Fig. 32-1). Plasma water is about 5% of body weight. The blood volume, given a hematocrit of 40%, is usually 8% of body weight, although it is higher in newborns and young infants. In premature newborns, it is around 10% of body weight. The volume of plasma water can be altered by pathologic conditions, including dehydration, anemia, polycythemia, heart failure,

abnormal plasma osmolality, and hypoalbuminemia. The interstitial fluid, normally 15% of body weight, can increase dramatically in diseases associated with edema, such as heart failure, protein-losing enteropathy, liver failure, and nephrotic syndrome.

The composition of solutes in the ICF and ECF is different. Sodium and chloride are the dominant cation and anion in the ECF. Potassium is the most abundant cation in the ICF, and proteins, organic anions, and phosphate are the most plentiful anions in the ICF. The dissimilarity between the anions in the ICF and the ECF is determined largely by the presence of intracellular molecules that do not cross the cell membrane, the barrier separating the ECF and the ICF. In contrast, the difference in the distribution of cations—sodium and potassium—is due to the activity of the $Na^+$, $K^+$-ATPase pump, which uses cellular energy to actively extrude sodium from cells and move potassium into cells.

## REGULATION OF INTRAVASCULAR VOLUME AND OSMOLALITY

Proper cell functioning requires close regulation of plasma osmolality and intravascular volume; these are controlled by independent systems for water balance, which determines osmolality, and sodium balance, which determines volume status. Maintenance of a normal **osmolality** depends on control of water balance. Control of **volume status** depends on regulation of sodium balance.

The plasma osmolality is tightly regulated between 285 and 295 mOsm/kg. Modification of water intake and excretion maintains a normal plasma osmolality. In the steady state, water intake and water produced from oxidation balances water losses from the skin, lungs, urine, and gastrointestinal tract. Only water intake and urinary losses can be regulated. A small increase in the plasma osmolality stimulates thirst. Urinary water losses are regulated by the secretion of **antidiuretic hormone** (ADH), which increases in response to an increasing plasma osmolality. ADH, by stimulating renal tubular reabsorption of water, decreases urinary water losses. Control of osmolality is subordinate to maintenance of an adequate intravascular volume. When significant volume depletion

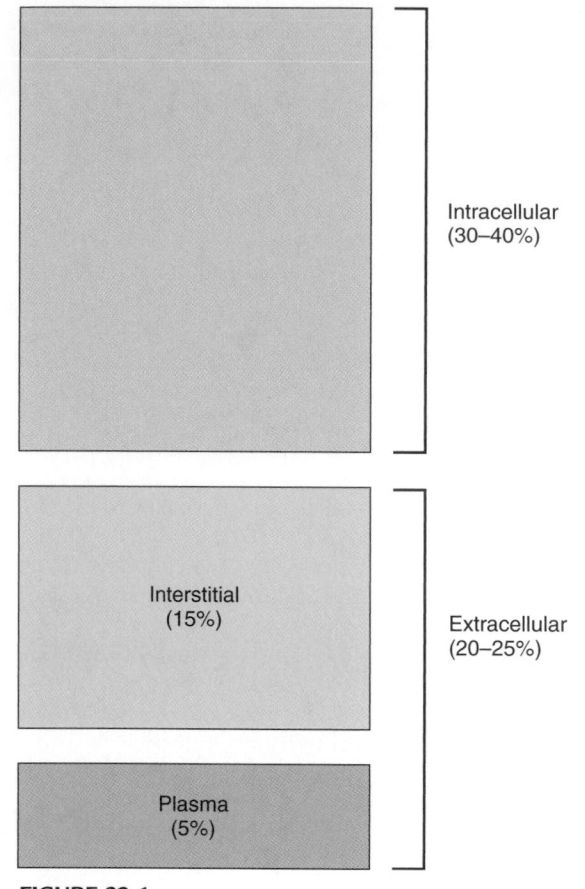

**FIGURE 32-1**

Compartments of total body water, expressed as percentage of body weight, in an older child or adult. (From Greenbaum LA: Pathophysiology of body fluids and fluid therapy. In Kliegman RM, Behrman RE, Jenson HB, et al: Nelson Textbook of Pediatrics, 18th ed. Philadelphia, 2007, *Elsevier Science*, p 268.)

is present, ADH secretion and thirst are stimulated, regardless of the plasma osmolality.

Volume depletion and volume overload may cause significant morbidity and mortality. Because sodium is the principal extracellular cation and is restricted to the ECF, adequate body sodium is necessary for maintenance of intravascular volume. The kidney determines sodium balance because there is little homeostatic control of sodium intake, although salt craving occasionally occurs, typically in children with chronic renal salt loss. The kidney regulates sodium balance by altering the percentage of filtered sodium that is reabsorbed along the nephron. The **renin-angiotensin system** is an important regulator of renal sodium reabsorption and excretion. The juxtaglomerular apparatus produces renin in response to decreased effective intravascular volume. Renin cleaves angiotensinogen, producing angiotensin I, which angiotensin-converting enzyme converts into angiotensin II. The actions of angiotensin II include direct stimulation of the proximal tubule to increase sodium reabsorption and stimulation of the adrenal gland to increase aldosterone secretion, which increases sodium reabsorption in the distal nephron.

Volume expansion stimulates the synthesis of **atrial natriuretic peptide**, which is produced by the atria in response to atrial wall distention. Along with increasing glomerular filtration rate, atrial natriuretic peptide inhibits sodium reabsorption, facilitating an increase in urinary sodium excretion.

## MAINTENANCE FLUIDS

Maintenance intravenous (IV) fluids are used in children who cannot be fed enterally. Along with maintenance fluids, children may require concurrent **replacement fluids** if they have excessive **ongoing losses**, such as may occur with drainage from a nasogastric tube. In addition, if dehydration is present, the patient also needs to receive deficit replacement (see Chapter 33).

Maintenance fluids are composed of a solution of water, glucose, sodium, potassium, and chloride. This solution replaces electrolyte losses from the urine and stool, as well as water losses from the urine, stool, skin, and lungs. The glucose in maintenance fluids provides approximately 20% of the normal caloric needs of the patient. This percentage is enough to prevent the development of starvation ketoacidosis and diminishes the protein degradation that would occur if the patient received no calories. Glucose also provides added osmoles, avoiding the administration of hypotonic fluids, which may cause hemolysis.

Maintenance fluids do not provide adequate calories, protein, fat, minerals, or vitamins. Because of inadequate calories, a child on maintenance IV fluids loses 0.5% to 1% of real weight each day. Patients should not remain on maintenance therapy indefinitely; parenteral nutrition (see Chapter 34) should be used for children who cannot be fed enterally for more than a few days. Parenteral nutrition is especially important in a patient with underlying malnutrition.

Daily water losses are measurable (urine and stool) and not measurable (*insensible losses* from the skin and lungs). Failure to replace these losses leads to a thirsty, uncomfortable child and, ultimately, a dehydrated child. Table 32-1 provides a system for calculating **24-hour maintenance water** needs based on the patient's weight. Sodium and potassium are given in maintenance fluids to replace losses from urine and stool.

| TABLE 32-1 Body Weight Method for Calculating Maintenance Fluid Volume and Rate | | |
|---|---|---|
| **Body Weight (kg)** | **Volume Per Day** | **Hourly Rate** |
| 0–10 | 100 mL/kg | 4 mL/kg/hr |
| 11–20 | 1000 mL 50 mL/kg for each 1 kg >10 kg | 40 mL/hr 2 mL/kg/hr × (wt − 10) |
| >20 | 1500 mL 20 mL/kg for each 1 kg >20 kg* | 60 mL/hr 1 mL/kg/hr × (wt − 20)[†] |

*The maximum total fluid per day is normally 2400 mL.
[†]The maximum fluid rate is normally 100 mL/hr.

After calculation of water needs and electrolyte needs, children typically receive either 5% dextrose (D5) in ¼ normal saline (NS) plus 20 mEq/L of potassium chloride (KCl) or D5 in ½ NS plus 20 mEq/L of KCl. Children weighing less than 10 kg do best with the solution containing ¼ NS (38.5 mEq/L) because of their high water needs per kilogram. In contrast, larger children and adults may receive the solution with ½ NS (77 mEq/L). These guidelines assume that there is no disease process present that would require an adjustment in either the volume or the electrolyte composition of maintenance fluids. (Children with renal insufficiency may be hyperkalemic or unable to excrete potassium and may not tolerate 20 mEq/L of KCl.) In children with complicated pathophysiologic derangements, it may be necessary to adjust the electrolyte composition and rate of maintenance fluids empirically based on electrolyte measurements and assessment of fluid balance.

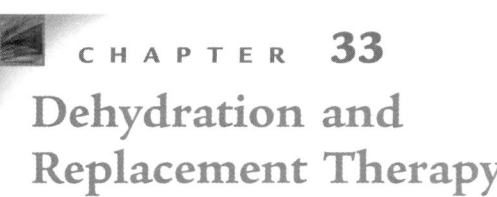

# CHAPTER 33

# Dehydration and Replacement Therapy

## REPLACEMENT THERAPY

Table 33-1 lists the three sources of normal water loss—the components of maintenance water (see Chapter 32). **Insensible losses**, composed of evaporative losses from the skin and lungs, represent approximately one third of total maintenance water. Sweating is not insensible and, in contrast to evaporative losses, sweat contains water and electrolytes.

A variety of clinical situations modify normal maintenance water balance (Table 33-2). Evaporative skin water losses can be significant in neonates, especially premature infants who are under radiant warmers or undergoing phototherapy. Burns can result in massive losses of water and electrolytes (see Chapter 44). Fever leads to a predictable increase in insensible losses, causing a 10% to 15% increase in maintenance water needs for each 1°C increase in temperature greater than 38°C. Tachypnea or a tracheostomy increases evaporative losses from the lungs.

The gastrointestinal tract is potentially a source of considerable water and electrolyte losses. A child who has large amounts of gastrointestinal losses should have these losses measured and replaced with an appropriate **replacement solution**. It is impossible to predict gastrointestinal losses

### TABLE 33-1  Components of Maintenance Water

| | |
|---|---|
| Urine | 60% |
| Insensible losses (skin and lungs) | 35% |
| Stool | 5% |

### TABLE 33-2  Adjustments in Maintenance Water

| Source | Causes of Increased Water Needs | Causes of Decreased Water Needs |
|---|---|---|
| Skin | Radiant warmer<br>Phototherapy<br>Fever<br>Sweat<br>Burns | Mist tent<br>Incubator (premature infants) |
| Lungs | Tachypnea<br>Tracheostomy | Humidified ventilator<br>Mist tent |
| Gastrointestinal | Diarrhea<br>Emesis<br>Nasogastric suction | |
| Renal | Polyuria | Oliguria/anuria |
| Miscellaneous | Surgical drain<br>Third space losses | Hypothyroidism |

for the next 24 hours. Hence, losses should be replaced after they occur, using a solution with the same approximate electrolyte concentration as the gastrointestinal fluid. Electrolyte content can be measured directly, or a solution can be selected based on the typical electrolyte composition of diarrhea or gastric losses (Table 33-3). The losses usually are replaced every 1 to 6 hours, depending on the rate of loss, with rapid losses being replaced more frequently. The child should also receive an appropriate maintenance fluid (see Chapter 32).

### TABLE 33-3  Adjusting Fluid Therapy for Gastrointestinal Losses

| Average Composition | Approach to Replacement |
|---|---|
| **Diarrhea**<br>Sodium: 55 mEq/L<br>Potassium: 25 mEq/L<br>Bicarbonate: 15 mEq/L | **Replacement of Ongoing Stool Losses**<br>Solution: 5% dextrose in ¼ normal saline + 20 mEq/L sodium bicarbonate + 20 mEq/L potassium chloride<br>Replace stool mL/mL every 1–6 hr |
| **Gastric Fluid**<br>Sodium: 60 mEq/L<br>Potassium: 10 mEq/L<br>Chloride: 90 mEq/L | **Replacement of Ongoing Gastric Losses**<br>Solution: normal saline + 10 mEq/L potassium chloride<br>Replace output mL/mL every 1–6 hr |

Urine output is normally the largest cause of water loss. Diseases such as renal failure and the syndrome of inappropriate antidiuretic hormone (SIADH), can lead to a decrease in urine volume. Continuation of maintenance fluids in a patient with oliguria or anuria produces fluid overload. In contrast, other conditions produce an increase in urine volume; these include the polyuric phase of acute tubular necrosis, diabetes mellitus, and diabetes insipidus. The patient must receive more than standard maintenance fluids when the urine output is excessive to prevent dehydration.

The approach to decreased or increased urine output is similar (Table 33-4). Insensible losses are replaced by a solution that is administered at a rate one third of the normal maintenance rate. Placing the **anuric** child on "insensibles" theoretically maintains an even fluid balance, with the caveat that one third of maintenance fluid is only an *estimate* of insensible losses. In the individual patient, this rate may need to be adjusted based on monitoring of the patient's weight and hydration status. An **oliguric** child needs to receive a urine replacement solution.

Most children with **polyuria** (except for children with diabetes mellitus [see Chapter 171]) should be placed on insensible fluids plus urine replacement. When urine output is excessive, it is important to measure the sodium and potassium concentration of the urine to determine the electrolyte composition of the urine replacement solution.

Output from surgical drains and chest tubes, when significant, should be measured and replaced. **Third space losses** manifest with edema and ascites and are due to a shift of fluid from the intravascular space into the interstitial space. Third space losses cannot be quantitated easily. Nonetheless, these losses can be large and lead to intravascular volume depletion, despite weight gain. Replacement of third space fluid is empirical but should be anticipated in patients who are at risk, such as children who have burns or abdominal surgery. Third space losses and chest tube output are isotonic and usually require replacement with an **isotonic fluid**, such as normal saline or Ringer's lactate. Adjustments in the amount of replacement fluid for third space losses are based on continuing assessment of the patient's intravascular volume status.

## TABLE 33-4 Adjusting Fluid Therapy for Altered Renal Output

| Oliguria/Anuria | Polyuria |
| --- | --- |
| Place the patient on insensible fluids (1/3 maintenance) | Place the patient on insensible fluids (1/3 maintenance) |
| Replace urine output mL/mL with half normal saline | Measure urine electrolytes |
| | Replace urine output mL/mL with a solution that is based on the measured urine electrolytes |

# DEHYDRATION

Dehydration, most often due to gastroenteritis, is common in children. The first step in caring for a child with dehydration is to assess the degree of dehydration. The degree of dehydration dictates the urgency of the situation and the volume of fluid needed for rehydration. Table 33-5 summarizes the clinical features that are present with varying degrees of dehydration.

An infant with **mild dehydration** (3% to 5% of body weight dehydrated) has few clinical signs or symptoms. The infant may be thirsty; the alert parent may notice a decline in urine output. The history describes decreased intake and increased fluid losses. An infant with **moderate dehydration** has demonstrable physical signs and symptoms. Intravascular space depletion is evident by an increased heart rate and reduced urine output. The patient is 10% dehydrated and needs fairly prompt intervention. An infant with **severe dehydration** is gravely ill. The decrease in blood pressure indicates that vital organs may be receiving inadequate perfusion (shock) (see Chapter 40). The infant is at least 15% dehydrated and should receive immediate and aggressive intravenous (IV) therapy. Mild, moderate, and severe dehydration represent 3%, 6%, and 9% of body weight lost in older children and adults. This difference is because water is a higher percentage of body weight in infants (see Chapter 32). Clinical assessment of dehydration is only an estimate; the patient must be continually re-evaluated during therapy. The degree of dehydration is underestimated in hypernatremic dehydration because the osmotically driven shift of water from the intracellular space to the extracellular space helps to preserve the intravascular volume.

## Laboratory Evaluation

Serum blood urea nitrogen (BUN) and creatinine concentrations are useful in assessing a child with dehydration. Volume depletion without renal insufficiency may cause a disproportionate increase in the BUN, with little or no change in the creatinine concentration. This situation is secondary to increased passive reabsorption of urea in the proximal tubule caused by appropriate renal conservation of sodium and water. This increase in the BUN may be absent or blunted in a child with poor protein intake because urea production depends on protein degradation. Conversely, the BUN may be disproportionately increased in a child with increased urea production, as occurs in a child with a gastrointestinal bleed or a child who is receiving glucocorticoids. A significant elevation of the creatinine concentration suggests renal injury.

The urine specific gravity is usually elevated ($\geq 1.025$) in cases of significant dehydration but decreases after rehydration. With dehydration, a urinalysis may show hyaline and granular casts, a few white blood cells and red blood cells, and 30 to 100 mg/dL of proteinuria. These findings usually are not associated with significant renal pathology, and they remit with therapy. Hemoconcentration from dehydration causes an increase in the hematocrit and hemoglobin.

| TABLE 33-5 Assessment of Degree of Dehydration | | | |
|---|---|---|---|
| | **Mild** | **Moderate** | **Severe** |
| Infant | 5% | 10% | 15% |
| Adolescent | 3% | 6% | 9% |
| Infants and young children | Thirsty, alert; restless | Thirsty; restless or lethargic; irritable | Drowsy; limp, cold, sweaty, cyanotic extremities; may be comatose |
| Older children | Thirsty, alert | Thirsty, alert (usually) | Usually conscious (but at reduced level), apprehensive; cold, sweaty, cyanotic extremities; wrinkled skin on fingers and toes; muscle cramps |
| **SIGNS AND SYMPTOMS** | | | |
| Tachycardia | Absent | Present | Present |
| Palpable pulses | Present | Present (weak) | Decreased |
| Blood pressure | Normal | Orthostatic hypotension | Hypotension |
| Cutaneous perfusion | Normal | Normal | Reduced and mottled |
| Skin turgor | Normal | Slight reduction | Reduced |
| Fontanel | Normal | Slightly depressed | Sunken |
| Mucous membrane | Moist | Dry | Very dry |
| Tears | Present | Present or absent | Absent |
| Respirations | Normal | Deep, may be rapid | Deep and rapid |
| Urine output | Normal | Oliguria | Anuria and severe oliguria |

Data from World Health Organization.

## Calculation of Fluid Deficit

A child with dehydration has lost water; there is usually a concurrent loss of sodium and potassium. The fluid deficit is the percentage of dehydration multiplied by the patient's weight (for a 10-kg child, 10% of 10 kg >1 L deficit).

## Approach to Dehydration

The child with dehydration requires acute intervention to ensure that there is adequate tissue perfusion (see Chapter 40). This resuscitation phase requires rapid restoration of the circulating intravascular volume which should be done with an isotonic solution, such as normal saline (NS) or Ringer's lactate. Blood is an appropriate fluid choice for a child with acute blood loss. The child is given a fluid bolus, usually 20 mL/kg of the isotonic solution, over about 20 minutes. A child with severe dehydration may require multiple fluid boluses and may need to receive fluid at a faster rate. The initial resuscitation and rehydration is complete when the child has an adequate intravascular volume. Typically the child has some general clinical improvement, including a lower heart rate, normalization of the blood pressure, improved perfusion, and a more alert affect.

With adequate intravascular volume, it is now appropriate to plan the fluid therapy for the next 24 hours (Table 33-6). In order to assure that the intravascular volume is restored, the patient receives an additional 20 mL/kg bolus of isotonic fluid over 2 hours. The child's total fluid needs are added together (maintenance + deficit). The volume of isotonic fluids the patient has received as acute resuscitation is subtracted from this total. The remaining fluid volume is then administered over 24 hours. Potassium usually is not included in the IV fluids until the patient voids, unless significant hypokalemia is present. Children with significant ongoing losses need to receive an appropriate replacement solution.

## Monitoring and Adjusting Therapy

All calculations in fluid therapy are only approximations. Thus, the patient needs to be monitored during treatment with therapy modifications based on the clinical situation (Table 33-7).

**Hyponatremic dehydration** occurs in children who have diarrhea and consume a hypotonic fluid (water or diluted formula). Volume depletion stimulates secretion of antidiuretic hormone, preventing the water excretion that should correct the hyponatremia. Some patients develop symptoms, predominantly neurologic, from the hyponatremia (see Chapter 35). Most patients with hyponatremic

| TABLE 33-6 Fluid Management of Dehydration |
|---|
| Restore intravascular volume |
|     Normal saline: 20 mL/kg over 20 minutes |
|     Repeat as needed |
| Rapid volume repletion: 20 mL/kg normal saline (maximum = 1 L) over 2 hours |
| Calculate 24-hour fluid needs: maintenance + deficit volume |
| Subtract isotonic fluid already administered from 24-hour fluid needs |
| Administer remaining volume over 24 hours using D5 ½ normal saline + 20 mEq/L KCl |
| Replace ongoing losses as they occur |

| TABLE 33-7 Monitoring Therapy |
| --- |
| Vital signs |
|     Pulse |
|     Blood pressure |
| Intake and output |
|     Fluid balance |
|     Urine output and specific gravity |
| Physical examination |
|     Weight |
|     Clinical signs of depletion or overload |
| Electrolytes |

| TABLE 33-8 Treatment of Hypernatremic Dehydration |
| --- |
| Restore intravascular volume |
|     Normal saline: 20 mL/kg over 20 minutes (repeat until intravascular volume restored) |
| Determine time for correction based on initial sodium concentration |
|     [Na] 145–157 mEq/L: 24 hr |
|     [Na] 158–170 mEq/L: 48 hr |
|     [Na] 171–183 mEq/L: 72 hr |
|     [Na] 184–196 mEq/L: 84 hr |
| Administer fluid at a constant rate over the time for correction |
|     Typical fluid: D5 1/2 normal saline (with 20 mEq/L potassium chloride unless contraindicated) |
|     Typical rate: 1.25–1.5 times maintenance |
| Follow serum sodium concentration |
| Adjust fluid based on clinical status and serum sodium concentration |
|     Signs of volume depletion: administer normal saline (20 mL/kg) |
|     Sodium decreases too rapidly |
|         Increase sodium concentration of IV fluid *or* |
|         Decrease rate of IV fluid |
|     Sodium decreases too slowly |
|         Decrease sodium concentration of IV fluid *or* |
|         Increase rate of IV fluid |
| Replace excessive ongoing losses as they occur |

IV, intravenous.

dehydration do well with the same general approach outlined in Table 33-6. Overly rapid correction of hyponatremia (>12 mEq/L/24 hr) should be avoided because of the remote risk of **central pontine myelinolysis**.

**Hypernatremic dehydration** is usually a consequence of an inability to take in fluid, because of a lack of access, a poor thirst mechanism (neurologic impairment), intractable emesis, or anorexia. The movement of water from the intracellular space to the extracellular space during hypernatremic dehydration partially protects the intravascular volume. Urine output may be preserved longer, and there may be less tachycardia. Children with hypernatremic dehydration are often lethargic and irritable. Hypernatremia may cause fever, hypertonicity, and hyperreflexia. More severe neurologic symptoms may develop if cerebral bleeding or thrombosis occurs.

Overly rapid treatment of hypernatremic dehydration may cause significant morbidity and mortality. **Idiogenic osmoles** are generated within the brain during the development of hypernatremia. These idiogenic osmoles increase the osmolality within the cells of the brain, providing protection against brain cell shrinkage secondary to movement of water out of cells into the hypertonic extracellular fluid. These idiogenic osmoles dissipate slowly during correction of hypernatremia. With rapid lowering of the extracellular osmolality during correction of hypernatremia, there may be a new gradient created that causes water movement from the extracellular space into the cells of the brain, producing **cerebral edema**. Possible manifestations of the resultant cerebral edema include seizures, brain herniation, and death.

To minimize the risk of cerebral edema during correction of hypernatremic dehydration, the serum sodium concentration should not decrease more than 12 mEq/L every 24 hours. The deficits in severe hypernatremic dehydration may need to be corrected over 2 to 4 days (Table 33-8). The choice and rate of fluid are not nearly as important as vigilant monitoring of the serum sodium concentration and adjustment of the therapy based on the result. Nonetheless, the initial resuscitation-rehydration phase of therapy remains the same as for other types of dehydration.

## Oral Rehydration

Mild to moderate dehydration from diarrhea of any cause can be treated effectively using a simple, oral rehydration solution (ORS) containing glucose and electrolytes (see

Chapter 112). The ORS relies on the coupled transport of sodium and glucose in the intestine. Oral rehydration therapy has significantly reduced the morbidity and mortality from acute diarrhea but is underused in developed countries. It should be attempted for most patients with mild to moderate diarrheal dehydration. Oral rehydration therapy is less expensive than IV therapy and has a lower complication rate. IV therapy may still be required for patients with severe dehydration; patients with uncontrollable vomiting; patients unable to drink because of extreme fatigue, stupor, or coma; or patients with gastric or intestinal distention.

As a guideline for oral rehydration, 50 mL/kg of the ORS should be given within 4 hours to patients with mild dehydration, and 100 mL/kg should be given over 4 hours to patients with moderate dehydration. Supplementary ORS is given to replace ongoing losses from diarrhea or emesis. An additional 10 mL/kg of ORS is given for each stool. Fluid intake should be decreased if the patient appears fully hydrated earlier than expected or develops periorbital edema. After rehydration, patients should resume their usual diet (breast milk, formula),

When rehydration is complete, maintenance therapy should be started, using 100 mL of ORS/kg in 24 hours until the diarrhea stops. Breastfeeding or formula-feeding should be maintained and not delayed for more than 24 hours. Patients with more severe diarrhea require continued supervision. The volume of ORS ingested should equal the volume of stool losses. If stool volume cannot be measured, an intake of 10 to 15 mL of ORS/kg/hr is appropriate.

# Parenteral Nutrition

Parenteral nutrition (PN) is necessary when enteral feeding is inadequate to meet the nutritional needs of a patient. Enteral nutrition is always preferred because it is more physiologic, less expensive, and associated with fewer complications. In some children, PN supplements enteral nutrition. In other children, PN is the only source of nutrition, although there are fewer complications if some nutrition can be provided enterally.

## INDICATIONS

A variety of clinical situations necessitate PN (Table 34-1). Acute PN is frequently given in an intensive care unit when there is poor tolerance of enteral feeds, potentially secondary to a transient ileus, or concerns regarding bowel ischemia or the risk of aspiration pneumonia. **Short bowel syndrome** is the most common indication for long-term PN; it may be caused by a congenital gastrointestinal anomaly or acquired after necrotizing enterocolitis (see Chapter 63). Some patients with a chronic indication for PN eventually may be transitioned to partial or full enteral feedings.

## ACCESS FOR PARENTERAL NUTRITION

PN can be given via either a peripheral intravenous (IV) line or a central venous line. Long-term PN should be given via a central venous line. Acute PN may be given peripherally, although a temporary central venous line often is used. Most children with cancer or receiving a bone marrow transplant have a central venous line. A **peripherally inserted central catheter** is an excellent source of central access for acute PN because there are fewer complications than with a standard central venous line.

A peripheral IV line has two major limitations. First, it frequently fails, necessitating interruption of PN and potentially painful placement of a new line. Second,

**TABLE 34-1 Indications for Parenteral Nutrition**

| ACUTE |
| --- |
| Prematurity |
| Trauma |
| Burns |
| Bowel surgery |
| Multiorgan system failure |
| Bone marrow transplantation |
| Malignancy |

| CHRONIC |
| --- |
| Short bowel |
| Intractable diarrhea syndromes |
| Intestinal pseudo-obstruction |
| Inflammatory bowel disease |
| Immunodeficiency |

high-osmolality solutions cause **phlebitis** of peripheral veins; this limits the dextrose and amino acid content of peripheral PN. The dextrose content of peripheral PN cannot be greater than 12%, with a lower limit if the amino acid concentration is high. Lipid emulsion has a low osmolality, therefore it can be administered peripherally via the same IV line as the dextrose and amino acid solution. Patients can receive adequate nutrition via a peripheral IV line, but the volume of PN needs to be higher than is necessary when central access is available because of the limitations on dextrose and amino acid concentration. This situation may be problematic in patients who cannot tolerate larger fluid volumes.

## COMPOSITION OF PARENTERAL NUTRITION

PN provides calories, amino acids, electrolytes, minerals, essential fatty acids, vitamins, iron, and trace elements. The **calories** in PN are from dextrose and fat. The amino acids in PN are a potential source of calories, but they should be used predominantly for protein synthesis. PN is given as two separate solutions: a dextrose plus amino acid solution and a 20% lipid emulsion. The dextrose solution has all of the other components of PN except for fat.

The dextrose concentration of peripheral PN is typically 10% to 12%, whereas central PN has a concentration of about 20%, although it may be increased to 25% to 30% in patients who are fluid restricted. To avoid hyperglycemia, the dextrose delivery is increased gradually when starting PN. Protein delivery in PN is via amino acids in the dextrose solution. The goal is 0.8 to 2 g protein/kg/24 hr for older children, 1.5 to 3 g/kg/24 hr for full-term and older infants, and 2.5 to 3.5 g/kg/24 hr for preterm infants.

The electrolyte and mineral composition of PN, which includes sodium, potassium, chloride, acetate, calcium, phosphate, and magnesium, is based on the patient's age, the volume of PN, and the nature of the underlying disease process. Vitamins, iron, and trace element delivery depend on age, with some adjustment necessary in certain diseases (decreased in renal failure or increased if stool losses). The 20% lipid emulsion provides essential fatty acids and calories. The lipid emulsion is started at a rate of 0.5 to 1 g/kg/24 hr, gradually increasing the rate so that the patient receives adequate calories; this typically requires 2.5 to 3.5 g/kg/24 hr. The lipid emulsion usually provides 30% to 40% of the required calories; it should not exceed 60%. The serum triglyceride concentration is monitored as the rate of lipid emulsion is increased, with reduction of the lipid emulsion rate if significant hypertriglyceridemia develops.

## COMPLICATIONS

There are many potential complications of PN. Central venous lines are associated with complications during insertion (pneumothorax or bleeding) and long-term issues (thrombosis). **Catheter-related sepsis**, most commonly due to coagulase-negative staphylococci, is common and on occasion necessitates catheter removal. Other potential pathogens are *Staphylococcus aureus,* gram-negative bacilli, and fungi. Electrolyte abnormalities, nutritional deficiencies, hyperglycemia, and complications from excessive protein intake (azotemia or hyperammonemia) can be detected with careful monitoring.

The most concerning complication of long-term PN is **cholestatic liver disease**, which can lead to cirrhosis and liver failure. Current PN decreases the risk of liver disease by including reduced amounts of hepatotoxic amino acids. The best preventive strategy is early use of the gastrointestinal tract, even if only trophic feeds are tolerated.

# CHAPTER 35
# Sodium Disorders

The kidney regulates sodium balance and is the principal site of sodium excretion. Sodium is unique among electrolytes because **water balance**, not sodium balance, usually determines its concentration. When the sodium concentration increases, the resultant higher plasma osmolality causes increased thirst and increased secretion of antidiuretic hormone (ADH), which leads to renal conservation of water. Both of these mechanisms increase the water content of the body, and the sodium concentration returns to normal. During hyponatremia, the fall in plasma osmolality decreases ADH secretion, and consequent renal water excretion leads to an increase in sodium concentration. Although water balance usually is regulated by osmolality, volume depletion stimulates thirst, ADH secretion, and renal conservation of water. Volume depletion takes precedence over osmolality;

volume depletion stimulates ADH secretion, even if a patient has hyponatremia.

The excretion of sodium by the kidney is not regulated by the plasma osmolality. The patient's effective plasma volume determines the amount of sodium in the urine. Effective plasma volume is controlled by a variety of regulatory systems, including the renin-angiotensin-aldosterone system and intrarenal mechanisms. In hyponatremia or hypernatremia, the underlying pathophysiology determines the urinary sodium concentration, not the serum sodium concentration.

## HYPONATREMIA

### Etiology

Different mechanisms can cause hyponatremia (Fig. 35-1). **Pseudohyponatremia** is a laboratory artifact that is present when the plasma contains high concentrations of protein or lipid. It does not occur when a direct ion-selective electrode determines the sodium concentration, a technique that is increasingly used in clinical laboratories. In true hyponatremia, the *measured* osmolality is low, whereas it is normal in pseudohyponatremia. **Hyperosmolality**, resulting from mannitol infusion or hyperglycemia, causes a low serum sodium concentration because water moves down its osmotic gradient from the intracellular space into the extracellular space, diluting the sodium concentration. For every 100 mg/dL-increment of the serum glucose, the serum sodium decreases by 1.6 mEq/L. Because the manifestations of hyponatremia are due to the low plasma osmolality, patients with hyponatremia caused by hyperosmolality do not have symptoms of hyponatremia and do not require correction of hyponatremia.

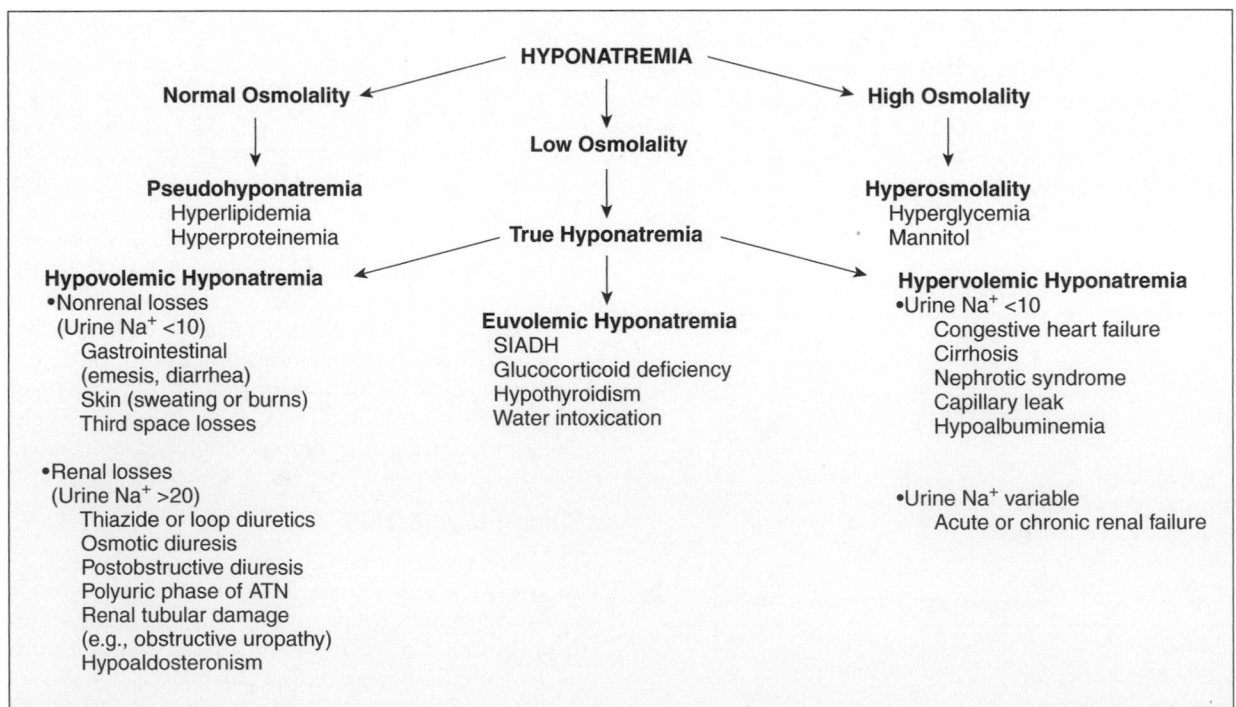

**FIGURE 35-1**

Differential diagnosis of hyponatremia. Assessment of hyponatremia is a three-step process: (1) Determine if the osmolality is low; if yes, the patient has true hyponatremia. (2) Evaluate the patient's volume status. (3) Determine the urine sodium concentration to help narrow the differential diagnosis. ATN, acute tubular necrosis; SIADH, syndrome of inappropriate secretion of antidiuretic hormone.

Classification of true hyponatremia is based on the patient's volume status (see Fig. 35-1). In **hypovolemic hyponatremia**, the child has lost sodium from the body. Water balance may be positive or negative, but there has been a higher net sodium loss than water loss; this is due to oral or intravenous (IV) water intake, with water retention by the kidneys to compensate for the intravascular volume depletion. If the sodium loss is due to a nonrenal disease, the urine sodium concentration is very low, as the kidneys attempt to preserve the intravascular volume by conserving sodium. In renal diseases, the urine sodium is inappropriately elevated.

Patients with hyponatremia and no evidence of volume overload or volume depletion have **euvolemic hyponatremia**. These patients typically have an excess of total body water and a slight decrease in total body sodium. Some of these patients have an increase in weight, implying that they are volume overloaded. Nevertheless, they usually appear normal or have only subtle signs of fluid overload. In **syndrome of inappropriate ADH (SIADH)**, there is secretion of ADH that is not inhibited by either low serum osmolality or expanded intravascular volume. Retention of water causes hyponatremia, and the expansion of the intravascular volume results in an increase in renal sodium excretion. Hyponatremia in hospitalized patients is often due to inappropriately produced ADH secondary to stress in the presence of hypotonic fluids. SIADH is associated with pneumonia, mechanical ventilation, meningitis, and other central nervous system disorders (trauma). Ectopic (tumor) production of ADH is rare in children. Infants also can develop euvolemic hyponatremia as a result of excessive water consumption or inappropriately diluted formula.

In **hypervolemic hyponatremia**, there is an excess of total body water and sodium, although the increase in water is greater than the increase in sodium. In renal failure, there is an inability to excrete sodium or water; the urine sodium may be low or high, depending on the cause of the renal insufficiency. In other causes of hypervolemic hyponatremia, there is a decrease in the effective blood volume because of either third space fluid loss or poor cardiac output (see Chapter 145). Regulatory systems sense this decrease in effective blood volume and retain water and sodium to correct the problem. ADH causes renal water retention, and the kidneys, under the influence of aldosterone and other intrarenal mechanisms, retain sodium, leading to a low urine sodium concentration. The patient's serum sodium concentration decreases because water intake exceeds sodium intake, and ADH prevents the normal loss of excess water.

## Clinical Manifestations

Hyponatremia causes a fall in the osmolality of the extracellular space. Because the intracellular space then has a higher osmolality, water moves from the extracellular space to the intracellular space to maintain osmotic equilibrium. The increase in intracellular water may cause cells to swell. **Brain cell swelling** is responsible for most of the symptoms of hyponatremia. Neurologic symptoms of hyponatremia include anorexia, nausea, emesis, malaise, lethargy, confusion, agitation, headache, seizures, coma, and decreased reflexes. Patients may develop hypothermia and Cheyne-Stokes respirations. Hyponatremia can cause muscle cramps and weakness. Symptoms are more severe when hyponatremia develops rapidly; chronic hyponatremia can be asymptomatic because of a compensatory decrease in brain cell osmolality, which limits cerebral swelling.

## Treatment

Rapid correction of hyponatremia can produce **central pontine myelinolysis**. Avoiding more than a 12-mEq/L increase in the serum sodium every 24 hours is prudent, especially if the hyponatremia developed gradually. Treatment of hypovolemic hyponatremia requires administration of IV fluids with sodium to provide maintenance requirements and deficit correction, as well as to replace ongoing losses (see Chapter 33). For children with SIADH, water restriction is the cornerstone of therapy. Children with hypothyroidism or cortisol deficiency need specific hormone replacement. **Acute water intoxication** rapidly self-corrects with transient restriction of water intake, which is followed by introduction of a normal diet. Treatment of hypervolemic hyponatremia centers on restriction of water and sodium intake, but disease-specific measures, such as dialysis in renal failure, also may be necessary.

Emergency treatment of **symptomatic hyponatremia**, such as seizures, uses IV hypertonic saline to increase the serum sodium concentration rapidly, which leads to a decrease in brain edema. One milliliter per kilogram of 3% sodium chloride increases the serum sodium by approximately 1 mEq/L. A child often improves after receiving 4 to 6 mL/kg of 3% sodium chloride.

# HYPERNATREMIA

## Etiology

There are three basic mechanisms of hypernatremia (Fig. 35-2). **Sodium intoxication** is frequently iatrogenic in a hospital setting resulting from correction of metabolic acidosis with sodium bicarbonate. In hyperaldosteronism, there is renal retention of sodium and resultant hypertension; the hypernatremia is mild.

Hypernatremia resulting from water losses develops only if the patient does not have access to water or cannot drink adequately because of neurologic impairment, emesis, or anorexia. Infants are at high risk because of their inability to control their own water intake. Ineffective breastfeeding, often in a primiparous mother, can cause severe hypernatremic dehydration. High insensible losses of water are especially common in premature infants; the losses increase further as a result of radiant warmers or phototherapy for hyperbilirubinemia. Children with extrarenal causes of water loss have high levels of ADH and very concentrated urine.

Children with diabetes insipidus have inappropriately diluted urine. Hereditary **nephrogenic diabetes insipidus** causes massive urinary water losses. Because it is most commonly an X-linked disorder, it usually occurs in boys, who may have episodes of severe hypernatremic dehydration and failure to thrive. The defect is in the gene for the ADH receptor in the X-linked form of nephrogenic

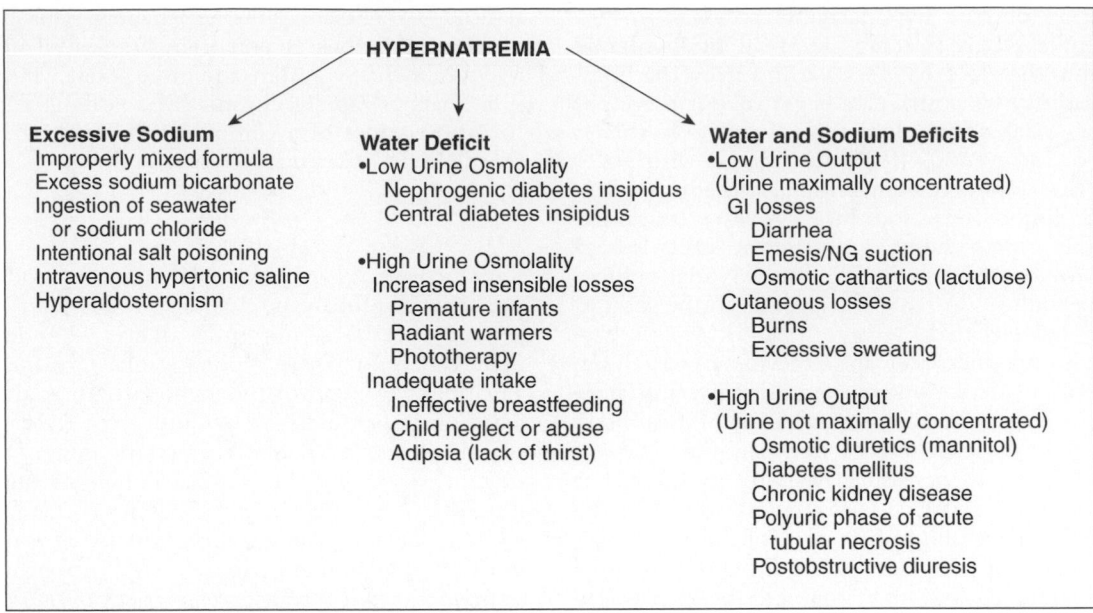

**FIGURE 35-2**

Differential diagnosis of hypernatremia by mechanism. GI, gastrointestinal; NG, nasogastric.

diabetes insipidus. *Acquired nephrogenic diabetes insipidus* may be secondary to interstitial nephritis, sickle cell disease, hypercalcemia, hypokalemia, or medications (lithium or amphotericin). If the defect is due to **central diabetes insipidus**, the urine output decreases, and the urine osmolality increases in response to administration of an ADH analog. Central causes of ADH deficiency include tumor, infarction, or trauma. There is no response to an ADH analog in a child with nephrogenic diabetes insipidus.

Diarrhea results in sodium and water depletion. Most children with gastroenteritis do not develop hypernatremia because they drink enough hypotonic fluid to compensate at least partially for stool water losses. Hypernatremia is most likely in a child with diarrhea who has inadequate intake because of emesis, lack of access to water, or anorexia. Some renal diseases, including obstructive uropathy, renal dysplasia, and juvenile nephronophthisis, can cause losses of sodium and water, potentially producing hypernatremia if the patient consumes insufficient water.

In situations with combined sodium and water deficits, analysis of the urine differentiates renal and nonrenal etiologies. When the losses are extrarenal, the kidney responds to volume depletion with low urine volume, a concentrated urine, and sodium retention (urine sodium <10 mEq/L). With renal causes, the urine volume is not appropriately low, the urine is not maximally concentrated, and the urine sodium may be inappropriately elevated.

## Clinical Manifestations

Most children with hypernatremia are dehydrated and have the typical signs and symptoms of dehydration (see Chapter 33). Children with hypernatremic dehydration tend to have better preservation of intravascular volume owing to the shift of water from the intracellular space to the extracellular space. Blood pressure and urine output are maintained, and hypernatremic infants potentially

become more dehydrated before seeking medical attention. Probably because of intracellular water loss, the pinched abdominal skin of a dehydrated, hypernatremic infant has a *doughy* feel.

Hypernatremia, even without dehydration, causes central nervous system symptoms that tend to parallel the degree of sodium elevation and the acuity of the increase. Patients are irritable, restless, weak, and lethargic. Some infants have a high-pitched cry and hyperpnea. Alert patients are very thirsty, although nausea may be present. Hypernatremia causes fever, although many patients have an underlying process that contributes to the fever. Hypernatremia is associated with hyperglycemia and mild hypocalcemia; the mechanisms are unknown.

Brain hemorrhage is the most devastating consequence of hypernatremia. As the extracellular osmolality increases, water moves out of brain cells, resulting in a decrease in brain volume. This decrease in volume can result in tearing of intracerebral veins and bridging blood vessels as the brain moves away from the skull and the meninges. Patients may have subarachnoid, subdural, and parenchymal hemorrhage. Seizures and coma are possible sequelae of the hemorrhage.

## Treatment

As hypernatremia develops, the brain generates idiogenic osmoles to increase the intracellular osmolality and prevent the loss of brain water. This mechanism is not instantaneous and is most prominent when hypernatremia has developed gradually. If the serum sodium concentration is lowered rapidly, there is movement of water from the serum into the brain cells to equalize the osmolality in the two compartments. The resultant brain swelling manifests as seizures or coma.

Because of the dangers of overly rapid correction, hypernatremia should be corrected slowly. The goal is to decrease the serum sodium by less than 12 mEq/L every 24 hours, a rate of 0.5 mEq/L/hr. The most important component of correcting moderate or severe hypernatremia is frequent monitoring of the serum sodium to allow adjustment of fluid therapy and provide adequate correction that is neither too slow nor too fast. If a child develops seizures from brain edema secondary to rapid correction, administration of hypotonic fluid should be stopped, and an infusion of 3% saline should be used to increase the serum sodium acutely.

In a child with hypernatremic dehydration, as in any child with dehydration, the first priority is restoration of intravascular volume with isotonic fluid. Table 33-8 outlines a general approach for correcting hypernatremic dehydration secondary to gastroenteritis. If the hypernatremia and dehydration are secondary to water loss, as occurs with diabetes insipidus, a more hypotonic IV fluid is appropriate. A child with central diabetes insipidus should receive an ADH analog to prevent further excessive water loss. A child with nephrogenic diabetes insipidus requires a urine replacement solution to offset ongoing water losses. Chronically, reduced sodium intake, thiazide diuretics, and nonsteroidal anti-inflammatory drugs can decrease water losses in nephrogenic diabetes insipidus.

Acute, severe hypernatremia, usually secondary to sodium administration, can be corrected more rapidly because idiogenic osmoles have not had time to accumulate; this balances the high morbidity and mortality from severe, acute hypernatremia with the dangers of overly rapid correction. When hypernatremia is due to sodium intoxication, and the hypernatremia is severe, it may be impossible to administer enough water to correct the hypernatremia rapidly without worsening volume overload. Some patients require use of a loop diuretic or dialysis.

# CHAPTER 36
# Potassium Disorders

The kidneys are the principal regulator of potassium balance, adjusting excretion based on intake. Factors affecting renal potassium excretion include aldosterone, acid-base status, serum potassium concentration, and renal function. The intracellular potassium concentration is approximately 30 times the extracellular potassium concentration. A variety of conditions alter the distribution of potassium between the intracellular and extracellular compartments, potentially causing either hypokalemia or hyperkalemia. The plasma concentration does not always reflect the total body potassium content.

## HYPOKALEMIA
### Etiology
Hypokalemia is common in children, with most cases related to gastroenteritis. Spurious hypokalemia occurs in patients with leukemia and elevated white blood cell counts if plasma for analysis is left at room temperature, permitting the white blood cells to take up potassium from the plasma. There are four basic mechanisms of hypokalemia (Table 36-1). Low intake, nonrenal losses, and renal losses all are associated with total body potassium depletion. With a **transcellular shift**, there is no change in total body potassium, although there may be concomitant potassium depletion secondary to other factors.

The transcellular shift of potassium after initiation of insulin therapy in children with diabetic ketoacidosis (see Chapter 171) can be dramatic. These patients have reduced total body potassium because of urinary losses, but they often have a normal serum potassium level before insulin therapy from a transcellular shift into the extracellular space secondary to insulin deficiency and metabolic acidosis. Children receiving aggressive doses of β-adrenergic agonists (albuterol) for asthma can have hypokalemia resulting from the intracellular movement of potassium. Poor intake is an unusual cause of hypokalemia, unless also associated with significant weight loss (anorexia nervosa).

Diarrhea has a high concentration of potassium, and the resulting hypokalemia usually is associated with a metabolic acidosis secondary to stool losses of bicarbonate. Urinary potassium wasting may be accompanied by a metabolic acidosis (proximal or distal renal tubular acidosis (see Chapter 37). With emesis or nasogastric suction, there is gastric loss of potassium, but this is fairly minimal given the low potassium content of gastric fluid (approximately 10 mEq/L). More important is the gastric loss of hydrochloride, leading to a metabolic alkalosis and a state of volume depletion. Metabolic alkalosis and volume depletion increase urinary losses of potassium.

Loop and thiazide diuretics lead to hypokalemia and a metabolic alkalosis. **Bartter syndrome** and **Gitelman syndrome** are autosomal recessive disorders resulting from defects in tubular transporters. Both disorders are associated with hypokalemia and a metabolic alkalosis. Bartter syndrome usually is associated with hypercalciuria, often with nephrocalcinosis, whereas children with Gitelman syndrome have low urinary calcium losses, but hypomagnesemia secondary to urinary losses.

In the presence of a high aldosterone level, there is urinary loss of potassium, hypokalemia, and a metabolic alkalosis. There also is renal retention of sodium, leading to hypertension. A variety of genetic and acquired disorders can cause high aldosterone levels. **Liddle syndrome**, an autosomal dominant disorder caused by constitutively active sodium channels, has the same clinical features as hyperaldosteronism, but the serum aldosterone level is low.

### Clinical Manifestations
The heart and skeletal muscle are especially vulnerable to hypokalemia. **Electrocardiographic (ECG) changes** include a flattened T wave, a depressed ST segment, and the appearance of a U wave, which is located between the T wave (if still visible) and P wave. Ventricular fibrillation and torsades de pointes may occur, although usually only in the context of underlying heart disease. Hypokalemia makes the heart especially susceptible to digitalis-induced arrhythmias, such as supraventricular tachycardia, ventricular tachycardia, and heart block.

**TABLE 36-1 Causes of Hypokalemia**

Spurious
  High white blood cell count
Transcellular shifts
  Alkalemia
  Insulin
  β-Adrenergic agonists
  Drugs/toxins (theophylline, barium, toluene)
  Hypokalemic periodic paralysis
Decreased intake
Extrarenal losses
  Diarrhea
  Laxative abuse
  Sweating
Renal losses
  With metabolic acidosis
    Distal RTA
    Proximal RTA
    Ureterosigmoidostomy
    Diabetic ketoacidosis
  Without specific acid-base disturbance
    Tubular toxins (amphotericin, cisplatin, aminoglycosides)
    Interstitial nephritis
    Diuretic phase of acute tubular necrosis
    Postobstructive diuresis
    Hypomagnesemia
    High urine anions (e.g., penicillin or penicillin derivatives)
  With metabolic alkalosis
    Low urine chloride
      Emesis/nasogastric suction
      Pyloric stenosis
      Chloride-losing diarrhea
      Cystic fibrosis
      Low-chloride formula
      Posthypercapnia
      Previous loop or thiazide diuretic use
    High urine chloride and normal blood pressure
      Gitelman syndrome
      Bartter syndrome
      Loop and thiazide diuretics
    High urine chloride and high blood pressure
      Adrenal adenoma or hyperplasia
      Glucocorticoid-remediable aldosteronism
      Renovascular disease
      Renin-secreting tumor
      17α-Hydroxylase deficiency
      11β-Hydroxylase deficiency
      Cushing syndrome
      11β-Hydroxysteroid dehydrogenase deficiency
      Licorice ingestion
      Liddle syndrome

RTA, renal tubular acidosis.

The clinical consequences in skeletal muscle include muscle weakness and cramps. **Paralysis** is a possible complication (generally only at potassium levels <2.5 mEq/L). Paralysis usually starts with the legs, followed by the arms. Respiratory paralysis may require mechanical ventilation.

Some patients develop **rhabdomyolysis**; the risk increases with exercise. Hypokalemia slows gastrointestinal motility; potassium levels less than 2.5 mEq/L may cause an ileus. Hypokalemia impairs bladder function, potentially leading to urinary retention. Hypokalemia causes polyuria by producing secondary nephrogenic diabetes insipidus. Chronic hypokalemia may cause kidney damage, including interstitial nephritis and renal cysts. In children, chronic hypokalemia, as in Bartter syndrome, leads to poor linear growth.

### Diagnosis

It is important to review the child's diet, history of gastrointestinal losses, and medications. Emesis and diuretic use can be surreptitious. The presence of hypertension suggests excess mineralocorticoids. Concomitant electrolyte abnormalities are useful clues. The combination of hypokalemia and metabolic acidosis is characteristic of diarrhea, distal renal tubular acidosis, and proximal renal tubular acidosis. A concurrent metabolic alkalosis is characteristic of gastric losses, aldosterone excess, diuretics, and Bartter syndrome or Gitelman syndrome. Alkalosis also causes a transcellular shift of potassium and increased urinary losses of potassium.

### Treatment

Factors that influence the therapy of hypokalemia include the potassium level, clinical symptoms, renal function, presence of transcellular shifts of potassium, ongoing losses, and the patient's ability to tolerate oral potassium. Severe, symptomatic hypokalemia requires aggressive treatment. Supplementation is more cautious if renal function is decreased because of the kidney's limited ability to excrete excessive potassium. The plasma potassium level does not always provide an accurate estimation of the total body potassium deficit because there may be shifts of potassium from the intracellular space to the plasma. Clinically, this shift occurs most commonly with metabolic acidosis and as a result of the insulin deficiency of diabetic ketoacidosis; the plasma potassium underestimates the degree of total body potassium depletion. When these problems are corrected, potassium moves into the intracellular space, and these patients require more potassium supplementation to correct the hypokalemia. Patients who have ongoing losses of potassium need correction of the deficit and replacement of the ongoing losses.

Because of the risk of hyperkalemia, intravenous (IV) potassium should be used cautiously. Oral potassium is safer, albeit not as rapid in urgent situations. The dose of IV potassium is 0.5 to 1 mEq/kg, usually given over 1 hour. The adult maximum dose is 40 mEq. Conservative dosing is generally preferred. For patients with excessive urinary losses, potassium-sparing diuretics are effective, but they need to be used cautiously in patients with renal insufficiency. When hypokalemia, metabolic alkalosis, and volume depletion are present, restoration of intravascular volume decreases urinary potassium losses. Disease-specific therapy is effective in many of the genetic tubular disorders.

# HYPERKALEMIA

## Etiology

Three basic mechanisms cause hyperkalemia (Table 36-2). In the individual patient, the etiology is sometimes multifactorial. **Fictitious hyperkalemia** is common in children because of the difficulties in obtaining blood specimens. This hyperkalemia is usually due to hemolysis during phlebotomy, but it can be the result of prolonged tourniquet application or fist clenching, which causes local potassium release from muscle. Falsely elevated serum potassium levels can occur when serum levels are measured in patients with markedly elevated white blood cell counts; a promptly analyzed plasma sample usually provides an accurate result.

Because of the kidney's ability to excrete potassium, it is unusual for excessive intake, by itself, to cause hyperkalemia. This mechanism can occur in a patient who is receiving large quantities of IV or oral potassium for excessive losses that are no longer present. Frequent or rapid blood transfusions can increase the potassium level acutely secondary to the high potassium content of blood. Increased intake may precipitate hyperkalemia if there is an underlying defect in potassium excretion.

The intracellular space has a high potassium concentration, so a **shift of potassium from the intracellular space** to the extracellular space can have a significant impact on the plasma potassium. This shift occurs with acidosis, cell destruction (rhabdomyolysis or tumor lysis syndrome), insulin deficiency, medications (succinylcholine, β-blockers), malignant hyperthermia, and hyperkalemic periodic paralysis.

Hyperkalemia secondary to decreased excretion occurs with renal insufficiency. Aldosterone deficiency or unresponsiveness to aldosterone causes hyperkalemia, often with associated metabolic acidosis (see Chapter 37) and hyponatremia. A form of congenital adrenal hyperplasia, **21-hydroxylase deficiency**, is the most frequent cause of aldosterone deficiency in children. Male infants typically present with hyperkalemia, metabolic acidosis, hyponatremia, and volume depletion. Female infants with this disorder usually are diagnosed as newborns because of ambiguous genitalia; treatment prevents the development of electrolyte problems.

Renin, via angiotensin II, stimulates aldosterone production. A deficiency in renin, resulting from kidney damage, can lead to decreased aldosterone production. These patients typically have hyperkalemia and a metabolic acidosis, without hyponatremia. Some patients have impaired renal function, partially accounting for the hyperkalemia, but the impairment in potassium excretion is more extreme than expected for the degree of renal insufficiency.

Children with **pseudohypoaldosteronism type 1** have hyperkalemia, metabolic acidosis, and salt wasting, leading to hyponatremia and volume depletion; aldosterone levels are elevated. In the autosomal recessive variant, there is a defect in the renal sodium channel that is normally activated by aldosterone. In the autosomal dominant form, patients have a defect in the aldosterone receptor, and the disease is milder, often remitting in adulthood. Pseudohypoaldosteronism type 2, also called **Gordon syndrome**, is an autosomal dominant disorder characterized by hypertension secondary to salt retention and impaired excretion

| TABLE 36-2  Causes of Hyperkalemia |
|---|
| Spurious laboratory value |
|     Hemolysis |
|     Tissue ischemia during blood drawing |
|     Thrombocytosis |
|     Leukocytosis |
| Increased intake |
|     IV or PO |
|     Blood transfusions |
| Transcellular shifts |
|     Acidemia |
|     Rhabdomyolysis |
|     Tumor lysis syndrome |
|     Tissue necrosis |
|     Hemolysis/hematomas/gastrointestinal bleeding |
|     Succinylcholine |
|     Digitalis intoxication |
|     Fluoride intoxication |
|     β-Adrenergic blockers |
|     Exercise |
|     Hyperosmolality |
|     Insulin deficiency |
|     Malignant hyperthermia |
|     Hyperkalemic periodic paralysis |
| Decreased excretion |
|     Renal failure |
|     Primary adrenal disease |
|         Acquired Addison disease |
|         21-Hydroxylase deficiency |
|         3β-Hydroxysteroid-dehydrogenase deficiency |
|         Lipoid congenital adrenal hyperplasia |
|         Adrenal hypoplasia congenita |
|         Aldosterone synthase deficiency |
|         Adrenoleukodystrophy |
|     Hyporeninemic hypoaldosteronism |
|         Urinary tract obstruction |
|         Sickle cell disease |
|         Kidney transplant |
|         Lupus nephritis |
|     Renal tubular disease |
|         Pseudohypoaldosteronism type 1 |
|         Pseudohypoaldosteronism type 2 |
|         Urinary tract obstruction |
|         Sickle cell disease |
|         Kidney transplant |
|     Medications |
|         ACE inhibitors |
|         Angiotensin II blockers |
|         Potassium-sparing diuretics |
|         Cyclosporine |
|         NSAIDs |
|         Trimethoprim |

ACE, angiotensin-converting enzyme; IV, intravenous; NSAIDs, nonsteroidal anti-inflammatory drugs; PO, oral.

of potassium and acid leading to hyperkalemia and metabolic acidosis. The risk of hyperkalemia secondary to medications that decrease renal potassium excretion is greatest in patients with underlying renal insufficiency.

## Clinical Manifestations

The most import effects of hyperkalemia are due to the role of potassium in membrane polarization. The cardiac conduction system is usually the dominant concern. **ECG changes** begin with peaking of the T waves. As the potassium level increases, an increased P-R interval, flattening of the P wave, and widening of the QRS complex occur; this eventually can progress to ventricular fibrillation. Asystole also may occur. Some patients have paresthesias, weakness, and tingling, but cardiac toxicity usually precedes these clinical symptoms.

## Diagnosis

The etiology of hyperkalemia is often readily apparent. Spurious hyperkalemia is common in children, so a repeat potassium level is often appropriate. If there is a significant elevation of the white blood cells, the repeat sample should be from plasma that is evaluated promptly. The history initially should focus on potassium intake, risk factors for transcellular shifts of potassium, medications that cause hyperkalemia, and the presence of signs of renal insufficiency, such as oliguria or an abnormal urinalysis. Initial laboratory evaluation should include serum creatinine and assessment of acid-base status. Many causes of hyperkalemia, such as renal insufficiency and aldosterone insufficiency or resistance, cause a metabolic acidosis, worsening hyperkalemia by the transcellular shift of potassium out of cells. Cell destruction, as seen in rhabdomyolysis or tumor lysis syndrome, can cause concomitant hyperphosphatemia, hyperuricemia, and an elevated serum lactate dehydrogenase.

## Treatment

The plasma potassium level, the ECG, and the risk of the problem worsening determine the aggressiveness of the therapeutic approach. A high serum potassium level with ECG changes requires more vigorous treatment. An additional source of concern is a patient with increasing plasma potassium despite minimal intake. This situation can occur if there is cellular release of potassium (tumor lysis syndrome), especially in the setting of diminished excretion (renal failure).

The first action in a child with a concerning elevation of plasma potassium is to stop all sources of additional potassium (oral and IV). If the potassium level is greater than 6 to 6.5 mEq/L, an ECG should be obtained to help assess the urgency of the situation. Therapy of hyperkalemia has two basic goals:

1. Prevent life-threatening arrhythmias.
2. Remove potassium from the body (Table 36-3).

Treatments that acutely prevent arrhythmias all work quickly (within minutes), but do not remove potassium from the body. Measures that remove potassium from the body do not act quickly but should be started as soon as possible.

Long-term management of hyperkalemia includes reducing intake via dietary changes and eliminating or reducing medications that cause hyperkalemia. Some patients require medications, such as sodium polystyrene sulfonate and loop

| TABLE 36-3 Treatment of Hyperkalemia |
|---|
| Rapidly decrease the risk of life-threatening arrhythmias |
|     Shift potassium intracellularly |
|         Sodium bicarbonate administration (IV) |
|         Insulin and glucose (IV) |
|         β-Agonist (albuterol via nebulizer) |
|     Cardiac membrane stabilization |
|         IV calcium |
| Remove potassium from the body |
|     Loop diuretic (IV or PO) |
|     Sodium polystyrene (PO or rectal) |
|     Dialysis |

IV, intravenous; PO, oral.

or thiazide diuretics, to increase potassium losses. The disorders due to a deficiency in aldosterone respond to replacement therapy with fludrocortisone, a mineralocorticoid.

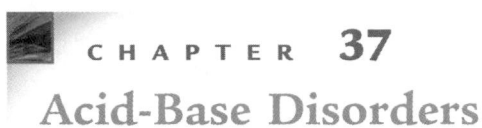

CHAPTER **37**

# Acid-Base Disorders

Close regulation of pH is necessary for cellular enzymes and other metabolic processes, which function optimally at a normal pH (7.35 to 7.45). Chronic, mild derangements in acid-base status may interfere with normal growth and development, whereas acute, severe changes in pH can be fatal. Control of acid-base balance depends on the kidneys, the lungs, and intracellular and extracellular buffers.

The lungs and the kidneys maintain a normal acid-base balance. Carbon dioxide ($CO_2$) generated during normal metabolism is a weak acid. The lungs prevent an increase in the partial pressure of $CO_2$ ($Pco_2$) in the blood by excreting the $CO_2$ that the body produces. $CO_2$ production varies depending on the body's metabolic needs. The rapid pulmonary response to changes in $CO_2$ concentration occurs via central sensing of the $Pco_2$ and a subsequent increase or decrease in ventilation to maintain a normal $Pco_2$ (35 to 45 mm Hg).

The kidneys excrete endogenous acids. An adult normally produces about 1 to 2 mEq/kg/day of hydrogen ions. Children normally produce 2 to 3 mEq/kg/day of hydrogen ions. The hydrogen ions from endogenous acid production are neutralized by bicarbonate, potentially causing the bicarbonate concentration to fall. The kidneys regenerate this bicarbonate by secreting hydrogen ions, maintaining the serum bicarbonate concentration in the normal range (20 to 28 mEq/L).

## CLINICAL ASSESSMENT OF ACID-BASE DISORDERS

**Acidemia** is a pH below normal (<7.35), and **alkalemia** is a pH above normal (>7.45). An **acidosis** is a pathologic process that causes an increase in the hydrogen ion concentration, and an **alkalosis** is a pathologic process that causes a decrease in the hydrogen ion concentration. A **simple acid-base disorder** is a single primary disturbance. During a simple metabolic disorder, there is respiratory compensation; the $P_{CO_2}$ decreases during a metabolic acidosis and increases during a metabolic alkalosis. With metabolic acidosis, the decrease in the pH increases the ventilatory drive, causing a decrease in the $P_{CO_2}$. The fall in the $CO_2$ concentration leads to an increase in the pH. This **appropriate respiratory compensation** for a metabolic process happens quickly and is complete within 12 to 24 hours.

During a primary respiratory process, there is a slower metabolic compensation, mediated by the kidneys. The kidneys respond to a respiratory acidosis by increasing hydrogen ion excretion, increasing bicarbonate generation, and raising the serum bicarbonate concentration. The kidneys increase bicarbonate excretion to compensate for a respiratory alkalosis; the serum bicarbonate concentration decreases. In contrast to a rapid respiratory compensation, it takes 3 to 4 days for the kidneys to complete **appropriate metabolic compensation**. However, there is a small and rapid compensatory change in the bicarbonate concentration during a primary respiratory process. The expected appropriate metabolic compensation for a respiratory disorder depends on whether the process is acute or chronic.

A **mixed acid-base disorder** is present when there is more than one primary acid-base disturbance. An infant with bronchopulmonary dysplasia may have a respiratory acidosis from chronic lung disease and a metabolic alkalosis from a diuretic used to treat the chronic lung disease. Formulas are available for calculating the appropriate metabolic or respiratory compensation for the six primary simple acid-base disorders (Table 37-1). Appropriate compensation is expected in a simple disorder; it is not optional. If a patient does not have appropriate compensation, a mixed acid-base disorder is present.

## TABLE 37-1  Appropriate Compensation During Simple Acid-Base Disorders

| Disorder | Expected Compensation* |
|---|---|
| Metabolic acidosis | $P_{CO_2} = 1.5 \times [HCO_3^-]\ 8 \pm 2$ |
| Metabolic alkalosis | $P_{CO_2}$ increases by 7 mm Hg for each 10-mEq/L increase in the serum $[HCO_3^-]$ |
| Respiratory acidosis | |
| Acute | $[HCO_3^-]$ increases by 1 for each 10-mm Hg increase in the $P_{CO_2}$ |
| Chronic | $[HCO_3^-]$ increases by 3.5 for each 10-mm Hg increase in the $P_{CO_2}$ |
| Respiratory alkalosis | |
| Acute | $[HCO_3^-]$ falls by 2 for each 10-mm Hg decrease in the $P_{CO_2}$ |
| Chronic | $[HCO_3^-]$ falls by 4 for each 10-mm Hg decrease in the $P_{CO_2}$ |

*$[HCO_3^-]$ is expressed in mEq/L.

## METABOLIC ACIDOSIS

Metabolic acidosis occurs frequently in hospitalized children; diarrhea is the most common cause. For a patient with an unknown medical problem, the presence of a metabolic acidosis is often helpful diagnostically because it suggests a relatively narrow differential diagnosis (Table 37-2).

### Etiology

Diarrhea causes a loss of bicarbonate from the body. The amount of bicarbonate lost in the stool depends on the volume of diarrhea and the bicarbonate concentration of the stool, which tends to increase with more severe diarrhea. Diarrhea often causes volume depletion because of losses of sodium and water, potentially exacerbating the acidosis by causing hypoperfusion (shock) and a lactic acidosis.

There are three forms of renal tubular acidosis (RTA):

● Distal (type I)
● Proximal (type II)
● Hyperkalemic (type IV)

In **distal RTA**, children may have accompanying hypokalemia, hypercalciuria, nephrolithiasis, and nephrocalcinosis; rickets is a less common finding. Failure to thrive, resulting from chronic metabolic acidosis, is the most common presenting complaint. Autosomal dominant and autosomal recessive forms of distal RTA exist. The autosomal dominant form is relatively mild. Autosomal recessive distal RTA is more severe and often associated with deafness secondary to a defect in the gene for a $H^+$-ATPase that is present in the kidney and the inner ear. Distal RTA also may be secondary to medications or congenital or acquired renal disease. Patients with distal RTA cannot acidify their urine and have a urine pH greater than 5.5, despite a metabolic acidosis.

**Proximal RTA** is rarely present in isolation. In most patients, proximal RTA is part of **Fanconi syndrome**, a generalized dysfunction of the proximal tubule. Along with renal wasting of bicarbonate, Fanconi syndrome causes glycosuria, aminoaciduria, and excessive urinary losses of phosphate and uric acid. The chronic hypophosphatemia is more clinically significant because it ultimately leads

## TABLE 37-2  Causes of Metabolic Acidosis

| NORMAL ANION GAP |
|---|
| Diarrhea |
| Renal tubular acidosis |
| Urinary tract diversions |
| Posthypocapnia |
| Ammonium chloride intake |

| INCREASED ANION GAP |
|---|
| Lactic acidosis (shock) |
| Ketoacidosis (diabetic, starvation, or alcoholic) |
| Kidney failure |
| Poisoning (e.g., ethylene glycol, methanol, or salicylates) |
| Inborn errors of metabolism |

to rickets in children. Rickets or failure to thrive may be the presenting complaint. Fanconi syndrome is rarely an isolated genetic disorder, with pediatric cases usually secondary to an underlying genetic disorder, most commonly **cystinosis**. Toxic medications, such as ifosfamide or valproate, may cause Fanconi syndrome. The ability to acidify the urine is intact in proximal RTA, and untreated patients have a urine pH less than 5.5. However, bicarbonate therapy increases bicarbonate losses in the urine, and the urine pH increases.

In **hyperkalemic RTA**, renal excretion of acid and potassium is impaired due to either an absence of aldosterone or an inability of the kidney to respond to aldosterone. In severe aldosterone deficiency, as occurs with congenital adrenal hyperplasia secondary to 21α-hydroxylase deficiency, the hyperkalemia and metabolic acidosis are accompanied by hyponatremia and volume depletion from renal salt wasting. Incomplete aldosterone deficiency causes less severe electrolyte disturbances; children may have isolated hyperkalemic RTA, hyperkalemia without acidosis, or isolated hyponatremia.

**Lactic acidosis** most commonly occurs when inadequate oxygen delivery to the tissues leads to anaerobic metabolism and excess production of lactic acid. Lactic acidosis may be secondary to shock, severe anemia, or hypoxemia. Inborn errors of carbohydrate metabolism produce a severe lactic acidosis (see Chapter 52). In diabetes mellitus, inadequate insulin leads to hyperglycemia and diabetic ketoacidosis (see Chapter 171). Renal failure (see Chapter 165) causes a metabolic acidosis because the kidneys are unable to excrete the acid produced by normal metabolism.

A variety of **toxic ingestions** cause a metabolic acidosis. Acute **salicylate** intoxication occurs after a large overdose. Chronic salicylate intoxication is possible because of the gradual buildup of the drug. In addition to a metabolic acidosis, some patients may have a respiratory alkalosis. Other symptoms of salicylate intoxication include fever, seizures, lethargy, and coma. Hyperventilation may be particularly marked. Tinnitus, vertigo, and hearing impairment are more likely with chronic salicylate intoxication. **Ethylene glycol**, a component of antifreeze, is converted in the liver to glyoxylic and oxalic acids, causing a severe metabolic acidosis. Excessive oxalate excretion causes calcium oxalate crystals to appear in the urine, and calcium oxalate precipitation in the kidney tubules can cause renal failure. The toxicity of **methanol** ingestion also depends on liver metabolism; formic acid is the toxic end product that causes the metabolic acidosis and other sequelae, which include damage to the optic nerve and central nervous system.

There are many **inborn errors of metabolism** that may cause a metabolic acidosis (see Section 10). The metabolic acidosis may be due to excessive production of ketoacids, lactic acid, or other organic anions. Some patients have accompanying hyperammonemia. In most patients, acidosis occurs only episodically during acute decompensations, which may be precipitated by ingestion of specific dietary substrates (proteins), the stress of a mild illness (fasting, catabolism), or poor compliance with dietary or medical therapy.

## Clinical Manifestations

The underlying disorder usually produces most of the signs and symptoms in children with a mild or moderate metabolic acidosis. The clinical manifestations of the acidosis are related to the degree of acidemia; patients with appropriate respiratory compensation and less severe acidemia have fewer manifestations than patients with a concomitant respiratory acidosis. At a serum pH less than 7.20, there is impaired cardiac contractility and an increased risk of arrhythmias, especially if underlying heart disease or other predisposing electrolyte disorders are present. With acidemia, there is a decrease in the cardiovascular response to catecholamines, potentially exacerbating hypotension in children with volume depletion or shock. Acidemia causes vasoconstriction of the pulmonary vasculature, which is especially problematic in newborns with persistent fetal circulation (see Chapter 61). The normal respiratory response to metabolic acidosis—compensatory hyperventilation—may be subtle with mild metabolic acidosis, but it causes discernible increased respiratory effort with worsening acidemia. Chronic metabolic acidosis causes failure to thrive.

## Diagnosis

The plasma anion gap is useful for evaluating patients with a metabolic acidosis. It divides patients into two diagnostic groups: normal anion gap and increased anion gap. The following formula determines the anion gap:

$$\text{Anion gap} = [Na^+] - [Cl^-] - [HCO_3^-]$$

A normal anion gap is 3 to 11. A decrease in the albumin concentration of 1 g/dL decreases the anion gap by roughly 4 mEq/L. Similarly, albeit less commonly, an increase in unmeasured cations, such as calcium, potassium, or magnesium, decreases the anion gap. Conversely, a decrease in unmeasured cations is a rare cause of an increased anion gap. Because of these variables, the broad range of a normal anion gap, and other factors, the presence of a normal or increased anion gap is not always reliable in differentiating the causes of a metabolic acidosis, especially when the metabolic acidosis is mild. Some patients have more than one explanation for their metabolic acidosis, such as a child with diarrhea and lactic acidosis secondary to hypoperfusion. The anion gap should not be interpreted in dogmatic isolation; consideration of other laboratory abnormalities and the clinical history improves its diagnostic utility.

## Treatment

The most effective therapeutic approach for patients with a metabolic acidosis is correction of the underlying disorder, if possible. The administration of insulin in diabetic ketoacidosis or restoration of adequate perfusion in lactic acidosis eventually results in normalization of acid-base balance. The use of bicarbonate therapy is indicated when the underlying disorder is irreparable; examples include RTA and chronic renal failure. In other disorders, the cause of the metabolic acidosis eventually resolves, but base therapy may be necessary during the acute illness.

In salicylate poisoning, alkali administration increases renal clearance of salicylate and decreases the amount of salicylate in brain cells. Short-term base therapy is often necessary in other poisonings and inborn errors of metabolism.

## METABOLIC ALKALOSIS

### Etiology

The causes of a metabolic alkalosis are divided into two categories based on the urinary chloride (Table 37-3). The alkalosis in patients with a low urinary chloride is maintained by volume depletion. They are called **chloride responsive** because volume repletion with fluid containing sodium chloride and potassium chloride is necessary to correct the metabolic alkalosis. Emesis, which causes loss of hydrochloride and volume depletion, is the most common cause of a metabolic alkalosis. Diuretic use increases chloride excretion in the urine. Consequently, while a patient is receiving diuretics, the urinary chloride is typically high (>20 mEq/L). After the diuretic effect has worn off, the urinary chloride is low (<15 mEq/L), because of appropriate renal chloride retention in response to volume depletion. Categorization of diuretics based on urinary chloride depends on the timing of the measurement. The metabolic alkalosis from diuretics is clearly chloride responsive; it corrects only after adequate volume repletion. This is the rationale for including it among the chloride-responsive causes of a metabolic alkalosis.

**TABLE 37-3  Causes of Metabolic Alkalosis**

**CHLORIDE RESPONSIVE (URINARY CHLORIDE <15 MEQ/L)**

Gastric losses (emesis or nasogastric suction)
Pyloric stenosis
Diuretics (loop or thiazide)
Chloride-losing diarrhea
Chloride-deficient formula
Cystic fibrosis (sweat losses of chloride)
Posthypercapnia (chloride loss during respiratory acidosis)

**CHLORIDE RESISTANT (URINARY CHLORIDE >20 MEQ/L)**

**High blood pressure**
  Adrenal adenoma or hyperplasia
  Glucocorticoid-remediable aldosteronism
  Renovascular disease
  Renin-secreting tumor
  17α-Hydroxylase deficiency
  11β-Hydroxylase deficiency
  Cushing syndrome
  11β-Hydroxysteroid dehydrogenase deficiency
  Licorice ingestion
  Liddle syndrome
**Normal blood pressure**
  Gitelman syndrome
  Bartter syndrome
  Base administration

The **chloride-resistant** causes of metabolic alkalosis can be subdivided based on blood pressure. Patients with the rare disorders that cause a metabolic alkalosis and hypertension either have increased aldosterone or act like they have increased aldosterone (owing to a genetic defect causing overproduction of another mineralocorticoid or a constitutively overactive sodium channel, as occurs in Liddle syndrome). Patients with Bartter syndrome or Gitelman syndrome (Chapter 36) have metabolic alkalosis, hypokalemia, and normal blood pressure secondary to renal tubular defects that cause continuous urinary losses of chloride.

### Clinical Manifestations

The symptoms in patients with a metabolic alkalosis often are related to the underlying disease and associated electrolyte disturbances. Hypokalemia is often present, and occasionally severe, in all the diseases that cause a metabolic alkalosis (see Chapter 36). Children with chloride-responsive causes of metabolic alkalosis often have symptoms related to volume depletion (see Chapter 33). In contrast, children with chloride-unresponsive causes may have symptoms related to hypertension. Alkalemia may cause arrhythmias, hypoxia secondary to hypoventilation, or decreased cardiac output.

### Diagnosis

Measurement of the urinary chloride concentration is the most helpful test in differentiating among the causes of a metabolic alkalosis. The history usually suggests a diagnosis, although no obvious explanation may be present in the patient with bulimia, surreptitious diuretic use, or an undiagnosed genetic disorder, such as Bartter syndrome or Gitelman syndrome.

### Treatment

The approach to therapy of metabolic alkalosis depends on the severity of the alkalosis and the underlying etiology. In children with a mild metabolic alkalosis ([$HCO_3^-$] <32 mEq/L), intervention is often unnecessary. Patients with chloride-responsive metabolic alkalosis respond to correction of hypokalemia and volume repletion with sodium and potassium chloride, but aggressive volume repletion may be contraindicated if mild volume depletion is medically necessary in the child receiving diuretic therapy. In children with chloride-resistant causes of a metabolic alkalosis that are associated with hypertension, volume repletion is contraindicated because it exacerbates the hypertension and does not repair the metabolic alkalosis. Treatment focuses on eliminating or blocking the action of the excess mineralocorticoid. In children with Bartter syndrome or Gitelman syndrome, therapy includes oral potassium supplementation and potassium-sparing diuretics.

## RESPIRATORY ACID-BASE DISTURBANCES

During a respiratory acidosis, there is a decrease in the effectiveness of $CO_2$ removal by the lungs. The causes of a respiratory acidosis are either pulmonary or nonpulmonary

| TABLE 37-4  Causes of Respiratory Acidosis |
| --- |
| Central nervous system depression (encephalitis or narcotic overdose) |
| Disorders of the spinal cord, peripheral nerves, or neuromuscular junction (botulism or Guillain-Barré syndrome) |
| Respiratory muscle weakness (muscular dystrophy) |
| Pulmonary disease (pneumonia or asthma) |
| Upper airway disease (laryngospasm) |

| TABLE 37-5  Causes of Respiratory Alkalosis |
| --- |
| Hypoxemia or tissue hypoxia (carbon monoxide poisoning or cyanotic heart disease) |
| Lung receptor stimulation (pneumonia or pulmonary embolism) |
| Central stimulation (anxiety or brain tumor) |
| Mechanical ventilation |
| Hyperammonemias |

(Table 37-4). A respiratory alkalosis is an inappropriate reduction in the blood $CO_2$ concentration. A variety of stimuli can increase the ventilatory drive and cause a respiratory alkalosis (Table 37-5). Treatment of respiratory acid-base disorders focuses on correction of the underlying disorder. Mechanical ventilation may be necessary in a child with a refractory respiratory acidosis.

 SUGGESTED READING

Fry AC, Karet FE: Inherited renal acidosis, *Physiology* 22:202–211, 2007.

Greenbaum LA: Pathophysiology of body fluids and fluid therapy. In: Kliegman RE, Behrman RE, Jenson HB, et al: Nelson Textbook of Pediatrics, 18th ed, Philadelphia, 2007, *Elsevier Science*, pp 267–319.

Kleta R, Bockenhauer D: Bartter syndromes and other salt-losing tubulopathies, *Nephron Physiol* 104:73–80, 2006.

Schaefer TJ, Wolford RW: Disorders of potassium, *Emerg Med Clin North Am* 23:723–747, 2005.

Spandorfer PR, Alessandrini EA, Joffe MD, et al: Oral versus intravenous rehydration of moderately dehydrated children: a randomized, controlled trial, *Pediatrics* 115:295–301, 2005.

Wessel JJ, Kocoshis SA: Nutritional management of infants with short bowel syndrome, *Semin Perinatol* 31:104–111, 2007.

# THE ACUTELY ILL OR INJURED CHILD

K. Jane Lee and Karen J. Marcdante

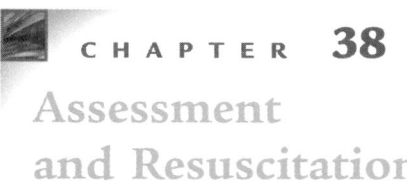

CHAPTER **38**

## Assessment and Resuscitation

## INITIAL ASSESSMENT

Initial assessment (the **ABCs—airway, breathing, and circulation**) of an acutely ill or injured child requires rapid identification of physiologic derangements in **tissue perfusion and oxygenation**. Once identified, immediate resuscitation must be implemented before pursuing the usual information needed to develop a differential diagnosis. Initial resuscitation measures are directed at improving and maintaining normal tissue perfusion and oxygenation. **Oxygen delivery** depends on cardiac output, hemoglobin concentration, and hemoglobin-oxygen saturation. The last-mentioned depends on air movement, alveolar gas exchange, pulmonary blood flow, and oxygen-hemoglobin binding characteristics.

## HISTORY

In the resuscitation phase, access to historical information may be limited. Characterization of onset of symptoms, details of events, and a brief identification of underlying medical problems should be sought by members of the team not actively involved in the resuscitation. Attempts at identifying historical issues that affect the ABCs are useful but should not delay intervention if tissue oxygenation and perfusion are markedly impaired.

## PHYSICAL EXAMINATION

Initial examination must focus rapidly on the **ABCs** (Table 38-1) to address the issues of oxygen delivery to tissues systematically. Airway patency is the first to be addressed, including assessment of the neurologically injured child's ability to protect the airway. Protection of the cervical spine also should be initiated at this step in any child with traumatic injury or who presents with altered mental status of uncertain etiology. Assessment of breathing

includes auscultation of air movement and application of a pulse oximeter (when available) to identify current oxygenation status. Circulatory status is assessed by palpation for distal and central pulses, focusing on the presence and quality of the pulses. Bounding pulses and a wide pulse pressure are often the first sign of the vasodilatory phase of shock and require immediate resuscitation measures. Weak, thready, or absent pulses are indicators for fluid resuscitation, initiation of chest compressions, or both. When assessment of the **ABCs** is complete and measures have been taken to achieve an acceptable level of tissue oxygenation, a more complete physical examination is performed. The sequence of this examination depends on whether the situation involves an acute medical illness or trauma. In trauma patients, the examination follows the **ABCDE pathway**. **D** stands for disability and prompts assessment of the neurologic system and evaluation for major traumatic injuries. **E** stands for exposure; the child is disrobed and searched for evidence of any life-threatening or limb-threatening problems. For the acutely ill and the injured child, the subsequent physical examination should identify evidence of organ dysfunction starting with areas suggested in the chief complaint and progressing to a thorough and systematic investigation of the entire patient.

## COMMON MANIFESTATIONS

The physiologic responses to acute illness and injury are mechanisms that attempt to correct inadequacies of tissue oxygenation and perfusion. When initial changes, such as increasing heart and respiratory rates, fail to meet the body's needs, other manifestations of impending cardiopulmonary failure occur (Table 38-2). **Respiratory failure**, the most common cause of acute deterioration in children, may result in inadequate tissue oxygenation and in respiratory acidosis. Signs and symptoms of respiratory failure (tachypnea, tachycardia, increased work of breathing, abnormal mentation) progress as tissue oxygenation becomes more inadequate. Inadequate perfusion (shock) leads to inadequate oxygen delivery and a resulting metabolic acidosis. **Shock** is characterized by signs of inadequate tissue perfusion (pallor, cool skin, poor pulses, delayed capillary refill, oliguria, and abnormal mentation). The presence of any of these symptoms demands careful assessment and intervention to correct the abnormality and to prevent further deterioration.

## TABLE 38-1 Rapid Cardiopulmonary Assessment

### AIRWAY PATENCY

Able to be maintained independently
Maintainable with positioning, suctioning
Unmaintainable, requires assistance

### BREATHING

Rate
Mechanics
    Retractions
    Grunting
    Use of accessory muscles
    Nasal flaring
Air movement
    Chest expansion
    Breath sounds
    Stridor
    Wheezing
    Paradoxical chest motion
Color

### CIRCULATION

Heart rate
Peripheral and central pulses
    Present/absent
    Volume/strength
Skin perfusion
    Capillary refill time
    Skin temperature
    Color
    Mottling
Blood pressure

### CENTRAL NERVOUS SYSTEM PERFUSION

Responsiveness (AVPU)
Recognition of parents or caregivers
Pupil size
Posturing

AVPU, *a*lert, responds to *v*oice, responds to *p*ain, *u*nresponsive.

## TABLE 38-2 Warning Signs and Symptoms Suggesting the Potential Need for Resuscitative Intervention*

| System | Signs and Symptoms |
|---|---|
| Central nervous system | Lethargy, agitation, delirium, obtundation, confusion |
| Respiratory | Apnea, grunting, nasal flaring, dyspnea, retracting, tachypnea, poor air movement, stridor, wheezing |
| Cardiovascular | Arrhythmia, bradycardia, tachycardia, weak pulses, poor capillary refill, hypotension |
| Skin and mucous membranes | Mottling, pallor, cyanosis, diaphoresis, poor membrane turgor, dry mucous membranes |

*Action would seldom be taken only if one or two of these signs and symptoms were present, but the occurrence of several in concert foreshadows grave consequences. Intervention should be directed at the primary disorder.

## TABLE 38-3 Elements of Acute Care

### EXAMINE

Perform an initial assessment followed by complete and systematic evaluation
Focus examination on areas of chief complaints; determine life-threatening and organ-threatening conditions

### MONITOR

Monitor vital signs
Monitor the physiologic parameters required to
1. Make a diagnosis
2. Ascertain response to therapy or progression of disease

### INTERVENE

Before initiating therapy, determine therapeutic goals and endpoints
Prioritize life-threatening and organ-threatening conditions
Initiate therapy based on recognized pathophysiologic derangements

### ANTICIPATE

Anticipation requires understanding of the underlying pathophysiology
Always plan for the "worst-case" scenario

## INITIAL DIAGNOSTIC EVALUATION

### Screening Tests

During the initial phase of resuscitation, monitoring vital signs and physiologic status is the key screening activity (Table 38-3). Continuous monitoring with attention to changes may indicate response to therapy or further deterioration requiring additional intervention. During the initial rapid assessment, diagnostic evaluation often is limited to pulse oximetry and bedside measurement of glucose levels. The latter is important in any child with altered mental status or at risk for inadequate glycogen stores (infants, malnourished patients). After resuscitation measures, further diagnostic tests and imaging are often necessary.

### Diagnostic Tests and Imaging

The choice of appropriate diagnostic tests and imaging is determined by the mechanism of disease and results of evaluation after initial resuscitation. The initial evaluation of major trauma patients is focused on identifying evidence of hemorrhage and organ and tissue injury. For an acutely ill child with respiratory distress, a chest x-ray is important. Appropriate cultures should be obtained when sepsis is suspected. A complete blood count may also be helpful despite poor sensitivity and specificity of the white blood cell and band counts. Children with historical or physical evidence of inadequate intravascular volume should have serum electrolyte levels obtained, including bicarbonate, blood urea nitrogen, and creatinine.

# RESUSCITATION

Resuscitation is focused on correcting identified abnormalities of oxygenation and perfusion and preventing further deterioration. **Oxygen supplementation** may improve oxygen saturation but may not completely correct tissue oxygenation. When oxygen supplementation is insufficient or air exchange is inadequate, assisted ventilation must be initiated. Inadequate perfusion is best managed initially by providing a fluid bolus. **Isotonic crystalloids** (normal saline, lactated Ringer solution) are the initial fluid of choice. A bolus of 10 to 20 mL/kg should be delivered in monitored conditions. Improvement, but not correction, after an initial bolus should prompt repeated boluses until circulation has been re-established. Because most children with shock have noncardiac causes, fluid administration of this magnitude is well tolerated. If hemorrhage is known or highly suspected, administration of packed red blood cells is appropriate. Monitoring for deteriorating physiologic status during fluid resuscitation (increase in heart rate, decrease in blood pressure) identifies children who may have cardiogenic shock. Fluid resuscitation increases preload, which may worsen pulmonary edema and cardiac function. If deterioration occurs, fluid administration should be interrupted, and resuscitation should be aimed at improving cardiac function.

When respiratory support and fluid resuscitation are insufficient, introduction of **vasoactive substances** is the next step. The choice of which agent to use depends on the type of shock present. Hypovolemic shock (when further volume is contraindicated) and distributive shock benefit from drugs that increase systemic vascular resistance (drugs with α-agonist activity, such as epinephrine or norepinephrine). The treatment of cardiogenic shock is more complex. To improve cardiac output by increasing the heart rate, drugs with positive chronotropy are used (epinephrine, norepinephrine, and dopamine). Afterload reduction, using drugs such as dobutamine, nitroprusside, or milrinone, also may be needed. Measuring mixed venous oxygen saturation, central venous pressure, and regional oxygen saturations helps guide therapy.

# CARDIOPULMONARY ARREST

Children who need cardiopulmonary resuscitation (CPR) usually have a primary respiratory arrest. The outcome of cardiopulmonary arrest in children is poor; only 2% to 10% survive, and most survivors have permanent neurologic disability. The ability to anticipate or recognize pre–cardiopulmonary arrest conditions and initiate prompt and appropriate therapy not only is lifesaving, but also preserves the quality of life (see Table 38-2).

**Hypoxia** has a central role in most of the events leading to cardiopulmonary arrest in children. Hypoxia also produces organ dysfunction or damage (Table 38-4). The approach to cardiopulmonary arrest extends beyond CPR and includes efforts to preserve vital organ function. The goal in resuscitating a pediatric patient following a cardiopulmonary arrest should be to optimize **cardiac output** and tissue oxygen delivery, which may be accomplished by using artificial ventilation and chest compression and by the judicious administration of pharmacologic agents.

**TABLE 38-4 Target Organs for Hypoxic-Ischemic Damage**

| Organ | Effect |
|---|---|
| Brain | Seizures, cerebral edema, infarction, herniation, anoxic damage, SIADH, diabetes insipidus |
| Cardiovascular | Heart failure, myocardial infarct |
| Lung and pulmonary vasculature | Acute respiratory distress syndrome, pulmonary hypertension |
| Liver | Infarction, necrosis, cholestasis |
| Kidney | Acute tubular necrosis, acute cortical necrosis |
| Gastrointestinal tract | Gastric ulceration, mucosal damage |
| Hematologic | Disseminated intravascular coagulation |

SIADH, syndrome of inappropriate secretion of antidiuretic hormone.

## Airway

The physician first should ensure that there is a **patent airway**. In children, airway patency often is compromised by a loss of muscle tone, allowing the mandibular block of tissue, including the tongue, bony mandible, and the soft surrounding tissues, to rest against the posterior pharyngeal wall. The head tilt-chin lift maneuver should be used to open the airway in children with no sign of head or neck trauma. In children with signs of head or neck trauma, the jaw thrust maneuver should be used.

Pediatric patients requiring resuscitation should be endotracheally intubated. Before intubation, the patient should be ventilated with 100% oxygen using a bag and mask. Cricoid pressure should be used to minimize inflation of the stomach. Many conscious patients may benefit from the use of induction medications (sedatives, analgesics, and paralytics) to assist intubation, but caution is necessary to prevent further cardiovascular compromise from vasodilating effects of many sedatives. The correct size of the tube may be estimated according to the size of the child's mid-fifth phalanx or the following formula: $4 + ($patient age in years$/4)$.

When the endotracheal tube is in place, the adequacy of ventilation and the position of the tube must be assessed. Use of end-tidal carbon dioxide ($CO_2$) monitoring devices may assist with validation of endotracheal placement, but low levels of detected $CO_2$ may be secondary to lack of pulmonary circulation. Adequate chest wall movement and auscultation of the chest to detect bilateral and symmetric breath sounds provide information on adequacy of air entry. If air exchange is not heard or cyanosis continues, the position or patency of the tube must be re-evaluated through direct visualization of tube location via laryngoscopy or, in patients with sufficient circulation, indirectly through the use of end-tidal $CO_2$ measurement.

## Breathing

The major role of endotracheal intubation is to protect or maintain the airway and ensure the delivery of adequate oxygen to the patient. Because hypoxemia is the final common pathway in pediatric cardiopulmonary arrests, providing oxygen is more important than correcting the respiratory acidosis. The clinician should deliver 100% oxygen at an initial rate of 12 to 20 breaths/min through the endotracheal tube, using a tidal volume necessary to produce adequate chest rise and relieve cyanosis. Care should be taken not to hyperventilate the patient.

## Circulation

When a patent airway is established and oxygenation and ventilation are maintained, **cardiac output** is re-established in many children. Carefully reassessing the patient before proceeding with other mechanical and pharmacologic maneuvers is essential. If cyanosis persists or the brachial or femoral pulses remain weak or absent, adequate circulation has not been re-established.

**Chest compressions** should be initiated if a pulse cannot be palpated or if the heart rate is less than 60 beats/min with signs of poor systemic perfusion. For compressions to be optimal, the child should be supine on a hard, flat surface. In infants and children, the area for compression is the lower half of the sternum. If two health care providers are available, encircling the chest with both hands to provide compressions is preferable for infants. Effective CPR requires a compression depth of one third to one half of the anterior-posterior diameter of the chest with complete recoil after each compression. The compression rate should be at least 100/min with breaths delivered 8 to 10 times per minute. If an advanced airway is in place compressions should not pause for ventilation; both should continue simultaneously.

The availability of **automated external defibrillators** outside the hospital setting may be useful in the relatively small number of children who are in ventricular fibrillation or pulseless ventricular tachycardia. Current recommendations include use in children older than 1 year of age.

## Drugs

When mechanical means fail to re-establish adequate circulation, pharmacologic intervention is essential (Table 38-5). Administration of drugs through a central venous line is preferred, although this is difficult to achieve in cases of unanticipated cardiopulmonary arrest. The effectiveness of peripheral intravenous administration is limited by poor circulation. If intravascular access is not present or rapidly established, administration through an intraosseous route is recommended. Some drugs can also be administered effectively through the endotracheal tube (epinephrine, lidocaine).

### TABLE 38-5  Drug Doses for Cardiopulmonary Resuscitation

| Drug | Indication | Dose |
| --- | --- | --- |
| Adenosine | Supraventricular tachycardia | 0.1–0.2 mg/kg maximum 12 mg |
| Amiodarone | Pulseless VF/VT | 5 mg/kg over 20–60 min, maximum 300 mg |
|  | Perfusing tachyarrhythmias | Maximum dose is 15 mg/kg/day |
| Atropine | Supraventricular or junctional bradycardia Asystole? | 0.02 mg/kg (minimum dose 0.1 mg); up to 0.5 mg (child), 1 mg (adolescent); higher doses needed in anticholinesterase poisoning |
| Bicarbonate | Metabolic acidosis? Hyperkalemia | 0.5–1 mEq/kg bolus; ensure adequate ventilation; use 4.2% solution in neonates; monitor ABGs, can repeat every 10 min |
| Calcium chloride | Hypocalcemia Hyperkalemia Wide QRS pattern? | 120 mg/kg; stop if bradycardia occurs |
| Dobutamine | Inotropy | 2–30 µg/kg/min |
| Dopamine | Inotropy | 0.5–2 µg/kg/min splanchnic, renal dilation; 2–7 µg/kg/min inotrope; 7–20 µg/kg/min inotrope and pressor |
| Epinephrine | Chronotropy Inotropy Hypotension | 0.01 mg/kg bolus every 5 min; 0.1–1 µg/kg/min drip, inotrope + pressor; may cause subendocardial ischemia and arrhythmias |
| Fluid | Hypovolemia Sepsis | Use crystalloid tailored to patient's physiologic needs |
| Glucose | Hypoglycemia | 5–10 mL/kg 10% dextrose; follow Dextrostix |
| Lidocaine | VT | 1 mg/kg/bolus followed by 20–50 µg/kg/min continuous infusion; monitor serum concentration and widening of QRS for toxicity |
| Nitroprusside | Reduce systemic vascular resistance Hypertensive crisis | 0.05–10.0 µg/kg/min by continuous infusion |
| Oxygen | Hypoxia | 100%, humidified |

?, Controversial, uncertain, or unproved efficacy; ABG, arterial blood gas; VF, ventricular fibrillation; VT, ventricular tachycardia.
Data from 2005 American Heart Association Guidelines for Cardiopulmonary Resuscitation and Emergency Cardiovascular Care. Part 12: Pediatric Advanced Life Support. *Circulation* 2005;112[Suppl 1]:IV167–IV187.

Perhaps the most important agent used during CPR is **oxygen**. Short periods of exposure to high oxygen tensions cause little pulmonary toxicity, and high oxygen tensions may be required to reverse some of the reactive pulmonary vascular responses to poor cardiac output.

**Epinephrine**, a catecholamine with mixed α-agonist and β-agonist properties constitutes the mainstay of drug therapy for CPR. The α-adrenergic effects are most important during acute phases of resuscitation, causing an increase in systemic vascular resistance that improves coronary blood flow. Standard dose therapy is recommended for the first and subsequent boluses. There is no benefit offered by high dose epinephrine, and it may be detrimental. Vasopressin, an endogenous hormone, causes constriction of capillaries and small arterioles and may be useful. Insufficient data support its routine use, but vasopressin may be considered in children failing standard medication administration.

The use of **sodium bicarbonate** is currently not recommended as a first-line approach. In pediatric patients, acidosis is more often respiratory, rather than metabolic, and administration of sodium bicarbonate can exacerbate the acidosis by inducing production of $CO_2$. Sodium bicarbonate may be judiciously used to correct identified excessive intake of acids or losses of bases, however oxygen delivery and elimination of $CO_2$ must be established first. Side effects include hypernatremia, hyperosmolality, hypokalemia, metabolic alkalosis (shifting the oxyhemoglobin curve to the left and impairing tissue oxygen delivery), reduced ionized calcium level, and impaired cardiac function.

Prompt electrical **defibrillation** is indicated when ventricular fibrillation or pulseless ventricular tachycardia is noted (Table 38-6). CPR should continue until just before defibrillation and resume immediately afterward, minimizing interruptions in compressions. If a second attempt at defibrillation is necessary, it should be followed by a dose of epinephrine. Children failing two episodes of defibrillation may benefit from administration of amiodarone. Defibrillation should be distinguished from **cardioversion** of supraventricular tachycardias, which also may compromise cardiac output. Cardioversion requires a lower starting dose and synchronization of the discharge to the electrocardiogram to prevent discharging during a susceptible period, which may convert supraventricular tachycardia to ventricular tachycardia or fibrillation.

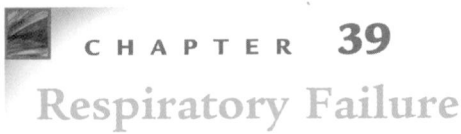

# CHAPTER 39
# Respiratory Failure

## ETIOLOGY

Acute respiratory failure occurs when the pulmonary system is unable to maintain adequate gas exchange to meet metabolic demands. The resulting failure can be classified as hypercarbic ($Paco_2$ >50 mm Hg in previously healthy children), hypoxemic ($Pao_2$ <60 mm Hg in previously healthy children without an intracardiac shunt), or both. **Hypoxemic respiratory failure** is frequently caused by ventilation-perfusion mismatch (perfusion of lung that is not adequately ventilated) and shunting (deoxygenated blood bypasses ventilated alveoli). **Hypercarbic respiratory failure** results from inadequate alveolar ventilation secondary to decreased minute ventilation (tidal volume × respiratory rate) or an increase in dead space ventilation (ventilation of areas receiving no perfusion).

Respiratory failure may occur with **acute lung injury (ALI)** or **acute respiratory distress syndrome (ARDS)**. ALI has the following four clinical features: acute onset, bilateral pulmonary edema, no clinical evidence of elevated left atrial pressure, and a ratio of $PaO_2$ to $FiO_2$ between 201 and 300 mm Hg regardless of the level of positive end-expiratory pressure (PEEP). The definition of ARDS is the same as ALI but with more severe hypoxemia ($PaO_2/FiO_2$ of ≤200 mm Hg). These syndromes can be triggered by a variety of insults, including sepsis, pneumonia, shock, burns, or traumatic injury, all resulting in inflammation and increased vascular permeability leading to pulmonary edema. Numerous mediators of inflammation (tumor necrosis factor, interferon-γ, nuclear factor κB, and adhesion molecules) may be involved in the development of ARDS. Surfactant action also may be affected.

## EPIDEMIOLOGY

Respiratory failure is frequently caused by bronchiolitis (often caused by respiratory syncytial virus), asthma, pneumonia, upper airway obstruction, and sepsis/ARDS. Respiratory failure requiring mechanical ventilation develops in approximately 5% of patients hospitalized for respiratory syncytial virus.

Asthma is increasing in prevalence and is the most common reason for unplanned hospital admissions in children 3 to 12 years of age in the United States. Environmental

---

| **TABLE 38-6 Recommendations for Defibrillation and Cardioversion in Children** |
|---|
| **DEFIBRILLATION** |
| Place self-adhesive defibrillation pads, gel pads, or electrode cream/paste at apex and upper right sternal border |
|     If not using self-adhesive pads, use infant paddles for children <10 kg; adult paddles for children >10 kg |
| Notify all participating personnel before discharging paddles so that no one is in contact with patient or bed |
| Begin with 2 J/kg, resume chest compressions immediately |
| If unsuccessful, double current (4 J/kg) and repeat |
| **CARDIOVERSION** |
| Consider sedation if possible |
| For symptomatic supraventricular tachycardia* or ventricular tachycardia with a pulse, synchronize signal with ECG |
| Choose paddles, position pads, and notify personnel as above |
| Begin with 0.5–1 J/kg |
| If unsuccessful, use 2 J/kg |

*Consider adenosine first (see Table 38-5).
ECG, electrocardiogram.

factors (exposure to cigarette smoke) and prior disease characteristics (severity of asthma, exercise intolerance, delayed start of therapy, and previous intensive care unit admissions) affect hospitalization and near-fatal episodes. The mortality rate of asthma for children younger than 19 years of age has increased by nearly 80% since 1980. Deaths are three times more common in African-American children.

Chronic respiratory failure (with acute exacerbations) is often due to chronic lung disease (bronchopulmonary dysplasia, cystic fibrosis), neurologic or neuromuscular abnormalities, and congenital anomalies.

## CLINICAL MANIFESTATIONS

Early signs of hypoxic respiratory failure include **tachypnea and tachycardia** as attempts are made to improve minute ventilation and cardiac output and to maintain delivery of oxygenated blood to the tissues. Further progression of disease may result in dyspnea, nasal flaring, grunting, use of accessory muscles of respiration, and diaphoresis. Late signs of inadequate oxygen delivery include **cyanosis** and **altered mental status** (initially confusion and agitation). Signs and symptoms of hypercarbic respiratory failure include attempts to increase minute ventilation (tachypnea and increased depth of breathing), and altered mental status (somnolence).

## LABORATORY AND IMAGING STUDIES

A chest radiograph may show evidence of the etiology of respiratory failure. The detection of atelectasis, hyperinflation, infiltrates, or pneumothoraces assists with ongoing management. Diffuse infiltrates or pulmonary edema may suggest ARDS. The chest radiograph may be normal when upper airway obstruction or impaired respiratory controls are the etiology. In patients presenting with stridor or other evidence of upper airway obstruction, a lateral neck film or computed tomography (CT) may delineate anatomic defects. Direct visualization through flexible bronchoscopy allows identification of dynamic abnormalities of the anatomic airway. Helical CT helps diagnose a pulmonary embolus.

**Pulse oximetry** allows noninvasive, continuous assessment of oxygenation but is unable to provide information about ventilation abnormalities. Determination of $CO_2$ levels requires a blood gas measurement (arterial, venous, or capillary). An **arterial blood gas** allows measurement of $CO_2$ levels and analysis of the severity of oxygenation defect through calculation of an alveolar-arterial oxygen difference. A normal $Pco_2$ in a patient who is hyperventilating should heighten concern about the risk of further deterioration.

## DIFFERENTIAL DIAGNOSIS

Hypoxic respiratory failure resulting from impairment of the alveolar-capillary function is seen in ARDS; cardiogenic pulmonary edema; interstitial lung disease; aspiration pneumonia; bronchiolitis; bacterial, fungal, or viral pneumonia; and sepsis. It also can be due to intrapulmonary or intracardiac shunting seen with atelectasis and embolism.

Hypercarbic respiratory failure occurs when the respiratory center fails as a result of drug use (opioids, barbiturates, anesthetic agents), neurologic or neuromuscular junction abnormalities (cervical spine trauma, demyelinating diseases, anterior horn cell disease, Guillain-Barré syndrome, botulism), chest wall injuries, or diseases that cause increased resistance to airflow (croup, vocal cord paralysis, postextubation edema). Maintenance of ventilation requires adequate function of the chest wall. Disorders of the neuromuscular pathways, such as muscular dystrophy, myasthenia gravis, and botulism, result in inadequate chest wall movement, development of atelectasis, and respiratory failure. Scoliosis rarely results in significant chest deformity that leads to restrictive pulmonary function. Similar impairments of air exchange may result from distention of the abdomen (postoperatively or due to ascites, obstruction, or a mass) and thoracic trauma (flail chest).

Mixed forms of respiratory failure are common and occur when disease processes result in more than one pathophysiologic change. Increased secretions seen in asthma often lead to atelectasis and hypoxia, whereas restrictions of expiratory airflow may lead to hypercarbia. Progression to respiratory failure results from peripheral airway obstruction, extensive atelectasis, and resultant hypoxemia and retention of $CO_2$. The identification of respiratory failure for patients with asthma includes a $Pao_2$ less than 60 mm Hg (as in other forms) but a $Paco_2$ greater than 45 mm Hg.

## TREATMENT

Initial treatment of patients in respiratory distress includes addressing the ABCs (see Chapter 38). **Bag/mask ventilation** must be initiated for patients with apnea or with signs of respiratory fatigue. In other patients, oxygen therapy is administered using appropriate methods (e.g., simple mask). Administration of oxygen by nasal cannula allows the patient to entrain room air and oxygen, making it an insufficient delivery method for most children in respiratory failure. Delivery methods, including intubation and mechanical ventilation, should be escalated if there is inability to increase oxygen saturation appropriately.

Patients presenting with hypercarbic respiratory failure are often hypoxic as well. When oxygenation is established, measures should be taken to address the underlying cause of hypercarbia (reversal of drug action, control of fever, or seizures). Patients who are hypercarbic without signs of respiratory fatigue or somnolence may not require intubation based on the $Pco_2$ alone; however, patients with marked increase in the work of breathing or inadequate respiratory effort may require assistance with ventilation.

After identification of the etiology of respiratory failure, specific interventions and treatments are tailored to the needs of the patient. External support of oxygenation and ventilation may be provided by **noninvasive ventilation** methods (continuous positive airway pressure, biphasic positive airway pressure, or negative pressure ventilation) or through invasive methods (traditional **mechanical ventilation**, high-frequency oscillatory ventilation, or extracorporeal membrane oxygenation). Elimination of $CO_2$ is achieved through manipulation of minute ventilation (tidal volume and respiratory rate). Oxygenation is improved by altering variables that affect oxygen delivery (fraction of inspired oxygen) or mean airway pressure (PEEP, peak inspiratory pressure, inspiratory time, gas flow).

## COMPLICATIONS

The major complication of hypoxic respiratory failure is the development of organ dysfunction. **Multiple organ dysfunction** includes the development of two or more of the following: respiratory failure, cardiac failure, renal insufficiency/failure, gastrointestinal or hepatic insufficiency, disseminated intravascular coagulation, and hypoxic-ischemic brain injury. Mortality rates increase with increasing numbers of involved organs (see Table 38-4).

Complications associated with mechanical ventilation include pressure-related and volume-related lung injury. Both overdistention and insufficient lung distention (loss of functional residual capacity) are associated with lung injury. Pneumomediastinum and pneumothorax are potential complications of the disease process and overdistention. Inflammatory mediators may play a role in the development of chronic fibrotic lung diseases in ventilated patients.

## PROGNOSIS

Prognosis varies with the etiology of respiratory failure. Less than 1% of previously healthy children with bronchiolitis die, whereas 3.5% of children with underlying respiratory or cardiac disease who develop bronchiolitis die. Asthma mortality rates, although still low, have increased. Despite advances in support and understanding of the pathophysiology of ARDS, the mortality rate remains approximately 30%. However, respiratory failure is the cause of death for only 15% of patients with ARDS.

## PREVENTION

Prevention strategies are explicit to the etiology of respiratory failure. Some infectious causes can be prevented through active immunization against organisms causing primary respiratory disease (pertussis, pneumococcus, *Haemophilus influenzae* type b) and sepsis (pneumococcus, *H. influenzae* type b). Passive immunization with respiratory syncytial virus immunoglobulins prevents severe illness in highly susceptible patients (prematurity, bronchopulmonary dysplasia). Primary prevention of traumatic injuries may decrease the incidence of ARDS. Compliance with appropriate therapies for asthma may decrease the number of episodes of respiratory failure (see Chapter 78).

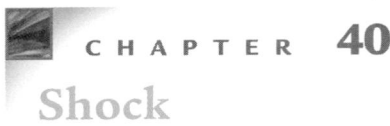 C H A P T E R    **40**

## Shock

## ETIOLOGY AND EPIDEMIOLOGY

Shock is the inability to provide sufficient perfusion of oxygenated blood and substrate to tissues to maintain organ function. **Oxygen delivery** is directly related to the arterial oxygen content (oxygen saturation and hemoglobin concentration) and to cardiac output (stroke volume and heart rate). Changes in metabolic needs are met primarily by adjustments in cardiac output. Stroke volume is related to myocardial end-diastolic fiber length (preload), myocardial contractility (inotropy), and resistance of blood ejection from the ventricle (afterload) (see Chapter 139). In a young infant whose myocardium possesses relatively less contractile tissue, increased demand for cardiac output is met primarily by a neurally mediated increase in heart rate. In older children and adolescents, cardiac output is most efficiently augmented by increasing stroke volume through neurohormonally mediated changes in vascular tone, resulting in increased venous return to the heart (increased preload), decreased arterial resistance (decreased afterload), and increased myocardial contractility.

## HYPOVOLEMIC SHOCK

Acute hypovolemia is the most common cause of shock in children. It results from loss of fluid from the intravascular space secondary to inadequate intake or excessive losses (vomiting and diarrhea, blood loss, capillary leak syndromes, or pathologic renal fluid losses) (Table 40-1). Reduced blood volume decreases preload, stroke volume, and cardiac output. Hypovolemic shock results in increased sympathoadrenal activity, producing an increased heart rate and enhanced myocardial contractility. Neurohormonally mediated constriction of the arterioles and capacitance vessels maintains blood pressure, augments venous return to the heart to improve preload, and redistributes blood flow from nonvital to vital organs. If hypovolemic shock remains untreated, the increased heart rate may impair coronary blood flow and ventricular filling, while elevated systemic vascular resistance increases myocardial oxygen consumption, resulting in worsening myocardial function. Ultimately, intense systemic vasoconstriction and hypovolemia produce tissue ischemia, impairing cell metabolism and releasing potent vasoactive mediators from injured cells. Cytokines and other vasoactive peptides can change myocardial contractility and vascular tone and promote release of other inflammatory mediators that increase capillary permeability and impair organ function further.

## DISTRIBUTIVE SHOCK

Abnormalities in the distribution of blood flow may result in profound inadequacies in tissue perfusion, even in the presence of a normal or high cardiac output. This maldistribution of flow usually results from abnormalities in vascular tone. Septic shock is the most common type of distributive shock in children. Other causes include anaphylaxis, neurologic injury, and drug-related causes (see Table 40-1).

Distributive shock may present with the **systemic inflammatory response syndrome** (SIRS), defined as two or more of the following: temperature greater than 38° C or less than 36° C; heart rate greater than 90 beats/min or more than two standard deviations above normal for age; tachypnea; or white blood count greater than 12,000 cells/mm$^3$, less than 4000 cells/mm$^3$, or greater than 10% immature forms.

| **TABLE 40-1  Classification of Shock and Common Underlying Causes** | | |
|---|---|---|
| Type | Primary Circulatory Derangement | Common Causes |
| Hypovolemic | Decreased circulating blood volume | Hemorrhage<br>Diarrhea<br>Diabetes insipidus<br>Diabetes mellitus<br>Burns<br>Adrenogenital syndrome<br>Capillary leak |
| Distributive | Vasodilation → venous pooling → decreased preload<br>Maldistribution of regional blood flow | Sepsis<br>Anaphylaxis<br>CNS/spinal injury<br>Drug intoxication |
| Cardiogenic | Decreased myocardial contractility | Congenital heart disease<br>Severe heart failure<br>Arrhythmia<br>Hypoxic/ischemic injuries<br>Cardiomyopathy<br>Metabolic derangements<br>Myocarditis<br>Drug intoxication<br>Kawasaki disease |
| Obstructive | Mechanical obstruction to ventricular outflow | Cardiac tamponade<br>Massive pulmonary embolus<br>Tension pneumothorax<br>Cardiac tumor |
| Dissociative | Oxygen not released from hemoglobin<br>Methemoglobinemia | Carbon monoxide poisoning |

CNS, central nervous system.

## CARDIOGENIC SHOCK

Cardiogenic shock is caused by an abnormality in myocardial function and is expressed as depressed myocardial contractility and cardiac output with poor tissue perfusion. Compensatory mechanisms may contribute to the progression of shock by depressing cardiac function further. Neurohormonal vasoconstrictor responses increase afterload and add to the work of the failing ventricle. Tachycardia may impair coronary blood flow, which decreases myocardial oxygen delivery. Increased central blood volume caused by sodium and water retention and by incomplete emptying of the ventricles during systole results in elevated left ventricular volume and pressure, which impair subendocardial blood flow. As compensatory mechanisms are overcome, the failing left ventricle produces increased ventricular end-diastolic volume and pressure, which leads to increased left atrial pressure, resulting in pulmonary edema. This sequence also contributes to right ventricular failure because of increased pulmonary artery pressure and increased right ventricular afterload.

Primary cardiogenic shock may occur in children who have congenital heart disease. Cardiogenic shock also may occur in previously healthy children secondary to viral myocarditis, dysrhythmias, or toxic or metabolic abnormalities or after hypoxic-ischemic injury (see Chapters 141, 142, 145, and 147, as well as Table 40-1).

## OBSTRUCTIVE SHOCK

Obstructive shock results from mechanical obstruction of ventricular outflow. Causes include congenital lesions such as coarctation of the aorta, interrupted aortic arch, and severe aortic valvular stenosis, along with acquired diseases (e.g., hypertrophic cardiomyopathy) (see Table 40-1). For neonates presenting in shock, obstructive lesions must be considered.

## DISSOCIATIVE SHOCK

Dissociative shock refers to conditions in which tissue perfusion is normal, but cells are unable to use oxygen because the hemoglobin has an abnormal affinity for oxygen, preventing its release to the tissues (see Table 40-1).

## CLINICAL MANIFESTATIONS

All forms of shock produce evidence that tissue perfusion and oxygenation are insufficient (increased heart rate, abnormal blood pressure, alterations of peripheral pulses). The etiology of shock may alter the initial presentation of these signs and symptoms.

## Hypovolemic Shock

Hypovolemic shock is distinguished from other causes of shock by history and the absence of signs of heart failure or sepsis. In addition to the signs of sympathoadrenal activity (tachycardia, vasoconstriction), clinical manifestations include signs of dehydration (dry mucous membranes, decreased urine output) or blood loss (pallor). Recovery depends on the degree of hypovolemia, the patient's preexisting status, and rapid diagnosis and treatment. The prognosis is good, with a low mortality (<10%) in uncomplicated cases.

## Distributive Shock

Patients with distributive shock usually have tachycardia and alterations of peripheral perfusion. In early stages, when cytokine release results in vasodilation, pulses may be bounding, and vital organ function may be maintained (an alert patient, with rapid capillary refill and some urine output in *warm shock*). As the disease progresses untreated, extremities become cool and mottled with a delayed capillary refill time. At this stage, the patient has hypotension and vasoconstriction. If the etiology of distributive shock is sepsis, the patient often has fever, lethargy, petechiae, or purpura, and he or she may have an identifiable source of infection.

## Cardiogenic Shock

Cardiogenic shock results when the myocardium is unable to supply the cardiac output required to support tissue perfusion and organ function. Because of this self-perpetuating cycle, heart failure progressing to death may be rapid. Patients with cardiogenic shock have tachycardia and tachypnea. The liver is usually enlarged, a gallop is often present, and jugular venous distention may be noted. Because renal blood flow is poor, sodium and water are retained, resulting in oliguria and peripheral edema.

## Obstructive Shock

Restriction of cardiac output results in an increase in heart rate and an alteration of stroke volume. The pulse pressure is narrow (making pulses harder to feel), and capillary refill is delayed. The liver is often enlarged, and jugular venous distention may be evident.

## Dissociative Shock

The principal abnormality in dissociative shock is the inability to deliver oxygen to tissues. Symptoms include tachycardia, tachypnea, alterations in mental status, and ultimately cardiovascular collapse.

## LABORATORY AND IMAGING STUDIES

Shock requires immediate resuscitation before obtaining laboratory or diagnostic studies. Following initial stabilization (including glucose administration if hypoglycemia is present), the type of shock dictates the necessary laboratory studies. All patients with shock may benefit from determination of a baseline arterial blood gas and blood lactate level to assess the impairment of tissue oxygenation. Measurement of **mixed venous oxygen saturation** aids in the assessment of the adequacy of oxygen delivery. In contrast to other forms of shock, patients with sepsis often have high mixed venous saturation values because of impairment of mitochondrial function and inability of tissues to extract oxygen. A complete blood count can potentially assess intravascular blood volume after equilibration following a hemorrhage. Electrolyte measurements in patients with hypovolemic shock may identify abnormalities from losses. Patients presenting in distributive shock require appropriate bacterial and viral cultures to identify a cause of infection. If cardiogenic or obstructive shock is suspected, an echocardiogram assists with the diagnosis and, in the case of tamponade, assists with placement of a pericardial drain to relieve the fluid. Patients with dissociative shock require detection of the causative agent (carbon monoxide, methemoglobin). The management of shock also requires monitoring of arterial blood gases for oxygenation, ventilation ($CO_2$), and acidosis, and frequently assessing the levels of serum electrolytes, calcium, magnesium, phosphorus, and blood urea nitrogen (BUN).

## DIFFERENTIAL DIAGNOSIS

▶ SEE TABLE 40-1.

## TREATMENT

### General Principles

The key to therapy is the recognition of shock in its early, partially compensated state, when many of the hemodynamic and metabolic alterations may be reversible. Initial therapy for shock follows the ABCs of resuscitation. Later therapy can then be directed at the underlying cause. Therapy should minimize cardiopulmonary work, while ensuring cardiac output, blood pressure, and gas exchange. Intubation, combined with mechanical ventilation with oxygen supplementation, improves oxygenation and decreases or eliminates the work of breathing but may impede venous return if distending airway pressures (positive end-expiratory pressure [PEEP] or peak inspiratory pressure) are excessive (see Chapter 61). Blood pressure support is crucial because the vasodilation in sepsis may reduce perfusion despite supranormal cardiac output.

Monitoring a child in shock requires maintaining access to the arterial and central venous circulation to record pressure measurements, perform blood sampling, and measure systemic blood pressure continuously. These measurements facilitate the estimation of preload and afterload. Regional monitoring with near infrared spectroscopy may allow early, noninvasive detection of alterations in perfusion.

### Organ-Directed Therapeutics

#### Fluid Resuscitation

Alterations in preload have a dramatic effect on cardiac output. In hypovolemic and distributive shock, decreased preload significantly impairs cardiac output. In these cases, early and aggressive fluid resuscitation is important and greatly affects outcome. In cardiogenic shock, an elevated preload contributes to pulmonary edema.

Selection of fluids for resuscitation and ongoing use is dictated by clinical circumstances. Crystalloid volume expanders generally are recommended as initial choices because they are effective and inexpensive. Most acutely ill children with signs of shock may safely receive, and usually benefit greatly from, a 20-mL/kg bolus of an isotonic crystalloid over 5 to 15 minutes. This dose may be repeated until a response is noted. Colloids contain larger molecules that may stay in the intravascular space longer than crystalloid solutions and exert oncotic pressure, drawing fluid out of the tissues into the vascular compartment. However, long-term risks of colloids may exceed benefits. Care must be exercised in treating cardiogenic shock with volume expansion because the ventricular filling pressures may rise without improvement of the cardiac performance. Carefully monitoring cardiac output or central venous pressure guides safe volume replacement.

## Cardiovascular Support

In an effort to improve cardiac output after volume resuscitation or when further volume replacement may be dangerous, a variety of inotropic and vasodilator drugs may be useful (Table 40-2). Therapy is directed first at increasing myocardial contractility, then at decreasing left ventricular afterload. The hemodynamic status of the patient dictates the choice of the agent.

Therapy usually is initiated with dopamine at 3 to 15 μg/kg/min. In children who fail to respond to several increments of an initial pressor, a more potent cardiotonic agent, such as epinephrine or norepinephrine, may be indicated. In addition to improving contractility, certain catecholamines cause an increase in systemic vascular resistance. The addition of a vasodilator drug may improve cardiac performance by decreasing the resistance against which the heart must pump (afterload). Afterload reduction may be achieved with dobutamine, milrinone, amrinone, nitroprusside, nitroglycerin, and angiotensin-converting enzyme inhibitors. The use of these drugs may be particularly important in late shock, when vasoconstriction is prominent.

## Respiratory Support

The lung is a target organ for inflammatory mediators in shock and SIRS. Respiratory failure may develop rapidly and become progressive. Intervention requires endotracheal intubation and mechanical ventilation accompanied by the use of supplemental oxygen and PEEP. Care must be taken with the process of intubation, because a child with compensated shock may suddenly decompensate on administration of sedative medications that reduce systemic vascular resistance. Severe cardiopulmonary failure may be managed with inhaled nitric oxide and, if necessary, extracorporeal membrane oxygenation (see Chapter 61).

## Renal Salvage

Poor cardiac output accompanied by decreased renal blood flow may cause prerenal azotemia and oliguria/anuria. Severe hypotension may produce **acute tubular necrosis** and **acute renal failure**. Prerenal azotemia is corrected when blood volume deficits are replaced or myocardial contractility is improved, but acute tubular necrosis does not improve immediately when shock is corrected. Prerenal azotemia is associated with a serum BUN-to-creatinine ratio of greater than 10:1 and a urine sodium level less than 20 mEq/L; acute tubular necrosis has a BUN-to-creatinine ratio of 10:1 or less and a urine sodium level between 40 and 60 mEq/L (see Chapter 165). Aggressive fluid replacement is often necessary to improve oliguria associated with prerenal azotemia. Because the management of shock requires administering large volumes of fluid, maintaining urine output greatly facilitates patient management.

Prevention of acute tubular necrosis and the subsequent complications associated with acute renal failure (hyperkalemia, acidosis, hypocalcemia, edema) is important. The use of pharmacologic agents to augment urine output is indicated when the intravascular volume has been replaced. The use of loop diuretics, such as furosemide, or combinations of a loop diuretic and a thiazide agent may enhance urine output. Infusion of low-dose dopamine, which produces renal artery vasodilation, also may improve urine output. Nevertheless, if hyperkalemia, refractory acidosis, hypervolemia, or altered mental status associated with uremia occurs, dialysis or hemofiltration should be initiated.

## COMPLICATIONS

Shock results in impairment of tissue perfusion and oxygenation and activation of inflammation and cytokine pathways. The major complication of shock is multiple organ system failure, defined as the dysfunction of more than one organ, including respiratory failure, renal failure, liver dysfunction, coagulation abnormalities, or cerebral dysfunction. Patients with shock and multiple organ failure have a higher mortality rate and, for survivors, a longer hospital stay.

| **TABLE 40-2 Catecholamines Used for Cardiopulmonary Resuscitation and in Shock** | | | | | |
|---|---|---|---|---|---|
| | Positive Inotrope | Positive Chronotrope | Direct Pressor | Indirect Pressor | Vasodilator |
| Dopamine | ++ | + | ± | ++ | ++* |
| Dobutamine | ++ | ± | − | − | + |
| Epinephrine | +++ | +++ | +++ | − | − |
| Isoproterenol | +++ | +++ | − | − | +++ |
| Norepinephrine | +++ | +++ | +++ | − | − |

*Primarily splanchnic and renal in low doses (3–5 μg/kg/min).

## PROGNOSIS

Early recognition and **goal-directed intervention** in patients with shock improve survival. Mortality rates for septic shock in children have decreased from greater than 90% in the 1960s to 8% to 9%. Specific mortality rates for other forms of shock are not readily available. However, delays in treatment of hypotension increase the incidence of multiple organ failure and mortality. Goal-directed therapy focused on maintaining mixed venous oxygen saturation may improve survival.

## PREVENTION

Prevention strategies for shock are focused, for the most part, on shock associated with sepsis and hypovolemia. Some forms of septic shock can be prevented through use of immunizations (*Haemophilus influenzae* type b, meningococcal, pneumococcal vaccines). Decreasing the risk of sepsis in a critically ill patient requires adherence to strict handwashing, isolation practices, and minimizing the duration of indwelling catheters. Measures to decrease pediatric trauma do much to minimize hemorrhage-induced shock.

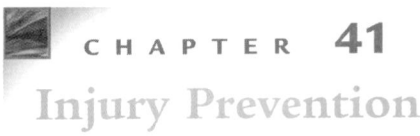

CHAPTER **41**

## Injury Prevention

## EPIDEMIOLOGY AND ETIOLOGY

Injury is the leading cause of death in children 1 to 18 years of age. Approximately 47% of these deaths are caused by motor vehicle crashes. Most remaining injury-related deaths are the result of homicide/suicide (34%) and drowning (5%). Geography, climate, population density (access to care), and population traits vary by region and affect the frequency, etiology, and severity of injuries.

Injury prevention requires evaluation of factors that affect the **host** (child), the **agent** (e.g., car and driver), and the **environment** (e.g., roadways, weather). The age of the child may determine the exposure to various agents and environments. For example, most injuries in infants and toddlers occur in the home as the result of exposure to agents found there (hot water heaters, bathtubs, soft bedding). Gender affects exposure to injury, with boys having a fatal injury rate more than twice that of girls.

More than 50% of trauma fatalities occur at the scene of the injury, in patients who receive injuries to the brainstem, head, aorta, heart, and upper cervical spine. Another 30% of deaths occur within 48 hours of the injury. Survival depends on the severity of shock at the time of hospital arrival and the length of time shock has been present. Taking an injured child to a center at which definitive care and stabilization occurs within 1 hour of the time of injury optimizes the outcome. A final peak in mortality occurs days to weeks after the initial injury and results from multisystem organ failure or other severe, life-threatening complications that have not responded to medical and surgical management.

## EDUCATION FOR PREVENTING INJURIES

The recognition that much of the morbidity and mortality are determined at the scene of an injury has stimulated the development of prevention measures. The **Haddon matrix** combines the epidemiologic components (host, agent, physical and social environments) with time factors (before, during, and after the event) to identify effective interventions focused on different aspects of the injury event. Primary strategies (preventing the event), secondary strategies (minimizing the severity of injury), and tertiary strategies (minimizing long-term impact) can be targeted for each epidemiologic component. Such strategies typically fall into one of three areas: education, enforcement, and environment (including engineering).

Education is often the first strategy considered but requires behavioral change and actions on the part of people. Most educational strategies are not well evaluated.

Despite the reliance on an action by the individuals involved, some active strategies benefit from enforcement. Children wearing bicycle helmets experience a significantly lower incidence of traumatic brain injury and death. Enforcement of seatbelt laws increases seatbelt use and may decrease injuries.

Automatic strategies require no action on the part of the population and often change the environment (speed bumps) or involve engineering (child-resistant pill bottles, air bags). Automatic strategies have more consistently resulted in a significant reduction in injuries. The most successful approaches to preventing injury have combined strategies (education, environmental changes, and engineering changes focused on the host, agent, and environment in all three time phases).

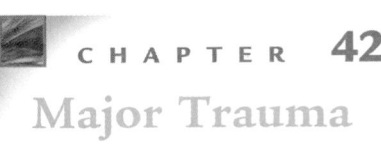

CHAPTER **42**

## Major Trauma

## ASSESSMENT AND RESUSCITATION

The general goal of **prehospital trauma care** is rapid assessment, support of the ABCs, immobilization, and transportation. Outcomes of patients with major or life-threatening trauma (Table 42-1) are significantly improved in a pediatric trauma center or in an adult center with pediatric trauma certification compared with level I or II adult trauma centers.

**TABLE 42-1 Children Requiring Pediatric Trauma Center Care**

Patients with serious injury to more than one organ or system

Patients with one-system injury who require critical care or monitoring in an intensive care unit

Patients with signs of shock who require more than one transfusion

Patients with fracture complicated by suspected neurovascular or compartment injury

Patients with fracture of axial skeleton

Patients with two or more long-bone fractures

Patients with potential replantation of an extremity

Patients with suspected or actual spinal cord or column injuries

Patients with head injury with any one of the following:

> Orbital or facial bone fracture
> Cerebrospinal fluid leaks
> Altered state of consciousness
> Changing neural signs
> Open head injuries
> Depressed skull fracture
> Requiring intracranial pressure monitoring

Patients suspected of requiring ventilator support

Once the injured child arrives at the emergency department, the trauma team must initiate an organized and synchronized response. The initial assessment of a seriously injured child should involve a systematic approach, including a primary survey, resuscitation, secondary survey, postresuscitation monitoring, and definitive care. The **primary survey** focuses on the **ABCDEs** of emergency care, as modified for trauma from the ABCs of cardiopulmonary resuscitation (see Chapter 38). The assessment of the airway and breathing components should include meticulous control of the cervical spine (especially if the patient has an altered mental status), evaluation for anatomic injuries that could impair air entry or gas exchange, and consideration of the likelihood of a full stomach (risk of aspiration pneumonia). Circulation can be assessed via observation (heart rate, skin color, mental status) and palpation (pulse quality, capillary refill, skin temperature) and restored (via two peripheral intravenous lines, when possible) while control of bleeding is accomplished through the use of direct pressure. Assessment for **disabilities** (D), including neurologic status, includes examination of pupil size and reactivity, a brief mental status assessment (*AVPU*—*a*lert; responds to *v*oice; responds to *p*ain; *u*nresponsive), and examination of extremity movement to assess for spinal cord injury. The **Glasgow Coma Scales** can direct decisions regarding the initiation of cerebral resuscitation in patients with suspected closed head injuries (Table 42-2). **E**, which stands for *exposure*, requires a full assessment of the patient by completely disrobing the child for a detailed examination of the entire body. The examiner should ensure a neutral thermal environment to prevent hypothermia.

On completion of the primary survey, a more detailed head-to-toe examination (the **secondary survey**) should ensue. The purpose of this careful re-examination is to identify life-threatening and limb-threatening injuries and less serious injuries. Coincident with the secondary survey and depending, in part, on the assessed physiologic status of the patient, certain procedures and resuscitative measures are initiated. The prioritization of definitive care needs is determined by the injury findings collected from the primary and secondary surveys, the child's physiologic response to resuscitation, and data from continuous monitoring. A **tertiary survey**, including repeat primary and secondary surveys along with review of laboratory tests and radiologic studies, should be performed within 24 hours.

## ETIOLOGY AND EPIDEMIOLOGY

▶ SEE CHAPTER 41.

## LABORATORY AND IMAGING STUDIES

Screening laboratory studies during initial resuscitation often include the tests listed in Table 42-3. Obtaining an arterial blood gas, serum lactate, base deficit, and mixed venous oxygen saturation assists in determining adequacy

**TABLE 42-2 Glasgow Coma Scales**

| Glasgow Coma Scale | | | Modified Coma Scale for Infants | | |
|---|---|---|---|---|---|
| Activity | Best Response | Score | Activity | Best Response | Score |
| Eye opening | Spontaneous | 4 | Eye opening | Spontaneous | 4 |
| | To verbal stimuli | 3 | | To speech | 3 |
| | To pain | 2 | | To pain | 2 |
| | None | 1 | | None | 1 |
| Verbal | Oriented | 5 | Verbal | Coos, babbles | 5 |
| | Confused | 4 | | Irritable, cries | 4 |
| | Inappropriate words | 3 | | Cries to pain | 3 |
| | Nonspecific sounds | 2 | | Moans to pain | 2 |
| | None | 1 | | None | 1 |
| Motor | Follows commands | 6 | Motor | Spontaneous movements | 6 |
| | Localizes pain | 5 | | Withdraws to touch | 5 |
| | Withdraws to pain | 4 | | Withdraws to pain | 4 |
| | Flexion to pain | 3 | | Abnormal flexion | 3 |
| | Extension to pain | 2 | | Abnormal extension | 2 |
| | None | 1 | | None | 1 |

**TABLE 42-3  Initial Laboratory Evaluation of the Major Trauma Patient**

### HEMATOLOGY

Complete blood count
Platelet count
Type and cross-match

### URINALYSIS

Gross
Microscopic

### CLINICAL CHEMISTRY

Amylase
AST/ALT

### RADIOLOGY

Cervical spine films
Anteroposterior chest radiograph
Radiographs of all apparent fractures
Computed tomography scans where indicated for head, chest, and abdominal trauma

AST/ALT, aspartate aminotransferase/alanine aminotransferase.

of resuscitation in many patients. Radiographic studies are determined by the pattern of injuries. A head computed tomography (CT) scan should be obtained in patients with evidence of head trauma or a history of loss of consciousness. Patients with obvious injury to the thorax or abdomen or who have pulmonary or abdominal symptoms may benefit from a CT scan. The focused abdominal sonography for trauma is gaining popularity because of concerns about radiation exposure. Diagnostic peritoneal lavage has limited utility. A spiral enhanced CT scan should be performed if there is concern about aortic injuries.

## CLINICAL MANIFESTATIONS AND TREATMENT

Head injuries and injuries to the limbs are the most common. Multiple organ involvement is also common, with 30% to 45% of pediatric trauma patients having multiple injuries and at least one skeletal fracture. Penetrating trauma is becoming more frequent and now accounts for 10% to 20% of all pediatric trauma admissions. After the initial evaluation and stabilization, the team focuses on the involved organ systems.

### Head Trauma

▶ SEE CHAPTER 184.

### Spinal Cord Trauma

Although spinal cord injury is not common in pediatric trauma patients, it is potentially devastating when it occurs. Cervical spine immobilization should be maintained until a spinal cord injury is ruled out. Cervical spine radiographs are not sufficient to rule out a spinal cord injury because the immature vertebral column in children may allow stretching of the cord or nerve roots with no radiologic abnormality (spinal cord injury without radiologic abnormality [SCIWORA]). SCIWORA may occur in 10% to 20% of children with a spinal cord injury; when it is suspected, magnetic resonance imaging should be performed. Controversy exists regarding the use of methylprednisolone for children with blunt spinal cord injury. It is not indicated for penetrating spinal cord injury.

### Thoracic Trauma

Thoracic injury occurs in only about 5% of children hospitalized for trauma, yet it is the second leading cause of death. Pulmonary contusion, pneumothorax, and rib fractures occur most commonly, and patients may present without external signs of trauma. Patients with pulmonary parenchymal injury should receive supportive treatment to ensure adequate oxygenation and ventilation. Most pediatric blunt thoracic injuries can be managed without surgery. Injury to the heart and great vessels is rare but requires urgent diagnosis and treatment. Great vessel injury should be suspected if a widened mediastinum is seen on chest radiograph.

### Abdominal Trauma

Injury to the abdomen occurs in approximately 8% of pediatric trauma patients. The relative size and closer proximity of intra-abdominal organs in children increase the risk of significant injury after blunt trauma. Penetrating trauma, which accounts for less than 10% of pediatric abdominal trauma, may result in a child who is asymptomatic or who presents in hypovolemic shock.

Performing serial physical examinations is the primary method of obtaining information on which to base decisions regarding operative intervention. Abdominal wall bruising is an important physical examination finding and is associated with significant intra-abdominal injury (often a hollow viscus) in more than 10% of patients. Operative intervention may be required in patients whose vital signs are persistently unstable in the face of aggressive fluid resuscitation, even in the absence of extravascular volume loss or an enlarging abdomen. The presence of peritoneal irritation or abdominal wall discoloration, together with signs of intravascular volume loss, indicates the need for laparotomy.

Abdominal CT is invaluable for assessing hemodynamically stable children with intra-abdominal trauma. Operative exploration is based on CT and physical findings and may be indicated when peritoneal irritation, hypovolemia, or free air on plain film is present.

Most blunt solid organ injury is handled nonoperatively. Clinical observation is important, because most failures with nonoperative management occur in the first 12 hours.

### Injury to the Spleen

The most frequently injured abdominal organ in children is the spleen. Suspicion of a splenic injury should be heightened if there are left upper quadrant abrasions or tenderness. A positive *Kehr* sign (pressure on the left upper quadrant eliciting left shoulder pain) is due to diaphragmatic irritation by the ruptured spleen and strongly suggests splenic injury. CT scans are used to grade splenic injury from 1 to 5 (grade 1, capsular tear or nonexpanding subcapsular hemorrhage, to grade 5, completely ruptured spleen).

Nonoperative management is the treatment of choice for most serious splenic injuries, unless there is continued large blood loss (transfusion requirement: >25-40 mL/kg/day) or hemodynamic instability. If a splenectomy is performed, patients should receive penicillin prophylaxis and should receive pneumococcal and *Haemophilus influenzae* vaccines to decrease the increased risk of overwhelming sepsis.

## Liver Trauma

Major trauma to the liver is a serious cause of morbidity and accounts for 40% of all deaths associated with blunt abdominal trauma in children. Severe hemorrhage is more common in patients with liver injury than with other abdominal injuries because of its dual blood supply. Without significant vascular injury, hepatic injury presents and behaves clinically like a splenic injury. Nonoperative management is recommended but requires close clinical observation for signs of ongoing blood loss or hemodynamic instability. Like splenic injury, there is a grading system based on the pattern of injury.

## Renal Injury

The kidney is injured in 10% to 20% of cases of blunt abdominal trauma, and more than 40% of children with injured kidneys have other internal injuries. A young child's kidney is more vulnerable to trauma than an adult's because of its anterior position in the peritoneal cavity, a more compliant rib cage, and relatively immature abdominal muscle development. The diagnosis of renal injury is based on history and physical examination coupled with urinalysis showing blood and increased protein levels. An intravenous pyelogram, ultrasound, or CT may also be useful. Low-grade renal injury is usually managed conservatively, consisting of bed rest, catheter drainage, and monitoring for resolution of injury by ultrasound or CT. Surgery may be required for falling hemoglobin levels, refractory shock, or urinary obstruction caused by clots.

## Pancreatic Injury

Injuries of the pancreas are less common in children than in adults but are seen in bicycle handlebar injuries, motor vehicle crashes, and nonaccidental trauma. The diagnosis is difficult unless there is obvious injury to overlying structures, such as the stomach or duodenum. Diffuse abdominal tenderness, pain, and vomiting may be accompanied by elevations of amylase and lipase but may not occur until several days after the injury. Hemodynamic instability secondary to retroperitoneal hemorrhage may be the presenting sign. Nasogastric suction and parenteral nutrition are indicated in the management of these patients. Nonoperative management is appropriate for contusions, but surgical intervention may be required in patients with distal transection. Drainage of pseudocysts

in patients who develop them may be required if they are unresponsive to bowel rest and parenteral nutrition.

## Intestinal Injury

Injury to the intestine occurs less frequently than injury to solid intra-abdominal organs and varies with the amount of intestinal contents. A full bowel is likely to shear more easily than an empty bowel. Shearing occurs at points of fixation (the ligament of Treitz, the ileocecal valve, and the ascending and descending peritoneal reflections). Intestinal/hollow viscus injuries are the most common intra-abdominal injuries in restrained children involved in motor vehicle crashes.

Abdominal tenderness is a common finding with intestinal perforation. Peritoneal signs are seen in less than 50% of children. Pneumoperitoneum occurs in only 20% of patients, but when present it should prompt surgical exploration. Serial physical examinations are useful when the clinical picture is uncertain.

Duodenal hematoma can occur in the absence of perforation. Duodenal hematomas result from blunt injury to the abdomen, and affected patients often present with persistent pain and bilious emesis. Most hematomas respond to nonoperative management with gastric decompression and parenteral nutrition.

## COMPLICATIONS

Patients requiring hospitalization for multiple trauma are at risk for a variety of complications based on the type and severity of injury. Sepsis and multiple organ failure may occur in children with multiple trauma. Delays in enteral nutrition because of an ileus may further increase the risk of sepsis secondary to translocation of bacteria across the intestinal mucosa.

Renal failure secondary to myoglobinuria may be seen in children who sustain crushing or electrical injuries and burns. Deep venous thrombosis is unusual in the pediatric population, but prophylaxis for older children (>14 years of age), who will be immobilized because of injury, is often provided.

## PROGNOSIS

Injuries are the largest cause of morbidity and mortality in children, accounting for more than 60% of deaths in children 1 to 19 years of age. Mortality rates for patients with head injuries range from 6% to 16%, with younger children having higher mortality rates. Isolated thoracic injury has a mortality rate of 5%, which increases to 25% if there is a concurrent head or abdominal injury. Penetrating trauma accounts for 10% to 20% of pediatric trauma admissions. Penetrating injuries caused by firearms have significant mortality, with 30% of victims dying in the field and another 12% in the emergency department. Morbidities are numerous and include hypoxic-ischemic brain injury, loss of limbs, and psychological dysfunction.

## PREVENTION

▶ SEE CHAPTER 41.

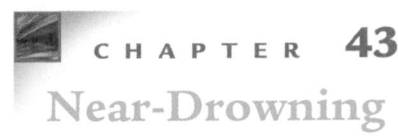

CHAPTER **43**

# Near-Drowning

## ETIOLOGY

Drowning, by definition, is fatal, and near-drowning is sometimes fatal. Drowning has been defined as death within 24 hours of submersion in water; victims of near-drowning survive for at least 24 hours. Initially, submersion results in aspiration of small amounts of fluid into the larynx, triggering breath holding or laryngospasm. In many cases, the laryngospasm resolves, and larger volumes of water or gastric contents are aspirated into the lungs, destroying surfactant and causing alveolitis and dysfunction of the alveolar-capillary gas exchange. The resulting hypoxemia leads to hypoxic brain injury that is exacerbated by ischemic injury after circulatory collapse. From 10% to 15% of patients become asphyxiated without aspirating.

## EPIDEMIOLOGY

Drowning is the third leading cause of death for children 1 to 18 years of age. Boys are four times as likely as girls to sustain a submersion injury. Boys younger than 4 years of age and those between 15 and 19 years of age have the highest rate of drowning. In the United States, most drowning occurs in freshwater. Most infants drown in bathtubs. It is estimated that for every child who drowns, four children are hospitalized for near-drowning.

## CLINICAL MANIFESTATIONS

**Hypoxemia** is the result of laryngospasm and aspiration during drowning. Victims may also develop respiratory distress secondary to **pulmonary endothelial injury**, **increased capillary permeability**, and **destruction of surfactant**. Clinical manifestations include tachypnea, tachycardia, increased work of breathing, and decreased breath sounds with or without crackles. The hypoxic-ischemic injury that may occur can lead to depressed myocardial function resulting in tachycardia, impaired perfusion, and potentially cardiovascular collapse. After resuscitation, acute respiratory distress syndrome is common. Altered mental status may be present and requires frequent monitoring of neurologic status. Following submersion in cold water, hypothermia may result in relative bradycardia and hypotension and place the child at risk for cardiac dysrhythmias.

## LABORATORY AND IMAGING STUDIES

After resuscitation, arterial blood gas measurement assists in assessing pulmonary gas exchange. A chemistry profile may reveal elevated liver enzymes if hypoxemia and ischemia were of long duration and provide baseline renal functions. Electrolytes are often obtained, although alterations of serum electrolytes are minimal, even in freshwater drowning.

## TREATMENT

Resuscitation of a near-drowning victim includes the basic ABCs. Victims of unwitnessed submersions require stabilization of the cervical spine because of the possibility of a fall or diving injury. Optimizing oxygenation and maintaining cerebral perfusion are two of the major foci of treatment. Rewarming the hypothermic patient requires careful attention to detail, including acid-base and cardiac status. Further treatment is based on the patient response to initial resuscitation. Some children begin breathing spontaneously and awaken before arrival at an emergency department. If submersion was significant, these children still require careful observation for pulmonary complications over the subsequent 6 to 12 hours. Children who have evidence of lung injury, cardiovascular compromise, or neurologic compromise should be monitored in an intensive care unit. Pulmonary dysfunction often results in hypoxemia. Oxygen supplementation should be implemented to maintain normal oxygen saturations. Mechanical ventilation may be needed in patients with significant pulmonary or neurologic dysfunction. Cardiovascular compromise is often the result of impaired contractility because of hypoxic-ischemic injury. The use of intracranial pressure monitoring devices and medical management with hypothermia and sedation is controversial and has not been shown to improve outcomes. Prophylactic antibiotics have not been shown to be beneficial and may increase the selection of resistant organisms.

## PROGNOSIS

The outcome of a near-drowning event is determined by the severity of the **hypoxic-ischemic injury** to the brain. Unfavorable prognostic markers for victims of near-drowning episodes include three or more of the following: age 3 years or older, submersion time of more than 5 minutes, greater than 10-minute delay in resuscitation efforts, coma on admission to emergency department, and pH less than 7.10.

## PREVENTION

Despite the decreased incidence of drowning since the 1990s, few prevention strategies have been shown to be effective. Exceptions include implementation of mandatory four-sided fencing around pools (decreased the number of children <5 years of age who drown) and immediate provision of cardiopulmonary resuscitation to children who are submerged. The use of safety flotation devices in older children during water sport activities may be beneficial. Enhanced supervision is required to reduce the incidence of infants drowning in bathtubs.

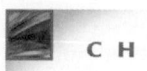

CHAPTER **44**

# Burns

## ETIOLOGY

The pathophysiology of burn injury is caused by disruption of the three key functions of the skin: regulation of heat loss, preservation of body fluids, and barrier to infection. Burn injury releases inflammatory and vasoactive mediators resulting in increased capillary permeability, decreased plasma volume, and decreased cardiac output. For treatment of severe burns, admission to a qualified burn center is necessary. Burns usually are classified on the basis of four criteria:

1. Depth of injury
2. Percent of body surface area involved
3. Location of the burn
4. Association with other injuries

## EPIDEMIOLOGY

Nearly 1% (>400,000) of all children sustains a burn injury each year. More than 25,000 require hospitalization, and more than 400 children 1 to 14 years of age die as a result of their burns each year. Scald burns are most common, comprising up to 85% of burns in children. Flame burns account for another 13%. Boys are more likely to sustain a burn injury, with the highest rate of injury occurring in boys younger than 5 years of age.

Most fire-related childhood deaths and injuries occur in homes without working smoke detectors. Mortality is primarily associated with burn severity (extent of body surface area and depth), although the presence of inhalation injury and young age also predict mortality.

## CLINICAL MANIFESTATIONS

The depth of injury should be assessed by the clinical appearance. **First-degree burns** are red, painful, and dry. Commonly seen with sun exposure or mild scald injuries, these burns involve injury to the epidermis only. They heal in 5 to 10 days without scarring and are not included in burn surface area calculations. **Second-degree burns**, or partial-thickness burns, involve portions of the dermis; some dermis remains viable. Healing is dependent on the uninjured dermis. Severe second-degree burns may take about a month to heal, and scarring results. **Third-degree burns**, or full-thickness burns, require grafts if they are more than 1 cm in diameter. They are avascular, lack sensation, and have a dry, leathery appearance. **Fourth-degree burns** involve underlying fascia, muscle, or bone. **Inhalation injuries** should be suspected if there are facial burns, singed nasal hairs, or carbonaceous sputum. Inhalation injuries may result in bronchospasm, airway inflammation, and impaired pulmonary function.

Burns can be classified as major or minor for treatment purposes. Major burns consist of those covering more than 15% of body surface area (>10% in infants), involving the face or perineum, or those involving inhalation injury. Second-degree and third-degree burns of the hands or feet and circumferential burns of the extremities also are classified as major. A method for estimating the percentage of skin surface area involved in burns in children of various ages is presented in Figure 44-1. The extent of skin involvement of older adolescent and adult patients is estimated as follows: each upper extremity, 9%; each lower extremity, 18%; anterior trunk, 18%; posterior trunk, 18%; head, 9%; and perineum, 1%.

The location of the burn is important in assessing the risk of disability. The risk is greatest when the face, eyes, ears, feet, perineum, or hands are involved. Inhalation injuries not only cause respiratory compromise but also may result in difficulty in eating and drinking.

## LABORATORY AND IMAGING STUDIES

Initial laboratory testing, including complete blood count, type and crossmatch for blood, coagulation studies, basic chemistry profile, arterial blood gas, and chest radiograph, can be helpful for patients with major burns. A **carboxyhemoglobin** assessment should be performed for any suspected inhalation exposure (a house or closed-space fire or a burn victim who requires cardiopulmonary resuscitation).

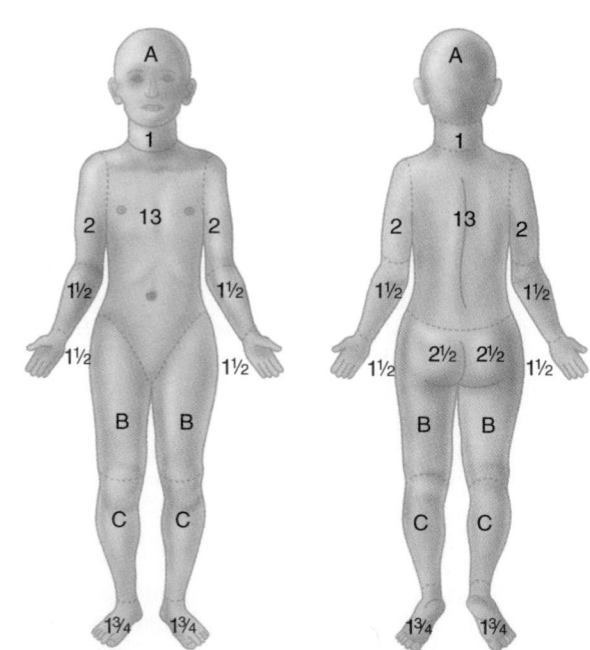

PERCENTAGE OF SURFACE AREA OF HEAD AND LEGS AT VARIOUS AGES

| | AGE IN YEARS | | | | |
|---|---|---|---|---|---|
| AREA IN DIAGRAM | 0 | 1 | 5 | 10 | 15 |
| A = ½ of head | 9½ | 8½ | 6½ | 5½ | 4½ |
| B = ½ of one thigh | 2¾ | 3¼ | 4 | 4¼ | 4½ |
| C = ½ of one lower leg | 2½ | 2½ | 2¾ | 3 | 3¼ |

**FIGURE 44-1**

This chart of body areas, together with the table inserted in the figure showing the percentage of surface area of head and legs at various ages, can be used to estimate the surface area burned in a child. (From Solomon JR: Pediatric burns. *Crit Care Clin* 1:159–174, 1985.)

Cyanide levels should be considered in children who sustain smoke inhalation and have altered mental status. Unusual patterns of burns may increase suspicion of child abuse and result in appropriate evaluation to rule out nonaccidental trauma to the skeleton or central nervous system.

## TREATMENT

The triage decision is based on:

1. Extent of the burn
2. Body surface area involved
3. Type of burn
4. Associated injuries
5. Any complicating medical or social problems
6. Availability of ambulatory management

Initial treatment should follow the ABCs of resuscitation. Airway management should include assessment for the presence of airway or inhalation injury. Smoke inhalation may be associated with carbon monoxide toxicity; 100% humidified oxygen should be given if hypoxia or inhalation is suspected. Hoarseness on vocalization also is consistent with a supraglottic injury. Some children with inhalation burns require endoscopy, an artificial airway, and mechanical ventilation.

The **systemic capillary leak** that occurs after a serious burn makes initial fluid and electrolyte support of a burned child crucial. The first priority is to support the circulating blood volume, which requires the administration of intravenous fluids to provide maintenance fluid and electrolyte requirements and to replace ongoing burn-related losses. No formula accurately predicts the fluid needs of every burn patient. Children with a significant burn should receive a rapid bolus of 20 mL/kg of lactated Ringer solution. The resuscitation formula for fluid therapy is determined by the percent of body surface burned. Total fluids are 2 to 4 mL/kg/percent burn/24 hour, with half the estimated burn requirement administered during the first 8 hours. (If resuscitation is delayed, half of the fluid replacement should be completed by the end of the eighth hour postinjury.) The goal of this fluid replacement is maintenance equal to or greater than 1 mL/kg/hour of urine output. Fluids should be titrated to accomplish this goal. Controversy exists over whether and when to administer colloid during fluid resuscitation. Colloid therapy may be needed for burns covering more than 30% of body surface area and may be provided after 24 hours of successful resuscitation with crystalloids.

Because burn injury produces a **hypermetabolic** response, children with significant burns require immediate nutritional support. Although enteral feeding may be resumed on day 2 or 3 of therapy, children with critical burn injury may require parenteral nutrition if unable to tolerate full enteral feeds. The hypermetabolic state can be modulated through the effective management of anxiety and pain as well as prevention of hypothermia by maintenance of a neutral thermal environment.

**Wound care** requires careful surgical management. Initial management includes relief of any pressure on peripheral circulation caused by eschar and débridement to allow classification of burns. Coverage with topical agents aids pain control and decreases insensible losses. Burns generally are covered with silver sulfadiazine (1%) applied to fine-mesh gauze or, if the burn is shallow, with polymyxin B/bacitracin/neomycin (Neosporin) ointment. Silver nitrate (0.5%) and 11.1% mafenide acetate (which is painful, produces metabolic acidosis, and penetrates eschar) are alternative antimicrobial agents. These agents inhibit but do not prevent bacterial growth. Various grafts, such as cadaver allografts, porcine xenografts, artificial bilaminate (cross-linked chondroitin-6-sulfate and silicone) skin substitute, and cultured patient's keratinocytes, have been used initially to cover wounds. For full-thickness burns, skin autografting and artificial skin substitutes are required for eventual closure. Burn management and rehabilitation are highly specialized skills, involving the recognition of many complications of burns (Table 44-1) and evaluation of the wound and its cause for suspected child abuse or neglect. Tetanus toxoid should be provided for patients with incomplete immunization status; immune globulin is indicated in the nonimmunized patient.

## COMPLICATIONS

▶ SEE TABLE 44-1.

**TABLE 44-1  Complications of Burns**

| Problem | Treatment |
|---|---|
| Sepsis | Monitor for infection, avoid prophylactic antibiotics |
| Hypovolemia | Fluid replacement |
| Hypothermia | Adjust ambient temperature: dry blankets in field |
| Laryngeal edema | Endotracheal intubation, tracheostomy |
| Carbon monoxide poisoning | 100% oxygen, hyperbaric $O_2$ |
| Cyanide poisoning | 100% $O_2$ plus amyl nitrate, sodium nitrate, and sodium thiosulfate |
| Cardiac dysfunction | Inotropic agents, diuretics |
| Gastric ulcers | $H_2$-receptor antagonist, antacids |
| Compartment syndrome | Escharotomy incision |
| Contractures | Physical therapy |
| Hypermetabolic state | Enteral and parenteral nutritional support |
| Renal failure | Supportive care, dialysis |
| Transient antidiuresis | Expectant management |
| Anemia | Transfusions as indicated |
| Psychological trauma | Psychological rehabilitation |
| Pulmonary infiltrates | PEEP, ventilation, $O_2$ |
| Pulmonary edema | Avoid overhydration, give diuretics |
| Pneumonia | Antibiotics |
| Bronchospasm | β-agonist aerosols |

PEEP, positive end-expiratory pressure.

## PROGNOSIS

Most children who sustain burns recover without significant disability; however, burns remain the third leading cause of injury-related pediatric deaths. Estimation of morbidity is difficult to ascertain from databases. Physical scarring and emotional impact of disfiguring burns are long-term consequences of burn injuries.

## PREVENTION

About 92% of burns occur in the home. Prevention is possible by using smoke and fire alarms, having identifiable escape routes and a fire extinguisher, and reducing hot water temperature to 49°C (120°F). Immersion full-thickness burns develop after 1 second at 70°C (158°F), after 5 seconds at 60°C (140°F), after 30 seconds at 54.5°C (130°F), and after 10 minutes at 49°C (120°F).

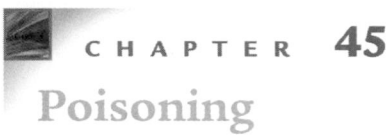

CHAPTER **45**

# Poisoning

## ETIOLOGY

The most common agents ingested by young children include cosmetics, personal hair products, cleaning solutions, and analgesics. The most common poisonings that lead to hospitalization involve acetaminophen, lead, and antidepressant medications. Fatal childhood poisonings are commonly caused by carbon monoxide, hydrocarbons, medications (analgesics, iron, cardiovascular drugs, cyclic antidepressants), drugs of abuse, and caustic ingestions.

## EPIDEMIOLOGY

Poisoning and ingestions account for more than 130,000 visits to emergency departments and approximately 1% of all pediatric hospitalizations each year. Unintentional ingestions are most common in the 1- to 5-year-old age group. In older children, drug overdoses (poisonings) most often are associated with suicide attempts. Most ingestions are unintentional (83%), occur in the home (90%), and result in no toxicity (72%) or minor toxicity (15%). Only 0.1% of cases are fatal.

## CLINICAL MANIFESTATIONS

Unless the ingested drug is revealed, poisoning is often a diagnosis of exclusion. A comatose child should be considered to have ingested a poison until proven otherwise. The history and physical examination by someone who understands the signs and symptoms of various ingestions often provide sufficient clues to distinguish between toxic ingestion and organic disease (Table 45-1). Determination of all substances that the child was exposed to, type of medication, amount of medication, and time of exposure is crucial in directing interventions. Available data often are incomplete or inaccurate, requiring a careful physical examination and laboratory approach. A complete physical examination, including vital signs, is necessary. Certain complexes of symptoms and signs are relatively specific to a given class of drugs (toxidrome) (Table 45-2).

## COMPLICATIONS

A poisoned child can exhibit any one of six basic clinical patterns: coma, toxicity, metabolic acidosis, heart rhythm aberrations, gastrointestinal symptoms, and seizures.

### Coma

Coma is perhaps the most striking symptom of a poison ingestion, but it also may be seen as a result of trauma, a cerebrovascular accident, asphyxia, or meningitis. A careful history and clinical examination are needed to distinguish among these alternatives.

### Systemic and Pulmonary Toxicity

Hydrocarbon ingestion occasionally may result in systemic toxicity, but more often it leads to pulmonary toxicity. Hydrocarbons with low viscosity, low surface tension, and high volatility pose the greatest risk of producing aspiration pneumonia; however, when swallowed, they pose no risk unless emesis is induced. Emesis or lavage should *not* be initiated in a child who has ingested volatile hydrocarbons.

Caustic ingestions may cause dysphagia, epigastric pain, oral mucosal burns, and low-grade fever. Patients with esophageal lesions may have no oral burns or may have significant signs and symptoms. Treatment depends on the agent ingested and the presence or absence of esophageal injury. Alkali agents may be solid, granular, or liquid. Liquid agents are tasteless and produce full-thickness liquefaction necrosis of the esophagus or oropharynx. When the esophageal lesions heal, strictures form. Ingestion of these agents also creates a long-term risk of esophageal carcinoma. Treatment includes antibiotics if there are signs of infection and dilation of late-forming (2 to 3 weeks later) strictures.

Ingested button batteries also may produce a caustic mucosal injury. Batteries that remain in the esophagus may cause esophageal burns and erosion and should be removed with an endoscope. Acid agents can injure the lungs (with hydrochloric acid fumes), oral mucosa, esophagus, and stomach. Because acids taste sour, children usually stop drinking the solution, limiting the injury. Acids produce a coagulation necrosis, which limits the chemical from penetrating into deeper layers of the mucosa and damages tissue less severely than alkali. The signs, symptoms, and therapeutic measures are similar to those for alkali ingestion.

### Metabolic Acidosis

A poisoned child may also have a high anion gap metabolic acidosis (mnemonic *MUDPIES*) (Table 45-3), which is assessed easily by measuring arterial blood gases, serum electrolyte levels, and urine pH. An osmolar gap, if present, strongly suggests the presence of an unmeasured component, such as methanol or ethylene glycol. These ingestions require thorough assessment and prompt intervention.

## TABLE 45-1 Historical and Physical Findings in Poisoning

### ODOR

| | |
|---|---|
| Bitter almonds | Cyanide |
| Acetone | Isopropyl alcohol, methanol, paraldehyde, salicylate |
| Alcohol | Ethanol |
| Wintergreen | Methyl salicylate |
| Garlic | Arsenic, thallium, organophosphates |
| Violets | Turpentine |

### OCULAR SIGNS

| | |
|---|---|
| Miosis | Narcotics (except meperidine), organophosphates, muscarinic mushrooms, clonidine, phenothiazines, chloral hydrate, barbiturates (late), PCP |
| Mydriasis | Atropine, alcohol, cocaine, amphetamines, antihistamines, cyclic antidepressants, cyanide, carbon monoxide |
| Nystagmus | Phenytoin, barbiturates, ethanol, carbon monoxide |
| Lacrimation | Organophosphates, irritant gas or vapors |
| Retinal hyperemia | Methanol |
| Poor vision | Methanol, botulism, carbon monoxide |

### CUTANEOUS SIGNS

| | |
|---|---|
| Needle tracks | Heroin, PCP, amphetamine |
| Bullae | Carbon monoxide, barbiturates |
| Dry, hot skin | Anticholinergic agents, botulism |
| Diaphoresis | Organophosphates, nitrates, muscarinic mushrooms, aspirin, cocaine |
| Alopecia | Thallium, arsenic, lead, mercury |
| Erythema | Boric acid, mercury, cyanide, anticholinergics |

### ORAL SIGNS

| | |
|---|---|
| Salivation | Organophosphates, salicylate, corrosives, strychnine |
| Dry mouth | Amphetamine, anticholinergics, antihistamine |
| Burns | Corrosives, oxalate-containing plants |
| Gum lines | Lead, mercury, arsenic |
| Dysphagia | Corrosives, botulism |

### INTESTINAL SIGNS

| | |
|---|---|
| Cramps | Arsenic, lead, thallium, organophosphates |
| Diarrhea | Antimicrobials, arsenic, iron, boric acid |
| Constipation | Lead, narcotics, botulism |
| Hematemesis | Aminophylline, corrosives, iron, salicylates |

### CARDIAC SIGNS

| | |
|---|---|
| Tachycardia | Atropine, aspirin, amphetamine, cocaine, cyclic antidepressants, theophylline |
| Bradycardia | Digitalis, narcotics, mushrooms, clonidine, organophosphates, β-blockers, calcium channel blockers |
| Hypertension | Amphetamine, LSD, cocaine, PCP |
| Hypotension | Phenothiazines, barbiturates, cyclic antidepressants, iron, β-blockers, calcium channel blockers |

### RESPIRATORY SIGNS

| | |
|---|---|
| Depressed respiration | Alcohol, narcotics, barbiturates |
| Increased respiration | Amphetamines, aspirin, ethylene glycol, carbon monoxide, cyanide |
| Pulmonary edema | Hydrocarbons, heroin, organophosphates, aspirin |

### CENTRAL NERVOUS SYSTEM SIGNS

| | |
|---|---|
| Ataxia | Alcohol, antidepressants, barbiturates, anticholinergics, phenytoin, narcotics |
| Coma | Sedatives, narcotics, barbiturates, PCP, organophosphates, salicylate, cyanide, carbon monoxide, cyclic antidepressants, lead |
| Hyperpyrexia | Anticholinergics, quinine, salicylates, LSD, phenothiazines, amphetamine, cocaine |
| Muscle fasciculation | Organophosphates, theophylline |
| Muscle rigidity | Cyclic antidepressants, PCP, phenothiazines, haloperidol |
| Paresthesia | Cocaine, camphor, PCP, MSG |
| Peripheral neuropathy | Lead, arsenic, mercury, organophosphates |
| Altered behavior | LSD, PCP, amphetamines, cocaine, alcohol, anticholinergics, camphor |

LSD, lysergic acid diethylamide; MSG, monosodium glutamate; PCP, phencyclidine.

**TABLE 45-2 Toxic Syndromes**

| Agent | Manifestations |
| --- | --- |
| Acetaminophen | Nausea, vomiting, pallor, delayed jaundice–hepatic failure (72–96 hr) |
| Amphetamine, cocaine, and sympathomimetics | Tachycardia, hypertension, hyperthermia, psychosis and paranoia, seizures, mydriasis, diaphoresis, piloerection, aggressive behavior |
| Anticholinergics | Mania, delirium, fever, red dry skin, dry mouth, tachycardia, mydriasis, urinary retention |
| Carbon monoxide | Headache, dizziness, coma, skin bullae, other systems affected |
| Cyanide | Coma, convulsions, hyperpnea, bitter almond odor |
| Ethylene glycol (antifreeze) | Metabolic acidosis, hyperosmolarity, hypocalcemia, oxalate crystalluria |
| Iron | Vomiting (bloody), diarrhea, hypotension, hepatic failure, leukocytosis, hyperglycemia, radiopaque pills on KUB, late intestinal stricture, *Yersinia* sepsis |
| Narcotics | Coma, respiratory depression, hypotension, pinpoint pupils, hyporeflexia |
| Cholinergics (organophosphates, nicotine) | Miosis, salivation, urination, diaphoresis, lacrimation, bronchospasm (bronchorrhea), muscle weakness and fasciculations, emesis, defecation, coma, confusion, pulmonary edema, bradycardia, reduced erythrocyte and serum cholinesterase, late peripheral neuropathy |
| Phenothiazines | Tachycardia, hypotension, muscle rigidity, coma, ataxia, oculogyric crisis, miosis, radiopaque pills on KUB |
| Salicylates | Tachypnea, fever, lethargy, coma, vomiting, diaphoresis, alkalosis (early), acidosis (late) |
| Cyclic antidepressants | Coma, convulsions, mydriasis, hyperreflexia, arrhythmia (prolonged Q-T interval), cardiac arrest, shock |

KUB, kidney-ureter-bladder radiograph.

## Dysrhythmias

Dysrhythmias may be prominent signs of a variety of toxic ingestions, although ventricular arrhythmias are rare. Prolonged Q-T intervals may suggest phenothiazine or antihistamine ingestion, and widened QRS complexes are seen with ingestions of cyclic antidepressants and quinidine. Because many drug and chemical overdoses may lead to sinus tachycardia, this is not a useful or discriminating sign; however, sinus bradycardia suggests digoxin, cyanide, a cholinergic agent, or β-blocker ingestion (Table 45-4).

## Gastrointestinal Symptoms

Gastrointestinal symptoms of poisoning include emesis, nausea, abdominal cramps, and diarrhea. These symptoms may be the result of direct toxic effects on the intestinal mucosa or of systemic toxicity after absorption.

## Seizures

Seizures are the sixth major mode of presentation for children with toxic ingestions, but poisoning is an uncommon cause of afebrile seizures. When seizures do occur with intoxication, they may be life-threatening and require aggressive therapeutic intervention.

## LABORATORY AND IMAGING STUDIES

Laboratory studies helpful in initial management include specific toxin-drug assays; measurement of arterial blood gases and electrolytes, osmoles, and glucose; and calculation of the anion or osmolar gap. A full 12-lead electrocardiogram should be part of the initial evaluation in all patients suspected of ingesting toxic substances. Urine screens for drugs of abuse or to confirm suspected ingestion of medications in the home may be revealing.

Quantitative toxicology assays are important for some agents (Table 45-5), not only for identifying the specific drug, but also for providing guidance for therapy, anticipating complications, and estimating the prognosis. The timing of measurement of the plasma level relative to the time of the patient's ingestion of the drug also is useful in predicting the severity of illness for acetaminophen (Fig. 45-1). Patients with drug levels (related to the time after ingestion) in the serious zone require immediate treatment.

## TREATMENT

### Supportive Care

Prompt attention must be given to protecting and maintaining the airway, establishing effective breathing, and supporting the circulation. This management sequence takes precedence over other diagnostic or therapeutic procedures. If the level of consciousness is depressed, and a toxic substance is suspected, glucose (1 g/kg intravenously), 100% oxygen, and naloxone should be administered.

### Gastrointestinal Decontamination

The intent of gastrointestinal decontamination is to prevent the absorption of a potentially toxic ingested substance and, in theory, to prevent the poisoning. There has been great controversy about which methods are the

## TABLE 45-3 Screening Laboratory Clues in Toxicologic Diagnosis

### METABOLIC ACIDOSIS (MNEMONIC = MUDPIES)

**M**ethanol,* carbon monoxide
**U**remia*
**D**iabetes mellitus*
**P**araldehyde,* phenformin
**I**soniazid, iron
**E**thanol,* ethylene glycol*
**S**alicylates, starvation, seizures

### HYPOGLYCEMIA

Ethanol
Isoniazid
Insulin
Propranolol
Oral hypoglycemic agents

### HYPERGLYCEMIA

Salicylates
Isoniazid
Iron
Phenothiazines
Sympathomimetics

### HYPOCALCEMIA

Oxalate
Ethylene glycol
Fluoride

### RADIOPAQUE SUBSTANCE ON KUB (MNEMONIC = CHIPPED)

**C**hloral hydrate, calcium carbonate
**H**eavy metals (lead, zinc, barium, arsenic, lithium, bismuth as in Pepto-Bismol)
**I**ron
**P**henothiazines
**P**lay-Doh, potassium chloride
**E**nteric-coated pills
**D**ental amalgam

*Indicates hyperosmolar condition.
KUB, kidney-ureter-bladder radiograph.

## TABLE 45-4 Drugs Associated with Major Modes of Presentation

### COMMON TOXIC CAUSES OF CARDIAC ARRHYTHMIA

Amphetamine
Antiarrhythmics
Anticholinergics
Antihistamines
Arsenic
Carbon monoxide
Chloral hydrate
Cocaine
Cyanide
Cyclic antidepressants
Digitalis
Freon
Phenothiazines
Physostigmine
Propranolol
Quinine, quinidine
Theophylline

### CAUSES OF COMA

Alcohol
Anticholinergics
Antihistamines
Barbiturates
Carbon monoxide
Clonidine
Cyanide
Cyclic antidepressants
Hypoglycemic agents
Lead
Lithium
Methemoglobinemia*
Methyldopa
Narcotics
Phencyclidine
Phenothiazines
Salicylates

### COMMON AGENTS CAUSING SEIZURES (MNEMONIC = CAPS)

**C**amphor
Carbamazepine
Carbon monoxide
Cocaine
Cyanide
**A**minophylline
Amphetamine
Anticholinergics
Antidepressants (cyclic)
**P**b (lead) (also lithium)
Pesticide (organophosphate)
Phencyclidine
Phenol
Phenothiazines
Propoxyphene
**S**alicylates
Strychnine

*Causes of methemoglobinemia: amyl nitrite, aniline dyes, benzocaine, bismuth subnitrate, dapsone, primaquine, quinones, spinach, sulfonamides.

safest and most efficacious. In light of this controversy, the American Academy of Clinical Toxicology (AACT) and the European Association of Poison Centres and Clinical Toxicologists (EAPCCT) have written several position papers on the subject. Their most recent recommendations (2004) follow. **Syrup of ipecac** should not be administered routinely to poisoned patients because of potential complications and lack of evidence that it improves outcome. Likewise, **gastric lavage** should not be used routinely, if ever, in the management of poisoned patients because of lack of efficacy and potential complications. **Single-dose activated charcoal** decreases drug absorption when used within 1 hour of ingestion; however, it has not been shown to improve outcome.

### TABLE 45-5 Drugs Amenable to Therapeutic Monitoring for Drug Toxicity

#### ANTIBIOTICS

Aminoglycosides—gentamicin, tobramycin, and amikacin
Chloramphenicol
Vancomycin

#### IMMUNOSUPPRESSION

Methotrexate
Cyclosporine

#### ANTIPYRETICS

Acetaminophen
Salicylate

#### OTHER

Digoxin
Lithium
Theophylline
Anticonvulsant drugs
Serotonin uptake inhibitor agent

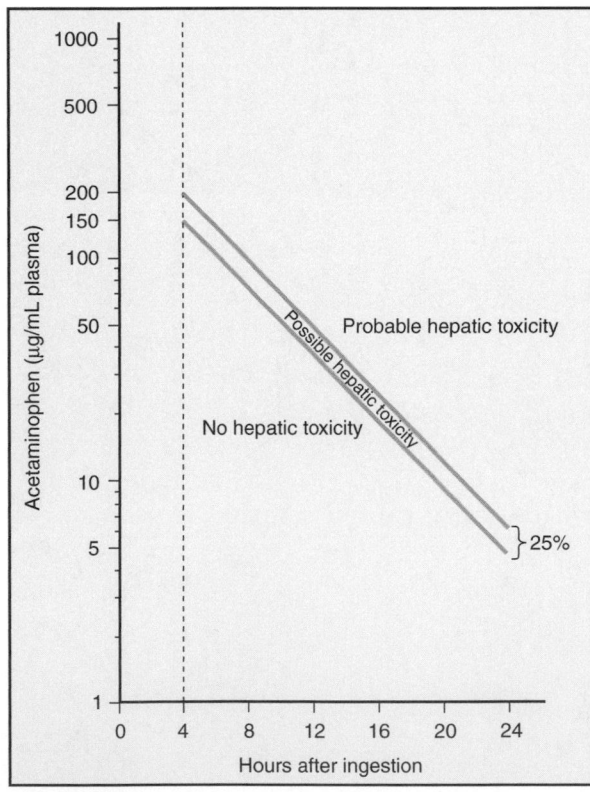

**FIGURE 45-1**

Semilogarithmic plot of plasma acetaminophen levels versus time. Rumack-Matthews nomogram for acetaminophen poisoning. Cautions for use of this chart are as follows: (1) The time coordinates refer to time of ingestion; (2) serum levels drawn before 4 hours may not represent peak levels; (3) the graph should be used only in relation to a single, acute ingestion; and (4) the lower solid line, 25% below the standard nomogram, is included to allow for possible errors in acetaminophen plasma assays and estimated time from ingestion of an overdose. (Adapted from Rumack BH, Matthew H: Acetaminophen poisoning and toxicity. *Pediatrics* 55:871–876, 1975.)

Thus, it should be used selectively in the management of a poisoned patient. Charcoal is ineffective against caustic or corrosive agents, hydrocarbons, heavy metals (arsenic, lead, mercury, iron, lithium), glycols, and water-insoluble compounds. **Multiple-dose activated charcoal** should be considered only if a patient has ingested a life-threatening amount of carbamazepine, dapsone, phenobarbital, quinine, or theophylline.

Also, the administration of a cathartic (sorbitol or magnesium citrate) alone has no role in the management of the poisoned patient. The AACT has stated that based on available data, the use of a cathartic in combination with activated charcoal is not recommended.

In addition, whole bowel irrigation using polyethylene glycol (GoLYTELY) as a nonabsorbable cathartic may be effective for toxic ingestion of sustained-release or enteric-coated drugs. The AACT does not recommend the routine use of whole bowel irrigation. However, there is theoretical benefit in its use for potentially toxic ingestions of iron, lead, zinc, or packets of illicit drugs.

### Additional Therapy

After initial resuscitation and gastrointestinal decontamination (if indicated) have been achieved, determining whether further therapy is needed is often difficult. There are three basic choices in the subsequent care of a child with a significant ingestion:

1. Providing continued supportive care
2. Using specific antidotes where available (Table 45-6)
3. Actively removing the toxin from the bloodstream

To make a rational decision regarding these options, a judgment should be made as to whether the drug causes tissue damage (e.g., methyl alcohol, aspirin, acetaminophen, theophylline, iron, ethylene glycol). Tissue damage is defined as an irreversible or slowly reversible structural or functional change in an organ system as a direct result of ingestion of a poison; this definition precludes indirect effects, such as respiratory depression or hypotension.

The decision about further therapy should take into consideration the amount of poison ingested; the diagnostic assessment, including the condition of the patient at the time of presentation; and the natural history of the suspected type of ingestion. All of these variables may be influenced by the child's prior clinical status or underlying medical problems (e.g., underlying hepatic or renal impairment). In the presence of a chronic ingestion, an acute overdose may cause significant clinical toxicity with a lower dose of the drug.

For most common ingestions in healthy individuals, continued supportive care and treatment directed toward specific complications are appropriate. Specific antidotes should be used according to prescribed guidelines (see Table 45-6). Active removal (hemoperfusion or dialysis) should be undertaken only for toxins that may cause tissue damage, for toxins that have been ingested by a patient already exhibiting confounding medical problems or to avoid prolonged supportive care. When in doubt, contacting one of the U.S. Poison Control Centers (1-800-222-1222) can help determine what additional treatment is necessary.

## TABLE 45-6 Emergency Antidotes

| Poison | Antidote | Dosage | Comments |
|---|---|---|---|
| Acetaminophen | N-Acetyl cysteine | 140 mg/kg PO initial dose, then 70 mg/kg PO q4h × 17 doses | Most effective within 16 hr of ingestion |
| Benzodiazepine | Flumazenil | 0.01–0.02 mg/kg IV; 0.2 mg max | Possible seizures, arrhythmias |
| β-Blocking agents | Atropine<br>Isoproterenol<br>Glucagon | 0.01–0.10 mg/kg IV<br>0.05–1.5 µg/kg/min IV infusion<br>0.05–0.1 mg/kg IV | Minimum dose 0.1 mg |
| Calcium channel blockers | Glucagon | 0.05–0.1 mg/kg IV | Increases cAMP, resulting in positive inotropy and chronotropy |
| Carbon monoxide | Oxygen | 100%; hyperbaric $O_2$ | Half-life of carboxyhemoglobin is 5 hr in room air but 1.5 hr in 100% $O_2$ |
| Cyclic antidepressants | Sodium bicarbonate | 0.5–1.0 mEq/kg IV, titrated to produce pH of 7.5–7.55 | — |
| Iron | Deferoxamine | Initial dose 10–15 mg/kg/hr IV | Deferoxamine Mesylate forms excretable ferrioxamine complex; hypotension |
| Lead | Edetate calcium (calcium disodium versenate [EDTA]) | 50–75 mg/kg/day × 5 days; divided q4h to q8h | |
| | BAL (British anti-Lewisite [dimercaprol]) | 3–5 mg/kg/dose q4h × 4–11 days; | May cause hypertension and sterile abscesses |
| | Penicillamine | 20–30 mg/kg/day PO divided q6h | Requires weekly monitoring for hepatic and bone marrow toxicity; should not be used in the presence of ongoing ingestion |
| | Succimer (2,3-Dimercaptosuccinic acid ([DMSA]) | 10 mg/kg/day PO tid × 5 days then 10 mg/kg/day PO bid × 14 days | Few toxic effects, requires lead-free home plus compliant family |
| Nitrites/ methemoglobinemia* | Methylene blue | 1–2 mg/kg, repeat in 1–4 hr if needed; treat for levels >30% | Exchange transfusion may be needed for severe methemoglobinemia; methylene blue overdose also causes methemoglobinemia |
| Opiates, Darvon, Lomotil | Naloxone | 0.10 mg/kg IV, ET, SC, IM<br>For children, up to 2 mg | Naloxone causes no respiratory depression |
| Organophosphates | Atropine | Initial dose 0.02–0.05 mg/kg IV | Physiologic: blocks acetylcholine; up to 5 mg IV every 15 min may be necessary in a critically ill adult |
| | Pralidoxime (2 PAM; Protopam) | Initial dose 25–50 mg/kg IV; 2g max follow with infusion of 10–20 mg/kg/hr | Specific: disrupts phosphate-cholinesterase bond; up to 500 mg/hr may be necessary in a critically ill adult |
| Sympathomimetic agents | Blocking agents: phentolamine; β-blocking agents; other antihypertensives | | Must be used in a setting in which vital signs can be monitored effectively |

*See Table 45-4 for causes of methemoglobinemia.
ET, endotracheal; IV, intravenous; PO, oral.
Data from Kulig K: Initial management of ingestions of toxic substances. *N Engl J Med* 326:1677–1681, 1992; Liebelt EL: Newer antidotal therapies for pediatric poisonings. *Clin Pediatr Emerg Med* 1:234–243, 2000; and Leikin JB, Paloucek EP, editors: Poisoning and toxicology compendium, Cleveland, 1998, *Lexi-Comp*.

## PROGNOSIS

Mortality from poisoning is rare. The most common exposures resulting in death include carbon monoxide, hydrocarbons, and opioids (all of which interfere with oxygen delivery to tissues). Medications that affect cardiac function (calcium channel antagonists, β-adrenergic sustained-release medications, tricyclic antidepressants, and adrenergic ingestions) also are in the top 10 causes of death from poisoning.

## PREVENTION

Properly educating parents regarding safe storage of medications and household toxins is necessary for preventing ingestions. If a child has ingested poison, a poison control center should be called.

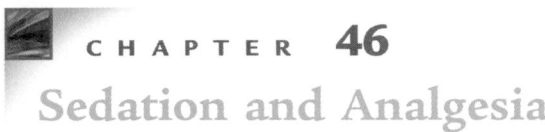

CHAPTER 46

# Sedation and Analgesia

An acutely ill pediatric patient may have pain, discomfort, and anxiety resulting from injury, surgery, and invasive procedures (intubation, bone marrow aspiration, venous access placement) or during life-sustaining mechanical ventilation. Clear goals should be identified to allow provision of optimal analgesia or sedation without compromising the physiologic status of the patient. Anxiolysis, cooperation, amnesia, immobility, and lack of awareness all are goals of sedation and can be accomplished with various drugs (Table 46-1). Many of these goals can be achieved with behavioral techniques (preprocedural teaching), but sedation is often a necessary adjunct for painful procedures. Pain may be expressed by verbal or visible discomfort, crying, agitation, tachycardia, hypertension, and tachypnea. A variety of scales have been developed in an attempt to quantify pain and allow more directed therapy. Few of these scales are well validated, especially in populations of acutely ill children with physiologic derangements

secondary to the underlying pathology. Pain caused by procedural interventions should always be treated with analgesics in addition to sedation (Table 46-2).

## ASSESSMENT

### Procedural Sedation

A medical evaluation must be performed for any patient receiving procedural sedation to identify underlying medical conditions that may affect the choice of sedative agents. Specific attention must be paid to assessment of the airway (for ability to maintain a patent airway) and respiratory system (asthma, recent respiratory illness, loose teeth), cardiovascular status (especially adequacy of volume status), factors affecting drug metabolism (renal or liver disease), and risk of aspiration (adequate nothing-by-mouth status, gastroesophageal reflux). During the administration of procedural sedation, assessment of status must include monitoring of oxygen saturation, heart rate, and respiratory rate, as well as some assessment of effectiveness of ventilation. This assessment must be performed by someone who is not involved in the procedure; this person is also responsible for recording vital signs and drugs administered on a time-based graph. Monitoring must be continued until the child has returned to baseline. Patients who are receiving long-term sedation (e.g., to maintain endotracheal tube placement) may need only local anesthesia for painful procedures but may benefit from additional sedation or analgesia as well.

### Nonprocedural Sedation

Many ventilated pediatric patients require sedation and some analgesia while intubated. The most common choice is a combination of a longer acting benzodiazepine and an opioid. Avoidance of oversedation is important. Use of appropriate pain and sedation scores allows for titration of medications to achieve goals of the sedation plan. Long-term use of benzodiazepines and opioids leads to tolerance, a problematic occurrence that must be considered as medications are added and weaned. True addiction is a rare occurrence, especially when medications are provided at the minimum level needed to achieve adequate sedation and pain control.

| **TABLE 46-1  Agents That Produce Sedation** | | |
|---|---|---|
| **Sedative-Hypnotics** | **Effect** | **Concerns** |
| Midazolam | Anxiolysis, sedation, muscle relaxation, amnesia | Tolerance is possible; apnea, hypotension, depressed myocardial function; short action |
| Lorazepam | Anxiolysis, sedation, muscle relaxation, amnesia | Same as midazolam; long action |
| Ketamine | Anesthesia, analgesia, amnesia | Dissociative reactions, tachycardia, hypertension, increased bronchial secretions, emergent delirium, hallucinations; increases intracranial pressure |
| Chloral hydrate | Sedative | Emesis, hypotension, arrhythmias, hepatic dysfunction, possible carcinogen |
| Propofol | Rapid-onset sedative for induction and maintenance of anesthesia | Metabolic acidosis in children; may depress cardiac function |

**TABLE 46-2  Agents That Produce Analgesia**

| Analgesic | Effect | Complications |
|---|---|---|
| Acetaminophen and NSAIDs | Moderate analgesia, antipyresis | Ceiling effect, requires PO administration; NSAIDs—gastrointestinal bleed, ulceration |
| **Opioids** | | **No ceiling effect, respiratory depression, sedation, pruritus, nausea/vomiting, decreased gastric motility, urinary retention, tolerance with abuse potential** |
| Morphine | Analgesia | May cause myocardial depression |
| Codeine | Analgesia | Nausea/vomiting |
| Fentanyl, alfentanil, sufentanil | Analgesia, sedation | No adverse effects on cardiovascular system; stiff chest syndrome |
| **Partial agonists/ agonist-antagonist** | **Dysphoria, withdrawal symptoms** | |
| Propoxyphene | Analgesia | Dizziness, sedation |
| Meperidine | Analgesia, sedation | May increase intracranial pressure, respiratory depressant, hypotension |
| Methadone | Analgesia | |

NSAIDs, nonsteroidal anti-inflammatory drugs; PO, oral.

## PAIN AND ANALGESIA

The subjective aspect of pain requires that self-reporting be used for assessment. Visual analog scales, developed for adult patients (allowing patients to rate pain on a scale of 1 to 10), have been used for older children. Pain scales for younger children often incorporate behavioral and physiologic parameters, despite the imprecision of physiologic responses.

Local anesthetics, such as lidocaine, can be used for minor procedures. However, lidocaine requires subcutaneous or intradermal injection. The use of EMLA, a cream containing lidocaine and prilocaine, is less effective than intradermal lidocaine but is preferred by many patients.

Patient-controlled analgesia is an effective method for providing balanced analgesia care in older children and adolescents. Children using patient-controlled analgesia have better pain relief and experience less sedation than patients receiving intermittent, nurse-controlled, bolus analgesics. Analgesics can be administered through the patient-controlled analgesia pump with continuous basal infusions, bolus administration, or both. Morphine is the most frequent opioid used for patient-controlled analgesia. Monitoring of oxygen saturations and respiratory rate are crucial with continuous opioid infusions because of the shift in $CO_2$ response curve and potential to decrease ventilatory response to hypoxia.

Epidural analgesia decreases the need for inhalation anesthetics during surgery and can provide significant analgesia without sedation in the postoperative period. Decreased costs and length of stay also may be benefits of epidural analgesic approaches. Medications used in epidurals include bupivacaine and morphine. Adverse effects include nausea and vomiting, motor blockade, and technical problems requiring catheter removal. Infection and permanent neurologic deficits are rare.

# SUGGESTED READING

American Heart Association: Guidelines for Cardiopulmonary Resuscitation and Emergency Cardiovascular Care. Part 11: Pediatric Basic Life Support, *Circulation* 112(Suppl 1):IV-156–IV-166, 2005.

American Heart Association: Guidelines for Cardiopulmonary Resuscitation and Emergency Cardiovascular Care. Part 12: Pediatric Advanced Life Support, *Circulation* 112(Suppl 1):IV-167–IV-187, 2005.

Kliegman RM, Behrman RE, Jenson HB: Nelson Textbook of Pediatrics, 18th ed, Philadelphia, 2007, *Saunders.*

Kliegman RM, Greenbaum LA, Lye PS: Practical Strategies in Pediatric Diagnosis and Therapy, 2nd ed, Philadelphia, 2004, *Saunders.*

# HUMAN GENETICS AND DYSMORPHOLOGY

**Paul A. Levy and Robert W. Marion**

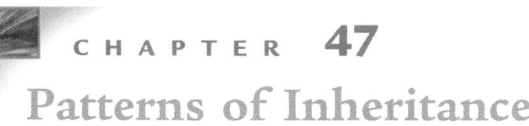

CHAPTER **47**

## Patterns of Inheritance

### TYPES OF GENETIC DISORDERS

Among infants born in the United States, 2% to 4% have **congenital malformations**, abnormalities of form or function identifiable at birth. At 1 year of age, the number approaches 7%, because some anomalies, such as ventriculoseptal defects, may not be identifiable until after the neonatal period. The incidence of congenital malformations is much greater in inpatient pediatric populations; 30% to 50% of hospitalized children have congenital anomalies or genetic disorders.

The clinical geneticist attempts to identify the etiology, mode of inheritance, and risk that a disorder might occur in the affected child's siblings. In evaluating children with congenital malformations, the clinical geneticist attempts to classify the patient's condition into one of five different categories:

1. Single gene mutations, accounting for 6% of children with congenital anomalies
2. Chromosomal disorders, accounting for approximately 7.5%
3. Multifactorially inherited conditions, accounting for 20%
4. Disorders that show an unusual pattern of inheritance, accounting for 2% to 3%
5. Conditions caused by exposure to teratogens, accounting for 6%

### INTRODUCTION TO GENETICS AND GENOMICS

DNA is composed of four nucleotide building blocks: adenine, guanine, cytosine, and thymine. Each nucleotide is linked to other nucleotides, forming a chain. The DNA molecule consists of two chains of nucleotides held together by hydrogen bonds. The purine nucleotides, adenine and guanine, cross-link by hydrogen bonds to the pyrimidines, thymine and cytosine. Because of this cross-linking, the nucleotide sequence of one strand sets the other strand's sequence. Separating the two strands permits complementary nucleotides to bind to each DNA strand; this copies the DNA and replicates the sequence.

DNA exists as multiple fragments that, together with a protein skeleton (chromatin), form chromosomes. Human cells have 23 pairs of chromosomes, with one copy of each chromosome inherited from each parent. Twenty-two pairs of chromosomes are **autosomes**; the remaining pair is called the **sex chromosomes**. Females have two X chromosomes; males have one X and one Y.

Spread along the chromosomes, like beads on a string, DNA sequences form **genes**, the basic units of heredity. A typical gene contains a promoter sequence, an untranslated region, and an open reading frame, all arrayed from the 5' to the 3' end of the DNA. In the open reading frame, every three nucleotides represent a single **codon**, coding for a particular amino acid. In this way, the sequence of bases dictates the sequence of amino acids in the corresponding protein. Some codons, rather than coding for a specific amino acid, act as a "start" signal, whereas others serve as "stop" signals. Between the start and stop codons, genes consist of two major portions: **exons**, regions containing the code that ultimately corresponds to a sequence of amino acids, and **introns** (intervening sequence), which do not become part of the amino acid sequence.

Genes are **transcribed** into messenger RNA (mRNA), then **translated** into proteins. During transcription, RNA is processed to remove introns. The mRNA serves as a template to construct the protein.

Human genetic material contains 3.1 billion bases. Less than 2% of the DNA codes for proteins, comprising the genome's approximately 20,000 genes. Through a mechanism called **alternative splicing**, these 20,000 genes may create more than 100,000 proteins. The remainder of the DNA, the portion not involved in protein formation, has been termed *junk DNA*; more than 50% appears as repeat sequences, in which two or three bases are repeated. The purpose of these repeat sequences and of the junk DNA is not yet known. However, it is believed to play a role in regulation of the remainder of the genome.

Disease may be caused by changes or **mutations** in the DNA sequence, with the **point mutation**, a change in a single DNA base, being the most common type. A point mutation that changes a codon and the resulting amino acid that goes into the protein is referred to as a

**missense mutation**. A **nonsense mutation** is a point mutation that changes the codon to a "stop" codon so that transcription stops prematurely. A **frameshift mutation** often stems from the loss or addition of one or more DNA bases; this causes a shift in how the DNA is transcribed and generally leads to premature stop codons.

**Single gene mutations** have an autosomal dominant (AD), autosomal recessive (AR), or X-linked pattern of inheritance. If a mutation in only one of the two copies of a gene is sufficient to cause disease, that disorder is considered **AD** (Table 47-1); if mutation in both copies of the gene must be present for disease to result, the condition is termed **AR** (Table 47-2). If a condition results from a mutation in a gene on the X chromosome, it usually causes disease in males, but generally not in females. This pattern of inheritance is termed **X-linked** (Table 47-3). Occasionally, as a result of skewing of inactivation of the X chromosome, an X-linked disorder may manifest symptoms of a disease in a heterozygous female. Genetic disorders also may result from abnormalities in the amount of genetic material present (termed *chromosomal disorders*), from interplay between genetic factors and environmental factors (called *multifactorial inheritance*), from unusual modes of inheritance, and as the result of exposure to certain drugs and chemicals known to cause birth defects (called *teratogens*).

## Pedigree Drawing

To identify specific patterns of inheritance, geneticists construct and analyze pedigrees, which are pictorial representations of a family history. Males are represented by squares and females by circles. Matings are connected with a solid line between each partner's symbols. Unmarried couples are often connected by a dashed line. Children from a couple are represented below their parents and are the next generation.

Grandparents, uncles, and aunts are added in similar fashion. Children of aunts and uncles also may be included. Ages or birthdays may be written next to or underneath each symbol. The proband (the patient who is the initial contact) is indicated with an arrow. Affected individuals are indicated by shading, or some other technique, which should be explained in a key. Carriers for a disorder (e.g., sickle cell disease) usually are indicated by a dot in the center of their symbol (Fig. 47-1).

To be useful, pedigrees should include representatives of at least three generations of family members.

| TABLE 47-1 Autosomal Dominant Diseases | | |
|---|---|---|
| **Disease** | **Frequency** | **Comments** |
| Achondroplasia<br>Thanatophoric dysplasia<br>Crouzon syndrome with acanthosis nigricans<br>Nonsyndromic craniosynostosis | ~1:12,000 | Mutations are in the gene for *fibroblast growth factor receptor-3* on chromosome 4p16.3<br>40% of cases are new mutations (different mutations in the same gene cause achondroplasia, thanatophoric dysplasia, Crouzon syndrome with acanthosis, and nonsyndromic craniosynostosis) |
| Neurofibromatosis 1 | 1:3500 | About 50% of cases result from new mutations in the gene for neurofibromin, a tumor suppressor gene located at 17q11.2. Expression is quite variable |
| Neurofibromatosis 2 (NF2, bilateral acoustic neuromas, Merlin) | Genotype at birth, 1:33,000<br>Phenotype prevalence, 1:200,000 | The NF2 gene is a tumor suppressor gene located at 22q12.2. The protein is called "Merlin" |
| Huntington disease (HD) | Variable in populations, 1:5000–1:20,000 | The disease is caused by a (CAG) repeat expansion in the "Huntington" protein gene on chromosome 4p16.3 |
| Myotonic dystrophy (DM, Steinert disease) | 1:500 in Quebec<br>1:25,000 Europeans | The disease is caused by a (CTG) repeat expansion in the DM kinase gene at chromosome 19q13.2. The condition shows genetic anticipation with successive generations |
| Marfan syndrome (FBN-1) | 1:10,000 | The syndrome is caused by mutations in the fibrillin 1 (FBN 1) gene on chromosome 15q21.1; there is variable expression |
| Hereditary angioneurotic edema (HANE) (C-1 esterase inhibitor that regulates the C-1 component of complement) | 1:10,000 | The gene is located on chromosome 11q11-q13.2. The phenotype of episodic and variable subcutaneous and submucosal swelling and pain is caused by diminished or altered esterase inhibitor protein, which can result from any one of many mutations in the gene |

**TABLE 47-2 Autosomal Recessive Diseases**

| Disease | Frequency | Comments |
|---|---|---|
| Adrenal hyperplasia, congenital (CAH, 21-hydroxylase deficiency, CA21H, CYP21, cytochrome P450, subfamily XXI) | 1:5000 | Phenotype variation corresponds roughly to allelic variation. A deficiency causes virilization in females. The gene is located at 6p21.3 within the HLA complex and within 0.005 centimorgans (cM) of HLA B |
| Phenylketonuria (PKU, phenylalanine hydroxylase deficiency, PAH) | 1:12,000– 1:17,000 | There are hundreds of disease-causing mutations in the PAH gene located on chromosome 12q22-q24.1. The first population-based newborn screening was a test for PKU because the disease is treatable by diet. Women with elevated phenylalanine have infants with damage to the CNS because high phenylalanine is neurotoxic and teratogenic |
| Cystic fibrosis (CF) | 1:2500 whites | The gene *CF transmembrane conductance regulator* (CFTR) is on chromosome 7q31.2 |
| Friedreich ataxia (FA, frataxin) | 1:25,000 | Frataxin is a mitochondrial protein involved with iron metabolism and respiration. The gene is on chromosome 9q13-q21, and the common mutation is a GAA expanded triplet repeat located in the first *intron* of the gene. FA does not show anticipation |
| Gaucher disease, all types (glucocerebrosidase deficiency, acid β-glucosidase deficiency) (a lysosomal storage disease) | 1:2500 Ashkenazi Jews | The gene is located on chromosome 1q21. There are many mutations; some mutations lead to neuropathic disease, but most are milder in expression. The phenotypes correspond to the genotypes, but the latter are difficult to analyze |
| Sickle cell disease (hemoglobin beta locus, beta 6 glu → val mutation) | 1:625 African Americans | This is the first condition with a defined molecular defect (1959). A single base change results in an amino acid substitution of valine for glutamic acid at position 6 of the beta chain of hemoglobin with resulting hemolytic anemia. The gene is on chromosome 11p15.5. Penicillin prophylaxis reduces death from pneumococcal infections in affected persons, especially in infants |

**TABLE 47-3 X-Linked Recessive Diseases**

| Disease | Frequency | Comments |
|---|---|---|
| Fragile X syndrome (FRAXA; numerous other names) | 1:4000 males | The gene is located at Xq27.3 The condition is attributable to a CGG triplet expansion that is associated with localized methylation (inactivation) of distal genes. Females may have some expression. Instability of the site may lead to tissue mosaicism; lymphocyte genotype and phenotype may not correlate |
| Duchenne muscular dystrophy (DMD, pseudohypertrophic progressive MD, dystrophin, Becker variants) | 1:4000 males | The gene is located at Xp21 The gene is relatively large, with 79 exons, and mutations and deletions may occur anywhere. The gene product is called *dystrophin*. Dystrophin is absent in DMD but abnormal in Becker MD |
| Hemophilia A (factor VIII deficiency, classic hemophilia) | 1:5000–1:10,000; males | The gene is located at Xq28 Factor VIII is essential for normal blood clotting. Phenotype depends on genotype and the presence of any residual factor VIII activity |
| Rett syndrome (RTT, RTS autism, dementia, ataxia, and loss of purposeful hand use); gene MECP2 (methyl-CpG-binding protein 2) | 1:10,000–1:15,000; girls | The gene is located at locus Xq28 These diseases are a subset of autism. There is a loss of regulation (repression) for other genes, including those in *trans* positions. The disease is lethal in males. Cases represent new mutations or parental gonadal mosaicism |

*Continued*

| Disease | Frequency | Comments |
|---|---|---|
| Colorblindness (partial deutan series, green color blindness [75%]; partial protan series, red color blindness [25%]) | 1:12; males | The gene is located at Xq28 (proximal) for deutan color blindness and at Xq28 (distal) for protan color blindness |
| Adrenoleukodystrophy (ALD, XL-ALD, Addison disease, and cerebral sclerosis) | Uncommon | The gene is located at Xq28<br><br>The disease involves a defect in peroxisome function relating to *very long-chain fatty acid CoA synthetase* with accumulation of C-26 fatty acids. Phenotype is variable, from rapid childhood progression to later onset and slow progression |
| Glucose-6-phosphate dehydrogenase deficiency (G6PD) | 1:10 African Americans<br>1:5 Kurdish Jews<br>A heteromorphism in these and other populations | The gene is located at Xq28<br><br>There are numerous variants in which oxidants cause hemolysis. Variants can confer partial resistance to severe malaria |

**TABLE 47-3 X-Linked Recessive Diseases—cont'd**

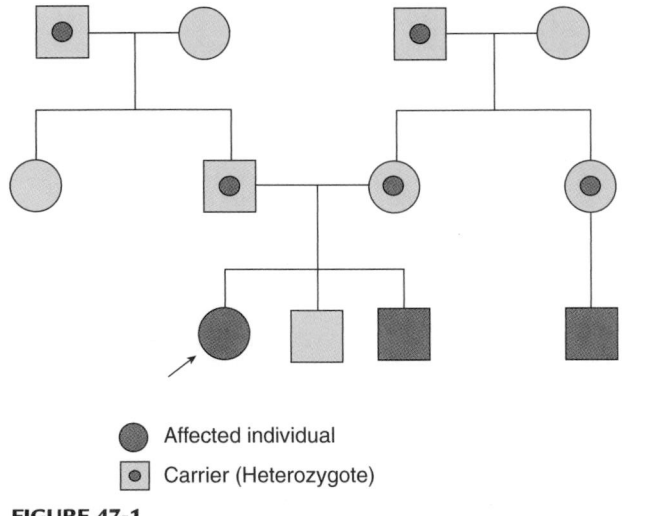

○ Affected individual
◉ Carrier (Heterozygote)

**FIGURE 47-1**

Pedigree showing affected individuals and carriers.

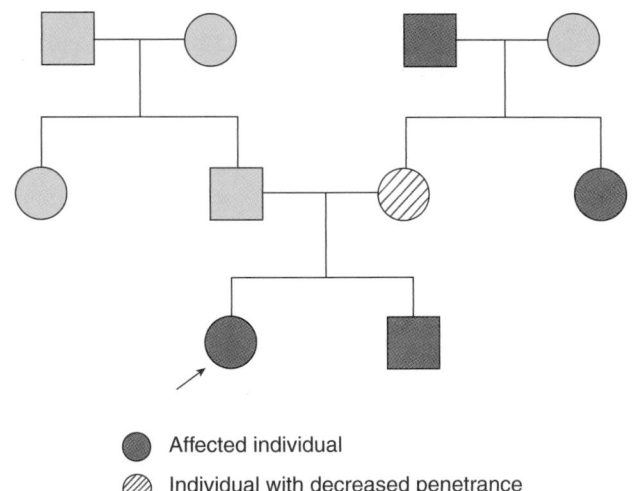

● Affected individual
◯ Individual with decreased penetrance

**FIGURE 47-2**

Pedigree showing decreased penetrance for an autosomal dominant disorder. Proband (*arrow*) is affected. Maternal grandfather also is affected. The individual's mother is presumed to be the carrier of the gene, even though she may show only slight symptoms of disease.

## Autosomal Dominant Disorders

If a single copy of a gene bearing a mutation is sufficient to cause disease, that condition is inherited in an AD fashion (see Table 47-1). In AD disorders, an affected parent may have one or more children who are affected with the same disorder. The parent, who has a mutation in one gene, has a 50% chance of passing the mutated gene to each child (Fig. 47-2). Possessing one *working* gene and one *nonworking* gene is termed **heterozygous**. If both copies are the same, they are referred to as **homozygous** (Table 47-4).

Some people who are obligate carriers of a mutation known to cause an AD disorder may not show clinical signs of the disorder, whereas other such individuals manifest symptoms. This phenomenon is referred to as **penetrance**. If all individuals who carry a mutation for an AD disorder show signs of that disorder, the gene is said to have complete penetrance. Many AD disorders show decreased penetrance.

Often, AD disorders show variability in symptoms expressed in different individuals carrying the same mutated

gene. Some individuals have only mild clinical symptoms, whereas others have more severe disease. This phenomenon is referred to as **variable expressivity**. To illustrate the differences between penetrance and expressivity, consider the condition neurofibromatosis type 1 (NF1). Caused by a mutation in the *NF1* gene on chromosome 17, NF1 is an AD disorder that causes café au lait macules, neurofibromas, and other findings. Although 100% penetrant, NF1 has marked variability in expression: some affected individuals have only café au lait spots, whereas others in the same family may experience life-threatening complications.

Sometimes, seemingly unrelated clinical findings, such as café au lait spots and neurofibromas in NF1, may be caused by a mutation in a single gene or gene pair. Known as **pleiotropy**, this phenomenon occurs in numerous single gene disorders.

## TABLE 47-4 Rules of Autosomal Dominant Inheritance

Trait appears in every generation
Each child of an affected parent has a one in two chance
  of being affected
Males and females are equally affected
Male-to-male transmission occurs
Traits generally involve mutations in genes that code for
  regulatory or structural proteins (collagen)

AD disorders sometimes appear in a child of unaffected parents because of a **spontaneous mutation**. Known in some cases to be associated with advanced paternal age (>35 years of age), spontaneous mutations may account for most individuals with some disorders. Approximately 80% of patients with achondroplasia are believed to have experienced a mutation in the fibroblast growth factor receptor type 3 (*FGFR3*) gene.

## Examples of Some Autosomal Dominant Disorders

### Achondroplasia

Caused by a defect in cartilage-derived bone, achondroplasia (ACH) is the most common skeletal dysplasia in humans. The bony abnormalities lead to short stature, macrocephaly, a flat midface with a prominent forehead, and rhizomelic shortening of the limbs. The disorder occurs in approximately 1 in 12,000 births.

ACH is caused by mutations in the *FGFR3* gene. Early in development, *FGFR3* is expressed during endochondral bone formation. More than 95% of cases of ACH are caused by one of two mutations in the same base pair (site 1138). This site, extremely active for mutations, is known as a mutational **hot spot.**

As they grow, children with ACH often develop associated medical and psychological problems. Hydrocephalus and central apnea may occur due to narrowing of the foramen magnum and compression of the brainstem. Bowing of the legs may occur later in childhood because of unequal growth of the tibia and fibula. Dental malocclusion, obstructive apnea, and hearing loss due to middle ear dysfunction are common in later childhood. During later childhood and adolescence, the psychological effects of the short stature may manifest. In adulthood, further complications include compression of nerve roots and sciatica. People with ACH have normal life spans and normal intelligence.

The diagnosis of ACH is made on the basis of clinical findings; characteristic x-ray abnormalities confirm the diagnosis. Molecular testing is available but is usually reserved for cases that are difficult to diagnose or those in which prenatal diagnosis is requested. Prenatal diagnosis is possible by molecular testing, using fetal cells obtained through amniocentesis or chorionic villus sampling.

### Neurofibromatosis Type 1

One of the most common AD disorders, NF1 is estimated to be present in 1 in 3500 individuals. NF1 is caused by a mutation in the gene *NF1*, which codes for the protein neurofibromin (see Chapter 186).

Although the penetrance of NF1 is 100%, the expression is extremely variable. Many affected individuals have features so mild that they are never diagnosed; such individuals may manifest only café au lait spots, axillary or inguinal freckling (smaller and darker than the café au lait spots and always found in clusters), Lisch nodules (pigmented hamartomas of the iris, best seen on slit-lamp examination), and neurofibromas (Schwann cell tumors). Between 10% and 20% of individuals have more severe symptoms, including brain tumors (optic gliomas and astrocytomas), renal vascular hypertension, skeletal involvement (scoliosis, pseudarthrosis of the tibia), and craniofacial disfigurement. Although diagnosis is made using clinical criteria, molecular diagnostic testing is also available. It is usually reserved for special cases.

### Marfan Syndrome

A condition that occurs in approximately 1 in 10,000 individuals, Marfan syndrome (MS) shows pleiotropy. Caused by a mutation in the *FBN1* gene, clinical symptoms mostly involve three systems: **cardiac, ophthalmologic,** and **skeletal.** Skeletal findings include a tall, thin body habitus (dolichostenomelia), spider-like fingers and toes (arachnodactyly), abnormalities of the sternum (pectus excavatum or carinatum), scoliosis, pes planus, and joint laxity. Eye findings include high myopia, which can lead to vitreoretinal degeneration; an abnormal suspensory ligament of the lens, which can lead to ectopia lentis (dislocation of the lens); and cataracts. Cardiac findings include progressive dilation of the aortic root. Aortic insufficiency followed by aortic dissection is a common complication. Other clinical features of MS include dural ectasia, abnormal pulmonary septation, and striae. Diagnostic criteria for MS are summarized in Table 47-5.

New mutations in *FBN1* account for 25% of cases of MS. The gene is large and complex; more than 200 mutations have been identified in affected individuals, making molecular diagnosis difficult.

Treatment had previously focused on providing beta-blockers to lower preload and decrease wear-and-tear on the aorta and, when the aortic root reaches 5.5 cm in diameter, to surgically place a composite graft to replace the aortic valve and ascending aorta. It is now understood that the cardiovascular effects of MS are caused not by the defect in the fibrillin protein itself but rather by an excess in transforming growth factor-beta (TGF-β), a protein usually bound by fibrillin. Losartan, an angiotensin II receptor antagonist that also lowers levels of TGF-β, has shown great efficacy in preventing aneurysms in animal models of MS.

## Autosomal Recessive Disorders

Disorders that are inherited in an AR manner manifest only when *both* copies of a gene pair have a mutation (Table 47-6). Affected children usually are born to unaffected parents, each of whom carries one copy of the mutation. If both members of a couple are carriers (or heterozygotes) for this mutation, each of their offspring has a 25% chance of being affected (Fig. 47-3).

**TABLE 47-5 Diagnostic Criteria for Marfan Syndrome\***

| System | Major Criteria | Minor Criteria |
|---|---|---|
| Skeletal | *Presence of at least 4 of the following manifestations:*<br>Pectus carinatum<br>Pectus excavatum requiring surgery<br>Reduced upper-to-lower segment ratio or arm span-to-height ratio >1.05<br>Wrist and thumb signs<br>Scoliosis >20° or spondylolisthesis present<br>Reduced extension at the elbows (<170°)<br>Medial displacement of medial malleolus causing pes planus<br>Protrusio acetabuli of any degree (as ascertained on radiographs) | Pectus excavatum of moderate severity<br>Joint hypermobility<br>Highly arched palate with crowding of teeth<br>Facial appearance (dolichocephaly, malar hypoplasia, enophthalmos, retrognathia, downslanting palpebral fissures) |
| Ocular | Ectopia lentis (dislocated lens) | Abnormally flat cornea (as measured by keratometry)<br>Increased axial length of globe (as measured by ultrasound) |
| Cardiac | Dilation of the ascending aorta with or without aortic regurgitation and involving at least the sinuses of Valsalva, *or*<br>Dissection of the ascending aorta | Mitral valve prolapse with or without mitral valve regurgitation<br>Dilation of the main pulmonary artery, in the absence of valvular or peripheral pulmonic stenosis or any other obvious cause (<40 years of age)<br>Calcification of the mitral annulus (<40 years of age)<br>Dilation or dissection of the descending thoracic or abdominal aorta (<50 years of age) |
| Pulmonary | None | Spontaneous pneumothorax<br>Apical blebs (ascertained by chest x-ray) |
| Skin | None | Stretch marks not associated with marked weight changes, pregnancy, or repetitive stress<br>Recurrent incisional hernias |
| Dura | Lumbosacral dural ectasia by CT or MRI | None |
| Family genetic history | Having a parent, child, or sibling who meets these diagnostic criteria independently<br>Presence of a haplotype around *FBN1*, inherited by descent, known to be associated with unequivocally diagnosed Marfan syndrome in the family | None |

\*If there is an affected family member, only one major criterion is necessary for diagnosis. If no family history, two major criteria (organ systems) and one minor criterion (involvement of a third organ system) are necessary.
CT, computed tomography; MRI, magnetic resonance imaging.

---

**TABLE 47-6 Rules of Autosomal Recessive Inheritance**

Trait appears in siblings, not in their parents or their offspring

On average, 25% of siblings of the proband are affected (at the time of conception, each sibling has a 25% chance of being affected)

A *normal* sibling of an affected individual has a two thirds chance of being a carrier (heterozygote)

Males and females are likely to be affected equally

Rare traits are likely to be associated with parental consanguinity

Traits generally involve mutations in genes that code for enzymes (e.g., phenylalanine hydroxylase–deficient in PKU) and are associated with serious illness and shortened life span

PKU, phenylketonuria.

## Sickle Cell Disease

▶ SEE CHAPTER 150.

## Tay-Sachs Disease

▶ SEE CHAPTERS 55 AND 185.

## X-Linked Disorders

More than 500 genes have been identified on the X chromosome, whereas only about 50 are believed to be present on the Y chromosome. Females, whose cells have two copies of an X chromosome, possess two copies of each gene on the X chromosome, whereas males, who have one X chromosome and a Y chromosome, have only one copy of these genes. Early in female embryonic development, one X chromosome is randomly inactivated in

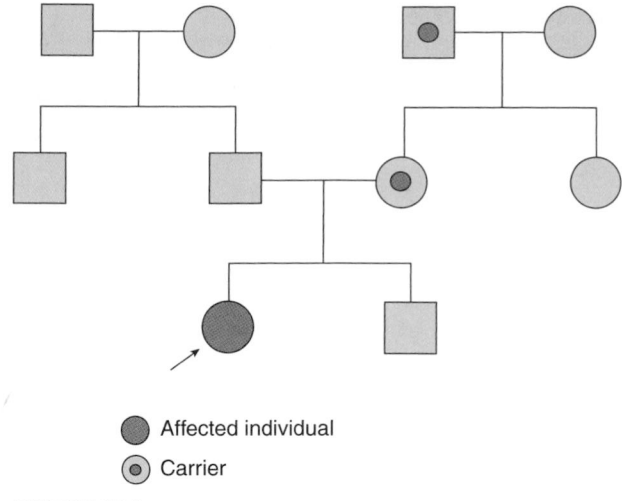

Affected individual

Carrier

**FIGURE 47-3**

Pedigree of family showing autosomal recessive inheritance.

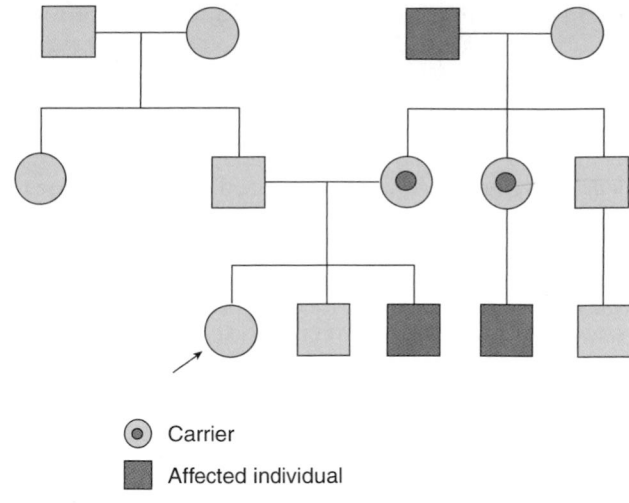

Carrier

Affected individual

**FIGURE 47-4**

Pedigree showing X-linked recessive inheritance.

each cell. There are many X-linked disorders (colorblindness, Duchenne muscular dystrophy, hemophilia A) in which heterozygous females show some manifestations of the disorder. Selective (skewed) inactivation of the normal gene produces symptoms in *carrier* women.

## X-Linked Recessive Inheritance

Most disorders involving the X chromosome are recessive. With only one copy of the X chromosome, males are more likely to manifest these diseases than females. Each son born to a female carrier of an X-linked recessive trait has a 50% chance of inheriting the trait, but none of this woman's daughters would be affected (each daughter has a 50% chance of being a carrier). An affected father transmits the mutation to all of his daughters, who are carriers, but not to his sons; having received their father's Y chromosome, they would not be affected (as such, there is no male-to-male transmission) (Table 47-7 and Fig. 47-4).

### Duchenne Muscular Dystrophy.
▶ SEE CHAPTER 182.

### Hemophilia A.
▶ SEE CHAPTER 151.

### TABLE 47-7 Rules of X-Linked Recessive Inheritance

Incidence of the trait is higher in males than in females

Trait is passed from carrier females, who may show mild expression of the gene, to half of their sons, who are more severely affected

Each son of a carrier female has a one in two chance of being affected

Trait is transmitted from affected males to all of their daughters; it is never transmitted father to son

Because the trait can be passed through multiple carrier females, it may *skip* generations

## X-Linked Dominant Inheritance

Only a few X-linked dominant disorders have been described. It might be expected that males and females would be equally affected, with females being less severely affected than males, the result of X inactivation. This is the case for **X-linked vitamin D–resistant rickets** (hypophosphatemic rickets), a disorder in which the kidney's ability to reabsorb phosphate is impaired. Phosphate levels and resulting rickets are not as severe in females as in males.

However, another group of X-linked dominant disorders are lethal in males. Affected mothers can have affected or normal daughters and normal sons. Affected sons die in utero. **Incontinentia pigmenti** involves a characteristic swirling skin pattern of hyperpigmentation that develops after a perinatal skin rash with blistering. Affected females also have variable involvement of the central nervous system, hair, nails, teeth, and eyes. In **Rett syndrome**, females are normal at birth, but later in the first year of life, they develop microcephaly and developmental regression and plateau. About 50% of patients develop seizures. Girls often are diagnosed with autism and, by 2 years of age, adopt a *handwashing* posture that causes them to lose all purposeful hand movements.

## OTHER TYPES OF GENETIC DISORDERS

### Multifactorial Disorders

Often termed **polygenic inheritance**, multifactorially inherited disorders result from the interplay of genetic and environmental factors. In addition to 20% of congenital malformations, including cleft lip and palate and spina bifida, most common disorders of childhood and adult life, such as asthma, atherosclerosis, diabetes, and cancer, result from an interaction between genes and the environment. These disorders do not follow simple mendelian modes of inheritance; rather, affected individuals tend to cluster in families. The disorders occur more often in first- and second-degree relatives than would be expected by chance, and they are more likely to be concordant (although not 100%) in monozygotic twins than in dizygotic twins.

## Hypertrophic Pyloric Stenosis

Occurring in about 1 in 300 children, hypertrophic pyloric stenosis (HPS) is five times more likely to occur in males than in females. When a child with HPS is born, the recurrence risk in future progeny is 5% to 10% for males and 1.5% to 2% for females. In adulthood, the risk of an affected male having an affected child is markedly increased over the general population: 4% of sons and 1% of daughters of such men would be likely to be affected. Even more striking is the risk to children born to affected females: 17% to 20% of sons and 7% of daughters are affected.

The thickness of the pyloric muscle may be distributed across a bell-shaped curve; the position on the bell-shaped curve is determined by many factors, including the expression of multiple, unknown genes. HPS may result when an individual's genetic and environmental influences cause him or her to fall to an extreme position on this curve, past a certain point, which is called a **threshold**. In HPS, this threshold is farther to the left for males than it is for females.

## Neural Tube Defects

Prior to 1998, myelomeningocele affected 1 in 1000 liveborn infants in the United States. Anencephaly occurred with a similar frequency, although most infants were either stillborn or died in the neonatal period. Since 1998, because of the supplementation of food staples with folic acid, both of these conditions have become far less frequent. Multiple genetic and nongenetic factors dictate the speed with which the neural tube closes, as follows:

1. The frequency of neural tube defects (NTDs) varies greatly in different ethnic groups. NTDs are more common in the British Isles, where, in 1990, they occurred in 1 in 250 live births, and far less common in Asia, where the frequency was 1 in 4000. These ethnic differences suggest a **genetic** component.
2. Couples from the British Isles who move to the United States have a risk intermediate between the risks in the United Kingdom and the United States, suggesting an **environmental** component.
3. The occurrence of NTDs exhibits seasonality. In the United States, affected infants are more likely to be born during the late fall and early winter, again suggesting an **environmental** component.
4. Periconceptual supplementation with folic acid has significantly lowered the risk of having an infant with an NTD. This nutritional influence suggests an **environmental** component.
5. Parents who have one child with an NTD are 20 to 40 times more likely to have a second affected child; this provides further evidence of a **genetic** component.

## Disorders with Unusual Patterns of Inheritance

### Mitochondrial Inheritance

Human cells contain non-nuclear DNA; a single chromosome is present in each mitochondrion and mutations within this DNA are associated with a group of diseases. Mitochondrial DNA (mtDNA), which is circular and 16.5 kb in length, replicates independently of nuclear DNA. Involved in energy production used to run the cell, mtDNA codes for a few respiratory chain proteins (most mitochondrial proteins are coded on nuclear DNA) and for a set of transfer RNAs unique to mitochondrial protein synthesis. Virtually all mitochondria are supplied by the oocyte, which means that mtDNA is maternally derived. A woman with a mutation in mtDNA passes this mutation to all of her children. More than one population of mitochondria may be present in the oocyte, a phenomenon called **heteroplasmy**. The mtDNA mutation may be present in a few or many mitochondria. When the fertilized egg divides, mitochondria are distributed randomly. The presence of symptoms in the offspring, and their severity depends on the ratio of mutant to wild-type mtDNA present in that tissue. If an abundance of mutant mitochondria exists in tissue that has high energy requirements (brain, muscle, and liver), clinical symptoms occur. If fewer mutant mitochondria are present, few clinical symptoms may be seen.

**MELAS** (**m**itochondrial **e**ncephalomyopathy with **l**actic **a**cidosis and **s**trokelike episodes) is an example of a mitochondrial disorder. Normal in early childhood, individuals affected with MELAS develop episodic vomiting, seizures, and recurrent cerebral insults that resemble strokes between 5 and 10 years of age. In 80% of cases, analysis of the mtDNA reveals a specific mutation (A3243G) in the *MTTL1* gene (a gene that codes for a mitochondrial transfer RNA).

In families in which MELAS occurs, a range of symptoms is seen in first-degree relatives, including **progressive external ophthalmoplegia**, hearing loss, cardiomyopathy, and diabetes mellitus. Although all offspring of a woman who carries a mutation would be affected, because of heteroplasmy, the severity of disease varies, depending on the percentage of mitochondria bearing the mutation that are present.

### Uniparental Disomy

Evaluation of a child with uniparental disomy (UPD) reveals a normal karyotype. However, chromosomal markers for one particular chromosome are identical to the markers found on the chromosomes of the patient's mother or father (but not both). In UPD, the patient inherits two copies of one parent's chromosome and no copy from the other parent.

UPD probably occurs through a few mechanisms, but the most common results from a spontaneous *rescue* mechanism. At the time of conception, through nondisjunction, the fertilized egg is trisomic for a particular chromosome, with two copies of one parent's chromosome and one copy of the other parent's chromosome; conceptuses with trisomy often miscarry early in development. Patients with UPD survive because they spontaneously lose one of three copies of the affected chromosome. If the single chromosome from one parent is lost, the patient has UPD.

An alternate explanation involves monosomy for a chromosome rather than trisomy. Had the patient, at the time of conception, inherited only a single copy of a chromosome, spontaneous duplication of the single chromosome would lead to UPD.

### Prader-Willi and Angelman Syndromes

**Prader-Willi syndrome (PWS)**, which occurs in approximately 1 in 10,000 infants, is characterized by hypotonia of prenatal onset; postnatal growth delay; a characteristic appearance, including almond-shaped eyes and small hands and feet; developmental disability; hypogonadotropic hypogonadism; and obesity after infancy. Early in life, affected infants are so hypotonic that they cannot take in enough calories to maintain their weight. Nasogastric feeding is invariably necessary, and failure to thrive is common. During the first year of life, muscle tone improves and children develop a voracious appetite. Some 60% to 70% of patients with PWS have a small deletion of chromosome 15 (15q11). In patients without a deletion, 20% have UPD of chromosome 15.

**Angelman syndrome (AS)** is a condition with moderate to severe mental retardation, absence of speech, ataxic movements of the arms and legs, a characteristic craniofacial appearance, and a seizure disorder that is characterized by inappropriate laughter. AS is also characterized by a deletion in the 15q11 region in 70% of affected individuals; UPD for chromosome 15 can be demonstrated in approximately 10% of AS patients.

If the deletion occurs in paternal chromosome 15, the affected individual has PWS, whereas AS results from a deletion occurring only in the maternal chromosome 15. When UPD is responsible, maternal UPD results in PWS, whereas paternal UPD results in AS. To summarize, if the patient lacks a copy of paternal chromosome 15q11.2, PWS will occur; if maternal chromosome 15q11.2 is lacking, AS results.

This phenomenon is explained by **genomic imprinting**. Imprinting is an epigenetic phenomenon, a nonheritable change in the DNA that causes an alteration in gene expression based on parental origin of the gene. PWS is caused by deficiency of the protein product of the gene *SNRPN* (small nuclear ribonucleoprotein). Although *SNRPN* is present on both maternally derived and paternally derived chromosome 15, it is expressed only in the paternally derived chromosome. Expression is normally blocked in the maternal chromosome because the bases of the open reading frame are methylated; this physical change in the DNA prevents gene expression. PWS results whenever a paternal chromosome 15 is missing, either through deletion or through UPD.

AS results from a lack of expression of ubiquitin-protein ligase E3A (*UBE3A*), a second gene in the chromosome 15q11.2 region. *UBE3A* is normally expressed only in the maternally derived chromosome 15. Although the gene is present in paternal chromosome 15, *UBE3A* is methylated, and gene expression is blocked. Therefore, if either the critical region of maternal chromosome 15 is deleted, or paternal UPD occurs, the individual will manifest symptoms of AS.

### Expansion of a Trinucleotide Repeat

More than 50% of human DNA appears as repeat sequences, two or three bases repeated over and over again. Disorders caused by expansion of trinucleotide repeats include **fragile X syndrome**, **Huntington disease**, **myotonic dystrophy**, **Friedreich ataxia**, and the **spinocerebellar ataxias**. Although an increase in the number of the three repeated bases is at the heart of each disorder, the molecular mechanism differs.

**Fragile X syndrome (FRAX)**, which occurs with a frequency of approximately 1 in 2000 children, is the most common cause of inherited mental retardation. Features include characteristic craniofacial findings (large head; prominent forehead, jaw, and ears); macro-orchidism with testicular volume twice normal in adulthood; a mild connective tissue disorder, including joint laxity, patulous eustachian tubes, and mitral valve prolapse; and a characteristic neurobehavioral profile, including mental retardation (ranging from mild to profound), autism spectrum disorder, and pervasive developmental disorder.

Positional cloning in the Xq27 region has identified a triplet repeat region composed of one cytosine and two guanine residues (CGG). Occurring in the CpG island, a part of the promoter region of a gene that has been called *FMR-1*, unaffected individuals who have no family history of FRAX have 0 to 45 CGG repeats (most have 25 to 35). In individuals with FRAX, the number of repeats is greater than 200; such people are said to have a *full mutation*. Between these two categories, a third group has 56 to 200 repeats; always phenotypically normal, these individuals are **premutation carriers**.

FRAX results from a failure to express the FMRP, the protein product of the *FMR-1* gene. Fragile X mental retardation protein (FMRP) is a carrier protein that shuttles mRNA between the nucleus and cytoplasm in the central nervous system and other areas (e.g., the developing testis) during early embryonic development. Although FMRP is produced in unaffected individuals and premutation carriers, in those with the full mutation, FMRP transcription of the protein is blocked because the large number of CGG repeats in the CPG island become methylated (an epigenetic phenomenon). Thus, FRAX occurs as a consequence of a **loss-of-function mutation**—the failure of expression of FMRP because of methylation of the promoter sequence.

In female premutation carriers, an expansion in the number of repeats from the premutation to the full mutation range may occur during gametogenesis. The cause of this expansion is not understood. Although these females do not have symptoms and signs of FRAX, premutation carriers may manifest ovarian failure and/or a neurologic condition known as fragile X tremor/ataxia syndrome later in life.

## TERATOGENIC AGENTS

Approximately 6.5% of all birth defects are attributed to teratogens, which are chemical, physical, or biologic agents that have the potential to damage embryonic tissue and result in one or more congenital malformations. Agents known to be teratogenic include drugs (prescription and nonprescription); intrauterine infections (rubella); maternal diseases, such as diabetes mellitus; and environmental substances, such as heavy metals. Knowledge of teratogenic agents and their effect on the developing fetus is important, because limiting exposure to these agents is an effective way to prevent birth defects (see Chapters 58, 59, and 60).

## Maternal Infections

Rubella was the first maternal infection known to cause a pattern of malformations in fetuses affected in utero. Cytomegalovirus, *Toxoplasma gondii*, herpes simplex, and varicella are additional potentially teratogenic in utero infections (see Chapter 66).

## Maternal Disease

Maternal diabetes mellitus and maternal phenylketonuria can result in congenital anomalies in the fetus. Strict control of these disorders before and during pregnancy protects the developing child (see Chapter 59).

## Medications and Chemicals

**Fetal alcohol spectrum disorder**, which occurs in 10 to 20 per 1000 children, may be the most common teratogenic syndrome. Features include prenatal and postnatal growth deficiency, developmental disabilities, microcephaly, skeletal and cardiac anomalies, and a characteristic facial appearance. To cause the full-blown fetal alcohol syndrome, pregnant women must drink at least 6 ounces of alcohol each day during the pregnancy. Lesser consumption during all or part of the gestation will lead to milder symptoms. Warfarin, retinoic acid, and phenytoin are additional teratogenic agents (see Chapter 59).

## Radiation

High-dose radiation exposure during pregnancy in Hiroshima, Japan, and Nagasaki, Japan, was shown to increase the rate of spontaneous abortion and result in children born with microcephaly, mental retardation, and skeletal malformations. Estimates of exposure to cause these effects were approximately 25 rad. The dose from routine radiologic diagnostic examinations is in the millirad range.

## Methyl Mercury

An inadvertent spill of methyl mercury into the water supply of Minamata, Japan, led to an outbreak of congenital malformations. Children were born with neurologic abnormalities, including mental retardation, cerebral palsy–like movement disorders, and blindness. This incident raised concern about exposure of fetuses to heavy metals (especially mercury) from contaminated fish in the diets of pregnant women.

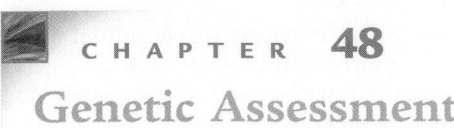

# CHAPTER 48
# Genetic Assessment

Individuals referred to a geneticist because of suspicion of a genetic disorder are called **probands**, and individuals who come for genetic counseling are **consultands**. Referral for genetic evaluation may be made for a wide variety of reasons and at different stages of life (fetus, neonate, childhood, pregnancy).

# PRECONCEPTION AND PRENATAL COUNSELING

## Familial Factors

Families with relatives affected with genetic disorders may have questions about how a disorder is inherited. The inheritance pattern and the risk of having an affected child can be discussed with a geneticist.

In some cultures, it is common for relatives to mate. **Consanguinity** does not increase the likelihood of offspring having any particular single genetic disorder, but it may increase the chance that a child will be born with a rare autosomal recessive (AR) condition, the mutated gene for which segregates through that family. Generally, the closer the relation between the partners, the greater the chance that the couple shares one or more mutated genes in common, increasing the risk that offspring will have an AR disorder. The risk of first cousins producing a child with an AR disorder is 1 in 64. In evaluating these couples, it is important to determine which ethnic group they belong to and to test for conditions commonly found in that group.

## Screening

It is common for couples to be screened for disorders that may occur in their ethnic group. People of Ashkenazi Jewish background may choose to be screened for heterozygosity for a panel of AR disorders, including Tay-Sachs disease, Niemann-Pick disease, Bloom syndrome, Canavan disease, Gaucher syndrome, cystic fibrosis, Fanconi anemia, and familial dysautonomia. People of African-American ancestry may choose to be screened for sickle cell anemia. People whose ancestors originated in the Mediterranean basin may be screened for thalassemia.

**Maternal serum screening** is offered to pregnant women during the first or second trimester of pregnancy (see Chapter 58) to assess the risk of both neural tube defects (NTDs) and fetal chromosomal abnormalities. **Alpha-fetoprotein (AFP)** is a protein secreted during fetal life by the liver, gastrointestinal tract, and yolk sac. If there is an open NTD, such as anencephaly or myelomeningocele, or any other defect in which the fetus' skin is disrupted, such as an omphalocele, abnormally high levels of AFP will be found in the amniotic fluid. Some of the AFP crosses the placenta and enters the maternal circulation. Levels of AFP are highest during 14 to 18 weeks of gestation, but some level of AFP generally can be detected in maternal blood samples at almost any time during the pregnancy. If the fetus has an NTD, high levels of AFP generally are detected in the maternal serum, but there is overlap between normal levels and levels detected in fetuses with NTDs. About 80% of fetuses with NTDs can be detected in this manner.

Lower than normal levels of AFP may be associated with a fetal chromosomal defect. Approximately 50% of fetuses with autosomal trisomies (Down syndrome, trisomy 18, trisomy 13) will be detected by low maternal serum AFP levels. Three other proteins—unconjugated estriol (uE3), inhibin A, and human chorionic gonadotropin (HCG)—are added to the maternal serum screening to compose the **quad screen**. The addition of these compounds increases the detection rate to about 80%.

There is an increased risk of Down syndrome (trisomy 21) when levels of uE3 and AFP are both low and there is an increased level of HCG. The risk of trisomy 18 is greatly increased when AFP, uE3, and HCG are low. Women with an abnormal maternal serum screen are offered genetic counseling, fetal sonography, and amniocentesis, which is the definitive test for identifying chromosomal abnormalities. A negative screening test does not eliminate the risk that the fetus has a chromosomal abnormality or an NTD.

It is common for pregnant women to have a *screening* sonogram at 18 weeks' gestation. An anatomy scan is done to look for congenital anomalies. Brain, heart, kidneys, lungs, and spine are examined.

## Maternal Factors

The presence of either acute or chronic maternal illness during pregnancy may lead to complications in the developing fetus. Chronic conditions may expose the fetus to maternal medications that are potentially teratogenic. Acute illnesses such as varicella, Lyme disease, and cytomegalovirus expose the fetus to infectious agents that may cause birth defects. Other factors, such as maternal smoking, alcohol use, and maternal exposure to radiation or chemicals, also may necessitate genetic counseling. Advanced maternal age is defined as a mother who is 35 years of age or older at the time of delivery. These women have an increased risk of a nondisjunctional event and are at risk for having an infant born with a trisomy.

**Amniocentesis** may be recommended for reasons other than advanced maternal age. Known chromosomal problems in the family, a family history of a NTD, a past history of multiple pregnancy losses, and a history of one or more family members with a known genetic disorder that requires biochemical or DNA testing for prenatal diagnosis are common reasons for referral for amniocentesis. The procedure typically is performed in the early midtrimester, between 15 and 18 weeks of gestation. Under ultrasound guidance, a needle is inserted transabdominally into the amniotic cavity, and 20 to 30 mL of amniotic fluid is withdrawn for diagnostic studies. Generally, cytogenetic studies are done on the amniotic cells, but biochemical or DNA testing also may be performed.

An alternative to amniocentesis is **chorionic villus sampling (CVS)**. Also performed under ultrasound guidance, CVS can be performed either transabdominally or transcervically. A small sample of the chorionic villi is taken by needle biopsy. CVS can be performed earlier than amniocentesis, usually between 10 and 12 weeks of gestation; however, it introduces a greater risk of pregnancy loss than amniocentesis. CVS is associated with an approximately 1% risk of spontaneous pregnancy loss, whereas the risk inherent in amniocentesis is approximately 1 in 1000.

## Postnatal—Newborn and Infant

Two to 4% of newborns have a genetic abnormality or birth defect. This broad definition of a birth defect includes not only a visible malformation but also functional defects that might not be apparent at birth.

Birth defects have a significant impact on childhood morbidity and mortality. Almost 11% of childhood deaths can be traced to a genetic cause. If contributing genetic factors related to childhood deaths are considered, this increases to almost 25%. Consultation with a geneticist for a newborn or infant may be prompted by many different findings, including the presence of a malformation, abnormal results on a routine newborn screening test, abnormalities in growth (e.g., failure to gain weight, increase in length, or abnormal head growth), developmental delay, blindness or deafness, and the knowledge of a family history of a genetic disorder or chromosomal abnormality or (as a result of prenatal testing) the presence of genetic disorder or chromosomal abnormality in the infant.

## Adolescent and Adult

Adolescents and adults may be seen by a geneticist for evaluation of a genetic disorder that has late onset. Some neurodegenerative disorders, such as Huntington disease and adult-onset spinal muscular atrophy, present later in life. Some forms of hereditary blindness (retinal degenerative diseases) and deafness (Usher syndrome, neurofibromatosis type 2) may not show significant symptoms until adolescence or early adulthood. Genetic consultation also may be prompted for a known family history of a **hereditary cancer syndrome** (breast and ovarian cancer, hereditary nonpolyposis colon cancer). Individuals may wish to have testing done to determine if they carry a mutation for these syndromes and would be at risk for developing certain types of cancers. A known family history or personal history of a genetic disorder or chromosomal abnormality might prompt testing in anticipation of pregnancy planning.

# GENERAL APPROACH TO PATIENTS

## Family History

A pedigree usually is drawn to help visualize various inheritance patterns. Answers to questions about the family help determine if there is an autosomal dominant (AD), AR, X-linked, or sporadic disorder. When a child is affected with the new onset of an AD disorder, it is necessary to closely examine the parents to check for the presence of manifestations. If the parents are unaffected, the child's condition is most likely the result of a new mutation, and the risk of recurrence in the condition is extremely low (although not 0, because of the possibility of gonadal mosaicism in one of the parents). When one parent is affected (even mildly so due to varying penetrance), the recurrence risk rises to 50%. With X-linked disorders, the focus is on the maternal family history to determine if there is a significant enough risk to warrant testing.

Questions about the couple's age are important to ascertain the risk related to advanced maternal age for chromosome abnormalities and increased paternal age for new mutations leading to AD and X-linked disorders. A history of more than two spontaneous abortions increases the risk that one of the parents has a balanced translocation and the spontaneous abortions are due to chromosomal abnormalities in the fetus.

## Pregnancy

During a genetic consultation, it is important to gather information about the pregnancy (see Chapters 58, 59, and 60). A maternal history of a chronic medical condition, such as a seizure disorder or diabetes, has known consequences in the fetus. Medication used in pregnancy can be teratogenic; the pregnant woman's exposure to toxic chemicals (work related) or use of alcohol, cigarettes, or drugs of abuse can have serious effects on the developing fetus. Maternal infection during pregnancy with varicella, *Toxoplasma*, cytomegalovirus, and parvovirus B19, among others, has been found to cause malformations in the fetus.

Follow-up is needed if an amniocentesis or CVS reveals abnormal results. A fetal ultrasound may have detected a malformation that needs follow-up when the infant is born. Often hydronephrosis is detected prenatally. These infants need a repeat ultrasound soon after birth.

## Delivery and Birth

An infant born prematurely is likely to have more complications than a term infant. An infant can be small, appropriate, or large for his or her gestational age; each of these has implications for the child (see Chapters 58, 59, and 60). In general, the finding that an infant is small for gestational age is suggestive of exposure to a teratogen or the presence of a chromosomal abnormality.

## Past Medical History

Children with inborn errors of metabolism who have intermittent symptoms often have a history of multiple hospitalizations for dehydration or vomiting. Neuromuscular disorders may have a normal period followed by increasing weakness or ataxia. Children with lysosomal storage diseases, such as the mucopolysaccharidoses, often have recurrent ear infections and can develop sleep apnea.

## Development

Many genetic disorders are associated with developmental disabilities. However, the onset of the disability may not always be present from the newborn period; many inborn errors of metabolism, including storage disorders, cause developmental manifestations after a period of normal development (see Chapters 7 and 8). Some adult-onset disorders have no symptoms until the teens or later. Assessing school problems is important. The type of learning problem, age at onset, and whether there is improvement with intervention or continued decline all are important for proper assessment.

## Physical Examination

A careful and thorough physical examination is necessary for all patients with signs, symptoms, or suspicion of genetic disease. Sometimes subtle clues may lead to an unsuspected diagnosis. Features suggestive of a syndrome are discussed in more detail in Chapter 50.

## Laboratory Evaluation

### Chromosome Analysis

An individual's chromosomal material, known as the karyotype, can be analyzed using cells capable of dividing. In pediatrics, lymphocytes obtained from peripheral blood are the usual source for such cells, but cells obtained from bone marrow aspiration, skin biopsy (fibroblasts), or, prenatally, from amniotic fluid or chorionic villi also can be used. Cells are placed in culture medium and stimulated to grow, their division is arrested in either metaphase or prophase, slides are made, the chromosomes are stained with Giemsa or other dyes, and the chromosomes are analyzed.

In metaphase, chromosomes are short, squat, and easy to count. Metaphase analysis should be ordered in children whose features suggest a known aneuploidy syndrome, such as a trisomy or monosomy. Chromosomes analyzed in prophase are long, thin, and drawn out; analysis gives far more details than are seen in metaphase preparations. Prophase analysis is ordered in individuals with multiple congenital anomalies without an obvious disorder.

### Fluorescent In Situ Hybridization

Fluorescent in situ hybridization (FISH) allows the identification of the presence or absence of a specific region of DNA. A complementary DNA probe specific for the region in question is generated, and a fluorescent marker is attached. The probe is incubated with cells from the subject and viewed under a microscope. The bound probe fluoresces, allowing the number of copies of DNA segment in question to be counted. This technique is useful in Prader-Willi syndrome and Angelman syndrome, in which a deletion in a segment of 15q11.2 occurs, and in velocardiofacial (DiGeorge) syndrome, which is associated with a deletion of 22.q11.2.

### Microarray Comparative Genomic Hybridization

Microarray comparative genomic hybridization (array CGH) has begun to supplant prophase analysis in cases in which a subtle chromosomal deletion or duplication (copy number variant) is suspected. In array CGH, DNA from the individual being studied and a normal control is labeled with fluorescent markers and hybridized to thousands of FISH-like probes for sequences spread around the genome. The probes are derived from known genes and noncoding regions. By analyzing the ratio of intensity of the fluorescent marker at each site, it is possible to determine whether the individual in question has any difference in copy number compared with the control DNA. Array CGH may be four to five times more sensitive in identifying copy number variants than high-resolution chromosome analysis.

### Direct DNA Analysis

Direct DNA analysis allows identification of mutations in a growing number of genetic disorders. Using a polymerase chain reaction, the specific gene in question can be amplified and analyzed. The website www.genetests.org lists disorders in which direct DNA analysis is available and identifies laboratories performing such testing.

# Chromosomal Disorders

Errors that occur in meiosis during the production of the gametes can lead to abnormalities of chromosome structure or number. Syndromes caused by chromosomal abnormalities include Down syndrome (DS), trisomy 13, trisomy 18, Turner syndrome (TS), and Klinefelter syndrome (KS), as well as rarer chromosomal duplications, deletions, or inversions.

Chromosomal abnormalities occur in approximately 8% of fertilized ova but only in 0.6% of liveborn infants. Fifty percent of spontaneous abortuses have chromosomal abnormalities, the most common being 45,X (TS); an estimated 99% of 45,X fetuses are spontaneously aborted). The fetal loss rate for DS, the most viable of the autosomal aneuploidies, approaches 80%. Most other chromosomal abnormalities also adversely affect fetal viability. In newborns and older children, many features suggest the presence of a chromosome anomaly, including low birth weight (small for gestational age), failure to thrive, developmental delay, and the presence of three or more congenital malformations.

## ABNORMALITIES IN NUMBER (ANEUPLOIDY)

During meiosis or mitosis, failure of a chromosomal pair to separate properly results in nondisjunction. **Aneuploidy** is a change in the number of chromosomes that occurs as a result of nondisjunction. A cell may have one (**monosomy**) or three (**trisomy**) copies of a particular chromosome.

### Trisomies

### Down Syndrome

DS is the most common abnormality of chromosomal number. It occurs in 1 of every 800 births. Most cases (92.5%) are due to nondisjunction; in 80%, the nondisjunctional event occurs in maternal meiosis phase I. As a result of nondisjunction, there are three copies of chromosome 21 (trisomy 21); using standard cytogenetic nomenclature, trisomy 21 is designated 47,XX,+21 or 47,XY,+21. In 4.5% of cases, the extra chromosome is part of a robertsonian translocation, which occurs when the long arms (q) of two acrocentric chromosomes (numbers 13, 14, 15, 21, or 22) fuse at the centromeres, and the short arms (p), containing copies of ribosomal RNA, are lost. The most common robertsonian translocation leading to DS involves chromosomes 14 and 21; standard nomenclature is 46,XX,t (14q21q) or 46,XY,t (14q21q).

In approximately 3% of children with DS, mosaicism occurs. These individuals have two populations of cells: one with trisomy 21 and one with a normal chromosome complement. Mosaicism results from a either a nondisjunctional event that occurs after fertilization and after a few cell divisions, or from what is referred to as **trisomic rescue**. The loss of this aneuploidy returns the cell to 46, XX or 46,XY. In either case, the individual is referred to as a mosaic for these two populations of cells and according to standard nomenclature is designated 47,XX,+21/46XX or 47,XY,+21/46,XY. Although it is widely believed that individuals with mosaic DS are more mildly affected, there are wide variations in the clinical findings.

Children with DS are most likely diagnosed in the newborn period. These infants tend to have normal birth weight and length, and they are hypotonic. The characteristic facial appearance, with brachycephaly, flattened occiput, hypoplastic midface, flattened nasal bridge, upslanting palpebral fissures, epicanthal folds, and large protruding tongue, is apparent at birth. Infants also have short broad hands, often with a transverse palmar crease, and a wide gap between the first and second toes. The severe hypotonia may cause feeding problems and decreased activity.

Approximately 40% of children with DS have **congenital heart disease**. These anomalies include atrioventricular canal, ventriculoseptal or atrioseptal defects, and valvular disease. Approximately 10% of newborns with DS have **gastrointestinal tract anomalies**. The three most common defects are duodenal atresia, annular pancreas, and imperforate anus.

One percent of infants with DS are found to have congenital hypothyroidism, which is identified as part of the newborn screening program. Acquired hypothyroidism is a more common problem. Thyroid function testing must be monitored periodically during the child's life.

Polycythemia at birth (hematocrit levels >70%) is common and may require treatment. Some infants with DS show a leukemoid reaction, with markedly elevated white blood cell counts. Although this resembles congenital leukemia, it is a self-limited condition, resolving on its own over the first month of life. Nonetheless, children with DS have an increased risk of **leukemia**, with a 10- to 18-fold increase in risk compared with individuals without DS. In children with DS younger than 1 year of age, congenital and infantile leukemia is generally acute nonlymphoblastic leukemia; in individuals older than 3 years of age, the types of leukemia are similar to those of other children, with acute lymphoblastic leukemia being the predominant type.

Children with DS are more susceptible to infection, more likely to develop cataracts, and approximately 10% have atlantoaxial instability, an increased distance between the first and second cervical vertebrae that may predispose to spinal cord injury. Many individuals older than 35 years of age develop Alzheimer-like features.

Seventy-five percent of infants with DS are born to women younger than 35 years of age. However, because only 5% of all infants are born to women older than 35, and 25% of infants are born to women older than 35, the risk of having a child with DS increases with increasing maternal age. Thus, prenatal testing using amniocentesis or chorionic villus sampling should be offered to any woman who will be 35 years of age or older at the time of delivery. In women who are younger than 35 years of age, to identify those whose risk may approach that of a woman of 35, maternal serum screening for alpha-fetoprotein, unconjugated estriol, inhibin A, and human chorionic gonadotropin should be offered; those in whom the risk is assessed to be as high as that of a woman of 35 should be offered amniocentesis.

The recurrence risk for parents who have had a child with DS depends on the child's cytogenetic findings. If the child has trisomy 21, the empiric recurrence risk is 1% (added to the age-specific risk for women <35 years of age; use just the age-specific risk for women >35 years of age) for subsequent pregnancies. If the child is found to have a robertsonian translocation, chromosomal analysis of both parents must be performed. In approximately 65% of cases, the translocation is found to have arisen de novo (i.e., spontaneously, with both parents having normal karyotypes), and in 35% of cases, one parent has a balanced translocation. The recurrence risk depends on which parent is the carrier: if the mother is the carrier, the risk of recurrence is 10% to 15%; if the father is the carrier, the recurrence risk is 2% to 5%.

## Trisomy 18

Trisomy 18 (47,XX,+18 or 47,XY,+18) is the second most common autosomal trisomy, occurring in approximately 1 in 7500 live births. Greater than 95% of conceptuses with trisomy 18 are spontaneously aborted in the first trimester. Trisomy 18 is usually lethal; less than 10% of affected infants survive until their first birthday. Most infants with trisomy 18 are small for gestational age. Clinical features include hypertonia, prominent occiput, receding jaw, low-set and malformed ears, short sternum, rocker-bottom feet, hypoplastic nails, and characteristic clenching of fists—the second and fifth digits overlap the third and fourth digits (Table 49-1).

## Trisomy 13

The third of the *common trisomies*, trisomy 13 (47,XX,+13 or 47,XY,+13) occurs in 1 in 12,000 live births. It is usually fatal in the first year of life; only 8.6% of infants survive beyond their first birthday.

Infants with trisomy 13 have numerous malformations (see Table 49-1). These infants are small for gestational age and microcephalic. Midline facial defects, such as cyclopia (single orbit), cebocephaly (single nostril), and cleft lip and palate are common, as are midline central nervous system anomalies, such as alobar holoprosencephaly. The forehead is generally sloping, ears are often small and malformed, and microphthalmia or anophthalmia may occur. Postaxial polydactyly of the hands is common, as is clubfeet or rocker-bottom feet. Hypospadias and cryptorchidism are common in boys, whereas girls generally have hypoplasia of the labia minora. Most infants with trisomy 13 also have congenital heart disease. Many infants with this condition have a punched-out scalp lesion over the left or right occiput called **aplasia cutis congenita**; when seen in conjunction with polydactyly and some or all of the previously mentioned facial findings, this finding is essentially pathognomonic for the diagnosis of trisomy 13.

## Klinefelter Syndrome (KS)

Occurring in 1 in 500 male births, KS is the most common genetic cause of hypogonadism and infertility in men. It is caused by the presence of an extra X chromosome (47,XXY) (see Chapter 174). The extra X chromosome

---

**TABLE 49-1 Possible Clinical Findings in Trisomy 13 and Trisomy 18**

|  | Trisomy 13 | Trisomy 18 |
|---|---|---|
| Head and face | Scalp defects (e.g., cutis aplasia) | Small and premature appearance |
|  | Microphthalmia, corneal abnormalities | Tight palpebral fissures |
|  | Cleft lip and palate in 60%–80% of cases | Narrow nose and hypoplastic nasal alae |
|  | Microcephaly | Narrow bifrontal diameter |
|  | Sloping forehead | Prominent occiput |
|  | Holoprosencephaly (arrhinencephaly) | Micrognathia |
|  | Capillary hemangiomas | Cleft lip or palate |
|  | Deafness |  |
| Chest | Congenital heart disease (e.g., VSD, PDA, and ASD) in 80% of cases | Congenital heart disease (e.g., VSD, PDA, and ASD) |
|  | Thin posterior ribs (missing ribs) | Short sternum, small nipples |
| Extremities | Overlapping of fingers and toes (clinodactyly) | Limited hip abduction |
|  | Polydactyly | Clinodactyly and overlapping fingers; index over third, fifth over fourth |
|  | Hypoplastic nails, hyperconvex nails | Rocker-bottom feet |
|  |  | Hypoplastic nails |
| General | Severe developmental delays and prenatal and postnatal growth retardation | Severe developmental delays and prenatal and postnatal growth retardation |
|  | Renal abnormalities | Premature birth, polyhydramnios |
|  | Nuclear projections in neutrophils | Inguinal or abdominal hernias |
|  | Only 5% live >6 mo | Only 5% live >1 yr |

ASD, atrial septal defect; PDA, patent ductus arteriosus; VSD, ventricular septal defect.

arises from a nondisjunction in either the sperm or the egg. About 15% of boys with features of KS are found to be mosaic, with 46,XY/47,XXY mosaicism being the most common finding. Before puberty, boys with KS are phenotypically indistinguishable from the rest of the population.

The diagnosis is most often made when the boy is 15 or 16 years of age. At that point, the finding of the progressive development of pubic and axillary hair in the presence of testes that remain infantile in volume should alert the clinician to the disorder. Adolescents and young adults with KS tend to be tall, with long limbs. During adolescence or adulthood, gynecomastia occurs.

Because of failure of growth and maturation of the testes, males with KS have testosterone deficiency and failure to produce viable sperm. Production of testicular testosterone is low; this results in failure to develop later secondary sexual characteristics, such as development of facial hair, deepening of the voice, and libido. In adulthood, osteopenia and osteoporosis develop. Because of these findings, testosterone supplementation is indicated.

Most men with KS are infertile because they produce few viable sperm. Through the use of isolation of viable sperm through testicular biopsy, coupled with in vitro fertilization and intracytoplasmic sperm injection, it is possible for men with KS to father children; all children born to these men using this technology have had a normal chromosome complement.

## Monosomies

### Turner Syndrome

TS is the only condition in which a monosomic conceptus survives to term; however, 99% of embryos with 45,X are spontaneously aborted. The most common aneuploidy found in conceptuses (accounting for 1.4%,), 45,X is seen in 13% of first-trimester pregnancy losses. Occurring in 1 in 3200 liveborn females, TS is notable for its spectrum of relatively mild physical and developmental findings. Affected women tend to have normal intelligence and life expectancy.

Females with TS typically have a characteristic facial appearance with low-set, mildly malformed ears, a triangular-appearing face, flattened nasal bridge, and epicanthal folds. There is webbing of the neck, with or without cystic hygroma, a shieldlike chest with widened internipple distance, and puffiness of the hands and feet. Internal malformations may include congenital heart defect (in 45%, coarctation of the aorta is the most common anomaly, followed by bicuspid aortic valve; later in life, poststenotic aortic dilation with aneurysm may develop). Renal anomalies, including horseshoe kidney, are seen in more than 50% of patients. Short stature is a cardinal feature of this condition, and hypothyroidism is estimated to occur five times more frequently in women with TS than in the general population.

The presence of streak gonads (gonadal dysgenesis) instead of well-developed ovaries leads to estrogen deficiency, which prevents these women from developing secondary sexual characteristics and results in amenorrhea. Although 10% of women with TS may have normal pubertal development and are even fertile, most affected women require estrogen replacement to complete secondary sexual development.

Infertility in these women is not corrected by estrogen replacement. Assisted reproductive technology using donor ova has allowed women with TS to bear children. During pregnancy, these women must be followed carefully, because poststenotic dilatation of the aorta, leading to dissecting aneurysm, may occur.

Many girls with TS escape detection during the newborn period because phenotypic features are subtle. About 33% of children with TS are diagnosed in the newborn period, because of the presence of heart disease and physical features, another 33% are diagnosed in childhood, often during a workup for short stature (and receive growth hormone therapy); the final 33% are diagnosed during adolescence, when they fail to develop secondary sexual characteristics.

The karyotypic spectrum in girls with TS is wide. Only 50% have a 45,X karyotype; 15% have an isochromosome Xq [46,X,i(Xq)], in which one X chromosome is represented by two copies of the long arm (leading to a trisomy of Xq and a monosomy of Xp); and approximately 25% are mosaic (45,X/46,XX or 45,X/46,XY). Deletions involving the short (p) arm of the X chromosome (Xp22) produce short stature and congenital malformations, whereas deletions of the long arm (Xq) cause gonadal dysgenesis.

Although monosomy X is caused by nondisjunction, TS is not associated with advanced maternal age. Rather, it is believed that 45,X karyotype results from a loss of either an X or a Y chromosome after conception; that is, it is a postconceptual mitotic (rather than meiotic) nondisjunctional event.

## SYNDROMES INVOLVING CHROMOSOMAL DELETIONS

### Cri du Chat Syndrome

A deletion of the short arm of chromosome 5 is responsible for cri du chat syndrome, with its characteristic catlike cry during early infancy, which is the result of tracheal hypoplasia. Other clinical features include low birth weight and postnatal failure to thrive, hypotonia, developmental delay, microcephaly, and craniofacial dysmorphism, including ocular hypertelorism, epicanthal folds, downward obliquity of the palpebral fissures, and low-set malformed ears. Clefts of the lip and plate, congenital heart disease, and other malformations may be seen.

The clinical severity of cri du chat syndrome depends on the size of the chromosomal deletion. Larger deletions are associated with more severe expression. Most cases arise de novo; the deletion is usually in the chromosome 5 inherited from the father. This phenomenon is believed to be due to imprinting.

### Williams Syndrome

Williams syndrome is due to a small deletion of chromosome 7q11. Congenital heart disease is seen in 80% of affected children, with supravalvar aortic and pulmonic stenosis and peripheral pulmonic stenosis being the most common anomalies. Although these children often have normal birth weight, they have growth delay, manifesting short stature. They have a distinctive facial appearance ("elfin facies"), with median flare of the eyebrows, fullness of the perioral and periorbital region, blue irides with a stellate pattern of pigment, and depressed nasal bridge with anteversion of the nares. Moderate mental retardation (average IQ in the 50 to 60 range) is common, but developmental testing reveals strength in personal social skills and deficiencies in cognitive areas. Hypercalcemia is present in neonates.

Individuals with Williams syndrome have a striking personality. Loquacious and gregarious, they are frequently described as having a *cocktail party* personality. However, approximately 10% of children with Williams syndrome have features of autism. Patients occasionally have unusual musical ability (about 20% have absolute or perfect pitch). Most children with Williams syndrome have a de novo deletion. In rare cases, the deletion is inherited from a parent in an autosomal dominant pattern.

## Aniridia Wilms Tumor Association

WAGR syndrome (**W**ilms tumor, **a**niridia, **g**enitourinary anomalies, and mental **r**etardation) is caused by a deletion of 11p13 and is generally a de novo deletion. Genitourinary abnormalities include cryptorchidism and hypospadias. Patients often have short stature, and half may have microcephaly. Wilms tumor develops in 50% of patients with aniridia, genitourinary abnormalities, and mental retardation (see Chapter 159).

## Prader-Willi Syndrome

▶ SEE CHAPTER 47.

## Angelman Syndrome

▶ SEE CHAPTER 47.

## Chromosome 22 Deletion Syndromes

Deletions of chromosome 22q11.2 are responsible for a group of findings that have been called by several names, including **velocardiofacial syndrome, conotruncal anomaly face syndrome, Shprintzen syndrome, DiGeorge syndrome**, and **CATCH 22** (Cardiac defects, Abnormal facial features, Thymic hypoplasia, Cleft palate, and Hypocalcemia). These conditions represent a continuum of findings, virtually all of which are due to the chromosomal deletion.

Chromosome 22 deletions are inherited in an autosomal dominant fashion. Common features include clefting of the palate with velopharyngeal insufficiency; conotruncal cardiac defects (including aortic coarctation, truncus arteriosus, ventriculoseptal defect, and tetralogy of Fallot); and a characteristic facial appearance, including a prominent nose and a broad nasal root. Speech and language difficulties are common, as is mild intellectual impairment. More than 200 additional abnormalities have been identified in individuals with these conditions. Some 70% of individuals with the deletion have immunodeficiencies, largely related to T-cell dysfunction. A wide spectrum of psychiatric disturbances, including schizophrenia and bipolar disorder, has been seen in more than 33% of affected adults.

Damage to the third and fourth pharyngeal pouches, embryonic structures that form parts of the cranial portion of the developing embryo, leads to abnormalities in the developing face (clefting of the palate, micrognathia), the thymus gland, the parathyroid glands, and the conotruncal region of the heart. This spectrum of findings, called the DiGeorge malformation sequence, is an important chromosome 22 deletion syndrome.

The deletion that occurs in chromosome 22 is usually too small to see with routine or high-resolution chromosome analysis; in 75% of cases, fluorescent in situ hybridization is needed to identify the missing piece of the chromosome. A gene called *TBX1* is within the deleted sequence. It is believed that deletion of one copy of *TBX1* is responsible for many of the features of the various conditions.

# SYNDROMES INVOLVING CHROMOSOME DUPLICATION

Duplications and deletions occur secondary to misalignment and unequal crossing over during meiosis. Small extra chromosomes are found in a small percentage of the population (0.06%). These "marker" chromosomes sometimes are associated with mental retardation and other abnormalities, and other times they have no apparent phenotypic effects.

## Inverted Duplication Chromosome 15

Chromosome 15 is the most common of all marker chromosomes, and its inverted duplication accounts for almost 40% of this group of chromosomal abnormalities. Features seen in children with 47,XX, +inv dup (15q) or 47,XY, inv dup (15q) depend on the size of the extra chromosomal material present: the larger the region, the worse the prognosis. Children with this disorder tend to have a variable degree of developmental delay; seizures are common, as are behavior problems. The phenotype shows minimal dysmorphic features, with a sloping forehead, short and downward slanting palpebral fissures, a prominent nose with a broad nasal bridge, a long and well-defined philtrum, a midline crease in the lower lip, and micrognathia.

## Cat Eye Syndrome

Named for the iris coloboma that gives patients' eyes a catlike appearance, cat eye syndrome is due to a marker chromosome with an interstitial duplication of 22q11. Although the colobomas name the syndrome, they occur in less than 50% of individuals with the marker chromosome. Other clinical features include mild mental retardation, behavioral disturbances, mild ocular hypertelorism, downward slanting palpebral fissures, micrognathia, auricular pits and/or tags, anal atresia with rectovestibular fistula, and renal agenesis.

# The Approach to the Dysmorphic Child

Dysmorphology is the recognition of the pattern of congenital malformations (often multiple congenital malformations) and dysmorphic features that characterize a particular syndrome. **Syndromes** are collections of abnormalities, including **malformations**, **deformations**, dysmorphic features, and abnormal behaviors that have a unifying, identifiable etiology. This etiology may be the presence of a mutation in a single gene, as is the case in **Rett syndrome**, a disorder that is caused by a mutation in the *MECP2* gene on Xq28; deletion or duplication of chromosomal material, such as is the case in **Prader-Willi syndrome**, which is caused by the deletion of the paternal copy of the imprinted *SNRPN* gene; or exposure to a teratogenic substance during embryonic development, as in fetal alcohol syndrome.

## DEFINITIONS

Congenital **malformations** are defined as clinically significant abnormalities in either form or function. They result from localized **intrinsic** defects in morphogenesis, which were caused by an event that occurred in embryonic or early fetal life. This event may have been a disturbance of development from some unknown cause, but often mutations in developmental genes led to the abnormality. **Extrinsic** factors may cause **disruptions** of development by disturbing the development of apparently normal tissues. These disruptions may include amniotic bands, interruption or disruption of blood supply to developing tissues, or exposure to teratogens. A **malformation sequence** is the end result of a malformation that has secondary effects on later developmental events. An example is the **Pierre Robin sequence**. The primary malformation, failure of the growth of the mandible during the first weeks of gestation, results in micrognathia, which forces the normal-sized tongue into an unusual position. The abnormally placed tongue blocks the fusion of the palatal shelves, which normally come together in the midline to produce the hard and soft palate; this leads to the presence of a U-shaped cleft palate. After delivery, the normal-sized tongue in the smaller than normal oral cavity leads to airway obstruction, a potentially life-threatening complication.

**Deformations** arise as a result of environmental forces acting on normal structures. They occur later in pregnancy or after delivery. Oligohydramnios may inhibit lung growth and cause compression of fetal structures, producing clubfoot, dislocated hips, and flattened facies (Potter's syndrome) (see Chapter 196). Deformations often resolve with minimal intervention, but malformations often require surgical and medical management.

**Minor malformations**, variants of normal that occur in less than 3% of the population, include findings such as transverse palmar creases, low-set ears, or hypertelorism;

when isolated they have no clinical significance. A **multiple malformation syndrome** is the recognizable pattern of anomalies that results from a single identifiable underlying cause. It may involve a series of malformations, malformation sequences, and deformations. These syndromes often prompt a consultation with a clinical geneticist. **Dysmorphology** is the specialty focusing on recognition of patterns of malformations that occur in syndromes (Table 50-1).

An **association** differs from a syndrome in that in the former, no single underlying etiology explains the recognizable pattern of anomalies that occur together more than would be expected by chance alone. The **VACTERL** association (**v**ertebral anomalies, **a**nal atresia, **c**ardiac defects, **t**racheoesophageal fistula, **r**enal anomalies, and **l**imb anomalies) is an example of a group of malformations that occur more commonly together than might be expected by chance. No single unifying etiology explains this condition, so it is considered an association.

In approximately half of children noted to have one or more congenital malformations, only a single malformation is identifiable; in the other half, multiple malformations are present. About 6% of infants with congenital malformations have chromosomal defects, 7.5% have a single gene disorder, 20% are multifactorial, and approximately 7% are due to exposure to a teratogen. In more than 50% of cases, no cause can be identified.

## HISTORY AND PHYSICAL EXAMINATION

### Pregnancy History

The history of the pregnancy and birth can reveal multiple risk factors that are associated with dysmorphology. Small for gestational age infants may have a chromosome anomaly or may have been exposed to a teratogen. Large for gestational age infants may be infants of diabetic mothers or have an overgrowth syndrome, such as Beckwith-Wiedemann syndrome. When evaluating an older child with developmental disabilities, complications of extreme prematurity may account for the child's problems. Postmaturity also is associated with some chromosome anomalies (e.g., trisomy 18) and anencephaly. Infants born from breech presentation are more likely to have congenital malformations.

Advanced maternal age is associated with an increased risk of nondisjunction leading to trisomies. Advanced paternal age may be associated with an increased risk of a new mutation leading to an autosomal dominant trait. Maternal medical problems and exposures (medications, drugs, cigarette smoking, and alcohol use) are associated with malformations (see Chapters 47 and 48).

An increased amount of amniotic fluid may be associated with intestinal obstruction or a central nervous system anomaly that leads to poor swallowing. A decreased amount of fluid may point to a urinary tract abnormality, leading to failure to produce urine or a chronic amniotic fluid leak.

### Family History

A pedigree should be constructed, searching for similar or dissimilar abnormalities in first-degree and second-degree relatives. A history of pregnancy or neonatal losses should

## TABLE 50-1 Glossary of Selected Terms Used in Dysmorphology

### TERMS PERTAINING TO THE FACE AND HEAD

*Brachycephaly*: Condition in which head shape is shortened from front to back along the sagittal plane; the skull is rounder than normal

*Canthus*: The lateral or medial angle of the eye formed by the junction of the upper and lower lids

*Columella*: The fleshy tissue of the nose that separates the nostrils

*Glabella*: Bony midline prominence of the brows

*Nasal alae*: The lateral flaring of the nostrils

*Nasolabial fold*: Groove that extends from the margin of the nasal alae to the lateral aspects of the lips

*Ocular hypertelorism*: Increased distance between the pupils of the two eyes

*Palpebral fissure*: The shape of the eyes based on the outline of the eyelids

*Philtrum*: The vertical groove in the midline of the face between the nose and the upper lip

*Plagiocephaly*: Condition in which head shape is asymmetric in the sagittal or coronal planes; can result from asymmetry in suture closure or from asymmetry of brain growth

*Scaphocephaly*: Condition in which the head is elongated from front to back in the sagittal plane; most normal skulls are scaphocephalic

*Synophrys*: Eyebrows that meet in the midline

*Telecanthus*: A wide space between the medial canthi

### TERMS PERTAINING TO THE EXTREMITIES

*Brachydactyly*: Condition of having short digits

*Camptodactyly*: Condition in which a digit is bent or fixed in the direction of flexion (a "trigger finger"-type appearance)

*Clinodactyly*: Condition in which a digit is crooked and curves toward or away from adjacent digits

*Hypoplastic nail*: An unusually small nail on a digit

*Melia*: Suffix meaning "limb" (e.g., amelia—missing limb; brachymelia—short limb)

*Polydactyly*: The condition of having six or more digits on an extremity

*Syndactyly*: The condition of having two or more digits at least partially fused (can involve any degree of fusion, from webbing of skin to full bony fusion of adjacent digits)

---

be documented. For a complete discussion of pedigrees, see Chapter 47.

## Physical Examination

When examining children with dysmorphic features, the following approach should be used.

### Growth

The height (length), weight, and head circumference should be measured carefully and plotted on appropriate growth curves. Small size or growth restriction may be secondary to a chromosomal abnormality, skeletal dysplasia, or exposure to toxic or teratogenic agents. Larger than expected-size suggests an overgrowth syndrome (Sotos or Beckwith-Wiedemann syndrome), or, if in the newborn period, it might suggest a diabetic mother.

The clinician should note if the child is proportionate. Limbs that are too short for the head and trunk imply the presence of a short-limbed bone dysplasia, such as achondroplasia. A trunk and head that are too short for the extremities suggest a disorder affecting the vertebrae, such as spondyloepiphyseal dysplasia.

### Craniofacial

Careful examination of the head and face is crucial for the diagnosis of many congenital malformation syndromes. Head shape should be carefully assessed; if the head is not normal in size and shape (normocephalic), it may be long and thin (dolichocephalic), short and wide (brachycephalic), or asymmetric or lopsided (plagiocephalic).

Facial features should be assessed next. Any asymmetry should be noted; asymmetry may be due to a deformation related to intrauterine position or a malformation of one side of the face. The face should be divided into four regions, which are evaluated separately. The **forehead** may show overt prominence (achondroplasia) or deficiency (often described as a sloping appearance, which occurs in children with primary microcephaly). The **midface**, extending from the eyebrows to the upper lip and from the outer canthi of the eyes to the commissures of the mouth, is especially important. Careful assessment of the distance between the eyes (inner canthal distance) and the pupils (interpupil distance) may confirm the impression of hypotelorism (eyes that are too close together), which suggests a defect in midline brain formation, or **hypertelorism** (eyes that are too far apart). The length of the palpebral fissure should be noted and may help define whether the opening for the eye is short, as is found with fetal alcohol syndrome, or excessively long, as in Kabuki makeup syndrome (short stature, mental retardation, long palpebral fissures with eversion of lateral portion of lower lid).

Other features of the eyes should be noted. The obliquity (slant) of the palpebral fissures may be upward (as seen with Down syndrome) or downward (as in Treacher Collins syndrome). The presence of epicanthal folds (Down syndrome and fetal alcohol syndrome) is also important. Features of the nose—especially the nasal bridge, which can be flattened in Down syndrome, fetal alcohol syndrome, and many other syndromes, or prominent as in velocardiofacial syndrome—should be noted.

The **malar** region of the face is examined next. It extends from the ear to the midface. The ears should be checked for size (measured and checked against appropriate growth charts), shape, position (low-set ears are below a line drawn from the outer canthus to the occiput), and orientation (posterior rotation is where the ear appears turned toward the rear of the head). Ears may be low set because they are small (or microtic) or because of a malformation of the mandibular region.

The **mandibular region** is the area from the lower portion of the ears bounded out to the chin by the mandible. In most newborns, the chin is often slightly retruded (that is slightly behind the vertical line extending from the forehead to the philtrum). If this retrusion is pronounced, the child may have the Pierre Robin malformation sequence. In addition, the mouth should be examined. The number and appearance of the teeth should be noted, the tongue should be observed for abnormalities, and the palate and uvula checked for defects.

## Neck

Examination of the neck may reveal webbing, a common feature in Turner syndrome and Noonan syndrome, or shortening, as is seen occasionally in some skeletal dysplasias and in conditions in which anomalies of the cervical spine occur, such as Klippel-Feil syndrome. The position of the posterior hairline also should be evaluated. The size of the thyroid gland should be assessed.

## Trunk

The chest may be examined for shape (shieldlike chest in Noonan syndrome and Turner syndrome) and symmetry. The presence of a pectus deformity should be noted and is common in Marfan syndrome. The presence of scoliosis should be assessed; it is common in Marfan syndrome and many other syndromes.

## Extremities

Many congenital malformation syndromes have anomalies of the extremities. All joints should be examined for range of motion. The presence of single or multiple joint contractures suggests either intrinsic neuromuscular dysfunction, as in some forms of muscular dystrophy, or external deforming forces that limited motion of the joint in utero. Multiple contractures also are found with arthrogryposis multiplex congenita and are due to a variety of causes. **Radioulnar synostosis**, an inability to pronate or supinate the elbow, occurs in fetal alcohol syndrome and in some X chromosome aneuploidy syndromes.

Examination of the hands is important. **Polydactyly** (the presence of extra digits) usually occurs as an isolated autosomal dominant trait but also can be seen in trisomy 13. **Oligodactyly** (a deficiency in the number of digits) is seen in Fanconi syndrome (anemia, leukopenia, thrombocytopenia, and associated heart, renal, and limb anomalies—usually radial aplasia and thumb malformation or aplasia), in which it is generally part of a more severe limb reduction defect, or secondary to intrauterine amputation, which may occur with amniotic band disruption sequence. **Syndactyly** (a joining of two or more digits) is common to many syndromes, including Smith-Lemli-Opitz syndrome (see Chapters 199 and 201).

**Dermatoglyphics** include palmar crease patterns. A transverse palmar crease, indicative of hypotonia during early fetal life, is seen in approximately 50% of children with Down syndrome (and 10% of individuals in the general population). A characteristic palmar crease pattern is seen in fetal alcohol syndrome.

## Genitalia

Genitalia should be examined closely for abnormalities in structure. In boys, if the penis appears short, it should be measured and compared with known age-related data. Ambiguous genitalia often are associated with endocrinologic disorders, such as congenital adrenal hyperplasia (girls have masculinized external genitalia, but male genitalia may be unaffected), or chromosomal disorders such as 45,X/46,XY mosaicism or possibly secondary to a multiple congenital anomaly syndrome (see Chapters 174 and 177). Although hypospadias, which occurs in 1 in 300 newborn boys, is a common congenital malformation that often occurs as an isolated defect, if it is associated with other anomalies, especially cryptorchidism, there is a strong possibility of a syndrome.

## LABORATORY EVALUATION

**Chromosome analysis**, either metaphase or prophase, should be ordered for children with multiple congenital anomalies, the involvement of one major organ system and the presence of multiple dysmorphic features, or the presence of mental retardation. For a complete discussion of chromosome analysis, see Chapter 48. **Fluorescent in situ hybridization** (FISH) should be requested when a syndrome with a known chromosomal defect for which probes are available is suspected. Disorders such as velocardiofacial syndrome, Williams syndrome, and Prader-Willi syndrome are included in this group. **Direct DNA** analysis can be performed to identify specific mutations. It is necessary to use Web-based resources to keep up-to-date. An extremely helpful website is www.genetests.org, which provides information about the availability of testing for specific conditions and identifies laboratories performing the testing.

**Radiologic imaging** plays an important role in the evaluation of children with dysmorphic features. Individuals found to have multiple external malformations should have a careful evaluation to search for the presence of internal malformations. Testing might include **ultrasound evaluations** of the head and abdomen to look for anomalies in the brain, kidney, bladder, liver, and spleen. **Skeletal radiographs** should be performed if there is concern about a possible skeletal dysplasia. The presence of a heart murmur should trigger a cardiology consultation; an **electrocardiogram** and **echocardiogram**

may be indicated. **Magnetic resonance imaging** may be indicated in children with neurologic abnormalities or a spinal defect. The presence of craniosynostosis may indicate a **computed tomography scan** of the head.

## DIAGNOSIS

Although the presence of characteristic findings may make the diagnosis of a malformation syndrome straightforward, in most cases no specific diagnosis is immediately evident. Some constellations of findings are rare, and finding a "match" may prove difficult. In many cases, all laboratory tests are normal, and confirmation relies on subjective findings. Clinical geneticists have attempted to resolve this difficulty by developing scoring systems, cross-referenced tables of anomalies that help in the development of a differential diagnosis, and computerized diagnostic programs. An accurate diagnosis is important for the following reasons:

1. It offers an explanation to the family why their child was born with congenital anomalies. This may help allay guilt because parents often believe that they are responsible for their child's problem.

2. The natural history of many disorders is well described, so a diagnosis allows the physician to anticipate medical problems associated with a particular syndrome and perform appropriate screening. It also provides reassurance that other medical problems are no more likely to occur than they might with other children who do not have the diagnosis.

3. It permits genetic counseling to be done so that the parents can understand the risk to future children and also permits prenatal testing to be done for the disorders for which it is available.

Diagnosis enables the clinician to provide the family with educational materials about the diagnosis and for contact with support groups for particular disorders. The Internet has become an important source for such information, but care should be exercised as information on the Internet is not subject to editorial control. Some of the information may be inaccurate. A good site is the National Organization for Rare Disorders (www.rarediseases.org), a clearinghouse for information about rare diseases and their support groups. Genetic testing information is available at the Genetests website (www.genetests.org). This site provides information on available clinical and research testing for many diseases.

## SUGGESTED READING

Baldini A: Dissecting contiguous gene defects: *TBX1. Curr Opin Gen Dev* 15:279–284, 2005.

Crissman BG, Worley G, Roizen N, et al: Current perspectives on Down syndrome: selected medical and social issues. *Am J Med Genet C Semin Med Genet* 142C:127–130, 2006.

Feuk L, Marshall CR, Wintle RF, et al: Structural variants: changing the landscape of chromosomes and design of disease studies. *Hum Mol Genet* 15(Spec No 1): R57–R66, 2006.

Guttmacher AE, Porteous ME, McInerney JD: Educating health-care professionals about genetics and genomics. *Nat Rev Genet* 8:151–157, 2007.

Hobbs CA, Cleves MA, Simmons CJ: Genetic epidemiology and congenital malformations. *Arch Pediatr Adolesc Med* 156:315–320, 2002.

Kliegman RM, Behrman RE, Jenson HB, et al: Nelson Textbook of Pediatrics, 18th ed, Philadelphia, 2007, *WB Saunders.*

McPherson E: Genetic diagnosis and testing in clinical practice. *Clin Med Res* 4(2):123–129, 2006.

McCandless SE, Brunger JW, Cassidy SB: The burden of genetic disease on inpatient care in a children's hospital. *Am J Hum Genet* 74:121–127, 2004.

Online Mendelian Inheritance in Man: *http://www.ncbi.nlm.nih.gov/sites/entrez?db=omim.*

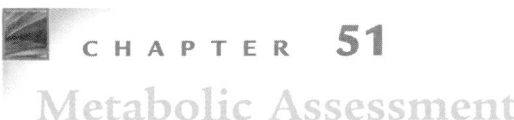

CHAPTER **51**

Metabolic Assessment

Although each inborn error of metabolism is rare, in the aggregate, they significantly contribute to the causes of mental retardation, seizures, sudden infant death, and neurologic impairment. Inborn errors of metabolism are a cause of acute neonatal illness in which prompt diagnosis and treatment make a difference in outcome and even survival. They affect all age groups. Prompt recognition is the responsibility of primary care physicians, who then need the expertise of metabolic teams that specialize in the diagnosis and management of these disorders.

Inborn errors of metabolism result from a genetic deficiency in a metabolic pathway; signs and symptoms result from the accumulation of metabolites related to the pathway. These metabolites may be toxic or may destroy cells because of storage in organelles. Deficiency of downstream metabolites also plays a role in pathogenesis. The process can involve one or multiple systems (Fig. 51-1). All mechanisms of inheritance occur (see Section 9).

The approach to diagnosis and management requires knowledge of the pathophysiology, the typical presentations in each age group, and the clinical consequences in body organs and systems. Evaluation includes clinical and laboratory assessment, as well as specific laboratory testing. **Management strategies** depend on understanding the pathophysiology and use of laboratory analyses to provide the best clinical control.

## SIGNS AND SYMPTOMS THAT SHOULD SUGGEST AN INBORN ERROR OF METABOLISM

The signs and symptoms of an inborn error are protean. Any organ system can be involved; the presentation varies among different age groups. Inborn errors of metabolism usually do not present immediately after birth but often occur after a few days to weeks, during which the infant appears well. Infants who survive the neonatal period without developing recognized symptoms often experience intermittent illness separated by periods of being well. Family history may be helpful, if positive. A history of early infant deaths is particularly suggestive. A negative family history does not exclude an inborn error of metabolism because this may be the first affected child in the family. The presentations may include toxicity, specific organ involvement, energy deficiency, dysmorphic findings, and appearance of organ storage.

## TYPES OF CLINICAL PRESENTATION OF INBORN ERRORS

### Toxic Presentation

Although some aspects of the presentation are specific to the abnormal pathway, many features are nonspecific and occur in a wide range of disorders. The toxic presentation often presents as an **encephalopathy**. Fever, infection, fasting, or other catabolic stresses may precipitate the symptom complex. A **metabolic acidosis**, vomiting, lethargy, and other neurologic findings may be present. During the acute presentation, diagnostic testing is most effective when metabolites are present in highest concentration in blood and urine during this time. Abnormal metabolism of amino acids, organic acids, ammonia, or carbohydrates may be at fault. **Hyperammonemia** is an important diagnostic possibility if an infant or child presents with features of toxic encephalopathy. Symptoms and signs depend on the underlying cause of the hyperammonemia, the age at which it develops, and its degree. The severity of hyperammonemia may provide a clue to the etiology (Tables 51-1 and 51-2).

### Severe Neonatal Hyperammonemia

Infants with genetic defects in urea synthesis, transient neonatal hyperammonemia, and impaired synthesis of urea and glutamine secondary to genetic disorders of organic acid metabolism can have levels of blood ammonia ($>1000\ \mu mol/L$) more than 10 times normal in the neonatal period. Poor feeding, hypotonia, apnea, hypothermia, and vomiting rapidly give way to **coma** and occasionally to intractable seizures. Respiratory alkalosis is common. Death occurs within days if the condition remains untreated.

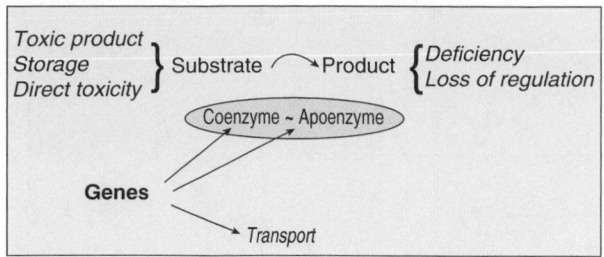

**FIGURE 51-1**

Depiction of the basic paradigm in inherited disorders of metabolism. Deficiency of an enzyme complex results in accumulation of metabolites proximal to the blocked metabolism and deficiency of the product of the reaction. Sites of genetic control are indicated.

## Moderate Neonatal Hyperammonemia

Moderate neonatal hyperammonemia (range, 200 to 400 µmol/L) is associated with depression of the central nervous system, poor feeding, and vomiting. Seizures are not characteristic. Respiratory alkalosis may occur. This type of hyperammonemia may be caused by partial blocks in urea synthesis and commonly is caused by disorders of organic acid metabolism that secondarily interfere with the elimination of nitrogen.

## Clinical Hyperammonemia in Later Infancy and Childhood

Infants who are affected by defects in the urea cycle may continue to do well while receiving the low-protein intake of breast milk, only to develop clinical hyperammonemia when dietary protein is increased or when catabolic stress occurs. Vomiting and lethargy frequently progress to coma. As protein intake is restricted by anorexia and vomiting or if intravenous glucose is given, the sensorium clears, and the infant recovers, but symptoms may recur again when metabolically stressed or ingesting an increased protein intake. Seizures are not typical. During a crisis, the plasma ammonia level is usually 200 to 500 µmol/L, but as it decreases with decreased intake the condition may go unrecognized for years, especially in the absence of central nervous system symptoms. If a crisis occurs during an epidemic of influenza, the child mistakenly may be thought to have **Reye syndrome**. Older children may have neuropsychiatric or behavioral abnormalities (Fig. 51-2).

## Specific Organ Presentation

Any organ or system can be injured by toxic accumulation of any of the metabolites involved in inborn errors. Symptoms relate to organ-specific or system-specific toxicity

---

**TABLE 51-1  Inborn Errors of Metabolism Presenting with Neurologic Signs in Infants <3 Months of Age**

| Generalized Seizures | Encephalopathic Coma with or without Seizures |
|---|---|
| All disorders that cause hypoglycemia | Maple syrup urine disease |
|   Most hepatic glycogen storage diseases | Nonketotic hyperglycinemia |
|   Galactosemia, hereditary fructose intolerance | Diseases producing extreme hyperammonemia |
|   Fructose-1,6-bisphosphatase deficiency |   Disorders of the urea cycle |
|   Disorders of fatty acid beta oxidation | |
| Disorders of the propionate pathway | Disorders of the propionate pathway |
| HMG-lyase deficiency | Disorders of beta oxidation |
| | Congenital lactic acidosis (PCD) |
| Pyruvate carboxylase deficiency (PCD) | |
| Maple syrup urine disease | |

**SEIZURES AND/OR POSTURING**

Nonketotic hyperglycinemia
Maple syrup urine disease

---

**TABLE 51-2  Etiologies of Hyperammonemia in Infants**

| Etiology of Hyperammonemia | Comments |
|---|---|
| Disorders of the urea cycle | Lethal hyperammonemia is common |
| Disorders of the propionate pathway | Severe hyperammonemia may precede acidosis |
| Disorders of fatty acid catabolism and of ketogenesis | Reye-like syndrome possible |
| Transient neonatal hyperammonemia | Idiopathic, self-limited |
| Portal-systemic shunting | Thrombosis of portal vein, cirrhosis, hepatitis |
| Idiopathic Reye syndrome | Rare |
| Drug intoxication: salicylate, valproic acid, acetaminophen | Obtain drug levels |
| Hyperinsulinism/hyperammonemia syndrome | Clinical hypoglycemia, subclinical hyperammonemia |

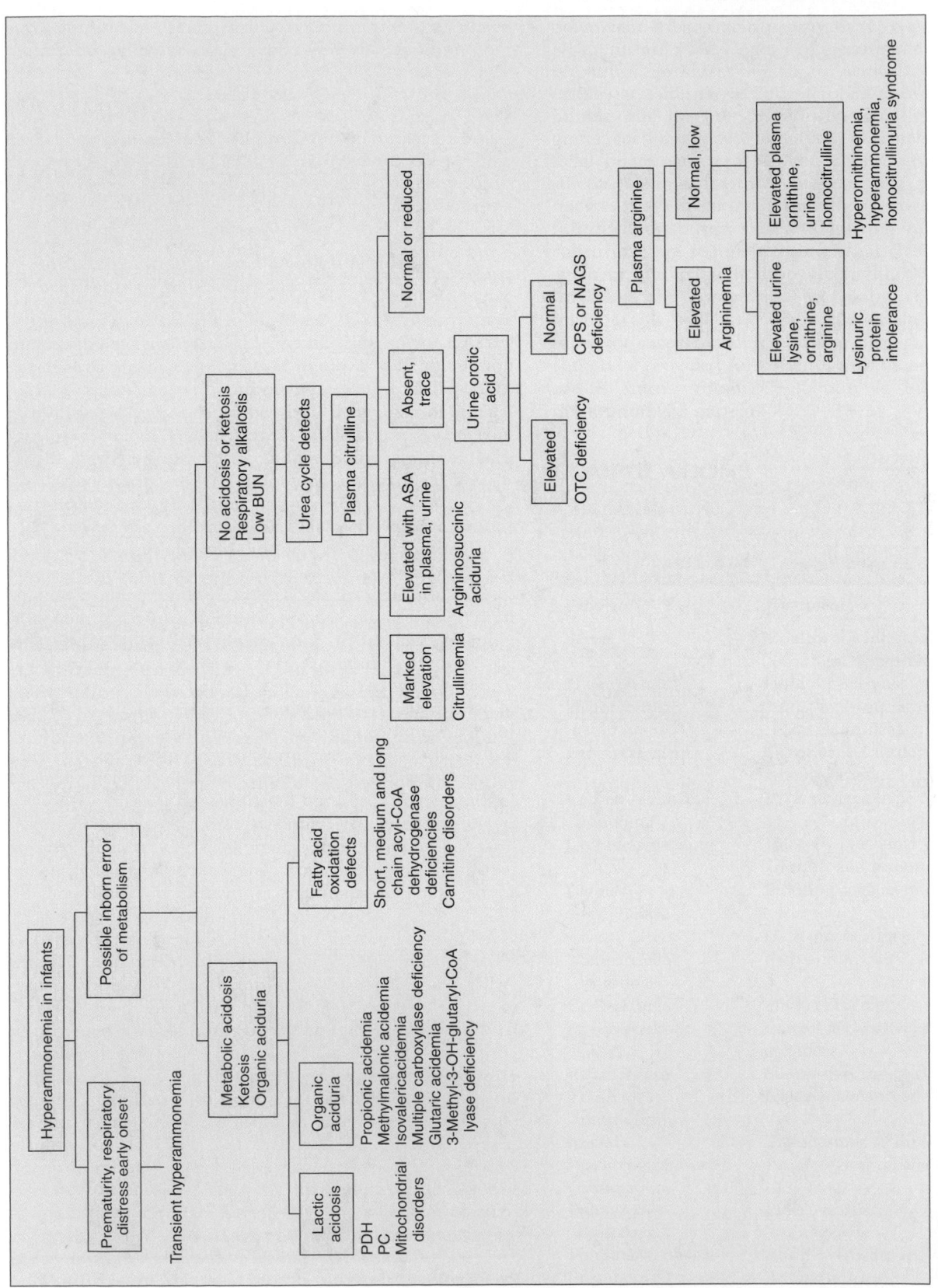

**FIGURE 51-2**

Algorithm for the approach to hyperammonemia in infants. ASA, argininosuccinic acid; CPS, carbamyl phosphate synthase; NAGS, N-acetylglutamate synthase; OTC, ornithine transcarbamylase; PC, pyruvate carboxylase deficiency; PDH, pyruvate dehydrogenase deficiency.

**TABLE 51-3 Inborn Errors of Metabolism Presenting with Hepatomegaly or Hepatic Dysfunction in Infants**

| Hepatomegaly | Hepatic Failure | Jaundice |
|---|---|---|
| GSD I | Galactosemia | Galactosemia |
| GSD III | Hereditary fructose intolerance | Hereditary fructose intolerance |
| Mucopolysaccharidosis I and II | Tyrosinemia type 1 (fumarylacetoacetate hydrolase deficiency) | Infantile tyrosinemia (fumarylacetoacetate hydrolase deficiency) |
| Gaucher and Niemann-Pick diseases | GSD IV (slowly evolving) | Crigler-Najjar disease |
| | | Rotor, Dubin-Johnson syndromes |

GSD, glycogen storage disease.

and injury. Examples include nervous system (seizures, coma, ataxia), liver (hepatocellular damage), eye (cataracts, dislocated lenses), renal (tubular dysfunction, cysts), and heart (cardiomyopathy, pericardial effusion) (Table 51-3; see Table 51-1).

## Energy Deficiency

Disorders whose pathophysiology results in energy deficiency may manifest myopathy; central nervous system dysfunction, including mental retardation and seizures; cardiomyopathy; vomiting; hypoglycemia; or renal tubular acidosis. Examples include disorders of fatty acid oxidation, disorders of mitochondrial function/oxidative phosphorylation, and disorders of carbohydrate metabolism.

## Ketosis and Ketotic Hypoglycemia

Acidosis is often found in children without metabolic diseases, with fasting associated with anorexia, vomiting, and diarrhea in the course of a viral illness. The clinical manifestations of the causative illness result in mild acidosis and ketonuria; administration of carbohydrate restores balance. In this normal response to fasting, the blood glucose level is relatively low. Severe ketosis may also be the result of disorders of ketone utilization such as ketothiolase deficiency (see Fig. 54-1) or glycogen synthase deficiency, a disorder of glycogen synthesis. In these conditions, hypoglycemia is significant, and the ketosis clears slowly, requiring significant amounts of intravenous glucose. These disorders frequently present in the context of fasting, infection with fever, or decreased intake secondary to vomiting and diarrhea. **Ketotic hypoglycemia** is a common condition in which tolerance for fasting is impaired to the extent that symptomatic hypoglycemia with seizures or coma occurs when the child encounters a ketotic stress. The stress may be significant (viral infection with vomiting) or minor (a prolongation by several hours of the normal overnight fast). Ketotic hypoglycemia first appears in the second year of life and occurs in otherwise healthy children. It is treated by frequent snacks and the provision of glucose during periods of stress. The pathophysiology is poorly understood (see Chapter 172). Although ketonuria is a normal response to prolonged (not overnight) fasting in older infants and children, it indicates metabolic disease in neonates. **A high anion gap metabolic acidosis with or without** ketosis suggests a metabolic disorder (Table 51-4). Although ketone production may not be robust in fatty acid oxidation disorders, the presence of ketonuria does not exclude this group of disorders.

**TABLE 51-4 Etiologies of Metabolic Acidosis Caused by Inborn Errors of Metabolism in Infants**

| Disorder | Comment |
|---|---|
| Methylmalonic acidemia (MMA) | Hyperammonemia, ketosis, neutropenia, thrombocytopenia |
| Propionic acidemia | Similar to MMA |
| Isovaleric acidemia | Similar to MMA; odor of *sweaty feet* |
| Pyruvate dehydrogenase deficiency | Lactic acidosis, hyperammonemia |
| Pyruvate carboxylase deficiency | Lactic acidosis, hypoglycemia, and ketosis |
| Respiratory chain (mitochondrial) disorders | Lactic acidosis, ketosis |
| Medium-chain acyl-CoA dehydrogenase deficiency (MCAD) | Moderate acidosis, hypoglycemia, decreased ketosis, possible hyperammonemia |
| Other fatty acid oxidation defects | Similar to MCAD |
| Galactosemia | Renal tubular acidosis, *Escherichia coli* sepsis, hypoglycemia |
| 3-Hydroxy-3-methyl-glutaryl-CoA lyase deficiency | Severe lactic acidosis, hyperammonemia, hypoglycemia |
| 3-Methylcrotonyl-CoA carboxylase deficiency | Severe lactic acidosis, hyperammonemia, hypoglycemia, ketosis |
| Multiple acyl-CoA dehydrogenase deficiency (glutaric aciduria 2) | Metabolic acidosis, hypoglycemia, lethal renal malformations |

## Disorders Associated with Dysmorphic Findings

Congenital malformations or dysmorphic features are not intuitively thought of as symptoms and signs of inborn errors. Conditions that cause congenital malformations include carbohydrate-deficient glycoprotein syndrome, disorders of cholesterol biosynthesis (Smith-Lemli-Opitz syndrome), disorders of copper transport (Menkes syndrome, occipital horn syndrome), maternal phenylketonuria syndrome, glutaric aciduria II (also called multiple acyl-coenzyme A [CoA] dehydrogenase deficiency), and several storage diseases.

## Storage Disorders

Storage disorders are caused by accumulation of incompletely metabolized large molecules. This storage often occurs in subcellular organelles, such as lysosomes. The glycogen storage diseases and mucopolysaccharide disorders are examples of storage disorders.

## Different Age Groups and Differing Clinical Phenotypes

A neonate no longer has the protective functions of the placenta to detoxify metabolites that accumulate because of an inborn error. In addition, maternal metabolism no longer provides nutrition to the neonate who cannot metabolize substrates such as glycogen and fatty acids. Introduction of new foods in older infancy and frequency of metabolic stress with fasting and fever in that age group make the infant vulnerable. Increased protein intake associated with growth in older children and adolescents may stress deficient pathways that previously were compensated. Hormonal factors in adolescence influence intermediary metabolism in unpredictable ways. In neonates, galactosemia may present with the introduction of milk, fatty acid disorders during fasting or breastfeeding, and organic acid and urea cycle disorders following the loss of maternal detoxification. In infants, hereditary fructose intolerance occurs after introduction of fructose or sucrose in the diet, and fatty acid disorders present with fasting or illness. In children, increased protein intake may unmask disorders of ammonia detoxification. In adolescents, hormonal changes may trigger changes that allow diagnosis of cobalamin C methylmalonic aciduria (cblC MMA).

## CLINICAL ASSESSMENT AND CLINICAL LABORATORY TESTING

The assessment begins with a careful history and clinical evaluation. Clinical laboratory testing can define the metabolic derangement (Table 51-5). The results generate a differential diagnosis and a list of more specific laboratory testing to confirm the diagnosis.

The combination of symptoms and abnormal clinical laboratory findings demands urgent metabolic evaluation. A metabolic emergency often presents with vomiting, acidosis, hypoglycemia, ketosis (or *lack of appropriate ketosis*), intercurrent infection, anorexia/failure to feed, lethargy proceeding to coma, and hyperventilation or hypoventilation.

| TABLE 51-5 Initial Diagnostic Evaluation for a Suspected Inborn Error of Metabolism* | |
|---|---|
| **Blood and Plasma** | **Urine** |
| Arterial blood gas | Glucose |
| Electrolytes—anion gap | pH |
| Glucose | Ketones |
| Ammonia | Reducing substances |
| Liver enzymes | Organic acids |
| Complete blood count, differential,† and platelet count | Acylglycines |
| Lactate, pyruvate | Orotic acid |
| Organic acids | |
| Amino acids | |
| Acylcarnitines | |
| Carnitine | |

*Organ-specific evaluation is indicated for specific symptoms (e.g., cranial magnetic resonance imaging for coma or seizures; echocardiography for cardiomyopathy; cerebrospinal fluid amino acids by column chromatography if nonketotic hyperglycemia is suspected).
†Thrombocytopenia and neutropenia are seen in organic acidurias; vacuolated lymphocytes and metachromatic granules are seen in lysosomal disorders.

Clinical evaluation should focus on the cardiac, renal, neurologic, and developmental assessment and look for change in mental status, seizures, abnormal tone, visual symptoms, poor developmental progress, global developmental delay, loss of milestones, cardiomyopathy, cardiac failure, cystic renal malformation, and renal tubular dysfunction.

**Clinical laboratory testing** should begin with tests that are available in most hospital clinical laboratories. Care in the collection and handling of laboratory specimens is crucial to obtaining accurate results. Plasma measurements of lactate and ammonia are particularly subject to spurious results if not handled correctly. Significant ketosis in the neonate is unusual and suggests an organic acid disorder. Ketosis out of proportion to fasting status in an older child occurs in disorders of ketone usage. Lack of severe ketosis in an older child under conditions of metabolic stress is a feature of fatty acid oxidation disorders.

## GENETIC ASPECTS OF INBORN ERRORS

### Mechanisms of Inheritance

Although all of the classic mechanisms of inheritance are represented, most inborn errors of metabolism are autosomal recessive (Table 51-6). Isolation or founder effect may make a specific recessive condition common in some populations (e.g., maple syrup urine disease in the Old Order Mennonite population in Pennsylvania). X-linked conditions exhibit the usual increased prevalence in males. Carriers of recessive genes or X-linked genes (females) are usually asymptomatic except in a few conditions. In ornithine transcarbamylase deficiency, females can be symptomatic if they have a significant distribution of abnormal cells in the liver. Mitochondrial inheritance, caused by

**TABLE 51-6 Inheritance Patterns: Genotypes and Phenotypes**

| | Examples | Phenotypes | Clinical Problems |
|---|---|---|---|
| **AUTOSOMAL GENES** | | | |
| Dominant inheritance | Familial hypercholesterolemia | Heterozygous—affected | Xanthomas and heart disease in adult life |
| | | Homozygous—affected markedly by *gene dose effect* | Xanthomas and heart disease in childhood |
| Recessive inheritance | Phenylketonuria | Heterozygous—normal | Normal |
| | Galactosemia | Homozygous—affected | Severe developmental delay |
| | | Heterozygous—normal | ? Cataracts (adult) |
| | | Homozygous—affected | Neonatal liver failure, cataracts; ovarian failure (adult) |
| **X-LINKED GENES** | | | |
| | Ornithine transcarbamylase deficiency | Male—affected | Severe infantile hyperammonemia |
| | | Female—variably affected depending on X-chromosome inactivation | Normal phenotype, postpartum hyperammonemia, recurrent Reye syndrome, neonatal hyperammonemia |
| **MITOCHONDRIAL GENES** | | | |
| | Mutant leucine transfer RNA (*A3243G*) | Both sexes affected equally, but clinical manifestations variable among family members | Lactic acidosis, skeletal myopathy, cardiomyopathy, seizures, mental retardation, ataxia, deafness in various syndromic combinations |
| | Depletion/duplication | Both sexes affected; genetics variable | Liver failure, myopathy, external ophthalmoplegia |

a mutation in 1 of 13 mitochondrial genes coding for proteins involved in oxidative phosphorylation, shows a maternal pattern of inheritance. The clinical disorders produced by abnormalities of these maternal genes depend on the specific defects and the tissue distribution of affected and normal mitochondria over time. Dominantly inherited diseases may be sporadic or evident in the family. When parents are closely related (**consanguineous**), there is a significant chance that a child has inherited two copies of the same abnormal allele, acquired from a common ancestor and resulting in a recessive condition.

## Identification of Molecular Pathology

If the molecular basis of an inborn error of metabolism is known (i.e., the gene or genes has/have been mapped and mutations defined), specific molecular testing may be clinically available. A defined set of mutations comprises most of the mutations for many disorders. In other conditions, there may be many hundreds of different mutations. In recessive disorders, it is common for a patient to be doubly heterozygous for two different mutations at the gene locus involved. There is a good correlation between specific mutations and clinical outcome for some disorders; the result of this testing can be an additional

guide to treatment. The ability to perform genetic testing in other at-risk family members can provide important genetic information for them, enabling decision making throughout the rest of the family.

## IDENTIFICATION OF INBORN ERRORS BY NEONATAL SCREENING

### Disorders Identified by Neonatal Screening

Nearly all states screen for at least eight or nine disorders. In most states, tandem mass spectrometry is used, and 30 metabolic disorders may be identifiable (Table 51-7). The **disorders of amino acid metabolism**, phenylketonuria, homocystinuria, maple syrup urine disease, and tyrosinemia all need to be treated early in infancy for treatment to be effective. The disorders of **organic acid metabolism**, propionic acidemia, methylmalonic acidemia, and isovaleric academia may result in vomiting and ketoacidosis early in life; some forms of methylmalonic acidemia present later, but central nervous system damage already may have occurred. **Galactosemia** is the disorder of carbohydrate metabolism that can be detected by screening. The initial presentation of galactosemia not identified by screening includes jaundice, bleeding, cataract, sepsis,

**TABLE 51-7 Disorders Identified in Newborn Screening Programs in the United States**

| Disorder | Methods | Optimal Age of Treatment | Confirmatory Testing |
|---|---|---|---|
| | | **AMINO ACID** | |
| PKU | Guthrie*, MS/MS | First weeks of life | Plasma phenylalanine, mutation testing |
| Tyrosinemia | Guthrie, MS/MS | First week of life | Plasma amino acid profile, urine succinylacetone |
| MSUD | Guthrie, MS/MS | First week of life | Plasma amino acid profile, look for alloisoleucine |
| | | **ORGANIC ACID** | |
| Propionic acidemia | MS/MS | First week of life | Urine organic acid profile |
| Methylmalonic acidemia | MS/MS | First weeks of life | Urine organic acid profile, plasma amino acid profile, plasma homocysteine |
| Isovaleric acidemia | MS/MS | First weeks of life | Urine organic acid profile |
| Biotinidase deficiency | Enzyme measurement | First weeks of life | Quantitative biotinidase measurement, DNA mutations |
| | | **FATTY ACID** | |
| MCAD | MS/MS | First weeks of life | Urine organic acid profile, urine acylglycine profile, plasma acylcarnitine profile |
| LCHAD | MS/MS | First weeks of life | Urine organic acid profile, urine acylglycine profile, plasma acylcarnitine profile |
| VLCAD | MS/MS | First weeks of life | Urine organic acid profile, urine acylglycine profile, plasma acylcarnitine profile |
| | | **CARBOHYDRATE** | |
| Galactosemia | GALT enzyme measurement | First few days of life | GALT enzyme measurement, DNA mutations, galactose-1-P measurement |
| | | **UREA CYCLE** | |
| | MS/MS | First few days of life | Plasma amino acid profile, DNA mutations |

*Guthrie test used rarely now, if at all.
GALT, galactose-1-p-uridyltransferase; LCHAD, long-chain 3-hydroxyacyl coenzyme A dehydrogenase; MCAD, medium-chain acyl-coenzyme A dehydrogenase; MS/MS, tandem mass spectrometry; MSUD, maple syrup urine disease; PKU, phenylketonuria; VLCAD; very long chain acyl-coenzyme A dehydrogenase.

and liver failure. **Biotinidase deficiency** is screened for by enzyme measurement. Presymptomatic treatment affects outcome in all of these conditions; in some it is lifesaving.

## Strategy of Neonatal Screening

The purpose of neonatal screening is the **early detection** and **rapid treatment** of disorders before onset of symptoms, early enough to prevent the morbidity and mortality of the disorders. The screening tests for inborn errors of metabolism historically have used microbiologic (Guthrie) assays for single analytes or semiquantitative fluorometric methods. The adaptation of tandem mass spectrometry of blood specimens to neonatal screening has been adopted in most states, allowing rapid neonatal diagnosis of numerous metabolic diseases with a single blood specimen.

In most states, infants are tested just before discharge or by 7 days of age if the infant remains hospitalized (see Chapter 58). A positive test demands prompt evaluation. Specific follow-up testing and treatment of an affected child depends on the disorder. Many infants who have a positive neonatal screening test do not have a metabolic disorder. Parents may need to be reassured that this *false-positive* test in no way reflects the infant's health and is the result of establishing cutoff values for the screening test to ensure that no affected infant is missed.

## Confirmatory Testing Principles

Neonatal screening is designed not to miss affected infants but is not diagnostic. Cutoff values for each analyte are established carefully to identify all infants with an elevated concentration of the analyte or decreased activity of an enzyme without having an unacceptable number of false-positive results. A positive screening test must be followed by specific clinical evaluation and laboratory testing to confirm the disorder. Protocols for the evaluation of an infant with an abnormal screening result clarify which infants need to be treated and which have had a false-positive test.

A positive screening test result causes anxiety for new parents. Definitive testing must be carried out promptly and accurately. If the diagnosis is confirmed, treatment must be begun immediately. If an inborn error of metabolism is excluded, parents need a thorough explanation and reassurance that the infant is well. Widespread newborn screening for these new disorders has shown that there are milder forms of these conditions than previously recognized by clinical presentation. Clarifying this after a positive newborn screening test requires access to molecular testing to define specific mutations. Some of these milder forms do not need aggressive treatment.

## Specialized Laboratory and Clinical Testing

Specialized testing for inherited disorders of metabolism is effective in confirming a diagnosis suspected on the basis of an abnormal newborn screening result or on the basis of clinical suspicion. The analytes that are helpful and examples of diagnoses made using these measurements depend on the deficient pathway in the disorder under consideration (Table 51-8).

Amino acid analysis is performed in plasma, urine, and cerebrospinal fluid. The plasma amino acid profile is most useful in identifying disorders of amino acid catabolism. Amino acids in the deficient pathway of the organic acid disorders may be abnormal, but often they are normal or may not be diagnostic.

The urine amino acid profile is helpful in diagnosing primary disorders of renal tubular function, such as Lowe syndrome and cystinuria, as well as secondary disorders of renal tubular function, such as cystinosis and Fanconi syndrome of any cause. The urine amino acid profile is not the test of choice for diagnosing disorders of amino acid or organic acid metabolism.

Markers of disordered fatty acid oxidation are measured in urine and plasma. Excessive intermediates of fatty acid oxidation and organic acid catabolism are conjugated with glycine and carnitine. The urine acylglycine profile and the plasma acylcarnitine profile reflect this accumulation. In organic acid disorders and fatty acid oxidation disorders, measurement of plasma carnitine reveals the secondary deficiency of carnitine and abnormal distribution of free and acylated carnitine. The plasma free fatty acid profile is helpful in diagnosis of disorders of fatty acid oxidation. Excess 3-OH-butyrate suggests a disorder of ketone metabolism; absence of ketones or decreased amounts of 3-OH-butyrate suggest a fatty acid oxidation disorder. Profiling of fatty acid intermediates in cultured skin fibroblasts may be informative.

The urine organic acid profile is a useful test. Disorders of organic acid metabolism, such as propionic acidemia and methylmalonic acidemia, have typical urine organic acid profiles. Although the analytes in blood and urine usually suggest the specific diagnosis, more targeted testing may be needed, in which enzymatic activity in the pathway is measured, or molecular abnormalities in the gene are sought.

Disorders of creatine biosynthesis are reflected by an increase in guanidinoacetic acid in blood and urine. Disorders of purine and pyrimidine metabolism are suggested by the presence of an abnormal urinary profile of purines, such as xanthine, hypoxanthine, inosine, guanosine, adenosine, adenine, and succinyladenosine. Similarly, disorders of pyrimidine metabolism are identified by an abnormal profile of pyrimidines, including uracil, uridine, thymine, thymidine, orotic acid, orotidine, dihydrouracil, dihydrothymine, pseudouridine, N-carbamoyl-β-alanine, and N-carbamoyl-β-amino-isobutyrate, in the urine.

Storage disorders show abnormalities in urine mucopolysaccharides (glycosaminoglycans, glycoproteins), sialic acid, heparan sulfate, dermatan sulfate, and chondroitin sulfate. Specific enzymology depends on the disorder; tissue can be either white blood cells or cultured skin fibroblasts, depending on assay. In several disorders, cerebrospinal fluid is the most helpful specimen, including glycine encephalopathy (amino acid profile), disorders of neurotransmitter synthesis

### TABLE 51-8 Specialized Metabolic Testing

| Test | Analytes Measured | Test Helpful in Identifying Disorders |
|---|---|---|
| Plasma amino acid profile | Amino acids, including alloisoleucine | PKU, tyrosinemias, MSUD, homocystinuria |
| Plasma total homocysteine | Protein-bound and free homocysteine | Homocystinuria, some forms of methylmalonic acidemia |
| Urine amino acid profile | Amino acids | Disorders of amino acid renal transport |
| Plasma acylcarnitine profile | Acylcarnitine derivatives of organic and fatty acid catabolism | Organic acid disorders, fatty acid oxidation disorders |
| Urine acylglycine profile | Acylglycine derivatives of organic and fatty acid catabolism | Organic acid disorders, fatty acid oxidation disorders |
| Plasma carnitines | Free, total, and acylated carnitine | Primary and secondary carnitine deficiency; abnormal in many organic acid and fatty acid disorders |
| Urine organic acid profile | Organic acids | Organic acid, mitochondrial and fatty acid disorders |
| Urine or blood succinylacetone | Succinylacetone | Tyrosinemia I |
| Urine oligosaccharide chromatography | Glycosaminoglycans, mucopolysaccharides | Lysosomal storage disorders |

MSUD, maple syrup urine disease; PKU, phenylketonuria.

(biogenic amine profile), glucose transporter (GLUT1) deficiency (plasma–to–cerebrospinal fluid glucose ratio), and serine synthesis defect (amino acid profile).

In many disorders, an abnormal metabolic profile is consistently present during illness and when the child is well. In some cases, during an episode of illness is the time when metabolic profiles are most likely to be diagnostic.

## OVERVIEW OF TREATMENT

There are several basic principles to treatment of inborn errors of metabolism. Syndromes with toxicity often present with encephalopathy, and the removal of toxic compounds is the first goal of therapy. Strategies include hemodialysis, hemovenovenous filtration, and administration of trapping agents (see Chapter 53). A second strategy is to enhance deficient enzyme activity through administration of enzyme cofactors (e.g., pyridoxine in homocystinuria). If deficiency of a pathway product plays an important role, providing missing products is helpful (e.g., tyrosine in the treatment of phenylketonuria). A major principle is to decrease flux through the deficient pathway by restricting precursors in the diet. Examples include the restriction of phenylalanine in phenylketonuria, of protein in disorders of ammonia detoxification, and of amino acid precursors in the organic acid disorders.

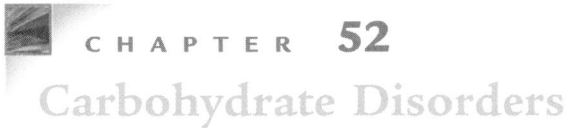

C H A P T E R  **52**

## Carbohydrate Disorders

## GLYCOGEN STORAGE DISEASES

Many glycogen storage diseases are characterized by **hypoglycemia** and **hepatomegaly** (Table 52-1). Glycogen, the storage form of glucose, is found most abundantly in the liver, where it modulates blood glucose levels, and in muscles, where it facilitates anaerobic work. Glycogen is synthesized from uridine diphosphoglucose through the concerted action of glycogen synthetase and brancher enzyme (Fig. 52-1). The accumulation of glycogen is stimulated by insulin. Glycogenolysis occurs through a cascade initiated by epinephrine or glucagon. It results in rapid phosphorolysis of glycogen to yield glucose-1-phosphate, accompanied by a lesser degree of hydrolysis of glucose residues from the branch points in glycogen molecules. In the liver and kidneys, glucose-1-phosphate is converted to glucose-6-phosphate through the actions of phosphoglucomutase; glucose-6-phosphatase hydrolyses glucose-6-phosphate to produce glucose. The latter enzyme is not present in muscles. Glycogen storage diseases fall into the following four categories:

1. Diseases that predominantly affect the liver and have a direct influence on blood glucose (types I, VI, and VIII)
2. Diseases that predominantly involve muscles and affect the ability to do anaerobic work (types V and VII)
3. Diseases that can affect the liver and muscles and directly influence blood glucose and muscle metabolism (type III)
4. Diseases that affect various tissues but have no direct effect on blood glucose or on the ability to do anaerobic work (types II and IV)

The **diagnosis** of glycogen storage disease can often be confirmed by DNA mutation testing in blood cells. When this is feasible, invasive procedures, such as muscle and liver biopsy, can be avoided. When mutation testing is not available, enzyme measurements in the tissue suspected to be affected confirm the diagnosis. If the diagnosis cannot be established, metabolic challenge and exercise testing may be needed. **Treatment** of hepatic glycogen storage disease is aimed at maintaining satisfactory blood glucose levels or supplying alternative energy sources to muscle. In glucose-6-phosphatase deficiency (type I), the treatment usually requires nocturnal intragastric feedings of glucose during the first 1 or 2 years of life. Thereafter, snacks or nocturnal intragastric feedings of uncooked cornstarch may be satisfactory; hepatic tumors (sometimes malignant) are a threat in adolescence and adult life. No specific treatment exists for the diseases of muscle that impair skeletal muscle ischemic exercise. Enzyme replacement early in life is effective in Pompe disease (type II), which involves cardiac and skeletal muscle.

## GALACTOSEMIA

Galactosemia is an autosomal recessive disease caused by deficiency of galactose-1-phosphate uridyltransferase (Fig. 52-2). Clinical manifestations are most striking in a neonate who, when fed milk, generally exhibits evidence of **liver failure** (hyperbilirubinemia, disorders of coagulation, and hypoglycemia), disordered **renal tubular function** (acidosis, glycosuria, and aminoaciduria), and **cataracts**. The neonatal screening test must have a rapid turnaround time because affected infants may die in the first week of life. Affected infants are at increased risk for severe neonatal *Escherichia coli* sepsis. Major effects on liver and kidney function and the development of cataracts are limited to the first few years of life; older children have learning disorders. Girls usually develop premature ovarian failure despite treatment.

**Laboratory manifestations** of galactosemia depend on dietary galactose intake. When galactose is ingested (as lactose), levels of plasma galactose and erythrocyte galactose-1-phosphate are elevated. Hypoglycemia is frequent, and albuminuria is present. Galactose frequently is present in the urine and can be detected by a positive reaction for reducing substances (Clinitest tablets) without a reaction with glucose oxidase on urine strip tests. The absence of urinary reducing substances cannot be relied on to exclude the diagnosis. The diagnosis is made by showing extreme reduction in erythrocyte galactose-1-phosphate uridyltransferase. DNA testing for the mutations in galactose-1-phosphate uridyltransferase confirms the diagnosis. Renal tubular dysfunction may be evidenced by a normal anion gap hyperchloremic metabolic acidosis. **Treatment** by the elimination of dietary galactose results in rapid correction of abnormalities, but infants who are extremely ill before treatment may die before therapy is effective. The concentration of galactose-1-phosphate rarely returns to normal even after treatment is begun.

## TABLE 52-1 Glycogen Storage Diseases*

| Disease | Affected Enzyme | Organs Affected | Clinical Syndrome | Neonatal Manifestations | Prognosis |
|---|---|---|---|---|---|
| Type I: von Gierke | Glucose-6-phosphatase | Liver, kidney, GI tract, platelets | Hypoglycemia, lactic acidosis, ketosis, hepatomegaly, hypotonia, slow growth, diarrhea, bleeding disorder, gout, hypertriglyceridemia, xanthomas | Hypoglycemia, lactic acidemia, liver may not be enlarged | Early death from hypoglycemia, lactic acidosis; may do well with supportive management; hepatomas occur in late childhood |
| Type II: Pompe | Lysosomal α-glucosidase | All, notably striated muscle, nerve cells | Symmetrical profound muscle weakness, cardiomegaly, heart failure, shortened P-R interval | May have muscle weakness, cardiomegaly, or both | Very poor; death in the first year of life is usual; variants exist; therapy with recombinant human α-glucosidase is promising |
| Type III: Forbes | Debranching enzyme | Liver, muscles | Early in course hypoglycemia, ketonuria, hepatomegaly that resolves with age; may show muscle fatigue | Usually none | Very good for hepatic disorder; if myopathy present, it tends to be like that of type V |
| Type IV: Andersen | Branching enzyme | Liver, other tissues | Hepatic cirrhosis beginning at several months of age; early liver failure | Usually none | Very poor; death from hepatic failure before 4 years of age |
| Type V: McArdle | Muscle phosphorylase | Muscle | Muscle fatigue beginning in adolescence | None | Good, with sedentary lifestyle |
| Type VI: Hers | Liver phosphorylase | Liver | Mild hypoglycemia with hepatomegaly, ketonuria | Usually none | Probably good |
| Type VII: Tarui | Muscle phosphofructokinase | Muscle | Clinical findings similar to type V | None | Similar to that of type V |
| Type VIII | Phosphorylase kinase | Liver | Clinical findings similar to type III, without myopathy | None | Good |

*Except for one form of hepatic phosphorylase kinase, which is X-linked, these disorders are autosomal recessive.
GI, gastrointestinal.

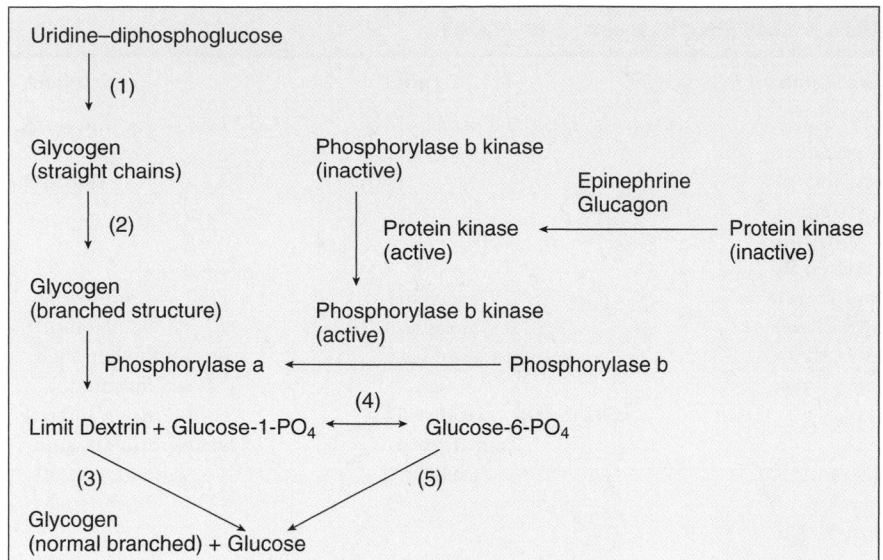

**FIGURE 52-1**

Glycogen synthesis and degradation. (1) Glycogen synthetase, (2) brancher enzyme, (3) debrancher enzyme, (4) phosphoglucomutase, (5) glucose-6-phosphatase.

**Galactokinase deficiency**, an autosomal recessive disorder, also leads to the accumulation of galactose in body fluids (see Fig. 52-2), which results in the formation of galactitol (dulcitol) through the action of aldose reductase. Galactitol, acting as an osmotic agent, can be responsible for cataract formation and, rarely, for increased intracranial pressure. These are the only clinical manifestations. Individuals homozygous for galactokinase deficiency usually develop cataracts after the neonatal period, whereas heterozygous individuals may be at risk for cataracts as adults. **Treatment** consists of lifelong elimination of galactose from the diet.

**Hereditary fructose intolerance,** in many ways, is analogous to galactosemia. When fructose is ingested, deficiency of fructose-1-phosphate aldolase leads to the intracellular accumulation of fructose-1-phosphate with resultant emesis, hypoglycemia, and severe liver and kidney disease. Elimination of fructose and sucrose from the diet cures the clinical disease. Affected patients sometimes spontaneously avoid fructose-containing foods and thus have no dental caries. **Fructosuria** is analogous to galactokinase deficiency in that it is caused by fructokinase deficiency, but the defect in fructosuria is harmless.

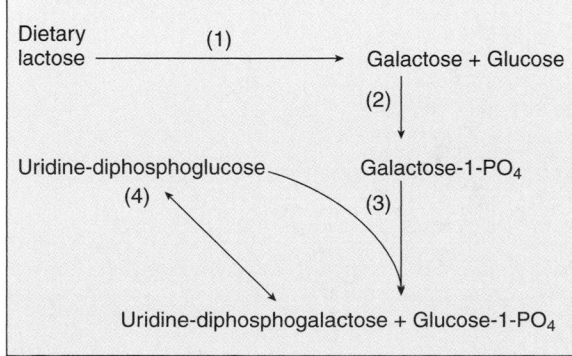

**FIGURE 52-2**

Pathway of galactose metabolism. (1) Lactase (intestinal), (2) galactokinase, (3) galactose-1-phosphate uridyltransferase, (4) uridine diphosphoglucose 4-epimerase.

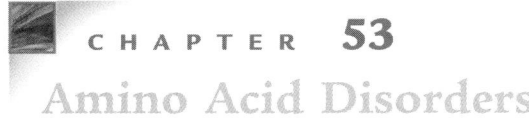

# CHAPTER 53
## Amino Acid Disorders

## DISORDERS OF AMINO ACID METABOLISM

Disorders of amino acid metabolism are the result of the inability to catabolize specific amino acids derived from protein. Usually a single amino acid pathway is involved. This amino acid accumulates in excess and is toxic to various organs, such as the brain, eyes, skin, or liver. Treatment is directed at the specific pathway, and usually involves dietary restriction of the offending amino acid and supplementation with special medical foods (formulas) that provide the other amino acids and other nutrients. Confirmatory testing includes quantitative specific plasma amino acid profiles along with specific mutation testing and sometimes enzymology.

## PHENYLKETONURIA

Phenylketonuria (PKU), an autosomal recessive disease, primarily affects the brain and occurs in 1:10,000 persons. Classic PKU is the result from a defect in the hydroxylation of phenylalanine to form tyrosine (Fig. 53-1); the activity of phenylalanine hydroxylase in the liver is absent or greatly reduced. Affected infants are normal at birth, but severe mental retardation (IQ 30) develops in the first year of life. The clinical syndrome in the untreated child classically includes blond hair, blue eyes, eczema, and mousy odor of the urine but is rarely seen because of universal neonatal screening for PKU. A positive newborn screening test must be followed up by performing quantitative plasma amino acid analysis, measuring phenylalanine and tyrosine. A plasma phenylalanine value of greater than 360 μM (6 mg/dL) is consistent with the diagnosis of one of the hyperphenylalaninemias and demands

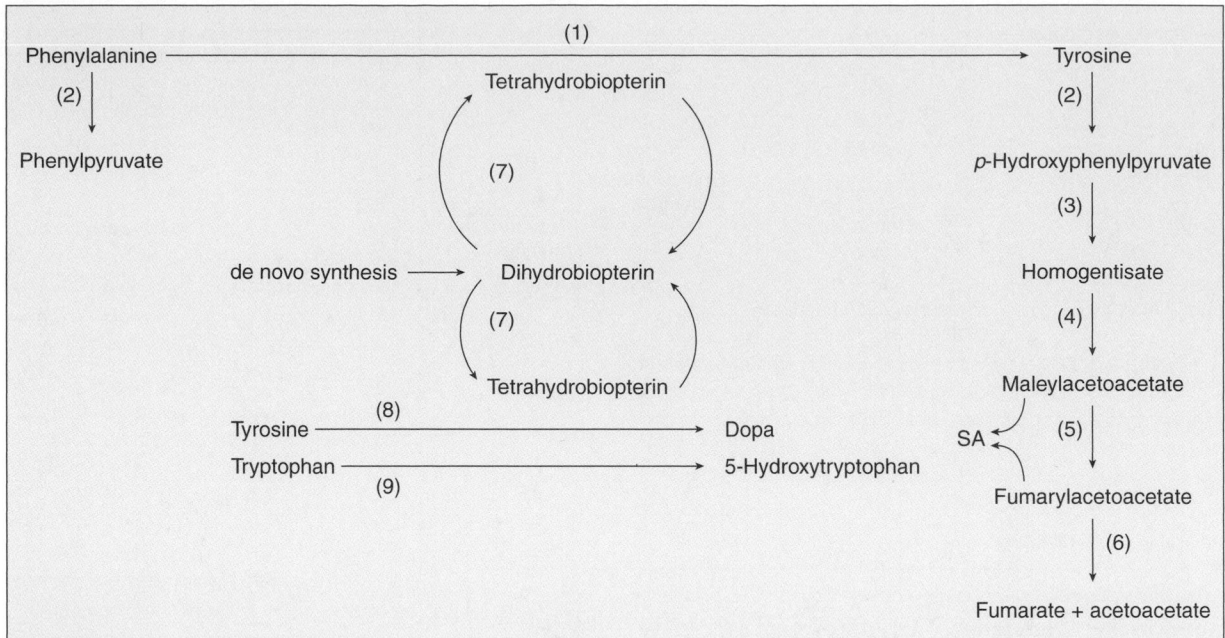

**FIGURE 53-1**

Metabolism of aromatic amino acids. (1) Phenylalanine hydroxylase, (2) transaminase, (3) p-hydroxyphenylpyruvate oxidase, (4) homogentisate oxidase, (5) maleylacetoacetate isomerase, (6) fumarylacetoacetate hydrolase, (7) dihydrobiopterin reductase, (8) tyrosine hydroxylase, (9) tryptophan hydroxylase. SA, succinylacetone.

prompt evaluation and treatment. Untreated, classic PKU is characterized by blood phenylalanine concentrations higher than 600 μM. Milder forms of hyperphenylalaninemia are indicated by values of plasma phenylalanine lower than this but higher than 360 μM. A significant percentage of premature infants and a few full-term infants have transient elevations in phenylalanine. Short-term follow-up usually identifies these infants promptly. Mutation testing of the *PAH* gene reveals more than 400 mutations. Some mutations are associated with mild hyperphenylalaninemia.

**Treatment** is designed to maintain plasma phenylalanine values in the therapeutic range of 120 to 360 μM, at least for the first 10 years of life. However, many persons have difficulty achieving this level of control consistently, particularly in adolescence and adulthood.

A small percentage of infants diagnosed with PKU (≤2% in the United States) have a defect in the synthesis or metabolism of tetrahydrobiopterin, the cofactor for phenylalanine hydroxylase and for other enzymes involved in the intermediary metabolism of aromatic amino acids. In these infants, a progressive, lethal central nervous system disease develops, reflecting abnormalities in other neurotransmitter metabolism for which tetrahydrobiopterin is necessary. Disorders in **biopterin metabolism** are diagnosed by measuring dihydrobiopterin reductase in erythrocytes and by analyzing biopterin metabolites in urine. This testing is carried out in all hyperphenylalaninemic infants.

**Outcome** of treatment in classic PKU is excellent. Most infants with classic PKU who are treated using a diet specifically restricted in phenylalanine and begun within the first 10 days of life achieve normal intelligence. Learning problems and problems with executive function are reported; early and consistent dietary control provides

the best chance for optimal outcome. In the disorders of biopterin biosynthesis, restriction of dietary phenylalanine reduces plasma phenylalanine, but does not ameliorate the clinical symptoms. This condition must be treated by replacement of the cofactor or by neuropharmacologic agents. Outcome is less predictable than in classic PKU.

Sustained control is difficult to achieve after the first 10 years of life. The safe concentration of phenylalanine in older children and adults with PKU has not been clearly established. Reversible cognitive dysfunction is associated with acute elevations of plasma phenylalanine in adults and children with PKU. If the elevated level has been sustained, the dysfunction may not be reversible. Treatment with modified preparation of tetrahydrobiopterin has shown good responses in some individuals with PKU. **Maternal hyperphenylalaninemia** requires rigorous management before conception and throughout pregnancy to prevent fetal brain damage, congenital heart disease, and microcephaly.

## TYROSINEMIAS

Tyrosinemia is identified in neonatal screening programs using tandem mass spectrometry methods. Elevated tyrosine levels also occur as a nonspecific consequence of severe liver disease or transient tyrosinemia of the newborn, which responds to ascorbic acid treatment. The inherited disorders of tyrosine metabolism are the target of neonatal screening. **Tyrosinemia I**, which is due to fumarylacetoacetate hydrolase deficiency (see Fig. 53-1), is a rare disease in which accumulated metabolites produce severe liver disease associated with bleeding disorder, hypoglycemia, hypoalbuminemia, elevated transaminases, and defects in renal tubular function. Hepatocellular carcinoma may occur eventually. Quantitative measurement of plasma tyrosine and blood or urine succinylacetone is performed after a positive neonatal screening test for hypertyrosinemia. The **diagnosis** of tyrosinemia I is confirmed by an increased concentration of succinylacetone; DNA testing is available for some mutations. **Treatment** with nitisinone (NTBC) (an inhibitor of the oxidation of parahydroxyphenylpyruvic acid) effectively eliminates the production of the toxic succinylacetone. A low-phenylalanine, low-tyrosine diet may also play a role. These treatments have supplanted liver transplantation in many children identified by neonatal screening. Whether they completely eliminate the occurrence of hepatocellular carcinoma is unknown.

Tyrosinemias **II** and **III** are more benign forms of hereditary tyrosinemia. Blocked metabolism of tyrosine at earlier steps in the pathway is responsible, and succinylacetone is not produced. The clinical features include hyperkeratosis of palms and soles and keratitis, which can cause severe visual disturbance. Treatment with a phenylalanine-restricted and tyrosine-restricted diet is effective.

## HOMOCYSTINURIA

Homocystinuria, an autosomal recessive disease (1:200,000 live births) involving connective tissue, the brain, and the vascular system, is caused by a deficiency of cystathionine β-synthase. In the normal metabolism of the sulfur amino acids, methionine gives rise to cystine; homocysteine is a pivotal intermediate (Fig. 53-2). When cystathionine β-synthase is deficient, homocysteine accumulates in the blood and appears in the urine. Another result is enhanced reconversion of homocysteine to methionine, resulting in an increase in the concentration of methionine in the blood. The neonatal screening test most commonly used

measures methionine. An excess of homocysteine produces a slowly evolving **clinical syndrome** that includes dislocated ocular lenses; long, slender extremities; malar flushing; and livedo reticularis. Arachnodactyly, scoliosis, pectus excavatum or carinatum, and genu valgum are skeletal features. Mental retardation, psychiatric illness, or both may be present. Major arterial or venous thromboses are a constant threat.

Homocystinuria has no neonatal manifestations. Confirmation of the **diagnosis** requires demonstration of elevated total homocysteine in the blood. A plasma amino acid profile reveals hypermethioninemia. Measurement of cystathionine β-synthase is not clinically available, but numerous mutations in the gene are known and can be tested.

There are two clinical forms of homocystinuria. In one form, activity of the deficient enzyme can be enhanced by the administration of large doses of pyridoxine (100 to 1000 mg/day). Folate supplementation is added to overcome folate deficiency if folate is trapped in the process of remethylation of homocysteine to methionine. This pyridoxine-responsive form comprises about 50% of cases and is the more likely form to be missed by neonatal screening because the methionine concentrations are not always above the screening cutoff. The second form is not responsive to pyridoxine therapy. The accumulation of homocysteine is controlled with a methionine-restricted diet and cystine and folate supplementation. The use of supplemental betaine (trimethylglycine), a donor of methyl groups for remethylation of homocysteine to methionine, also has a role in the management of pyridoxine-unresponsive patients. Sometimes diet and betaine are required to control plasma homocysteine, even in pyridoxine-responsive patients. The prognosis is good for infants whose plasma homocysteine concentration is controlled.

## MAPLE SYRUP URINE DISEASE

Maple syrup urine disease (MSUD) is an autosomal recessive disease, more properly named **branched chain ketoaciduria**. A deficiency of the decarboxylase initiates the degradation of the ketoacid analogs of the three branched chain amino acids—leucine, isoleucine, and valine (Fig. 53-3). MSUD is rare (1:250,000) in the general population but much more common in some population isolates (Pennsylvania Mennonites 1:150). Neonatal screening programs commonly include MSUD.

Although MSUD does have intermittent-onset and late-onset forms, **clinical manifestations** of the classic form typically begin within 1 to 4 weeks of birth. Poor feeding, vomiting, and tachypnea commonly are noted, but the hallmark of the disease is profound depression of the central nervous system, associated with alternating hypotonia and hypertonia (extensor spasms), opisthotonos, and seizures. The urine has the odor of maple syrup.

Laboratory manifestations of MSUD include hypoglycemia and a variable presence of metabolic acidosis, with elevation of the undetermined anions; the acidosis is caused, in part, by plasma branched chain organic acids and, in part, by the usual *ketone bodies*, β-hydroxybutyrate and acetoacetate. Branched chain ketoacids (but not β-hydroxybutyrate or acetoacetate) react immediately with 2,4-dinitrophenylhydrazine to form a copious, white precipitate.

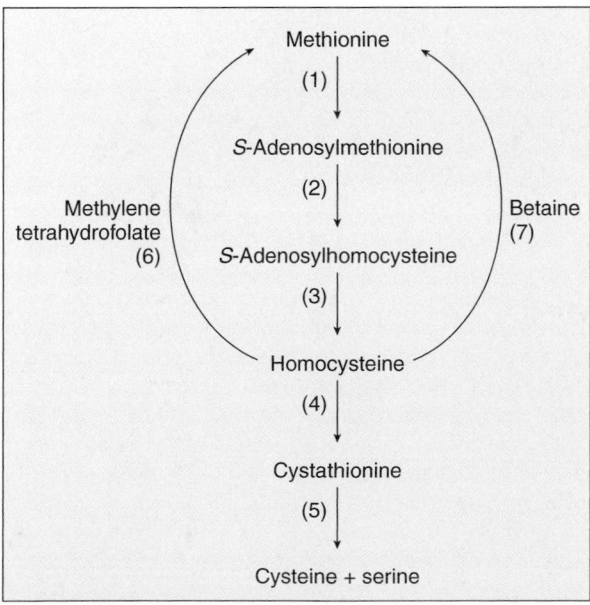

**FIGURE 53-2**

Metabolism of methionine and homocysteine. (1) Methionine adenosyltransferase, (2) S-methyltransferase, (3) S-adenosylhomocysteine hydrolase, (4) cystathionine β-synthase, (5) cystathionase, (6) homocysteine methyltransferase, (7) betaine-homocysteine methyltransferase.

**FIGURE 53-3**

Metabolism of the branched chain amino acids.
(1) Aminotransferases, (2) α-ketoacid
dehydrogenase complex.

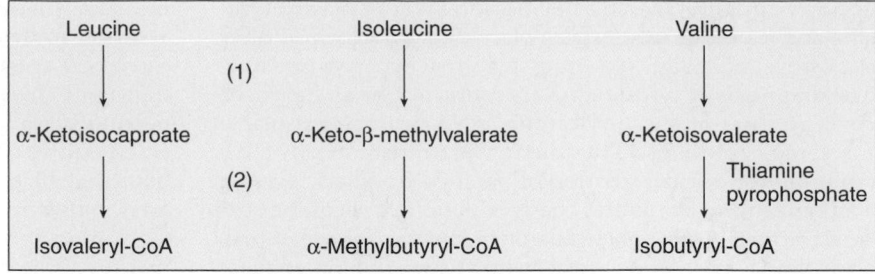

The **definitive diagnosis** of MSUD generally is made by showing large increases in plasma leucine, isoleucine, and valine concentrations and identification of alloisoleucine in the plasma in excess. The urinary organic acid profile is usually abnormal and shows the ketoacid derivatives of the branched chain amino acids.

Provision of adequate calories and protein, **excluding branched chain amino acids**, is also crucial. The intake of branched chain amino acids (all three are essential amino acids) is restricted to the amounts required for growth in severely affected infants; restriction must be continued for life. Hemodialysis, hemofiltration, or peritoneal dialysis can be lifesaving during acidotic crises. Ordinary catabolic stresses, such as moderate infections or labor and delivery in a pregnant mother with MSUD, can precipitate clinical crises. Liver transplantation effectively treats MSUD.

## DISORDERS OF AMMONIA DISPOSAL

Inherited enzymatic deficiencies have been described for each of the steps of urea synthesis (Fig. 53-4). Neonatal screening does not currently detect all of the disorders in the urea cycle.

Ornithine Carbamoyltransferase Deficiency: Ornithine carbamoyltransferase (OTC) deficiency is unique among the defects in the urea cycle in that it is X-linked. The number of known gene mutations is quite large and includes both deletions and point mutations. If the enzyme is nonfunctional, there is no OTC activity in affected males, who are likely to die in the neonatal period. Affected females are heterozygous and, because of lyonization, may have a significant degree of enzyme deficiency and may be clinically affected. **Clinical manifestations** range through lethal disease in the male (coma, encephalopathy) to clinical normalcy in a high percentage of females. Late-onset forms in males also occur. Manifestations in clinically affected females include recurrent emesis, lethargy, seizures, developmental delay, and mental retardation. Affected females may spontaneously limit their protein intake.

Confirmatory testing for OTC includes a plasma amino acid profile, which may show deficient citrulline and arginine concentrations. A urine organic acid profile shows increased excretion of orotic acid. Mutation testing and sequencing of the entire coding region of the related genes are available as clinical tests.

## Treatment of Hyperammonemia

During episodes of symptomatic hyperammonemia, protein intake is eliminated, and intravenous glucose is given in sufficient quantity to suppress catabolism of endogenous protein. Ammonia can be eliminated by use of the **ammonia scavenger** agents, **sodium benzoate** and **sodium phenylacetate**, which are excreted in the urine as conjugates of glycine and glutamine. Arginine, which is usually deficient, is supplied. Sterilization of the intestine and/or treatment with lactulose can provide brief benefit during acute episodes of hyperammonemia. When hyperammonemia is extreme, direct removal of ammonia, usually using hemodialysis or hemofiltration, is more effective than exchange transfusion or peritoneal dialysis. Despite successful management of hyperammonemic crises, the long-term outcome for males with severe neonatal hyperammonemia is guarded. Early liver transplantation has increased survival, especially in males with severe OTC deficiency.

A reduction of dietary protein intake is the mainstay of ongoing treatment for hyperammonemia. Crystalline essential amino acids can be supplied in amounts just sufficient to support new protein synthesis. Arginine is an essential amino acid when arginine synthesis via the urea cycle is

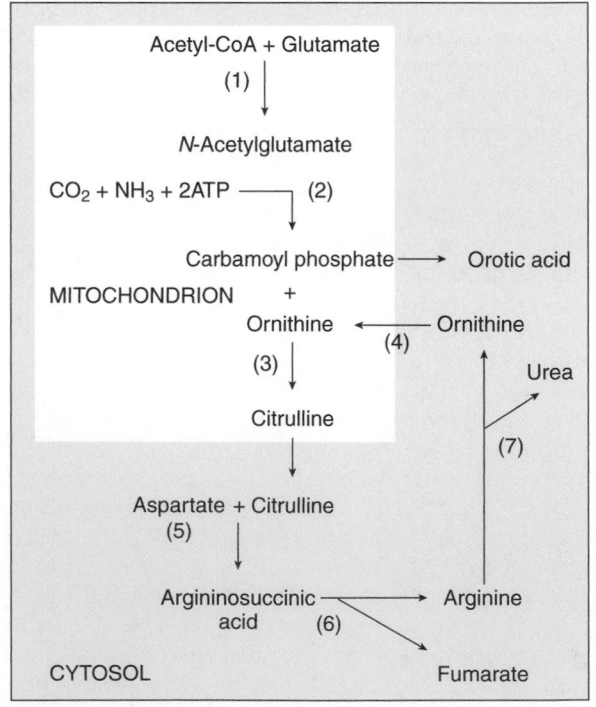

**FIGURE 53-4**

The urea cycle. (1) *N*-acetylglutamate synthase,
(2) carbamoylphosphate synthetase, (3) ornithine
carbamoylphosphate synthetase, (3) ornithine
carbamoyltransferase, (4) ornithine translocator,
(5) argininosuccinic acid synthetase, (6) argininosuccinic acid
lyase, (7) arginase.

grossly impaired, thus arginine must be supplied. Citrulline needs to be supplied for some urea cycle disorders. For OTC deficiency and carbamoyl phosphate synthase deficiency, treatment with phenylbutyrate (which is metabolized to phenylacetate) prevents accumulation of ammonia.

## DISORDERS OF AMINO ACID TRANSPORT THAT AFFECT SPECIFIC TRANSPORT MECHANISMS IN THE KIDNEY AND INTESTINE

**Cystinuria** is a disorder of renal tubular transport of cystine, lysine, arginine, and ornithine. Although intestinal transport is affected in some genetic forms, the symptoms are largely due to the renal transport abnormality. The concentration of cystine exceeds its solubility product and results in significant renal stones. Evaluation and diagnosis is based on the pattern of amino acid excretion in the urine. Mutation testing can be done. **Treatment** is based on increasing the solubility of cystine by complexing it with compounds such as penicillamine.

Intestinal transport of tryptophan is impaired in **Hartnup syndrome**; pellagra-like symptoms result from this deficiency. Diagnosis is based on the amino acid pattern in urine, and treatment with tryptophan is successful.

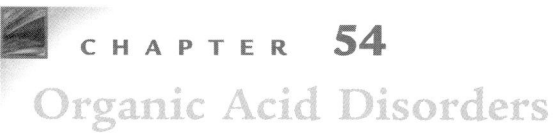

# CHAPTER 54
# Organic Acid Disorders

## DISORDERS OF ORGANIC ACID METABOLISM

Organic acid disorders result from a block in the pathways of amino acid catabolism. Occurring after the amino moiety has been removed, they result in the accumulation of specific organic acids in the blood and urine. Treatment is directed at the specific abnormality, with restriction in precursor substrates and administration of enzyme cofactors, when available. Outcome is influenced by frequency and severity of ketoacidotic crises and is optimal when diagnosis is made before the onset of the first episode. Liver transplantation has been used in some patients, but long-term outcome after liver transplantation has not been well studied. Confirmatory testing begins with a urine organic acid profile and plasma amino acid profile. When abnormal results confirm the specific disorder, DNA testing may identify the mutations involved. More specific testing if a mutation is not found requires enzyme measurements in appropriate tissues.

## PROPIONIC ACIDEMIA AND METHYLMALONIC ACIDEMIA

Propionic acidemia and methylmalonic acidemia result from defects in a series of reactions called the propionate pathway (Fig. 54-1). Defects in these steps produce **ketosis** and **hyperglycinemia**. Propionic acidemia and methylmalonic

acidemia are identified by neonatal screening with tandem mass spectometry methods. The **clinical manifestations** of both of these disorders in the neonatal period consist of tachypnea, vomiting, lethargy, coma, intermittent ketoacidosis, hyperglycinemia, neutropenia, thrombocytopenia, hyperammonemia, and hypoglycemia. If these disorders are not identified by neonatal screening, intermittent episodes of metabolic acidosis occur. Crises occur during periods of catabolic stress, such as fever, vomiting, and diarrhea; they also may occur without an apparent precipitating event. During periods of neutropenia, the risk of serious bacterial infection is increased. Failure to thrive and impaired development are common.

**Propionic acidemia** results from deficiency in propionyl CoA-carboxylase, an enzyme that has two pairs of identical subunits. All forms of propionic acidemia are inherited in an autosomal recessive manner and are due to mutations in one of the subunits. **Methylmalonic acidemia** results from deficiency in methylmalonyl mutase; this may be caused by mutations in the gene for the mutase protein itself or in one of the steps of the synthesis of the cobalamin cofactors for the enzyme. A complex set of defects in cobalamin metabolism results in other forms of methylmalonic acidemia, some of which are associated with hyperhomocystinemia. **Treatment** with massive doses of hydroxycobalamin (the active form of vitamin $B_{12}$) is helpful in some cases of methylmalonic acidemia.

For propionic acidemia and the vitamin $B_{12}$–unresponsive forms of methylmalonic acidemia, management includes the restriction of dietary protein and addition of a medical food deficient in the specific amino acid precursors of propionyl-CoA (isoleucine, valine, methionine, and threonine). Carnitine supplementation is often needed because it is lost in the urine as acylcarnitines. Intestinal bacteria produce a significant quantity of propionate; thus, antibacterial treatment to reduce the population of bacteria in the gut has some beneficial effect in propionic acidemia and vitamin $B_{12}$–unresponsive methylmalonic acidemia.

## ISOVALERIC ACIDEMIA

Isovaleric acidemia results from a block in the catabolism of leucine. Its clinical manifestations are similar to those of defects in the propionate pathway. The strong odor of isovaleric acid results in *sweaty feet* **odor** in untreated infants. Restricting the intake of leucine, glycine therapy enhances the formation of isovalerylglycine, a relatively harmless conjugate of isovaleric acid (Fig. 54-2), which is excreted in the urine. Patients identified by newborn screening may have a milder phenotype; genotype-phenotype correlation studies are in progress to determine whether some forms do not need aggressive treatment.

## GLUTARIC ACIDEMIA I

Glutaric acidemia I results from a deficiency at the end of the lysine catabolic pathway. It is an autosomal recessive disease produced by deficiency of glutaryl-CoA dehydrogenase activity (Fig. 54-3). **Clinical manifestations** include **macrocephaly**, which may be present at birth, and **dystonia**, which characteristically develops after the first 18 months of

**FIGURE 54-1**

The propionate pathway. (1) β-Ketothiolase,
(2) propionyl-CoA carboxylase, (3) methylmalonyl-CoA
isomerase, (4) methylmalonyl-CoA mutase,
(5) cobalamin metabolic pathway. CoA, coenzyme A.

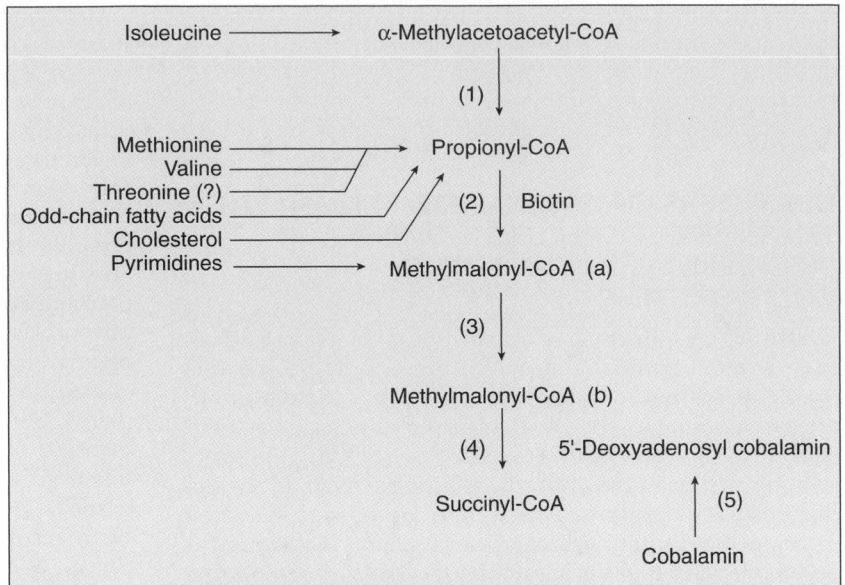

**FIGURE 54-2**

Metabolism in isovaleric acidemia. (1) Leucine catabolic
pathway (transamination and decarboxylation),
(2) isovaleryl-CoA dehydrogenase, (3) glycine
acyltransferase. CoA, coenzyme A.

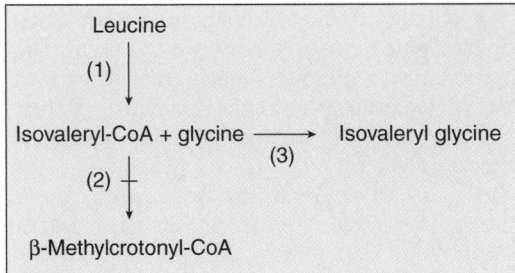

## BIOTINIDASE DEFICIENCY AND HOLOCARBOXYLASE DEFICIENCY

Biotin is a ubiquitous vitamin that is covalently linked to many carboxylases and cannot be recycled from its attachment to the carboxylases. Thus, inherited biotinidase deficiency greatly increases the dietary requirement for biotin. Affected individuals become biotin deficient while consuming normal diets. Clinical disease can appear in the neonatal period or be delayed until later infancy, depending on the degree of deficiency.

**Clinical manifestations** of biotin deficiency vary greatly (seizures, hypotonia, sensory neural deafness, alopecia, skin rash, metabolic acidosis, and immune deficits) and, undoubtedly, depend on which enzymes in which tissues have the most biotin depletion. Carboxylation is a crucial reaction in the metabolism of organic acids; most patients with biotinidase deficiency excrete abnormal amounts of several organic acids, among which β-methylcrotonylglycine is prominent. In addition to biotinidase deficiency, an inherited deficiency of holocarboxylase synthetase gives rise to severe disease and to similar patterns of organic aciduria. Both conditions respond well to **treatment** with large doses of biotin (10 to 40 mg/day). Confirmatory testing is accomplished with quantitative measurement of biotinidase activity.

life, after an episode of intercurrent illness associated with fever and metabolic distress. Clinical features include *metabolic* strokelike episodes associated with infarction of the basal ganglia. **Treatment** includes a protein-restricted diet accompanied by a medical food deficient in lysine. Despite this treatment, as many as one third of children still develop brain damage. Improved outcome may occur when episodes of metabolic distress are managed aggressively.

**FIGURE 54-3**

Scheme of flavoprotein metabolism with reference to glutaric aciduria types I and II. (1) Glutaryl-CoA dehydrogenase (deficient in glutaric aciduria type1), (2) fatty acyl-CoA dehydrogenases, (3) other flavoprotein dehydrogenases, (4) ETF (deficiency results in glutaric aciduria type II), (5) ETF-ubiquinone oxidoreductase (deficiency results in glutaric aciduria type II). CoA, coenzyme A; ETF, electron transfer flavoprotein.

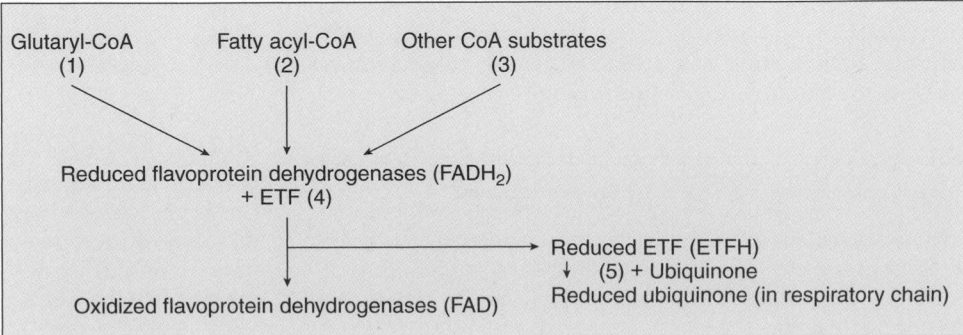

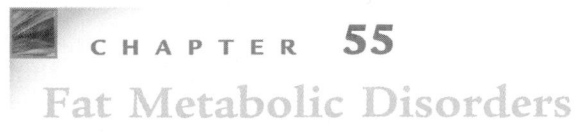

CHAPTER **55**

# Fat Metabolic Disorders

## DISORDERS OF FATTY ACID OXIDATION

Fatty acids are derived from hydrolysis of triglycerides and catabolism of fat. The catabolism of fatty acids (Fig. 55-1) proceeds through the serial, oxidative removal of two carbons at a time as acetyl groups (each as acetyl-CoA). The reactions are catalyzed by a group of enzymes that exhibit specificities related to the chain length and other properties of the fatty acids: very long chain acyl-CoA dehydrogenase (VLCAD), long-chain hydroxyacyl-CoA dehydrogenase (LCHAD) or trifunctional protein, medium-chain acyl-CoA dehydrogenase (MCAD), and short-chain acyl-CoA dehydrogenase (SCAD). MCAD deficiency is the most common inborn error of β-oxidation. Hypoketotic hypoglycemia is a common manifestation, as is Reye syndrome–like illness with hypoglycemia and elevated liver enzymes. Fatty infiltration of the liver also occurs. True hepatic failure is rare. Episodes may be recurrent in the patient or the family. **Sudden infant death syndrome** is reported in infants with MCAD deficiency, perhaps related to hypoglycemia. **Treatment** requires avoidance of fasting and provision of calories with fever or other metabolic stress. Medium-chain triglycerides must be avoided.

VLCAD deficiency and LCHAD (trifunctional protein) deficiency result in significant myopathy and cardiomyopathy, and LCHAD deficiency is accompanied by a retinopathy in later childhood. In all of the disorders of β-oxidation, carnitine depletion can occur through excessive urinary excretion of carnitine esters of the incompletely oxidized fatty acids. Measurement of plasma carnitine is helpful in monitoring for this deficiency, which results in weakness and muscle pain, along with myoglobinuria in some people.

**Hydroxymethylglutaryl-CoA lyase deficiency**, although not a disorder of β-oxidation, interferes profoundly with hepatic adaptation to fasting by impairing ketogenesis (see Fig. 55-1). The clinical manifestations are those of MCAD deficiency, except that carnitine depletion is less prominent.

The **diagnosis** of disorders involving a deficiency of β-oxidation is suggested by the clinical picture and by hypoketotic hypoglycemia. The diagnosis is confirmed by analysis of urinary organic acid and acylglycine profiles, along with plasma acylcarnitine and free fatty acid profiles. Enzyme measurements and DNA testing complete the confirmatory testing. The profile of acylcarnitines in cultured skin fibroblasts may be helpful if other testing is not conclusive. In MCAD deficiency, a single mutation, 985A-G, accounts for a significant percentage of cases. **Treatment** includes avoidance of fasting, and fluid and calorie supplementation during periods of metabolic stress, such as fever. In MCAD deficiency, medium-chain triglycerides must be avoided. In the long-chain fatty acid metabolic disorders, provision of medium-chain fatty acids improves muscle energy metabolism. SCAD deficiency has a variable and poorly understood phenotype that can include little in the way of symptoms or, in other patients, muscle weakness and hypoglycemia when fasting. Avoidance of fasting is recommended. Carnitine supplementation may be helpful. Careful monitoring is recommended.

## GLUTARIC ACIDURIA TYPE II

Glutaric aciduria type II (multiple acyl-CoA dehydrogenase deficiency) is a clinical disease produced by a defect in the transfer of electrons from flavine adenine nucleotides to the electron transport chain (electron transfer flavoprotein [ETF], or ETF dehydrogenase); this defect results in

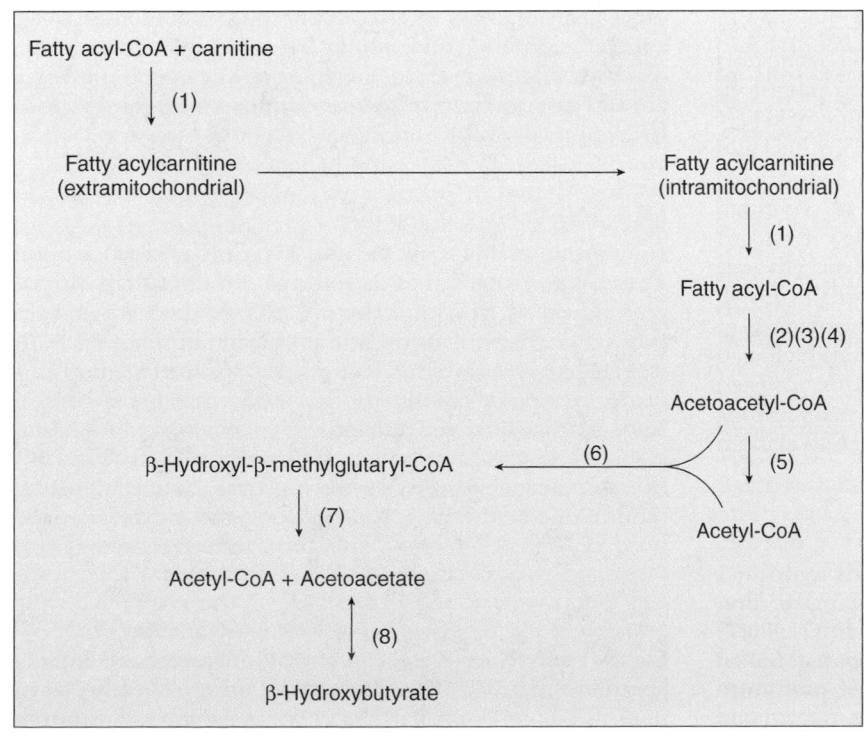

**FIGURE 55-1**

Scheme of fatty acid and catabolism and ketone body formation. (1) Carnitine acyl-CoA dehydrogenases, (2) long-chain fatty acyl-CoA dehydrogenase (trifunctional protein), (3) medium-chain fatty acyl-CoA dehydrogenase, (4) short-chain fatty acyl-CoA dehydrogenase, (5) β-ketothiolase, (6) β-hydroxy-β-methylglutaryl-CoA synthase, (7) β-hydroxy-β-methylglutaryl-CoA lyase, (8) β-hydroxybutyrate dehydrogenase. CoA, coenzyme A.

a deficiency of multiple fatty acyl CoA dehydrogenases (see Fig. 55-1). It should not be confused with glutaric acidemia type I (see Chapter 54). When the enzyme essentially is nonfunctional, congenital anomalies are common, including renal cysts, facial abnormalities, rocker-bottom feet, and hypospadias. Severely affected infants have nonketotic hypoglycemia, metabolic acidosis, and the odor of sweaty feet soon after birth; these infants may die within the neonatal period. Less severely affected infants may have a more episodic, Reye syndrome–like illness. Skeletal and cardiac myopathy can be prominent in this complex, multisystemic disease. Onset in later childhood may be marked by recurrent hypoglycemia and myopathy. **Treatment** has not been effective in infants with complete deficiency. Milder forms respond to avoidance of fasting and caloric support during metabolic stress. Some patients respond to administration of riboflavin. Glutaric aciduria type II exhibits autosomal recessive inheritance. Confirmatory testing is similar to that for the other fatty acid oxidation disorders.

## CARNITINE DEFICIENCY

Carnitine is a crucial cofactor in the transport of long-chain fatty acids across the mitochondrial inner membrane (see Fig. 55-1). It is synthesized from lysine by humans and is present in dietary red meat and dairy products. Carnitine deficiency is either primary (caused by failure of intake, synthesis, or transport of carnitine) or secondary (caused by the excretion of excessive amounts of carnitine as carnityl esters in patients with other inborn errors of metabolism or treatment with drugs that complex carnitine, such as valproic acid). Primary systemic carnitine deficiency results from inadequate renal reabsorption of carnitine secondary to a mutation in the sodium-dependent carnitine transporter. It responds well to carnitine supplementation. There are numerous examples of secondary carnitine deficiency among the organic acidurias, most prominently in disorders of the propionate pathway and in disorders of the β-oxidation of long-chain and medium-chain fatty acids. Clinical manifestations of carnitine deficiency include hypoketotic hypoglycemia, lethargy, lassitude, muscle weakness, and cardiomyopathy.

## CHAPTER 56

# Lysosomal and Peroxisomal Disorders

## PEROXISOMAL DISORDERS

Peroxisomes are subcellular organelles involved in metabolism and biosynthesis of bile acids, membrane phospholipids, and some β-oxidation of long-chain fatty acids. Disorders include conditions caused by abnormal peroxisomal enzyme function and abnormal peroxisomal biogenesis. **Clinical symptoms** are protean and nearly always include **developmental delay** and **dysmorphic features** that can involve the skeleton and the head. Zellweger syndrome, neonatal adrenoleukodystrophy, and infantile Refsum disease are examples of disorders of peroxisome biogenesis. **Zellweger syndrome**, an autosomal recessive disease (1:100,000 births), is also called *cerebrohepatorenal syndrome*. Peroxisomes are virtually absent, as are normal peroxisomal functions, which include the oxidation of very long chain fatty acids. Affected infants have high foreheads, flat orbital ridges, widely open fontanelles, hepatomegaly, and hypotonia. Other anomalies are common. Failure to thrive, seizures, and nystagmus develop early, and death occurs within the first year. Refsum disease, neonatal adrenoleukodystrophy, and malonic aciduria are examples of peroxisomal single enzyme disorders. Diagnostic testing includes measurement of very long chain fatty acids in plasma and pipecolic acid in urine. Specific molecular testing, particularly for the disorders involving one in the series of *PEX* genes, is available for some disorders. Most of these conditions are untreatable; bone marrow transplant can be helpful in X-linked adrenoleukodystrophy.

## LYSOSOMAL STORAGE DISORDERS

Lysosomes are subcellular organelles that contain degradative enzymes for complex **glycosaminoglycans**, also called **mucopolysaccharides**. Glycosaminoglycans are macromolecules that play a number of roles within cells. Genetic disorders result from abnormal formation of the lysosome itself or from deficiency in specific hydrolytic enzymes, in the mechanisms that protect intralysosomal enzymes from hydrolytic destruction, in the transport of materials into the lysosome and of metabolites out of the lysosome. These materials are stored in cells and ultimately result in their destruction, especially in the nervous system. The clinical disorders are diverse, reflecting tissue specificity of lysosomal function and the intrinsic turnover rates of the compounds whose cycling is affected (Table 56-1). Some disorders affect many tissues but spare the brain. Some are apparent only during adult life. Storage in solid organs results in organomegaly. In many of these disorders, developmental delay, corneal clouding, and limitation of joint mobility are common features. Storage in tissues of the upper and lower airways may result in respiratory compromise. Nonimmune hydrops fetalis occurs in several lysosomal disorders.

## DIAGNOSTIC TESTING

Diagnostic testing includes measurement of glycosaminoglycans in urine and an enzyme assay for lysosomal enzyme activity in white blood cells. If the urine test is positive, it helps direct specific enzyme measurement. If it is negative, it does not exclude a lysosomal storage disorder, and other testing modalities are needed if clinical signs are convincing. In disorders in which specific mutations are known, molecular testing refines the diagnosis. Specific diagnosis, carrier testing, and prenatal testing require one of these approaches. Enzyme analysis is complex; experienced laboratories are the best source of this testing. If this testing is to be used for prenatal diagnosis, the details about the expression of the enzyme during fetal life must be known. For this reason, molecular testing is more specific for prenatal diagnosis. Making a specific diagnosis is even more important because treatment for some lysosomal disorders is available. Treatment strategies are arduous, so specific diagnosis is crucial.

## TREATMENT STRATEGIES

Treatment for many of these conditions is supportive. Careful attention to respiratory status and physical therapy is very important. Specific treatment directed at the metabolic abnormality is available for some lysosomal disorders. For some, bone marrow (stem cell) transplantation can restore lysosomal function. For others, replacement of the missing hydrolytic enzyme by systemic administration of the enzyme allows degradation of stored material. The disorders caused by deficient α-L-iduronidase (Hurler syndrome, Scheie syndrome, and their variants) respond to treatment with intravenous human recombinant α-L-iduronidase (laronidase). Other disorders for which enzyme therapy is available include MPS VI (Maroteaux-Lamy syndrome), Gaucher disease, Fabry disease, and MPS II (Hunter syndrome). Stem cell transplantation has been helpful or is under investigation in the following disorders: MPS type IH (Hurler syndrome), MPS type VI (Marateaux-Lamy syndrome), MPS type VII (Sly syndrome), Krabbe disease, metachromatic leukodystrophy, alpha-fucosidosis, alpha-mannosidosis, Gaucher disease, and Niemann-Pick disease type B.

Treatment needs to begin before clinical signs appear, because central nervous system manifestations are not improved by these approaches.

## TABLE 56-1 Lysosomal Storage Diseases

| Disease (Eponym) | Enzyme Deficiency | Clinical Onset | Dysostosis Multiplex | Cornea | Retina |
|---|---|---|---|---|---|
| **MUCOPOLYSACCHARIDOSES (MPS)** | | | | | |
| MPS I (Hurler) | α-L-Iduronidase | ~1 yr | Yes | Cloudy | — |
| MPS II (Hunter) | Iduronate-2-sulfatase | 1–2 yr | Yes | Clear | Retinal degeneration, papilledema |
| MPS III (Sanfilippo) | One of several degrading heparan $SO_4$s | 2–6 yr | Mild | Clear | — |
| MPS IV (Morquiro) | Galactose-6-sulfatase or β-galactosidase | 2 yr | No, dwarfism deformities | Faint clouding | — |
| MPS VI (Maroteaux-Lamy) | N-Acetylga-lactosamine-4-sulfatase | 2 yr | Yes | Cloudy | — |
| MPS VII (Sly) | β-glucuronidase | Variable neonatal | Yes | ± Cloudy | — |
| **LIPIDOSES** | | | | | |
| Glucosylcer-amide lipidosis (Gaucher 1) | Glucocerebro-sidase | Any age | No | Clear | Normal |
| Glucosylcer-amide lipidosis 2 (Gaucher 2) | Glucocerebro-sidase | Fetal life to 2nd year | No | Clear | Normal |
| Sphingomyelin lipidosis A (Niemann-Pick A) | Sphingomy-elinase | 1st mo | No | Clear | Cherry-red spots (50%) |
| Sphingomyelin lipidosis B (Niemann-Pick B) | Sphingomy-elinase | 1st mo or later | No | Clear | Normal |
| Niemann-Pick C | Lysosomal cholesterol; trafficking (NPC1 gene) | Fetal life to adolescence | No | Clear | Normal |
| $GM_2$ gangliosidosis (Tay-Sachs) | Hexosaminidase A | 3–6 mo | No | Clear | Cherry-red spots |
| Generalized gangliosidosis (infantile) ($GM_1$) | β-Galactosidase | Neonatal to 1st mo | Yes | Clear | Cherry-red spots (50%) |
| Metachromatic leukodystrophy | Arylsulfatase A | 1–2 yr | No | Clear | Normal |
| Fabry disease | α-Galactosidase A (cerebrosidase) | Childhood, adolescence | No | Cloudy by slit lamp | — |
| Galactosyl ceramide lipidosis (Krabbe) | Galacto-cerebroside β-galactosidase | Early months | No | Clear | Optic atrophy |
| Wolman disease | Acid lipase | Neonatal | No | Clear | Normal |
| Farber lipogranulo-matosis | Acid ceramidase | 1st 4 mo | No | Usually clear | Cherry-red spots (12%) |

| Liver, Spleen | CNS Findings | Stored Material in Urine | WBC/Bone Marrow | Comment | Multiple Forms |
|---|---|---|---|---|---|
| Both enlarged | Profound loss of function | Acid mucopoly-saccharide | Alder-Reilly bodies (WBC) | Kyphosis | Yes—Scheie and compounds |
| Both enlarged | Slow loss of function | Acid mucopoly-saccharide | Alder-Reilly bodies (WBC) | X-linked | Yes |
| Liver ± enlarged | Rapid loss of function | Acid mucopoly-saccharide | Alder-Reilly bodies (WBC) | — | Several types biochemically |
| — | Normal | Acid mucopoly-saccharide | Alder-Reilly bodies (WBC) | — | Yes |
| Normal in size | Normal | Acid mucopoly-saccharide | Alder-Reilly bodies (WBC) | — | Yes |
| Both enlarged | ± Affected | Acid mucopoly-saccharide | Alder-Reilly bodies (WBC) | Nonimmune hydrops | Yes |
| Both enlarged | Normal | No | Gaucher cells in marrow | Bone pain fractures | Variability is the rule |
| Both enlarged | Profound loss of function | No | Gaucher cells in marrow | — | Yes |
| Both enlarged | Profound loss of function | No | Foam cells in marrow | — | No |
| Both enlarged | Normal | No | Foam cells in marrow | — | Yes |
| Enlarged | Vertical ophthalmo-plegia, dystonia, cataplexy, seizures | No | Foam cells and sea-blue histiocytes in marrow | Pathogenesis not as for NP-A and NP-B | Lethal neonatal to adolescent onset |
| Normal | Profound loss of function | No | Normal | Sandhoff disease related | Yes |
| Both enlarged | Profound loss of function | No | Inclusion in WBC | — | Yes |
| Normal | Profound loss of function | No | Normal | — | Yes |
| Liver may be enlarged | Normal | No | Normal | X-linked | No |
| Normal | Profound loss of function | No | Normal | Storage not lysosomal | Yes |
| Both enlarged | Profound loss of function | No | Inclusion in WBC | — | Yes |
| May be enlarged | Normal or impaired | Usually not | — | Arthritis, nodules, hoarseness | Yes |

*Continued*

## TABLE 56-1 Lysosomal Storage Diseases—cont'd

| Disease (Eponym) | Enzyme Deficiency | Clinical Onset | Dysostosis Multiplex | Cornea | Retina |
|---|---|---|---|---|---|
| **MUCOLIPIDOSES (ML) AND CLINICALLY RELATED DISEASE** | | | | | |
| Sialidosis II (formerly ML I) | Neuraminidase | Neonatal | Yes | Cloudy | Cherry-red spot |
| Sialidosis I (formerly ML I) | Neuraminidase | Usually second decade | No | Fine opacities | Cherry-red spot |
| Galactosialidosis | Absence of PP/CathA causes loss of neuraminidase and β-galactosidase | Usually second decade | Frequent | Clouding | Cherry-red spot |
| ML II (I-cell disease) | Mannosyl phospho-transferase | Neonatal | Yes | Clouding | — |
| ML III (pseudo-Hurler polydys-trophy) | Mannosyl phospho-transferase | 2–4 yr | Yes | Late clouding | Normal |
| Multiple sulfatase deficiency | Many sulfatases | 1–2 yr | Yes | Usually clear | Usually normal |
| Aspartylglyco-saminuria | Aspartylglucos-aminidase | 6 mo | Mild | Clear | Normal |
| Mannosidosis | α-Mannosidase | 1st mo | Yes | Cloudy | — |
| Fucosidosis | α-L-Fucosidase | 1st mo | Yes | Clear | May be pigmented |
| **STORAGE DISEASES CAUSED BY DEFECTS IN LYSOSOMAL PROTEOLYSIS** | | | | | |
| Neuronal ceroid lipofuscinosis (NCL), Batten disease | Impaired lysosomal proteolysis—various specific etiologies | 6 mo–10 yr, adult form | No | Normal | May have brown pigment |
| **STORAGE DISEASES CAUSED BY DEFECTIVE SYNTHESIS OF THE LYSOSOMAL MEMBRANE** | | | | | |
| Cardiomyopathy, myopathy, mental retardation, Danon disease | Lamp-2, a structural protein of lysosomes, is deficient | Usually 5–6 yr | No | Normal | Normal |
| **STORAGE DISEASES CAUSED BY DYSFUNCTION OF LYSOSOMAL TRANSPORT PROTEINS** | | | | | |
| Nephropathic cystinosis | Defect in cystine transport from lysosome to cytoplasm | 6 mo–1 yr | No | Cystine crystals | Pigmentary retinopathy |
| Salla disease | Defect in sialic acid transport from lysosome to cytoplasm | 6–9 mo | No | Normal | Normal |

CNS, central nervous system; WBC, white blood cell.

| Liver, Spleen | CNS Findings | Stored Material in Urine | WBC/Bone Marrow | Comment | Multiple Forms |
|---|---|---|---|---|---|
| Both enlarged | Yes | Oligosaccharides | Vacuolated lymphocytes | — | Yes (also see galactosialidosis) |
| Normal | Myoclonus, seizures | Oligosaccharides | Usually none | Cherry-red spot/myoclonus syndrome | Severity varies |
| Occasionally enlarged | Myoclonus, seizures Mental retardation | Oligosaccharides | Foamy lymphocytes | Onset from 1–40 yr | Congenital and infantile forms such as sialidosis 2 |
| Liver often enlarged | Profound loss of function | Oligosaccharides | No | Gingival hyperplasia | No |
| Normal in size? | Modest loss of function | Oligosaccharides | No | — | No |
| Both enlarged | Profound loss of function | Acid mucopolysaccharide | Alder-Reilly bodies (WBC) | Ichthyosis | Yes |
| Early, not late | Profound loss of function | Aspartylglucosamine | Inclusions in lymphocytes | Develop cataracts | No |
| Liver enlarged | Profound loss of function | Generally no | Inclusions in lymphocytes | Cataracts | Yes |
| Both enlarged commonly | Profound loss of function | Oligosaccharides | Inclusions in lymphocytes | — | Yes |
| Normal, distinct | Optic atrophy, seizures, dementia | | | Clinical picture consistent, time course variable | Etiologies for age-related forms |
| Hepatomegaly | Delayed development, seizures | | | X-linked pediatric disease in males only | Variability in time course of signs |
| Hepatomegaly common | Normal CNS function | Generalized aminoaciduria | Elevated cystine in WBCs | Treatment with cysteamine is effective | Yes |
| Normal | Delayed development, ataxia, nystagmus, exotropia | Sialic aciduria | Vacuolated lymphocytes may be found | Growth retarded in some | Lethal infantile form |

CHAPTER **57**

Mitochondrial Disorders

## MITOCHONDRIAL FUNCTION

Mitochondria generate energy from oxidative phosphorylation to produce ATP by transferring electrons formed by glycolysis and the Krebs cycle to a cascade that generates NADH and $FADH_2$ (Fig. 57-1). Mitochondria reside in most organs, so signs and symptoms of mitochondrial dysfunction can affect multiple organ systems. The more dependent on energy production an organ is, the more profound the symptoms of deficiency of mitochondrial function in that organ will be. Taken together, mitochondrial disorders may affect as many as 1 in 5000 people.

## SIGNS AND SYMPTOMS OF GENETIC DISORDERS OF MITOCHONDRIAL FUNCTION

The signs and symptoms of mitochondrial disorders are protean. Symptoms depend on how an organ is affected by energy deficiency. Muscle function that is compromised will result in muscle pain, fatigue, and weakness. Myopathy is common and may show ragged red fibers on a muscle biopsy (Table 57-1). Rhabdomyolysis can occur. Brain dysfunction may be expressed as seizures, loss of intellectual function, headache, or signs consistent with stroke. Spastic paraplegia may occur. Ataxia and basal ganglia symptoms are features of some disorders. Vision and eye muscle movement may be compromised. Cardiomyopathy is frequent, and cardiac rhythm disturbances occur. Liver dysfunction may be expressed as both synthetic deficiencies and liver failure. Diabetes may signal pancreatic involvement. Renal tubular abnormalities and renal failure both occur.

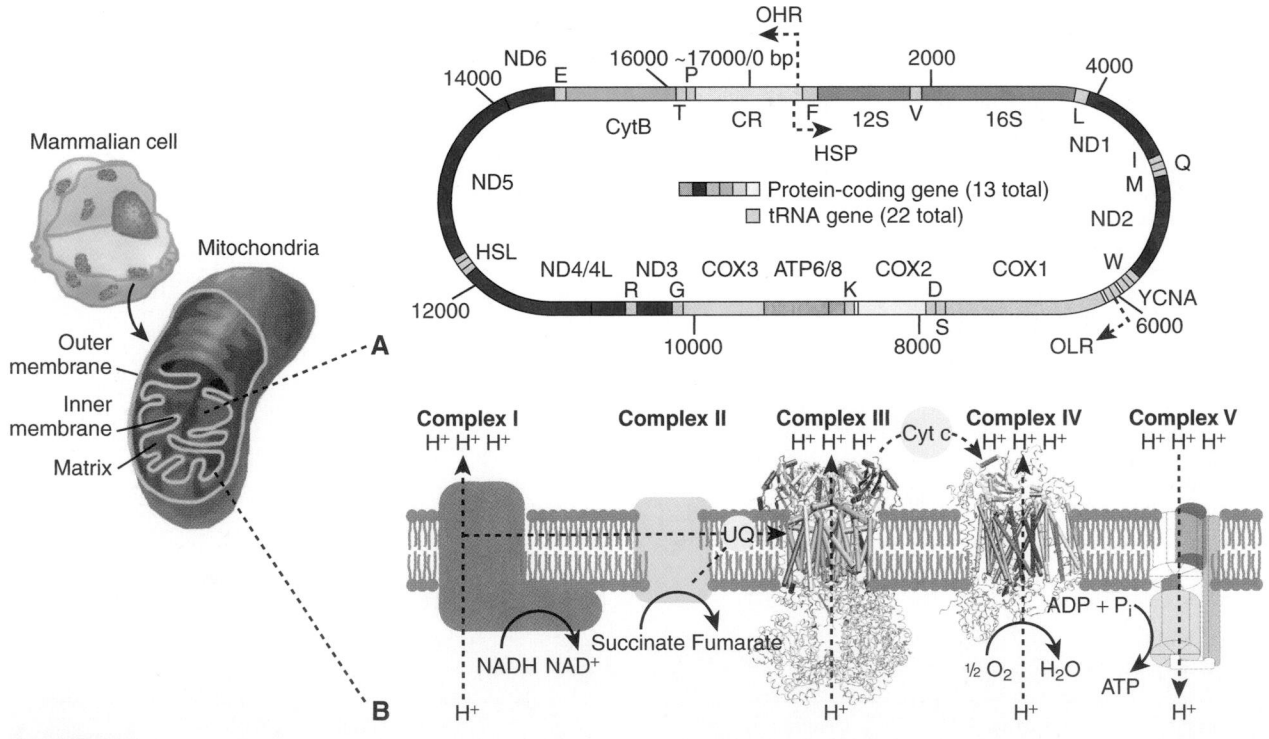

**FIGURE 57-1**

The mammalian mitochondrial genome and its protein-coding gene repertoire involved in the oxidative phosphorylation pathway. **(A)** Schematic representation of genes within mammalian mitochondrial genome (~7000 bp). Genes on the outer circle are transcribed from the light-strand. Location of the tRNAs (*red boxes*) conform to the canonical placental mammalian arrangement. **(B)** Simplified view of the mitochondrial oxidative phosphorylation machinery. Complexes I (NADH dehydrogenase) and II (succinate dehydrogenase) receive electrons from either NADH or $FADH_2$. Electrons are then carried between complexes by the carrier molecules coenzyme Q/ubiquinone (UQ) and cytochrome c (CYC). The potential energy of these electron transfer events is used to pump protons against the gradient, from the mitochondrial matrix into the intermembrane space [complexes I and III (cytochrome $bc_1$) and IV (cytochrome c oxidase)]. ATP synthesis by complex V (ATP synthase) is driven by the proton gradient and occurs in the mitochondrial matrix. HSP, putative heavy-strand promoter; IM, intermembrane space; MM, mitochondria matrix; OHR, origin of heavy-strand replication; OLR, origin of light-strand replication. (From da Fonseca RR, Johnson WE, O'Brien SJ, et al: The adaptive evolution of the mammalian mitochondrial genome. *BMC Genomics* 9:119, 2008.)

**TABLE 57-1 Signs and Symptoms of Mitochondrial Disorders**

| Mitochondrial Complex | Clinical Presentation |
|---|---|
| Complex I | Leigh, Alpers, leukodystrophy, cardiomyopathy, lactic acidosis |
| Complex II | Neurodegeneration, Leigh syndrome, paraganglioma |
| Complex III | Tubulopathy and encephalopathy, GRACILE syndrome |
| Complex IV (COX) | Leigh syndrome, infantile cardiomyopathy, neonatal liver failure |
| Complex V | Malformation syndrome, neonatal lactic acidosis |
| Mitochondrial translation | Macrocystic leukodystrophy, lactic acidosis, myopathy |
| mtDNA maintenance | mtDNA depletion syndromes: Alpers, Leigh, hepatopathy, ataxia |

GRACILE syndrome, growth retardation, aminoaciduria, cholestasis, iron overload, lactic acidosis, early death; mtDNA, mitochondrial DNA.

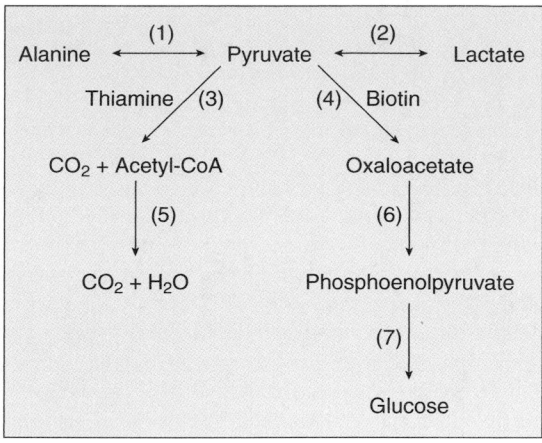

**FIGURE 57-2**

Metabolism of pyruvate and lactate. (1) Alanine aminotransferase, (2) lactate dehydrogenase, (3) pyruvate dehydrogenase, (4) pyruvate carboxylase, (5) Krebs cycle, (6) phosphoenolpyruvate carboxykinase, (7) reverse glycosis. CoA, coenzyme A.

Gastrointestinal symptoms include both diarrhea and constipation that are difficult to treat. **Alper disease** (cerebral degeneration and liver disease) and **Leigh disease** (subacute necrotizing encephalomyelopathy) show similar brain lesions but in distinctly different areas of the brain. Because the signs and symptoms involve multiple organs and may seem nonspecific, physicians may not suspect a mitochondrial disorder until significant progression has occurred.

## BIOCHEMICAL ABNORMALITIES IN MITOCHONDRIAL FUNCTION

Defects in the mitochondrial respiratory chain produce lactic acidosis. Given the complexity of the respiratory chain, it is not surprising that the described defects are varied as to cause, intensity, and tissues affected. However, not all patients with mitochondrial disorders exhibit lactic acidosis. The metabolism of glucose to carbon dioxide and water, with pyruvate as an intermediate (Fig. 57-2), occurs as part of the energy cycle in many tissues. Interference with mitochondrial oxidative metabolism results in the accumulation of pyruvate. Because lactate dehydrogenase is ubiquitous, and because the equilibrium catalyzed by this enzyme greatly favors lactate over pyruvate, the accumulation of pyruvate results in lactic acidosis. The most common cause of such lactic acidosis is oxygen deficiency caused by anoxia or poor perfusion. Lactic acidosis also occurs when specific reactions of pyruvate are impaired. In the liver, pyruvate undergoes carboxylation to form oxaloacetate using the enzyme pyruvate carboxylase; deficiency in this enzyme causes severe lactic acidosis. In many tissues, lactate is catabolized to form acetyl coenzyme A (CoA) by the pyruvate dehydrogenase complex; deficiency in pyruvate dehydrogenase also can cause lactic acidosis. Because these reactions also play a role in gluconeogenesis, hypoglycemia can be a feature of these disorders. These disorders comprise forms of primary lactic acidosis. They frequently present as intractable, lethal acidosis in the first days or weeks of life and are difficult to treat. Some of the enzymes in this pathway can be measured and specific diagnosis can be made. This may require white blood cells or tissue biopsy.

## GENETICS OF MITOCHONDRIAL DISORDERS

Mitochondrial function is carried out by proteins that are coded for by both nuclear and mitochondrial genes. These enzymes are extremely complicated, and several are quite large. The mitochondrial genome encodes 13 subunits of the enzymes involved in mitochondrial oxidative phosphorylation. More than 85 autosomal genes code for the rest of the subunits of these enzymes. In children, only about 20% of cases of mitochondrial disease are caused by mutations in mitochondrial DNA (mtDNA); the rest are due to mutations in nuclear genes. Depletion of mtDNA itself often results from mutations in nuclear genes that maintain mtDNA (e.g., polymerase [DNA directed], gamma [*POLG*]. Most disorders show autosomal recessive inheritance. A few are passed on by maternal mtDNA mutation (Table 57-2).

## TREATMENT OF MITOCHONDRIAL DISORDERS

Repairing the basic energy deficit and getting the appropriate drugs and cofactors to the appropriate location within the mitochondrion are difficult. Nevertheless, a number of strategies are used, including judicious physical therapy and exercise with adequate rest, adequate nutrition, and cofactors for the deficient pathway. Treatment is limited for most mitochondrial defects. Vitamin cofactors for the respiratory chain, such as riboflavin and vitamin E, and pharmaceutical forms of coenzyme Q are often used. When a single organ bears most of the damage, organ transplant may be effective. Identification of family members at risk may allow earlier diagnosis and treatment.

**TABLE 57-2 Inheritance in Mitochondrial Disorders**

| Mitochondrial Complex | Genes | Inheritance |
|---|---|---|
| Complex I | 43 subunits, 7 mtDNA mtDNA maintenance genes | Autosomal recessive (>90%) |
| Complex II | SDH | Autosomal recessive and dominant (rare) |
| Complex III | Assembly factor for complex III | Autosomal recessive |
| Complex IV (COX) | 23 genes; autosomal and mitochondrial and assembly factors | Autosomal recessive |
| Complex V | ATP synthase | Maternally inherited |
| Mitochondrial translation | Myopathy and anemia | Autosomal recessive |
| mtDNA maintenance | mtDNA depletion, Alpers, Leigh, failure to thrive, and myopathy | Autosomal recessive |

mtDNA, mitochondrial DNA; SDH, succinate dehydrogenase.

# SUGGESTED READING

de Baulny HO, Benoist JF, Rigal O, et al: Methylmalonic and propionic acidaemias: management and outcome, *J Inherit Metab Dis* 28(3):415–423, 2005.

Debray FG, Lambert M, Mitchell G: Disorders of mitochondrial function, *Curr Opin Pediatr* 20(4):471–482, 2008.

Heese BA: Current strategies in the management of lysosomal storage diseases, *Semin Pediatr Neurol* 15(3):119–126, 2008.

Kayser MA: Inherited metabolic diseases in neurodevelopmental and neurobehavioral disorders, *Semin Pediatr Neurol* 15(3):127–131, 2008.

Kliegman RM, Behrman RE, Jenson HB, et al: Nelson Textbook of Pediatrics, 18th ed, Philadelphia, 2007, *Saunders*.

Koeberl DD, Kishnani PS, Chen YT: Glycogen storage disease types I and II: treatment updates, *J Inherit Metab Dis* 30(2):159–164, 2007.

Kompare M, Rizzo WB: Mitochondrial fatty-acid oxidation disorders, *Semin Pediatr Neurol* 15(3):140–149, 2008.

Longo N: Inborn errors of metabolism: new challenges with expanded newborn screening programs, *Am J Med Genet C Semin Med Genet* 142C(2):61–63, 2006.

Maillot F, Lilburn M, Baudin J, et al: Factors influencing outcomes in the offspring of mothers with phenylketonuria during pregnancy: the importance of variation in maternal blood phenylalanine, *Am J Clin Nutr* 88(3):700–705, 2008.

Stea TH, Mansoor MA, Wandel M, et al: Changes in predictors and status of homocysteine in young male adults after a dietary intervention with vegetables, fruits and bread, *Eur J Nutr* 47(4):201–209, 2008.

Tuchman M, Lee B, Lichter-Konecki U, et al: Cross-sectional multicenter study of patients with urea cycle disorders in the United States, *Mol Genet Metab* 94 (4):397–402, 2008.

Vockley J, Ensenauer R: Isovaleric acidemia: new aspects of genetic and phenotypic heterogeneity, *Am J Med Genet C Semin Med Genet* 142C(2):95–103, 2006.

# FETAL AND NEONATAL MEDICINE

**Clarence W. Gowen, Jr.**

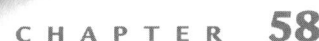

CHAPTER **58**

## Assessment of the Mother, Fetus, and Newborn

### ASSESSMENT OF THE MOTHER

The optimal care of the newborn requires knowledge of the family history, prior and current pregnancies, and events of labor and delivery. Neonatal medicine requires a comprehensive understanding of the physiology of normal pregnancy; placental and fetal growth, function, and maturity; and any extrauterine or intrauterine pathologic events that affect the mother, placenta, or fetus. These latter adverse effects may result in an unfavorable neonatal outcome and include such significant maternal influences as poor nutrition, cigarette smoking, poverty, physical or psychological stresses, extremes of age (<16 years, >35 years), race, medical illness present before pregnancy, and medications as well as obstetric complications during the antepartum and intrapartum periods, perinatal infections, exposure to toxins and illicit drugs, and the inherent genetic predisposition of the fetus.

Pregnancies associated with perinatal morbidity or mortality are considered high risk. Identification of high-risk pregnancies is essential to the care of the infant because they may result in intrauterine fetal death, intrauterine growth restriction (IUGR), congenital anomalies, excessive fetal growth, birth asphyxia and trauma, prematurity (birth at <38 weeks) or postmaturity (birth at ≥42 weeks), neonatal disease, or long-term risks of cerebral palsy, mental retardation, and chronic sequelae of neonatal intensive care. Ten percent to 20% of women may be high risk at some time during their pregnancy. Although some obstetric complications are first seen during labor and delivery and cannot be predicted, more than 50% of perinatal mortality and morbidity results from problems identified before delivery as high risk. After a high-risk pregnancy is identified, measures can be instituted to prevent complications, provide intensive fetal surveillance, and initiate appropriate treatments of the mother and fetus.

A history of previous premature birth, intrauterine fetal death, multiple gestation, IUGR, congenital malformation, explained or unexplained neonatal death (e.g., group B streptococcal sepsis), birth trauma, preeclampsia, gestational diabetes, grand multipara status (five or more pregnancies), or cesarean section is associated with additional risk in subsequent pregnancies.

**Pregnancy complications** that increase the risk of a poor outcome can be secondary to maternal or fetal causes or both. Complications include placenta previa; abruptio placentae; preeclampsia; diabetes; oligohydramnios or polyhydramnios; multiple gestation; blood group sensitization; abnormal levels of unconjugated estriols, chorionic gonadotropin, or alpha-fetoprotein; abnormal fetal ultrasound; hydrops fetalis; maternal trauma or surgery; abnormal fetal presentation (breech); exposure to prescribed or illicit drugs; prolonged labor; cephalopelvic disproportion; prolapsed cord; fetal distress; prolonged or premature rupture of membranes; short cervical length (<25 mm) and the presence of fetal fibronectin in cervical secretions at less than 35 weeks' gestation (a predictor of preterm labor); cervical infections and vaginosis; and congenital infections, including rubella, cytomegalovirus, herpes simplex, human immunodeficiency virus (HIV), toxoplasmosis, syphilis, and gonorrhea.

**Maternal medical complications** associated with increased risk of maternal and fetal morbidity and mortality include diabetes, chronic hypertension, congenital heart disease (especially with right-to-left shunting and Eisenmenger complex), glomerulonephritis, collagen vascular disease (especially systemic lupus erythematosus with or without antiphospholipid antibodies), lung disease (cystic fibrosis), severe anemia (sickle cell anemia), hyperthyroidism, myasthenia gravis, idiopathic thrombocytopenic purpura, inborn errors of metabolism (maternal phenylketonuria), and malignancy.

**Obstetric complications** often are associated with increased fetal or neonatal risk. Vaginal bleeding in the first trimester or early second trimester may be caused by a threatened or actual spontaneous abortion and is associated with increased risk of congenital malformations or chromosomal disorders. Painless vaginal bleeding that is not associated with labor and occurs in the late second or (more likely) third trimester often is the result of **placenta previa**. Bleeding develops when the placental mass overlies the internal cervical os; this may produce maternal hemorrhagic shock, necessitating transfusions. Bleeding also may result in premature delivery. Painful vaginal bleeding is often the result of retroplacental hemorrhage or **placental abruption**. Associated findings may be advanced maternal age and parity, maternal chronic hypertension, maternal cocaine use, preterm rupture of membranes, polyhydramnios, twin gestation, and preeclampsia. Fetal asphyxia ensues as the retroplacental hematoma causes placental separation that interferes with fetal oxygenation. Both types of bleeding are associated with fetal blood loss. Neonatal anemia may be more common with placenta previa.

Abnormalities in the volume of amniotic fluid, resulting in oligohydramnios or polyhydramnios, are associated with increased fetal and neonatal risk. **Oligohydramnios** (amniotic ultrasound fluid index ≤2 cm) is associated with IUGR and major congenital anomalies, particularly of the fetal kidneys, and with chromosomal syndromes. Bilateral renal agenesis results in diminished production of amniotic fluid and a specific deformation syndrome (**Potter syndrome**), which includes clubfeet, characteristic compressed facies, low-set ears, scaphoid abdomen, and diminished chest wall size accompanied by pulmonary hypoplasia and, often, pneumothorax. Uterine compression in the absence of amniotic fluid retards lung growth, and patients with this condition die of respiratory failure rather than renal insufficiency. Twin-to-twin transfusion syndrome (donor) and complications from amniotic fluid leakage also are associated with oligohydramnios. Oligohydramnios increases the risk of fetal distress during labor (meconium-stained fluid and variable decelerations); the risk may be reduced by saline amnioinfusion during labor.

**Polyhydramnios** may be acute and associated with premature labor, maternal discomfort, and respiratory compromise. More often, polyhydramnios is chronic and is associated with diabetes, immune or nonimmune hydrops fetalis, multiple gestation, trisomy 18 or 21, and major congenital anomalies. Anencephaly, hydrocephaly, and meningomyelocele are associated with reduced fetal swallowing. Esophageal and duodenal atresia, as well as cleft palate, interfere with swallowing and gastrointestinal fluid dynamics. Additional causes of polyhydramnios include Werdnig-Hoffmann and Beckwith-Wiedemann syndromes, conjoined twins, chylothorax, cystic adenomatoid lung malformation, diaphragmatic hernia, gastroschisis, sacral teratoma, placental chorioangioma, and myotonic dystrophy. **Hydrops fetalis** may be a result of Rh or other blood group incompatibilities and anemia caused by intrauterine hemolysis of fetal erythrocytes by maternal IgG-sensitized antibodies crossing the placenta. Hydrops is characterized by fetal edema, ascites, hypoalbuminemia, and congestive heart failure. Causes of **nonimmune hydrops** include fetal arrhythmias (supraventricular tachycardia, congenital heart block), fetal anemia (bone marrow suppression, nonimmune hemolysis, or twin-to-twin transfusion), severe congenital malformation, intrauterine infections, congenital neuroblastoma, inborn errors of metabolism (storage diseases), fetal hepatitis, nephrotic syndrome, and pulmonary lymphangiectasia. Twin-to-twin transfusion syndrome

(recipient) also may be associated with polyhydramnios. Polyhydramnios is often the result of unknown causes. If severe, polyhydramnios may be managed with bed rest, indomethacin, or serial amniocenteses.

**Premature rupture of the membranes**, which occurs in the absence of labor, and **prolonged rupture of the membranes** (>24 hours) are associated with an increased risk of maternal or fetal infection (chorioamnionitis) and preterm birth. In the immediate newborn period, group B streptococcus and *Escherichia coli* are the two most common pathogens associated with sepsis. *Listeria monocytogenes* is a less common cause. *Mycoplasma hominis, Ureaplasma urealyticum, Chlamydia trachomatis*, and anaerobic bacteria of the vaginal flora also have been implicated in infection of the amniotic fluid. Infection with community-acquired methicillin-resistant *Staphylococcus aureus* must be considered for infants with skin infections or with known exposures. The risk of serious fetal infection increases, as the duration between rupture and labor (latent period) increases, especially if the period is greater than 24 hours. Intrapartum antibiotic therapy decreases the risk of neonatal sepsis.

**Multiple gestations** are associated with increased risk resulting from polyhydramnios, premature birth, IUGR, abnormal presentation (breech), congenital anomalies (intestinal atresia, porencephaly, and single umbilical artery), intrauterine fetal demise, birth asphyxia, and twin-to-twin transfusion syndrome. **Twin-to-twin transfusion syndrome** is associated with a high mortality and is seen only in monozygotic twins who share a common placenta and have an arteriovenous connection between their circulations. The fetus on the arterial side of the shunt serves as the blood donor, resulting in fetal anemia, growth retardation, and oligohydramnios for this fetus. The recipient, or venous-side twin, is larger or discordant in size, is plethoric and polycythemic, and may show polyhydramnios. Weight differences of 20% and hemoglobin differences of 5 g/dL suggest the diagnosis. Ultrasonography in the second trimester reveals discordant amniotic fluid volume with oliguria/oligohydramnios and hypervolemia/polyuria/polyhydramnios with a distended bladder, with or without hydrops and heart failure. Mortality is high if presentation occurs in the second trimester; however, most monochorionic twins have bidirectional balanced shunts and are not affected. Treatment includes amniocentesis and attempts to ablate the arteriovenous connection (using a laser). The birth order of twins also affects morbidity by increasing the risk of the second-born twin for breech position, birth asphyxia, birth trauma, and respiratory distress syndrome.

Overall, twinning is observed in 1:80 pregnancies; 80% of all twin gestations are dizygotic twins. The diagnosis of the type of twins can be determined by placentation, sex, fetal membrane structure, and, if necessary, tissue and blood group typing or DNA analysis.

Toxemia of pregnancy, or **preeclampsia/eclampsia**, is a disorder of unknown but probably vascular etiology that may lead to maternal hypertension, uteroplacental insufficiency, IUGR, intrauterine asphyxia, maternal seizures, and maternal death. Toxemia is more common in nulliparous women and in women with twin gestation, chronic hypertension, obesity, renal disease, positive family history of toxemia, or diabetes mellitus. A subcategory of pre-eclampsia, the *HELLP* syndrome (**h**emolysis, **e**levated **l**iver enzyme levels, **l**ow **p**latelets), is more severe and is often associated with a fetal inborn error of fatty acid oxidation (long-chain hydroxyacyl–coenzyme A dehydrogenase of the trifunctional protein complex).

## FETUS AND NEWBORN

The late fetal–early neonatal period has the highest mortality rate of any age interval. **Perinatal mortality** refers to fetal deaths occurring from the 20th week of gestation until the 28th day after birth and is expressed as number of deaths per 1000 live births. Intrauterine fetal death accounts for 40% to 50% of the perinatal mortality rate. Such infants, defined as **stillborn**, are born without a heart rate and are apneic, limp, pale, and cyanotic. Many stillborn infants exhibit evidence of maceration; pale, peeling skin; corneal opacification; and soft cranial contents.

Mortality rates around the time of birth are expressed as number of deaths per 1000 live births. The **neonatal mortality rate** includes all infants dying during the period from after birth to the first 28 days of life. Modern neonatal intensive care allows many newborns with life-threatening diseases to survive the neonatal period, only to die of their original diseases or of complications of therapy after 28 days of life. This delayed mortality and mortality caused by acquired illnesses occur during the **postneonatal period**, which begins after 28 days of life and extends to the end of the first year of life.

The **infant mortality rate** encompasses the neonatal and the postneonatal periods. In the United States, it declined to 6.7:1000 in 2006. The rate for African-American infants was approximately 13:6000. The most common causes of perinatal and neonatal death are listed in Table 58-1. Overall, congenital anomalies and diseases of the premature infant are the most significant causes of neonatal mortality.

**Low birth weight** (LBW) infants, defined as infants having birth weights of less than 2500 g, represent a disproportionately large component of the neonatal and infant mortality rates. Although LBW infants make up only about 6% to 7% of all births, they account for more than 70% of neonatal deaths. IUGR is the most common cause of LBW in developing countries, whereas prematurity is the cause in developed countries.

**Very low birth weight** (VLBW) infants, weighing less than 1500 g at birth, represent about 1% of all births but account for 50% of neonatal deaths. Compared with infants weighing 2500 g or more, LBW infants are 40 times more likely to die in the neonatal period; VLBW infants have a 200-fold higher risk of neonatal death. The LBW rate has not improved in recent years and is one of the major reasons that the U.S. infant mortality rate is high compared with other large, modern, industrialized countries.

Maternal factors associated with a LBW caused by premature birth or IUGR include a previous LBW birth, low socioeconomic status, low level of maternal education, no antenatal care, maternal age younger than 16 years or older than 35 years, short interval between pregnancies, cigarette smoking, alcohol and illicit drug use, physical (excessive standing or walking) or psychological (poor social support)

### TABLE 58-1 Major Causes of Perinatal and Neonatal Mortality

**FETUS**

Abruptio placentae
Chromosomal anomalies
Congenital malformations (heart, CNS, renal)
Hydrops fetalis
Intrauterine asphyxia*
Intrauterine infection*
Maternal underlying disease (chronic hypertension, autoimmune disease, diabetes mellitus)
Multiple gestation*
Placental insufficiency*
Umbilical cord accident

**PRETERM INFANT**

Respiratory distress syndrome/bronchopulmonary dysplasia (chronic lung disease)*
Severe immaturity*
Congenital anomalies
Infection
Intraventricular hemorrhage*
Necrotizing enterocolitis

**FULL-TERM INFANT**

Birth asphyxia*
Birth trauma
Congenital anomalies*
Infection*
Macrosomia
Meconium aspiration pneumonia
Persistent pulmonary hypertension

*Common.
CNS, central nervous system.

stresses, unmarried status, low prepregnancy weight (<45 kg), poor weight gain during pregnancy (<10 lb), and African-American race. LBW and VLBW rates for African-American women are twice the rates for white women. The neonatal and infant mortality rates are twofold higher among African-American infants. These racial differences are only partly explained by poverty.

In addition to the sociodemographic variables associated with LBW, specific, identifiable medical causes of preterm birth exist. Factors such as uterine anomalies, hydrops fetalis, and most medical illnesses are not seen more frequently in African Americans or in patients of lower socioeconomic status. Prematurity may be caused by spontaneous labor (50% of cases), spontaneous rupture of membranes (25%), or premature delivery for maternal or fetal indications (25%).

## ASSESSMENT OF THE FETUS

**Fetal size** can be determined accurately by ultrasound techniques. **Fetal growth** can be assessed by determining the fundal height of the uterus through bimanual examination of the gravid abdomen. Ultrasound measurements of the fetal biparietal diameter, femur length, and abdominal circumference are used to estimate fetal growth. A combination of these measurements predicts fetal weight. Deviations from the normal fetal growth curve are associated with high-risk conditions.

**IUGR** is present when fetal growth stops and, over time, declines to less than the fifth percentile of growth for gestational age or when growth proceeds slowly, but absolute size remains less than the fifth percentile. Growth restriction may result from fetal conditions that reduce the innate growth potential, such as fetal rubella infection, primordial dwarfing syndromes, chromosomal abnormalities, and congenital malformation syndromes. Reduced fetal production of insulin and insulin-like growth factor I is associated with fetal growth restriction. Placental causes of IUGR include villitis (congenital infections), placental tumors, chronic abruptio placentae, twin-to-twin transfusion syndrome, and placental insufficiency. Maternal causes include severe peripheral vascular diseases that reduce uterine blood flow (chronic hypertension, diabetic vasculopathy, and preeclampsia/eclampsia), reduced nutritional intake, alcohol or drug abuse, cigarette smoking, and uterine constraint (noted predominantly in mothers of small stature with a low prepregnancy weight) and reduced weight gain during pregnancy. The outcome of IUGR depends on the cause of the reduced fetal growth and the associated complications after birth (Table 58-2). Fetuses subjected to chronic intrauterine hypoxia as a result of uteroplacental insufficiency are at an increased risk for the comorbidities of birth asphyxia, polycythemia, and hypoglycemia. Fetuses with reduced tissue mass due to chromosomal, metabolic, or multiple congenital anomaly syndromes have poor outcomes based on the prognosis for the particular syndrome. Fetuses born to small mothers and fetuses with poor nutritional intake usually show catch-up growth after birth.

Fetal size does not always correlate with functional or structural maturity. Determining **fetal maturity** is crucial when making a decision to deliver a fetus because of fetal or maternal disease. Fetal gestational age may be determined accurately on the basis of a correct estimate of the last menstrual period. Clinically relevant landmark dates can be used to determine gestational age; the first audible heart tones by fetoscope are detected at 18 to 20 weeks (12 to 14 weeks by Doppler methods), and quickening of fetal movements usually is perceived at 18 to 20 weeks. However, it is not always possible to determine fetal maturity by such dating, especially in a high-risk situation, such as preterm labor or a diabetic pregnancy.

**Surfactant**, a combination of surface-active phospholipids and proteins, is produced by the maturing fetal lung and eventually is secreted into the amniotic fluid. The amount of surfactant in amniotic fluid is a direct reflection of surface-active material in the fetal lung and can be used to predict the presence or absence of **pulmonary maturity**. Because phosphatidylcholine, or lecithin, is a principal component of surfactant, the determination of lecithin in amniotic fluid is used to predict a mature fetus. Lecithin concentration increases with increasing gestational age, beginning at 32 to 34 weeks.

Methods used to assess **fetal well-being** before the onset of labor are focused on identifying a fetus at risk for asphyxia or a fetus who already is compromised by uteroplacental insufficiency. The **oxytocin challenge test** simulates uterine contractions through an infusion of oxytocin sufficient to produce three contractions in a 10-minute period. The development of periodic fetal bradycardia out of phase with uterine contractions (late deceleration) is a positive test result and predicts an at-risk fetus.

The **nonstress test** examines the heart rate response to fetal body movements. Heart rate increases of more than 15 beats/min, lasting 15 seconds, are reassuring. If two such episodes occur in 30 minutes, the test result is considered reactive (versus nonreactive), and the fetus is not at risk. Additional signs of fetal well-being are fetal breathing movements, gross body movements, fetal tone, and the presence of amniotic fluid pockets of greater than 2 cm, detected by ultrasound. The **biophysical profile** combines the nonstress test with these four parameters and offers the most accurate fetal assessment.

**Doppler examination** of the fetal aorta or umbilical arteries permits identification of decreased or reversed

| TABLE 58-2 Problems of Intrauterine Growth Restriction and Small for Gestational Age | |
|---|---|
| Problem* | Pathogenesis |
| Intrauterine fetal demise | Placental insufficiency, hypoxia, acidosis, infection, lethal anomaly |
| Temperature instability | Cold stress, ↓ fat stores, hypoxia, hypoglycemia |
| Perinatal asphyxia | ↓ Uteroplacental perfusion during labor with or without chronic fetal hypoxia-acidosis, meconium aspiration syndrome |
| Hypoglycemia | ↓ Tissue glycogen stores; ↓ gluconeogenesis, hyperinsulinism, ↑ glucose needs of hypoxia, hypothermia, relatively large brain |
| Polycythemia-hyperviscosity | Fetal hypoxia with ↑ erythropoietin production |
| Reduced oxygen consumption/hypothermia | Hypoxia, hypoglycemia, starvation effect, poor subcutaneous fat stores |
| Dysmorphology | Syndrome anomalads, chromosomal-genetic disorders, oligohydramnios-induced deformations |
| Pulmonary hemorrhage | Hypothermia, polycythemia, hypoxia |

*Other problems are common to the gestational age–related risks of prematurity if born before 37 weeks.
Modified from Stoll BJ, Kliegman RM: The high-risk infant. In Behrman RE, Kliegman RM, Jenson HB, editors: Nelson Textbook of Pediatrics, 16th ed, Philadelphia, 2000, *Saunders*.

diastolic blood flow associated with increased peripheral vascular resistance, fetal hypoxia with acidosis, and placental insufficiency. **Cordocentesis** (percutaneous umbilical blood sampling) can provide fetal blood for $Po_2$, pH, lactate, and hemoglobin measurements to identify a hypoxic, acidotic, or anemic fetus who is at risk for intrauterine fetal demise or birth asphyxia. Cordocentesis also can be used to determine fetal blood type, platelet count, microbial culture, antibody titer, and rapid karyotype.

In a high-risk pregnancy, the fetal heart rate should be monitored continuously during labor, as should uterine contractions. Fetal heart rate abnormalities may indicate baseline tachycardia (>160 beats/min as a result of anemia, β-sympathomimetic drugs, maternal fever, hyperthyroidism, arrhythmia, or fetal distress), baseline **bradycardia** (<120 beats/min as a result of fetal distress, complete heart block, or local anesthetics), or reduced beat-to-beat variability (flattened tracing resulting from fetal sleep, tachycardia, atropine, sedatives, prematurity, or fetal distress). Periodic changes of the heart rate relative to uterine pressure help determine the presence of hypoxia and acidosis caused by uteroplacental insufficiency or maternal hypotension (late or type II decelerations) or by umbilical cord compression (variable decelerations). In the presence of severe decelerations (late or repeated prolonged variable), a fetal scalp blood gas level should be obtained to assess **fetal acidosis**. A scalp pH of less than 7.20 indicates fetal hypoxic compromise. A pH between 7.20 and 7.25 is in a borderline zone and warrants repeat testing.

Fetal anomalies may be detected by ultrasonography. Emphasis should be placed on visualization of the genitourinary tract; the head (for anencephaly or hydrocephaly), neck (for thickened nuchal translucency), and back (for spina bifida); skeleton; gastrointestinal tract; and heart. Four-chamber and great artery views are required for detection of heart anomalies. **Chromosomal anomaly syndromes** may reveal choroid cysts, hypoplasia of the middle phalanx of the fifth digit, nuchal fluid, retrognathism, and low-set ears. In addition, chromosomal syndromes often are associated with an abnormal "triple test" (low estriols, low maternal serum alpha-fetoprotein levels, and elevated placental chorionic gonadotropin levels). If a fetal abnormality is detected, fetal therapy or delivery with therapy in the neonatal intensive care unit may be lifesaving.

## ASSESSMENT OF THE NEWBORN

The approach to the birth of an infant requires a detailed history (Table 58-3). Knowing the mother's risk factors enables the delivery room team to anticipate problems that may occur after birth. The history of a woman's labor and delivery can reveal events that might lead to complications affecting either the mother or the neonate, even when the pregnancy was previously considered low risk. Anticipating the need to resuscitate a newborn as a result of fetal distress increases the likelihood of successful resuscitation.

The **transition from fetal to neonatal physiology** occurs at birth. Oxygen transport across the placenta results in a gradient between the maternal and fetal

---

### TABLE 58-3 Components of the Perinatal History

#### DEMOGRAPHIC SOCIAL INFORMATION

Age
Race
Sexually transmitted infections, hepatitis, AIDS
Illicit drugs, cigarettes, ethanol, cocaine
Immune status (syphilis, rubella, hepatitis B, blood group)
Occupational exposure

#### PAST MEDICAL DISEASES

Chronic hypertension
Heart disease
Diabetes mellitus
Thyroid disorders
Hematologic/malignancy
Collagen-vascular disease (SLE)
Genetic history—inborn errors of metabolism, bleeding, jaundice
Drug therapy

#### PRIOR PREGNANCY

Abortion
Intrauterine fetal demise
Congenital malformation
Incompetent cervix
Birth weight
Prematurity
Twins
Blood group sensitization/neonatal jaundice
Hydrops
Infertility

#### PRESENT PREGNANCY

Current gestational age
Method of assessing gestational age
Fetal surveillance (OCT, NST, biophysical profile)
Ultrasonography (anomalies, hydrops)
Amniotic fluid analysis (L/S ratio)
Oligohydramnios-polyhydramnios
Vaginal bleeding
Preterm labor
Premature (prolonged) rupture of membranes (duration)
Preeclampsia
Urinary tract infection
Colonization status (herpes simplex, group B streptococcus)
Medications/drugs
Acute medical illness/exposure to infectious agents
Fetal therapy

#### LABOR AND DELIVERY

Duration of labor
Presentation—vertex, breech
Vaginal versus cesarean section
Spontaneous labor versus augmented or induced with oxytocin (Pitocin)
Forceps delivery
Presence of meconium-stained fluid

*Continued*

## TABLE 58-3 Components of the Perinatal History—cont'd

Maternal fever/amnionitis
Fetal heart rate patterns (distress)
Scalp pH
Maternal analgesia, anesthesia
Nuchal cord
Apgar score/methods of resuscitation
Gestational age assessment
Growth status (AGA, LGA, SGA)

AGA, average for gestational age; AIDS, acquired immunodeficiency syndrome; LGA, large for gestational age; L/S, lecithin-to-sphingomyelin ratio; NST, nonstress test; OCT, oxytocin challenge test; SGA, small for gestational age; SLE, systemic lupus erythematosus.

$Pao_2$. Although fetal oxygenated blood has a low $Pao_2$ level compared with that of adults and infants, the fetus is not anaerobic. Fetal oxygen uptake and consumption are similar to neonatal rates, even though the thermal environments and activity levels of fetuses and neonates differ. The oxygen content of fetal blood is almost equal to the oxygen content in older infants and children because fetal blood has a much higher concentration of hemoglobin.

Fetal hemoglobin (two alpha and two gamma chains) has a higher affinity for oxygen than adult hemoglobin, facilitating oxygen transfer across the placenta. The fetal hemoglobin-oxygen dissociation curve is shifted to the left of the adult curve (Fig. 58-1); at the same $Pao_2$ level, fetal hemoglobin is more saturated than adult hemoglobin. Because fetal hemoglobin functions on the steep, lower end of the oxygen saturation curve ($Pao_2$, 20 to 30 mm Hg), however, oxygen unloading to the tissue is not deficient. In contrast, at the higher oxygen concentrations present in the placenta, oxygen loading is enhanced. In the last trimester, fetal hemoglobin production begins to decrease as adult hemoglobin production begins to increase, becoming the only hemoglobin available to the infant by 3 to 6 months of life. At this time, the fetal hemoglobin dissociation curve has shifted to the adult position.

A portion of well-oxygenated umbilical venous blood returning to the heart from the placenta perfuses the liver. The remainder bypasses the liver through a shunt (the **ductus venosus**) and enters the inferior vena cava. This oxygenated blood in the vena cava constitutes 65% to 70% of venous return to the right atrium. The crista dividens in the right atrium directs one third of this blood across the patent foramen ovale to the left atrium, where it subsequently is pumped to the coronary, cerebral, and upper extremity circulations by the left ventricle. Venous return from the upper body combines with the remaining two thirds of the vena caval blood in the right atrium and is directed to the right ventricle. This mixture of venous low-oxygenated blood from the upper and lower body enters the pulmonary artery. Only 8% to 10% of it is pumped to the pulmonary circuit; the remaining 80% to 92% of the right ventricular output bypasses the lungs through a **patent ductus arteriosus** and enters the descending aorta. The amount of blood flowing to the pulmonary system is low because vasoconstriction produced by medial muscle hypertrophy of the pulmonary arterioles and fluid in the fetal lung increases resistance to blood flow. Pulmonary artery tone also responds to hypoxia, hypercapnia, and acidosis with vasoconstriction, a response that may increase pulmonary vascular resistance further. The ductus arteriosus remains patent in the fetus because of low $Pao_2$ levels and dilating prostaglandins. In utero, the right ventricle is the dominant ventricle, pumping 65% of the combined ventricular output, which is a high volume (450 mL/kg/min) compared with that pumped by an older infant's right ventricle (200 mL/kg/min).

The **transition of the circulation** occurring between the fetal and neonatal periods involves the removal of the low-resistance circulation of the placenta, the onset of breathing, reduction of pulmonary arterial resistance, and closure of in utero shunts. Clamping the umbilical cord eliminates the low-pressure system of the placenta and increases systemic blood pressure. Decreased venous return from the placenta decreases right atrial pressure. As breathing begins, air replaces lung fluid, maintaining the functional residual capacity. Fluid leaves the lung, in part, through the trachea; it is either swallowed or squeezed out during vaginal delivery. The pulmonary lymphatic and venous systems reabsorb the remaining fluid.

Most normal infants require little pressure to spontaneously *open* the lungs after birth (5 to 10 cm $H_2O$). A few infants require assistance with greater opening pressures (20 to 30 cm $H_2O$). With the onset of breathing, pulmonary vascular resistance decreases, partly a result of the mechanics of breathing and partly a result of the elevated arterial oxygen tensions. The increased blood flow to the lungs increases the volume of pulmonary venous

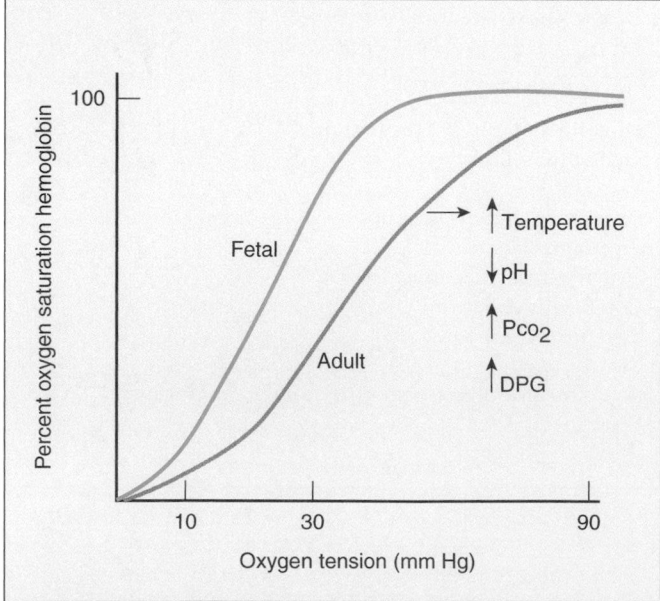

**FIGURE 58-1**

Hemoglobin-oxygen dissociation curves. The position of the adult curve depends on the binding of adult hemoglobin to 2,3-diphosphoglycerate (DPG), temperature, $Pco_2$, and hydrogen ion concentration (pH).

blood returning to the left atrium; left atrial pressure now exceeds right atrial pressure, and the foramen ovale closes. As the flow through the pulmonary circulation increases and arterial oxygen tensions rise, the ductus arteriosus begins to constrict. In a term infant, this constriction functionally closes the ductus arteriosus within 1 day after birth. A permanent closure requires thrombosis and fibrosis, a process that may take several weeks. In a premature infant, the ductus arteriosus is less sensitive to the effects of oxygen; if circulating levels of vasodilating prostaglandins are elevated, the ductus arteriosus may remain patent. This patency is a common problem in a premature infant with respiratory distress syndrome.

Ventilation, oxygenation, and normal pH and $Pco_2$ levels immediately reduce pulmonary artery vasoconstriction by causing smooth muscle relaxation. Remodeling of the medial muscle hypertrophy begins at birth and continues for the next 3 months, resulting in a further reduction of pulmonary vascular resistance and a further increase of pulmonary blood flow. Persistence or aggravation of pulmonary vasoconstriction caused by acidosis, hypoxia, hypercapnia, hypothermia, polycythemia, asphyxia, shunting of blood from the lungs, or pulmonary parenchymal hypoplasia results in **persistent pulmonary hypertension of the newborn (PPHN)**. Failure to replace pulmonary alveolar fluid completely with air can lead to respiratory distress **(transient tachypnea of the newborn)**.

## Routine Delivery Room Care and Resuscitation

Silver nitrate (1%) instilled into both eyes without being washed out is an indicated effective therapy for the prevention of neonatal gonococcal ophthalmia, which can result in severe panophthalmitis and subsequent blindness. Silver nitrate may produce a chemical conjunctivitis with a mucopurulent discharge and is not effective against *C. trachomatis*. Many hospitals use erythromycin drops to prevent neonatal gonococcal and chlamydial eye disease.

Bacterial colonization of a newborn may begin in utero if the fetal membranes have been ruptured. Most infants undergo colonization after birth and acquire the bacteria present in the mother's genitourinary system, such as group B streptococci, staphylococci, *E. coli*, and clostridia. Colonization is common at the umbilicus, skin, nasopharynx, and intestine. Antiseptic skin or cord care is routine in most nurseries to prevent the spread of pathologic bacteria from one infant to another and to prevent disease in the individual infant. Staphylococcal bullous impetigo, omphalitis, diarrhea, and systemic disease may result from colonization with virulent *S. aureus*. For term infants, washing of the skin with 3% hexachlorophene is not routinely recommended but may prevent serious staphylococcal disease; preterm infants may absorb hexachlorophene, and neurotoxicity may develop. Triple antibiotic ointment (polymyxin B, neomycin, and bacitracin) or bacitracin may be applied to the umbilical cord to reduce its colonization with gram-positive bacteria. Epidemics of *S. aureus* nursery infections are managed with strict infectious disease control measures (cohorting, hand washing, and monitoring for colonization).

**Vitamin K prophylaxis (intramuscular)** should be given to all infants to prevent hemorrhagic disease of the newborn. Before discharge, infants should receive the hepatitis B vaccine and be screened for various diseases (Tables 58-4 and 58-5).

Fetal or neonatal hypoxia, hypercapnia, poor cardiac output, and a metabolic acidosis can result from numerous conditions affecting the fetus, the placenta, or the mother. Whether in utero or after birth, asphyxia-caused **hypoxic-ischemic brain injury** is the result of reduced gaseous exchange through the placenta or through the lungs. Asphyxia associated with severe bradycardia or cardiac insufficiency reduces or eliminates tissue blood flow, resulting in ischemia. The fetal and neonatal circulatory systems respond to reduced oxygen availability by shunting the blood preferentially to the brain, heart, and adrenal glands and away from the intestine, kidneys, lungs, and skin.

Metabolic acidosis during asphyxia is caused by the combined effects of poor cardiac output secondary to hypoxic depression of myocardial function, systemic hypoxia, and tissue anaerobic metabolism. With severe or prolonged intrauterine or neonatal asphyxia, multiple vital organs are affected (Table 58-6).

---

**TABLE 58-4  Approximate Frequencies of Disorders Included in or Considered for Newborn Screening in the United States**

| Disorder | Estimated Frequency | Disorder | Estimated Frequency |
|---|---|---|---|
| Congenital hypothyroidism | 1:4000 | Sickle cell disease | 1:4000 |
| Phenylketonuria | 1:12,000 | Cystic fibrosis | 1:4000 |
| Medium-chain acyl-CoA dehydrogenase | 1:10,000 | Duchenne muscular dystrophy | 1:8000* |
| Galactosemia | 1:60,000 | Congenital toxoplasmosis | 1:10,000 |
| Maple syrup urine disease | 1:200,000 | Hyperlipidemia | 1:500 |
| Homocystinuria | 1:200,000 | $\alpha_1$-Antitrypsin deficiency | 1:8000 |
| Biotinidase deficiency | 1:70,000 | | |
| Congenital adrenal hyperplasia | 1:19,000 | | |

*For males, 1:4000.

From Kim SZ, Levy HL: Newborn screening. In Taeusch HW, Ballard RA, editors: Avery's Diseases of the Newborn, 7th ed, Philadelphia, 1998, *Saunders*.

**TABLE 58-5  Abnormal Newborn Screening Results: Possible Implications and Initial Action to Be Taken**

| Newborn Screening Finding | Differential Diagnosis | Initial Action |
|---|---|---|
| ↑ Phenylalanine | PKU, non-PKU hyperphenylalaninemia, pterin defect, galactosemia, transient hyperphenylalaninemia | Repeat blood specimen |
| ↓ $T_4$, ↑ TSH | Congenital hypothyroidism, iodine exposure | Repeat blood specimen or thyroid function testing, begin thyroxine treatment |
| ↓ $T_4$, normal TSH | Maternal hyperthyroidism, thyroxine-binding globulin deficiency, secondary hypothyroidism, congenital hypothyroidism with delayed TSH elevation | Repeat blood specimen |
| ↑ Galactose (1-P) transferase | Galactosemia, liver disease, reducing substance, repeat deficiency variant (Duarte), transient | Clinical evaluation, urine for blood specimen. If reducing substance positive, begin lactose-free formula |
| ↓ Galactose-1-phosphate uridyltransferase | Galactosemia, transferase deficiency variant (Duarte), transient | Clinical evaluation, urine for reducing substance, repeat blood specimen. If reducing substance positive, begin lactose-free formula |
| ↑ Methionine | Homocystinuria, isolated liver dysfunction, tyrosinemia type I, transient hypermethioninemia | Repeat blood and urine specimen |
| ↑ Leucine | Maple syrup urine disease, transient elevation | Clinical evaluation including urine for ketones, acid-base status, amino acid studies, immediate neonatal ICU care if urine ketones positive |
| ↑ Tyrosine | Tyrosinemia type I or type II, transient tyrosinemia, liver disease | Repeat blood specimen |
| ↑ 17α-Hydroxyprogesterone | Congenital adrenal hyperplasia, prematurity, transient (residual fetal adrenal cortex), stress in neonatal period, early specimen collection | Clinical evaluation including genital examination, serum electrolytes, repeat blood specimen |
| S-hemoglobin | Sickle cell disease, sickle cell trait | Hemoglobin electrophoresis |
| ↑ Trypsinogen | Cystic fibrosis, transient, intestinal anomalies, perinatal stress, trisomies 13 and 18, renal failure | Repeat blood specimen, possible sweat test and DNA testing |
| ↑ Creatinine phosphokinase | Duchenne muscular dystrophy, other type of muscular dystrophy, birth trauma, invasive procedure | Repeat blood test |
| ↓ Biotinidase | Biotinidase deficiency | Serum biotinidase assay, biotin therapy |
| ↓ G6PD | G6PD deficiency | Complete blood count, bilirubin determination |
| ↓ α₁-Antitrypsin | $\alpha_1$-Antitrypsin deficiency | Confirmatory test |
| Toxoplasma antibody (IgM) | Congenital toxoplasmosis | Infectious disease consultation |
| HIV antibody (IgG) | Maternally transmitted HIV, possible AIDS | Infectious disease consultation |
| ↑ Organic acids | Fatty acid oxidation defects (medium-chain acyl-CoA dehydrogenase deficiency) | Perform specific assay (tandem mass spectroscopy); frequent feeds |

G6PD, glucose-6-phosphate dehydrogenase; ICU, intensive care unit; PKU, phenylketonuria; $T_4$, thyroxine; TSH, thyroid-stimulating hormone.

From Kim SZ, Levy HL: Newborn screening. In Taeusch HW, Ballard RA, editors: Avery's Diseases of the Newborn, 7th ed, Philadelphia, 1998, Saunders.

Many conditions that contribute to **fetal or neonatal asphyxia** are the same medical or obstetric problems associated with high-risk pregnancy (Table 58-7). Maternal diseases that interfere with uteroplacental perfusion (chronic hypertension, preeclampsia, and diabetes mellitus) place the fetus at risk for intrauterine asphyxia. Maternal epidural anesthesia and the development of the vena caval compression syndrome may produce maternal hypotension, which decreases uterine perfusion. Maternal medications given to relieve pain during labor may cross the placenta and depress the infant's respiratory center, resulting in apnea at the time of birth.

Fetal conditions associated with asphyxia usually do not become manifested until delivery, when the infant must initiate and sustain ventilation. In addition, the upper and lower airways must be patent and

**TABLE 58-6 Effects of Asphyxia**

| System | Effect |
|---|---|
| Central nervous system | Hypoxic-ischemic encephalopathy, IVH, PVL, cerebral edema, seizures, hypotonia, hypertonia |
| Cardiovascular | Myocardial ischemia, poor contractility, tricuspid insufficiency, hypotension |
| Pulmonary | Persistent pulmonary hypertension, respiratory distress syndrome |
| Renal | Acute tubular or cortical necrosis |
| Adrenal | Adrenal hemorrhage |
| Gastrointestinal | Perforation, ulceration, necrosis |
| Metabolic | Inappropriate ADH, hyponatremia, hypoglycemia, hypocalcemia, myoglobinuria |
| Integument | Subcutaneous fat necrosis |
| Hematology | Disseminated intravascular coagulation |

ADH, antidiuretic hormone; IVH, intraventricular hemorrhage; PVL, periventricular leukomalacia.

**TABLE 58-7 Etiology of Birth Asphyxia**

| Type | Example |
|---|---|
| **INTRAUTERINE** | |
| Hypoxia-ischemia | Uteroplacental insufficiency, abruptio placentae, prolapsed cord, maternal hypotension, unknown |
| Anemia-shock | Vasa previa, placenta previa, fetomaternal hemorrhage, erythroblastosis |
| **INTRAPARTUM** | |
| Birth trauma | Cephalopelvic disproportion, shoulder dystocia, breech presentation, spinal cord transection |
| Hypoxia-ischemia | Umbilical cord compression, tetanic contraction, abruptio placentae |
| **POSTPARTUM** | |
| Central nervous system | Maternal medication, trauma, previous episodes of fetal hypoxia–acidosis |
| Congenital neuromuscular disease | Congenital myasthenia gravis, myopathy, myotonic dystrophy |
| Infection | Consolidated pneumonia, shock |
| Airway disorder | Choanal atresia, severe obstructing goiter, laryngeal webs |
| Pulmonary disorder | Severe immaturity, pneumothorax, pleural effusion, diaphragmatic hernia, pulmonary hypoplasia |
| Renal disorder | Pulmonary hypoplasia, pneumothorax |

unobstructed. Alveoli must be free from foreign material, such as meconium, amniotic fluid debris, and infectious exudates, which increases airway resistance, reduces lung compliance, and leads to respiratory distress and hypoxia. Some extremely immature infants weighing less than 1000 g at birth may be unable to expand their lungs, even in the absence of other pathology. Their compliant chest walls and surfactant deficiency may result in poor air exchange, retractions, hypoxia, and apnea.

The newborn (particularly a preterm infant) responds paradoxically to hypoxia with apnea rather than tachypnea as occurs in adults. Episodes of intrauterine asphyxia also may depress the neonatal central nervous system. If recovery of the fetal heart rate occurs as a result of improved uteroplacental perfusion, fetal hypoxia and acidosis may resolve. Nonetheless, if the effect on the respiratory center is more severe, a newborn may not initiate an adequate ventilatory response at birth and may undergo another episode of asphyxia.

The **Apgar examination**, a rapid scoring system based on physiologic responses to the birth process, is a good method for assessing the need to resuscitate a newborn (Table 58-8). At intervals of 1 minute and 5 minutes after birth, each of the five physiologic parameters is observed or elicited by a qualified examiner. Full-term infants with a normal cardiopulmonary adaptation should score 8 to 9 at 1 and 5 minutes. Apgar scores of 4 to 7 warrant close attention to determine whether the infant's status will improve and to ascertain whether any pathologic condition is contributing to the low Apgar score.

By definition, an Apgar score of 0 to 3 represents either a cardiopulmonary arrest or a condition caused by severe bradycardia, hypoventilation, or central nervous system depression. Most low Apgar scores are caused by difficulty in establishing adequate ventilation and not by primary cardiac pathology. In addition to an Apgar score of 0 to 3, most infants with asphyxia severe enough to cause neurologic injury also manifest fetal acidosis (pH <7); seizures, coma, or hypotonia; and multiorgan dysfunction. Low Apgar scores may be caused by fetal hypoxia or other factors listed in Table 58-7. Most infants with low Apgar scores respond to assisted ventilation by face mask or by endotracheal intubation and usually do not need emergency medication.

**Resuscitation** of a newborn with a low Apgar score follows the same systematic sequence as that for resuscitation of older patients, but in the newborn period this simplified *ABCD* approach requires some qualification (Fig. 58-2). In the ABCD approach, **A** stands for securing a patent airway by clearing amniotic fluid or meconium by suctioning; **A** is also a reminder of *anticipation* and the need for knowing the events of pregnancy, labor, and delivery. Evidence of a diaphragmatic hernia and a low Apgar score indicate that immediate endotracheal intubation is required. If a mask and bag are used, gas enters the lung and the stomach, and the latter may act as an expanding mass in the chest that compromises respiration. If fetal hydrops has occurred with pleural effusions, a bilateral thoracentesis to evacuate the pleural effusions may be needed to establish adequate ventilation.

**B** represents **breathing**. If the neonate is apneic or hypoventilates and remains cyanotic, artificial ventilation

**TABLE 58-8  Apgar Score**

| Signs | Points | | |
|---|---|---|---|
| | 0 | 1 | 2 |
| Heart rate | 0 | <100/min | >100/min |
| Respiration | None | Weak cry | Vigorous cry |
| Muscle tone | None | Some extremity flexion | Arms, legs well flexed |
| Reflex irritability | None | Some motion | Cry, withdrawal |
| Color of body | Blue | Pink body, blue extremities | Pink all over |

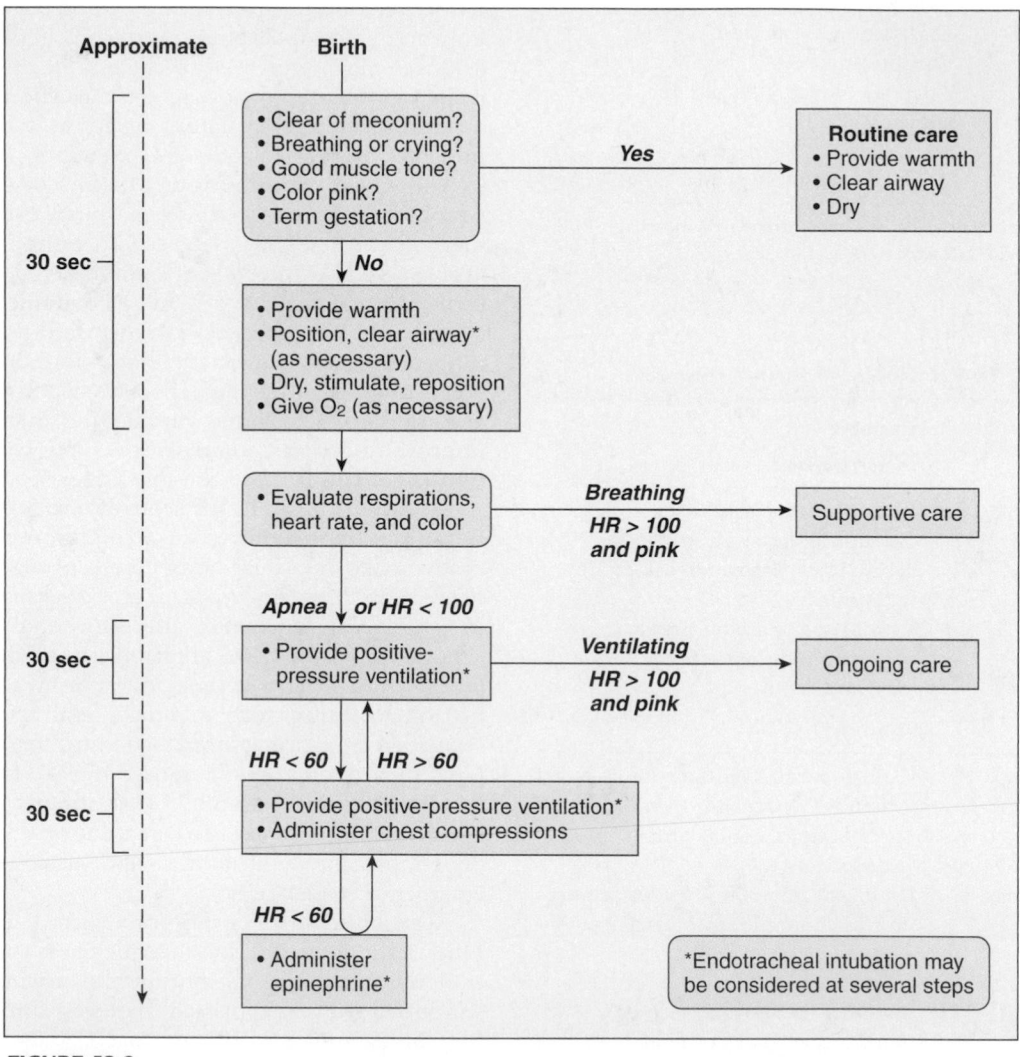

**FIGURE 58-2**

Algorithm for resuscitation of the newborn infant. HR, heart rate. (From National guidelines for neonatal resuscitation. *Pediatrics* 106:E29, 2000.)

should be initiated. Ventilation should be performed with a well-fitted mask attached to an anesthesia bag and a manometer to prevent extremely high pressures from being given to the newborn; 100% oxygen should be administered through the mask. If the infant does not revive, an endotracheal tube should be placed, attached to the anesthesia bag and manometer, and 100% oxygen should be administered. The pressure generated should begin at 20 to 25 cm $H_2O$, with a rate of 40 to 60 breaths/min. An adequate response to ventilation includes good chest rise, return of breath sounds, well-oxygenated color, heart rate returning to the normal range (120 to 160 beats/min), normal end-tidal carbon dioxide, and, later, increased muscle activity and wakefulness. The usual recovery after a cardiac arrest first involves a return to a normal heart rate followed by disappearance of cyanosis, and noticeably improved perfusion. An infant may remain limp and be apneic for a prolonged time after return of cardiac output and correction of acidosis.

Breathing initially should be briefly delayed if meconium-stained amniotic fluid is present to avoid dissemination of meconium into the lungs, producing severe aspiration pneumonia. If meconium is noted in the amniotic fluid, the oropharynx should be suctioned when the head is delivered. After the birth of a **depressed infant**, the oral cavity should be suctioned again; the vocal cords should be visualized and the infant intubated, with suction applied while the tube is below the vocal cords. If meconium is noted below the cords, intubation should be repeated quickly to clear the remaining meconium. During this time, the infant should not be stimulated to breathe, and positive-pressure ventilation should not be applied.

**C** represents **circulation** and external cardiac massage. If artificial ventilation does not improve bradycardia, if asystole is present, or if peripheral pulses cannot be palpated, external cardiac massage should be performed at a rate of 120 compressions/min with compressions and breaths given at a ratio of 3:1. External cardiac massage usually is not needed because most infants in the delivery room respond to ventilation.

**D** represents the **administration of drugs**. If bradycardia is unresponsive to ventilation or if asystole is present, resuscitation drugs should be administered. Intravenous (IV) epinephrine (1:10,000), 0.1 to 0.3 mL/kg, should be given through an umbilical venous line or injected into the endotracheal tube. Additional medications for resuscitation include 2 mEq/kg of IV sodium bicarbonate if acidosis is prolonged and a rapid infusion of fluids (normal saline, or O-negative red blood cells if anemia is present) if poor perfusion suggests hypovolemia. Sodium bicarbonate should be given only if severe metabolic acidosis is suspected or is proven by blood gas analysis. Sodium bicarbonate should not be given unless the lungs are adequately ventilated. Before medications are administered in the presence of electrical cardiac activity with poor pulses, it is important to determine whether there is a **pneumothorax**. Transillumination of the thorax, involving the use of a bright light through each side of the thorax and over the sternum, may suggest pneumothorax if one side transmits more light than the other. Breath sounds may be decreased over a pneumothorax and there may be a shift of the heart tones away from the side of a tension pneumothorax.

If central nervous system depression in the infant may be due to a narcotic medication given to the mother, 0.1 mg/kg of naloxone (Narcan) can be given to the infant intravenously or endotracheally. Before this drug is administered, the ABCs should be followed carefully. Naloxone should not be given to a newborn of a mother who is suspected of being addicted to narcotics or is on methadone maintenance because the newborn may experience severe withdrawal seizures.

## Physical Examination and Gestational Age Assessment

The first physical examination of a newborn may be a general physical examination of a well infant, an examination to confirm fetal diagnoses or to determine the cause of various manifestations of neonatal diseases. Problems in the transition from fetal to neonatal life may be detectable immediately in the delivery room or during the first day of life. Physical examination also may reveal effects of the labor and delivery resulting from asphyxia, drugs, or birth trauma. The first newborn examination is an important way to detect congenital malformations or deformations (Table 58-9). Significant congenital malformations may be present in 1% to 3% of all births.

### Appearance

The general appearance of the infant should be evaluated first. Signs such as cyanosis, nasal flaring, intercostal retractions, and grunting suggest pulmonary disease. Meconium staining of the umbilical cord, nails, and skin suggest fetal distress and the possibility of aspiration pneumonia. The level of spontaneous activity, passive muscle tone, quality of the cry, and apnea are useful screening signs to evaluate the state of the nervous system.

### TABLE 58-9 Life-Threatening Congenital Anomalies

| Name | Manifestations |
| --- | --- |
| Choanal atresia (stenosis) | Respiratory distress in delivery room, apnea, unable to pass nasogastric tube through nares |
| Pierre Robin syndrome | Micrognathia, cleft palate, airway obstruction |
| Diaphragmatic hernia | Scaphoid abdomen, bowel sounds present in left chest, heart shifted to right, respiratory distress, polyhydramnios |
| Tracheoesophageal fistula | Polyhydramnios, aspiration pneumonia, excessive salivation, unable to place nasogastric tube in stomach |
| Intestinal obstruction: volvulus, duodenal atresia, ileal atresia | Polyhydramnios, bile-stained emesis, abdominal distention |
| Gastroschisis/omphalocele | Polyhydramnios; intestinal obstruction |
| Renal agenesis/Potter syndrome | Oligohydramnios, anuria, pulmonary hypoplasia, pneumothorax |
| Hydronephrosis | Bilateral abdominal masses |
| Neural tube defects: anencephalus, meningomyelocele | Polyhydramnios, elevated α-fetoprotein; decreased fetal activity |
| Down syndrome (trisomy 21) | Hypotonia, congenital heart disease, duodenal atresia |
| Ductal-dependent congenital heart disease | Cyanosis, murmur, shock |

## Vital Signs

The examination should proceed with an assessment of vital signs, particularly heart rate (normal rate, 120 to 160 beats/min); respiratory rate (normal rate, 30 to 60 breaths/min); temperature (usually done per rectum and later as an axillary measurement); and blood pressure (often reserved for sick infants). Length, weight, and head circumference should be measured and plotted on growth curves to determine whether growth is normal, accelerated, or retarded for the specific gestational age.

## Gestational Age

Gestational age is determined by an assessment of various physical signs (Fig. 58-3) and neuromuscular characteristics (Fig. 58-4) that vary according to fetal age and maturity. **Physical criteria** mature with advancing fetal age, including increasing firmness of the pinna of the ear; increasing size of the breast tissue; decreasing fine, immature lanugo hair over the back; and decreasing opacity of the skin. **Neurologic criteria** mature with gestational age, including increasing flexion of the legs, hips, and arms; increasing tone of the flexor muscles of the neck; and decreasing laxity of the joints. These signs are determined during the first day of life and are assigned scores. The cumulative score is correlated with a gestational age, which is usually accurate to within 2 weeks (Fig. 58-5).

Gestational age assessment permits the detection of abnormal fetal growth patterns, aiding in predicting the neonatal complications of largeness or smallness for gestational age (Fig. 58-6). Infants born at a weight greater than the 90th percentile for age are considered **large for gestational age**. Among the risks associated with being large for gestational age are all the risks of the infant of a diabetic mother and risks associated with postmaturity. Infants born at a weight less than 10th percentile for age (some growth curves use <2 standard deviations or the fifth percentile) are **small for gestational age** and have IUGR. Problems associated with small for gestational age infants include congenital malformations, in addition to the problems listed in Table 58-2.

## Skin

The skin should be evaluated for pallor, plethora, jaundice, cyanosis, meconium staining, petechiae, ecchymoses, congenital nevi, and neonatal rashes. Vasomotor instability with cutis marmorata, telangiectasia, phlebectasia (intermittent

| Physical maturity | −1 | 0 | 1 | 2 | 3 | 4 | 5 |
|---|---|---|---|---|---|---|---|
| Skin | Sticky, friable, transparent | Gelatinous, red, translucent | Smooth, pink, visible veins | Superficial peeling or rash, few veins | Cracking, pale areas, rare veins | Parchment, deep cracking, no vessels | Leathery, cracked, wrinkled |
| Lanugo | None | Sparse | Abundant | Thinning | Bald areas | Mostly bald | |
| Plantar surface | Heel–toe 40-50 mm: −1 Less than 40 mm: −2 | <50 mm, no crease | Faint red marks | Anterior transverse crease only | Creases on anterior 2/3 | Creases over entire sole | |
| Breast | Imperceptible | Barely perceptible | Flat areola– no bud | Stripped areola, 1-2 mm bud | Raised areola, 3-4 mm bud | Full areola, 5-10 mm bud | |
| Eye/ear | Lids fused, loosely (−1), tightly (−2) | Lids open, pinna flat, stays folded | Slightly curved pinna; soft, slow recoil | Well-curved pinna, soft but ready recoil | Formed and firm; instant recoil | Thick cartilage, ear stiff | |
| Genitals male | Scrotum flat, smooth | Scrotum empty, faint rugae | Testes in upper canal, rare rugae | Testes descending, few rugae | Testes down, good rugae | Testes pendulous, deep rugae | |
| Genitals female | Clitoris prominent, labia flat | Prominent clitoris, small labia minora | Prominent clitoris, enlarging minora | Majora and minora equally prominent | Majora large, minora small | Majora cover clitoris and minora | |

**FIGURE 58-3**

Physical criteria for assessment of maturity and gestational age. Expanded New Ballard Score (NBS) includes extremely premature infants and has been refined to improve accuracy in more mature infants. (From Ballard JL, et al: New Ballard Score, expanded to include extremely premature infants. *J Pediatr* 119:417, 1991.)

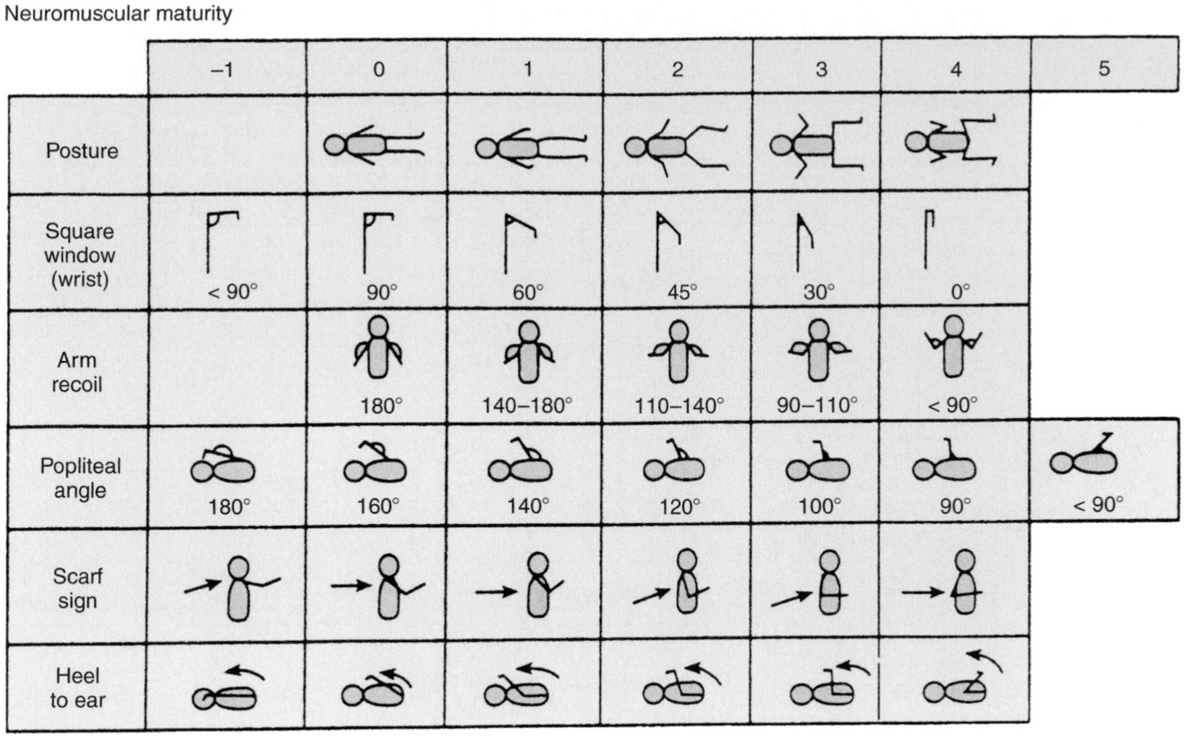

Neuromuscular maturity

| | −1 | 0 | 1 | 2 | 3 | 4 | 5 |
|---|---|---|---|---|---|---|---|
| Posture | | | | | | | |
| Square window (wrist) | < 90° | 90° | 60° | 45° | 30° | 0° | |
| Arm recoil | | 180° | 140–180° | 110–140° | 90–110° | < 90° | |
| Popliteal angle | 180° | 160° | 140° | 120° | 100° | 90° | < 90° |
| Scarf sign | | | | | | | |
| Heel to ear | | | | | | | |

**FIGURE 58-4**

Neuromuscular criteria for assessment of maturity and gestational age. Expanded New Ballard Score (NBS) includes extremely premature infants and has been refined to improve accuracy in more mature infants. (From Ballard JL, et al: New Ballard Score, expanded to include extremely premature infants. *J Pediatr* 119:417, 1991).

Maturity rating

| Score | Weeks |
|---|---|
| −10 | 20 |
| −5 | 22 |
| 0 | 24 |
| 5 | 26 |
| 10 | 28 |
| 15 | 30 |
| 20 | 32 |
| 25 | 34 |
| 30 | 36 |
| 35 | 38 |
| 40 | 40 |
| 45 | 42 |
| 50 | 44 |

**FIGURE 58-5**

Maturity rating as calculated by adding the physical and neurologic scores, calculating the gestational age. (From Ballard JL, et al: New Ballard Score, expanded to include extremely premature infants. *J Pediatr* 119:417, 1991).

mottling with venous prominence), and acrocyanosis (feet and hands) is normal in a premature infant. Acrocyanosis also may be noted in a healthy term infant in the first days after birth. The harlequin color change is a striking, transient, but normal sign of vasomotor instability and divides the body from head to pubis, through the midline, into equal halves of pink and pale color.

The skin is covered with lanugo hair, which disappears by term gestation. **Hair tufts** over the lumbosacral spine suggest a spinal cord defect. **Vernix caseosa**, a soft, white, creamy layer covering the skin in preterm infants, disappears by term. Post-term infants often have peeling, parchment-like skin. **Mongolian spots** are transient, dark blue to black pigmented macules seen over the lower back and buttocks in 90% of African-American, Indian, and Asian infants. **Nevus simplex** (*salmon patch*), or pink macular hemangiomas, is common, usually transient, and noted on the back of the neck, eyelids, and forehead. **Nevus flammeus**, or **port-wine stain**, is seen on the face and should cause the examiner to consider Sturge-Weber syndrome (trigeminal angiomatosis, convulsions, and ipsilateral intracranial *tram-line* calcifications).

**Congenital melanocytic nevi** are pigmented lesions of varying size noted in 1% of neonates. **Giant pigmented nevi** are uncommon but have malignant potential. **Capillary hemangiomas** are raised, red lesions, whereas **cavernous hemangiomas** are deeper, blue masses. Both lesions increase in size after birth, then resolve when the child is 1 to 4 years of age. When enlarged, these hemangiomas may produce high-output heart failure or platelet

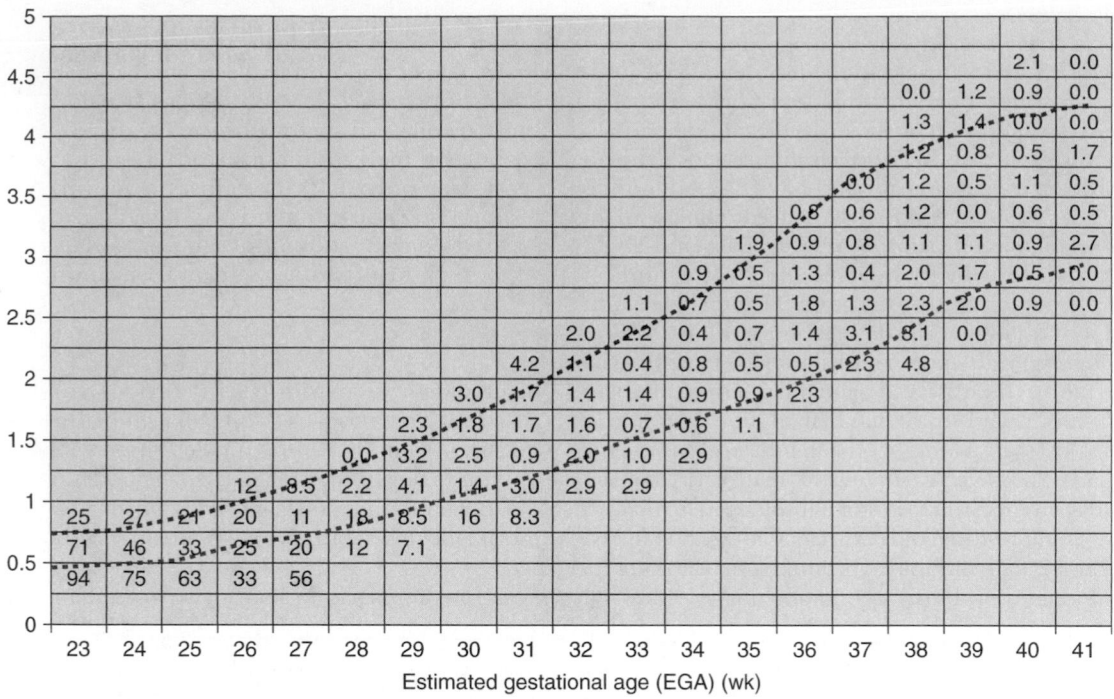

**FIGURE 58-6**

Birth weight–specific and estimated gestational age–specific mortality rates. The dashed lines of the figure represent the 10th and 90th percentile weights. The grid lines are plotted by each gestational age and in 250-g weight increments. Each number in the box is the percent mortality rate for the grid defined by gestational age and birth weight range. (From Thomas P, Peabody J, Turnier V, et al: A new look at intrauterine growth and impact of race, attitude, and gender. *Pediatrics* 106:E21, 2000.)

trapping and hemorrhage. **Erythema toxicum** is an erythematous, papular-vesicular rash common in neonates that develops after birth and involves eosinophils in the vesicular fluid. **Pustular melanosis**, more common in African-American infants, may be seen at birth and consists of a small, dry vesicle on a pigmented brown macular base. Erythema toxicum and pustular melanosis are benign lesions, but may mimic more serious conditions, such as the vesicular rash of disseminated herpes simplex or the bullous eruption of *S. aureus* impetigo. Tzanck smear, Gram stain, Wright stain, direct fluorescent antibody stain, polymerase chain reaction for herpes DNA, and appropriate cultures may be needed to distinguish these rashes. Other common characteristic rashes are **milia** (yellow-white epidermal cysts of the pilosebaceous follicles that are noted on the nose) and **miliaria** (prickly heat), which is caused by obstructed sweat glands. **Edema** may be present in preterm infants, but also suggests hydrops fetalis, sepsis, hypoalbuminemia, or lymphatic disorders.

## Skull

The skull may be elongated and molded after a prolonged labor, which resolves 2 to 3 days after birth. The sutures should be palpated to determine the width and the presence of premature fusion or cranial synostosis. The anterior and posterior fontanelles should be soft and nonbulging, with the anterior larger than the posterior. A large fontanelle is associated with hydrocephalus, hypothyroidism, rickets, and other disorders. Soft areas away from the fontanelle are **craniotabes**; these lesions feel like a ping-pong ball when they are palpated. They may be a result of in utero compression. The skull should be examined carefully for signs of trauma or lacerations from internal fetal electrode sites or fetal scalp pH sampling; abscess formation may develop in these areas.

## Face, Eyes, and Mouth

The face should be inspected for dysmorphic features, such as epicanthal folds, hypertelorism, preauricular tags or sinuses, low-set ears, long philtrum, and cleft lip or palate. Facial asymmetry may be a result of seventh nerve palsy; head tilt may be caused by torticollis.

The eyes should open spontaneously, especially in an upright position. Before 28 weeks' gestational age, the eyelids may be fused. Coloboma, megalocornea, and microphthalmia suggest other malformations or intrauterine infections. A cloudy cornea greater than 1 cm in diameter also may be seen in congenital glaucoma, uveal tract dysgenesis, and storage diseases. Conjunctival and retinal hemorrhages are common and usually of no significance. The pupillary response to light is present at 28 weeks of gestation. The **red reflex** of the retina is shown easily. A white reflex, or **leukokoria**, is abnormal and may be the result of cataracts, ocular tumor, severe chorioretinitis, persistent hyperplastic primary vitreous, or retinopathy of prematurity.

The mouth should be inspected for the presence of natal teeth, clefts of the soft and hard palate and uvula, and micrognathia. A bifid uvula suggests a submucosal cleft. White, shiny, multiple transient epidermal inclusion cysts (Epstein pearls) on the hard palate are normal. Hard, marble-sized masses in the buccal mucosa are usually transient idiopathic fat necrosis. The **tympanic membranes** are dull, gray, opaque, and immobile in the first 1 to 4 weeks. These findings should not be confused with otitis media.

## Neck and Chest

The neck appears short and symmetrical. Abnormalities include midline clefts or masses caused by thyroglossal duct cysts or by goiter and lateral neck masses (or sinuses), which are the result of branchial clefts. Cystic hygromas and hemangiomas may be present. Shortening of the sternocleidomastoid muscle with a fibrous *tumor* over the muscle produces head tilt and asymmetrical facies (neonatal torticollis). Arnold-Chiari malformation and cervical spine lesions also produce torticollis. Edema and webbing of the neck suggest Turner syndrome. Both clavicles should be palpated for fractures.

Examination of the **chest** includes inspection of the chest wall to identify asymmetry resulting from absence of the pectoralis muscle and inspection of the breast tissue to determine gestational age and detect a breast abscess. Boys and girls may have breast engorgement and produce milk; milk expression should not be attempted. **Supernumerary nipples** may be bilateral and may be associated with renal anomalies.

## Lungs

Examination of the lungs includes observations of the rate, depth, and nature of intercostal or sternal retractions. Breath sounds should be equal on both sides of the chest, and rales should not be heard after the first 1 to 2 hours of life. Diminished or absent breath sounds on one side suggest pneumothorax, collapsed lung, pleural effusion, or diaphragmatic hernia. Shift of the cardiac impulse away from a tension pneumothorax and diaphragmatic hernia and toward the collapsed lung is a helpful physical finding for differentiating these disorders. Subcutaneous emphysema of the neck or chest also suggests a pneumothorax or pneumomediastinum, whereas bowel sounds auscultated in the chest in the presence of a scaphoid abdomen suggest a diaphragmatic hernia.

## Heart

The position of the heart in infants is more midline than in older children. The first heart sound is normal, whereas the second heart sound may not be split in the first day of life. Decreased splitting of the second heart sound is noted in PPHN, transposition of the great vessels, and pulmonary atresia. Heart murmurs in newborns are common in the delivery room and during the first day of life. Most of these murmurs are transient and are due to closure of the ductus arteriosus, peripheral pulmonary artery stenosis, or a small ventral septal defect. Pulses should be palpated in the upper and lower extremities (over the brachial and femoral arteries). Blood pressure in the upper and lower extremities should be measured in all patients with a murmur or heart failure. An upper-to-lower extremity gradient of more than 10 to 20 mm Hg suggests coarctation of the aorta.

## Abdomen

The liver may be palpable 2 cm below the right costal margin. The spleen tip is less likely to be palpable. A left-sided liver suggests situs inversus and asplenia syndrome. Both kidneys should be palpable in the first day of life with gentle, deep palpation. The first urination occurs during the first day of life in more than 95% of normal term infants.

Abdominal masses usually represent hydronephrosis or dysplastic-multicystic kidney disease. Less often, masses indicate ovarian cysts, intestinal duplication, neuroblastoma, or mesoblastic nephroma. Masses should be evaluated immediately with ultrasound. Abdominal distention may be caused by intestinal obstructions, such as ileal atresia, meconium ileus, midgut volvulus, imperforate anus, or Hirschsprung disease. Meconium stool is passed normally within 48 hours of birth in 99% of term infants. The anus should be patent. An imperforate anus is not always visible; the first temperature taken with a rectal thermometer should be taken carefully. The abdominal wall musculature may be absent, as in prune-belly syndrome, or weak, resulting in diastasis recti. **Umbilical hernias** are common in African-American infants. The umbilical cord should be inspected to determine the presence of two arteries and one vein and the absence of an urachus or a herniation of abdominal contents, as occurs with an **omphalocele**. The latter is associated with extraintestinal problems, such as genetic trisomies and hypoglycemia (Beckwith-Wiedemann syndrome). Bleeding from the cord suggests a coagulation disorder, and a chronic discharge may be a granuloma of the umbilical stump or, less frequently, a draining omphalomesenteric cyst. Erythema around the umbilicus is **omphalitis** and may cause portal vein thrombophlebitis and subsequent extrahepatic portal hypertension. The herniation of bowel through the abdominal wall 2 to 3 cm lateral to the umbilicus is a **gastroschisis**.

## Genitalia

The appearance of the genitalia varies with gestational age. At term, the testes should be descended into a well-formed pigmented and rugated scrotum. The testes occasionally are in the inguinal canal; this is more common among preterm infants, as is cryptorchidism. Scrotal swelling may represent a hernia, transient hydrocele, in utero torsion of the testes, or, rarely, dissected meconium from meconium ileus and peritonitis. Hydroceles are clear and readily seen by transillumination, whereas testicular torsion in the newborn may present as a painless, dark swelling. The urethral opening should be at the end of the penis. Epispadias or hypospadias alone should not raise concern about pseudohermaphroditism. However, if no testes are present in the scrotum and hypospadias is present, problems of sexual development should be suspected (see Chapter 177). Circumcision should be deferred with hypospadias because the foreskin is often needed for the repair. The normal prepuce is often too tight to retract in the neonatal period.

The female genitalia normally may reveal a milky white or blood-streaked vaginal discharge as a result of maternal hormone withdrawal. Mucosal tags of the labia majora are common. Distention of an imperforate hymen may produce hydrometrocolpos and a lower midline abdominal mass as a result of an enlarged uterus. Clitoral enlargement with fusion of the labial-scrotal folds (labia majora) suggests adrenogenital syndrome or exposure to masculinizing maternal hormones.

## Extremities

Examination of the extremities should involve assessment of length, symmetry, and presence of hemihypertrophy, atrophy, polydactyly, syndactyly, simian creases, absent fingers, overlapping fingers, rocker-bottom feet, clubfoot, congenital bands, fractures, and amputations.

## Spine

The spine should be examined for evidence of sacral hair tufts, a dermal sinus tract above the gluteal folds, congenital scoliosis (a result of hemivertebra), and soft tissue masses such as lipomas or meningomyeloceles.

## Hips

The hips should be examined for congenital dysplasia (dislocation). Gluteal fold asymmetry or leg length discrepancy is suggestive of dysplasia, but the examiner should perform the Barlow test and the Ortolani maneuver to evaluate the stability of the hip joint. These tests determine whether the femoral head can be displaced from the acetabulum (**Barlow test**) and then replaced (**Ortolani maneuver**) (see Chapter 198). The examiner's long finger is placed over the greater trochanter, and the thumb is placed medially, just distal to the long finger. With the thighs held in midabduction, the examiner attempts to pull the femoral head gently out of the acetabulum with lateral pressure of the thumb and by rocking the knee medially. The reverse maneuver is performed by pressing the long finger on the greater trochanter and rocking the knee laterally. A *clunking* sensation is palpated when the femoral head leaves and returns to the acetabulum.

## NEUROLOGIC ASSESSMENT

The neurologic examination should include assessment of active and passive tone, level of alertness, primary neonatal (primitive) reflexes, deep tendon reflexes, spontaneous motor activity, and cranial nerves (involving retinal examination, extraocular muscle movement, masseter power as in sucking, facial motility, hearing, and tongue function). The Moro reflex, present at birth and gone in 3 to 6 months, is one of the primary newborn reflexes. It is elicited by sudden, slight dropping of the supported head from a slightly raised supine position, which should elicit opening of the hands and extension and abduction of the arms, followed by upper extremity flexion and a cry. The palmar grasp is present by 28 weeks of age and gone by 4 months. Deep tendon reflexes may be brisk in a normal newborn; 5 to 10 beats of ankle clonus are normal. The Babinski sign is extensor or upgoing. The sensory examination can be evaluated by withdrawal of an extremity, grimace, and cry in response to painful stimuli. The rooting reflex (turning of the head toward light tactile stimulation of the perioral area) is present by 32 weeks of age.

## Special Conditions Requiring Resuscitation in the Delivery Room

### Cyanosis

**Acrocyanosis** (blue color of the hands and feet with pink color of the rest of the body) is common in the delivery room and is usually normal. **Central cyanosis** of the trunk, mucosal membranes, and tongue can occur at any time after birth and is always a manifestation of a serious underlying condition. Cyanosis is noted with 4 to 5 g/dL of deoxygenated hemoglobin. Central cyanosis can be caused by problems in many different organ systems, although cardiopulmonary diseases are the most common (Table 58-10). Respiratory distress syndrome, sepsis, and cyanotic heart disease are the three most common causes of cyanosis in infants admitted to a neonatal intensive care unit. A systematic evaluation of these and other causes of cyanosis is required for every cyanotic infant after prompt administration of oxygen, with or without assisted ventilation.

### Life-Threatening Congenital Malformations

Various congenital anomalies can interfere with vital organ function after birth (see Table 58-9). Some malformations, such as choanal atresia and other lesions obstructing the airway, may complicate ventilation. Intrathoracic lesions, such as cysts or diaphragmatic hernia, interfere with respiration. Other malformations that obstruct the gastrointestinal system at the level of the esophagus, duodenum, ileum, or colon may lead to aspiration pneumonia, intestinal perforation, or gangrene. Gastroschisis and omphalocele are associated with exposed bowel on the abdominal wall. Omphalocele also is often associated with other malformations, whereas intestinal necrosis is more common in gastroschisis.

Many congenital malformations are obvious in the delivery room. Fetal ultrasound can detect many serious congenital anomalies in utero. Immediate palliative medical or surgical treatment or corrective surgery must be planned for most infants with major congenital malformations.

### Shock

Shock in the delivery room is manifested by pallor, poor capillary refill time, lack of palpable pulses, hypotonia, cyanosis, and eventually cardiopulmonary arrest. Blood loss before or during labor and delivery is a common cause of shock in the delivery room. Blood loss may be caused by fetal-maternal hemorrhage, placenta previa, vasa previa, twin-to-twin transfusion syndrome, or displacement of blood from the fetus to the placenta as during asphyxia (*asphyxia pallida*). Hemorrhage into a viscus, such as the liver or spleen, may be noted in macrosomic infants, and hemorrhage into the cerebral ventricles

**TABLE 58-10 Differential Diagnosis of Neonatal Cyanosis**

| System/Disease | Mechanism |
|---|---|
| **PULMONARY** | |
| Respiratory distress syndrome | Surfactant deficiency |
| Sepsis, pneumonia | Inflammation, pulmonary hypertension, ARDS |
| Meconium aspiration pneumonia | Mechanical obstruction, inflammation, pulmonary hypertension |
| Persistent pulmonary hypertension of the newborn | Pulmonary hypertension |
| Diaphragmatic hernia | Pulmonary hypoplasia, pulmonary hypertension |
| Transient tachypnea | Retained lung fluid |
| **CARDIOVASCULAR** | |
| Cyanotic heart disease with decreased pulmonary blood flow | Right-to-left shunt as in pulmonary atresia, tetralogy of Fallot |
| Cyanotic heart disease with increased pulmonary blood flow | Mixing lesion as in single ventricle or truncus arteriosus |
| Cyanotic heart disease with congestive heart failure | Right-to-left shunt with pulmonary edema and poor cardiac output as in hypoplastic left heart and coarctation of aorta |
| Heart failure alone | Pulmonary edema and poor cardiac contractility as in sepsis, myocarditis, supraventricular tachycardia, or complete heart block; high-output failure as in PDA or vein of Galen or other arteriovenous malformations |
| **CENTRAL NERVOUS SYSTEM (CNS)** | |
| Maternal sedative drugs | Hypoventilation, apnea |
| Asphyxia | CNS depression |
| Intracranial hemorrhage | CNS depression, seizure |
| Neuromuscular disease | Hypotonia, hypoventilation, pulmonary hypoplasia |
| **HEMATOLOGIC** | |
| Acute blood loss | Shock |
| Chronic blood loss | Congestive heart failure |
| Polycythemia | Pulmonary hypertension |
| Methemoglobinemia | Low-affinity hemoglobin or red blood cell enzyme defect |
| **METABOLIC** | |
| Hypoglycemia | CNS depression, congestive heart failure |
| Adrenogenital syndrome | Shock (salt-losing) |

ARDS, acute respiratory distress syndrome; PDA, patent ductus arteriosus.

may produce shock and apnea in preterm infants. Anemia, hypoalbuminemia, hypovolemia, and shock at birth are common manifestations of Rh immune hydrops.

Severe intrauterine bacterial sepsis may present with shock in the delivery room or immediately after the infant is transferred to the nursery. Typically these infants are mottled, hypotonic, and cyanotic and have diminished peripheral pulses. They have a normal hemoglobin concentration but may manifest neutropenia, thrombocytopenia, and disseminated intravascular coagulation. Peripheral symmetrical gangrene (purpuric rash) often is a sign of hypotensive shock in infants with severe congenital bacterial infections. Congenital left ventricular cardiac obstruction (critical aortic stenosis or hypoplastic left heart syndrome) also produces shock, although not usually in the delivery room.

**Treatment** of newborn infants with shock should involve the management approaches used for the sick infant. Problems may be anticipated through knowledge of the infant's immune status, evidence of hydrops, or suspicion of intrauterine infection or anomalies. Stabilization of the airway and institution of respiratory support are essential. Hypovolemic shock should be managed with repeated boluses of 10 to 15 mL/kg of normal saline or lactated Ringer solution. If severe immune hemolysis is predicted, blood typed against the mother's blood should be available in the delivery room and should be given to the newborn if signs of anemia and shock are present. Thereafter, all blood should be crossmatched with the infant's and mother's blood before transfusion. Drugs such as dopamine, dobutamine, epinephrine, or cortisol may improve cardiac output and tissue perfusion.

## Birth Injury

Birth injury refers to avoidable and unavoidable injury to the fetus during the birth process. **Caput succedaneum** is a diffuse, edematous, often dark swelling of the soft tissue of the scalp that extends across the midline and suture lines. In infants delivered from a face presentation, soft tissue edema of the eyelids and face is an equivalent phenomenon. Caput succedaneum may be seen after prolonged labor in full-term and preterm infants. Molding of the head often is associated with caput succedaneum and is the result of pressure that is induced from overriding the parietal and frontal bones against their respective sutures.

A **cephalhematoma** is a subperiosteal hemorrhage that does not cross the suture lines surrounding the respective bones. A linear skull fracture rarely may be seen underlying a cephalhematoma. With time, the cephalhematoma may organize, calcify, and form a central depression.

Infants with cephalhematoma and caput succedaneum require no specific treatment. Occasionally a premature infant may develop a massive scalp hemorrhage. This **subgaleal bleeding** and the bleeding noted from a cephalhematoma may cause indirect hyperbilirubinemia requiring phototherapy. **Retinal and subconjunctival hemorrhages** are common but usually are small and insignificant. No treatment is necessary.

**Spinal cord** or **spine injuries** may occur in the fetus as a result of the hyperextended *star gazing* posture. Injuries also may occur in infants after excessive rotational (at C3–4) or longitudinal (at C7–T1) force is transmitted to the neck during vertex or breech delivery. Fractures of vertebrae are rare and may cause direct damage to the spinal cord, leading to transection and permanent sequelae, hemorrhage, edema, and neurologic signs. Rarely a snapping sound indicating cord transection rather than vertebral displacement is heard at the time of delivery. Neurologic dysfunction usually involves complete flaccid paralysis, absence of deep tendon reflexes, and absence of responses to painful stimuli below the lesion. Painful stimuli may elicit reflex flexion of the legs. Infants with spinal cord injury often are flaccid, apneic, and asphyxiated, all of which may mask the underlying spinal cord transection.

Injury to the nerves of the **brachial plexus** may result from excessive traction on the neck, producing paresis or complete paralysis. The mildest injury (neurapraxia) is edema; axonotmesis is more severe and consists of disrupted nerve fibers with an intact myelin sheath; neurotmesis, or complete nerve disruption or root avulsion, is most severe. **Erb-Duchenne paralysis** involves the fifth and sixth cervical nerves and is the most common and usually mildest injury. The infant cannot abduct the arm at the shoulder, externally rotate the arm, or supinate the forearm. The usual picture is one of painless adduction, internal rotation of the arm, and pronation of the forearm. The **Moro reflex** is absent on the involved side, and the hand grasp is intact. **Phrenic nerve palsy** (C3, C4, and C5) may lead to diaphragmatic paralysis and respiratory distress. Elevation of the diaphragm caused by nerve injury must be differentiated from elevation caused by eventration resulting from congenital weakness or absence of diaphragm muscle. **Klumpke paralysis** is caused by injury to the seventh and eighth cervical nerves and the first thoracic nerve, resulting in a paralyzed hand and, if the sympathetic nerves are injured, an ipsilateral **Horner syndrome** (ptosis, miosis). Complete arm and hand paralysis is noted with the most severe form of damage to C5, C6, C7, C8, and T1. **Treatment** of brachial plexus injury is supportive and includes positioning to avoid contractures. Active and passive range of motion exercises also may be beneficial. If the deficit persists, nerve grafting may be beneficial.

**Facial nerve injury** may be the result of compression of the seventh nerve between the facial bone and the mother's pelvic bones or the physician's forceps. This peripheral nerve injury is characterized by an asymmetric, crying face whose normal side, including the forehead, moves in a regular manner. The affected side is flaccid, the eye does not close, the nasolabial fold is absent, and the side of the mouth droops at rest. If there is a central injury to the facial nerve, only the lower two thirds of the face (not the forehead) are involved. Complete agenesis of the facial nucleus results in a central facial paralysis; when this is bilateral, as in **Möbius syndrome**, the face appears expressionless.

**Skull fractures** are rare, are usually linear, and require no treatment other than observation for very rare, delayed (1 to 3 months) complications (e.g., leptomeningeal cyst). Depressed skull fractures are unusual, but may be seen with complicated forceps delivery and may need surgical elevation. Fractures of the **clavicle** usually are unilateral and are noted in macrosomic infants after shoulder dystocia. Often a snap is heard after a difficult delivery, and the infant exhibits an asymmetrical Moro response and decreased movement of the affected side. The prognosis is excellent; many infants require no treatment or a simple figure of eight bandage to immobilize the bone.

**Extremity fractures** are less common than fractures of the clavicle and involve the humerus more often than the femur. **Treatment** involves immobilization and a triangular splint bandage for the humerus and traction suspension of the legs for femoral fractures. The prognosis is excellent.

Fractures of the **facial bones** are rare, but dislocation of the cartilaginous part of the nasal septum out of the vomeral groove and columella is common. Clinical manifestations include feeding difficulty, respiratory distress, asymmetrical nares, and a flattened, laterally displaced nose. Treatment reduces the dislocation by elevating the cartilage back into the vomeral groove.

**Visceral trauma** to the liver, spleen, or adrenal gland occurs in macrosomic infants and in extremely premature infants, with or without breech or vaginal delivery. Rupture of the liver with subcapsular hematoma formation may lead to anemia, hypovolemia, shock, hemoperitoneum, and disseminated intravascular coagulation. Infants with anemia and shock who are suspected to have an intraventricular hemorrhage but with a normal head ultrasound examination should be evaluated for hepatic or splenic rupture. Adrenal hemorrhage may be asymptomatic, detected only by finding calcified adrenal glands in normal infants. Infants with severe adrenal hemorrhage may exhibit a flank mass, jaundice, and hematuria, with or without shock.

## Temperature Regulation

In utero, thermoregulation of the fetus is performed by the placenta, which acts as an efficient heat exchanger. Fetal temperature is nonetheless higher than the mother's temperature. If maternal temperature becomes elevated during a febrile illness or on exposure to environmental heat, fetal temperature increases further. The immediate temperature at birth of an infant born to a febrile mother with chorioamnionitis is elevated regardless of the presence of infection in the infant, unless the infant has cooled in the delivery room.

After birth, a newborn remains covered by amniotic fluid and situated in a cold environment (20° C to 25° C). An infant's skin temperature may decrease 0.3° C/min, and the core temperature may decrease 0.1° C/min in the delivery room. In the absence of an external heat source, the infant must increase metabolism substantially to maintain body temperature.

Heat loss occurs through four basic mechanisms. In the cold delivery room, the wet infant loses heat predominantly by **evaporation** (cutaneous and respiratory loss when wet or in low humidity), **radiation** (loss to nearby cold, solid surfaces), and **convection** (loss to air current). When the infant is dry, radiation, convection, and **conduction** (loss to object in direct contact with infant) are important causes of heat loss. After birth, all high-risk infants should be dried immediately to eliminate evaporative heat losses. A radiant or convective heat source should be provided for these high-risk infants. Normal term infants should be dried and wrapped in a blanket.

The ideal environmental temperature is the **neutral thermal environment**, the ambient temperature that results in the lowest rate of heat being produced by the infant and maintains normal body temperature. The neutral thermal environmental temperature decreases with increasing gestational and postnatal age. Ambient temperatures less than the neutral thermal environment first result in increasing rates of oxygen consumption for heat production, which is designed to maintain normal body temperature. If the ambient temperature decreases further or if oxygen consumption cannot increase sufficiently (due to hypoxia, hypoglycemia, or drugs), the core body temperature decreases.

Heat production by a newborn is created predominantly by nonshivering thermogenesis in specialized areas of tissue containing brown adipose tissue. Brown fat is highly vascular, contains many mitochondria per cell, and is situated around large blood vessels, resulting in rapid heat transfer to the circulation. The vessels of the neck, thorax, and interscapular region are common locations of brown fat. These tissues also are innervated by the sympathetic nervous system, which serves as a primary stimulus for heat production by brown adipose cells. Shivering does not occur in newborns.

Severe **cold injury** in an infant is manifested by acidosis, hypoxia, hypoglycemia, apnea, bradycardia, pulmonary hemorrhage, and a pink skin color. The color is caused by trapping of oxygenated hemoglobin in the cutaneous capillaries. Many of these infants appear dead, but most respond to treatment and recover. Milder degrees of cold injury in the delivery room may contribute to metabolic acidosis and hypoxia after birth. Conversely, hypoxia delays heat generation in cold-stressed infants.

**Treatment** of severe hypothermia should involve resuscitation and rapid warming of core (e.g., lung and stomach) and external surfaces. Fluid resuscitation also is needed to treat the hypovolemia seen in many of these infants. Reduced core temperature (32° C to 35° C) in the immediate newborn period often requires only external warming with a radiant warmer, incubator, or both.

## Elevated Temperature

Exposure to ambient temperatures above the neutral thermal environment results in *heat stress* and an elevated core temperature. Sweating is uncommon in newborns and may be noted only on the forehead. In response to moderate heat stress, infants may increase their respiratory rate to dissipate heat. Excessive environmental temperatures may result in heatstroke or in hemorrhagic shock encephalopathy syndrome.

# MISCELLANEOUS DISORDERS

## Hypocalcemia

Hypocalcemia is common in sick and premature newborns. Calcium levels are higher in cord blood than in maternal blood because of active placental transfer of calcium to the fetus. Fetal calcium accretion in the third trimester approaches 150 mg/kg/24 hr, and fetal bone mineral content doubles between 30 and 40 weeks of gestation. All infants show a slight decline of serum calcium levels after birth, reaching a trough level at 24 to 48 hours, the point at which hypocalcemia usually occurs. Total serum calcium levels of less than 7 mg/dL and ionized calcium levels of less than 3 to 3.5 mg/dL are considered hypocalcemic.

The etiology of hypocalcemia varies with the time of onset and the associated illnesses of the child. **Early neonatal hypocalcemia** occurs in the first 3 days of life and is often asymptomatic. Transient hypoparathyroidism and a reduced parathyroid response to the usual postnatal decline of serum calcium levels may be responsible for hypocalcemia in premature infants and infants of diabetic mothers. Congenital absences of the parathyroid gland and DiGeorge syndrome also have been associated with hypocalcemia. **Hypomagnesemia** (<1.5 mg/dL) may be seen simultaneously with hypocalcemia, especially in infants of diabetic mothers. Treatment with calcium alone does not relieve symptoms or increase serum calcium levels until hypomagnesemia is also treated. Sodium bicarbonate therapy, phosphate release from cell necrosis, transient hypoparathyroidism, and hypercalcitoninemia may be responsible for early neonatal hypocalcemia associated with asphyxia. Early-onset hypocalcemia associated with asphyxia often occurs with seizures as a result of hypoxic-ischemic encephalopathy or hypocalcemia. **Late neonatal hypocalcemia**, or **neonatal tetany**, often is the result of ingestion of high phosphate–containing milk or the inability to excrete the usual phosphorus in commercial infant formula. Hyperphosphatemia (>8 mg/dL) usually occurs in infants with hypocalcemia after the first week of life. Vitamin D deficiency states and malabsorption also have been associated with late-onset hypocalcemia.

The clinical manifestations of hypocalcemia and hypomagnesemia include apnea, muscle twitching, seizures, laryngospasm, **Chvostek sign** (facial muscle spasm when the side of the face over the seventh nerve is tapped), and **Trousseau sign** (carpopedal spasm induced by partial inflation of a blood pressure cuff). The latter two signs are rare in the immediate newborn period.

Neonatal hypocalcemia may be prevented by administration of IV or oral calcium supplementation at a rate of 25 to 75 mg/kg/24 hr. Early asymptomatic hypocalcemia of preterm infants and infants of diabetic mothers often resolves spontaneously. Symptomatic hypocalcemia should be treated with 2 to 4 mL/kg of 10% calcium gluconate given intravenously and slowly over 10 to 15 minutes, followed by a continuous infusion of 75 mg/kg/ 24 hr of elemental calcium. If hypomagnesemia is associated with hypocalcemia, 50% magnesium sulfate, 0.1 mL/kg, should be given by intramuscular injection and repeated every 8 to 12 hours.

The **treatment** of late hypocalcemia includes immediate management, as in early hypocalcemia, plus the initiation of feedings with low phosphate formula. Subcutaneous infiltration of IV calcium salts can cause tissue necrosis; oral supplements are hypertonic and may irritate the intestinal mucosa.

## Neonatal Drug Addiction and Withdrawal

Infants may become passively and physiologically addicted to medications or to drugs of abuse (heroin, methadone, barbiturates, tranquilizers, amphetamines) taken chronically by the mother during pregnancy; these infants subsequently may have signs and symptoms of drug withdrawal. Many of these pregnancies are at high risk for other complications related to IV drug abuse, such as hepatitis, acquired immunodeficiency syndrome (AIDS), and syphilis. In addition, the LBW rate and the long-term risk for sudden infant death syndrome are higher in the infants of these high-risk women.

## Opiates

Neonatal withdrawal signs and symptoms usually begin at 1 to 5 days of life with maternal heroin use and at 1 to 4 weeks with maternal methadone addiction. Clinical manifestations of withdrawal include sneezing, yawning, ravenous appetite, emesis, diarrhea, fever, diaphoresis, tachypnea, high-pitched cry, tremors, jitteriness, poor sleep, poor feeding, and seizures. The illness tends to be more severe during methadone withdrawal. The initial treatment includes swaddling in blankets in a quiet, dark room. When hyperactivity is constant, and irritability interferes with sleeping and feeding, or when diarrhea or seizures are present, pharmacologic treatment is indicated. Seizures usually are treated with phenobarbital. The other symptoms may be managed with replacement doses of a narcotic (usually tincture of opium) to calm the infant; weaning from narcotics may be prolonged over 1 to 2 months.

## Cocaine

Cocaine use during pregnancy is associated with preterm labor, abruptio placentae, neonatal irritability, and decreased attentiveness. Infants may be small for gestational age and have small head circumferences. Usually no treatment is needed.

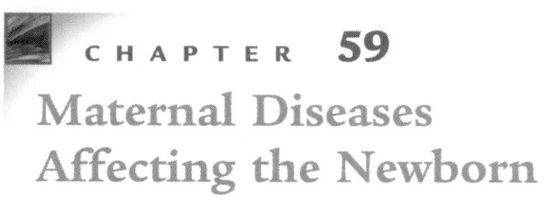

CHAPTER **59**

# Maternal Diseases Affecting the Newborn

Maternal diseases presenting during pregnancy can affect the fetus directly or indirectly (Table 59-1). Autoantibody-mediated diseases can have direct consequences on the fetus and neonate because the antibodies are usually of the IgG type and can cross the placenta to the fetal circulation.

## ANTIPHOSPHOLIPID SYNDROME

Antiphospholipid syndrome is associated with thrombophilia and recurrent pregnancy loss. Antiphospholipid antibodies are found in 2% to 5% of the general healthy population, but they also may be associated with systemic lupus erythematosus and other rheumatic diseases. Obstetric complications arise from the prothrombotic effects of the antiphospholipid antibodies on placental funcion. Vasculopathy, infarction, and thrombosis have been identified in mothers with antiphospholipid syndrome. Antiphospholipid syndrome can include fetal growth impairment, placental insufficiency, maternal preeclampsia, and premature birth.

## IDIOPATHIC THROMBOCYTOPENIA

Idiopathic thrombocytopenic purpura (ITP) is seen in approximately 1 to 2 per 1000 live births and is an immune process in which antibodies are directed against platelets. Platelet-associated IgG antibodies can cross the placenta and cause thrombocytopenia in the fetus and newborn. The severely thrombocytopenic fetus is at increased risk for intracranial hemorrhage. ITP during pregnancy requires close maternal and fetal management to reduce the risks of life-threatening maternal hemorrhage and trauma to the fetus at delivery. Postnatal management involves observation of the infant's platelet count. For infants who have evidence of hemorrhage, single-donor irradiated platelets may be administered to control the bleeding. The infant may benefit from an infusion of intravenous immunoglobulin. Neonatal thrombocytopenia usually resolves within 4 to 6 weeks.

**TABLE 59-1 Maternal Disease Affecting the Fetus or Neonate**

| Maternal Disorder | Fetal Effects | Mechanism |
| --- | --- | --- |
| Cyanotic heart disease | Intrauterine growth restriction | Low fetal oxygen delivery |
| Diabetes mellitus | | |
|   Mild | Large for gestational age, hypoglycemia | Fetal hyperglycemia—produces hyperinsulinemia promoting growth |
|   Severe | Growth retardation | Vascular disease, placental insufficiency |
| Drug addiction | Intrauterine growth restriction, neonatal withdrawal | Direct drug effect, plus poor diet |
| Endemic goiter | Hypothyroidism | Iodine deficiency |
| Graves' disease | Transient thyrotoxicosis | Placental immunoglobulin passage of thyrotropin receptor antibody |
| Hyperparathyroidism | Hypocalcemia | Maternal calcium crosses to fetus and suppresses fetal parathyroid gland |
| Hypertension | Intrauterine growth restriction, intrauterine fetal demise | Placental insufficiency, fetal hypoxia |
| Idiopathic thrombocytopenic purpura | Thrombocytopenia | Nonspecific platelet antibodies cross placenta |
| Infection | Neonatal sepsis (see Chapter 66) | Transplacental or ascending infection |
| Isoimmune neutropenia or thrombocytopenia | Neutropenia or thrombocytopenia | Specific antifetal neutrophil or platelet antibody crosses placenta after sensitization of mother |
| Malignant melanoma | Placental or fetal tumor | Metastasis |
| Myasthenia gravis | Transient neonatal myasthenia | Immunoglobulin to acetylcholine receptor crosses the placenta |
| Myotonic dystrophy | Neonatal myotonic dystrophy | Autosomal dominant with genetic anticipation |
| Phenylketonuria | Microcephaly, retardation, ventricular septal defect | Elevated fetal phenylalanine levels |
| Rh or other blood group sensitization | Fetal anemia, hypoalbuminemia, hydrops, neonatal jaundice | Antibody crosses placenta directed at fetal cells with antigen |
| Systemic lupus erythematosus | Congenital heart block, rash, anemia, thrombocytopenia, neutropenia, cardiomyopathy, stillbirth | Antibody directed at fetal heart, red and white blood cells, and platelets; lupus anticoagulant |

From Stoll BJ, Kliegman RM: The fetus and neonatal infant. In Behrman RE, Kliegman RM, Jenson HB, editors: Nelson Textbook of Pediatrics, 16th ed, Philadelphia, *WB Saunders*, 2000.

## SYSTEMIC LUPUS ERYTHEMATOSUS

Immune abnormalities in systemic lupus erythematosus (SLE) can lead to the production of anti-Ro (SS-A) and anti-La (SS-B) antibodies that can cross the placenta and injure fetal tissue. The most serious complication is damage to the cardiac conducting system, which results in **congenital heart block**. The heart block observed in association with maternal SLE tends to be complete (third degree), although less advanced blocks have been observed. The mortality rate is approximately 20%, and most surviving infants require pacing. Neonatal lupus may occur and is characterized by skin lesions (sharply demarcated erythematous plaques or central atrophic macules with peripheral scaling with predilection for the eyes, face, and scalp), thrombocytopenia, autoimmune hemolysis, and hepatic involvement.

## NEONATAL HYPERTHYROIDISM

Graves' disease is associated with thyroid-stimulating antibodies. The prevalence of clinical hyperthyroidism in pregnancy has been reported to be about 0.1% to 0.4% and is the most common endocrine disorder during pregnancy after diabetes. Neonatal hyperthyroidism is due to the transplacental passage of thyroid-stimulating antibodies; hyperthyroidism can appear rapidly within the first 12 to 48 hours. Symptoms may include intrauterine growth restriction, prematurity, goiter (may cause tracheal obstruction), exophthalmos, stare, craniosynostosis (usually coronal), flushing, congestive heart failure, tachycardia, arrhythmias, hypertension, hypoglycemia, thrombocytopenia, and hepatosplenomegaly. Treatment includes propylthiouracil, iodine drops, and propranolol. Autoimmune neonatal hyperthyroidism usually resolves in 2 to 4 months.

### TABLE 59-2 Problems of Diabetic Pregnancy

#### MATERNAL

Ketoacidosis
Hyperglycemia/hypoglycemia
Nephritis
Preeclampsia
Polyhydramnios
Retinopathy

#### NEONATAL

Birth asphyxia
Birth injury (macrosomia, shoulder dystocia)
Congenital anomalies (lumbosacral dysgenesis—caudal regression)
Congenital heart disease (ventricular and atrial septal defects, transposition of the great arteries, truncus arteriosus, double-outlet right ventricle, coarctation of the aorta)
Hyperbilirubinemia (unconjugated)
Hypocalcemia
Hypoglycemia
Hypomagnesemia
Neurologic disorders (neural tube defects, holoprosencephaly)
Organomegaly
Polycythemia (hyperviscosity)
Renal disorders (double ureter, renal vein thrombosis, hydronephrosis, renal agenesis)
Respiratory distress syndrome
Small left colon syndrome
Transient tachypnea of the newborn

### TABLE 59-3 Common Teratogenic Drugs

| Drug | Results |
| --- | --- |
| Alcohol | Fetal alcohol syndrome, microcephaly, congenital heart disease |
| Aminopterin | Mesomelia, cranial dysplasia |
| Coumarin | Hypoplastic nasal bridge, chondrodysplasia punctata |
| Fluoxetine | Minor malformations, low birth weight, poor neonatal adaptation |
| Folic acid antagonists* | Neural tube, cardiovascular, renal, and oral cleft defects |
| Isotretinoin (Accutane) and vitamin A | Facial and ear anomalies, congenital heart disease |
| Lithium | Ebstein anomaly |
| Methyl mercury | Microcephaly, blindness, deafness, retardation (Minamata disease) |
| Misoprostol | Arthrogryposis |
| Penicillamine | Cutis laxa syndrome |
| Phenytoin (Dilantin) | Hypoplastic nails, intrauterine growth restriction, typical facies |
| Radioactive iodine | Fetal hypothyroidism |
| Radiation | Microcephaly |
| Stilbestrol (DES) | Vaginal adenocarcinoma during adolescence |
| Streptomycin | Deafness |
| Testosterone-like drugs | Virilization of female |
| Tetracycline | Enamel hypoplasia |
| Thalidomide | Phocomelia |
| Toluene (solvent abuse) | Fetal alcohol–like syndrome, preterm labor |
| Trimethadione | Congenital anomalies, typical facies |
| Valproate | Spina bifida |
| Vitamin D | Supravalvular aortic stenosis |

*Trimethoprim, triamterene, phenytoin, primidone, phenobarbital, carbamazepine.

## DIABETES MELLITUS

Diabetes mellitus that develops during pregnancy (*gestational diabetes* is noted in about 5% of women) or diabetes that is present before pregnancy adversely influences fetal and neonatal well-being. The effect of diabetes on the fetus depends in part on the severity of the diabetic state: age of onset of diabetes, duration of treatment with insulin, and presence of vascular disease. Poorly controlled maternal diabetes leads to maternal and fetal hyperglycemia that stimulates the fetal pancreas, resulting in hyperplasia of the islets of Langerhans. Fetal hyperinsulinemia results in increased fat and protein synthesis and fetal macrosomia, producing a fetus that is large for gestational age. After birth, hyperinsulinemia persists, resulting in fasting neonatal hypoglycemia. Strictly controlling maternal diabetes during pregnancy and preventing hyperglycemia during labor and delivery prevent macrosomic fetal growth and neonatal hypoglycemia. Additional problems of the diabetic mother and her fetus and newborn are summarized in Table 59-2.

## OTHER CONDITIONS

Other maternal illnesses, such as severe pulmonary disease (cystic fibrosis), cyanotic heart disease, and sickle cell anemia, may reduce oxygen availability to the fetus. Severe hypertensive or diabetic vasculopathy can result in uteroplacental insufficiency. In addition to the fact that the fetus is directly affected by maternal illnesses, the fetus and the newborn may be adversely affected by the medications used to treat the maternal illnesses. These effects may appear as teratogenesis (Table 59-3) or as an adverse metabolic, neurologic, or cardiopulmonary adaptation to extrauterine life (Table 59-4). Acquired infectious diseases of the mother also may affect the fetus or newborn adversely.

**TABLE 59-4  Agents Acting on Pregnant Women That May Adversely Affect the Newborn Infant**

| Agent | Potential Condition(s) |
|---|---|
| Acebutolol | IUGR, hypotension, bradycardia |
| Acetazolamide | Metabolic acidosis |
| Adrenal corticosteroids | Adrenocortical failure (rare) |
| Amiodarone | Bradycardia, hypothyroidism |
| Anesthetic agents (volatile) | CNS depression |
| Aspirin | Neonatal bleeding, prolonged gestation |
| Atenolol | IUGR, hypoglycemia |
| Blue cohosh herbal tea | Neonatal heart failure |
| Bromides | Rash, CNS depression, IUGR |
| Captopril, enalapril | Transient anuric renal failure, oligohydramnios |
| Caudal-paracervical anesthesia with mepivacaine (accidental introduction of anesthetic into scalp of infant) | Bradypnea, apnea, bradycardia, convulsions |
| Cholinergic agents (edrophonium, pyridostigmine) | Transient muscle weakness |
| CNS depressants (narcotics, barbiturates, benzodiazepines) during labor | CNS depression, hypotonia |
| Cephalothin | Positive direct Coombs test reaction |
| Fluoxetine | Possible transient neonatal withdrawal, hypertonicity, minor anomalies |
| Haloperidol | Withdrawal |
| Hexamethonium bromide | Paralytic ileus |
| Ibuprofen | Oligohydramnios, PPHN |
| Imipramine | Withdrawal |
| Indomethacin | Oliguria, oligohydramnios, intestinal perforation, PPHN |
| Intravenous fluids during labor (e.g., salt-free solutions) | Electrolyte disturbances, hyponatremia, hypoglycemia |
| Iodide (radioactive) | Goiter |
| Iodides | Neonatal goiter |
| Lead | Reduced intellectual function |
| Magnesium sulfate | Respiratory depression, meconium plug, hypotonia |
| Methimazole | Goiter, hypothyroidism |
| Morphine and its derivatives (addiction) | Withdrawal symptoms (poor feeding, vomiting, diarrhea, restlessness, yawning and stretching, dyspnea and cyanosis, fever and sweating, pallor, tremors, convulsions) |
| Naphthalene | Hemolytic anemia (in G6PD-deficient infants) |
| Nitrofurantoin | Hemolytic anemia (in G6PD-deficient infants) |
| Oxytocin | Hyperbilirubinemia, hyponatremia |
| Phenobarbital | Bleeding diathesis (vitamin K deficiency), possible long-term reduction in IQ, sedation |
| Primaquine | Hemolytic anemia (in G6PD-deficient infants) |
| Propranolol | Hypoglycemia, bradycardia, apnea |
| Propylthiouracil | Goiter, hypothyroidism |
| Reserpine | Drowsiness, nasal congestion, poor temperature stability |
| Sulfonamides | Interfere with protein binding of bilirubin; kernicterus at low levels of serum bilirubin, hemolysis with G6PD deficiency |
| Sulfonylurea | Refractory hypoglycemia |
| Sympathomimetic (tocolytic-β agonist) agents | Tachycardia |
| Thiazides | Neonatal thrombocytopenia (rare) |

CNS, central nervous system; G6PD, glucose-6-phosphate dehydrogenase; IUGR, intrauterine growth restriction; PPHN, persistent pulmonary hypertension of the newborn.

From Stoll BJ, Kliegman RM: The fetus and neonatal infant. In Behrman RE, Kliegman RM, Jenson HB, editors: Nelson Textbook of Pediatrics, 16th ed, Philadelphia, 2000, *Saunders.*

CHAPTER **60**

# Diseases of the Fetus

The principal determinants of fetal disease include the fetal genotype and the maternal in utero environment. Variation in environmental factors rather than the fetal genetics plays a more significant role in determining overall fetal well-being, although a genetically abnormal fetus may not thrive as well or survive. The ability to assess a fetus genetically, biochemically, and physically is greatly enhanced through the development of amniocentesis, fetoscopy, chorionic villus sampling, fetal blood sampling, and real-time ultrasonography. These techniques permit the early diagnosis and recognition of many fetal disorders and the development of therapeutic interventions.

## INTRAUTERINE GROWTH RESTRICTION AND SMALL FOR GESTATIONAL AGE

Fetuses subjected to abnormal maternal, placental, or fetal conditions that restrain growth are a high-risk group and traditionally classified as having intrauterine growth restriction (IUGR). Small for gestational age (SGA) is used as a synonym for IUGR; however, the terms *IUGR* and *SGA* are not synonymous. IUGR represents a deviation from expected growth patterns. The decreased fetal growth associated with IUGR is an adaptation to unfavorable intrauterine conditions that result in permanent alterations in metabolism, growth, and development. IUGR most frequently occurs with a variety of maternal conditions that are associated with preterm delivery. SGA describes an infant whose birth weight is statistically less than the 10th percentile or two standard deviations below the mean birth weight for gestational age. The cause of SGA may be pathologic, as in an infant with IUGR, or nonpathologic, as in an infant who is small but otherwise healthy (Table 60-1).

Only about 50% of IUGR infants are identified before delivery. Measurement and recording of maternal fundal height in conjunction with serial ultrasound assessment of the fetus (growth rate, amniotic fluid volume, malformations, anomalies, and Doppler velocimetry of uterine, placental, and fetal blood flow) can aid detection. When suspected and identified, IUGR and SGA fetuses must be monitored for fetal well-being, and appropriate maternal care needs to be instituted (see Chapter 58).

At birth, infants who are mildly to moderately SGA appear smaller than normal with decreased subcutaneous fat. More severely affected infants may present with a *wasted appearance* with asymmetrical findings, including larger heads for the size of the body (central nervous system sparing), widened anterior fontanelles, small abdomen, thin arms and legs, decreased subcutaneous fat, dry and redundant skin, decreased muscle mass, and thin (often meconium-stained) umbilical cord. Gestational age is often difficult to assess when based on physical appearance and perceived advanced neurologic maturity. Physical examination should detail the presence of dysmorphic

| **TABLE 60-1 Etiologies for Intrauterine Growth Restriction and Small for Gestational Age at Birth** |
|---|
| **MATERNAL FACTORS** |
| Age (young and advanced) |
| Cigarette smoking |
| Genetics (short stature, weight) |
| Illnesses during pregnancy (preeclampsia, severe diabetes, chronic hypertension, connective tissue disease) |
| Infections (intrauterine) |
| Lack of good prenatal care |
| Oligohydramnios |
| Poor nutrition |
| Race (African American) |
| **FETAL FACTORS** |
| Chromosomal abnormality and nonchromosomal syndromes |
| Congenital infections |
| Inborn errors of metabolism |
| Multiple gestations |
| Insulin resistance or reduced insulin or insulin-like growth factor-1 production |
| **MATERNAL MEDICATIONS** |
| Antimetabolites (methotrexate) |
| Heavy metals (mercury, lead) |
| Hydantoin |
| Narcotics (morphine, methadone) |
| Steroids (prednisone) |
| Substance and illicit drug use (alcohol, cocaine) |
| Warfarin |
| **PLACENTAL AND UTERINE ABNORMALITIES** |
| Abruptio placentae |
| Abnormal implantation |
| Abnormal placental vessels |
| Chorioangioma |
| Circumvallate placenta |
| Fetal vessel thrombosis |
| Ischemic villous necrosis |
| Multiple gestations |
| True knots in umbilical cord |
| Villitis (congenital infection) |

features, abnormal extremities, or gross anomalies that might suggest underlying congenital malformations, chromosomal defects, or exposure to teratogens. Hepatosplenomegaly, jaundice, and skin rashes in addition to ocular disorders, such as chorioretinitis, cataracts, glaucoma, and cloudy cornea, suggest the presence of a congenital infection or inborn error of metabolism. Infants with severe IUGR or SGA, particularly in conjunction with fetal distress, may have problems at birth that include respiratory acidosis, metabolic acidosis, asphyxia, hypoxemia, hypotension, hypoglycemia, polycythemia, meconium aspiration syndrome, and persistent pulmonary hypertension of the newborn.

Management of IUGR and SGA infants is usually symptomatic and supportive. The diagnostic evaluation at birth should be directed at identifying the cause of the IUGR and SGA if possible. The consequences of IUGR and SGA depend on the etiology, severity, and duration of growth retardation. The mortality rates of infants who are severely affected are 5 to 20 times those of infants who are appropriate for gestational age. Postnatal growth and development depend in part on the etiology, the postnatal nutritional intake, and the social environment. Infants who have IUGR and SGA secondary to congenital infection, chromosomal abnormalities, or constitutional syndromes remain small throughout life. Infants who have growth inhibited late in gestation because of uterine constraints, placental insufficiency, or poor nutrition have catch-up growth and approach their inherited growth and development potential under optimal environmental conditions.

## HYDROPS FETALIS

Hydrops fetalis is caused by immune and nonimmune conditions. Hydrops fetalis is a fetal clinical condition of excessive fluid accumulation in the skin and one or more other body compartments, including the pleural space, peritoneal cavity, pericardial sac, or placenta with resultant high morbidity and mortality. Hydrops initially was described in association with Rhesus blood group isoimmunization. The use of Rho (D) immune globulin has reduced the incidence of isoimmune fetal hydrops. Concurrently the incidence of nonimmune hydrops has increased as a cause of this severe clinical condition.

Fetal hydrops results from an imbalance of interstitial fluid accumulation and decreased removal of fluid by the capillaries and lymphatic system. Fluid accumulation can be secondary to congestive heart failure, obstructed lymphatic flow, or decreased plasma oncotic pressure (hypoproteinemic states). Edema formation is the final common pathway for many disease processes that affect the fetus, including fetal cardiac, genetic, hematologic, metabolic, infections, or malformation syndromes.

The diagnostic workup of the hydropic fetus should focus on discovering the underlying cause. Maternal findings may include hypertension, anemia, multiple gestation, thickened placenta, and polyhydramnios, whereas fetal findings may include tachycardia, ascites, scalp and body wall edema, and pleural and pericardial effusion. Invasive fetal testing may be indicated. Amniocentesis provides amniotic fluid samples for karyotype, culture, alpha-fetoprotein, and metabolic and enzyme analysis. Percutaneous umbilical cord blood sampling can provide fetal blood for chromosomal analysis and hematologic and metabolic studies and provide a source for intervention (fetal transfusion for profound anemia).

Management depends on the underlying cause and the gestational age of the fetus. Resuscitative efforts at delivery are often required. It is often necessary to remove ascitic fluid from the abdomen or pleural fluid to improve ventilation. Profound anemia necessitates immediate transfusion with packed red blood cells.

The overall mortality for infants with nonimmune hydrops is approximately 50%. If the diagnosis is made before 24 weeks of gestation with subsequent premature delivery, the survival rate is approximately 4% to 6%.

## CHAPTER 61

# Respiratory Diseases of the Newborn

Respiratory distress that becomes manifested by tachypnea, intercostal retractions, reduced air exchange, cyanosis, expiratory grunting, and nasal flaring is a nonspecific response to serious illness. Not all of the disorders producing neonatal respiratory distress are primary diseases of the lungs. The differential diagnosis of respiratory distress includes pulmonary, cardiac, hematologic, infectious, anatomic, and metabolic disorders that may involve the lungs directly or indirectly. Surfactant deficiency causes **respiratory distress syndrome (RDS)**, resulting in cyanosis and tachypnea; **infection** produces pneumonia, shown by interstitial or lobar infiltrates; **meconium aspiration** results in a chemical pneumonitis with hypoxia and pulmonary hypertension; **hydrops fetalis** causes anemia and hypoalbuminemia with high-output heart failure and pulmonary edema; and congenital or acquired **pulmonary hypoplasia** causes pulmonary hypertension and pulmonary insufficiency. It also is clinically useful to differentiate the common causes of respiratory distress according to gestational age (Table 61-1).

In addition to the specific therapy for the individual disorder, the supportive care and evaluation of the infant with respiratory distress can be applied to all the problems mentioned earlier (Table 61-2). Blood gas monitoring and interpretation are key components of general respiratory care.

Treatment of hypoxemia requires knowledge of normal values. In term infants, the arterial $PaO_2$ level is 55 to 60 mm Hg at 30 minutes of life, 75 mm Hg at 4 hours, and 90 mm Hg at 24 hours. Preterm infants have lower values. $PacO_2$ levels should be 35 to 40 mm Hg, and the pH should be 7.35 to 7.40. It is imperative that arterial blood gas analysis be performed in all infants with significant respiratory distress, whether or not cyanosis is perceived. Cyanosis becomes evident when there is 5 g of unsaturated hemoglobin; anemia may interfere with the perception of cyanosis. Jaundice also may interfere with the appearance of cyanosis. Capillary blood gas determinations are useful in determining blood pH and the $PacO_2$ level. Because of the nature of the heel-stick capillary blood gas technique, venous blood may mix with arterial blood, resulting in falsely low blood $PaO_2$ readings. Serial blood gas levels may be monitored by an indwelling arterial catheter placed in a peripheral artery or through the umbilical artery to the aorta at the level of the T6–10 or the L4–5 vertebrae. This placement avoids catheter occlusion of the celiac (T12), superior mesenteric (T12-L1), renal (L1–2), and inferior mesenteric (L2-3) arteries. Another method for monitoring blood gas levels is to combine capillary blood gas techniques with noninvasive methods used to monitor oxygen (pulse oximetry or transcutaneous oxygen diffusion).

**TABLE 61-1 Etiology of Respiratory Distress**

**PRETERM INFANT**

Respiratory distress syndrome (RDS)*
Erythroblastosis fetalis
Nonimmune hydrops
Pulmonary hemorrhage

**FULL-TERM INFANT**

Primary pulmonary hypertension of the neonate*
Meconium aspiration pneumonia*
Polycythemia
Amniotic fluid aspiration

**PRETERM AND FULL-TERM INFANT**

Bacterial sepsis (GBS)*
Transient tachypnea*
Spontaneous pneumothorax
Congenital anomalies (e.g., congenital lobar emphysema,
  cystic adenomatoid malformation, diaphragmatic hernia)
Congenital heart disease
Pulmonary hypoplasia
Viral infection (e.g., herpes simplex, CMV)
Inborn metabolic errors

*Common.
CMV, cytomegalovirus; GBS, group B streptococcus.

**TABLE 61-2 Initial Laboratory Evaluation of Respiratory Distress**

| Test | Rationale |
| --- | --- |
| Chest radiograph | To determine reticular granular pattern of RDS; to determine presence of pneumothorax, cardiomegaly, life-threatening congenital anomalies |
| Arterial blood gas | To determine severity of respiratory compromise, hypoxemia, and hypercapnia and type of acidosis; the severity determines treatment strategy |
| Complete blood count | Hemoglobin/hematocrit to determine anemia and polycythemia; white blood cell count to determine neutropenia/sepsis; platelet count and smear to determine DIC |
| Blood culture | To recover potential pathogen |
| Blood glucose | To determine presence of hypoglycemia, which may produce or occur simultaneously with respiratory distress; to determine stress hyperglycemia |
| Echocardiogram, ECG | In the presence of a murmur, cardiomegaly, or refractory hypoxia; to determine structural heart disease or PPHN |

DIC, disseminated intravascular coagulation; ECG, electrocardiogram; PPHN, primary pulmonary hypertension of the newborn; RDS, respiratory distress syndrome.

**Metabolic acidosis**, defined as a reduced pH ($<7.25$) and bicarbonate concentration ($<18$ mEq/L) accompanied by a normal or low $P_{CO_2}$ level, may be caused by hypoxia or by insufficient tissue perfusion. The origin of the disorder may be pulmonary, cardiac, infectious, renal, hematologic, nutritional, metabolic, or iatrogenic. The initial approach to metabolic acidosis is to determine the cause and treat the pathophysiologic problem. This approach may include, as in the sequence of therapy for hypoxia, increasing the inspired oxygen concentration; applying continuous positive airway pressure nasally, using oxygen as the gas; or initiating mechanical ventilation using positive end-expiratory pressure and oxygen. Patients with hypotension produced by hypovolemia require fluids and may need inotropic or vasoactive drug support. If metabolic acidosis persists despite specific therapy, sodium bicarbonate (1 mEq/kg/dose) may be given by slow intravenous infusion. Near-normal or low $P_{CO_2}$ levels should be documented before sodium bicarbonate infusion. The buffering effect of sodium bicarbonate results in increased $P_{CO_2}$ levels, unless adequate ventilation is maintained.

**Respiratory acidosis**, defined as an elevated $P_{CO_2}$ level and reduced pH without a reduction in the bicarbonate concentration, may be caused by pulmonary insufficiency or central hypoventilation. Most disorders producing respiratory distress can lead to hypercapnia. Treatment involves assisted ventilation but not sodium bicarbonate. If central nervous system depression of respirations is caused by placental passage of narcotic analgesics, assisted ventilation is instituted first, then the central nervous system depression is reversed by naloxone.

# RESPIRATORY DISTRESS SYNDROME (HYALINE MEMBRANE DISEASE)

RDS occurs after the onset of breathing and is associated with an insufficiency of pulmonary surfactant.

## Lung Development

The lining of the alveolus consists of 90% type I cells and 10% type II cells. After 20 weeks of gestation, the type II cells contain vacuolated, osmophilic, lamellar inclusion bodies, which are packages of surface-active material (Fig. 61-1). This lipoprotein surfactant is 90% lipid and is composed predominantly of saturated phosphatidylcholine (lecithin), but also contains phosphatidylglycerol, other phospholipids, and neutral lipids. The surfactant proteins SP-A, SP-B, SP-C, and SP-D are packaged into the lamellar body and contribute to surface-active properties and recycling of surfactant. Surfactant prevents atelectasis by reducing surface tension at low lung volumes when it is concentrated at end expiration as the alveolar radius decreases; surfactant contributes to lung recoil by increasing surface tension at larger lung volumes when it is diluted during inspiration as the alveolar radius increases. Without surfactant, surface tension forces are not reduced, and atelectasis develops during end expiration as the alveolus collapses.

The timing of surfactant production in quantities sufficient to prevent atelectasis depends on an increase in fetal cortisol levels that begins between 32 and 34 weeks

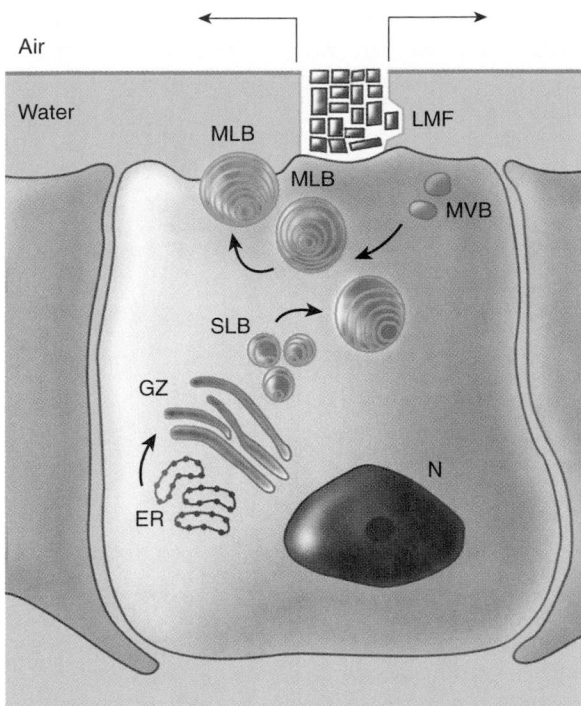

**FIGURE 61-1**

Proposed pathway of synthesis, transport, secretion, and reuptake of surfactant in the type II alveolar cell. Phospholipids are synthesized in the smooth endoplasmic reticulum (ER). The glucose/glycerol precursor may be derived from lung glycogen or circulating glucose. Phospholipids and surfactant proteins are packaged in the Golgi apparatus (GZ), emerge as small lamellar bodies (SLB), coalesce to mature lamellar bodies (MLB), migrate to the apical membrane, and are released by exocytosis into the liquid hypophase below the air-liquid interface. The tightly coiled lamellar body unravels to form the lattice (tubular) myelin figure (LMF), the immediate precursor to the phospholipid monolayer at the alveolar surface. Reuptake by endocytosis forms multivesicular bodies (MVB) that recycle surfactant. The enzymes, receptors, transporters, and surfactant proteins are controlled by regulatory processes at the transcriptional level in the nucleus (N). Corticosteroid and thyroid hormones are regulatory ligands that may accelerate surfactant synthesis. (From Hansen T, Corbet A: Lung development and function. In Taeusch HW, Ballard R, Avery ME, editors: Diseases of the Newborn, 6th ed, Philadelphia, 1991, *Saunders*, p 465.)

of gestation. By 34 to 36 weeks, sufficient surface-active material is produced by the type II cells in the lung, is secreted into the alveolar lumen, and is excreted into the amniotic fluid. The concentration of lecithin in amniotic fluid indicates fetal pulmonary maturity. Because the amount of lecithin is difficult to quantify, the ratio of lecithin (which increases with maturity) to sphingomyelin (which remains constant during gestation) (L/S ratio) is determined. An L/S ratio of 2:1 usually indicates pulmonary maturity. The presence of minor phospholipids, such as phosphatidylglycerol, also is indicative of fetal lung maturity and may be useful in situations in which the L/S ratio is borderline or possibly affected by maternal diabetes, which reduces lung maturity. The absence of phosphatidylglycerol suggests that surfactant might not be mature.

## Clinical Manifestations

A deficiency of pulmonary surfactant results in atelectasis, decreased functional residual capacity, arterial hypoxemia, and respiratory distress. Surfactant synthesis may be reduced as a result of hypovolemia, hypothermia, acidosis, hypoxemia, and rare genetic disorders of surfactant synthesis. These factors also produce pulmonary artery vasospasm, which may contribute to RDS in larger premature infants who have developed sufficient pulmonary arteriole smooth muscle to produce vasoconstriction. Surfactant deficiency–induced atelectasis causes alveoli to be perfused but not ventilated, which results in a pulmonary shunt and hypoxemia. As atelectasis increases, the lungs become increasingly difficult to expand, and lung compliance decreases. Because the chest wall of the premature infant is very compliant, the infant attempts to overcome decreased lung compliance with increasing inspiratory pressures, resulting in retractions of the chest wall. The sequence of decreased lung compliance and chest wall retractions leads to poor air exchange, an increased physiologic dead space, alveolar hypoventilation, and hypercapnia. A cycle of hypoxia, hypercapnia, and acidosis acts on type II cells to reduce surfactant synthesis and, in some infants, on the pulmonary arterioles to produce pulmonary hypertension.

Infants at greatest risk for RDS are premature and have an immature L/S ratio. The incidence of RDS increases with decreasing gestational age. RDS develops in 30% to 60% of infants between 28 and 32 weeks of gestation. Other risk factors include delivery of a previous preterm infant with RDS, maternal diabetes, hypothermia, fetal distress, asphyxia, male sex, white race, being the second born of twins, and delivery by cesarean section without labor.

RDS may develop immediately in the delivery room in extremely immature infants at 26 to 30 weeks of gestation. Some more mature infants (34 weeks' gestation) may not show signs of RDS until 3 to 4 hours after birth, correlating with the initial release of stored surfactant at the onset of breathing accompanied by the ongoing inability to replace the surfactant owing to inadequate stores. **Manifestations** of RDS include cyanosis, tachypnea, nasal flaring, intercostal and sternal retractions, and grunting. Grunting is caused by closure of the glottis during expiration, the effect of which is to maintain lung volume (decreasing atelectasis) and gas exchange during exhalation. Atelectasis is well documented by radiographic examination of the chest, which shows a ground-glass haze in the lung surrounding air-filled bronchi (the air bronchogram) (Fig. 61-2). Severe RDS may show an airless lung field or a *whiteout* on a radiograph, even obliterating the distinction between the atelectatic lungs and the heart.

During the first 72 hours, infants with RDS have increasing distress and hypoxemia. In infants with severe RDS, the development of edema, apnea, and respiratory failure necessitates assisted ventilation. Thereafter, uncomplicated cases show a spontaneous improvement that often is heralded by diuresis and a marked resolution of edema. Complications include the development of a pneumothorax, a patent ductus arteriosus (PDA), and bronchopulmonary dysplasia (BPD). The differential diagnosis of RDS includes diseases associated with cyanosis and respiratory distress (see Table 58-10).

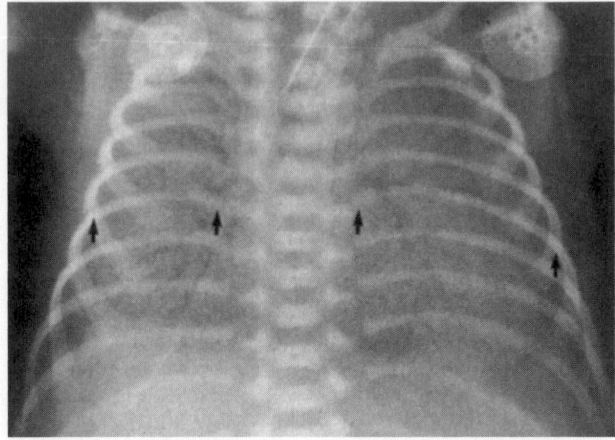

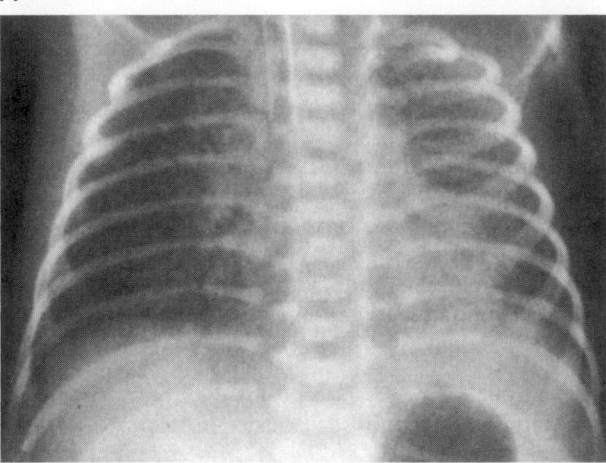

**FIGURE 61-2**

Respiratory distress syndrome. The infant is intubated, and the lungs show a dense reticulonodular pattern with air bronchograms (**A**). To evaluate rotation on the frontal chest, the lengths of the posterior ribs are compared from left to right (*arrows*). Because the infant is supine, the side of the longer ribs indicates to which side the thorax is rotated. In this case, the left ribs are longer, and this radiograph is a left posterior oblique view. Surfactant was administered, resulting in significant improvement in the density of the lung (**B**). The right lung is slightly better aerated than the left. Uneven distribution of clearing is common. (From Hilton S, Edwards D: Practical Pediatric Radiology, 2nd ed, Philadelphia, 1994, *Saunders.*)

## Prevention and Treatment

Strategies to prevent preterm birth include maternal cervical cerclage, bed rest, treatment of infections, and administration of tocolytic medications. Additionally, prevention of neonatal cold stress, birth asphyxia, and hypovolemia reduces the risk of RDS. If premature delivery is unavoidable, the antenatal administration of corticosteroids (e.g., betamethasone) to the mother (and thus to the fetus) stimulates fetal lung production of surfactant; this approach requires multiple doses for at least 48 hours.

After birth, RDS may be prevented or its severity reduced by intratracheal administration of exogenous surfactant immediately after birth in the delivery room or within a few hours of birth. A mammalian-derived surfactant is currently preferred. Exogenous surfactant can be administered repeatedly during the course of RDS in

patients receiving endotracheal intubation, mechanical ventilation, and oxygen therapy. Additional management includes the general supportive and ventilation care presented in Table 61-3.

The $PaO_2$ level should be maintained between 60 and 70 mm Hg (oxygen saturation 90%), and the pH should be maintained greater than 7.25. An increased concentration of warm and humidified inspired oxygen administered by an oxygen hood or nasal cannula may be all that is needed for larger premature infants. If hypoxemia ($PaO_2$ <50 mm Hg) is present, and the needed inspired oxygen concentration is 70% to 100%, nasal continuous positive airway pressure should be added at a distending pressure of 8 to 10 cm $H_2O$. If respiratory failure ensues ($Pco_2$ >60 mm Hg, pH <7.20, and $PaO_2$ <50 mm Hg with 100% oxygen), assisted ventilation using a respirator is indicated. Conventional rate (25 to 60 breaths/min), high-frequency jet (150 to 600 breaths/min), and oscillator (900 to 3000 breaths/min) ventilators all have been successful in managing respiratory failure caused by severe RDS. Suggested starting settings on a conventional ventilator are fraction of inspired oxygen, 60% to 100%; peak inspiratory pressure, 20 to 25 cm $H_2O$; positive end-expiratory pressure, 5 cm $H_2O$; and respiratory rate, 30 to 50 breaths/min.

In response to persistent hypercapnia, alveolar ventilation (tidal volume − dead space × rate) must be increased. Ventilation can be increased by an increase in the ventilator's rate or an increase in the tidal volume, which is the gradient between peak inspiratory pressure and positive end-expiratory pressure. In response to hypoxia, the inspired oxygen content may be increased. Alternatively, the degree of oxygenation depends on the mean airway pressure. Mean airway pressure is directly related to peak inspiratory pressure, positive end-expiratory pressure, flow, and inspiratory-to-expiratory ratio. Increased mean airway pressure may improve oxygenation by improving lung volume, enhancing ventilation-perfusion matching.

**TABLE 61-3  Potential Causes of Neonatal Apnea**

| | |
|---|---|
| Central nervous system | IVH, drugs, seizures, hypoxic injury |
| Respiratory | Pneumonia, obstructive airway lesions, atelectasis, extreme prematurity (<1000 g), laryngeal reflex, phrenic nerve paralysis, severe RDS, pneumothorax |
| Infectious | Sepsis, necrotizing enterocolitis, meningitis (bacterial, fungal, viral) |
| Gastrointestinal | Oral feeding, bowel movement, gastroesophageal reflux, esophagitis, intestinal perforation |
| Metabolic | ↓ Glucose, ↓ calcium, ↓ $Po_2$, ↓↑ sodium, ↑ ammonia, ↑ organic acids, ↑ ambient temperature, hypothermia |
| Cardiovascular | Hypotension, hypertension, heart failure, anemia, hypovolemia, change in vagal tone |
| Idiopathic | Immaturity of respiratory center, sleep state, upper airway collapse |

IVH, intraventricular hemorrhage; RDS, respiratory distress syndrome.

Because of the difficulty in distinguishing sepsis and pneumonia from RDS, broad-spectrum parenteral antibiotics (ampicillin and gentamicin) are administered for 48 to 72 hours, pending the recovery of an organism from a previously obtained blood culture.

## COMPLICATIONS OF RESPIRATORY DISTRESS SYNDROME

### Patent Ductus Arteriosus

PDA is a common complication that occurs in many low birth weight infants who have RDS. The incidence of PDA is inversely related to the maturity of the infant. In term newborns, the ductus closes within 24 to 48 hours after birth. However, in preterm newborns, the ductus frequently fails to close, requiring medical or surgical closure. The ductus arteriosus in a preterm infant is less responsive to vasoconstrictive stimuli, which when complicated with hypoxemia during RDS, may lead to a persistent PDA that creates a shunt between the pulmonary and systemic circulations.

During the acute phase of RDS, hypoxia, hypercapnia, and acidosis lead to pulmonary arterial vasoconstriction and increased pressure. The pulmonary and systemic pressures may be equal, and flow through the ductus may be small or bidirectional. When RDS improves and pulmonary vascular resistance declines, flow through the ductus arteriosus increases in a left-to-right direction. Significant systemic-to-pulmonary shunting may lead to heart failure and pulmonary edema. Excessive intravenous fluid administration may increase the incidence of symptomatic PDA. The infant's respiratory status deteriorates because of increased lung fluid, hypercapnia, and hypoxemia. In response to poor blood gas levels, the infant is subjected to higher inspired oxygen concentrations and higher peak inspiratory ventilator pressures, both of which can damage the lung and cause chronic lung disease.

**Clinical manifestations** of a PDA usually become apparent on day 2 to 4 of life. Because the left-to-right shunt directs flow to a low-pressure circulation from one of high pressure, the pulse pressure widens; a previously inactive precordium shows an extremely active precordial impulse, and peripheral pulses become easily palpable and bounding. The murmur of a PDA may be continuous in systole and diastole, but usually only the systolic component is auscultated. Heart failure and pulmonary edema result in rales and hepatomegaly. A chest radiograph shows cardiomegaly and pulmonary edema; a two-dimensional echocardiogram shows patency; and Doppler studies show markedly increased left-to-right flow through the ductus.

**Treatment** of a PDA during RDS involves initial fluid restriction and diuretic administration. If there is no improvement after 24 to 48 hours, indomethacin or ibuprofen, prostaglandin synthetase inhibitors, is administered. Contraindications to using indomethacin include thrombocytopenia (platelets <50,000/mm$^3$), bleeding, serum creatinine measuring more than 1.8 mg/dL, and oliguria. Because 20% to 30% of infants do not respond initially to indomethacin and because the PDA reopens in 10% to 20% of infants who do, a repeat course of indomethacin or surgical ligation is required in some patients.

### Pulmonary Air Leaks

Assisted ventilation with high peak inspiratory pressures and positive end-expiratory pressures may cause overdistention of alveoli in localized areas of the lung. Rupture of the alveolar epithelial lining may produce pulmonary interstitial emphysema as gas dissects along the interstitial space and the peribronchial lymphatics. Extravasation of gas into the parenchyma reduces lung compliance and worsens respiratory failure. Gas dissection into the mediastinal space produces a pneumomediastinum, occasionally dissecting into the subcutaneous tissues around the neck, causing subcutaneous emphysema.

Alveolar rupture adjacent to the pleural space produces a **pneumothorax** (Fig. 61-3). If the gas is under tension, the pneumothorax shifts the mediastinum to the opposite side of the chest, producing hypotension, hypoxia, and hypercapnia. The diagnosis of a pneumothorax may be based on unequal transillumination of the chest and may be confirmed by chest radiograph. Treatment of a symptomatic pneumothorax requires insertion of a pleural chest tube connected to negative pressure or to an underwater drain. Prophylactic or therapeutic use of exogenous surfactant has reduced the incidence of pulmonary air leaks.

Pneumothorax also is observed after vigorous resuscitation, meconium aspiration pneumonia, pulmonary hypoplasia, and diaphragmatic hernia. Spontaneous pneumothorax is seen in less than 1% of deliveries and may be associated with renal malformations.

### Bronchopulmonary Dysplasia (Chronic Lung Disease)

BPD is a clinical diagnosis defined by oxygen dependence at 36 weeks' postconceptual age and accompanied by characteristic clinical and radiographic findings that correspond to anatomic abnormalities. Oxygen concentrations

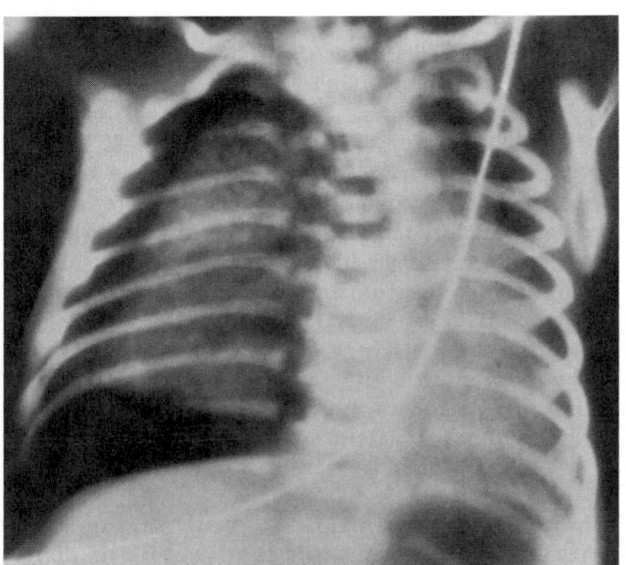

**FIGURE 61-3**

Pneumothorax. Right-sided hyperlucent pleural air is obvious. The findings of linear interstitial air and the resultant noncompliant but collapsed lung are noted. (From Heller RM, Kirchner SG: Advanced exercises in diagnostic radiology: The Newborn, Philadelphia, *WB Saunders*, 1979).

greater than 40% are toxic to the neonatal lung. Oxygen-mediated lung injury results from the generation of super-oxides, hydrogen peroxide, and oxygen free radicals, which disrupt membrane lipids. Assisted ventilation with high peak pressures produces barotrauma, compounding the damaging effects of highly inspired oxygen levels. In most patients, BPD develops after ventilation for RDS that may have been complicated by PDA or pulmonary interstitial emphysema. Inflammation from prolonged assisted ventilation and repeated systemic and pulmonary infections may play a major role. Failure of RDS to improve after 2 weeks, the need for prolonged mechanical ventilation, and oxygen therapy required at 36 weeks' postconception age are characteristic of patients with RDS in whom BPD develops. BPD also may develop in infants weighing less than 1000 g who require mechanical ventilation for poor respiratory drive in the absence of RDS. Fifty percent of infants of 24 to 26 weeks' gestational age require oxygen at 36 weeks' corrected age.

The **radiographic appearance** of BPD is characterized initially by lung opacification and subsequently by development of cysts accompanied by areas of overdistention and atelectasis, giving the lung a spongelike appearance. The histopathology of BPD reveals interstitial edema, atelectasis, mucosal metaplasia, interstitial fibrosis, necrotizing obliterative bronchiolitis, and overdistended alveoli.

The **clinical manifestations** of BPD are oxygen dependence, hypercapnia, compensatory metabolic alkalosis, pulmonary hypertension, poor growth, and development of right-sided heart failure. Increased airway resistance with reactive airway bronchoconstriction also is noted and is treated with bronchodilating agents. Severe chest retractions produce negative interstitial pressure that draws fluid into the interstitial space. Together with cor pulmonale, these chest retractions cause fluid retention, necessitating fluid restriction and the administration of diuretics.

Patients with severe BPD may need treatment with mechanical ventilation for many months. To reduce the risk of subglottic stenosis, a tracheotomy may be indicated. To reduce oxygen toxicity and barotrauma, ventilator settings are reduced to maintain blood gases with slightly lower $Pao_2$ (50 mm Hg) and higher $Paco_2$ (50 to 75 mm Hg) levels than for infants during the acute phase of RDS. Dexamethasone therapy may reduce inflammation, improve pulmonary function, and enhance weaning of patients from assisted ventilation. However, dexamethasone may increase the risk of cerebral palsy or abnormal neuromotor developmental outcome. Older survivors of BPD have hyperinflation, reactive airways, and developmental delay. They are at risk for severe respiratory syncytial virus pneumonia and as infants should receive prophylaxis against respiratory syncytial virus.

### Retinopathy of Prematurity (Retrolental Fibroplasia)

Retinopathy of prematurity (ROP) is caused by the acute and chronic effects of oxygen toxicity on the developing blood vessels of the premature infant's retina. The completely vascularized retina of the term infant is not susceptible to ROP. ROP is a leading cause of blindness in very low birth weight infants (<1500 g). Excessive arterial oxygen tensions produce vasoconstriction of immature retinal vasculature in the first stage of this disease. Vaso-obliteration follows if the duration and extent of hyperoxia are prolonged beyond the

time when vasoconstriction is reversible. Hypercarbia and hypoxia may contribute to ROP. The subsequent proliferative stages are characterized by extraretinal fibrovascular proliferation, forming a ridge between the vascular and avascular portions of the retina, and by the development of neovascular tufts. In mild cases, vasoproliferation is noted at the periphery of the retina. Severe cases may have neovascularization involving the entire retina, retinal detachment resulting from traction on vessels as they leave the optic disc, fibrous proliferation behind the lens producing leukokoria, and synechiae displacing the lens forward, leading to glaucoma. Both eyes usually are involved, but severity may be asymmetrical.

The incidence of ROP may be reduced by careful monitoring of arterial blood gas levels in all patients receiving oxygen. Although there is no absolutely safe $Pao_2$ level, it is wise to keep the arterial oxygen level between 50 and 70 mm Hg in premature infants. Infants who weigh less than 1500 g or who are born before 28 weeks' gestational age (some authors say 32 weeks) should be screened when they are 4 weeks of age or more than 34 weeks' corrected gestational age, whichever comes first. Laser therapy or (less often) cryotherapy may be used for vitreous hemorrhage or for severe, progressive vasoproliferation. Surgery is indicated for retinal detachment. Less severe stages of ROP resolve spontaneously and without visual impairment in most patients.

## TRANSIENT TACHYPNEA OF THE NEWBORN

Transient tachypnea of the newborn is a self-limited condition characterized by tachypnea, mild retractions, hypoxia, and occasional grunting, usually without signs of severe respiratory distress. Cyanosis, when present, usually requires treatment with supplemental oxygen in the range of 30% to 40%. Transient tachypnea of the newborn usually is noted in larger premature infants and in term infants born by precipitous delivery or cesarean section without prior labor. Infants of diabetic mothers and infants with poor respiratory drive as a result of placental passage of analgesic drugs are at risk. Transient tachypnea of the newborn may be caused by retained lung fluid or slow resorption of lung fluid. Chest radiographs show prominent central vascular markings, fluid in the lung fissures, overaeration, and occasionally a small pleural effusion. Air bronchograms and a reticulogranular pattern are not seen; their presence suggests another pulmonary process, such as RDS or pneumonia.

## MECONIUM ASPIRATION SYNDROME

Meconium-stained amniotic fluid is seen in 15% of predominantly term and post-term deliveries. Although the passage of meconium into amniotic fluid is common in infants born in the breech presentation, meconium-stained fluid should be considered clinically as a sign of fetal distress in all infants. The presence of meconium in the amniotic fluid suggests in utero distress with asphyxia, hypoxia, and acidosis.

Aspiration of amniotic fluid contaminated with particulate meconium may occur in utero in a distressed, gasping fetus; more often, meconium is aspirated into the lung immediately after delivery. Affected infants have abnormal chest radiographs, showing a high incidence of pneumonia and pneumothoraces.

**Meconium aspiration pneumonia** is characterized by tachypnea, hypoxia, hypercapnia, and small airway obstruction causing a ball-valve effect, leading to air trapping, overdistention, and extra-alveolar air leaks. Complete small airway obstruction produces atelectasis. Within 24 to 48 hours, a chemical pneumonia develops in addition to the mechanical effects of airway obstruction. Abnormal pulmonary function may be caused by the meconium in part through inactivation of surfactant. Primary pulmonary hypertension of the newborn (PPHN) frequently accompanies meconium aspiration, with right-to-left shunting caused by increased pulmonary vascular resistance. The chest radiograph reveals patchy infiltrates, overdistention, flattening of the diaphragm, increased anteroposterior diameter, and a high incidence of pneumomediastinum and pneumothoraces. Comorbid diseases include those associated with in utero asphyxia that initiated the passage of meconium.

**Treatment** of meconium aspiration includes general supportive care and assisted ventilation. Infants with a PPHN-like presentation should be treated for PPHN. If severe hypoxia does not subside with conventional or high-frequency ventilation, surfactant therapy, and inhaled nitric oxide, extracorporeal membrane oxygenation (ECMO) may be beneficial.

Prevention of meconium aspiration syndrome involves careful in utero monitoring to prevent asphyxia. When meconium-stained fluid is observed, the obstetrician should suction the infant's oropharynx before delivering the rest of the infant's body. If the infant is depressed with poor tone, minimal respiratory effort, and cyanosis, the infant's oropharynx should be suctioned, the vocal cords visualized, and the area below the vocal cords suctioned to remove any meconium from the trachea. This procedure can be repeated two to three times as long as meconium is present, before either stimulating the infant to breathe or initiating assisted ventilation. Saline intrauterine amnioinfusion during labor may reduce the incidence of aspiration and pneumonia.

## PRIMARY PULMONARY HYPERTENSION OF THE NEWBORN

PPHN occurs in post-term, term, or near-term infants. PPHN is characterized by severe hypoxemia, without evidence of parenchymal lung or structural heart disease that also may cause right-to-left shunting. PPHN is often seen with asphyxia or meconium-stained fluid. The chest radiograph usually reveals normal lung fields rather than the expected infiltrates and hyperinflation that may accompany meconium aspiration. Additional problems that may lead to PPHN are congenital pneumonia, hyperviscosity-polycythemia, congenital diaphragmatic hernia, pulmonary hypoplasia, congenital cyanotic heart disease, hypoglycemia, and hypothermia. Total anomalous venous return associated with obstruction of blood flow may produce a clinical picture that involves severe hypoxia and that is indistinguishable from PPHN; however, a chest radiograph reveals severe pulmonary venous engorgement and a small heart. Echocardiography or cardiac catheterization confirms the diagnosis.

Significant right-to-left shunting through a patent foramen ovale, through a PDA, and through intrapulmonary channels is characteristic of PPHN. The pulmonary vasculature often shows hypertrophied arterial wall smooth muscle, suggesting that the process of or predisposition to PPHN began in utero as a result of previous periods of fetal hypoxia. After birth, hypoxia, hypercapnia, and acidosis exacerbate pulmonary artery vasoconstriction, leading to further hypoxia and acidosis. Some infants with PPHN have extrapulmonary manifestations as a result of asphyxia. Myocardial injuries include heart failure, transient mitral insufficiency, and papillary muscle or myocardial infarction. Thrombocytopenia, right atrial thrombi, and pulmonary embolism also may be noted.

The **diagnosis** is confirmed by echocardiographic examination, which shows elevated pulmonary artery pressures and sites of right-to-left shunting. Echocardiography also rules out structural congenital heart disease and transient myocardial dysfunction.

**Treatment** involves general supportive care; correction of hypotension, anemia, and acidosis; and management of complications associated with asphyxia. If myocardial dysfunction is present, dopamine or dobutamine is needed. The most important therapy for PPHN is assisted ventilation. Reversible mild pulmonary hypertension may respond to conventional assisted ventilation. Patients with severe PPHN do not always respond to conventional therapy. Paralysis with pancuronium may be needed to assist such vigorous ventilation. Surfactant replacement seems to have no effect when PPHN is the primary diagnosis. If mechanical ventilation and supportive care are unsuccessful in improving oxygenation, inhaled nitric oxide, a selective pulmonary artery vasodilating agent, should be administered. If hypoxia persists, the patient may be a candidate for ECMO. Infants who require extremely high ventilator settings, marked by an alveolar-to-arterial oxygen gradient greater than 620 mm Hg, have a high mortality rate and benefit from ECMO if they do not respond to nitric oxide. In addition, the oxygenation index (OI) is used to assess the severity of hypoxemia and to guide the timing of interventions such as inhaled nitric oxide and ECMO. The OI is calculated using the equation: OI = [(mean airway pressure × fraction of inspired oxygen)/$PaO_2$] × 100. A high OI indicates severe hypoxemic respiratory failure.

## APNEA OF PREMATURITY

Although apnea typically is associated with immaturity of the respiratory control system, it also may be the presenting sign of other diseases or pathophysiologic states that affect preterm infants (see Table 61-3). A thorough consideration of possible causes is always warranted, especially with the onset or unexpected increase in the frequency of episodes of apnea (or bradycardia).

Apnea is defined as the cessation of pulmonary airflow for a specific time interval, usually longer than 10 to 20 seconds. Bradycardia often accompanies prolonged apnea. **Central apnea** refers to a complete cessation of airflow and respiratory efforts with no chest wall movement. **Obstructive apnea** refers to the absence of noticeable airflow but with the continuation of chest wall movements. **Mixed apnea**, a combination of these two events, is the most frequent type. It may begin as a brief episode of obstruction followed by a central apnea. Alternatively, central apnea may produce upper airway closure (passive pharyngeal hypotonia), resulting in mixed apnea.

A careful evaluation to determine the cause of apnea should be performed immediately in any infant with apnea. The incidence of apnea increases as gestational age decreases. Idiopathic apnea, a disease of premature infants, appears in the absence of any other identifiable disease states during the first week of life and usually resolves by 36 to 40 weeks of postconceptional age (gestational age at birth + postnatal age). The premature infant's process of regulating respiration is especially vulnerable to apnea. Preterm infants respond paradoxically to hypoxia by developing apnea rather than by increasing respirations as do mature infants. Poor tone of the laryngeal muscles also may lead to collapse of the upper airway, causing obstruction. Isolated obstructive apnea also may occur as a result of flexion or extreme lateral positioning of the premature infant's head, which obstructs the soft trachea.

**Treatment** of apnea of prematurity involves administration of oxygen to hypoxic infants, transfusion of anemic infants, and physical cutaneous stimulation for infants with mild apnea. Methylxanthines (caffeine or theophylline) are the mainstay of pharmacologic treatment of apnea. Xanthine therapy increases minute ventilation, improves the carbon dioxide sensitivity, decreases hypoxic depression of breathing, enhances diaphragmatic activity, and decreases periodic breathing. Treatment usually is initiated with a loading dose followed by maintenance therapy. High-flow nasal cannula therapy and nasal continuous positive airway pressure of 4 to 6 cm $H_2O$ also are effective and relatively safe methods of treating obstructive or mixed apneas; they may work by stimulating the infant and splinting the upper airway. Continuous positive airway pressure also probably increases functional residual capacity, improving oxygenation.

## MISCELLANEOUS RESPIRATORY DISORDERS

Pulmonary hypoplasia becomes manifested in the delivery room as severe respiratory distress that progresses rapidly to pulmonary insufficiency. The lungs, which are very small, develop pneumothoraces with normal resuscitative efforts. A small chest size radiographically, joint contractures, and early onset of pneumothoraces (often bilateral) are early clues to the diagnosis. Pulmonary hypertension results from the decreased lung mass and hypertrophy of pulmonary arteriole muscle.

**Pulmonary hypoplasia** may be a result of asphyxiating thoracic dystrophies (a small chest wall) or of decreased amniotic fluid volume that causes uterine compression of the developing chest wall, inhibiting lung growth. The latter failure of lung development may be associated with renal agenesis (Potter syndrome) or with a chronic leak of amniotic fluid from ruptured membranes. Isolated agenesis of one lung (usually the left lung) often is asymptomatic and familial. In contrast, serious pulmonary hypoplasia is noted in patients with a diaphragmatic hernia. Herniated bowel interferes with lung growth and leads to hypertrophy of the muscle layers of small pulmonary arteries, producing pulmonary hypertension. Pneumothoraces are common. Treatment of congenital diaphragmatic hernia involves surgical evacuation of the chest and repair of the diaphragmatic defect after the pulmonary hypertension is treated. Respiratory care is similar to that for patients with PPHN. **Neuromuscular diseases** that interfere with fetal breathing movements also may produce pulmonary hypoplasia

(e.g., congenital anterior horn cell disease [Werdnig-Hoffmann syndrome]). Another cause of bilateral pulmonary hypoplasia is hydrops fetalis (see Chapter 60). Hydrops from any cause is characterized by anasarca, ascites, and pleural and pericardial effusions. Bilateral pleural effusions act as space-occupying masses that interfere with lung growth, resulting in pulmonary hypoplasia.

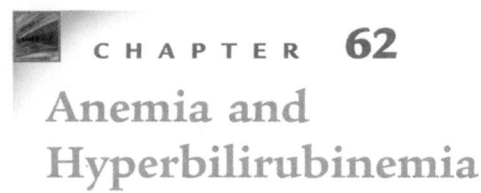

CHAPTER **62**

# Anemia and Hyperbilirubinemia

## ANEMIA

Embryonic hematopoiesis begins by the 20th day of gestation and is evidenced as blood islands in the yolk sac. In midgestation, erythropoiesis occurs in the liver and spleen; the bone marrow becomes the predominant site in the last trimester. Hemoglobin concentration increases from 8 to 10 g/dL at 12 weeks to 16.5 to 18 g/dL at 40 weeks. Fetal red blood cell (RBC) production is responsive to erythropoietin, and the concentration of this hormone increases with fetal hypoxia and anemia.

After birth, hemoglobin levels increase transiently at 6 to 12 hours, then decline to 11 to 12 g/dL at 3 to 6 months. A premature infant (<32 weeks' gestational age) has a lower hemoglobin concentration and a more rapid postnatal decline of hemoglobin level, which achieves a nadir 1 to 2 months after birth. Fetal and neonatal RBCs have a shorter life span (70 to 90 days) and a higher mean corpuscular volume (110 to 120 fL) than adult cells. In the fetus, hemoglobin synthesis in the last two trimesters of pregnancy produces fetal hemoglobin (hemoglobin F), composed of two alpha chains and two gamma chains. Immediately before term, the infant begins to synthesize beta-hemoglobin chains; the term infant should have some adult hemoglobin (two alpha chains and two beta chains). Fetal hemoglobin represents 60% to 90% of hemoglobin at term birth, and the levels decline to adult levels of less than 5% by 4 months of age.

For a term infant, blood volume is 72 to 93 mL/kg, and for a preterm infant, blood volume is 90 to 100 mL/kg. The placenta and umbilical vessels contain approximately 20 to 30 mL/kg of additional blood that can increase neonatal blood volume and hemoglobin levels transiently for the first 3 days of life if clamping or milking (*stripping*) of the umbilical cord is delayed at birth. Delayed clamping increases the risk of polycythemia, increased pulmonary vascular resistance, hypoxia, and jaundice, but it improves glomerular filtration. Early clamping may lead to anemia, a cardiac murmur, poor peripheral perfusion but lower pulmonary vascular pressures, and less tachypnea. Hydrostatic pressure affects blood transfer between the placenta and the infant at birth, and an undesired fetal-to-placental transfusion occurs if the infant is situated above the level of the placenta.

The physiologic anemia noted at 2 to 3 months of age in term infants and at 1 to 2 months of age in preterm infants is a normal process that does not result in signs of illness and does not require any treatment. It is a physiologic condition believed to be related to several factors, including increased tissue oxygenation experienced at birth, shortened RBC life span, and low erythropoietin levels.

### Etiology

Symptomatic anemia in the newborn period (Fig. 62-1) may be caused by decreased RBC production, increased RBC destruction, or blood loss.

### Decreased Red Blood Cell Production

Anemia caused by decreased production of RBCs appears at birth with pallor, a low reticulocyte count, and absence of erythroid precursors in the bone marrow. Potential causes of neonatal decreased RBC production include bone marrow failure syndromes (congenital RBC aplasia [Diamond-Blackfan anemia]), infection (congenital viral infections [parvovirus, rubella], acquired bacterial or viral sepsis), nutritional deficiencies (protein, iron, folate, vitamin $B_{12}$), and congenital leukemia.

### Increased Red Blood Cell Destruction

Immunologically mediated hemolysis in utero may lead to **erythroblastosis fetalis**, or the fetus may be spared, and **hemolytic disease** may appear in the newborn. Hemolysis of fetal erythrocytes is a result of blood group differences between the sensitized mother and fetus, which causes production of maternal IgG antibodies directed against an antigen on fetal cells.

**ABO blood group incompatibility** with neonatal hemolysis develops only if the mother has IgG antibodies from a previous exposure to A or B antigens. These IgG antibodies cross the placenta by active transport and affect the fetus or newborn. Sensitization of the mother to fetal antigens may have occurred by previous transfusions or by conditions of pregnancy that result in transfer of fetal erythrocytes into the maternal circulation, such as first trimester abortion, ectopic pregnancy, amniocentesis, manual extraction of the placenta, version (external or internal) procedures, or normal pregnancy.

ABO incompatibility with sensitization usually does not cause fetal disease other than extremely mild anemia. It may produce **hemolytic disease of the newborn**, however, which is manifested as significant anemia and hyperbilirubinemia. Because many mothers who have

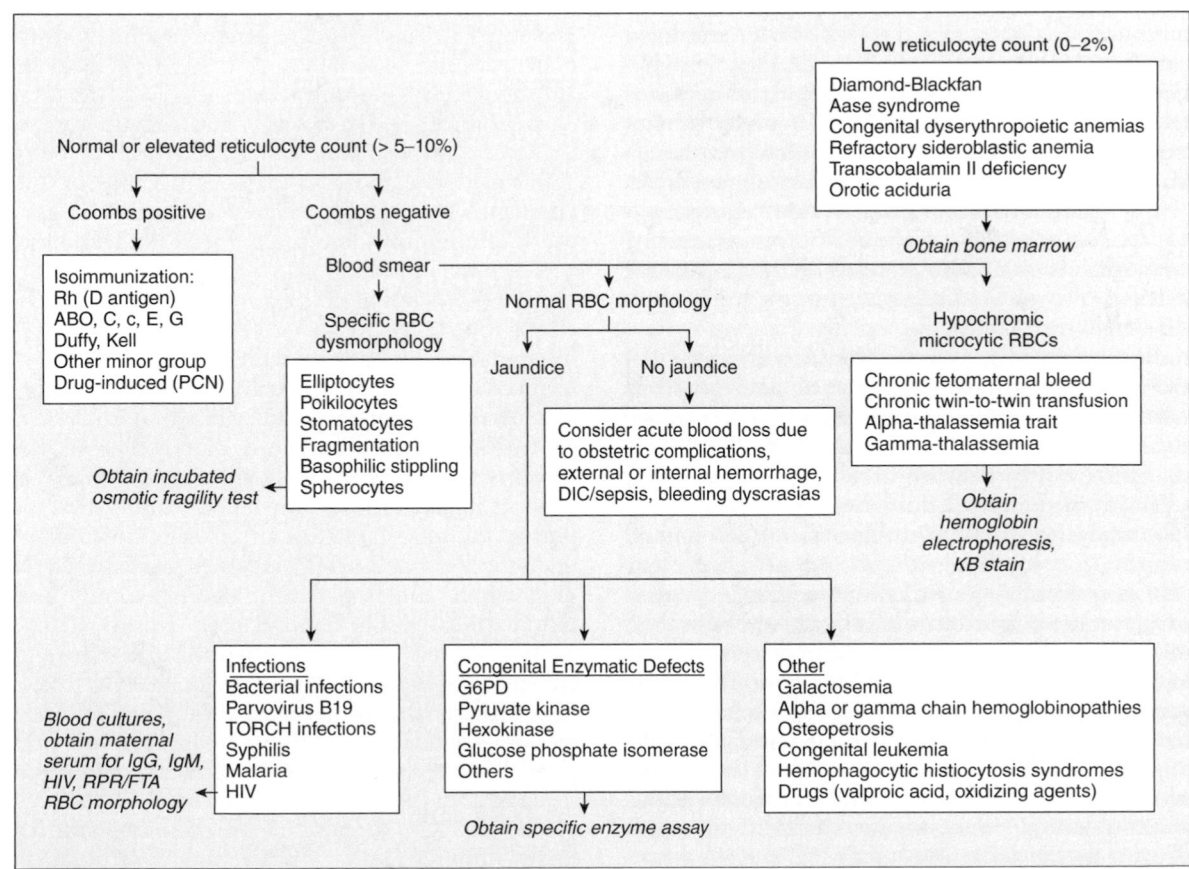

**FIGURE 62-1**

Differential diagnosis of neonatal anemia. The physician obtains information from the family, maternal and labor and delivery histories, and laboratory tests, including hemoglobin, reticulocyte count, blood type, direct Coombs test, peripheral smear, red blood cell (RBC) indices, and bilirubin concentration. DIC, disseminated intravascular coagulation; FTA, fluorescent treponemal antibody test; G6PD, glucose-6-phosphate dehydrogenase; KB, Kleihauer-Betke; PCN, penicillin; RPR, rapid plasma reagin tests. (From Ohls RK: Anemia in the neonate. In Christensen RD, editor: Hematologic Problems of the Neonate, Philadelphia, 2000, *Saunders*, p 162.)

blood group O have IgG antibodies to A and B before pregnancy, the firstborn infant of A or B blood type may be affected. In contrast to Rh disease, ABO hemolytic disease does not become more severe with subsequent pregnancies. Hemolysis with ABO incompatibility is less severe than hemolysis in Rh-sensitized pregnancy, either because the anti-A or anti-B antibody may bind to nonerythrocytic cells that contain A or B antigen or because fetal erythrocytes have fewer A or B antigenic determinants than they have Rh sites. With the declining incidence of Rh hemolytic disease, ABO incompatibility has become the most common cause of neonatal hyperbilirubinemia requiring therapy—currently accounting for approximately 20% of clinically significant jaundice in the newborn.

**Erythroblastosis fetalis** classically is caused by Rh blood group incompatibility. Most Rh-negative women have no anti-Rh antibodies at the time of their first pregnancy. The Rh antigen system consists of five antigens: C, D, E, c, and e; the d type is not antigenic. In most Rh-sensitized cases, the D antigen of the fetus sensitizes the Rh-negative (d) mother, resulting in IgG antibody production during the first pregnancy. Because most mothers are not sensitized to Rh antigens at the start of pregnancy, Rh erythroblastosis fetalis is usually a disease of the second and subsequent pregnancies. The first affected pregnancy results in an antibody response in the mother, which may be detected during antenatal screening with the Coombs test and determined to be anti-D antibody. The first affected newborn may show no serious fetal disease and may manifest hemolytic disease of the newborn only by the development of anemia and hyperbilirubinemia. Subsequent pregnancies result in an increasing severity of response because of an earlier onset of hemolysis in utero. Fetal anemia, heart failure, elevated venous pressure, portal vein obstruction, and hypoalbuminemia result in **fetal hydrops**, which is characterized by ascites, pleural and pericardial effusions, and anasarca (see Chapter 60). The risk of fetal death is high.

The **management** of a pregnancy complicated by Rh sensitization depends on the severity of hemolysis, its effects on the fetus, and the maturity of the fetus at the time it becomes affected. The severity of the hemolysis can be assessed by the quantity of bilirubin transferred from the fetus to the amniotic fluid, quantified by spectrophotometric analysis of the optical density (at 450 nm) of amniotic fluid.

Three zones of optical densities with decreasing slopes toward term gestation have been developed to predict the severity of the illness. The high optical density zone 3 is associated with severe hemolysis. Fetuses in the lower zones probably are not affected. If a fetus' optical density measurement for bilirubin falls into zone 3, and the fetus has pulmonary maturity as determined by the lecithin-to-sphingomyelin ratio, the infant should be delivered and treated in the neonatal intensive care unit. If the lungs are immature and the fetus is between 22 and 33 weeks of gestational age, an ultrasound-guided intrauterine transfusion with O-negative blood into the umbilical vein is indicated and may have to be repeated until pulmonary maturity is reached or fetal distress is detected. Indications for fetal intravascular transfusion in sensitized fetuses between 22 and 32 weeks of gestational age include a fetal hematocrit of less than 25% to 30%, fetal hydrops, and fetal distress too early in gestation for delivery. Intravascular intrauterine transfusion corrects fetal anemia, improves the outcome of severe hydrops, and reduces the need for postnatal exchange transfusion, but is associated with neonatal anemia as a result of continued hemolysis plus suppressed erythropoiesis.

**Prevention** of sensitization of the mother carrying an Rh-positive fetus is possible by treating the mother during gestation (>28 weeks' gestational age) and within 72 hours after birth with anti-Rh-positive immune globulin (RhoGAM). The dose of RhoGAM (300 μg) is based on the ability of this amount of anti-Rh-positive antibody to bind all the possible fetal Rh-positive erythrocytes entering the maternal circulation during the fetal-to-maternal transfusion at birth (approximately 30 mL). RhoGAM may bind Rh-positive fetal erythrocytes or interfere with maternal anti-Rh-positive antibody production by another, unknown mechanism. RhoGAM is effective only in preventing sensitization to the D antigen. Other blood group antigens that can cause immune hydrops and erythroblastosis include Rh C, E, Kell, and Duffy. Anti-Kell alloimmunity produces lower amniotic bilirubin levels and a lower reticulocyte count because in addition to hemolysis it inhibits erythropoiesis.

Nonimmune causes of hemolysis in the newborn include RBC enzyme deficiencies of the Embden-Meyerhof pathway, such as pyruvate kinase or glucose-6-phosphate dehydrogenase deficiency. RBC membrane disorders are another cause of nonimmune hemolysis. Hereditary spherocytosis is inherited as a severe autosomal recessive form or less severe autosomal dominant form and is the result of a deficiency of spectrin, a protein of the RBC membrane. Hemoglobinopathies, such as thalassemia, are another cause of nonimmunologically mediated hemolysis.

## Blood Loss

Anemia from blood loss at birth is manifested by two patterns of presentation, depending on the rapidity of blood loss. **Acute blood loss** after fetal-maternal hemorrhage, rupture of the umbilical cord, placenta previa, or internal hemorrhage (hepatic or splenic hematoma; retroperitoneal) is characterized by pallor, diminished peripheral pulses, and shock. There are no signs of extramedullary hematopoiesis and no hepatosplenomegaly. The hemoglobin content and serum iron levels initially are normal, but the hemoglobin levels decline during the subsequent 24 hours. Newborns with **chronic blood loss** caused by chronic fetal-maternal hemorrhage or a twin-to-twin transfusion present with marked pallor, heart failure, hepatosplenomegaly with or without hydrops, a low hemoglobin level at birth, a hypochromic microcytic blood smear, and decreased serum iron stores. Fetal-maternal bleeding occurs in 50% to 75% of all pregnancies, with fetal blood losses ranging from 1 to 50 mL; most blood losses are 1 mL or less, 1 in 400 are approximately 30 mL, and 1 in 2000 are approximately 100 mL.

The diagnosis of fetal-maternal hemorrhage is confirmed by the Kleihauer-Betke acid elution test. Pink fetal RBCs are observed and counted in the mother's peripheral blood smear because fetal hemoglobin is resistant to acid elution; adult hemoglobin is eluted, leaving discolored maternal cells (patients with sickle cell anemia or hereditary persistence of fetal hemoglobin may have a false-positive result, and ABO incompatibility may produce a false-negative result).

## Diagnosis and Management

Hemolysis in utero resulting from any cause may produce a spectrum of clinical manifestations at birth. Severe hydrops with anasarca, heart failure, and pulmonary edema may prevent adequate ventilation at birth, resulting in asphyxia. Infants affected with hemolysis in utero have hepatosplenomegaly and pallor and become jaundiced within the first 24 hours after birth. Less severely affected infants manifest pallor and hepatosplenomegaly at birth and become jaundiced subsequently. Patients with ABO incompatibility often are asymptomatic and show no physical signs at birth; mild anemia with jaundice develops during the first 24 to 72 hours of life.

Because hydrops, anemia, or jaundice are secondary to many diverse causes of hemolysis, a laboratory evaluation is needed in all patients with suspected hemolysis. A complete blood count, blood smear, reticulocyte count, blood type, and direct Coombs test (to determine the presence of antibody-coated RBCs) should be performed in the initial evaluation of all infants with hemolysis. Reduced hemoglobin levels, reticulocytosis, and a blood smear characterized by polychromasia and anisocytosis are expected with isoimmune hemolysis. Spherocytes commonly are observed in ABO incompatibility. The determination of the blood type and the Coombs test identify the responsible antigen and antibody in immunologically mediated hemolysis.

In the absence of a positive Coombs test and blood group differences between the mother and fetus, other causes of nonimmune hemolysis must be considered. RBC enzyme assays, hemoglobin electrophoresis, or RBC membrane tests (osmotic fragility, spectrin assay) should be performed. Internal hemorrhage also may be associated with anemia, reticulocytosis, and jaundice when the hemorrhage reabsorbs; ultrasound evaluation of the brain, liver, spleen, or adrenal gland may be indicated when nonimmune hemolysis is suspected. Shock is more typical in patients with internal hemorrhage, whereas in hemolytic diseases heart failure may be seen with severe anemia. Evaluation of a possible fetal-maternal hemorrhage should include the Kleihauer-Betke test.

The **treatment** of *symptomatic* neonatal anemia is transfusion of crossmatched packed RBCs. If immune hemolysis is present, the cells to be transfused must be crossmatched against maternal and neonatal plasma. Acute volume loss may necessitate resuscitation with nonblood products, such as saline if blood is not available; packed RBCs can be given subsequently. To correct anemia and any remaining blood volume deficit, 10 to 15 mL/kg of packed RBCs should be sufficient. Cytomegalovirus-seronegative blood should be given to cytomegalovirus-seronegative infants, and all blood products should be irradiated to reduce the risk of graft-versus-host disease; blood should be screened for HIV, hepatitis B and C, and syphilis. Recombinant erythropoietin may improve the hematocrit in infants with a hyporegenerative anemia after in utero transfusion.

## HYPERBILIRUBINEMIA

Hemolytic disease of the newborn is a common cause of neonatal jaundice. Nonetheless, because of the immaturity of the pathways of bilirubin metabolism, many newborn infants without evidence of hemolysis become jaundiced.

Bilirubin is produced by the catabolism of hemoglobin in the reticuloendothelial system. The tetrapyrrole ring of heme is cleaved by heme oxygenase to form equivalent quantities of biliverdin and carbon monoxide. Because no other biologic source of carbon monoxide exists, the excretion of this gas is stoichiometrically identical to the production of bilirubin. Biliverdin is converted to bilirubin by biliverdin reductase. One gram of hemoglobin produces 35 mg of bilirubin. Sources of bilirubin other than circulating hemoglobin represent 20% of bilirubin production; these sources include inefficient (shunt) hemoglobin production and lysis of precursor cells in bone marrow. Compared with adults, newborns have a twofold to threefold greater rate of bilirubin production (6 to 10 mg/kg/24 hr vs. 3 mg/kg/24 hr). This increased production is caused in part by an increased RBC mass (higher hematocrit) and a shortened erythrocyte life span of 70 to 90 days compared with the 120-day erythrocyte life span in adults.

Bilirubin produced after hemoglobin catabolism is lipid soluble and unconjugated and reacts as an indirect reagent in the van den Bergh test. Indirect-reacting, unconjugated bilirubin is toxic to the central nervous system and is insoluble in water, limiting its excretion. Unconjugated bilirubin binds to albumin on specific bilirubin binding sites; 1 g of albumin binds 8.5 mg of bilirubin in a newborn. If the binding sites become saturated or if a competitive compound binds at the site, displacing bound bilirubin, free bilirubin becomes available to enter the central nervous system. Organic acids such as free fatty acids and drugs such as sulfisoxazole can displace bilirubin from its binding site on albumin.

Bilirubin dissociates from albumin at the hepatocyte and becomes bound to a cytoplasmic liver protein Y (ligandin). Hepatic conjugation results in the production of bilirubin diglucuronide, which is water soluble and capable of biliary and renal excretion. The enzyme glucuronosyltransferase represents the rate-limiting step of bilirubin conjugation. The concentrations of ligandin and glucuronosyltransferase are lower in newborns, particularly in premature infants, than in older children.

Conjugated bilirubin gives a direct reaction in the van den Bergh test. Most conjugated bilirubin is excreted through the bile into the small intestine and eliminated in the stool. Some bilirubin may undergo hydrolysis back to the unconjugated fraction by intestinal glucuronidase, however, and may be reabsorbed (enterohepatic recirculation). In addition, bacteria in the neonatal intestine convert bilirubin to urobilinogen and stercobilinogen, which are excreted in urine and stool and usually limit bilirubin reabsorption. Delayed passage of meconium, which contains bilirubin, also may contribute to the enterohepatic recirculation of bilirubin.

Bilirubin is produced in utero by the normal fetus and by the fetus affected by erythroblastosis fetalis. Indirect, unconjugated, lipid-soluble fetal bilirubin is transferred across the placenta and becomes conjugated by maternal hepatic enzymes. The placenta is impermeable to conjugated water-soluble bilirubin. Fetal bilirubin levels become only mildly elevated in the presence of severe hemolysis, but may increase when hemolysis produces fetal hepatic inspissated bile stasis and conjugated hyperbilirubinemia. Maternal indirect (but not direct) hyperbilirubinemia also may increase fetal bilirubin levels.

## Etiology of Indirect Unconjugated Hyperbilirubinemia

**Physiologic jaundice** is a common cause of hyperbilirubinemia among newborns. It is a diagnosis of exclusion, made after careful evaluation has ruled out more serious causes of jaundice, such as hemolysis, infection, and metabolic diseases. Physiologic jaundice is the result of many factors that are normal physiologic characteristics of newborns: increased bilirubin production resulting from an increased RBC mass, shortened RBC life span, and hepatic immaturity of ligandin and glucuronosyltransferase. Physiologic jaundice may be exaggerated among infants of Greek and Asian ancestry.

The clinical pattern of physiologic jaundice in term infants includes a peak indirect-reacting bilirubin level of no more than 12 mg/dL on day 3 of life. In premature infants, the peak is higher (15 mg/dL) and occurs later (fifth day). The peak level of indirect bilirubin during physiologic jaundice may be higher in breast milk–fed infants than in formula-fed infants (15 to 17 mg/dL vs. 12 mg/dL). This higher level may be partly a result of the decreased fluid intake of infants fed breast milk. Jaundice is unphysiologic or pathologic if it is clinically evident on the first day of life, if the bilirubin level increases more than 0.5 mg/dL/hr, if the peak bilirubin is greater than 13 mg/dL in term infants, if the direct bilirubin fraction is greater than 1.5 mg/dL, or if hepatosplenomegaly and anemia are present.

**Crigler-Najjar syndrome** is a serious, rare, autosomal recessive, permanent deficiency of glucuronosyltransferase that results in severe indirect hyperbilirubinemia. Type II responds to enzyme induction by phenobarbital, producing an increase in enzyme activity and a reduction of bilirubin levels. Type I does not respond to phenobarbital and manifests as persistent indirect hyperbilirubinemia, often leading to kernicterus. Gilbert disease is caused by a mutation of the promoter region of glucuronosyltransferase and results in a mild indirect hyperbilirubinemia. In the presence of another icterogenic factor (hemolysis), more severe jaundice may develop.

**Breast milk jaundice** may be associated with unconjugated hyperbilirubinemia without evidence of hemolysis during the first to second week of life. Bilirubin levels rarely increase to more than 20 mg/dL. Interruption of breastfeeding for 1 to 2 days results in a rapid decline of bilirubin levels, which do not increase significantly after breastfeeding resumes. Breast milk may contain an inhibitor of bilirubin conjugation or may increase enterohepatic recirculation of bilirubin because of breast milk glucuronidase.

**Jaundice on the first day of life** is always pathologic, and immediate attention is needed to establish the cause. Early onset often is a result of hemolysis, internal hemorrhage (cephalhematoma, hepatic or splenic hematoma), or infection (Table 62-1). Infection also is often associated with direct-reacting bilirubin resulting from perinatal congenital infections or from bacterial sepsis.

Physical evidence of jaundice is observed in infants when bilirubin levels reach 5 to 10 mg/dL (vs. 2 mg/dL in adults). When jaundice is observed, the laboratory evaluation for hyperbilirubinemia should include a total bilirubin measurement to determine the magnitude of hyperbilirubinemia. Bilirubin levels greater than 5 mg/dL on the first day of life or greater than 13 mg/dL thereafter in term infants should be evaluated further with measurement of indirect and direct bilirubin levels, blood typing, Coombs test, complete blood count, blood smear, and reticulocyte count. These tests must be performed before treatment of hyperbilirubinemia with phototherapy or exchange transfusion. In the absence of hemolysis or evidence for either the common or the rare causes of nonhemolytic indirect hyperbilirubinemia, the diagnosis is either physiologic or breast milk jaundice. Jaundice present after 2 weeks of age is pathologic and suggests a direct-reacting hyperbilirubinemia.

## Etiology of Direct Conjugated Hyperbilirubinemia

Direct-reacting hyperbilirubinemia (defined as a direct bilirubin level >2 mg/dL or >20% of the total bilirubin) is never physiologic and should always be evaluated thoroughly according to the diagnostic categories (Table 62-2).

**TABLE 62-1 Etiology of Unconjugated Hyperbilirubinemia**

| | Hemolysis Present | Hemolysis Absent |
|---|---|---|
| Common | *Blood group incompatibility*: ABO, Rh, Kell, Duffy Infection | Physiologic jaundice, breast milk jaundice, internal hemorrhage, polycythemia, infant of diabetic mother |
| Rare | *Red blood cell enzyme defects*: glucose-6-phosphate dehydrogenase, pyruvate kinase *Red blood cell membrane disorders*: spherocytosis, ovalocytosis *Hemoglobinopathy*: thalassemia | Mutations of glucuronyl transferase enzyme (Crigler-Najjar syndrome, Gilbert disease), pyloric stenosis, hypothyroidism, immune thrombocytopenia |

**TABLE 62-2 Etiology of Conjugated Hyperbilirubinemia**

| COMMON |
| --- |
| Hyperalimentation cholestasis |
| CMV infection |
| Other perinatal congenital infections (TORCH) |
| Inspissated bile from prolonged hemolysis |
| Neonatal hepatitis |
| Sepsis |

| UNCOMMON |
| --- |
| Hepatic infarction |
| Inborn errors of metabolism (galactosemia, tyrosinemia) |
| Cystic fibrosis |
| Biliary atresia |
| Choledochal cyst |
| $\alpha_1$-Antitrypsin deficiency |
| Neonatal iron storage disease |
| Alagille syndrome (arteriohepatic dysplasia) |
| Byler disease |

CMV, cytomegalovirus; TORCH, toxoplasmosis, other, rubella, cytomegalovirus, herpes simplex.

Direct-reacting bilirubin (composed mostly of conjugated bilirubin) is not neurotoxic to the infant but signifies a serious underlying disorder involving cholestasis or hepatocellular injury. The diagnostic evaluation of patients with direct-reacting hyperbilirubinemia involves the determination of the levels of liver enzymes (aspartate aminotransferase, alkaline phosphatase, alanine aminotransferase, and γ-glutamyl transpeptidase), bacterial and viral cultures, metabolic screening tests, hepatic ultrasound, sweat chloride test, and occasionally liver biopsy. Additionally, the presence of dark urine and gray-white (acholic) stools with jaundice after the second week of life strongly suggests biliary atresia. The treatment of disorders manifested by direct bilirubinemia is specific for the diseases that are listed in Table 62-2. These diseases do not respond to phototherapy or exchange transfusion.

## Kernicterus (Bilirubin Encephalopathy)

Lipid-soluble, unconjugated, indirect bilirubin fraction is toxic to the developing central nervous system, especially when indirect bilirubin concentrations are high and exceed the binding capacity of albumin. Kernicterus results when indirect bilirubin is deposited in brain cells and disrupts neuronal metabolism and function, especially in the basal ganglia. Indirect bilirubin may cross the blood-brain barrier because of its lipid solubility. Other theories propose that a disruption of the blood-brain barrier permits entry of a bilirubin-albumin or free bilirubin–fatty acid complex.

Kernicterus usually is noted when the bilirubin level is excessively high for gestational age. It usually does not develop in term infants when bilirubin levels are less than 20 to 25 mg/dL, but the incidence increases as serum bilirubin levels exceed 25 mg/dL. Kernicterus may be noted at bilirubin levels less than 20 mg/dL in the presence of sepsis, meningitis, hemolysis, asphyxia, hypoxia, hypothermia, hypoglycemia, bilirubin-displacing drugs (sulfa drugs), and prematurity. Other risks for kernicterus in term infants are hemolysis, jaundice noted within 24 hours of birth, and delayed diagnosis of hyperbilirubinemia. Kernicterus has developed in extremely immature infants weighing less than 1000 g when bilirubin levels are less than 10 mg/dL because of a more permeable blood-brain barrier associated with prematurity.

The earliest clinical manifestations of kernicterus are lethargy, hypotonia, irritability, poor Moro response, and poor feeding. A high-pitched cry and emesis also may be present. Early signs are noted after day 4 of life. Later signs include bulging fontanelle, opisthotonic posturing, pulmonary hemorrhage, fever, hypertonicity, paralysis of upward gaze, and seizures. Infants with severe cases of kernicterus die in the neonatal period. Spasticity resolves in surviving infants, who may manifest later nerve deafness, choreoathetoid cerebral palsy, mental retardation, enamel dysplasia, and discoloration of teeth as permanent sequelae. Kernicterus may be prevented by avoiding excessively high indirect bilirubin levels and by avoiding conditions or drugs that may displace bilirubin from albumin. Early signs of kernicterus occasionally may be reversed by immediately instituting an exchange transfusion (see later).

## Therapy of Indirect Hyperbilirubinemia

**Phototherapy** is an effective and safe method for reducing indirect bilirubin levels, particularly when initiated before serum bilirubin increases to levels associated with kernicterus. In term infants, phototherapy is begun when indirect bilirubin levels are between 16 and 18 mg/dL. Phototherapy is initiated in premature infants when bilirubin is at lower levels, to prevent bilirubin from reaching the high concentrations necessitating exchange transfusion. Blue lights and white lights are effective in reducing bilirubin levels.

Under the effects of phototherapy light with maximal irradiance in the 425- to 475-nm wavelength band, bilirubin is transformed into isomers that are water soluble and easily excreted. Unconjugated bilirubin (IX) is in the 4Z, 15Z configuration. Phototherapy causes a photochemical reaction producing the reversible, more water-soluble isomer 4Z, 15E bilirubin IX. This isomer can be excreted easily, bypassing the liver's conjugation system. Another photochemical reaction results in the rapid production of lumirubin, a more water-soluble isomer than the aforementioned isomer, which does not spontaneously revert to unconjugated native bilirubin and can be excreted in urine.

Complications of phototherapy include an increased insensible water loss, diarrhea, and dehydration. Additional problems are macular-papular red skin rash, lethargy, masking of cyanosis, nasal obstruction by eye pads, and potential for retinal damage. Skin bronzing may be noted in infants with direct-reacting hyperbilirubinemia. Infants with mild hemolytic disease of the newborn occasionally may be managed successfully with phototherapy for hyperbilirubinemia, but care must be taken to follow these infants for the late occurrence of anemia from continued hemolysis.

**Exchange transfusion** usually is reserved for infants with dangerously high indirect bilirubin levels who are at risk for kernicterus. As a rule of thumb, a level of 20 mg/dL for indirect-reacting bilirubin is the *exchange number* for infants *with hemolysis* who weigh more than 2000 g. Asymptomatic infants with physiologic or breast milk jaundice may not require exchange transfusion, unless the indirect bilirubin level exceeds 25 mg/dL. The exchangeable level of indirect bilirubin for other infants may be estimated by calculating 10% of the birth weight in grams: the level in an infant weighing 1500 g would be 15 mg/dL. Infants weighing less than 1000 g usually do not require an exchange transfusion until the bilirubin level exceeds 10 mg/dL.

The exchange transfusion usually is performed through an umbilical venous catheter placed in the inferior vena cava or, if free flow is obtained, at the confluence of the umbilical vein and the portal system. The level of serum bilirubin immediately after the exchange transfusion declines to levels that are about half of those before the exchange; levels rebound 6 to 8 hours later as a result of continued hemolysis and redistribution of bilirubin from tissue stores.

**Complications** of exchange transfusion include problems related to the blood (transfusion reaction, metabolic instability, or infection), the catheter (vessel perforation or hemorrhage), or the procedure (hypotension or necrotizing enterocolitis [NEC]). Unusual complications include thrombocytopenia and graft-versus-host disease. Continuation of phototherapy may reduce the necessity for subsequent exchange transfusions.

## Polycythemia (Hyperviscosity Syndrome)

Polycythemia is an excessively high hematocrit (≥65%) and leads to hyperviscosity that produces symptoms related to vascular stasis, hypoperfusion, and ischemia. As the hematocrit increases from 40% to 60%, there is a small increase in blood viscosity. When the central hematocrit increases to greater than 65%, the blood viscosity begins to increase markedly, and symptoms may appear. Neonatal erythrocytes are less filterable or deformable than adult erythrocytes, which further contributes to hyperviscosity. A central venous hematocrit of 65% or greater is noted in 3% to 5% of infants. Infants at special risk for polycythemia are term and post-term small for gestational age infants, infants of diabetic mothers, infants with delayed cord clamping, and infants with neonatal hyperthyroidism, adrenogenital syndrome, trisomy 13, trisomy 18, trisomy 21, twin-to-twin transfusion syndrome (recipient), and Beckwith-Wiedemann syndrome. In some infants, polycythemia may reflect a compensation for prolonged periods of fetal hypoxia caused by placental insufficiency; these infants have increased erythropoietin levels at birth.

Polycythemic patients appear plethoric or ruddy and may develop acrocyanosis. Symptoms are a result of the increased RBC mass and of vascular compromise. Seizures, lethargy, and irritability reflect abnormalities of microcirculation of the brain, whereas hyperbilirubinemia may reflect the poor hepatic circulation or the increased

amount of hemoglobin that is being broken down into bilirubin. Additional problems include respiratory distress and primary pulmonary hypertension of the newborn (PPHN) that result in part from elevated pulmonary vascular resistance. The chest radiograph often reveals cardiomegaly, increased vascular markings, pleural effusions, and interstitial edema. Other problems are NEC, hypoglycemia, thrombocytopenia, priapism, testicular infarction, hemiplegic stroke, and feeding intolerance. Many of these complications also are related to the primary condition associated with polycythemia (small for gestational age infants are at risk for hypoglycemia and PPHN after periods of hypoxia in utero).

Long-term sequelae of neonatal polycythemia relate to neurodevelopmental abnormalities that may be prevented by treatment of symptomatic infants with partial exchange transfusion after birth. A partial exchange transfusion removes whole blood and replaces it with normal saline. The equation used to calculate the volume exchanged is based on the central venous hematocrit because peripheral hematocrits may be falsely elevated:

$$\text{Volume to exchange(mL)} = \frac{[\text{blood volume} \times (\text{observed hematocrit} - \text{desired hematocrit})]}{\text{observed hematocrit}}$$

The desired hematocrit is 50%, and the blood volume 85 mL/kg.

## COAGULATION DISORDERS

Disorders of coagulation are common in the neonatal period. Hemorrhage during this time may be a result of trauma, inherited permanent deficiency of coagulation factors, transient deficiencies of vitamin K–dependent factors, disorders of platelets, and disseminated intravascular coagulation (DIC) seen in sick newborns with shock or hypoxia. Thrombosis also is a potential problem in the newborn because of developmentally lower circulating levels of antithrombin III, protein C (a vitamin K–dependent protein that inhibits factors VIII and V), and the fibrinolytic system.

Coagulation factors do not pass through the placenta to the fetus, and newborn infants have relatively low levels of the vitamin K–dependent factors II, VII, IX, and X. Contact factors XI and XII, prekallikrein, and kininogen also are lower in newborns than in adults. Fibrinogen (factor I); plasma levels of factors V, VIII, and XIII; and platelet counts are within the adult normal range.

Because of the transient, relative deficiencies of the contact and vitamin K–dependent factors, the *partial thromboplastin time* (PTT), which is dependent on factors XII, IX, VIII, X, V, II, and I, is prolonged in the newborn period. Preterm infants have the most marked prolongation of the PTT (50 to 80 seconds) compared with term infants (35 to 50 seconds) and older, more mature infants (25 to 35 seconds). The administration of heparin and the presence of DIC, hemophilia, and severe vitamin K deficiency prolong the PTT.

The *prothrombin time* (PT), which is dependent on factors VII, X, V, II, and I, is a more sensitive test for vitamin K deficiency. The PT is only slightly prolonged in term infants (13 to 20 seconds) compared with pre-term infants (13 to 21 seconds) and more mature patients (12 to 14 seconds). Abnormal prolongations of the PT occur with vitamin K deficiency, hepatic injury, and DIC. Levels of *fibrinogen* and *fibrin degradation products* are similar in infants and adults. The *bleeding time*, which reflects platelet function and number, is normal during the newborn period in the absence of maternal salicylate therapy.

*Vitamin K* is a necessary cofactor for the carboxylation of glutamate on precursor proteins, converting them into the more active coagulation factors II, VII, IX, and X; γ-carboxyglutamic acid binds calcium, which is required for the immediate activation of factors during hemor-rhage. There is no congenital deficiency of hepatic syn-thesis of these precursor proteins, but in the absence of vitamin K their conversion to the active factor is not pos-sible. Levels of *protein induced by vitamin K absence* increase in vitamin K deficiency and are helpful diagnostic mar-kers; vitamin K administration rapidly corrects the coagu-lation defects, reducing protein induced by vitamin K absence to undetectable levels.

Although most newborns are born with reduced levels of vitamin K–dependent factors, hemorrhagic complica-tions develop only rarely. Infants at risk for **hemorrhagic disease of the newborn** have the most profound defi-ciency of vitamin K–dependent factors, and these factors decline further after birth. Because breast milk is a poor source of vitamin K, breastfed infants are at increased risk for hemorrhage that usually occurs between days 3 and 7 of life. Bleeding usually ensues from the umbilical cord, circumcision site, intestines, scalp, mucosa, and skin, but internal hemorrhage places the infant at risk for fatal complications, such as intracranial bleeding.

Hemorrhage on the first day of life resulting from a deficiency of the vitamin K–dependent factors often is associated with administration to the mother of drugs that affect vitamin K metabolism in the infant. This early pattern of hemorrhage has been seen with maternal war-farin or antibiotic (e.g., isoniazid or rifampin) therapy and in infants of mothers receiving phenobarbital and phenytoin. Bleeding also may occur 1 to 3 months after birth, particularly among breastfed infants. Vitamin K deficiency in breastfed infants also should raise suspi-cion about the possibility of vitamin K malabsorption resulting from cystic fibrosis, biliary atresia, hepatitis, or antibiotic suppression of the colonic bacteria that produce vitamin K.

Bleeding associated with vitamin K deficiency may be **prevented** by administration of vitamin K to all infants at birth. Before routine administration of vitamin K, 1% to 2% of all newborns have hemorrhagic disease of the newborn. One intramuscular dose (1 mg) of vitamin K prevents vitamin K–deficiency bleeding. **Treatment** of bleeding resulting from vitamin K deficiency involves intravenous administration of 1 mg of vitamin K. If severe, life-threatening hemorrhage is present, fresh fro-zen plasma also should be given. Unusually high doses of vitamin K may be needed for hepatic disease and for maternal warfarin or anticonvulsant therapy.

## Clinical Manifestations and Differential Diagnoses of Bleeding Disorders

Bleeding disorders in a newborn may be associated with cutaneous bleeding, such as cephalhematoma, subgaleal hemorrhage, ecchymosis, and petechiae. Facial petechiae are common in infants born by vertex presentation, with or without a nuchal cord, and usually are insignificant. Mucosal bleeding may appear as hematemesis, melena, or epistaxis. Internal hemorrhage results in organ-specific dysfunction, such as seizures, accompanied by intracranial hemorrhage. Bleeding from venipuncture or heel-stick sites, circumcision sites, or the umbilical cord also is common.

The differential diagnosis depends partly on the clinical circumstances associated with the hemorrhage. In a **sick newborn**, the differential diagnosis should include DIC, hepatic failure, and thrombocytopenia. Thrombocytopenia in an ill neonate may be secondary to consumption by trapping of platelets in a hemangioma (**Kasabach-Merritt syndrome**) or may be associated with perinatal, congeni-tal, or bacterial infections; NEC; thrombotic endocardi-tis; PPHN; organic acidemia; maternal preeclampsia; or asphyxia. Thrombocytopenia also may be due to periph-eral washout of platelets after an exchange transfusion. Treatment of a sick infant with thrombocytopenia should be directed at the underlying disorder, supplemented by infusions of platelets, blood, or both.

The etiology of DIC in a newborn includes hypoxia, hypotension, asphyxia, bacterial or viral sepsis, NEC, death of a twin while in utero, cavernous hemangioma, nonimmune hydrops, neonatal cold injury, neonatal neo-plasm, and hepatic disease. The treatment of DIC should be focused primarily on therapy for the initiating or underlying disorder. Supportive management of con-sumptive coagulopathy involves platelet transfusions and factor replacement with fresh frozen plasma. Heparin and factor C concentrate should be reserved for infants with DIC who also have thrombosis.

Disorders of hemostasis in a well child are not asso-ciated with systemic disease in a newborn but reflect coag-ulation factor or platelet deficiency. Hemophilia initially is associated with cutaneous or mucosal bleeding and no systemic illness. If bleeding continues, hypovolemic shock may develop. Bleeding into the brain, liver, or spleen may result in organ-specific signs and shock.

In a **well child**, thrombocytopenia may be part of a syndrome such as Fanconi anemia syndrome (involving hypoplasia and aplasia of the thumb), radial aplasia-thrombocytopenia syndrome (thumbs present), or Wiskott-Aldrich syndrome. Various maternal drugs also may reduce the neonatal platelet count without producing other adverse effects. These drugs include sulfonamides, quinidine, quinine, and thiazide diuretics.

The most common causes of thrombocytopenia in well newborns are transient isoimmune thrombocytopenia and transient neonatal thrombocytopenia in well infants born to mothers with idiopathic thrombocytopenic purpura (ITP). **Isoimmune thrombocytopenia** is caused by anti-platelet antibodies produced by the HPLA1-negative mother after her sensitization to specific paternal platelet antigen (HPA-1a and HPA-5b represent 85% and 10% of cases) expressed on the fetal platelet. The incidence is 1:1000 to 1:2000 births. This response to maternal-sensitized antibodies that produce isoimmune thrombocytopenia is analogous to the response that produces erythroblastosis fetalis. The maternal antiplatelet antibody does not produce maternal thrombocytopenia, but after crossing the placenta this IgG antibody binds to fetal platelets that are trapped by the reticuloendothelial tissue, resulting in thrombocytopenia. Infants with thrombocytopenia produced in this manner are at risk for development of petechiae, purpura, and intracranial hemorrhage (an incidence of 10% to 15%) before or after birth. Vaginal delivery may increase the risk of neonatal bleeding; cesarean section may be indicated.

Specific **treatment** for severe thrombocytopenia ($<20,000$ platelets/mm$^3$) or significant bleeding is transfusion of ABO-compatible and RhD-compatible, HPA-1a-negative and HPA-5b-negative maternal platelets. Because the antibody in isoimmune thrombocytopenia is directed against the fetal rather than the maternal platelet, plateletpheresis of the mother yields sufficient platelets for performing a platelet transfusion to treat the affected infant. After one platelet transfusion, the infant's platelet count dramatically increases and usually remains in a safe range. Without treatment, thrombocytopenia resolves during the first month of life as the maternal antibody level declines. *Treatment* of the mother with intravenous immunoglobulin or the thrombocytopenic fetus with intravascular platelet transfusion (cordocentesis) is also effective. Cesarean section reduces the risk of intracranial hemorrhage.

**Neonatal thrombocytopenia in infants born to women with ITP** also is a result of placental transfer of maternal IgG antibodies. In ITP, these autoantibodies are directed against all platelet antigens, and mother and newborn may have low platelet counts. The risks of hemorrhage in an infant born to a mother with ITP may be lessened by cesarean section and by treatment of the mother with corticosteroids.

**Treatment** of an affected infant born to a mother with ITP may involve prednisone and intravenous immunoglobulin. In an emergency, random donor platelets may be used and may produce a transient increase in the infant's platelet count. Thrombocytopenia resolves spontaneously during the first month of life as maternal-derived antibody levels decline. Elevated levels of platelet-associated antibodies also have been noted in thrombocytopenic infants with sepsis and thrombocytopenia of unknown cause who were born to mothers without demonstrable platelet antibodies.

The laboratory evaluation of an infant (well or sick) with bleeding must include a platelet count, blood smear, and evaluation of PTT and PT. Isolated thrombocytopenia in a well infant suggests immune thrombocytopenia. Laboratory evidence of DIC includes a markedly prolonged PTT and PT (minutes rather than seconds), thrombocytopenia, and a blood smear suggesting a microangiopathic hemolytic anemia (burr or fragmented blood cells). Further evaluation reveals low levels of fibrinogen ($<100$ mg/dL) and elevated levels of fibrin degradation products. Vitamin K deficiency prolongs the PT more than the PTT, whereas hemophilia resulting from factors VIII and IX deficiency prolongs only the PTT. Specific factor levels confirm the *diagnosis* of hemophilia.

CHAPTER 63

# Necrotizing Enterocolitis

**Necrotizing enterocolitis (NEC)** is a syndrome of intestinal injury and is the most common intestinal emergency occurring in preterm infants admitted to the neonatal intensive care unit. NEC occurs in 1 to 3 per 1000 live births and 1% to 7% of admissions to the neonatal intensive care unit. Prematurity is the most consistent and significant factor associated with neonatal NEC. The disease occurs in 10% of infants who weigh less than 1500 g at birth. NEC is infrequent in term infants ($<10\%$ of affected infants).

Most cases of NEC occur in premature infants born before 34 weeks' gestation who have been fed enterally. Prematurity is associated with immaturity of the gastrointestinal tract, including decreased integrity of the intestinal mucosal barrier, depressed mucosal enzymes, suppressed gastrointestinal hormones, suppressed intestinal host defense system, decreased coordination of intestinal motility, and differences in blood flow autoregulation, which is thought to play a significant role in the pathogenesis of NEC. More than 90% of infants diagnosed with NEC have been fed enterally; however, NEC has been reported in infants who have never been fed. Feeding with human milk has shown a beneficial role in reducing the incidence of NEC. In addition, probiotics may offer potential benefits for the preterm infant by increasing mucosal barrier function, improving nutrition, upregulating the immune system, and reducing mucosal colonization by potential pathogens. It also is theorized that compromised intestinal blood flow contributes to NEC.

Early clinical signs of NEC include abdominal distention, feeding intolerance/increased gastric residuals, emesis, rectal bleeding, and occasional diarrhea. As the disease progresses, patients may develop marked abdominal distention, bilious emesis, ascites, abdominal wall erythema, lethargy, temperature instability, increased episodes of apnea/bradycardia, disseminated intravascular coagulation, and shock. With abdominal perforation, the abdomen may develop a bluish discoloration.

The white blood cell count can be elevated, but often it is depressed. Thrombocytopenia is common. In addition, infants may develop coagulation abnormalities along with metabolic derangements, including metabolic acidosis, electrolyte imbalance, and hypoglycemia and hyperglycemia. No unique infectious agent has been associated with NEC; bacteriologic and fungal cultures may prove helpful but not conclusive.

**Radiographic imaging** is essential to the diagnosis of NEC. The earliest radiographic finding is intestinal ileus, often associated with thickening of the bowel loops and air-fluid levels. The pathognomonic radiographic finding is **pneumatosis intestinalis** caused by hydrogen gas production from pathogenic bacteria present between the subserosal and muscularis layers of the bowel wall. Radiographic findings also may include a fixed or persistent dilated loop of bowel, intrahepatic venous gas, and *pneumoperitoneum* seen with bowel perforation.

The **differential diagnosis** of NEC includes sepsis with intestinal ileus or a volvulus. Both conditions can present with systemic signs of sepsis and abdominal distention. The absence of pneumatosis on abdominal radiographs does not rule out the diagnosis of NEC; however, other causes of abdominal distention and perforation (gastric or ileal perforation) should be considered and investigated. Patients diagnosed with Hirschsprung enterocolitis or severe gastroenteritis may present with pneumatosis intestinalis.

The **management** of NEC includes the discontinuation of enteral feedings, gastrointestinal decompression with nasogastric suction, fluid and electrolyte replacement, total parenteral nutrition, and systemic broad-spectrum antibiotics. When the diagnosis of NEC is made, consultation with a pediatric surgeon should be obtained. Even with aggressive and appropriate medical management, 25% to 50% of infants with NEC require surgical intervention. The decision to perform surgery is obvious when the presence of a pneumoperitoneum is observed on abdominal radiograph. Other, not so obvious indications for surgical intervention include rapid clinical deterioration despite medical therapy, rapid onset and progression of pneumatosis, abdominal mass, and intestinal obstruction. The surgical procedure of choice is laparotomy with removal of the frankly necrotic and nonviable bowel. Many extremely small infants are managed initially with primary peritoneal drainage followed by surgical intervention as needed later when the infant is stable, and a laparotomy can be performed safely. The long-term outcome includes intestinal strictures requiring further surgical intervention, short bowel syndrome with poor absorption of enteral fluids and nutrients, associated cholestasis with resultant cirrhosis and liver failure from prolonged parenteral nutrition, and neurodevelopmental delay from prolonged hospitalization.

# CHAPTER 64

# Hypoxic-Ischemic Encephalopathy, Intracranial Hemorrhage, and Seizures

The neonatal central nervous system is anatomically and functionally immature. Although division of cerebral cortical neuronal cells stops during the second trimester of pregnancy, glial cell growth, dendritic arborization, myelination, and cerebellar neuronal cell number continue to increase beyond term gestation and into infancy. At birth, the human newborn spends more time asleep (predominantly in rapid eye movement or active sleep) than in a wakeful state and is totally dependent on adults. Primitive reflexes, such as the Moro, grasp, stepping, rooting, sucking, and crossed extensor reflexes, are readily elicited and are normal for this age. In addition, the newborn has a wealth of cortical functions that are less easily shown (e.g., the ability to extinguish repetitive or painful stimuli).

The newborn also has the capacity for attentive eye fixation and differential responses to the mother's voice. During the perinatal period, many pathophysiologic mechanisms can adversely and permanently affect the developing brain, including prenatal events, such as hypoxia, ischemia, infections, inflammation, malformations, maternal drugs, and coagulation disorders, and postnatal events, such as birth trauma, hypoxia-ischemia, inborn errors of metabolism, hypoglycemia, hypothyroidism, hyperthyroidism, polycythemia, hemorrhage, and meningitis.

## NEONATAL SEIZURES

Seizures during the neonatal period may be the result of multiple causes, with characteristic **historical and clinical manifestations**. **Seizures caused by hypoxic-ischemic encephalopathy** (postasphyxial seizures), a common cause of seizures in the full-term infant, usually occur 12 to 24 hours after a history of birth asphyxia and often are refractory to conventional doses of anticonvulsant medications. Postasphyxial seizures also may be caused by metabolic disorders associated with neonatal asphyxia, such as hypoglycemia and hypocalcemia. **Intraventricular hemorrhage** (**IVH**) is a common cause of seizures in premature infants and often occurs between 1 and 3 days of age. Seizures with IVH are associated with a bulging fontanelle, hemorrhagic spinal fluid, anemia, lethargy, and coma. Seizures caused by **hypoglycemia** often occur when blood glucose levels decline to the lowest postnatal value (at 1 to 2 hours of age or after 24 to 48 hours of poor nutritional intake). Seizures caused by **hypocalcemia** and **hypomagnesemia** develop in high-risk infants and respond well to therapy with calcium, magnesium, or both.

Seizures noted in the delivery room often are caused by direct *injection of local anesthetic agents* into the fetal scalp (associated with transient bradycardia and fixed dilated pupils), severe *anoxia*, or *congenital brain malformation*. Seizures after the first 5 days of life may be the result of *infection* or *drug withdrawal*. Seizures associated with lethargy, acidosis, and a family history of infant deaths may be the result of an *inborn error of metabolism*. An infant whose parent has a history of a neonatal seizure also is at risk for *benign familial seizures*. In an infant who appears well, a sudden onset on day 1 to 3 of life of seizures that are of short duration and that do not recur may be the result of a *subarachnoid hemorrhage*. Focal seizures often are the result of local cerebral infarction.

Seizures may be difficult to differentiate from benign jitteriness or from tremulousness in infants of diabetic mothers, in infants with narcotic withdrawal syndrome, and in any infants after an episode of asphyxia. In contrast to seizures, jitteriness and tremors are sensory dependent, elicited by stimuli, and interrupted by holding the extremity. Seizure activity becomes manifested as coarse, fast and slow clonic activity, whereas jitteriness is characterized by fine, rapid movement. Seizures may be associated with abnormal eye movements, such as tonic deviation to one side. The electroencephalogram often shows seizure activity when the clinical diagnosis is uncertain. Identifying seizures in the newborn period is often difficult because the infant, especially the low birth weight infant, usually

**TABLE 64-1  Clinical Characteristics of Neonatal Seizures**

| Designation | Characterization |
| --- | --- |
| Focal clonic | Repetitive, rhythmic contractions of muscle groups of the limbs, face, or trunk |
| | May be unilateral or multifocal |
| | May appear synchronously or asynchronously in various body regions |
| | Cannot be suppressed by restraint |
| Focal tonic | Sustained posturing of single limbs |
| | Sustained asymmetric posturing of the trunk |
| | Sustained eye deviation |
| | Cannot be provoked by stimulation or suppressed by restraint |
| Myoclonic | Arrhythmic contractions of muscle groups of the limbs, face, or trunk |
| | Typically not repetitive or may recur at a slow rate |
| | May be generalized, focal, or fragmentary |
| | May be provoked by stimulation |
| Generalized tonic | Sustained symmetric posturing of limbs, trunk, and neck |
| | May be flexor, extensor, or mixed extensor/flexor |
| | May be provoked by stimulation |
| | May be suppressed by restraint or repositioning |
| Ocular signs | Random and roving eye movements or nystagmus |
| | Distinct from tonic eye deviation |
| Orobuccolingual movements | Sucking, chewing, tongue protrusions |
| | May be provoked by stimulation |
| Progression movements | Rowing or swimming movements of the arms |
| | Pedaling or bicycling movements of the legs |
| | May be provoked by stimulation |
| | May be suppressed by restraint or repositioning |

From Mizrahi EM: Neonatal seizures. In Shinnar S, Branski D, editors: Pediatric and adolescent medicine, vol 6, Childhood seizures, Basel, 1995, S. Karger.

does not show the tonic-clonic major motor activity typical of the older child (Table 64-1). Subtle seizures are a common manifestation in newborns. The subtle signs of seizure activity include apnea, eye deviation, tongue thrusting, eye blinking, fluctuation of vital signs, and staring. Continuous bedside electroencephalogram monitoring can help identify subtle seizures.

The **diagnostic evaluation** of infants with seizures should involve an immediate determination of capillary blood glucose levels with a Chemstrip. In addition, blood concentrations of sodium, calcium, glucose, and bilirubin should be determined. When infection is suspected, cerebrospinal fluid and blood specimens should be obtained for culture. After the seizure has stopped, a careful examination should be done to identify signs of increased intracranial pressure, congenital malformations, and systemic illness. If signs of elevated intracranial pressure are absent, a lumbar puncture should be performed. If the diagnosis is not apparent at this point, further evaluation should involve magnetic resonance imaging, computed tomography, or cerebral ultrasound and tests to determine the presence of an inborn error of metabolism. Determinations of inborn errors of metabolism are especially important in infants with unexplained lethargy, coma, acidosis, ketonuria, or respiratory alkalosis (see Section 10).

The **treatment** of neonatal seizures may be specific, such as treatment of meningitis or the correction of

**hypoglycemia, hypocalcemia, hypomagnesemia, hyponatremia, or vitamin B$_6$** deficiency or dependency. In the absence of an identifiable cause, therapy should involve an anticonvulsant agent, such as 20 to 40 mg/kg of phenobarbital, 10 to 20 mg/kg of phenytoin (Dilantin), or 0.1 to 0.3 mg/kg of diazepam (Valium), followed by one of the two longer acting drugs. Treatment of status epilepticus requires repeated doses of phenobarbital and may require diazepam or midazolam, titrated to clinical signs. The long-term outcome for neonatal seizures usually is related to the underlying cause and to the primary pathology, such as hypoxic-ischemic encephalopathy, meningitis, drug withdrawal, stroke, or hemorrhage.

## INTRACRANIAL HEMORRHAGE

Intracranial hemorrhage may be confined to one anatomic area of the brain, such as the subdural, subarachnoid, periventricular, intraventricular, intraparenchymal, or cerebellar region. **Subdural hemorrhages** are seen in association with birth trauma, cephalopelvic disproportion, forceps delivery, large for gestational age infants, skull fractures, and postnatal head trauma. The subdural hematoma does not always cause symptoms immediately after birth; with time, however, the RBCs undergo hemolysis and water is drawn into the hemorrhage because of the high oncotic pressure of protein, resulting in an expanding symptomatic lesion. Anemia, vomiting, seizures, and macrocephaly may occur in an infant who is 1 to 2 months of age and has a subdural hematoma. **Child abuse** should be suspected and appropriate diagnostic evaluation undertaken to identify other possible signs of skeletal, ocular, or soft tissue injury. Occasionally, a massive subdural hemorrhage in the neonatal period is caused by rupture of the vein of Galen or by an inherited coagulation disorder, such as hemophilia. Infants with these conditions exhibit shock, seizures, and coma. The **treatment** of all symptomatic subdural hematomas is surgical evacuation.

**Subarachnoid hemorrhages** may be spontaneous, associated with hypoxia, or caused by bleeding from a cerebral arteriovenous malformation. Seizures are a common presenting manifestation, and the *prognosis* depends on the underlying injury. Treatment is directed at the seizure and the rare occurrence of posthemorrhagic hydrocephalus.

**Periventricular hemorrhage** and **IVH** are common in very low birth weight infants, and the risk decreases with increasing gestational age. Fifty percent of infants weighing less than 1500 g have evidence of intracranial bleeding. The pathogenesis for these hemorrhages is unknown (they usually are not caused by coagulation disorders), but the initial site of bleeding may be the weak blood vessels in the periventricular germinal matrix. The vessels in this area have poor structural support. These vessels may rupture and hemorrhage because of passive changes in cerebral blood flow occurring with the variations of blood pressure that sick premature infants often exhibit (failure of autoregulation). In some sick infants, these blood pressure variations are the only identifiable etiologic factors. In others, the disorders that may cause the elevation or depression of blood pressure or that interfere with venous return from the head (venous stasis) increase the risk of IVH; these disorders include asphyxia, pneumothorax, mechanical ventilation, hypercapnia, hypoxemia, prolonged labor, breech delivery, patent ductus arteriosus, heart failure, and therapy with hypertonic solutions such as sodium bicarbonate.

Most periventricular hemorrhages and IVHs occur in the first 3 days of life. It is unusual for IVH to occur after day 5 of life. The clinical manifestations of IVH include seizures, apnea, bradycardia, lethargy, coma, hypotension, metabolic acidosis, anemia not corrected by blood transfusion, bulging fontanelle, and cutaneous mottling. Many infants with small hemorrhages (grade 1 or 2) are asymptomatic; infants with larger hemorrhages (grade 4) often have a catastrophic event that rapidly progresses to shock and coma.

The diagnosis of IVH is confirmed and the severity graded by ultrasound or computed tomography examination through the anterior fontanelle. Grade 1 IVH is confined to the germinal matrix; grade 2 is an extension of grade 1, with blood noted in the ventricle without ventricular enlargement; grade 3 is an extension of grade 2 with ventricular dilation; and grade 4 has blood in dilated ventricles and in the cerebral cortex, either contiguous with or distant from the ventricle. Grade 4 hemorrhage has a poor prognosis, as does the development of periventricular, small, echolucent cystic lesions, with or without

porencephalic cysts and posthemorrhagic hydrocephalus. Periventricular cysts often are noted after the resolution of echodense areas in the periventricular white matter. The cysts may correspond to the development of **periventricular leukomalacia**, which may be a precursor to cerebral palsy. Extensive intraparenchymal echodensities represent hemorrhagic necrosis. They are associated with a high mortality rate and have a poor neurodevelopmental prognosis for survivors.

Treatment of an acute hemorrhage involves standard supportive care, including ventilation for apnea and blood transfusion for shock. Posthemorrhagic hydrocephalus may be managed with serial daily lumbar punctures, an external ventriculostomy tube, or a permanent ventricular-peritoneal shunt. Implementation of the shunt often is delayed because of the high protein content of the hemorrhagic ventricular fluid.

# HYPOXIC-ISCHEMIC ENCEPHALOPATHY

Conditions known to reduce uteroplacental blood flow or to interfere with spontaneous respiration lead to perinatal hypoxia, to lactic acidosis and, if severe enough to reduce cardiac output or cause cardiac arrest, to ischemia. The combination of the reduced availability of oxygen for the brain resulting from hypoxia and the diminished or absent blood flow to the brain resulting from ischemia leads to reduced glucose for metabolism and to an accumulation of lactate that produces local tissue acidosis. After reperfusion, hypoxic-ischemic injury also may be complicated by cell necrosis and vascular endothelial edema, reducing blood flow distal to the involved vessel. Typically, hypoxic-ischemic encephalopathy in the term infant is characterized by cerebral edema, cortical necrosis, and involvement of the basal ganglia, whereas in the preterm infant, it is characterized by periventricular leukomalacia. Both lesions may result in cortical atrophy, mental retardation, and spastic quadriplegia or diplegia.

The clinical manifestations and characteristic course of hypoxic-ischemic encephalopathy vary according to the severity of the injury (Table 64-2). Infants with severe stage 3 hypoxic-ischemic encephalopathy are usually hypotonic, although occasionally they initially appear hypertonic and hyperalert at birth. As cerebral edema develops, brain functions are affected in a descending order; cortical depression produces coma, and brainstem depression results in apnea. As cerebral edema progresses, refractory seizures begin 12 to 24 hours after birth. Concurrently the infant has no signs of spontaneous respirations, is hypotonic, and has diminished or absent deep tendon reflexes.

Survivors of stage 3 hypoxic-ischemic encephalopathy have a high incidence of seizures and serious neurodevelopmental handicaps. The prognosis of severe asphyxia also depends on other organ system injury (see Table 58-6). Another indicator of poor prognosis is time of onset of spontaneous respiration as estimated by Apgar score. Infants with Apgar scores of 0 to 3 at 10 minutes have a 20% mortality and a 5% incidence of cerebral palsy; if the score remains this low by 20 minutes, the mortality increases to 60%, and the incidence of cerebral palsy increases to 57%.

| TABLE 64-2  Hypoxic-Ischemic Encephalopathy in Term Infants | | | |
|---|---|---|---|
| Signs | Stage 1 | Stage 2 | Stage 3 |
| Level of consciousness | Hyperalert | Lethargic | Stuporous |
| Muscle tone | Normal | Hypotonic | Flaccid |
| Tendon reflexes/clonus | Hyperactive | Hyperactive | Absent |
| Moro reflex | Strong | Weak | Absent |
| Pupils | Mydriasis | Miosis | Unequal, poor light reflex |
| Seizures | None | Common | Decerebration |
| Electroencephalographic | Normal | Low voltage changing to seizure activity | Burst suppression to isoelectric |
| Duration | >24 hr if progresses, otherwise may remain normal | 24 hr to 14 days | Days to weeks |

Modified from Sarnat HB, Sarnat MS: Neonatal encephalopathy following fetal distress. *Arch Neurol* 33:696, 1976.

CHAPTER 65

# Sepsis and Meningitis

Systemic and local infections (lung, cutaneous, ocular, umbilical, kidney, bone-joint, and meningeal) are common in the newborn period. Infection may be acquired in utero through the transplacental or transcervical routes and during or after birth. Ascending infection through the cervix, with or without rupture of the amniotic fluid membranes, may result in amnionitis, funisitis (infection of the umbilical cord), congenital pneumonia, and sepsis. The bacteria responsible for ascending infection of the fetus are common bacterial organisms of the maternal genitourinary tract, such as group B streptococci, *Escherichia coli, Haemophilus influenzae,* and *Klebsiella.* Herpes simplex virus (HSV)-1 or more often HSV-2 also causes ascending infection that at times may be indistinguishable from bacterial sepsis. Syphilis and *Listeria monocytogenes* are acquired by transplacental infection.

Maternal humoral immunity may protect the fetus against some neonatal pathogens, such as group B streptococci and HSV. Nonetheless, various deficiencies of the neonatal antimicrobial defense mechanism probably are more important than maternal immune status as a contributing factor for neonatal infection, especially in the low birth weight infant. The incidence of sepsis is approximately 1:1500 in full-term infants and 1:250 in preterm infants. The sixfold-higher rate of sepsis in preterm infants compared with term infants relates to the more immature immunologic systems of preterm infants and to their prolonged periods of hospitalization, which increase risk of nosocomially acquired infectious diseases.

Preterm infants before 32 weeks of gestational age have not received the full complement of maternal antibodies (IgG), which cross the placenta by active transport predominantly in the latter half of the third trimester. In addition, although low birth weight infants may generate IgM antibodies, their own IgG response to infection is reduced. These infants also have deficiencies of the alternate and, to a smaller degree, the classic complement activation pathways, which results in diminished complement-mediated opsonization. Newborn infants also show a deficit in phagocytic migration to the site of infection (to the lung) and in the bone marrow reserve pool of leukocytes. In addition, in the presence of suboptimal activation of complement, neonatal neutrophils ingest and kill bacteria less effectively than adult neutrophils do. Neutrophils from sick infants seem to have an even greater deficit in bacterial killing capacity compared with phagocytic cells from normal neonates.

Defense mechanisms against viral pathogens also may be deficient in a newborn. Neonatal antibody-dependent, cell-mediated immunity by the natural killer lymphocytes is deficient in the absence of maternal antibodies and in the presence of reduced interferon production; reduced antibody levels occur in premature infants and in infants born during a primary viral infection of the mother, such as with enteroviruses, HSV-2, or cytomegalovirus. In addition, antibody-independent cytotoxicity may be reduced in lymphocytes of newborns.

Bacterial sepsis and meningitis often are linked closely in neonates. Despite this association, the incidence of meningitis relative to neonatal sepsis has been on a steady decline. The incidence of meningitis is approximately 1 in 20 cases of sepsis. The causative organisms isolated most frequently are the same as for neonatal sepsis: group B streptococci, *E. coli,* and *L. monocytogenes.* Gram-negative organisms, such as *Klebsiella* and *Serratia marcescens,* are more common in less developed countries, and coagulase-negative staphylococci need to be considered in very low birth weight infants. Male infants seem to be more susceptible to neonatal infection than female infants. Severely premature infants are at even greater risk secondary to less effective defense mechanisms and deficient transfer of antibodies from the mother to the fetus (which occurs mostly after 32 weeks' gestation). Neonates in the neonatal intensive care unit live in a hostile environment, with exposure to endotracheal tubes, central arterial and venous catheters, and blood draws all predisposing to bacteremia and meningitis. Genetic factors have been implicated in the ability of bacteria to cross the blood-brain barrier. This penetration has been noted for group B streptococci, *E. coli, Listeria, Citrobacter,* and *Streptococcus pneumoniae.*

Neonatal sepsis presents during three periods. **Early-onset sepsis** often begins in utero and usually is a result of infection caused by the bacteria in the mother's genitourinary tract. Organisms related to this sepsis include group B streptococci, *E. coli, Klebsiella, L. monocytogenes,* and nontypeable *H. influenzae.* Most infected infants are premature and show nonspecific cardiorespiratory signs, such as grunting, tachypnea, and cyanosis at birth. Risk factors for early-onset sepsis include vaginal colonization with group B streptococci, prolonged rupture of the membranes (>24 hours), amnionitis, maternal fever or leukocytosis, fetal tachycardia, and preterm birth. African-American race and male sex are unexplained additional risk factors for neonatal sepsis.

**Early-onset sepsis** (birth to 7 days) is an overwhelming multiorgan system disease frequently manifested as respiratory failure, shock, meningitis (in 30% of cases), disseminated intravascular coagulation, acute tubular necrosis, and symmetrical peripheral gangrene. Early manifestations—grunting, poor feeding, pallor, apnea, lethargy, hypothermia, or an abnormal cry—may be nonspecific. Profound neutropenia, hypoxia, and hypotension may be refractory to treatment with broad-spectrum antibiotics, mechanical ventilation, and vasopressors such as dopamine and dobutamine. In the initial stages of early-onset septicemia in a preterm infant, it is often difficult to differentiate sepsis from respiratory distress syndrome. Because of this difficulty, premature infants with respiratory distress syndrome receive broad-spectrum antibiotics.

The clinical manifestations of sepsis are difficult to separate from the manifestations of meningitis in the neonate. Infants with early-onset sepsis should be evaluated by blood and cerebrospinal fluid (CSF) cultures, CSF Gram stain, cell count, and protein and glucose levels. Normal newborns generally have an elevated CSF protein content (100 to 150 mg/dL) and may have 25 to 30/mm$^3$ white blood cells (mean, 9/mm$^3$), which are 75% lymphocytes in the absence of infection. Some infants with neonatal meningitis caused by group B streptococci do not have an elevated CSF leukocyte count but are seen to have microorganisms in the CSF on Gram stain. In addition to culture, other methods of identifying the pathogenic bacteria are the determination of bacterial antigen in samples of blood, urine, or CSF. In cases of neonatal meningitis, the ratio of CSF glucose to blood glucose usually is less than 50%. The polymerase chain reaction test primarily is used to identify viral infections. Serial complete blood counts should be performed to identify neutropenia, an increased number of immature neutrophils (bands), and thrombocytopenia. C-reactive protein levels are often elevated in neonatal patients with bacterial sepsis.

A chest radiograph also should be obtained to determine the presence of pneumonia. In addition to the traditional neonatal pathogens, pneumonia in very low birth weight infants may be the result of acquisition of maternal genital mycoplasmal agent (e.g., *Ureaplasma urealyticum* or *Mycoplasma hominis*). Arterial blood gases should be monitored to detect hypoxemia and metabolic acidosis that may be caused by hypoxia, shock, or both. Blood pressure, urine output, and peripheral perfusion should be monitored to determine the need to treat septic shock with fluids and vasopressor agents.

The mainstay of treatment for sepsis and meningitis is antibiotic therapy. Antibiotics are used to suppress bacterial growth, allowing the infant's defense mechanisms time to respond. In addition, support measures, such as assisted ventilation and cardiovascular support, are equally important to the management of the infant. A combination of ampicillin and an aminoglycoside (usually gentamicin) for 10 to 14 days is effective treatment against most organisms responsible for early-onset sepsis. The combination of ampicillin and cefotaxime also is proposed as an alternative method of treatment. If meningitis is present, the treatment should be extended to 21 days or 14 days after a negative result from a CSF culture. Persistently positive results from CSF cultures are common with neonatal meningitis caused by gram-negative organisms, even with appropriate antibiotic treatment, and may be present for 2 to 3 days after antibiotic therapy. If gram-negative meningitis is present, some authorities continue to treat with an effective penicillin derivative combined with an aminoglycoside, whereas most change to a third-generation cephalosporin. High-dose penicillin (250,000 to 450,000 U/kg/24 hr) is appropriate for group B streptococcal meningitis. Inhaled nitric oxide, extracorporeal membrane oxygenation (in term infants), or both, may improve the outcome of sepsis-related pulmonary hypertension. Intratracheal surfactant may reverse respiratory failure. Intrapartum penicillin empirical prophylaxis for group B streptococcal colonized mothers or mothers with risk factors (fever, preterm labor, previous infant with group B streptococci, and amnionitis) has reduced the rate of early-onset infection.

**Late-onset sepsis** (8 to 28 days) usually occurs in a healthy full-term infant who was discharged in good health from the normal newborn nursery. Clinical manifestations may include lethargy, poor feeding, hypotonia, apathy, seizures, bulging fontanelle, fever, and direct-reacting hyperbilirubinemia. In addition to bacteremia, hematogenous seeding may result in focal infections, such as meningitis (in 75% of cases), osteomyelitis (group B streptococci, *Staphylococcus aureus*), arthritis (gonococcus, *S. aureus, Candida albicans*, gram-negative bacteria), and urinary tract infection (gram-negative bacteria).

The evaluation of infants with late-onset sepsis is similar to that for infants with early-onset sepsis, with special attention given to a careful physical examination of the bones (infants with osteomyelitis may exhibit pseudoparalysis) and to the laboratory examination and culture of urine obtained by sterile suprapubic aspiration or urethral catheterization. Late-onset sepsis may be caused by the same pathogens as early-onset sepsis, but infants exhibiting sepsis late in the neonatal period also may have infections caused by the pathogens usually found in older infants (*H. influenzae, S. pneumoniae,* and *Neisseria meningitidis*). In addition, viral agents (HSV, cytomegalovirus, or enteroviruses) may manifest with a late-onset, sepsis-like picture.

Because of the increased rate of resistance of *H. influenzae* and pneumococcus to ampicillin, some centers begin treatment with ampicillin and a third-generation cephalosporin (and vancomycin if meningitis is present) when sepsis occurs in the last week of the first month of life. The treatment of late-onset neonatal sepsis and meningitis is the same as that for early-onset sepsis.

**Nosocomially acquired sepsis** (8 days to discharge) occurs predominantly in premature infants in the neonatal intensive care unit; many of these infants have been colonized with the multidrug-resistant bacteria indigenous to the neonatal intensive care unit. The risk of such serious bacterial infection is increased by frequent treatment with broad-spectrum antibiotics for sepsis and by the presence of central venous indwelling catheters, endotracheal tubes, umbilical vessel catheters, and electronic monitoring devices. Epidemics of bacterial (coagulase-negative staphylococci, fungi, enteric bacteria) or viral sepsis, bacterial or aseptic meningitis, staphylococcal bullous skin infections, cellulitis, pneumonia (bacterial or caused by adenovirus or respiratory syncytial virus), omphalitis (caused by *S. aureus* or gram-negative bacilli), and diarrhea (staphylococcal, enteroviral, or caused by rotavirus or enteropathogenic *E. coli*) are common in the neonatal intensive care unit and in the nursery for well infants.

The initial clinical manifestations of nosocomial infection in a premature infant may be subtle and include apnea and bradycardia, temperature instability, abdominal distention, and poor feeding. In the later stages, signs of infection are shock, disseminated intravascular coagulation, worsening respiratory status, and local reactions, such as omphalitis, eye discharge, diarrhea, and bullous impetigo.

The treatment of nosocomially acquired sepsis depends on the indigenous microbiologic flora of the particular hospital and the antibiotic sensitivities. Because *S. aureus* (occasionally methicillin-resistant), *Staphylococcus epidermidis* (methicillin-resistant), and gram-negative pathogens are common nosocomial bacterial agents in many nurseries, a combination of vancomycin or oxacillin/nafcillin (some use ampicillin) with an aminoglycoside (gentamicin or tobramycin) is appropriate. The dose and interval for administering all aminoglycosides, such as gentamicin, vary with postnatal age and birth weight. In addition, treatment with aminoglycosides for more than 3 days necessitates monitoring of the serum peak and trough concentrations to optimize therapy and to avoid ototoxicity and nephrotoxicity. Persistent signs of infection despite antibacterial treatment suggest candidal or viral sepsis.

# CHAPTER 66
# Congenital Infections

An infection acquired transplacentally during gestation is a congenital infection. Numerous pathogens that produce mild or subclinical disease in older infants and children can cause severe disease in neonates who acquire such infections prenatally or perinatally. Sepsis, meningitis, pneumonia, and other infections caused by numerous perinatally acquired pathogens are the cause of significant neonatal morbidity and mortality. Congenital infections include a well-known group of fungal, bacterial, and viral pathogens: toxoplasmosis, rubella, cytomegalovirus (CMV), herpes simplex virus (HSV), varicella-zoster virus, congenital syphilis, parvovirus, human immunodeficiency virus (HIV), hepatitis B, *Neisseria gonorrhoeae*, *Chlamydia*, and *Mycobacterium tuberculosis*.

Many of the clinical manifestations of congenital infections are similar, including intrauterine growth restriction, nonimmune hydrops, anemia, thrombocytopenia, jaundice, hepatosplenomegaly, chorioretinitis, and congenital malformations. Some unique manifestations and epidemiologic characteristics of these infections are listed in Table 66-1. Evaluation of patients thought to have a congenital infection should include attempts to isolate the organism by culture (for rubella, CMV, HSV, gonorrhea, and *M. tuberculosis*), to identify the antigen of the pathogen (for hepatitis B and *Chlamydia trachomatis*), to identify the pathogen's genome with polymerase chain reaction (PCR), and to identify specific fetal production of antibodies (IgM or increasing titer of IgG for *Toxoplasma*, syphilis, parvovirus, HIV, or *Borrelia*).

Treatment is not always available, specific, or effective. Nonetheless, some encouraging results have been reported for preventing the disease and for specifically treating the infant when the correct diagnosis is made (see Table 66-1).

## TOXOPLASMOSIS

Vertical transmission of *Toxoplasma gondii* occurs by transplacental transfer of the organism from the mother to the fetus after an acute maternal infection. Fetal infection rarely can occur after reactivation of disease in an immunocompromised pregnant mother. Transmission from an acutely infected mother to her fetus occurs in about 30% to 40% of cases, but the rate varies directly with gestational age. Transmission rates and the timing of fetal infection correlate directly with placental blood flow; the risk of infection increases throughout gestation to 90% or greater near term, and the time interval between maternal and fetal infection decreases.

The severity of fetal disease varies inversely with the gestational age at which maternal infection occurs. Most infants have subclinical infection with no overt disease at birth; however, specific ophthalmologic and central nervous system (CNS) evaluations may reveal abnormalities. The classic findings of hydrocephalus, chorioretinitis, and intracerebral calcifications suggest the diagnosis of congenital toxoplasmosis. Affected infants tend to be small for gestational age, develop early-onset jaundice, have hepatosplenomegaly, and present with a generalized maculopapular rash. Seizures are common, and skull films may reveal diffuse cortical calcifications in contrast to the periventricular pattern observed with CMV. These infants are at increased risk for long-term neurologic and neurodevelopmental complications.

Serologic tests are the primary means of diagnosis. IgG-specific antibodies achieve a peak concentration 1 to 2 months after infection and remain positive indefinitely. For infants with seroconversion or a fourfold increase in IgG titers, specific IgM antibody determinations should be performed in patients to confirm disease. Especially for congenital infections, measurement of IgA and IgE antibodies can be useful to confirm the disease. Thorough ophthalmologic, auditory, and neurologic evaluations (head computed tomography and cerebrospinal fluid [CSF] examination) are indicated.

## TABLE 66-1 Perinatal Congenital Infections (TORCH)

| Agent | Maternal Epidemiology | Neonatal Features |
|---|---|---|
| *Toxoplasma gondii* | Heterophil-negative mononucleosis<br>Exposure to cats or raw meat or immunosuppression<br>High-risk exposure at 10–24 wk gestation | Hydrocephalus, abnormal spinal fluid, intracranial calcifications, chorioretinitis, jaundice, hepatosplenomegaly, fever<br>Many infants asymptomatic at birth<br>*Treatment:* pyrimethamine plus sulfadiazine |
| Rubella virus | Unimmunized seronegative mother; fever ± rash<br>Detectable defects with infection:<br>  by 8 wk, 85%<br>  9–12 wk, 50%<br>  13–20 wk, 16%<br>Virus may be present in infant's throat for 1 yr<br>*Prevention:* vaccine | Intrauterine growth restriction, microcephaly, microphthalmia, cataracts, glaucoma, "salt and pepper" chorioretinitis, hepatosplenomegaly, jaundice, PDA, deafness, blueberry muffin rash, anemia, thrombocytopenia, leukopenia, metaphyseal lucencies, B-cell and T-cell deficiency<br>Infant may be asymptomatic at birth |
| CMV | Sexually transmitted disease: primary genital infection may be asymptomatic<br>Heterophil-negative mononucleosis; infant may have viruria for 1–6 yr | Sepsis, intrauterine growth restriction, chorioretinitis, microcephaly, periventricular calcifications, blueberry muffin rash, anemia, thrombocytopenia, neutropenia, hepatosplenomegaly, jaundice, deafness, pneumonia<br>Many asymptomatic at birth<br>*Prevention:* CMV-negative blood products<br>*Possible treatment:* ganciclovir? |
| Herpes simplex type 2 or 1 virus | Sexually transmitted disease: primary genital infection may be asymptomatic; intrauterine infection rare, acquisition at time of birth more common | *Intrauterine infection:* chorioretinitis, skin lesions, microcephaly<br><br>*Postnatal:* encephalitis, localized or disseminated disease, skin vesicles, keratoconjunctivitis<br>*Treatment:* acyclovir |
| Varicella-zoster virus | Intrauterine infection with chickenpox<br>Infant develops severe neonatal varicella with maternal illness 5 days before or 2 days after delivery | Microphthalmia, cataracts, chorioretinitis, cutaneous and bony aplasia/hypoplasia/atrophy, cutaneous scars<br>Zoster as in older child<br><br>*Prevention of neonatal* condition with VZIG<br>*Treatment of ill neonate:* acyclovir |
| *Treponema pallidum* (syphilis) | Sexually transmitted disease<br>Maternal primary asymptomatic: painless "hidden" chancre<br>Penicillin, not erythromycin, prevents fetal infection | Presentation *at birth* as nonimmune hydrops, prematurity, anemia, neutropenia, thrombocytopenia, pneumonia, hepatosplenomegaly<br><br>*Late neonatal* as snuffles (rhinitis), rash, hepatosplenomegaly, condylomata lata, metaphysitis, cerebrospinal fluid pleocytosis, keratitis, periosteal new bone, lymphocytosis, hepatitis<br>*Late onset:* teeth, eye, bone, skin, central nervous system, ear<br>*Treatment:* penicillin |
| Parvovirus | Etiology of fifth disease; fever, rash, arthralgia in adults | Nonimmune hydrops, fetal anemia<br><br>Treatment: in utero transfusion |
| HIV | AIDS; most mothers are asymptomatic and HIV positive; high-risk history; prostitute, drug abuse, married to bisexual, or hemophiliac | AIDS symptoms develop between 3 and 6 mo of age in 10%–25%; failure to thrive, recurrent infection, hepatosplenomegaly, neurologic abnormalities<br><br>*Management:* trimethoprim/sulfamethoxazole, AZT, other antiretroviral agents<br>*Prevention:* prenatal, intrapartum, postpartum AZT; avoid breastfeeding |

*Continued*

**TABLE 66-1  Perinatal Congenital Infections (TORCH)—cont'd**

| Agent | Maternal Epidemiology | Neonatal Features |
|---|---|---|
| Hepatitis B virus | Vertical transmission common; may result in cirrhosis, hepatocellular carcinoma | Acute neonatal hepatitis; many become asymptomatic carriers<br>*Prevention:* HBIG, vaccine |
| *Neisseria gonorrhoeae* | Sexually transmitted disease, infant acquires at birth<br><br>*Treatment:* cefotaxime, ceftriaxone | Gonococcal ophthalmia, sepsis, meningitis<br><br>*Prevention:* silver nitrate, erythromycin eye drops<br>*Treatment:* ceftriaxone |
| *Chlamydia trachomatis* | Sexually transmitted disease, infant acquires at birth<br><br>*Treatment:* oral erythromycin | Conjunctivitis, pneumonia<br><br>*Prevention:* erythromycin eye drops<br>*Treatment:* oral erythromycin |
| *Mycobacterium tuberculosis* | Positive PPD skin test, recent converter, positive chest radiograph, positive family member<br><br>*Treatment:* INH and rifampin ± ethambutol | Congenital rare septic pneumonia; acquired primary pulmonary TB; asymptomatic, follow PPD<br><br>*Prevention:* INH, BCG, separation<br>Treatment: INH, rifampin, pyrazinamide |
| *Trypanosoma cruzi* (Chagas disease) | Central South American native, immigrant, travel<br><br>Chronic disease in mother | Failure to thrive, heart failure, achalasia<br><br>*Treatment:* nifurtimox |

AZT, zidovudine (azidothymidine); BCG, bacille Calmette-Guérin; CMV, cytomegalovirus; HBIG, hepatitis B immune globulin; INH, isoniazid; PDA, patent ductus arteriosus; PPD, purified protein derivative; TB, tuberculosis; VZIG, varicella-zoster immune globulin.

For symptomatic and asymptomatic congenital infections, initial therapy should include pyrimethamine (supplemented with folic acid) combined with sulfadiazine. Duration of therapy is often prolonged even up to 1 year. Optimal dosages of medications and duration of therapy should be determined in consultation with appropriate specialists.

## RUBELLA

With the widespread use of vaccination, congenital rubella is rare in developed countries. Acquired in utero during early gestation, rubella can cause severe neonatal consequences. The occurrence of congenital defects approaches 85% if infection is acquired during the first 4 weeks of gestation; close to 40% spontaneously abort or are stillborn. If infection occurs during weeks 13 to 16, 35% of infants can have abnormalities. Infection after 4 months' gestation does not seem to cause disease.

The most common characteristic abnormalities associated with congenital rubella include ophthalmologic (cataracts, retinopathy, and glaucoma), cardiac (patent ductus arteriosus and peripheral pulmonary artery stenosis), auditory (sensorineural hearing loss), and neurologic (behavioral disorders, meningoencephalitis, and mental retardation) conditions. Additionally, infants can present with growth retardation, hepatosplenomegaly, early-onset jaundice, thrombocytopenia, radiolucent bone disease, and purpuric skin lesions ("blueberry muffin" appearance from dermal erythropoiesis).

Detection of rubella-specific IgM antibody usually indicates recent infection. Additionally, measurement of rubella-specific IgG over several months can be confirmatory.

Rubella virus can be isolated from blood, urine, CSF, and throat swab specimens. Infants with congenital rubella are chronically and persistently infected and tend to shed live virus in urine, stools, and respiratory secretions for 1 year. Infants should be isolated while in the hospital and kept away from susceptible pregnant women when sent home.

## CYTOMEGALOVIRUS

CMV is the most common congenital infection and the leading cause of sensorineural hearing loss, mental retardation, retinal disease, and cerebral palsy. Congenital CMV occurs in about 0.5% to 1.5% of births. When primary infection occurs in mothers during a pregnancy, the virus is transmitted to the fetus in approximately 35% of cases. Rates of CMV infection are three to seven times greater in infants born to adolescent mothers. The risk of transmission of CMV to the fetus is independent of gestational age at the time of maternal infection. The earlier in gestation that the primary maternal infection occurs, the more symptomatic the infant will be at birth. The most common sources of CMV for primary infections occurring in mothers during pregnancy are sexual contacts and contact with young children. It is well known that CMV can be transmitted to the fetus even when maternal infection occurred long before conception. This transmission can occur as the result of virus reactivation, chronic infection, or reinfection with a new strain.

More than 90% of infants who have congenital CMV infection exhibit no clinical evidence of disease at birth. Approximately 10% of infected infants are small for gestational age and have symptoms at birth. Findings include microcephaly, thrombocytopenia, hepatosplenomegaly, hepatitis, intracranial calcifications, chorioretinitis, and hearing abnormalities. Some infants can present with a blueberry muffin appearance as the result of dermal erythropoiesis. Skull films may reveal periventricular calcifications. An additional 10% of infected infants may not present until later in infancy or early childhood, when they are found to have sensorineural hearing loss and developmental delays. Mortality is 10% to 15% in symptomatic newborns. Perinatal CMV infection acquired during birth or from mother's milk is not associated with newborn illness or CNS sequelae.

Congenital CMV infection is diagnosed by detection of virus in the urine or saliva. Detection is often accomplished by traditional virus culture methods but can take several weeks to obtain a result. Rapid culture methods using centrifugation to enhance infectivity and monoclonal antibody to detect early antigens in infected tissue culture can give results in 24 hours. PCR also can be used to detect small amounts of CMV DNA in the urine. Detection of CMV within the first 3 weeks after birth is considered proof of congenital CMV infection.

There are no antiviral agents currently approved for the treatment of congenital CMV infection. Trial studies in severely symptomatic newborns of the antiviral agent, ganciclovir, have shown a lack of progression of hearing loss.

## HERPES SIMPLEX VIRUS

HSV-2 accounts for 90% of primary genital herpes. About 70% to 85% of neonatal herpes simplex infections are caused by HSV-2. Most commonly, neonatal infections are acquired from the mother shortly before (ascending infection) or during passage through the birth canal at delivery. The incidence of neonatal HSV is estimated to range from 1 in 3000 to 20,000 live births. Infants with HSV infections are more likely to be born prematurely (40% of affected infants are <36 weeks' gestation). The risk of infection at delivery in an infant born vaginally to a mother with primary genital herpes is about 33% to 50%. The risk to an infant born to a mother with a reactivated infection is less than 5%. More than 75% of infants who acquire HSV infection are born to mothers who have no previous history or clinical findings consistent with HSV infection.

Most infants are normal at birth, and symptoms of infection develop at 5 to 10 days of life. Symptoms of neonatal HSV infection include disseminated disease involving multiple organ systems, most notably the liver and lungs; localized infection to the CNS; or localized infection to the skin, eyes, and mouth. Symptoms may overlap, and in many cases of disseminated disease, skin lesions are a late finding. Disseminated infection should be considered in any infant with symptoms of sepsis, liver dysfunction, and negative bacteriologic cultures. HSV infection also should be suspected in any neonate who presents with fever, irritability, abnormal CSF findings, and seizures. Initial symptoms can occur anytime between birth and 4 weeks of age, although disseminated disease usually occurs during the first week of life. HSV infections are often severe, and a delay in treatment can result in significant morbidity and mortality.

For the diagnosis of neonatal HSV infection, specimens for culture should be obtained from any skin vesicle, nasopharynx, eyes, urine, blood, CSF, stool, or rectum. Positive cultures obtained from these sites more than 48 hours after birth indicate intrapartum exposure. PCR is a sensitive method for detecting HSV DNA in blood, urine, and CSF.

Parenteral acyclovir is the treatment of choice for neonatal HSV infections. Acyclovir should be administered to all infants suspected to have infection or diagnosed with HSV. The most benign outcome with regard to morbidity and mortality is observed in infants with disease limited to the skin, eyes, and mouth.

## VARICELLA-ZOSTER VIRUS

The incidence of congenital infection among infants born to mothers who have varicella is about 2% when infection occurs within the first 20 weeks of gestation. Fetal infection after maternal varicella can result in varicella embryopathy, which is characterized by *zigzag* skin scarring and limb atrophy. CNS manifestations (hydrocephalus and microcephaly) and eye abnormalities (cataracts and chorioretinitis) also may occur.

Varicella infection can be fatal for the infant of a mother who develops varicella 5 days before to 2 days after delivery. Clinical features include severe rash, pneumonia, hepatitis, and death in 20% to 30% of cases. Infants born to mothers who are infected before 5 days prior to delivery have less severe disease secondary to the placental transfer of varicella-specific IgG antibody.

Varicella-zoster virus can be isolated from scrapings of a vesicle base during the first 3 to 4 days of the eruptions, but rarely from secretions from other sites, such as the respiratory tract. A significant increase in serum varicella IgG antibody can confirm the diagnosis. PCR is a sensitive method for detecting varicella DNA in any body fluid or tissue.

## CONGENITAL SYPHILIS

Congenital syphilis most commonly results from transplacental infection of the fetus, although the fetus can acquire infection by contact with a chancre at birth. Additionally, hematogenous infection can occur throughout pregnancy. The longer the time elapsed between the mother's infection and pregnancy, the less likely she is to transmit the disease to the fetus.

Intrauterine infection can result in stillbirth, hydrops fetalis, or prematurity. Clinical symptoms vary but include hepatosplenomegaly, snuffles, lymphadenopathy, mucocutaneous lesions, osteochondritis, rash, hemolytic anemia, and thrombocytopenia. Untreated infants, regardless of whether they manifest symptoms at birth, may develop late symptoms, which usually appear after 2 years of age and involve the CNS, bones, joints, teeth, eyes, and skin. Some manifestations of disease may not become apparent until many years after birth, such as interstitial keratitis, eighth cranial nerve deafness, Hutchinson teeth, bowing of the skins, frontal bossing, mulberry molars, saddle nose, rhagades, and Clutton joints. The combination of interstitial keratitis, eighth cranial nerve deafness, and Hutchinson teeth is commonly referred to as the *Hutchinson triad.*

Many infants are asymptomatic at the time of diagnosis. If untreated, most infants develop symptoms within the first 5 weeks of life. The most striking lesions affect the mucocutaneous tissues and bones. Early signs of infection may be poor feeding and snuffles (syphilitic rhinitis). Snuffles are more severe and persistent than the common cold and are often bloody. A maculopapular desquamative rash develops over the palms and soles and around the mouth and anus. The rash may progress to become vesicular with bullae. Severely ill infants may be born with hydrops and have profound anemia. Severe consolidated pneumonia may be present at birth, and there may be laboratory findings consistent with a glomerulonephritis. CSF evaluation may reveal a pleocytosis and elevated protein. More than 90% of symptomatic infants exhibit radiographic abnormalities of the long bones consistent with osteochondritis and perichondritis.

No newborn should be discharged from the hospital without knowledge or determination of the mother's serologic status for syphilis. All infants born to seropositive mothers require a careful examination and a quantitative nontreponemal syphilis test. Darkfield examination of direct fluorescent antibody staining of organisms obtained by scraping a skin or mucous membrane lesion is the quickest and most direct method of diagnosis. More commonly, serologic testing is used. The nontreponemal reaginic antibody assays—the Venereal Disease Research Laboratory (VDRL) and the rapid plasma reagin—are helpful as indicators of disease. All infants born to seropositive mothers require a careful examination and a quantitative nontreponemal syphilis test. The test performed on the infant should be the same as that performed on the mother to enable comparison of results. An infant should be evaluated further if the maternal titer has increased fourfold, if the infant's titer is fourfold greater than the mother's titer, if the infant is symptomatic, or if the mother has inadequately treated syphilis. A mother infected later in pregnancy may deliver an infant who is incubating active disease. The mother and infant may have negative serologic testing at birth. When clinical or serologic tests suggest congenital syphilis, CSF should be examined microscopically, and a CSF VDRL test should be performed. An increased CSF white blood cell count and protein concentration suggests neurosyphilis; a positive CSF VDRL is diagnostic.

**Parenteral penicillin** is the preferred drug of choice for treatment of syphilis. Penicillin G for 10 to 14 days is the only documented effective therapy for infants who have congenital syphilis and neurosyphilis. Infants should have repeat nontreponemal antibody titers repeated at 3, 6, and 12 months to document falling titers. Infants with neurosyphilis must be followed carefully with serologic testing and CSF determinations every 6 months for at least 3 years or until CSF findings are normal.

## HUMAN PARVOVIRUS B19

Infection with parvovirus B19 is recognized most often as erythema infectiosum, which is characterized by mild systemic symptoms, fever, and commonly a distinctive "slapped cheek" facial rash. Approximately 30% to 60% of adults are seropositive for human parvovirus B19.

A significant proportion of childbearing women is potentially susceptible to infection.

Parvovirus B19 selectively infects erythropoietic precursors and inhibits their growth by inducing cell cycle arrest and apoptosis. Parvovirus infections often are associated with mild neutropenia and thrombocytopenia, but instances of transient pancytopenia also have been reported. Although the actual risk is probably low, the virus can infect the fetus, leading to fetal anemia, nonimmune hydrops, and fetal demise. Pathologic studies of parvovirus B19 human fetuses also have suggested that myocardial inflammation and subendocardial fibroelastosis may contribute to fetal hydrops.

Detection of serum parvovirus B19–specific IgM antibody is the preferred diagnostic test. A positive IgM test result indicates that infection probably occurred within the past 2 to 4 months. Antenatal treatment of parvovirus B19–infected fetuses with hydrops has included serial maternal ultrasound, fetal intrauterine blood transfusion, and maternal digitalization. Spontaneous resolution of fetal hydrops with normal outcome has been reported. Treatment for the infant after birth is mainly supportive and centered on the management of hydrops. Infants with aplastic crisis may require transfusions of blood products.

## HUMAN IMMUNODEFICIENCY VIRUS

▶ (SEE CHAPTER 125)

## HEPATITIS B

▶ (SEE CHAPTER 113)

## *NEISSERIA GONORRHOEAE*

*N. gonorrhoeae* infection in a newborn usually involves the eyes (ophthalmia neonatorum). Other sites of infection include scalp abscesses (often associated with fetal monitoring with scalp electrodes), vaginitis, and disseminated disease with bacteremia, arthritis, or meningitis. Transmission to the infant usually occurs during passage through the birth canal when mucous membranes come in contact with infected secretions.

Infection usually is present within the first 5 days of life and is characterized initially by a clear, watery discharge, which rapidly becomes purulent. There is marked conjunctival hyperemia and chemosis. Infection tends to be bilateral; however, one eye may be clinically worse than the other. Untreated infections can spread to the cornea (keratitis) and anterior chamber of the eye. This extension can result in corneal perforation and blindness.

**Recommended treatment** for isolated infection, such as ophthalmia neonatorum, is one intramuscular dose of ceftriaxone. Infants with gonococcal ophthalmia should receive eye irrigations with saline solution at frequent intervals before discharge. Topical antibiotic therapy alone is inadequate and is unnecessary when recommended systemic antimicrobial therapy is given. Infants with gonococcal ophthalmia should be hospitalized and evaluated for disseminated disease (sepsis, arthritis, meningitis). Disseminated disease should be treated with antimicrobial therapy (ceftriaxone or cefotaxime) for 7 days. Cefotaxime can be used in infants with hyperbilirubinemia. If documented, infants with meningitis should be treated for 10 to 14 days.

Tests for concomitant infection with *C. trachomatis*, congenital syphilis, and HIV should be performed. Results of the maternal test for hepatitis B surface antigen should be confirmed. Topical prophylaxis with silver nitrate, erythromycin, or tetracycline is recommended for all newborns for the prevention of gonococcal ophthalmia.

## CHLAMYDIA

*C. trachomatis* is the most common reportable sexually transmitted infection, with a high rate of infection among sexually active adolescents and young adults. Prevalence of the organism in pregnant women ranges from 6% to 12% and can be 40% in adolescents. *Chlamydia* can be transmitted from the genital tract of infected mothers to their newborns. Acquisition occurs in about 50% of infants born vaginally to infected mothers. Transmission also has been reported in some infants delivered by cesarean section with intact membranes. In infected infants, the risk of conjunctivitis is 25% to 50%, and the risk of pneumonia is 5% to 20%. The nasopharynx is the most commonly infected anatomic site.

Neonatal chlamydial conjunctivitis is characterized by ocular congestion, edema, and discharge developing 5 to 14 days to several weeks after birth and lasting for 1 to 2 weeks. Clinical manifestations vary from mild conjunctivitis to intense inflammation and swelling. Both eyes are almost always involved; however, one eye may appear to be more swollen and infected than the other. The cornea is rarely involved and preauricular adenopathy is rare.

Pneumonia in a young infant can occur between 2 and 19 weeks of age and is characterized by an afebrile illness with a repetitive staccato cough, tachypnea, and rales. Wheezing is uncommon. Hyperinflation with diffuse infiltrates can be seen on chest radiograph. Nasal stuffiness and otitis media can occur.

Diagnosis can be made by scraping the conjunctiva and culturing the material. Giemsa staining of the conjunctival scrapings revealing the presence of blue-stained intracytoplasmic inclusions within the epithelial cells is diagnostic. PCR is also available. Infants with conjunctivitis and pneumonia are treated with oral erythromycin for 14 days. Topical treatment of conjunctivitis is ineffective and unnecessary. The recommended topical prophylaxis with silver nitrate, erythromycin, or tetracycline for all newborns for the prevention of gonococcal ophthalmia does not prevent neonatal chlamydial conjunctivitis.

## MYCOBACTERIUM TUBERCULOSIS

▶ (SEE CHAPTER 124)

**SUGGESTED    READING**

De Almeida MFB, Draque CM: Neonatal jaundice and breastfeeding, *NeoReviews* 8:e282–e288, 2007.

Frankovich J, Sandborg C, Barnes P, et al: Neonatal lupus and related autoimmune disorders of infants, *NeoReviews* 9:e207–e217, 2008.

HAPO Study Cooperative Research Group: Hyperglycemia and adverse pregnancy outcomes, *N Engl J Med* 358(19):1991–2002, 2008.

Hoffman JD, Estrella EA: Newborn presentation of connective tissue disorders, *NeoReviews* 8:e110–e119, 2007.

Kates EH, Kates JS: Anemia and polycythemia in the newborn, *Pediatr Rev* 28:33–34, 2007.

Phillip AGS: Neonatal meningitis in the new millennium, *NeoReviews* 4:c73–c80, 2003.

Steinhorn RH, Farrow KN: Pulmonary hypertension in the neonate, *NeoReviews* 8:e14–e21, 2007.

Tumbaga PF, Philip AGS: Perinatal group B streptococcal infections and the new guidelines: an update, *NeoReviews* 7:e524–e530, 2006.

Wong RJ, Stevenson DK, Ahlfors CE, et al: Neonatal jaundice: bilirubin physiology and clinical chemistry, *NeoReviews* 8:e58–e67, 2007.

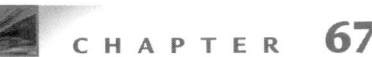

CHAPTER 67

# Overview and Assessment of Adolescents

The leading causes of mortality (Table 67-1) and morbidity (Table 67-2) in adolescents in the United States are behaviorally mediated. Motor vehicle injuries and other injuries account for more than 75% of all deaths. Unhealthy dietary behaviors and inadequate physical activity result in adolescent obesity with associated health complications (e.g., diabetes, hypertension).

It is the physician's responsibility to use every opportunity to inquire about risk-taking behaviors (Fig. 67-1), even when adolescents present to physicians with unrelated acute medical illnesses (e.g., sprained ankle, sore throat.) Physical symptoms in adolescents are often related to psychosocial problems.

## INTERVIEWING ADOLESCENTS

The adolescent interview differs through a shift of information gathering from the parent to the adolescent. Interviewing an adolescent alone and discussing confidentiality are the cornerstones of obtaining information regarding adolescent risk-taking behaviors and anticipatory guidance (see Chapters 7 and 9).

The interview should take into account the developmental age of the adolescent (Table 67-3). However, conversations about sports, friends, movies, and activities outside school can be useful for all ages and help develop a rapport (Fig. 67-2).

**Confidentiality** is a key element when interviewing an adolescent (Table 67-4). It is vital to engage the adolescent in an open discussion about risk-taking behavior, and this is more likely to happen when the adolescent is alone. Some issues cannot be kept confidential, such as suicidal

### TABLE 67-1 Leading Causes of Death in Adolescents

| Rank | Cause | Rate (per 100,000) |
|---|---|---|
| 1 | Unintentional injuries | 35.0 |
| 2 | Assault (homicide) | 9.3 |
| 3 | Suicide | 7.4 |
| 4 | Malignant neoplasms | 3.5 |
| 5 | Diseases of the heart | 2.0 |
| 6 | Congenital anomalies | 1.2 |
| 7 | Chronic respiratory disease | 0.5 |
| All others | Pulmonary disease, pneumonia, cerebrovascular disease | 8.9 |

From Centers for Disease Control and Prevention, National Center for Health Statistics: *Nat Vital Stat Rep* 53(17), 2005.

### TABLE 67-2 Prevalence of Common Chronic Illnesses of Children and Adolescents

| Illness | Prevalence |
|---|---|
| **PULMONARY** | |
| Asthma | 8%–12 % |
| Cystic fibrosis | 1:2500 white, 1:17,000 black |
| **NEUROMUSCULAR** | |
| Cerebral palsy | 2–3:1000 |
| Mental retardation | 1%–2% |
| Seizure disorder | 3.5:1000 |
| Any seizure | 3%–5% |
| Auditory-visual defects | 2%–3% |
| Traumatic paralysis | 2:1000 |
| Scoliosis | 3% males, 5% females |
| Migraine | 6%–27% (↑ with increasing age) |
| **ENDOCRINE/NUTRITION** | |
| Diabetes mellitus | 1.8:1000 |
| Obesity | 25%–30% |
| Anorexia nervosa | 0.5%–1% |
| Bulimia | 1% (young adolescence), 5%–10% (19–20 yr) |
| Dysmenorrhea | 20% |
| Acne | 65% |

intent, a positive human immunodeficiency virus (HIV) test (a duty to warn third parties), and disclosure of sexual or physical abuse. If there is an ambiguous situation, it is wise to obtain legal, ethical, or social worker consultation. When caring for a young adolescent, the health care provider should encourage open discussions with a parent, guardian, or other adult. Adolescents seek health care intermittently, and therefore it is important to take these opportunities to interview adolescents alone and discuss risk-taking issues (Table 67-5).

## Structured Communication Adolescent Guide (SCAG)

### Instructions for scoring this form

After your check-up, please score your doctor (or medical student) using this form.

*Examples:*

| 0 = Did Not | 1 = Did | 2 = Did Well |
|---|---|---|
| Dr. didn't ask at all. | Dr. asked as if reading a list. | Dr. established a relationship. |
| | Dr. asked as if embarrassed. | Dr. comfortable with questions. |
| | I felt judged. | Dr. did not judge. |
| | I felt a bit uncomfortable. | I felt comfortable. |

**General Rating:** Give a general impression of each section.
A = Excellent, B = Good, C = Average, D = Poor, F = Fail

| | Did Not 0 | Did 1 | Did Well 2 | Give examples of things that stood out in your interview, one positive and one negative. |
|---|---|---|---|---|
| **A. GETTING STARTED** | | | | *Example: I liked that you talked to me and not just my mom.* |
| 1. Greeted me. | 0 | 1 | 2 | |
| 2. Introduced self. | 0 | 1 | 2 | |
| 3. Discussed confidentiality. | 0 | 1 | 2 | |
| **GENERAL RATING**    A    B    C    D    F | | | | |

| | Did Not 0 | Did 1 | Did Well 2 | Give examples of things that stood out in your interview, one positive and one negative. |
|---|---|---|---|---|
| **B. GATHERING INFORMATION** | | | | *Example: I felt bad when you asked about smoking with my mom in the room.* |
| 4. Good body language. | 0 | 1 | 2 | |
| 5. Encouraged me to speak by asking questions other than ones with a yes/no answer. | 0 | 1 | 2 | |
| 6. Encouraged parent to speak (leave out if no parent present). | 0 | 1 | 2 | |
| 7. Listened and did not judge me. | 0 | 1 | 2 | |
| 8. Established relationship with me by appropriate choice of words. | 0 | 1 | 2 | |
| **GENERAL RATING**    A    B    C    D    F | | | | |

**FIGURE 67-1**

The Structured Communication Adolescent Guide (SCAG). The SCAG is an interviewing tool developed for learners to use with real or standardized adolescent patients. It incorporates the four major interview components: confidentiality, separation of the adolescent from the adult, psychosocial data gathering (using the HEADDSS mnemonic), and a nonjudgmental approach. The SCAG is at a grade 5 reading level and has demonstrated reliability and validity. A printable version is available through MedEdPORTAL.

*(Continued)*

|  | Did Not 0 | Did 1 | Did Well 2 | Give examples of things that stood out in your interview, one positive and one negative. |
|---|---|---|---|---|
| **C. TEEN ALONE** | | | | *Example: I was glad you talked about confidentially. I need lots of reassurance that you won't tell my mom.* |
| 9. Separated me and parent. *(Leave out if no parent present.)* | 0 | 1 | 2 | |
| 10. Discussed confidentiality. | 0 | 1 | 2 | |
| 11. Gave me a chance to talk about things other than what I came in to discuss. | 0 | 1 | 2 | |
| 12. Reflected on my feelings or concerns (example: You seem...) | 0 | 1 | 2 | |
| **LIFESTYLES:** Physician asks or talks about the following: | | | | |
| 13. **Home:** Family | 0 | 1 | 2 | |
| 14. **Education:** School | 0 | 1 | 2 | |
| 15.      Friends | 0 | 1 | 2 | |
| 16. **Activities** | 0 | 1 | 2 | |
| 17. **Alcohol:** Beer and hard liquor | 0 | 1 | 2 | |
| 18. **Drugs:** Cigarettes | 0 | 1 | 2 | |
| 19.      Marijuana | 0 | 1 | 2 | |
| 20.      Street drugs | 0 | 1 | 2 | |
| 21. **Diet:** Weight/diet/eating habits | 0 | 1 | 2 | |
| 22. **Sex:** Boyfriend/girlfriend | 0 | 1 | 2 | |
| 23.      Sexual activity | 0 | 1 | 2 | |
| 24.      Safe sex/ contraception | 0 | 1 | 2 | |
| 25. **Self:** Body image, self-esteem | 0 | 1 | 2 | *Example: You weren't embarrassed to talk about sex. OR You seemed embarrassed to talk about sex.* |
| 26.      Moods/depression/ suicide | 0 | 1 | 2 | |
| **GENERAL RATING**    A    B    C    D    F | | | | |

|  | Did Not 0 | Did 1 | Did Well 2 | Comments: Please give examples of things that stood out in your interview. |
|---|---|---|---|---|
| **D. WRAP UP** | | | | *Example: I wasn't sure what the next step would be.* |
| 27. Summary, recapped issues | 0 | 1 | 2 | |
| 28. Kept the confidentiality | 0 | 1 | 2 | |
| 29. Asked if there were any questions | 0 | 1 | 2 | |
| 30. Talked about what to do next (plan and follow-up) | 0 | 1 | 2 | |
| **GENERAL RATING**    A    B    C    D    F | | | | |

**FIGURE 67-1—Cont'd**

**TABLE 67-3 Adolescent Psychological Development**

| Stage | Age | Thinking | Characteristics |
|---|---|---|---|
| Early teens | 10–14 | Concrete ↓ | Appearance—"Am I normal?"<br>Invincible<br>Peer group<br>No tomorrow |
| Middle teens | 15–17 | | Risk-taking increased<br>Limit testing<br>"Who am I?"<br>Experiment with ideas |
| Late teens | 18–21 | Formal Operational | Future<br>Planning<br>Partner<br>Separation |

**TABLE 67-5 Interviewing the Adolescent Alone: Discussion of HEADDSS Topics***

| | |
|---|---|
| **H**OME/friends | Family, relationships, and activities. "What do you do for fun?" |
| **E**DUCATION | "What do you like best at school?" "How's school going?" |
| **A**LCOHOL | "Are any of your friends drinking?" "Are you drinking?" |
| **D**RUGS | Cigarettes, marijuana, street drugs. "Have you ever smoked?" "Many adolescents experiment with different drugs and substances. . . . have you tried anything?" |
| **D**IET* | Weight, diet/eating habits. "Many adolescents worry about their weight and try dieting. Have you ever done this?" |
| **S**EX | Sexual activity, contraception. "Are you going out with anybody?" "Have you dated in the past?" |
| **S**UICIDE/ DEPRESSION | Mood swings, depression, suicide attempts or thoughts, self-image. "Feeling down or depressed is common for everyone. Have you ever felt so bad that you wanted to harm yourself?" |

*The acronym HEADDSS can represent other terms, i.e., A = Activities, D = Depression. Also see Figure 67-1.

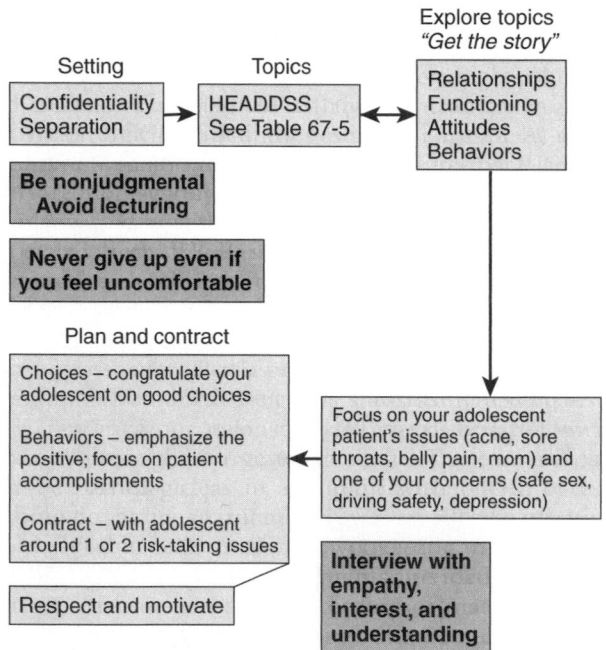

SETTING ~ TOPICS ~ EXPLORE ~ PLAN

**FIGURE 67-2**

STEP guide for adolescent interviewing.

The law confers certain rights on adolescents, depending on their health condition and personal characteristics, allowing them to receive health services without parental permission (Table 67-6). Usually adolescents can seek health care without parental consent for reproductive, mental, and emergency health services. Emancipated adolescents and *mature minors* may be treated without parental consent; such status should be documented in the record. The key characteristics of mature minors are their competence and capacity to understand, not their chronologic age. There must be a reasonable judgment that the health intervention is in the best interests of the minor.

During the physical examination, a choice between the parent or a chaperone being present needs to be offered.

**TABLE 67-4 Guidelines for Confidentiality**

Prepare the preadolescent and parent for confidentiality and being interviewed alone.
Discuss confidentiality at start of the interview.
Conversations with parents/guardians/adolescent are confidential (with exceptions*).
Reaffirm confidentiality when alone with your adolescent patient.

*Exceptions to confidentiality include major or impending harm to any person (i.e., abuse, suicide, homicide).

**TABLE 67-6 Legal Rights of Minors**

Age of majority (≥18 years of age in most states)
*Exceptions in which health care services can be provided to a minor**
  Emergency care (e.g., life-threatening condition or condition in which a delay in treatment would increase significantly the likelihood of morbidity)
  Diagnosis and treatment of sexuality-related health care
  Diagnosis and treatment of drug-related health care
  Emancipated minors (physically and financially independent of family; Armed Forces; married; childbirth)
  Mature minors (able to comprehend the risks and benefits of evaluation and treatment)
  ***All exceptions should be documented clearly in the patient's health record.***

*Determined by individual state laws.

# PHYSICAL GROWTH AND DEVELOPMENT OF ADOLESCENTS

## Girls

Breast budding under the areola (**thelarche**) and pubertal fine straight pubic hair over the mons pubis (**adrenarche** or **pubarche**) are early pubertal changes occurring around 11 years of age (range, 8 to 13 years) (see Chapter 174). These changes mark the sexual maturity rating, or Tanner stage, II of pubertal development (Figs. 67-3 and 67-4). Completion of the Tanner stages should take 4 to 5 years. The peak growth spurt usually occurs approximately 1 year after thelarche at sexual maturity rating stage III to IV breast development and before the onset of menstruation

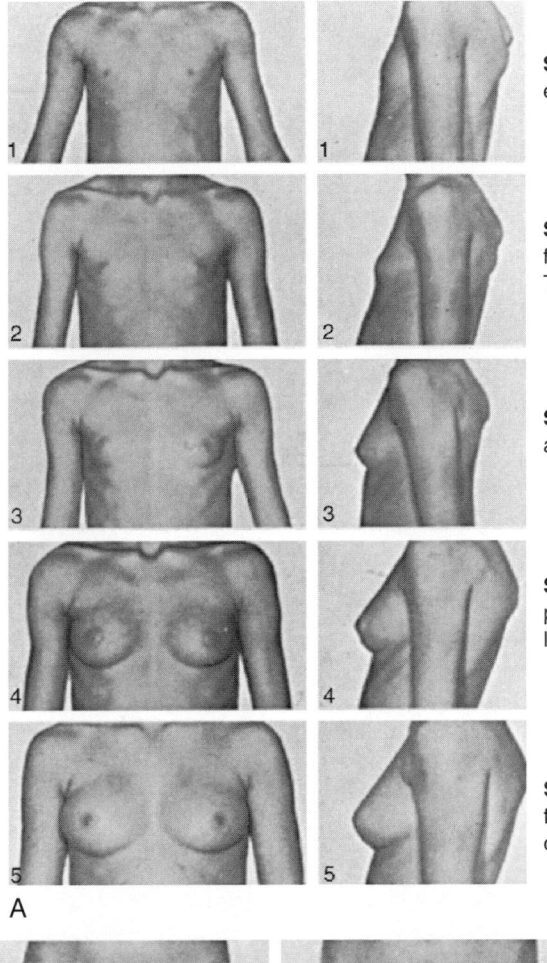

**Stage 1** The breasts are preadolescent. There is elevation of the papilla only.

**Stage 2** Breast bud stage. A small mound is formed by the elevation of the breast and papilla. The areolar diameter enlarges.

**Stage 3** There is further enlargement of breast and areola with no separation of their contours.

**Stage 4** There is a projection of the areola and papilla to form a secondary mound above the level of the breast.

**Stage 5** The breasts resemble those of a mature female as the areola has recessed to the general contour of the breast.

A

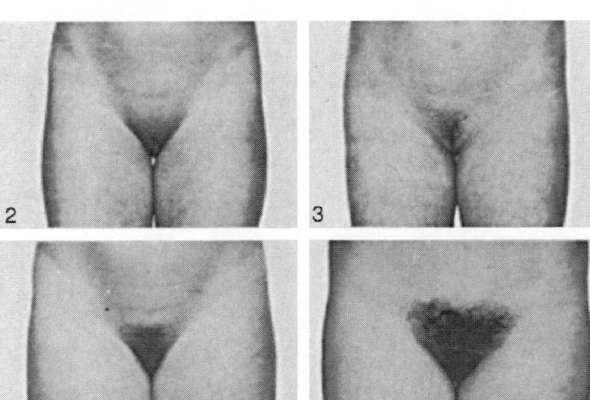

**Stage 2** There is sparse growth of long, slightly pigmented, downy hair, straight or only slightly curled, primarily along the labia.

**Stage 3** The hair is considerably darker, coarser, and more curled. The hair spreads sparsely over the junction of the pubes.

**Stage 4** The hair, now adult in type, covers a smaller area than in the adult and does not extend onto the thighs.

**Stage 5** The hair is adult in quantity and type, with extension onto the thighs.

B

**FIGURE 67-3**

Typical progression of female pubertal development, stages 1 to 5. **A,** Pubertal development in size of female breasts. **B,** Pubertal development of female pubic hair. Note that in stage 1 (not shown) there is no pubic hair. *(Courtesy of J.M. Tanner, MD, Institute of Child Health, Department of Growth and Development, University of London, London, England.)*

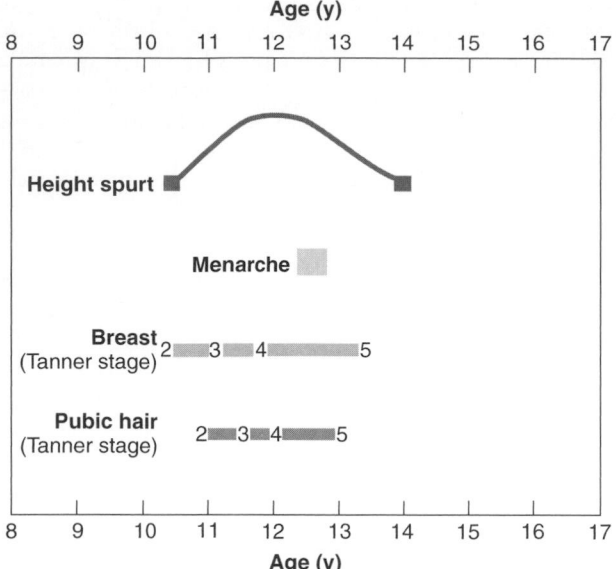

**FIGURE 67-4**

Sequence of pubertal events in the average American female. More recent studies suggest that onset of breast development may be 9 years of age for African-American girls and 10 years of age for white girls. (Adapted from Brookman RR, Rauh JL, Morrison JA, et al: The Princeton maturation study. 1976, unpublished data for adolescents in Cincinnati, Ohio. Reprinted from *Assessment of Pubertal Development.* Columbus, Ohio, Ross Laboratories, 1986.)

(**menarche**). Menarche is a relatively late pubertal event. Females grow only 2 to 5 cm in height before menarche (see Chapter 174).

The mean ages of thelarche and adrenarche are approximately 9 and 10 years for African-American and white girls, respectively. The mean ages of menarche are 12.2 and 12.9 years for African-American and white girls, respectively. The interval from the initiation of thelarche to the onset of menses (menarche) is 2.3 ± 1 years. Pubertal changes before 6 years of age in African-American and 7 years of age in white girls is considered precocious.

## Boys

Testicular enlargement (≥2.5 cm) corresponds to sexual maturity rating, or Tanner, stage I to II (Figs. 67-5 and 67-6). Testicular enlargement is followed by pubic hair development at the base of the penis (**adrenarche**) and then axillary hair within the year. The growth spurt is a relatively late event; it can occur from 10.5 years of age to 16 years of age. Deepening of the voice, facial hair, and acne indicate the early stages of puberty. See Chapter 174 for discussion of disorders of puberty.

## Changes Associated with Physical Maturation

Tanner stages mark biologic maturation that can be related to specific laboratory value changes and certain physical conditions. The higher hematocrit values in adolescent boys than in adolescent girls are the result of greater androgenic stimulation of the bone marrow and

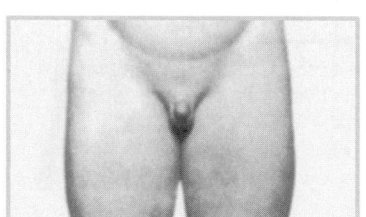

**Stage 1** The penis, testes, and scrotum are of childhood size.

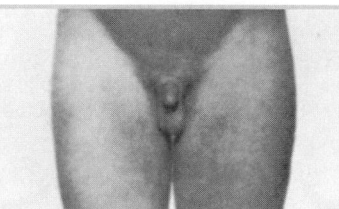

**Stage 2** There is enlargement of the scrotum and testes, but the penis usually does not enlarge. The scrotal skin reddens.

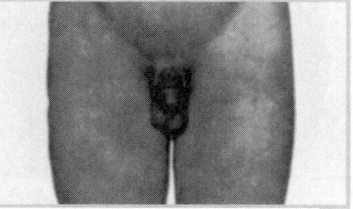

**Stage 3** There is further growth of the testes and scrotum and enlargement of the penis, mainly in length.

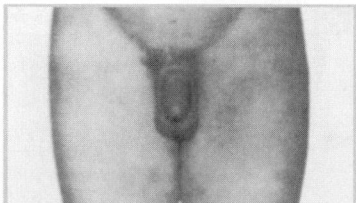

**Stage 4** There is still further growth of the testes and scrotum and increased size of the penis, especially in breadth.

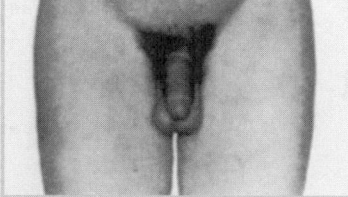

**Stage 5** The genitalia are adult in size and shape.

A

**FIGURE 67-5**

Typical progression of male pubertal development. **A,** Pubertal development in size of male genitalia. **B,** Pubertal development of male pubic hair. Note that in stage 1 there is no pubic hair. *(Courtesy of J.M. Tanner, MD, Institute of Child Health, Department of Growth and Development, University of London, London, England.)*

*(Continued)*

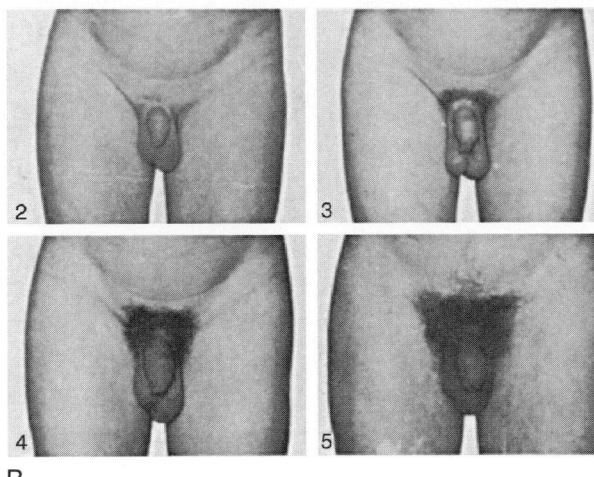

**Stage 2** There is sparse growth of long, slightly pigmented, downy hair, straight or only slightly curled, primarily at the base of the penis.

**Stage 3** The hair is considerably darker, coarser, and more curled. The hair spreads sparsely over the junction of the pubes.

**Stage 4** The hair, now adult in type, covers a smaller area than in the adult and does not extend onto the thighs.

**Stage 5** The hair is adult in quantity and type, with extension onto the thighs.

**FIGURE 67-5—Cont'd**

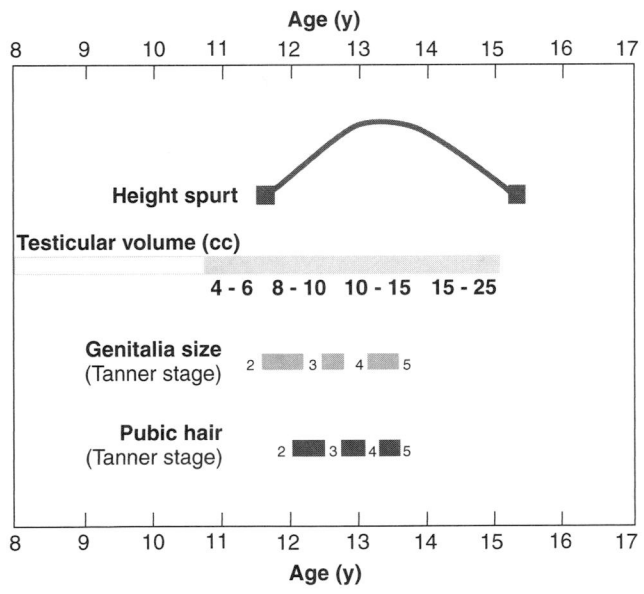

**FIGURE 67-6**

Sequence of pubertal events in the average American male. Testicular volume less than 4 mL using orchidometer (Prader Beads) represents prepubertal stage. (Adapted from Brookman RR, Rauh JL, Morrison JA, et al: The Princeton maturation study. 1976, unpublished data for adolescents in Cincinnati, Ohio. Reprinted from *Assessment of Pubertal Development.* Columbus, Ohio, Ross Laboratories, 1986.)

not loss through menstruation. Alkaline phosphatase levels in boys and girls increase during puberty because of rapid bone turnover, especially during the growth spurt. Worsening of mild scoliosis is common in adolescents during their growth spurt.

## PSYCHOLOGICAL GROWTH AND DEVELOPMENT OF ADOLESCENTS

▶ SEE TABLE 67-3 AND CHAPTERS 7 AND 9.

# Well-Adolescent Care

A nonjudgmental approach when history taking and collection of information in a friendly, open-minded manner produce a more accurate assessment of the adolescent. Keep questions to one at a time, and find some common ground to get the adolescent talking about himself or herself. The physician should be truthful and interested in the adolescent. The HEADDSS mnemonic can be used to remember the risk-taking elements of the history (see Table 67-5). Adolescents who experiment in one area of risk taking often have contemplated or tried multiple other risk-taking behaviors. It is important to collect the information before embarking on advice. When all the risk-taking information has been gathered, the physician should choose one or two health care issues to discuss, making it clear that the information is confidential and that he or she is there to help the adolescent in a partnership way. Although the focus in adolescent care is on psychosocial issues, a general examination also needs to be performed (Table 68-1). General pediatric issues, such as immunization (see Chapter 94) and health screening, should be included (see Table 9-5).

## EARLY ADOLESCENCE (AGE 10 TO 14 YEARS)

Rapid changes in physical appearance and behavior are the major characteristics of early adolescence, leading to a great deal of self-consciousness and need for privacy. The history focuses on an overall appraisal of the early adolescent's physical and psychosocial health.

**TABLE 68-1 Examination of the Adolescent**

### PHYSICAL EXAMINATION—CHECKLIST

Explain to your patient what you are going to do

Explain how you are going to do it

Ask if your adolescent wants his or her parent in the room*

Be sensitive to the adolescent's needs

Always use a sheet or blanket to provide privacy

Let the adolescent remain in his or her underwear with or without other clothes and work around clothing

Ask some questions as you go through the physical to keep the adolescent at ease. Give reassurance that elements of the physical are normal for this age

### ASSESSMENT

Examination can be used to offer reassurance about normalcy[†]

Assess

    Height/weight/body mass index and plot on percentile charts

    Skin for acne

    Mouth for periodontal disease

    Tanner staging

    Breasts and testicles

    Thyroid (palpation)

    Skeletal: scoliosis, Osgood-Schlatter disease, slipped capital femoral epiphysis

    Mental status for depression

    Signs of substance abuse, risk-taking behaviors, and trauma

*If not, you will need a chaperone.

[†]For example, 70% of boys can have breast enlargement (gynecomastia), and girls often have one breast larger than the other.

## MIDDLE ADOLESCENCE (AGE 15 TO 17 YEARS)

Autonomy and a global sense of identity are the major characteristics of middle adolescence. The history focuses on the middle adolescent's interactions with family, school, and peers. High-risk behaviors as a result of experimentation are common.

## LATE ADOLESCENCE (AGE 18 TO 21 YEARS)

Individuality and planning for the future are the major characteristics of late adolescence. Greater emphasis is placed on the late adolescent's responsibility for his or her health.

## PELVIC EXAMINATION

A full pelvic examination is rarely required in a virginal adolescent girl. A bimanual rectal-abdominal examination (all midline internal genitalia are immediately anterior to the rectal wall) is as efficient as a vaginal-abdominal examination. In some girls, especially virginal, anesthesia may be required for a full pelvic examination.

Before a pelvic examination, the patient should be informed about the importance of the assessment and what maneuvers will take place; she should be encouraged to ask questions before, during, or after the examination. In addition, a chaperone should be offered when a family caregiver is not present. The patient should be told that she has complete control over the examination and be supported to participate by using a mirror or to help guide the examiner. The patient can choose a supine or partially sitting position. The examiner should maintain eye contact during the examination. Before all maneuvers, the patient must be informed of what to expect and the sensations.

A padded examination table with the patient in a frog-leg position maximizes comfort of a pelvic examination. Stirrups can be used but are less comfortable. The examination room, lubricants, and instruments should be warm. The examination should be unhurried but efficient.

**Inspection** of the genitalia includes evaluation of the pubic hair, labia majora and minora, clitoris, urethra, and hymenal ring. When a **speculum examination** is required, it must be performed before bimanual palpation of internal genitalia because lubricants interfere with the evaluation of microscopic and microbiologic samples. The speculum allows visualization of the vaginal walls and cervical os for collection of appropriate specimens, such as cultures or Papanicolaou (Pap) smears. A Pap smear is not needed until the adolescent is sexually active, unless there is a history of sexual abuse or vulvar infection with human papillomavirus. In the rare circumstance that a vaginal examination is necessary in a virginal girl, a Huffman (0.5 inch × 4.5 inches) or Pedersen (0.9 inch × 4.5 inches) speculum should be used. A nonvirginal introitus frequently admits a small to medium-sized adult speculum.

## NORMAL VARIANTS OF PUBERTY

### Breast Asymmetry and Masses

It is not unusual for one breast to begin growth before, or to grow more rapidly than, the other, with resulting asymmetry. Some girls need to be reassured that after full maturation the asymmetry will be less obvious and that all women have some degree of asymmetry. The breast bud is a pea-sized mass below the nipple that is often tender. Occasionally, young women present with a breast mass; usually these are **benign fibroadenomas** or cysts (Table 68-2). Breast cancer is extremely rare in this age group. Ultrasound evaluation is better for evaluation of young, dense, breasts and avoids the radiation exposure of mammography.

### Physiologic Leukorrhea

Peripubertal girls (sexual maturity rating stage III) often complain of vaginal discharge. If the discharge is clear, without symptoms of pruritus or odor, it is most likely physiologic leukorrhea, due to ovarian estrogen stimulation of the uterus and vagina. Physical examination should reveal evidence of an estrogenized vulva and hymen without erythema or excoriation. The physician

| TABLE 68-2 Etiology of Breast Masses in Adolescents |
| --- |
| Classic or juvenile fibroadenoma (70%) |
| Fibrocystic disease |
| Breast cyst |
| Abscess/mastitis |
| Intraductal papilloma |
| Fat necrosis/lipoma |
| Cystosarcoma phyllodes (low-grade malignancy) |
| Adenomatous hyperplasia |
| Hemangioma, lymphangioma, lymphoma (rare) |
| Carcinoma (<1%) |

| TABLE 68-3 Etiology of Gynecomastia |
| --- |
| Idiopathic |
| Hypogonadism (primary or secondary) |
| Liver disease |
| Renal disease |
| Hyperthyroidism |
| Neoplasms |
|    Adrenal |
|    Ectopic human chorionic gonadotropin secreting |
|    Testicular |
| Drugs |
|    Antiandrogens |
|    Antibiotics (isoniazid, ketoconazole, metronidazole) |
|    Antacids ($H_2$ blockers) |
|    Cancer chemotherapy (especially alkylating agents) |
|    Cardiovascular drugs |
| Drugs of abuse |
|    Alcohol |
|    Amphetamines |
|    Heroin |
|    Marijuana |
| Hormones (for female sex) |
| Psychoactive agents (e.g., diazepam, phenothiazines, tricyclics) |

should always be alert for signs of abuse. If there are symptoms, cultures should be obtained. In these circumstances, vaginal cultures can be obtained without a speculum because **sexually transmitted infections** are vaginal until menarche, when cervical infections are the rule. Inspection of physiologic leukorrhea shows few white blood cells, estrogen maturation of vaginal epithelial cells, and no pathogens on culture.

## Irregular Menses

Menarche typically occurs approximately 2 years after thelarche, at the average age of 12.6 years. The initial menses are anovulatory and tend to be irregular in duration. This irregularity may persist for 2 to 5 years, so reassurance may be required. During this phase, estrogen feedback on the hypothalamus decreases gonadotropin secretion, which reduces estrogen production and induces an estrogen withdrawal bleed that can be prolonged and heavy. Anovulatory bleeding is usually painless. As the hypothalamic-pituitary-gonadal axis matures, the cycle becomes ovulatory, and menses are secondary to progesterone withdrawal. When ovulation is established, the average cycle length is 21 to 45 days. Some adolescents ovulate with their first cycle, as indicated by pregnancy before menarche.

## Gynecomastia

Breast enlargement in boys is usually a benign, self-limited condition. Gynecomastia is noted in 50% to 60% of boys during early adolescence. It is often idiopathic, but it may be noted in various conditions (Table 68-3). Typical findings include the appearance of a 1- to 3-cm, round, freely mobile, often tender, and firm mass immediately beneath the areola during sexual maturity rating stage III. Large, hard, or fixed enlargements and masses associated with any nipple discharge warrant further investigation. Reassurance is usually the only treatment required. If the condition worsens and is associated with psychological morbidity, it may be treated with bromocriptine. Surgical treatment with reduction mammoplasty can be helpful with massive hypertrophy.

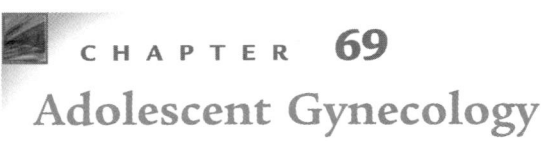

## CHAPTER 69

# Adolescent Gynecology

## MENSTRUAL DISORDERS

**Irregular menses** is the most common complaint of early adolescent girls. As regular, ovulatory cycles become established, pain with menstruation (**dysmenorrhea**) is a frequent complaint.

## Amenorrhea

**Primary amenorrhea** is the complete absence of menstruation by 16 years of age in the presence of breast development or by 14 years of age in the absence of breast development. **Secondary amenorrhea** refers to the cessation of menses for more than three consecutive months, any time after menarche, although irregular menses are the norm in the first 2 years after menarche.

Primary amenorrhea may be a result of functional or anatomic abnormalities of the hypothalamus, pituitary gland, ovaries, or uterus. Physiologic immaturity, stress, excessive exercise, and abnormal dietary patterns (anorexia/bulimia) are the most common causes of amenorrhea. Pregnancy should be considered in all cases of secondary amenorrhea, even if the patient denies sexual activity.

The **history** and **physical examination** usually point to a diagnosis and should guide the investigation. In adolescents with primary amenorrhea, abdominal pain, and secondary sexual characteristics, an outflow tract obstruction should be ruled out by ultrasound. There also may be an abdominal mass resulting from accumulated blood; imperforate hymen is visible on physical examination. For girls with primary amenorrhea without secondary sexual characteristics and an unremarkable history and physical examination, an endocrine evaluation is indicated. Follicle-stimulating hormone (FSH) and luteinizing hormone (LH) provide information about the origin of amenorrhea. A prolactinoma, although rare, must be ruled out. Elevated FSH and LH indicate primary ovarian failure, ovarian dysgenesis, or ovarian agenesis that warrants a karyotype. **Turner syndrome** is a common cause, but other chromosomal anomalies should be ruled out. Low levels of FSH and LH suggest hypothalamic dysfunction, which may be due to physiologic immaturity (often familial), isolated gonadotropin deficiency, or hypogonadotropic hypogonadism (chronic illness, low body weight, stressful life events). Additional hormone evaluation includes thyroid-stimulating hormone and prolactin. Hypothyroidism is a common cause of menstrual dysfunction.

Girls with secondary amenorrhea have secondary sexual characteristics. The most common causes are pregnancy, anorexia/stress (low LH, FSH, and estradiol), and **polycystic ovary syndrome**. In polycystic ovary syndrome, there may be symptoms of androgen excess, such as acne and hirsutism, and weight gain. If hirsutism or virilization is present, free and total testosterone, androstenedione, and dihydroepiandrosterone sulfate should be measured to rule out ovarian or adrenal tumors. 17-Hydroxyprogesterone rules out late-onset **congenital adrenal hyperplasia**. In polycystic ovary syndrome, the LH-to-FSH ratio is 2:1 or more; estradiol may be normal or low; and androgens, including dihydroepiandrosterone sulfate, are elevated, although not to the extent a tumor produces.

In a patient with amenorrhea (primary or secondary), normal secondary sex characteristics, negative pregnancy test, normal prolactin and thyroid-stimulating hormone, and no evidence of outflow tract obstruction, the total effect of estrogen on the uterus (rather than a single point estradiol level) can be determined by a **progesterone withdrawal test**. To achieve this, 5 to 10 mg of medroxyprogesterone (depending on body weight) is given daily for 5 days. If the uterus is normal and primed by estrogen (an intact hypothalamic-pituitary-gonadal axis) with no outflow tract obstruction, there should be bleeding within 1 week after the last progesterone tablet. If there is bleeding, the amenorrhea is secondary to anovulation, and cyclic progesterone withdrawal is recommended to induce uniform shedding to prevent endometrial hyperplasia and prolonged heavy bleeding secondary to asynchronous endometrial shedding. If there is no progesterone withdrawal bleeding, the uterus has been insufficiently exposed to estrogen, and there is systemic estrogen deficiency.

**Therapy** for the amenorrhea should be directed at the cause. Anovulation can be managed with either progesterone withdrawal or combined oral contraceptives (COCs). In hypothalamic amenorrhea and ovarian failure, there is an associated hypoestrogenism; therapy needs to be directed at replacing estrogen and progesterone, usually with a COC. Polycystic ovary syndrome usually can be treated effectively with weight loss, exercise, progesterone withdrawal, or COC. If there is evidence of androgen excess, COCs reduce androgen production from the ovaries and increases sex hormone–binding globulin to reduce the amount of available androgen. Spironolactone helps treat hirsutism, and when there is evidence of insulin insensitivity, metformin can restore ovulatory cycles.

## Abnormal Uterine Bleeding

Normal, ovulatory menses can occur 21 to 45 days apart, measuring from the first day of menstruation to the first day of the next menstruation. The average duration of flow is 3 to 7 days, with more than 7 days considered prolonged. More than 8 well-soaked pads or 12 tampons per day may be considered excessive, although classically blood loss is difficult to estimate because the frequency of pad change varies greatly among women. Table 69-1 defines menstrual disorders. If the menstrual problem is unclear and nonacute, observation and charting on a menstrual calendar are warranted. Excessively heavy, prolonged, or infrequent bleeding in the first year after menarche is often physiologic but should be investigated, especially if there is associated iron deficiency anemia.

In adolescents with heavy or prolonged menses, especially those presenting in early menarche, approximately 20% have a coagulation disorder, and 10% have other pathology. If an underlying pathology is discovered (**functional uterine bleeding**), treatment should be directed at the primary disorder and the secondary menstrual dysfunction.

**Dysfunctional uterine bleeding** is any abnormal pattern of endometrial shedding not caused by an underlying pathologic process. It is one of the few conditions in adolescent health care that is a diagnosis of exclusion (Table 69-2). **Anovulation** occurs in most of these cases. Without progesterone from the corpus luteum, unopposed estrogen causes endometrial hyperplasia and irregular endometrial shedding, which can be prolonged and heavy, sometimes life-threatening. Progesterone induces a secretory endometrium. When progesterone is withdrawn, the endometrium sheds in a synchronous fashion with myometrial and vascular contractions (causing dysmenorrhea but limiting blood loss). After 1 year of regular cycles, irregular bleeding usually indicates an organic abnormality.

A thorough history with a menstrual calendar indicating the amount of flow and associated symptoms is followed by physical examination, including a pelvic

---

**TABLE 69-1 Definition of Menstrual Disorders**

Amenorrhea—no menstruation
Oligomenorrhea—too few (episodes of bleeding)
Menorrhagia—too much (blood loss)
Metrorrhagia—too many (episodes of bleeding)
Menometrorrhagia—too much and too many

### TABLE 69-2 Differential Diagnosis of Abnormal Vaginal Bleeding*

Pregnancy, including ectopic pregnancy
Infection—usually sexually transmitted
Endocrine disorder—thyroid disorder, PCO, pituitary disorder
Systemic disease
Trauma
Medications
Blood dyscrasia
Vaginal, cervical, or uterine disorders
Ovarian tumor/cyst
Contraception
Foreign body

*When all excluded, the diagnosis of dysfunctional uterine bleeding can be made.
PCO, polycystic ovaries.

examination in a nonvirginal adolescent or an ultrasound in a virginal adolescent. A complete blood count, pregnancy test, thyroid function tests, and coagulation screen should be performed. In sexually active adolescents, **sexually transmitted infections (STIs)** should be ruled out.

Unpredictable, heavy, and prolonged menses may impair school attendance and social functioning; iron deficiency anemia is associated with lower academic scores. **Treatment** is indicated for heavy menses. Chronic and acute bleeding can be managed with COCs; multiple daily doses may be required until blood loss is controlled. Occasionally, uncontrollable bleeding requires hospitalization for intravenous fluids and high-dose estrogen. Uterine curettage is rarely indicated in adolescents. Iron therapy is also important. Use of COCs to regulate menstruation and allow the hypothalamic-pituitary-gonadal axis to mature is appropriate; only 6 to 12 months of therapy may be required. COCs are paramount in the management of menorrhagia in individuals with **bleeding disorders** (von Willebrand disease), although adjuvant therapy with tranexamic acid may be needed if the COC is given cyclically. Parents are often concerned that COC use will cause their daughter to become sexually active, but literature and experience do not support this.

## Dysmenorrhea

The most common gynecologic complaint of young women is painful menstruation, or dysmenorrhea, during the first 1 to 3 days of bleeding. **Primary dysmenorrhea** is defined as pelvic pain during menstruation in the absence of pelvic pathology and is a feature of ovulation, typically developing 1 to 3 years after menarche, with an increasing incidence to the age of 24, as ovulatory cycles are established. The etiology is the release of prostaglandins and leukotrienes from the degenerating endometrium after progesterone levels decline from the ovulatory follicle (corpus luteum). This release causes increased uterine tone and increased frequency and dysrhythmia of uterine contractions creating excessive uterine pressures and ischemia, which heightens the sensitivity of pain fibers to bradykinin and other physical stimuli.

Pain occurring at menarche should be investigated by ultrasound to rule out an underlying structural problem, such as an obstructive müllerian anomaly. Primary dysmenorrhea, the most common form of painful menses, is experienced by most adolescent girls and is a leading cause of short-term school absenteeism.

**Secondary dysmenorrhea** is menstrual pain associated with pelvic pathology and is caused most frequently by **endometriosis** or **pelvic inflammatory disease**. Adolescents with endometriosis usually have mild to moderate disease, but girls with obstructed outflow tracts tend to have severe endometriosis soon after menarche. Intrauterine device use and benign tumors of the uterus (leiomyomas or polyps) are a rare cause of acquired dysmenorrhea in adolescents. The types of dysmenorrhea usually can be distinguished by history and physical examination. Ultrasound is preferred to define obstructing genital tract lesions. Magnetic resonance imaging may be useful in complex reproductive tract anomalies. Laparoscopy is required to diagnose endometriosis and pelvic inflammatory disease with certainty, although it usually is reserved for patients who fail medical therapy.

**Treatment** of primary dysmenorrhea should be considered with symptoms causing significant distress. First-line therapy is with nonsteroidal anti-inflammatory drugs (NSAIDs), to inhibit the synthesis of prostaglandins (Table 69-3). To maximize pain relief, NSAIDs should be taken before or as soon as menstruation begins, and the dosing schedule should be followed closely. NSAIDs also decrease blood flow, but they do not regulate menstrual cycles. Typically, NSAIDs are needed for 2 to 3 days. If NSAIDs fail to provide adequate relief, COCs may be added.

If dysmenorrhea persists despite an adequate trial of COCs (>4 months), an alternative diagnosis, such as endometriosis, should be considered. Endometriosis can usually be managed with COCs. When they fail, a laparoscopy should be performed before advancing therapy to confirm the diagnosis and excise endometriotic lesions. Continuous COC therapy (84 days of active COC followed by a 5- to 7-day hormone-free interval) may control symptoms. An alternative is depot medroxyprogesterone acetate (150 mg) every 2 months until symptoms are controlled, then every 3 months. Because treatment for endometriosis is long-term, medications used in older

### TABLE 69-3 Treatment of Dysmenorrhea

NSAIDs
Over-the-counter
  Ibuprofen or naproxen sodium taken every 4 hr
Prescription
  Ibuprofen 400 mg PO qid
  Naproxen 500 mg PO stat then 250 PO qid
  Mefenamic acid 500 mg PO stat then 250 mg qid
Combined oral contraceptives—cyclic or continuous
Progesterone-only pill
Depo-Provera—150 mg IM every 13 wk

NSAIDs, nonsteroidal anti-inflammatory drugs.

women, such as danazol (a weak synthetic male hormone) or gonadotropin-releasing hormone agonists (nafarelin or leuprolide), are a last resort for symptom relief.

## PREGNANCY

The median age of first intercourse in the United States is 17 years for girls and 16 years for boys; this is similar to other developed countries. Although the age of coital initiation is similar among different socioeconomic groups, the prevalence of adolescent childbearing outside of marriage is greatest in the lower socioeconomic strata. Approximately 900,000 females 12 to 19 years of age become pregnant each year. In women younger than 20 years of age, there are 97 pregnancies, 54 births, and 29 abortions per 1000. Increased use of contraceptives has reduced adolescent pregnancy by up to 35%, since the peak year of 1990. Adolescents who continue their pregnancy have an increased incidence of premature births, small for gestational age infants, postneonatal mortality, child abuse, subsequent maternal unemployment, and poor maternal educational achievement. These risks are primarily due to behavior rather than inherent biologic risks within adolescents. With good prenatal care, nutrition, and social support, a pregnant adolescent has the same chance of delivering a healthy term infant as an adult of similar sociodemographic background.

### Diagnosis

Pregnancy should be considered and ruled out in any adolescent presenting with secondary amenorrhea. Frequently, pregnant adolescents delay seeking a diagnosis until several periods have been missed and initially may deny having intercourse. Early adolescents often present with other symptoms, such as vomiting, vague pains, or deteriorating behavior and may report normal periods. Because of the varied presentations of adolescent pregnancy, a thorough menstrual history should be obtained in all menstruating adolescents. Urine pregnancy tests are sensitive approximately 7 to 10 days after conception. Rape or incest should be ruled out in all cases of adolescent pregnancy.

When pregnancy is confirmed, immediate gestational dating is important to assist in planning. Options are to continue or terminate the pregnancy (if not beyond 20 to 24 weeks' gestation). With the former, the adolescent may choose to parent the child or have the child adopted. Pregnant adolescents should be encouraged to involve their families because the adolescent may not be mature enough to make the decision alone; parents may be more understanding than the adolescent expects.

### Continuation of the Pregnancy

Adolescents who continue the pregnancy need early, consistent, and comprehensive prenatal care by a team of health care providers. All aspects of their socioeconomic situation should be evaluated in an effort to optimize the infant's health and development. Although fewer than 5% of adolescents have their infants adopted, this option should be discussed. Pregnancy is the most common cause for females to drop out of school, so special attention should be given to keeping the adolescent in school during and after pregnancy.

### Termination

If a pregnant adolescent chooses to terminate her pregnancy, she should be referred immediately to a nonjudgmental abortion service. The options for pregnancy termination depend on the gestational age; there is increasing morbidity and mortality with increasing gestational age. Surgical procedures include manual vacuum aspiration (≤8 weeks' gestational age), suction curettage (≤12 to 14 weeks' gestational age depending on the provider), and dilation and evacuation (14 to 20 weeks' gestational age). Early pregnancy (<8 weeks' gestational age) can be terminated medically with oral mifepristone (RU-486) in combination with misoprostol, methotrexate with misoprostol, or misoprostol alone. Adolescents rarely present early enough to explore this option. In the second trimester (>12 weeks' gestational age), labor induction and delivery can be effected by vaginal misoprostol or the intra-amniotic instillation of prostaglandins or hypertonic saline. Psychosocial support and subsequent contraceptive counseling and implementation should be available for adolescents who choose abortion.

## CONTRACEPTION

Adolescents often begin intercourse without adequate birth control. Knowledge about sexuality and contraception is crucial. Because unintended pregnancy can be associated with significant psychosocial morbidity for the mother, father, and child, prevention should be a primary goal. All methods of contraception significantly reduce the risk of pregnancy when used in a consistent and correct fashion. The best form of contraception is the one an individual will use.

### Abstinence

Abstaining from sexual intercourse is the most commonly used and most effective form of adolescent birth control. A degree of self-control, self-assuredness, and self-esteem is necessary. Adolescents who choose to be sexually active should be offered birth control, because there is a 70% chance of pregnancy in 1 year of regular, unprotected intercourse.

### Steroidal Contraception

It is important to remind young women that steroidal contraception does not provide any protection from STIs, and condoms should be used to reduce the risk of infection.

### Combined Oral Contraceptives

COCs contain a synthetic estrogen and progesterone that suppress gonadotropin secretion and ovarian follicle development and ovulation. COCs also produce an

**TABLE 69-4  Absolute Contraindications to Combined Oral Contraceptives**

<6 wk postpartum
Smoking and age >35 yr
Hypertension (systolic ≥160 mm Hg or diastolic ≥100 mm Hg)
Current or past history of venous thromboembolism
Ischemic heart disease
History of cerebrovascular accident
Complicated valvular heart disease (pulmonary hypertension, atrial fibrillation, history of subacute bacterial endocarditis)
Migraine with focal neurologic symptoms
Breast cancer (current)
Diabetes with retinopathy/nephropathy/neuropathy
Severe cirrhosis
Liver tumor (adenoma or hepatoma)

atrophic endometrium (inhospitable for blastocyst implantation) and thicken cervical mucus to inhibit sperm penetration. COCs are 99% effective if taken regularly and have numerous noncontraceptive benefits (decreased acne, less dysmenorrhea, and smaller menstrual flow). After a history and physical examination, COCs can be started on the first day of the next menstrual period. Contraindications and relative contraindications to COCs are listed in Tables 69-4 and 69-5. Blood pressure measurement to rule out preexisting hypertension should be obtained before prescribing a COC. A Papanicolaou (Pap) smear and STI screening are not mandatory for the initiation of contraception because birth control and health screenings are separate issues and can be left to the next visit. Initially the adolescent should be seen monthly to reinforce good contraceptive use and safer sex (condom use to reduce STI). Counseling is the key to good contraceptive use and continuation. Until adolescents show the ability to take a pill daily, contraception with COCs should be avoided. When COCs are prescribed, 20 µg (or less) low-dose ethinyl estradiol pills in 28-day packets are recommended because they encourage a daily routine. One novel contraceptive regimen has packaged 84 active tablets to be taken sequentially followed by a 7-day hormone-free interval and the next package. Any COC can be used in such a fashion to induce long intervals between withdrawal bleeding.

**TABLE 69-5  Relative Contraindications to Combined Oral Contraceptives**

Adequately controlled hypertension
Hypertension (systolic 140–159 mm Hg, diastolic 90–99 mm Hg)
Migraine and age >35 yr
Currently symptomatic gallbladder disease
Mild cirrhosis
History of combined oral contraceptive–related cholestasis

Initially, **side effects**, such as nausea (pills should be taken at night to reduce this), breast tenderness, and breakthrough bleeding (especially if pills are missed), are common. The adolescent should be counseled that these symptoms are usually transient and not to discontinue COC use until discussion with a health care professional. Adolescents should be informed that COCs do not generally cause weight gain, but rather that as women mature, weight gain is normal. Usually 3 to 4 months on one COC is needed to determine acceptability. If there is breakthrough bleeding, before changing pills, the physician should determine how often pills are forgotten. If **a single pill is forgotten**, two pills should be taken on the subsequent day. **If 2 days were missed**, two pills may be taken on the 2 subsequent days. **If 3 or more days are missed**, the adolescent should consider emergency contraception, if at risk for pregnancy, and take a total of 7 days off, while using another form of birth control, then start a new cycle. If taken properly, COCs are effective in the first month of use, but health care providers usually suggest use of additional contraception in the first month.

## Progesterone-Only Pill or Minipill

Although not as widely used as COCs, the progestin-only pill, *norethindrone (Micronor)*, is a safe and effective form of contraception when used consistently. It is supplied in packages of 28 tablets, each containing 0.35 mg of norethindrone with no hormone-free interval. It prevents pregnancy through reduced volume, increased viscosity, and altered molecular structure of cervical mucus, resulting in little or no sperm penetration. In addition, endometrial changes reduce the potential for implantation, and ovulation is partially or completely suppressed. Approximately 40% of women using progestin-only contraceptives continue to ovulate. Progesterone-only contraception is indicated for women who have a contraindication to estrogen-based contraceptives (see Table 69-4) or have estrogen-related side effects.

## Contraceptive Vaginal Ring

The contraceptive vaginal ring (*NuvaRing*) is a flexible, Silastic ring with an outer diameter of 54 mm and a cross-sectional diameter of 4 mm. The ring releases a constant rate of 15 µg of ethinyl estradiol and 0.120 mg of etonogestrel per day. Each ring is used continuously for 3 weeks and then removed. A new ring is inserted 7 days later. Because the need for daily or coital use is circumvented, failure secondary to missed dosing is reduced. The contraindications and side effects are the same as with COCs.

## Contraceptive Patch

The contraceptive patch (*norelgestromin [Evra]*) is a 25-cm$^2$ pink patch that is applied, usually on the buttocks, for 1 week followed by removal and application of a new patch for a total of 3 weeks of patch use, then a patch-free week for a withdrawal bleed. The 4-week cycle is repeated. The daily dose is equivalent to a 35-µg ethinyl estradiol COC.

Because the need for daily or coital use is circumvented, failure secondary to missed dosing is reduced. In women weighing 90 kg or more, the contraceptive patch is less efficacious. Contraindications and side effects are the same as COCs.

## Hormonal Injections and Implants

Intramuscular injection of 150 mg of medroxyprogesterone acetate (*Depo-Provera*) every 13 weeks is an effective form of birth control. Progesterone-only contraception is associated with menstrual irregularities (70% amenorrhea and 30% metrorrhagia). Medroxyprogesterone acetate (*Depo-SubQ Provera 104*) is designed for subcutaneous use every 13 weeks and may be self-administered with minimal training. An implant containing the progestin etonogestrel (*Implanon*) is now available on the U.S. market. This single rod implant is inserted subcutaneously and is effective for 3 years. These forms of contraception are user and coital independent and reduce failure secondary to missed doses.

## Intrauterine Devices

Intrauterine devices (IUDs) are inserted into the uterus where they release either copper (*ParaGard*) that is spermicidal or levonorgestrel (*Mirena*) that prevents implantation by inducing an atrophic endometrium. The copper IUD, which lasts up to 10 years, may increase the amount and duration of bleeding as well as dysmenorrhea. Mirena is highly effective for up to 5 years while decreasing bleeding and dysmenorrhea, even causing amenorrhea. IUDs are not generally recommended for adolescents due to the risk of STI in this age group. IUDs do not increase the risk of infection but may worsen the outcome by increasing the incidence of upper tract disease (pelvic inflammatory disease), tubal obstruction, and infertility. In addition, it can be more difficult to insert an IUD in a nulliparous female. IUDs require no active involvement by the user and, thus, eliminate user error. Condoms should be encouraged to reduce the risk of STI.

## Emergency Postcoital Contraception

Emergency postcoital contraception should be discussed at every visit. A prescription should be given in advance of need when no over-the-counter access is available. Emergency contraception reduces the risk of pregnancy after unprotected intercourse if used within 72 hours, although efficacy is greatest when used as early as possible. There is some efficacy, although reduced, for up to 5 days. Other indications and contraindications to emergency postcoital contraception are listed in Table 69-6. There are two forms of emergency contraception: the **Yuzpe Regimen** consisting of two *Ovral* tablets (50 μg of ethinyl estradiol and 250 μg of norgestrel each) repeated in 12 hours (a total of four pills) and **Plan B** (0.75 mg of levonorgestrel), one pill taken twice, 12 hours apart or two tablets given once. Plan B is also associated with significantly less nausea and vomiting than

| TABLE 69-6 Emergency Contraception |
|---|
| **INDICATIONS** |
| No method of contraception being used |
| Condom breaks |
| Diaphragm dislodged/removed <6 hr |
| Missed birth control pills |
| >1 wk late for Depo-Provera |
| Ejaculation on external genitalia |
| Sexual assault |
| **CONTRAINDICATIONS** |
| Known pregnancy |
| If strong contraindications to estrogens, use progestin |

the Yuzpe Regimen. Mifepristone is also an effective postcoital contraceptive; however, it is not approved for this use in the United States. A copper IUD can be inserted 7 days from the act of unprotected intercourse and has an efficacy of greater than 99%. This method is not generally recommended for adolescents (see previous discussion).

## Barrier Methods

### Condoms and Foam

When condoms and spermicide (foam, gel, film, sponge) are used together in a consistent (each and every act of intercourse) and correct (film must be placed 10 minutes before intercourse) fashion, they are almost as effective as COCs in the prevention of pregnancy, especially in individuals who have infrequent intercourse. Advantages of this method are that the agents are available over-the-counter without the need for a physician visit or prescription and that they reduce the risk of STIs, including human immunodeficiency virus (HIV) (latex and polyurethane condoms). The female condom (*Reality*) is an additional barrier method made of polyurethane that affords females more control, but adolescents usually do not consider it aesthetically pleasing.

### Sponge, Caps, and Diaphragm

The vaginal sponge (*Protectaid*) is a spermicide-impregnated synthetic sponge that is effective for 24 hours of intercourse. The *FemCap* is a silicone cap fitted by a health care provider and then placed on the cervix by the user before intercourse. This method is technically difficult, especially for an adolescent. The *diaphragm* is fitted by a health care provider but is technically simpler to use than the cap because the edges go into the vaginal fornices. To be effective, the diaphragm should be used with spermicide applied to the cervical side and along the rim. The diaphragm needs additional spermicide with each act of intercourse. The *Leashield* is a silicone device, similar to a diaphragm that covers the cervix and adheres to the vaginal vault by a mild vacuum generated by its design. All of these methods need to be left in place for 6 hours after the last act of intercourse for optimal efficacy.

## Coitus Interruptus

Withdrawal is a common method of birth control used by sexually active adolescents, but it is ineffective because sperm are released into the vagina before ejaculation and withdrawal may occur after ejaculation has begun.

## Rhythm Method (Periodic Coital Abstinence)

The rhythm method is the practice of periodic abstinence just before, during, and just after ovulation. This method requires the user to have an accurate knowledge of her cycle, awareness of clues indicating ovulation, and discipline. Adolescents tend to have unpredictable cycles and consequently less predictable ovulation, so it is difficult to determine with any accuracy a time of the month that can be considered completely safe.

## Oral and Anal Sex

Some adolescents engage in oral or anal sex because they believe that it eliminates the need for contraception. Many do not consider this activity to mean *having sex.* Condoms generally are not used during oral or anal sex, but the risk of acquiring an STI is still present. Heterosexual adolescents who deny being sexually active should be asked specifically about nonvaginal forms of sexual activity, and adolescents who engage in oral and anal sex require STI and HIV counseling and screening.

## RAPE

*Rape* is a legal term for nonconsensual intercourse. Almost half of rape victims are adolescents, and the perpetrator is known in 50% of cases. Although gathering historical and physical evidence for a criminal investigation is important, the physician's primary responsibility is to perform these functions in a supportive, nonjudgmental manner. The history should include details of the sexual assault, time from the assault until presentation, whether the victim cleaned herself, date of last menstrual period, and previous sexual activity, if any.

For optimal results, forensic material should be collected within 72 hours of the assault. Clothes, especially undergarments, need to be placed in a paper bag for drying (plastic holds humidity, which allows organisms to grow, destroying forensic evidence). The patient should be inspected for bruising, bites, and oral, genital, and anal trauma. Photographs are the best record to document injuries. Specimens should be obtained from the fingernails, mouth, vagina, pubic hair, and anus. The sexual assault kit provides materials to obtain DNA from semen, saliva, blood, fingernail scrapings, and pubic hair. A wet mount of vaginal fluids shows the presence or absence

of sperm under the microscope. Cultures for STIs should be taken but are often negative (unless previously infected), because 72 hours are needed for the bacterial load to be sufficient for culture. Blood should be drawn for baseline HIV and syphilis (Venereal Disease Research Laboratories [VDRL] test). All materials must be maintained in a "chain of evidence" that cannot be called into question in court.

Therapy after a rape includes prophylaxis for emergency contraception and STI and, if indicated, hepatitis immune globulin and hepatitis vaccine. A single oral dose of cefixime, 400 mg, and azithromycin, 1 g, treats *Chlamydia,* gonorrhea, and syphilis. An alternative regimen is a single intramuscular dose of ceftriaxone, 125 mg, with a single oral dose of azithromycin, 1 g. For prophylaxis against bacterial vaginosis and *Trichomonas,* a single oral dose of metronidazole, 2 g, is recommended. Repeat cultures, wet mounts, and a pregnancy test should be performed 3 weeks after the assault, followed by serology for syphilis, hepatitis, and HIV at 12 weeks. Long-term sequelae are common; patients should be offered immediate and ongoing psychological support, such as that offered by local rape crisis services.

# CHAPTER 70
# Eating Disorders

Eating disorders are common chronic diseases in adolescents, especially in females. The *Diagnostic and Statistical Manual of Mental Disorders, fourth edition (DSM-IV),* classifies these psychiatric illnesses as *anorexia nervosa, bulimia nervosa, binge eating disorder (compulsive eating),* and *eating disorder not otherwise specified.* The diagnosis in young adolescents (pre–growth spurt, premenstrual) may not follow the classic DSM IV–diagnostic criteria. The normal developmental milestones of adolescence may be triggers for eating disorders (Table 70-1).

**TABLE 70-1 Normal Adolescent Milestones**

| Psychological Stages | Issues That Can Trigger Eating Disorders |
|---|---|
| Early adolescence—increased body awareness | Fear of growing up |
| Middle adolescence—increased self-awareness | Rebelliousness |
| | Competition and achievement |
| Late adolescence—identity | Anxiety and worry for the future |
| | Need for control |

# ANOREXIA NERVOSA

The prevalence of anorexia nervosa is 1.5% in teenage girls. The female-to-male ratio is approximately 20:1, and the condition shows a familial pattern. The cause of anorexia nervosa is unknown, but it involves a complex interaction between social, environmental, psychological, and biologic events (Fig. 70-1). Risk factors have been identified (Fig. 70-2).

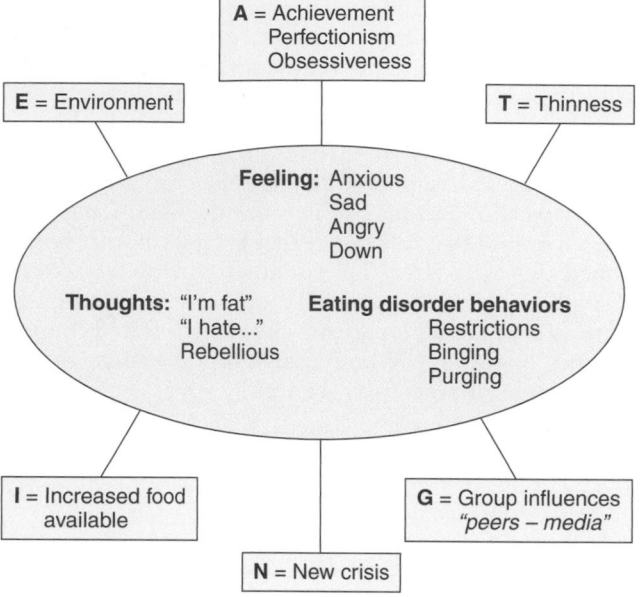

**FIGURE 70-1**

The slippery slope to eating disorders.

**FIGURE 70-2**

The EATING disorder cycle.

## Clinical Manifestations and Diagnosis

It is important to screen early for eating disorders. Screening is best done as a part of the larger psychosocial screen for risk-taking factors (see Fig. 67-1). It is recommended that the adolescent be interviewed alone. An adolescent with an eating disorder may minimize the problem. So interviewing the parent(s) alone is also important, the first event that a patient with anorexia or bulimia usually describes is a behavioral change in eating or exercise (food obsession, food-related ruminations, mood changes). The patient has an unrealistic body image and feels too fat despite appearing excessively thin. Parents' response to this situation can be anger, self-blame, focusing attention on the child, ignoring the disorder, or approving of the behavior.

The physician should be nonjudgmental, collect information, and work on a differential diagnosis. The **differential diagnosis** of weight loss includes gastroesophageal reflux, peptic ulcer, malignancy, chronic diarrhea, malabsorption, inflammatory bowel disease, increased energy demands, hypothalamic lesions, hyperthyroidism, diabetes mellitus, and Addison disease. Psychiatric disorders also need to be considered (drug abuse, depression, obsessive-compulsive disorders).

The **clinical features** of anorexia include the patient wearing oversized layered clothing to hide appearance, fine hair on the face and trunk (lanugo-like hair), rough and scaly skin, bradycardia, hypothermia, decreased body mass index, erosion of enamel of teeth (acid from emesis), and acrocyanosis of hands and feet. Signs of hyperthyroidism should not be present (see Chapter 175). The diagnostic criteria for anorexia nervosa are listed in Table 70-2.

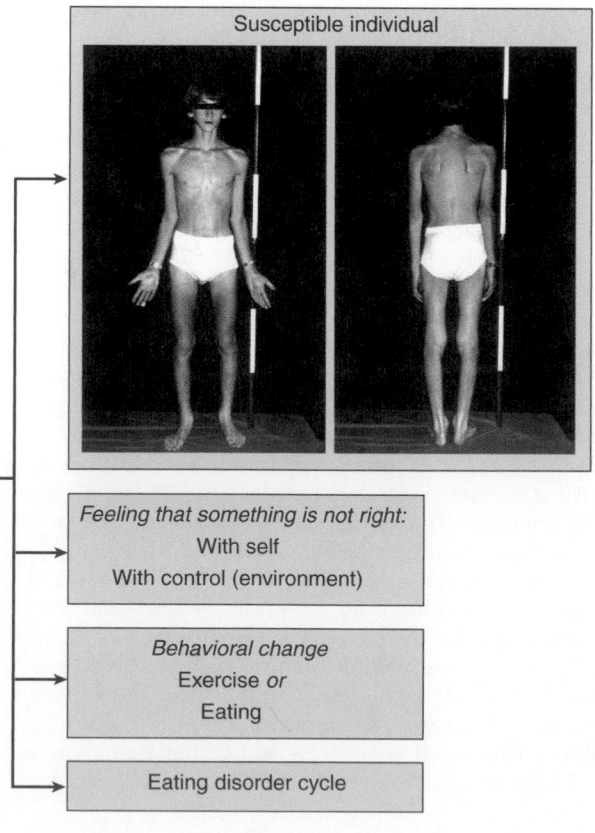

| TABLE 70-2 Diagnostic Criteria for Anorexia Nervosa |
|---|
| Refusal to maintain body weight at or above a minimally normal weight for age and height (e.g., weight loss leading to body weight <85% of ideal)* |
| Intense fear of gaining weight or becoming fat, even though underweight |
| Denial of the seriousness of the low body weight—a disturbance in the way in which one's body weight or shape is experienced |
| Amenorrhea in postmenarche females* |

*The diagnostic criteria may be difficult to meet in a young adolescent. Allow for a wide spectrum of clinical features.

| TABLE 70-4 Diagnostic Criteria for Bulimia Nervosa |
|---|
| Recurrent episodes of binge eating, at least twice a week for 3 months, characterized by the following: |
|   Eating in a discrete period an amount of food that is definitely larger than most people would eat during a similar period |
|   A sense of lack of control over eating during the episode (e.g., a feeling that one cannot stop eating or control what or how much one is eating) |
| Compensatory behavior to prevent weight gain (i.e., self-induced vomiting, misuse of laxatives or diuretics, excessive exercise) |
| Self-evaluation unduly influenced by body shape and weight |
| Disturbance does not occur exclusively during episodes of anorexia nervosa |

## Treatment and Prognosis

*Treatment* requires a multidisciplinary approach consisting of a feeding program as well as individual and family therapy. Feeding is accomplished through voluntary intake of regular foods or of a nutritional formula orally or by nasogastric tube. When vital signs are stable, discussion and negotiation of a detailed treatment contract with the patient and the parents are essential. The first step is to restore body weight. Hospitalization may be necessary (Table 70-3). When 80% of normal weight is achieved, the patient is given freedom to gain weight at a personal pace. The *prognosis* includes a 3% to 5% mortality (suicide, malnutrition) rate, the development of bulimic symptoms (30% of individuals), and persistent anorexia nervosa syndrome (20% of individuals).

## BULIMIA NERVOSA

Table 70-4 presents the diagnostic criteria for bulimia nervosa. The prevalence of bulimia nervosa is 5% in female college students. The female-to-male ratio is 10:1. Binge-eating episodes consist of large quantities of often forbidden foods or leftovers or both, consumed rapidly, followed by vomiting. Metabolic abnormalities result from the excessive vomiting or laxative and diuretic intake. Binge-eating episodes and the loss of control over eating often occur in young women who are slightly overweight with a history of dieting.

Nutritional, educational, and self-monitoring techniques are used to increase awareness of the maladaptive behavior, following which efforts are made to change the eating behavior. Patients with bulimia nervosa may respond to antidepressant therapy because they often have

personality disturbances, impulse control difficulties, and family histories of affective disorders. Patients feel embarrassed, guilty, and ashamed of their actions. Attempted suicide and completed suicide (5%) are an important concern.

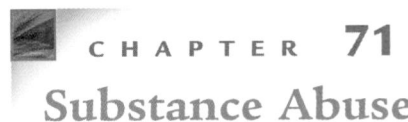

## CHAPTER 71

# Substance Abuse

The age at which street drugs are first used is decreasing (<12 years), and females are overtaking males in terms of substance use. Ninety percent of adult smokers begin their habit during their adolescent years. Marijuana and stimulant drug use is showing an upward trend. Inhalant use (glue solvents, aerosol products) is prevalent in younger adolescents and in Native Americans. The use of *club drugs* by adolescents from upper income groups at rave parties (3,4-methylenedioxymethamphetamine [Ecstasy]) and so-called date-rape drugs (gamma-hydroxybutyrate or flunitrazepam [Rohypnol]) has risen sharply. Anabolic steroid use has increased in adolescent boys seeking enhanced athletic performance.

A history of drug use should be taken in a nonjudgmental and supportive manner and include the types of substances, frequency, timing, circumstances, and outcomes of substance use. Table 71-1 is a helpful screening tool. There are few physical findings even with chronic adolescent substance use. An adolescent may present in an overdose or intoxicated state, or in a psychosis triggered by a hallucinogen, such as phencyclidine ("angel dust"). Club drugs have direct (coma and seizures) and indirect (sexual assault and dehydration) adverse effects. Anabolic steroids also have direct (gynecomastia and testicular atrophy) and indirect (mood swings and violence) adverse effects.

| TABLE 70-3 When to Hospitalize an Anorexic Patient |
|---|
| Weight loss >25% ideal body weight* |
| Risk of suicide |
| Bradycardia, hypothermia |
| Dehydration, hypokalemia, dysrhythmias |
| Outpatient treatment fails |

*Less weight loss accepted in young adolescent.

## TABLE 71-1 CRAFFT: A Screening Tool for Adolescent Substance Abuse

| | | |
|---|---|---|
| C | Car | Driving under the influence of drugs |
| R | Relax | Using drugs to relax, fit in, feel better |
| A | Alone | Drugs/alcohol consumption while alone |
| F | Forgetting | Forgetting things as a result of drugs/alcohol |
| F | Family/ Friends | Family and friends tell teen to stop/cut down |
| T | Trouble | Getting into trouble because of drugs/alcohol |

## ACUTE OVERDOSE

Many drugs (most commonly alcohol, amphetamines, opiates, and cocaine) can result in a toxicologic emergency. This situation most often occurs the first time an adolescent uses a substance and makes identification of the offending agent difficult (Table 71-2). Initial management should be directed at appropriate supportive medical treatment, with follow-up counseling after the toxic effects have diminished.

## TABLE 71-2 Substances Abused by Adolescents: Names and Acute Effects

| Substance (Street/Alternative Name) | Effects and Facts | Route of Administration (Time of Action) | Detection |
|---|---|---|---|
| Alcohol (Meths) | Disinhibition, ataxia, slurred speech, respiratory and CNS depression | Ingested (depends on amount and tolerance) | Urine and blood |
| Nicotine Snuff, dipping, chewed | Relaxation, CNS dependence, ↑ blood pressure, ↑ heart rate, ↓ temperature | Inhaled (minutes) | |
| Marijuana (Cannabis) (Hashish, joints) | Euphoria, relaxation, ↑ appetite, ↓ reaction time | Inhaled (minutes) Tablets (30 min +) | Urine up to 1 mo |
| **Stimulants** | Alertness, euphoria Insomnia, ↓ appetite | Inhaled and snorted (Quick high) Tablets (longer effect) | Urine up to 48 h |
| Cocaine (crack) Amphetamines (ice) | | | |
| **Hallucinogens** | Hallucination, anxiety | Oral | |
| Mescaline | Psychosis, dilated pupils | Injected, sniffed, ingested | Immunoassay |
| Psilocybin (magic mushrooms) | Dysphoria | | |
| LSD | "Artistic high" "Lucy in the sky with diamonds" | 2–12 hr "trip" | |
| Phencyclidine (PCP, angel dust) | Microdots in many colors Can induce suicide attempts | | Immunoassay for PCP |
| EDMA | | | |
| **Ecstasy** (club drugs: combinations, i.e., of hallucinogens and amphetamines) | | | Ecstasy *not* detected by urine screen |
| **Opiates** | Euphoria, ataxia, miosis, slurred speech | Oral, IV, smoked, snorted, and sniffed | |
| Heroin | | | |
| Opium and heroin (freebase) OxyContin (cotton, hillbilly)—new | A common adolescent mix | | |
| **Tranquilizers** | | Small white pills; dissolve easily, odorless, colorless, tasteless (often mixed in alcohol) | Urine 1–24 h |
| Flunitrazepam (Rohypnol, "roofies," "date rape" drugs) | | | |
| Sedatives (barbiturates, "downers") | | | |
| **Inhalants** (solvents, gasoline) | Like alcohol | Inhaled | |
| **Anabolic steroids** | To enhance athletic performance | Tablets | Urine |

Common side effects (treatment) of substance abuse drugs are paranoia (haloperidol), seizures (diazepam), hyperthermia (slow cooling), hypertension (β-blockers), and opiate overdose (naloxone).

CNS, central nervous system; EDMA, 3,4-ethylenedioxy-*N*-methylamphetamine; LSD, lysergic acid diethylamide.

From Office of the Surgeon General: www.surgeongeneral.gov (click on Reports and Publications, then click on Surgeon General's Reports, and then click on Reducing Tobacco Use: A Report of the Surgeon General.)

## ACUTE ILLNESS

Heavy alcohol use can cause acute gastritis and acute pancreatitis. Intravenous drug use can result in hepatitis B, bacterial endocarditis, osteomyelitis, septic pulmonary embolism, infection, or acquired immunodeficiency syndrome (AIDS). Chronic marijuana or tobacco use is associated with bronchoconstriction and bronchitis.

## CHRONIC USE

Compulsive drug or alcohol use results in an adolescent being unable to help himself or herself out of drug dependency and the psychosocial sequelae that attend such habituation (e.g., stealing, prostitution, drug dealing, unemployment, school failure, social isolation).

## TREATMENT

Specific management of substance use by adolescents depends on many individual patient factors. Because of the highly addictive (physical and psychological) nature of most substances, residential drug treatment facilities are being suggested, especially for younger adolescents.

## SUGGESTED READING

Blake K, Mann K, Kutcher M: *The Structured Communication Adolescent Guide (SCAG)* MedEdPORTAL; 2008. http://services.aamc.org/jsp/mededportal/retrieveSubmissionDetailById.do?subId=798.

Braverman PK: Sexually transmitted diseases in adolescents, *Med Clin North Am* 84:869–889, 2000.

Hazen E, Schlozman S, Beresin E: Adolescent psychological development: a review, *Pediatr Rev* 29:161–167, 2008.

Johnston LD, O'Malley PM, Bachman JG, et al: Monitoring the future: national results on adolescent drug use: overview of key findings, *National Institutes of Health Publication No. 06-5882,* 2006.

Le Grange D, Loeb K, Van Orman S, et al: Adolescent bulimia nervosa, *Arch Pediatr Adolesc Med* 158:478–482, 2004.

Minjarez DA, Bradshaw KD: Abnormal uterine bleeding in adolescents, *Obstet Gynecol Clin North Am* 27:63–78, 2000.

Mitan LA, Slap GB: Adolescent menstrual disorders: update, *Med Clin North Am* 84:851–868, 2000.

Munoz MT, Argente J: New concepts in anorexia nervosa, *J Pediatr Endocrinol Metab* (Suppl 3):473–480, 2004.

National Institute on Drug Abuse (NIDA): www.drugabuse.gov/.

Office of National Drug Control Policy: National Youth Anti-Drug Media Campaign: www.mediacampaign.org/.

Sacks D, Westwood M: An approach to interviewing adolescents, *Paediatr Child Health* 8:554–556, 2003.

The Emergency Contraception Website, Office of Population Research: Princeton, NJ. http://ec.princeton.edu/.

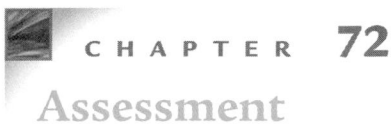

CHAPTER 72

Assessment

**Primary immunodeficiency diseases** result from gene defects that affect one or more components of the immune system. The hallmarks of immunodeficiency include increased susceptibility and frequent, chronic, or unusually severe infections. The major components of host defenses include an anatomic barrier, innate immunity, and adaptive immunity. Integrity of the **anatomic-mucociliary barrier** at the interface between the body and its environment (skin and mucous membranes) is essential for protection against infection (Table 72-1). The innate immune system initiates antigen-nonspecific mechanisms as a first line of defense against pathogens, before the development of more versatile adaptive immune responses involving antigen-specific T and B lymphocytes. The **innate immune system** responds rapidly to pathogens. Complement proteins activate sequentially, killing pathogens by facilitating uptake by phagocytic cells or by antibody-independent lysis of pathogens. Other important soluble factors of innate immunity are acute-phase proteins, cytokines, and chemokines (Table 72-2). Proinflammatory acute-phase proteins, including C-reactive protein and mannose-binding lectin, are involved in recognition of damaged cells and pathogens, and they activate complement and induce production of inflammatory cytokines. The pattern of chemokines produced determines the type and location of inflammatory infiltrate.

The cellular arm of innate immunity includes phagocytic cells that engulf and digest foreign antigens and microorganisms. Polymorphonuclear neutrophils ingest pyogenic bacteria and some fungi, especially *Aspergillus*. Macrophages, which develop from circulating monocytes, are effective in killing facultative intracellular organisms such as *Mycobacterium, Toxoplasma,* and *Legionella*. In addition, natural killer (NK) lymphocytes mediate cytotoxic activity against virus-infected cells and cancer cells. Recognition of pathogens by the innate immune system is facilitated by receptors on macrophages, NK cells, and neutrophils that recognize conserved pathogen motifs called **pathogen-associated molecular patterns,** including lipopolysaccharide of gram-negative bacteria, lipoteichoic acid of gram-positive bacteria, mannans of yeast, and specific nucleotide sequences of bacterial and viral DNA.

The key features of the **adaptive immune system** are antigen specificity and the development of immunologic memory, produced by expansion and maturation of antigen-specific T cells and B cells. Antibodies (immunoglobulin) produced by **B cells** neutralize toxins released by pathogens, facilitating opsonization of the pathogen by phagocytic cells, activating complement causing cytolysis of the pathogen, and directing NK cells to kill infected cells through antibody-mediated cytotoxicity. **T cells** kill virus-infected cells and cancer cells, delivering the necessary signals for B-cell antibody synthesis, memory B-cell formation, and activating macrophages to kill intracellular pathogens.

Immunodeficiency can result from defects in one or more components of innate or adaptive immunity, leading to recurrent, opportunistic, or life-threatening infections. Primary immunodeficiency diseases are relatively rare individually, but together cause significant chronic disease, morbidity, and mortality. To distinguish true immunodeficiency from an immunologically normal child who has recurrent infections, evaluation must be based on a comprehensive understanding of the immune system, the patient's age, the site, and the pathogens involved (Table 72-3).

## HISTORY

A **family history** of primary immunodeficiency disease, or of infants dying from infection, warrants an immunologic evaluation, especially in the presence of recurrent infections. The frequency, severity, and location of the infection and the pathogens involved can help differentiate infections in a normal host from infections in an immunodeficient patient (see Table 72-3). Patients with primary immunodeficiency acquire infection with opportunistic organisms that do not ordinarily cause disease. Antibody deficiency diseases initially manifest with common infections, such as otitis media and sinusitis, but at a higher frequency than in immunocompetent children. Eight or more episodes of otitis media, two or more serious sinus infections, or two or more episodes of pneumonia in 1 year suggest an antibody deficiency, especially if the infections

### TABLE 72-1 Anatomic and Mucociliary Defects That Result in Recurrent or Opportunistic Infections

#### ANATOMIC DEFECTS IN UPPER AIRWAYS

Aspiration syndromes (gastroesophageal reflux, ineffective cough, foreign body)
Cleft palate, eustachian tube dysfunction
Adenoidal hypertrophy
Nasal polyps
Obstruction of paranasal sinus drainage (osteomeatal complex disease), encephaloceles
Post-traumatic or congenital sinus tracts (CSF rhinorrhea)

#### ANATOMIC DEFECTS IN THE TRACHEOBRONCHIAL TREE

Tracheal esophageal fistula, bronchobiliary fistula
Pulmonary sequestration, bronchogenic cysts
Vascular ring
Tumor, foreign body, or enlarged nodes

#### PHYSIOLOGIC DEFECTS IN UPPER AND LOWER AIRWAYS

Primary ciliary dyskinesia syndromes, Young syndrome
Cystic fibrosis, bronchopulmonary dysplasia, bronchiectasis
Allergic disease (allergic rhinitis, asthma)
Chronic cigarette smoke exposure

#### OTHER DEFECTS

Burns
Chronic atopic dermatitis
Ureteral obstruction, vesicoureteral reflux
IV drug use
Central venous line, artificial heart value, CSF shunt, peritoneal dialysis catheter, urinary catheter
Dermal sinus tract

CSF, cerebrospinal fluid.

are difficult to treat. Recurrent sinopulmonary infections with encapsulated bacteria suggest antibody-mediated immunity because these pathogens evade phagocytosis. Failure to thrive, diarrhea, malabsorption, and fungal infections suggest T-cell immunodeficiency. Recurrent viral infections can result from T-cell or NK-cell deficiency. Opportunistic infections with organisms, such as *Pneumocystis jiroveci* (*carinii*), suggest a T-cell disorder, such as severe combined immunodeficiency (SCID), or T-cell dysfunction, as in X-linked hyper-IgM. Deep-seated abscesses and infections with *Staphylococcus aureus, Serratia marcescens,* and *Aspergillus* suggest a disorder of neutrophil function, such as chronic granulomatous disease (CGD). Delayed separation of the umbilical cord, especially in the presence of omphalitis, and periodontal disease, in addition to abscesses, indicate leukocyte adhesion deficiency, whereas hyper-IgE syndrome is associated with cold abscesses, eczema, and frequent fractures. The presence of deep-seated infections can help differentiate hyper-IgE syndrome from atopic dermatitis, which can be associated with extremely elevated levels of IgE. Onset of symptoms in adolescence or young adulthood suggests common variable immunodeficiency (CVID) rather than agammaglobulinemia, although milder phenotypes of primary immunodeficiency disease may not present until later in life. The presence of associated problems, such as congenital heart disease and hypocalcemia, suggests DiGeorge syndrome. Ataxia-telangiectasia is associated with abnormal gait and telangiectasia on the skin. Atopic dermatitis is present in patients with hyper-IgE syndrome and is associated with easy bruising or a bleeding disorder in patients with Wiskott-Aldrich syndrome.

## PHYSICAL EXAMINATION

Recurrent infection in immunologically deficient children is associated with incomplete recovery at sites of infection, (scarring of skin or tympanic membranes, abnormal hearing, persistent perforation of the tympanic membrane, persistent ear drainage, chronic lung disease, persistent cough, sputum production, failure to thrive, digital clubbing, or anemia). Substantial morbidity from repeated infections suggests the presence of significant immunologic disease. Height and weight percentiles, nutritional status, and presence of subcutaneous fat should be assessed. Oral thrush, purulent nasal or otic discharge, and chronic rales may be evidence of repeated or persistent infections. Lymphoid tissue (tonsils and lymph nodes) should be examined. Absence of tonsils suggests agammaglobulinemia or SCID, whereas increased size of lymphoid tissue suggests CVID, CGD, autosomal recessive hyper-IgM syndrome, or human immunodeficiency virus (HIV) infection. Cerebellar ataxia and telangiectasia indicate ataxia-telangiectasia. Eczema and petechiae or bruises suggest Wiskott-Aldrich syndrome.

## DIFFERENTIAL DIAGNOSIS

Separate episodes of infection must be differentiated from a recrudescence or relapse of a single episode, which may occur when infections are treated inadequately. Recurrent episodes of severe infection, such as meningitis or sepsis, are much more worrisome, but antibody deficiency states initially manifest with common infections, such as otitis media and sinusitis. In patients with antibody deficiency states, ciliary dyskinesia, T-cell deficiencies, or neutrophil disorders, infections develop at multiple sites (ears, sinuses, lungs, skin), whereas in individuals with anatomic problems (sequestered pulmonary lobe, ureteral reflux), infections are confined to a single anatomic site. Asplenia is associated with recurrent and severe infections, even in the presence of protective antibody titers. Infection with HIV should be considered in any patient presenting with a history suggesting a T-cell immunodeficiency. There are many secondary causes of immunodeficiency (Table 72-4).

## DIAGNOSTIC EVALUATION

The diagnosis of patients with primary immunodeficiency diseases depends on early recognition of signs and symptoms, followed by laboratory tests to evaluate immune function. Recognizing the patient who may have an immunodeficiency disease prompts evaluation and referral to an immunologist (see Table 72-3).

**TABLE 72-2 Cytokines and Chemotactic Cytokines and Their Functions**

| Factor | Source | Function |
|---|---|---|
| IL-1 | Macrophages | Costimulatory effect on T cells enhances antigen presentation |
| IL-2 | T cells | Primary T-cell growth factor; B-cell and NK-cell growth factor |
| IL-3 | T cells | Mast cell growth factor; multicolony-stimulating factor |
| IL-4 | T cells | T-cell growth factor; enhances IgE synthesis; enhances B-cell differentiation; mast cell growth |
| IL-5 | T cells | Enhances immunoglobulin synthesis; enhances IgA synthesis; enhances eosinophil differentiation |
| IL-6 | T cells, macrophages, fibroblasts, endothelium | Enhances immunoglobulin synthesis, antiviral activity, and hepatocyte-stimulating factor |
| IL-7 | Stromal cells | Enhances growth of pre-B cells and pre-T cells |
| IL-8 | T cells, macrophages, epithelium | Neutrophil-activating protein; T lymphocyte, neutrophil chemotactic factor |
| IL-9 | T cells | Acts in synergy with IL-4 to induce IgE production, mast cell growth |
| IL-10 | T cells, including regulatory T cells, macrophages | Cytokine synthesis inhibitory factor; suppresses macrophage function; enhances B-cell growth; inhibits IL-12 production |
| IL-12 | Macrophages, neutrophils | NK cell stimulatory factor; cytotoxic lymphocyte maturation factor; enhances IFN-$\gamma$ synthesis; inhibits IL-4 synthesis |
| IL-13 | T cells | Enhances IgE synthesis; enhances B-cell growth; inhibits macrophage activation; causes airway hyperreactivity |
| IL-17 | T cells | Induces IL-1$\beta$ and IL-6 synthesis, involved in autoimmunity |
| IL-18 | Macrophages | Enhances IFN-$\gamma$ synthesis |
| IFN-$\gamma$ | T cells | Macrophage activation; inhibits IgE synthesis; antiviral activity |
| TGF-$\beta$ | T cells including regulatory T cells, many other cells | Inhibits T-cell and B-cell proliferation and activation |
| RANTES | T cells, endothelium | Chemokine for monocytes, T cells, eosinophils |
| MIP-1$\alpha$ | Mononuclear cells, endothelium | Chemokine for T cells; enhances differentiation of CD4$^+$ T cells |
| Eotaxin 1, 2, and 3 | Epithelium, endothelium, eosinophils, fibroblasts, macrophages | Chemokine for eosinophils, basophils, and Th2 cells |
| IP-10 | Monocytes, macrophages, endothelium | Chemokine for activated T cells, monocytes, and NK cells; T cells activate NK cells |

IFN, interferon; NK, natural killer; RANTES, regulated on activation, normal T expressed and secreted; Th2, T helper 2.

## Laboratory Tests

A diagnosis of primary immunodeficiency disease cannot be established without the use of laboratory tests. The choice of test and the extent of testing depend on the clinical history. Several tests are used in the diagnosis of primary immunodeficiency disease (Table 72-5).

A **complete blood count with differential** should always be obtained to identify patients with neutropenia or lymphopenia (SCID) as well as the presence of eosinophils (allergic disease) and anemia (chronic disease).

**Serum immunoglobulin levels** vary with age, with normal adult values of IgG at full-term birth from transplacental transfer of maternal IgG, a physiologic nadir occurring at 6 to 8 months of age, and a gradual increase to adult values over several years. IgA can be absent at birth. IgA and IgM levels increase gradually over several years, with IgA taking the longest to reach normal adult values. Low albumin levels with low immunoglobulin levels suggest low synthetic rates for all proteins or increased loss of proteins, as in protein-losing enteropathy. High immunoglobulin levels suggest intact B-cell immunity and can be found in diseases with recurrent infections, such as CGD, immotile cilia syndrome, cystic fibrosis, and HIV infection. Elevated IgE levels can be found in hyper-IgE syndrome and in atopic dermatitis.

**Specific antibody titers** after childhood vaccination (tetanus, diphtheria, *Haemophilus influenzae* type b, or *Streptococcus pneumoniae* vaccines) reflect the capacity of the immune system to synthesize antibodies and to develop memory B cells. If titers are low, immunization with a specific vaccine and titers obtained 4 to 6 weeks later confirm response to the immunization. Poor response to bacterial polysaccharide antigens is normal before 24 months of age, but is also associated with IgG subclass deficiency or specific antibody deficiency with normal immunoglobulins in older children. The development of protein-conjugate polysaccharide vaccines has prevented infections with these organisms in early childhood.

## TABLE 72-3  Clinical Characteristics of Primary Immunodeficiencies

### B-CELL DEFECTS

Recurrent pyogenic infections with extracellular encapsulated organisms, such as *Streptococcus pneumoniae*, *Haemophilus influenzae* type b, and group A streptococcus

Otitis, sinusitis, recurrent pneumonia, bronchiectasis, and conjunctivitis

Few problems with fungal or viral infections (except enterovirus encephalitis and poliomyelitis)

Decreased levels of immunoglobulins in serum and secretions

Diarrhea common, especially secondary to infection with *Giardia lamblia*

Growth retardation not striking

Compatible with survival to adulthood or for several years after onset unless complications occur

### COMPLEMENT DEFECTS

Recurrent bacterial infections with extracellular encapsulated organisms, such as *S. pneumoniae* and *H. influenzae*

Susceptibility to recurrent infections with *Neisseria meningitidis*

Increased incidence of autoimmune disease

Severe or recurrent skin and respiratory tract infection

### T-CELL DEFECTS

Recurrent infections with less virulent or opportunistic organisms, such as fungi, mycobacteria, viruses, and protozoa

Growth retardation, malabsorption, diarrhea, and failure to thrive common

Anergy

Susceptible to graft-versus-host reactions if given unirradiated blood

Fatal reactions may occur from live virus or bacille Calmette-Guérin (BCG) vaccination

High incidence of malignancy

Poor survival beyond infancy or early childhood

### NEUTROPHIL DEFECTS

Recurrent dermatologic infections with bacteria such as *Staphylococcus, Pseudomonas,* and *Escherichia coli,* and fungi such as *Aspergillus*

Subcutaneous, lymph node, lung, and liver abscesses

Pulmonary infections common, including abscess and pneumatocele formation, contributing to chronic disease

Bone and joint infection common

Delayed separation of umbilical cord

Absence of pus at site(s) of infection

---

## TABLE 72-4  Causes of Secondary Immunodeficiency

### VIRAL INFECTIONS

HIV (destroys CD4 T cells)

### METABOLIC DISORDERS

Diabetes mellitus
Malnutrition
Uremia
Sickle cell disease
Zinc deficiency
Multiple carboxylase deficiency
Burns

### PROTEIN-LOSING STATES

Nephrotic syndrome
Protein-losing enteropathy

### OTHER CAUSES

Prematurity
Immunosuppressive agents (e.g., corticosteroids, radiation, and antimetabolites)
Malignancy (leukemia, Hodgkin disease, nonlymphoid cancer)
Acquired asplenia
Periodontitis
Chronic (acute) blood transfusions
Acquired neutropenia (autoimmune, viral, or drug-induced)
Stem cell transplantation/graft-versus-host disease
Systemic lupus erythematosus
Sarcoidosis

---

**Lymphocyte phenotyping** by flow cytometry enumerates the percentage and absolute numbers of T-cell, B-cell, and NK-cell subsets and the presence of surface proteins that are necessary for normal immunity, such as major histocompatibility complex molecules or adhesion molecules. Absent T cells in the presence or absence of B cells indicates SCID, whereas isolated deficiency of B cells characterizes agammaglobulinemia.

**Delayed-type hypersensitivity** skin tests to antigens such as tetanus, diphtheria, *Candida,* or mumps demonstrate the presence of antigen-specific memory T cells and functioning antigen-presenting cells. T cells recognize peptide fragments derived from antigens and presented by major histocompatibility complex molecules on the surface of antigen-presenting cells. If delayed-type hypersensitivity skin test results are negative, patients should receive a booster vaccination and be retested 4 weeks later. If the results remain negative, in vitro T-cell proliferation assays should be performed to confirm or exclude the lack of T-cell responsiveness.

**T-cell proliferation** assays to mitogens (phytohemagglutinin, concanavalin A, or pokeweed mitogen) or antigens (tetanus toxoid or *Candida*) are in vitro assays that confirm the capacity of T cells to proliferate in response to a nonspecific stimulus (mitogens) or the presence of antigen-specific memory T cells (antigens). Such presence requires prior vaccination (tetanus) or exposure (*Candida*) to the antigen.

This situation has made it difficult, however, to assess antibody responses to polysaccharide vaccines in children older than 2 years. Antibody responses to the *S. pneumoniae* serotypes found in the 23-valent polysaccharide vaccine, but not in the conjugate vaccine, can be used to test antibody responses to polysaccharide antigens. Low or absent specific antibody responses confirm the diagnosis of antibody deficiency even if B cells are present and serum immunoglobulin levels are in the normal range.

## TABLE 72-5 Tests for Suspected Immune Deficiency

### GENERAL

Complete blood count, including hemoglobin, differential white blood cell count and morphology, and platelet count

Radiographs to document infection in chest, sinus, mastoids, and long bones, if indicated by clinical history

Cultures, if appropriate

### ANTIBODY-MEDIATED IMMUNITY

Quantitative immunoglobulin levels: IgG, IgA, IgM, IgE

Isohemagglutinin titers (anti-A, anti-B): measures IgM function

Specific antibody levels:

Protein antigens: diphtheria, tetanus

Protein-conjugated antigens: *Haemophilus influenzae, Streptococcus pneumoniae* (conjugate vaccine)

Polysaccharide antigens: *S. pneumoniae* (unconjugated vaccine)

B-cell numbers and subsets by flow cytometry

### CELL-MEDIATED IMMUNITY

Lymphocyte count and morphology

Delayed hypersensitivity skin tests (*Candida*, tetanus toxoid, mumps): measure T-cell and macrophage function

T-cell and NK cell numbers and subsets by flow cytometry

T-lymphocyte function analyses

NK cell function assays

### PHAGOCYTOSIS

Neutrophil cell count and morphology

Nitroblue tetrazolium dye test/dihydrorhodamine 123 using flow cytometry

Staphylococcal killing, chemotaxis assay

Myeloperoxidase stain

### COMPLEMENT

Total hemolytic complement $CH_{50}$: measures classical pathway complement activity

$AP_{50}$: measures alternative pathway complement activity

Levels of individual complement components

C1-inhibitor level and function

NK, natural killer.

**Tests for cytokine synthesis or expression of activation markers** by T cells may be performed in specialized research laboratories and can help identify defects in T-cell function when, despite present T cells, the clinical history suggests a T-cell disorder.

**Complement assays** include the total hemolytic activity of serum ($CH_{50}$), which identifies presence of normal levels of the major components of complement. Activation of the alternative pathway of complement is performed by the $AP_{50}$ test. If the $CH_{50}$ or $AP_{50}$ level is abnormal, tests for individual complement components must be analyzed in specialized laboratories. Tests for C1-inhibitor antigen and function are used to diagnose hereditary or acquired angioneurotic edema. False-negative results for the commercially available test of C1-inhibitor function used by most clinical laboratories require testing by specialized laboratories if the diagnosis of angioneurotic edema is suspected. **Tests for neutrophil function** include the nitroblue tetrazolium test for CGD, in which a soluble yellow dye turns into an insoluble blue dye inside activated neutrophils that have generated oxygen radicals to kill bacteria. Patients with CGD have no blue-staining neutrophils, whereas, on average, half of the neutrophils turn blue in carriers. A more sensitive test for CGD is a flow cytometry–based assay using dihydrorhodamine 123. In vitro tests for evaluation of neutrophil phagocytosis, chemotaxis, and bacterial killing and for the presence of myeloperoxidase activity are available in some laboratories, and tests for the expression of adhesion molecules such as CD18 (leukocyte function–associated antigen type 1, LFA-1) can be performed by flow cytometry.

**Genetic testing** to confirm the diagnosis of a primary immunodeficiency disease can be performed in specialized laboratories and may be helpful for deciding on a course of treatment, determining the natural history and prognosis of the disease, genetic counseling, and prenatal diagnosis. In patients in whom DiGeorge syndrome is suspected, fluorescent in situ hybridization studies for deletions of chromosome 22 can be helpful. In patients in whom ataxia-telangiectasia is suspected, chromosomal studies for breakage in chromosomes 7 and 14 are useful.

## Diagnostic Imaging

The absence of a thymus on chest x-ray suggests DiGeorge syndrome. Abnormalities in the cerebellum are found in patients with ataxia-telangiectasia. Otherwise, the use of diagnostic imaging in the evaluation of immunodeficiency diseases is essentially limited to the diagnosis of infectious diseases.

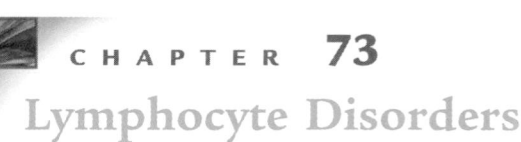

## CHAPTER 73

# Lymphocyte Disorders

Disorders that affect lymphocyte development or function result in significant immunodeficiency because lymphocytes provide antigen specificity and memory responses. Lymphocytes develop from hematopoietic stem cells through a series of stages that culminate in a common lymphoid progenitor, which gives rise to T lymphocytes, B lymphocytes, and natural killer (NK) lymphocytes. B cells complete their development in the bone marrow, and T cells develop in the thymus from bone marrow–derived precursors (Fig. 73-1). Isolated B-cell disorders result in **antibody deficiency diseases**, whereas T-cell disorders usually cause **combined immunodeficiency** because they are necessary for cell-mediated immunity, immunity to intracellular pathogens, and antibody synthesis by B cells. NK cells are an important component of the **innate immune response** and can kill virus-infected cells and tumor cells. Antibodies can enhance NK cell function by antibody-mediated cellular cytotoxicity.

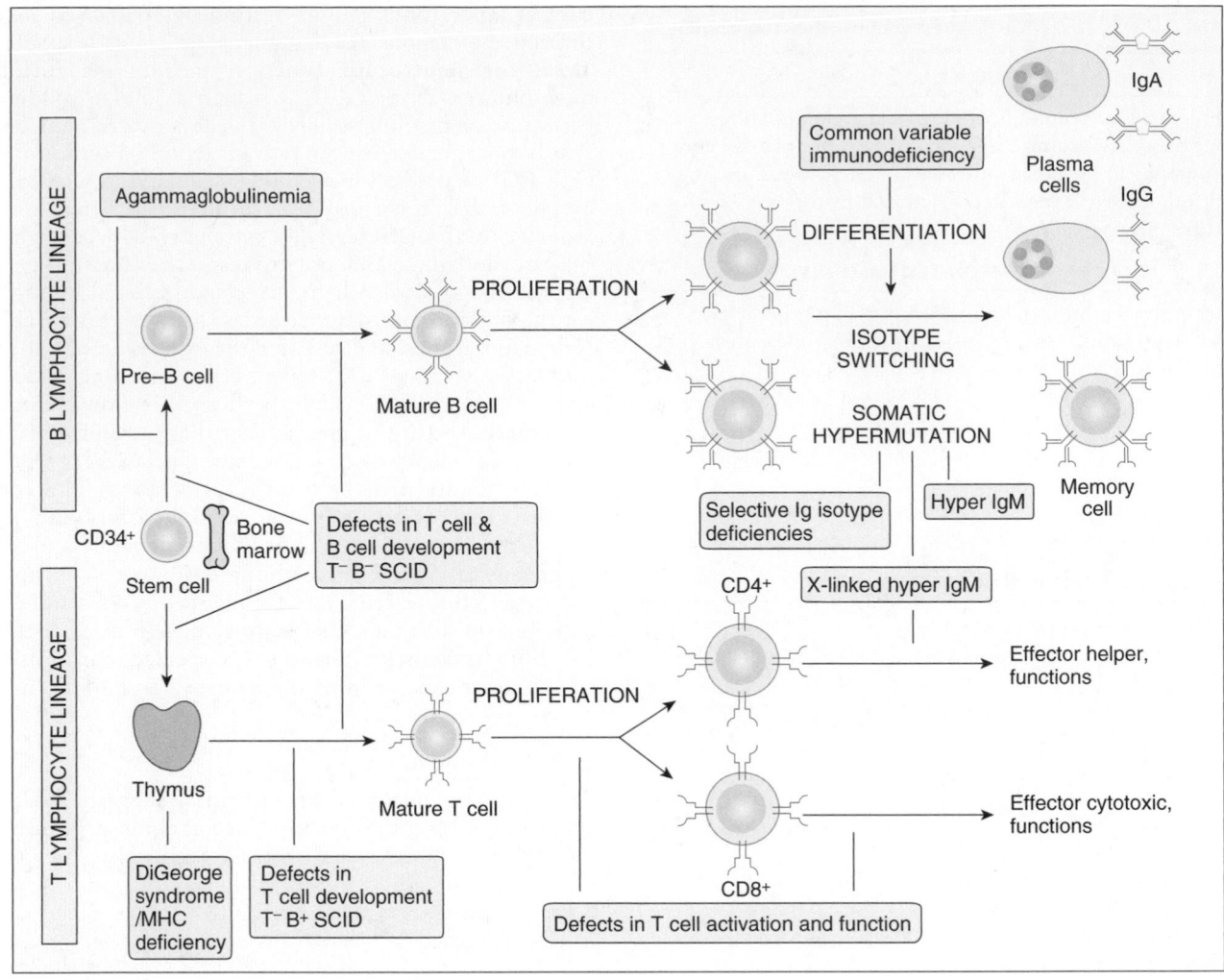

**FIGURE 73-1**

Sites of cellular abnormalities in congenital immunodeficiencies. In primary immunodeficiency diseases, the maturation or activation of B or T lymphocytes may be blocked at different stages. B, B lymphocyte; T, T lymphocyte. (Adapted from Abbas AK, Lichtman AH, Pober JS: Cellular and molecular immunology, 3rd ed, Philadelphia, *Saunders*, 1997.)

## ETIOLOGY AND CLINICAL MANIFESTATIONS

### Antibody Deficiency Diseases

B cells synthesize antibodies that can kill pathogens in conjunction with complement proteins, facilitate uptake of pathogens by phagocytic cells, and neutralize toxins secreted by pathogens. Disorders of B cells result in an increased susceptibility to infections by encapsulated bacteria because these pathogens resist uptake by phagocytic cells and require antibodies for their clearance. A variety of defects can affect the development or function of B cells.

**Agammaglobulinemia** results from the absence of B cells with subsequent absence or severe decrease in immunoglobulin levels and a total absence of specific antibody. **X-linked agammaglobulinemia** affects males and is characterized by a profound deficiency of B cells, severe hypogammaglobulinemia, and absence of lymphoid tissue (Table 73-1; see Fig. 73-1). The defect is caused by mutations in a gene encoding for the tyrosine kinase *Btk* on chromosome Xq22 that is involved in signaling via the pre–B-cell receptor and the B-cell antigen receptor. The B-cell antigen receptor complex consists of an immunoglobulin molecule in association with several transmembrane and cytoplasmic molecules that function in signal transduction. Defects in any of the genes that encode for structural or signaling molecules associated with the pre–B-cell and B-cell receptors can lead to agammaglobulinemia. These gene defects are inherited in an autosomal recessive manner and include mutations in the μ heavy chain gene on chromosomes 14 and λ5, and Vpre-B surrogate light chains, Igα, Igβ, and BLNK. X-linked agammaglobulinemia is more common than the autosomal recessive forms because, in affected males, only one copy of the gene needs to be defective to express the disease. Other unknown gene defects can also lead to agammaglobulinemia.

**TABLE 73-1 Antibody Deficiency Diseases**

| Disorder | Genetics | Onset | Manifestations | Pathogenesis | Associated Features |
|---|---|---|---|---|---|
| Agammaglobulinemia | X-linked (Xq22) | Infancy (6–9 mo) | Recurrent infections, sinusitis, pneumonia, meningitis (encapsulated bacteria, enteroviruses) | Arrest in B cell differentiation (pre-B level); mutations in: *Btk* gene (X-linked); μ chain, BLK, Igα, Igβ Vpre-B, and λ5 (AR) | Lymphoid hypoplasia |
| Common variable immunodeficiency | AR; AD | Second to third decade | Sinusitis, bronchitis, pneumonia, chronic diarrhea | Arrest in plasma cell differentiation, mutations in ICOS, TACI, CD19 | Autoimmune disease, RA, SLE, Graves' disease, ITP, malignancy |
| Transient hypogammaglobulinemia of infancy | | Infancy (3–7 mo) | Recurrent viral and pyogenic infections | Unknown; delayed plasma cell maturation | Frequently in families with other immunodeficiencies |
| IgA deficiency | Variable | Variable | Sinopulmonary infections | Failure of IgA expressing B-cell differentiation | IgG subclass common variable immunodeficiency, autoimmune diseases |
| IgG subclass deficiency | Variable | Variable | Sinopulmonary infections; may be normal | Defect in IgG isotype production | IgA deficiency, ataxia telangiectasia, polysaccharide antibody deficiency |
| IgM deficiency | Variable | First year | Variable (normal to recurrent sinopulmonary infections and meningitis) | Defective helper T cell–B cell interaction | Whipple disease, regional enteritis, lymphoid hyperplasia |
| Specific antibody deficiency, IgA deficiency | Variable | After 2 years of age | Sinopulmonary infections | Unknown | IgG subclass deficiency |
| Immunodeficiency | AR | Variable | Sinopulmonary infections | Defect in CD40 signaling, mutations in: AID, UNG | Autoimmunity with increased IgM |

AD, autosomal dominant; AR, autosomal recessive; ITP, idiopathic thrombocytopenic purpura; RA, rheumatoid arthritis; SLE, systemic lupus erythematosus.

Patients with agammaglobulinemia usually present during the first 6 to 12 months of life, as maternally derived antibodies wane, although some patients present with symptoms at 3 to 5 years of age. These patients develop infections with *Streptococcus pneumoniae, Haemophilus influenzae* type b, *Staphylococcus aureus,* and *Pseudomonas,* organisms for which antibody is an important opsonin. They also have increased susceptibility to giardiasis and enteroviral infections, leading to chronic enteroviral meningoencephalitis and vaccine–associated poliomyelitis (if immunized with oral live, attenuated poliovirus vaccine).

**Common variable immunodeficiency (CVID)** is a heterogeneous disorder characterized by hypogammaglobulinemia developing after an initial period of normal immune function, most commonly in the second and third decades of life (see Table 73-1). Serum IgG levels are less than 500 mg/dL (usually <300 mg/dL) with IgA levels less than 10 mg/dL and low IgM levels. Antibody titers to protein antigens, such as tetanus and diphtheria, and to polysaccharide antigens, such as pneumococcus, are absent. T-cell function is variable; patients may have decreased numbers of CD4 T cells, decreased lymphocyte proliferation to mitogens and antigens, or normal T-cell numbers and function. B cells may be present at low or normal numbers. Patients exhibit normal-sized or enlarged tonsils and lymph nodes and may have splenomegaly. They are susceptible to frequent respiratory tract infections; bronchiectasis; autoimmune diseases such as hemolytic anemia, thrombocytopenia, and neutropenia; gastrointestinal disease with malabsorption, chronic diarrhea, liver dysfunction, and *Helicobacter pylori* infection; granulomatous disease; and cancer, especially lymphoma. CVID is observed frequently in families with IgA deficiency. The gene defects leading to the majority of cases of CVID are unknown. Some patients have a defect in the gene encoding for ICOS, the "inducible costimulator" on activated T cells, TACI (transmembrane activator and calcium-modulating cyclophilin ligand interactor), or CD19. These patients have normal T-cell numbers and function but have a decrease in naive and memory B cells. Some patients who were thought to have CVID were found by genetic studies to have X-linked agammaglobulinemia, X-linked lymphoproliferative disease, or hyper-IgM syndrome. It is important to exclude these disorders and other causes of hypogammaglobulinemia, such as hypogammaglobulinemia associated with thymoma or secondary to immunoglobulin loss (intestinal loss), before making the diagnosis of CVID.

Selective **IgA deficiency** is defined as serum IgA levels less than 10 mg/dL with normal or increased levels of other immunoglobulins. The diagnosis cannot be confirmed until the patient is at least 4 years of age when IgA levels should reach adult levels. Selective IgA deficiency occurs in approximately 1 in 500 individuals. Many patients with selective IgA deficiency are asymptomatic. In others, it is associated with recurrent sinopulmonary infections, IgG$_2$ subclass deficiency, specific antibody deficiency, food allergy, autoimmune disease, or celiac disease. IgA deficiency occurs in families, suggesting autosomal inheritance. It also is seen in families with CVID.

**IgG subclass deficiency** occurs when the level of antibodies in one or more of the four IgG subclasses is selectively decreased while total IgG levels are normal or only slightly decreased. The IgG$_2$ subclass is the most prevalent of the IgG subclasses. Deficiency in IgG$_1$ usually is reflected as hypogammaglobulinemia. IgG$_2$ subclass deficiency is the most common of the IgG subclass deficiencies and often is associated with IgA deficiency, ataxia-telangiectasia, and reduced capacity to produce antibody against polysaccharide antigens. IgG$_3$ subclass deficiency also has been associated with recurrent infections. Absence of IgG$_4$ is not considered to be clinically significant. An inability to synthesize specific antibody titers to protein or polysaccharide antigens is the best marker of IgG subclass deficiency associated with recurrent infections and requiring therapy.

**Transient hypogammaglobulinemia of infancy** is a temporary condition characterized by delayed immunoglobulin production. The pathogenesis of this disorder is unknown but is thought to result from a prolongation of the physiologic hypogammaglobulinemia of infancy. The immunoglobulin nadir at 6 months of age is accentuated, with immunoglobulin levels less than 200 mg/dL. Immunoglobulin levels remain diminished throughout the first year of life and usually increase to normal, age-appropriate levels, generally by 2 to 4 years of age. Occasionally, low levels persist longer. The incidence of sinopulmonary infection is increased in some patients. The diagnosis is supported by normal levels of both B and T cells, and normal antibody responses to protein antigens such as diphtheria and tetanus toxoids. The transient nature of this disorder cannot be confirmed, however, until immunoglobulin levels return to normal ranges.

**Antibody deficiency syndrome** is characterized by recurrent infections with normal immunoglobulin levels and normal lymphocyte numbers and subsets, but an inability to synthesize specific antibody to polysaccharide antigens, such as to the 23-valent pneumococcal vaccine. The pathogenesis of this disorder is unknown. Lack of specific antibody titers explains the recurrent infections and justifies therapy.

## Combined Immunodeficiency Diseases

Disorders that affect T-cell development or function usually result in combined immunodeficiency because T cells provide necessary signals for B-cell differentiation. **Hyper-IgM syndrome** is usually classified under antibody deficiency diseases or B-cell disorders. However, the most common form of hyper-IgM, X-linked hyper-IgM, is a combined immunodeficiency disease with deficient T cell function. Hyper-IgM syndrome is characterized by a failure of immunoglobulin isotype switching from IgM and IgD to IgG, IgA, or IgE, and a lack of memory responses. Affected patients have normal or elevated serum levels of IgM with low or absent levels of IgG, IgA, and IgE. Immunoglobulin isotype switching allows a B cell to maintain antigen specificity while altering immunoglobulin function and is directed by cytokines, requiring direct interaction between CD40 ligand on a CD4 T cell and CD40 on a B cell (Fig. 73-2). Subsequent signal transduction via CD40 activates several signaling molecules and transcription factors, including

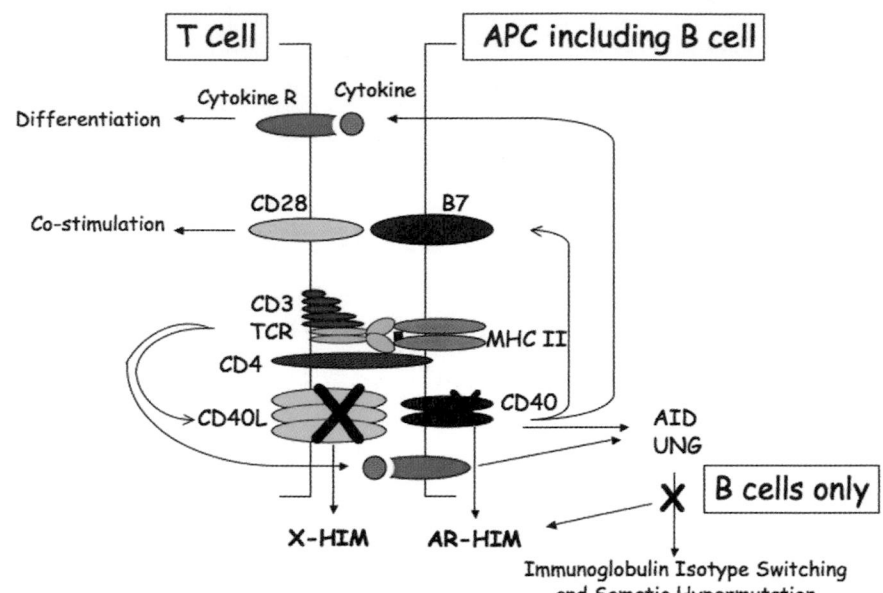

FIGURE 73-2

Schematic representation of the interaction between a CD4 T cell and a B cell. T cell activation follows T cell receptor (TCR) recognition of peptide antigen presented via MHC class II molecules resulting in CD40 ligand (CD40L) expression and cytokine synthesis. CD40L stimulates the B cell via CD40, resulting in expression of costimulatory molecules (B7) that are important in T cell priming and cytokine synthesis that drives T cell differentiation. CD40 signaling and signaling by cytokines in B cells activate activation-induced cytidine deaminase (AID) and uracil DNA-glycosylase (UNG) to promote immunoglobulin isotype switching and somatic hypermutation. Defects in CD40L cause X-linked hyper-IgM (X-HIM), and defects in CD40, AID, or UNG cause autosomal recessive hyper-IgM (AR-HIM). Defects in either CD40L or CD40 affect T cell costimulation and priming, leading to T cell defects, whereas defects in AID and UNG maintain normal T cell costimulation and function.

nuclear factor κB (NF-κB) and two enzymes, activation-induced cytidine deaminase (AID), and uracil DNA-glycosylase (UNG). In addition, signaling via CD40 on B cells and other antigen-presenting cells leads to upregulation of costimulatory molecules important for promoting T cell differentiation.

X-linked hyper-IgM results from defects in the CD40 ligand gene, inhibiting the capacity of the ligand to bind to CD40. As a result, no signal reaches the B cell for immunoglobulin isotype switching or antigen-presenting cells for upregulation of costimulatory molecules necessary for T-cell priming. Defects in CD40, inherited in an autosomal recessive manner, lead to a similar immunodeficiency due to a lack of signaling via CD40 (Fig. 73-2 and Table 73-2). Other forms of autosomal recessive hyper-IgM result from defects in B-cell AID or UNG and present with a failure of immunoglobulin isotype switching without any abnormality in T-cell function. These forms of hyper-IgM are an antibody deficiency disease and not a combined immunodeficiency disease (see Table 73-1). Patients with defects in CD40 ligand or CD40 have small lymph nodes with no germinal centers, whereas patients with defects in AID or UNG have large germinal centers and lymphadenopathy.

All of these patients have increased susceptibility to sinopulmonary infections; however, patients with defects in CD40 ligand or CD40 also are susceptible to opportunistic infections, such as *P. jiroveci* (*carinii*) and *Cryptosporidium parvum*. Autosomal recessive forms of hyper-IgM appear to increase susceptibility to autoimmune disease. The hyper-IgM phenotype is also found in an X-linked disorder associated with ectodermal dysplasia, resulting from the defects in the gene encoding the NF-κB essential modulator (NEMO) and results in low IgG, IgA, and IgE levels with normal or elevated IgM levels. Patients with defects in NEMO are susceptible to a wider spectrum of infectious organisms, especially meningitis and infection with atypical mycobacteria, because NF-κB signaling is important for

several functions of both innate and adaptive immune systems.

**Severe combined immunodeficiency (SCID)** is characterized by a profound lack of T-cell numbers or function and B-cell dysfunction resulting from absence of B cells from the gene defect itself or secondary to lack of T-cell function (see Fig. 73-1). T cells develop from bone marrow–derived precursors in the thymus (see Fig. 73-2), where they undergo several stages of development characterized by recombination of the variable region of T-cell antigen receptor chains α and β (or γ and δ). In addition, thymocytes differentiate into CD4 or CD8 T cells if they interact with major histocompatibility complex (MHC) class II or class I molecules, respectively. The T-cell antigen receptor recognizes peptide fragments only from antigens that are presented via MHC molecules: CD4 T cells by MHC class II molecules and CD8 T cells by MHC class I molecules. Because the variable region of the T-cell antigen receptor rearranges randomly to provide as much variability as possible, not all T-cell antigen receptors can interact with the MHC molecules present in the individual. A process of positive selection occurs in the thymus to select thymocytes with antigen receptors that can interact with the expressed MHC molecules (see Fig. 73-2), while all other thymocytes in the thymus die. Some of the positively selected thymocytes have antigen receptors, however, that recognize self-antigens presented by MHC molecules in the thymus. These cells are deleted in the thymus by a process of negative selection. Positive selection and negative selection in the thymus ensure that the mature T cells that leave the thymus for the peripheral lymphoid tissues can function with the individual's MHC molecules and do not mount autoimmune responses. SCID can result from any specific genetic mutation that interferes with T cell development in the thymus or T cell function in the periphery.

**X-linked SCID**, the most common form, is caused by mutations in the gene on chromosome Xq13.1 coding for

**TABLE 73-2 Combined Immunodeficiency Diseases**

| Disorder | Genetics | Onset | Manifestations | Pathogenesis | Associated Features |
|---|---|---|---|---|---|
| Immunodeficiency with increased IgM (see Table 73-1) | X-linked (Xq26), AR | First year | Sinopulmonary infections, opportunistic infections, *Pneumocystis jiroveci* | Defect in CD40 ligand (X-linked) or CD40 (AR) | Neutropenia, liver disease, cancer |
| DiGeorge anomaly | 22q11.2 (or 10p) deletion | Newborn, early infancy | Hypocalcemic tetany; pyogenic infections, partial or complete T-cell deficiency | Hypoplasia of third and fourth pharyngeal pouch | Congenital heart disease (aortic arch anomalies), hypoparathyroidism, micrognathia, hypertelorism |
| Severe combined immunodeficiency | X-linked AR | 1–3 mo | Candidiasis, all types of infections, failure to thrive, chronic diarrhea | Mutation in IL-2Rγ chain, Jak3 kinase, ZAP-70, IL-7Rα | GVHD from maternal-fetal transfusions, severe GVHD from nonirradiated blood transfusion |
| Severe combined immunodeficiency (T⁻ B⁺ SCID) | AR | 1–3 mo | Same as T⁻ B⁺ SCID | Mutation in RAG1/2, Artemis, ADA/PNP deficiency: dATP/dGTP-induced lymphocyte toxicity | Same as T⁻ B⁺ SCID<br>ADA deficiency: chondro-osseous dysplasia<br>PNP deficiency: neurologic disorders |
| Omenn syndrome | AR | 1–3 mo | Exfoliative erythroderma, same as T⁻ B⁻ SCID lymphadenopathy, hepatosplenomegaly | Hypomorphic mutations in SCID-causing genes (RAG1/2, Artemis, IL-7Rα) | Restricted T-cell receptor heterogeneity, eosinophilia, elevated IgE |
| Reticular dysgenesis (T⁻ B⁻ SCID) | AR | 1–3 mo | Same as T⁻ B⁻ SCID | Defective maturation of common stem cell affecting myeloid and lymphoid cells | Agammaglobulinemia, alymphocytosis, agranulocytosis |
| Bare lymphocyte syndrome (MHC class I deficiency) | AR | First decade | Sinopulmonary infections | Mutation in TAP1 or TAP2 (transporter associated with antigen processing) | Decreased CD8 T cells, chronic lung inflammation |
| Bare lymphocyte syndrome (MHC class II deficiency) | AR | Early infancy | Respiratory tract infections, chronic diarrhea, viral infections in central nervous system | Mutations in CIITA, RFX5, RFXAP, and RFX-B (DNA binding factors) | Decreased CD4 T cells, autoimmune disease |

AD, autosomal dominant; ADA, adenosine deaminase; AR, autosomal recessive; dATP, deoxyadenosine triphosphate; dGTP, deoxyguanosine triphosphate; GVHD, graft-versus-host disease; IL, interleukin; IL-2Rγ, interleukin-2 receptor gamma chain; MHC, major histocompatibility complex; PNP, purine nucleoside phosphorylase; SCID, severe combined immunodeficiency; T⁻ B⁺, T⁻ cells absent and B cells present; T⁺ B⁻, T cells absent and B cells absent.

the common gamma chain of the interleukin -2 (IL-2), IL-4, IL-7, IL-9, IL-15, and IL-21 receptors. Affected patients have no T cells or NK cells in the peripheral blood but have normal numbers of B cells. Immunoglobulin levels are low or undetectable. Lymph nodes and tonsils are absent. The defect in T cell and NK cell development results from a failure of signaling via the IL-7 and IL-15 receptors, respectively. Defects in the IL-7 receptor alpha chain also result in absent T cells but normal numbers of B cells and NK cells, whereas IL-15 is necessary for NK cell development.

**Autosomal recessive SCID** results from defects in signaling molecules, such as Janus tyrosine kinase 3 (Jak3), which signals downstream of the common gamma chain, or ZAP-70 kinase, necessary for CD4 T-cell signaling. In Jak3 deficiency, T cells and NK cells are absent, whereas nonfunctional B cells are present in normal numbers. In ZAP-70 deficiency, there is a marked decrease in CD8 T cells with normal numbers of nonfunctional CD4 T cells.

Recombination of the variable regions of the T-cell receptor and immunoglobulin molecules requires two genes called *recombinase activating gene (RAG) 1* and *2* as well as other genes important in DNA excision and repair such as *Artemis*. Defects in any of the genes that abolish its function result in autosomal recessive SCID with no T cells or B cells present. Mutations in *RAG1*, *RAG2*, or *Artemis* that preserve limited function result in **Omenn syndrome**, a variant form of SCID that is characterized by exfoliative erythroderma, lymphadenopathy, hepatosplenomegaly, marked eosinophilia, elevated serum IgE, and impaired T-cell function. Patients with Omenn syndrome have T cells in the periphery, but these T cells have a limited repertoire.

**Bare lymphocyte syndrome** results from defects in transcription factors that regulate expression of class II molecules or genes that affect transport of antigen peptides, which leads to absence of either MHC class I or MHC class II molecules. Lymphoid tissue and B cells may be present in normal amounts, but CD4 T cells are decreased or absent in class II deficiency, whereas CD8 cells are decreased or absent in class I deficiency. Some patients may have normal numbers of CD4 or CD8 T cells, but none of the T cells are functional because peptide antigens cannot be presented to T cells.

Deficiencies in **adenosine deaminase (ADA)** and **purine nucleoside phosphorylase**, two enzymes involved in the purine salvage pathway, also result in SCID. These deficiencies are caused by mutations in the ADA gene on chromosome 20q12-q13.1 or the purine nucleoside phosphorylase gene on chromosome 14q13. Accumulation of nucleoside substrates or their metabolic products in the plasma and urine is toxic to lymphocytes. T cells are particularly sensitive to the accumulation of toxic purine metabolites, especially deoxyadenosine triphosphate and deoxyadenosine, which results in absent or markedly reduced T-cell function, often with absent B cells or B-cell function. Most patients exhibit severe infection early in life, although the diagnosis in patients with partial immune function is not established until after 5 years of age or, occasionally, in adulthood. Patients with late-onset diagnosis are generally lymphopenic; they may have B cells and normal total immunoglobulin levels but little functional antibody (**Nezelof syndrome**). All patients

with ADA or purine nucleoside phosphorylase deficiency SCID have lymphopenia and loss of immune function over time.

**Clinical manifestations** of SCID include failure to thrive, severe bacterial infection in the first month of life, chronic candidiasis, infection with *P. jiroveci* (*carinii*) and other opportunistic organisms, and intractable diarrhea. Patients often have skin disease similar to eczema, possibly related to graft-versus-host disease (GVHD) from engraftment of maternal lymphocytes, which is not usually fatal. Patients with SCID are extremely susceptible to fatal GVHD, however, from lymphocytes in blood transfusions. Patients with T-cell disorders always should receive irradiated blood products.

**DiGeorge syndrome** is the classic example of T-cell deficiency and is the result of dysmorphogenesis of the third and fourth pharyngeal pouches, resulting in hypoplasia of the thymus required for T-cell maturation. Most, but not all, patients with DiGeorge syndrome have a field defect on chromosome 22q11.2, including the **velocardiofacial syndrome** and **CATCH 22 syndrome** (**c**ardiac anomalies, **a**bnormal facies, **t**hymic hypoplasia, **c**left palate, and **h**ypocalcemia). DiGeorge syndrome is classically characterized by hypocalcemic tetany, conotruncal and aortic arch anomalies, and increased infections. The diagnosis of CATCH 22 is established by fluorescent in situ hybridization with a DNA probe to detect deletions in chromosome 22q11.2. Most patients have partial immune defects with low T-cell numbers and function that improve with age. Severe T-cell deficiency is rare, but it results in SCID.

**Wiskott-Aldrich syndrome** is an X-linked disorder characterized by thrombocytopenia, eczema, defects in cell-mediated and humoral immunity, and a predisposition to lymphoproliferative disease (Table 73-3). It is caused by mutations of the gene on chromosome Xp11.22 coding for the 53-kD Wiskott-Aldrich syndrome protein, expressed in lymphocytes, platelets, and monocytes. Deficiency of this protein results in elevated levels of IgE and IgA, decreased IgM, poor responses to polysaccharide antigens, waning T-cell function, and profound thrombocytopenia. Opportunistic infections and autoimmune cytopenias become problematic in older children. **Isolated X-linked thrombocytopenia** also results from mutations of the identical gene. One third of patients with Wiskott-Aldrich syndrome die as a result of hemorrhage, and two thirds die as a result of recurrent infection caused by bacteria, cytomegalovirus, *P. jiroveci* (*carinii*), or herpes simplex virus. Stem cell transplantation has corrected the immunologic and hematologic problems in some patients.

**Ataxia-telangiectasia** is a syndrome caused by the *ATM* (ataxia-telangiectasia, mutated) gene on chromosome 11q22.3, which codes for a phosphatidylinositol-3 kinase (see Table 73-3). Patients have cutaneous and conjunctival telangiectasias and progressive cerebellar ataxia with degeneration of Purkinje cells. IgA deficiency, IgG$_2$ subclass deficiency of variable severity, low IgE levels, and variably depressed T-cell function may be seen. The normal function of the *ATM* gene is not clear but it seems to be involved in detecting DNA damage, blocking cell growth division until the damage is repaired, or both. Ataxia-telangiectasia cells are exquisitely sensitive

**TABLE 73-3  Other Immunodeficiency Diseases**

| Disorder | Genetics | Onset | Manifestations | Pathogenesis | Associated Features |
|---|---|---|---|---|---|
| Wiskott-Aldrich syndrome | X-linked, (Xp11.22) | Early infancy | Thrombocytopenia, atopic dermatitis, recurrent infections | 53-kD protein (WASP) defect | Polysaccharide antibody deficiency, small platelets, decreased cell-mediated immunity, lymphoproliferation |
| Ataxia-telangiectasia | AR (11q22.3) | 2–5 yr | Recurrent otitis media, pneumonia, meningitis with encapsulated organisms | *ATM* gene mutation Disorder of cell cycle checkpoint and of DNA double strand break repair | Neurologic and endocrine dysfunction, malignancy, telangiectasis; sensitivity to radiation |
| Nijmegen breakage syndrome | AR (8q21) | Infancy | Sinopulmonary infections, bronchiectasis, urinary tract infections | Defect in chromosomal repair mechanisms; hypomorphic mutation in *NBS1* (Nibrin) | Sensitivity to ionizing radiation; microcephaly with mild neurologic impairment; malignancy |
| Cartilage-hair hypoplasia (short-limbed dwarf) | AR (9p13-21) | Birth | Variable | Mutation in *RMRP* (RNase MRP RNA) | Metaphyseal dysplasia, short extremities |
| Chronic mucocutaneous candidiasis (APECED) | AR | 3–5 yr | Candidal infections of mucous membranes, skin, and nails | Mutations in *AIRE* gene | Autoimmune endocrinopathies |
| X-linked-lymphoproliferative syndrome | X-linked (Xq25) | Variable | Variable decrease in T, B, and NK cell function, absent NK T cells, hypogammaglobulinemia | Mutation in *SH2D1A* (*SAP*: SLAM-associated protein) | Life-threatening Epstein-Barr virus infection, lymphoma or Hodgkin disease, aplastic anemia, lymphohistiocytic disorder |
| Hyper-IgE syndrome | AD, AR | Variable | Skin and pulmonary abscesses, fungal infections, eczema, elevated IgE | Mutation in STAT3 (AD) mutation in TYK2 (AR) | Coarse facial features, failure to shed primary teeth, frequent fractures |

AD, autosomal dominant; AR, autosomal recessive; NK, natural killer.

to irradiation. Leukemias, lymphomas, and diabetes also may be present. Sexual maturation is delayed. There is no uniformly effective therapy, but antimicrobial therapy and intravenous immunoglobulin (IVIG) replacement therapy may be helpful.

**Chronic mucocutaneous candidiasis** (autoimmune-polyendocrinopathy-candidiasis-ectodermal dystrophy [APECED]) is characterized by chronic or recurrent candidal infections of the mucous membranes, skin, and nails (see Table 73-3). There is normal antibody production but significantly decreased or absent lymphocyte proliferation and delayed skin reactivity to *Candida*. Patients usually do not respond to topical antifungal therapy and must be treated with oral antifungal agents. In most patients, an autoimmune endocrine disorder, such as hypoparathyroidism and Addison disease, develops by early adulthood. Other autoimmune disorders have been reported. The insidious onset requires the need for frequent evaluation for autoimmune endocrine disorders. This disease results from a defect in the gene for the transcription factor autoimmune regulator *(AIRE),* which is necessary for expression of peripheral tissue antigens in the thymus, resulting in tolerance to these tissues in normal individuals.

Patients with **X-linked lymphoproliferative disease** (see Table 73-3) have a defect in immune responsiveness to Epstein-Barr virus (EBV). Boys with this disease are normal until infected with EBV, which is acutely fatal in 80% of patients. The disease is caused by a mutation in the gene called *SH2D1A* at chromosome Xq25, which codes for an adapter protein that normally inhibits signal transduction in proliferating T cells. With EBV infection, the mutation results in extensive expansion of CD8 T cells, hepatic necrosis, and death. Boys who survive initial EBV infection have significant hypogammaglobulinemia and are at high risk for developing aplastic anemia and lymphoma. Treatment of the acute EBV infection with prednisone and acyclovir may be helpful; VP-16 and anti-CD20 monoclonal antibody also may be of use. IVIG for hypogammaglobulinemia is indicated. Stem cell transplantation can prevent disease progression and provide a cure.

**Hyper-IgE syndrome** is characterized by markedly elevated serum IgE levels, a rash that resembles atopic dermatitis, eosinophilia, and staphylococcal abscesses of the skin, lungs, joints, and viscera (see Table 73-3). Infections with *H. influenzae* type b, *Candida,* and *Aspergillus* also may occur. These patients have coarse facial features, develop osteopenia, and may have giant pneumatoceles in the lungs after staphylococcal pneumonias. Although serum IgG, IgA, and IgM levels are normal, humoral immune responses to specific antigens are reduced, as is cell-mediated immunity. Long-term treatment with antistaphylococcal medications is indicated, and immunoglobulin replacement therapy may be helpful. Most patients have an autosomal dominant form of inheritance, whereas some patients appear to have an autosomal recessive inheritance. Defects in the *TYK2* gene have recently been found in a patient with an autosomal recessive hyper-IgE syndrome, and defects in the *STAT3* (signal transducer and activator of transcription 3) gene were identified in one with autosomal dominant hyper-IgE syndrome. Both of these genes

are involved in IL-6 signaling. Patients with *STAT3* defects have a deficiency of Th17 cells, proinflammatory cells that require IL-6 for their differentiation, secrete IL-17, and appear to be involved in immunity to bacterial and fungal pathogens as well as in the pathogenesis of autoimmune disease.

## TREATMENT

The approach to therapy of lymphocyte disorders depends on the diagnosis, clinical findings, and laboratory findings (Table 73-4). When immunodeficiency is suspected, and while the evaluation is in process, all blood products need to be irradiated and negative for cytomegalovirus. Lymphocytes present in blood products can cause fatal **GVHD** in patients with SCID. Cytomegalovirus infection can be fatal in an immunodeficiency patient undergoing stem cell transplantation. Live virus vaccines should be withheld from patients and household members until a diagnosis is established.

Infections should be treated with appropriate antibiotics. Prevention of recurrent infections provides a better quality of life and decreases possible consequences. Patients with milder forms of antibody deficiency diseases may benefit from **vaccination** with protein-conjugate vaccines to *H. influenzae* type b and *S. pneumoniae,* assaying postvaccination titers at least 1 month later. These vaccines are administered routinely to young children; however, older children and adults with antibody deficiency syndrome also should receive them to generate protective antibody levels. Other microorganisms, including nonvaccine *S. pneumoniae* serotypes, can cause infections in susceptible patients. In addition to immunization, antibiotic prophylaxis or IVIG may prevent recurrent infections.

**Antibiotic prophylaxis** can be provided with once-daily administration of trimethoprim-sulfamethoxazole or amoxicillin at one half of the total daily therapeutic

---

**TABLE 73-4  General Management of Patients with Immunodeficiency**

Avoid transfusions with blood products unless they are irradiated and cytomegalovirus negative

Avoid live virus vaccines, especially in patients with severe T-cell deficiencies or agammaglobulinemia, and in household members

Use prophylaxis to *Pneumocystis jiroveci* (*carinii*) in T-cell immunodeficiency and in X-linked hyper-IgM

Follow pulmonary function in patients with recurrent pneumonia

Use chest physiotherapy and postural drainage in patients with recurrent pneumonia

Use prophylactic antibiotics, because minor infections can quickly disseminate

Examine diarrheal stools for *Giardia lamblia* and *Clostridium difficile*

Avoid unnecessary exposure to individuals with infection

Use immunoglobulin for severe antibody deficiency states at a dose of 400–600 mg/kg q3–4 wk IV

dose, especially if the patient does not have a severe antibody deficiency and has not had severe or complicated infections. Therapy with antibiotics may be complicated by the development of immediate, autoimmune, immune complex, and delayed-type hypersensitivity drug reactions. Alternating prophylactic antibiotics on a monthly basis may help reduce the incidence of drug-resistant microorganisms.

**Immunoglobulin replacement therapy,** intravenously or subcutaneously, is a lifesaving therapy for patients with severe antibody deficiency diseases. It provides passive immunity against common microorganisms and reduces the frequency and severity of infection in most patients with antibody deficiency diseases. Immunoglobulin replacement therapy is indicated for patients with agammaglobulinemia, hyper-IgM syndrome, other antibody deficiency diseases and combined immunodeficiency diseases; for patients with infections requiring hospitalization, especially in intensive care units, or with infections that affect growth as well as hearing or speech development; and for patients who have failed antibiotic prophylaxis. Immunoglobulin replacement therapy is usually administered at a total monthly dose of 400 to 600 mg/kg of body weight administered every 3 to 4 weeks intravenously, or every 1 to 2 weeks subcutaneously by infusion pump. IVIG therapy should be monitored by regularly measuring trough immunoglobulin levels, antibody titers to *H. influenzae* type b, and, most importantly, the patient's clinical course. Patients who continue to have recurrent infections, especially in the last week before the administration of IVIG, may require higher doses or more frequent administration. A combination of prophylactic antibiotics and immunoglobulin replacement therapy may be indicated in patients who continue to have recurrent infections. Other causes of recurrent infections should be reconsidered, however. **Complications of IVIG** therapy include transfusion reactions with chills, fever, and myalgias. They usually can be prevented in subsequent infusions by pretreatment with an antihistamine and an antipyretic and by a slower rate of infusion. Headache from aseptic meningitis can develop after IVIG therapy, usually in the first 24 hours. It most often responds to treatment with ibuprofen. Thrombosis and acute renal failure have also been reported, usually in high-risk patients. Allergic reactions to IVIG can occur in patients with absent IgA. Allergic reactions are rare and should not occur in patients who have detectable serum IgA levels or patients who cannot synthesize any antibodies. Subcutaneous administration of immunoglobulin has fewer adverse effects but may be complicated by local reactions at the site(s) of infusion. The risk of transmission of infectious agents, despite preparation from large numbers of selected donors, is extremely low.

Therapy for severe T-cell disorders is stem cell transplantation, preferably from an human leukocyte antigen–matched sibling (see Chapter 76). Immunoglobulin replacement provides passive antibody-mediated immunity. Some patients continue to have poor B-cell function after stem cell transplantation and require immunoglobulin replacement therapy. **GVHD**, in which the transplanted cells initiate an immune response against the host tissues, is the main complication of stem cell transplantation. Patients with the ADA deficiency form of SCID who lack histocompatible sibling donors can receive repeated intramuscular replacement doses of ADA, stabilized by coupling to polyethylene glycol. Gene therapy has been performed in several patients with the common gamma chain deficiency form and ADA deficiency form of SCID by transfer of a normal gene into bone marrow stem cells, which are infused into the patient. Gene therapy for common gamma chain deficiency was successful in most of the treated patients; however, it was complicated by the development of leukemia in some patients.

## PREVENTION AND NEWBORN SCREENING

Prenatal diagnosis is possible for all immunodeficiency diseases with an identified gene defect. Testing can be performed by gene sequencing, especially when the mutation in the index case has been identified. Polymerase chain reaction amplification of T-cell receptor excision circles that are present in recent thymic emigrants is currently being tested as a newborn screening method to identify patients with SCID, which would allow the initiation of therapy before any serious infections or complications develop.

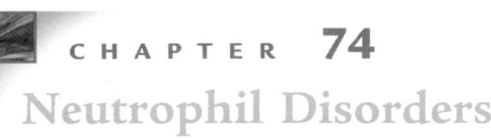

CHAPTER **74**

# Neutrophil Disorders

Neutrophils play important roles in immunity and wound healing; their primary function is ingesting and killing pathogens. Neutrophil disorders can result from deficient cell numbers, defective chemotaxis, or defective function (Table 74-1). Patients with neutrophil disorders are susceptible to infections with *Staphylococcus aureus,* certain fungi, and gram-negative bacteria. Suggestive signs include mucous membrane infections (gingivitis), abscesses in the skin and viscera, lymphadenitis, poor wound healing, delayed umbilical cord separation, or absence of pus. Neutrophils develop in the bone marrow from hematopoietic stem cells by the action of several colony-stimulating factors, including stem cell factor, granulocyte-monocyte colony-stimulating factor (GM-CSF), granulocyte colony-stimulating factor (G-CSF), and interleukin-3 (IL-3). On leaving the bone marrow, mature neutrophils are found in the circulation or reside in the marginating pool. Chemotactic factors, including the complement fragment C5a, IL-8, and bacterial formulated peptides, mobilize neutrophils to enter tissues and sites of infections. Adhesion molecules are necessary for neutrophils to roll and adhere to vascular endothelium and extravasate from the blood into sites of infection, where they encounter, phagocytose, and kill pathogens, especially those coated by complement or antibodies. Neutrophils kill ingested pathogens using granular enzymes or by activation of oxygen radicals.

## TABLE 74-1 Phagocytic Disorders

| Name | Defect | Comment |
|---|---|---|
| Chronic granulomatous disease | Bactericidal | X-linked recessive (66%), autosomal recessive (33%); eczema, osteomyelitis, granulomas, abscesses caused by *Staphylococcus aureus, Burkholderia cepacia, Aspergillus fumigatus* |
| Chédiak-Higashi syndrome (1q42I-44) | Bactericidal plus chemotaxis; poor natural killer function | Autosomal recessive; oculocutaneous albinism, neuropathy, giant neutrophilic cytoplasmic inclusions; malignancy, neutropenia |
| Hyperimmunoglobulin E (Job syndrome) | Chemotaxis, opsonization | Autosomal dominant (STAT3 mutation), autosomal recessive (TYK2 mutation), eczema, staphylococcal abscesses, granulocyte and monocyte chemotaxis affected |
| Myeloperoxidase deficiency | Bactericidal, fungicidal | Reduced chemiluminescence; autosomal recessive (1:4000); persistent candidiasis in diabetic patients |
| Glucose-6-phosphate dehydrogenase deficiency | Bactericidal | Phenotypically similar to chronic granulomatous disease |
| Burns, malnutrition | Bactericidal plus chemotaxis | Reversible defects |
| Lazy leukocyte syndrome | Chemotaxis | Normal bone marrow cells but poor migration; granulocytopenia |
| Leukocyte adhesion deficiency; CD18 deficiency (21q22.3) | Adherence, chemotaxis, phagocytosis; reduced lymphocyte cytotoxicity | Delayed separation or infection of umbilical cord; lethal bacterial infections without pus; autosomal recessive; neutrophilia; deficiency of LFA-1, Mac-1, CR3 |
| Shwachman-Diamond syndrome | Chemotaxis, neutropenia | Pancreatic insufficiency, metaphyseal chondrodysplasia; autosomal recessive |

## ETIOLOGY AND CLINICAL MANIFESTATIONS

### Disorders of Neutrophil Numbers

The normal neutrophil count varies with age. **Neutropenia** may be caused by decreased marrow production or peripheral neutrophil destruction and is defined as an absolute neutrophil count (ANC) less than 1500/mm³ for white children 1 year of age or older. African-American children normally have lower total white blood cell and neutrophil counts. The effect of neutropenia depends on its severity. The susceptibility to infection is minimally increased until the ANC is less than 1000/mm³. Most patients do well with an ANC greater than 500/mm³. At these levels, localized infections are more common than generalized bacteremia. Serious bacterial infections are more common with an ANC less than 200/mm³. In the absence of an adequate neutrophil count, migration of neutrophils to areas of damage in the skin and mucous membrane is delayed. Neutropenia may be congenital or acquired (Table 74-2) and may be associated with specific diseases, especially infections (Table 74-3), or result from drug reactions (Table 74-4). The major types of infections associated with neutropenia are cellulitis, pharyngitis, gingivitis, lymphadenitis, abscesses (cutaneous or perianal), enteritis (typhlitis), and pneumonia. The sites of the infection usually are colonized heavily with normal bacterial flora that becomes invasive in the presence of neutropenia.

There are several forms of congenital neutropenia. **Severe congenital neutropenia (Kostmann syndrome)** is an autosomal recessive disorder and may present in infancy. In severe congenital neutropenia, myeloid cells fail to mature beyond the early stages of the promyelocyte.

The peripheral blood may show an impressive monocytosis. The genetic defect in Kostmann syndrome is a mutation in the gene for HAX-1, a protein found in mitochondria, which protects myeloid cells from apoptosis. Endogenous G-CSF levels are increased; nevertheless, exogenous G-CSF produces a rise in the neutrophil count, improving the care of these children. Acute myeloid leukemia has developed in a few patients who have survived into adolescence. Stem cell transplantation may be curative.

Severe congenital neutropenia, that may be either persistent or cyclic, also is a component of **Shwachman-Diamond syndrome**, an autosomal recessive syndrome of pancreatic insufficiency accompanying bone marrow dysfunction. This is a panmyeloid disorder in which neutropenia is the most prominent manifestation. Patients may have all the common complications of neutropenia, including gingivitis, which may be severe and lead to serious oral infections, alveolar bone destruction, and loss of teeth at an early age. Metaphyseal dysostosis and dwarfism may occur. Patients usually respond to G-CSF.

Other congenital neutropenias caused by deficient neutrophil production vary in severity and are poorly characterized. A gain of function mutation in the Wiskott-Aldrich syndrome protein has also been associated with an X-linked form of severe congenital neutropenia. The Wiskott-Aldrich syndrome protein demonstrates how mutations in same gene, albeit at different locations, can result in different diseases: Wiskott-Aldrich syndrome, X-linked thrombocytopenia, and X-linked congenital neutropenia. **Benign congenital neutropenia** is a functional diagnosis for patients with significant neutropenia in whom major infectious complications do not develop. Many patients whose ANC ranges from 100 to 500/mm³ have an increased

## TABLE 74-2 Mechanisms of Neutropenia

### ABNORMAL BONE MARROW

*Marrow Injury*
Drugs: idiosyncratic, cytotoxic (myelosuppressive)
Radiation
Chemicals: DDT, benzene
Hereditary
Immune-mediated: T and B cell and immunoglobulin
Infection: HIV, hepatitis B
Infiltrative processes: tumor, storage disease
*Maturation Defects*
Folic acid deficiency
Vitamin $B_{12}$
Glycogen storage disease type Ib
Shwachman-Diamond syndrome
Organic acidemias
Clonal disorders: congenital
Cyclic neutropenia

### PERIPHERAL CIRCULATION

*Pseudoneutropenia: Shift to Bone Marrow*
Hereditary
Severe infection
*Intravascular*
Destruction: neonatal isoimmune, autoimmune, hypersplenism
Leukoagglutination: lung, after cardiac bypass surgery

### EXTRAVASCULAR MECHANISMS

Increased use: severe infection, anaphylaxis
Destruction: antibody-mediated, hypersplenism

Adapted from Moore JO, Oritel TL, Rosse WF: Disorders of granulocytes and monocytes. In Andreoli TE, Bennett JC, Carpenter CCJ, Plum F, editors: Cecil Essentials of Medicine, 4th ed, Philadelphia, 1997, *Saunders.*

## TABLE 74-3 Infections Associated with Neutropenia

### BACTERIAL

Typhoid-paratyphoid
Brucellosis
Neonatal sepsis
Meningococcemia
Overwhelming sepsis
Congenital syphilis
Tuberculosis

### VIRAL

Measles
Hepatitis B
HIV
Rubella
Cytomegalovirus
Influenza
Epstein-Barr virus

### RICKETTSIAL

Rocky Mountain spotted fever
Typhus
Ehrlichiosis
Rickettsialpox

gene encoding for neutrophil elastase, has been found in patients with sporadic, autosomal dominant, and autosomal recessive forms of cyclic neutropenia.

**Isoimmune neutropenia** occurs in neonates as the result of transplacental transfer of maternal antibodies to fetal neutrophil antigens. The mother is sensitized to specific neutrophil antigens on fetal leukocytes that are inherited from the father and are not present on maternal cells. Isoimmune neonatal neutropenia, similar to isoimmune anemia and thrombocytopenia, is a transient

## TABLE 74-4 Drugs Associated with Neutropenia

### CYTOTOXIC

Myelosuppressive, chemotherapeutic agents
Immunosuppressive agents

### IDIOSYNCRATIC

Chloramphenicol
Sulfonamides
Propylthiouracil
Penicillins
Trimethoprim-sulfamethoxazole
Carbamazepine
Phenytoin
Cimetidine
Methyldopa
Indomethacin
Chlorpromazine
Penicillamine
Gold salts

frequency of infections, particularly respiratory infections, but the major problem is the slow resolution of infections that develop. These disorders may be sporadic or familial and, in some instances, are transmitted as an autosomal dominant disorder. Severe congenital neutropenia may be associated with SCID in **reticular dysgenesis**, a disorder of hematopoietic stem cells affecting all bone marrow lineages.

**Cyclic neutropenia** is a stem cell disorder in which all marrow elements cycle. It may be transmitted as an autosomal dominant, recessive, or sporadic disorder. Because of the short half-life of neutrophils in the blood (6 to 7 hours) compared with platelets (10 days) and red blood cells (120 days), neutropenia is the only clinically significant abnormality. The usual cycle is 21 days, with neutropenia lasting 4 to 6 days, accompanied by monocytosis and often by eosinophilia. Stomatitis or oral ulcers, pharyngitis, lymphadenopathy, fever, and cellulitis are present at the time of neutropenia. Severe, debilitating bone pain is common when the neutrophil count is low. G-CSF results in increasing neutrophil numbers and a shorter duration of neutropenia. Defects in *ELA2*, the

process (see Chapters 62 and 151). Cutaneous infections are common, and sepsis is rare. Early treatment of infection while the infant is neutropenic is the major goal of therapy. Intravenous immune globulin may decrease the duration of neutropenia.

**Autoimmune neutropenia** usually develops in children 5 to 24 months of age and often persists for prolonged periods. Neutrophil autoantibodies may be IgG, IgM, IgA, or a combination of these. Usually, the condition resolves in 6 months to 4 years. Clinical symptoms may dictate treatment. Although intravenous immune globulin and corticosteroids have been used, most patients respond to G-CSF. Autoimmune neutropenia rarely may be an early manifestation of systemic lupus erythematosus or rheumatoid arthritis.

Neutropenia is common in stressed neonates. Virtually any major illness, including asphyxia, may precipitate transient neonatal neutropenia. Maternal conditions, such as hypertension and eclampsia, can induce neonatal neutropenia. Significant neutropenia may develop in infected neonates, in part, due to depletion of bone marrow stores, which are far less extensive in neonates than adults.

## Disorders of Neutrophil Migration

Neutrophils normally adhere to endothelium and migrate to areas of inflammation by the interaction of membrane proteins, called *integrins* and *selectins,* with endothelial cell adhesion molecules. A hallmark of defects in neutrophil migration is the absence of pus at sites of infection. In **leukocyte adhesion deficiency type I (LAD-I)**, infants lacking the $\beta_2$ integrin CD18 exhibit the condition early in infancy with failure of separation of the umbilical cord (often 2 months after birth) with attendant omphalitis and sepsis (see Table 74-1). The neutrophil count usually is greater than $20,000/mm^3$ because of failure of the neutrophils to adhere normally to vascular endothelium and to migrate out of blood to the tissues (Fig. 74-1). Cutaneous, respiratory, and mucosal infections occur. Children with this condition often have severe gingivitis. Sepsis usually leads to death in early childhood. This disorder is transmitted as an autosomal recessive trait. Stem cell transplantation may be lifesaving.

**LAD-II** results from impairment of neutrophil rolling along the vascular wall, which is the first step in neutrophil migration into tissues and sites of infection. Rolling is mediated by sialylated and fucosylated tetrasaccharides related to the sialylated Lewis X blood group found on the surface of neutrophils, monocytes, and activated lymphocytes binding to selectin molecules on vascular endothelium (see Fig. 74-1). LAD-II results from a general defect in fucose metabolism leading to the absence of sialylated Lewis X blood group on the surface of neutrophils and other leukocytes.

A variety of conditions are associated with chemotactic defects in neutrophils. **Hyper-IgE syndrome**, caused by defects in the IL-6 signaling pathway, is characterized by eczema, hyperimmunoglobulinemia E, an extrinsic chemotactic defect, absent T-cell and B-cell responses to antigens, and recurrent cold boils (usually caused by *S. aureus*) that do not become markedly red or drain (see Chapter 73 and Table 74-1).

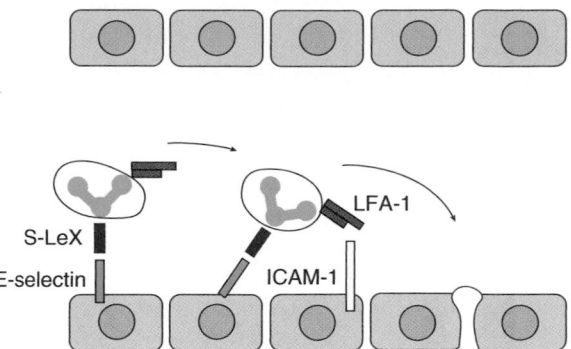

**FIGURE 74-1**

Schematic representation of neutrophil migration from the vascular space across the vascular endothelium into tissues. Neutrophils bind to selectin molecules on the surface of vascular endothelium via sialylated and fucosylated tetrasaccharides related to the sialylated Lewis X blood group (S-LeX) found on the surface of neutrophils. The bound neutrophils roll along the endothelium and become tightly bound by the interaction of the adhesion molecule leukocyte function–associated antigen type 1 (LFA-1) on the neutrophil and intercellular adhesion molecule type 1 (ICAM-1) on vascular endothelium, allowing neutrophils to move through the endothelium and into the tissue spaces. (Adapted from Janeway CA, Travers P, Walport M, Capra JD: Immunobiology: The Immune System in Health and Disease, 4th ed, New York, 1999, *Elsevier.*)

## Disorders of Neutrophil Function

Defects in neutrophil function are relatively rare inherited disorders and tend to be associated with a marked susceptibility to bacterial and fungal infection. **Chronic granulomatous disease (CGD)** is a rare disorder of white blood cells that results from defective intracellular killing of bacteria and intracellular pathogens by neutrophils and macrophages because of an inability to activate the "respiratory burst," the catalytic conversion of molecular oxygen to superoxide ($O_2^-$). Reduced nicotinamide adenine dinucleotide phosphate oxidase, the enzyme that catalyzes the respiratory burst, consists of four subunits, two subunits of cytochrome b558, gp91$^{phox}$ and p22$^{phox}$, and two cytosolic oxidase components, p47$^{phox}$ and p67$^{phox}$. Defects in any of these enzymes lead to an inability to kill catalase-positive pathogens such as *S. aureus* and enteric gram-negative bacteria and fungi (*Aspergillus fumigatus, Candida albicans, Torulopsis glabrata*). The gp91$^{phox}$ gene is located on chromosome Xp21.1 and is responsible for the more common form of the disease. Only one copy of the gene needs to be defective for the disease to be expressed in males. The other gene defects are inherited in an autosomal recessive manner. The chromosome locations for these genes are 16q24 for p22$^{phox}$, 7q11.23 for p47$^{phox}$, and 1q25 for p67$^{phox}$. Glucose-6-phosphate dehydrogenase also is involved in the production of superoxide; severe forms of glucose-6-phosphate dehydrogenase deficiency also result in CGD. Patients characteristically have lymphadenopathy, hypergammaglobulinemia, hepatosplenomegaly, dermatitis, failure to thrive, anemia, chronic diarrhea, and abscesses. Infections occur in the lungs, the middle ear, gastrointestinal tract, skin, urinary tract, lymph nodes, liver, and bones. Granulomas may obstruct the pylorus or ureters.

**Chédiak-Higashi syndrome**, an abnormality of secondary granules, is an autosomal recessive disorder caused by a mutation in a cytoplasmic protein (CHS1) of unknown function (thought to be involved in organellar protein trafficking) resulting in fusion of the primary and secondary granules in neutrophils. Giant granules are present in many cells, including lymphocytes, platelets, and melanocytes. Patients usually have partial oculocutaneous albinism. The defect in Chédiak-Higashi syndrome results in defective neutrophil and natural killer cell function, leading to recurrent and sometimes fatal infections with streptococci and staphylococci. Most patients progress to an accelerated phase associated with Epstein-Barr virus infection and characterized by a **lymphoproliferative syndrome** with generalized lymphohistiocytic infiltrates, fever, jaundice, hepatomegaly, lymphadenopathy, and pancytopenia. The condition resembles familial erythrophagocytic lymphohistiocytosis and virus-associated hemophagocytic syndrome more than a malignant lymphoma.

## LABORATORY DIAGNOSIS

The evaluation of a neutropenic child depends on clinical signs of infection, family and medication history, age of the patient, cyclic or persistent nature of the condition, signs of bone marrow infiltration (malignancy or storage disease), and evidence of involvement of other cell lines (Fig. 74-2). Neutropenia is confirmed by a complete blood count and differential. A bone marrow aspirate and biopsy may be necessary to determine whether the neutropenia is due to a failure of production in the bone marrow, infiltration of the bone marrow, or loss of neutrophils in the periphery. Antineutrophil antibodies help diagnose autoimmune neutropenia.

Neutrophil chemotactic defects can be excluded by the presence of neutrophils at the site of infection. The **Rebuck skin window** is a 4-hour in vivo test for neutrophil chemotaxis that is not performed routinely by most laboratories. Flow cytometry for the presence of adhesion molecules, such as CD18, can help diagnose leukocyte adhesion defects. Point mutations that affect the function of the adhesion molecule but do not alter antibody binding are missed using flow cytometry.

**FIGURE 74-2**

Algorithm for evaluation of neutropenia. SLE, systemic lupus erythematosus; TB, tuberculosis; WBC, white blood cell.

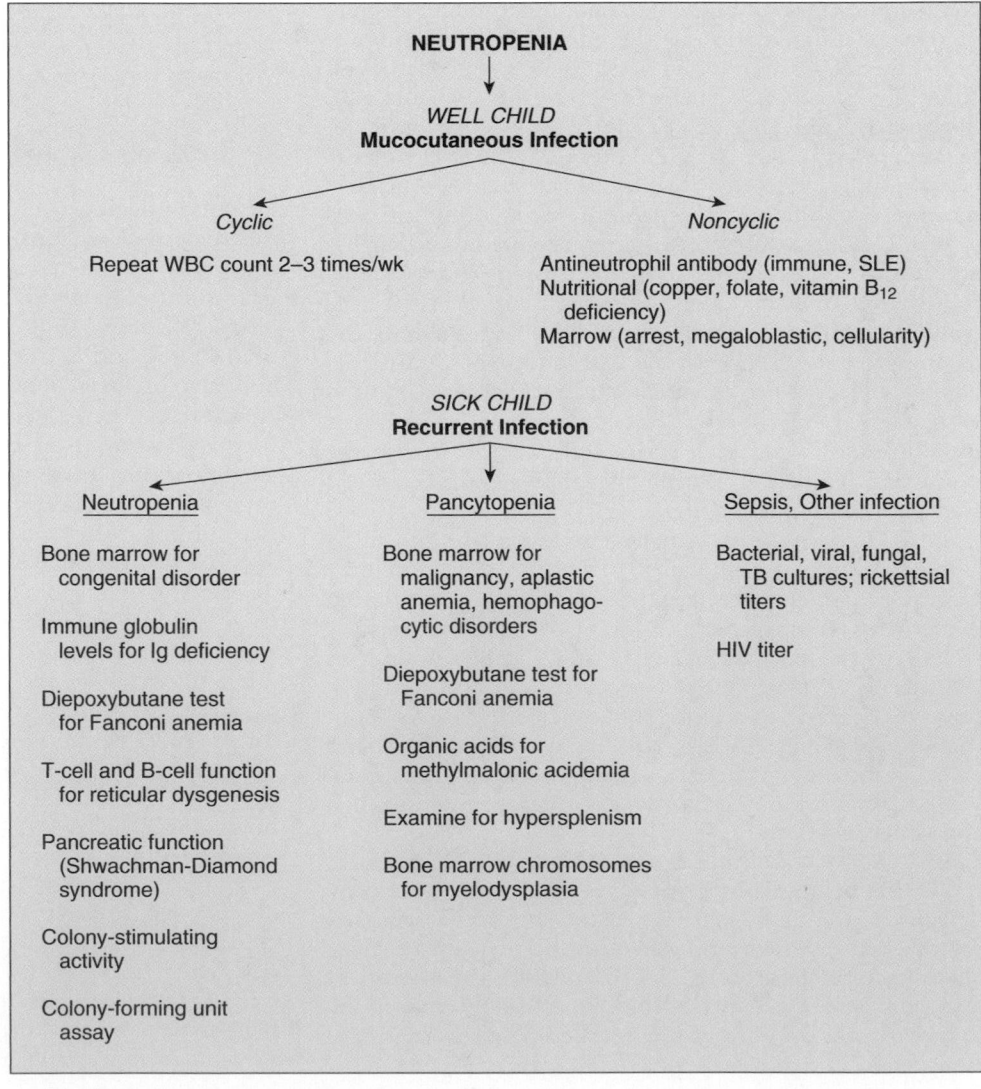

CGD can be diagnosed by the flow cytometry-based test using dihydrorhodamine 123 or the **nitroblue tetrazolium** test (see Chapter 72). Light microscopy of neutrophils for the presence of giant granules can help diagnose Chédiak-Higashi syndrome. The presence of an elevated IgE level, especially in association with poor antibody and T-cell responses to antigens, suggests hyper-IgE syndrome.

## TREATMENT

Therapy for neutropenia depends on the underlying cause. Patients with severe bacterial infections require broad-spectrum antibiotics; the resolution of neutropenia is the most important prognostic factor. Most patients with severe congenital neutropenia or autoimmune neutropenia respond to therapy with G-CSF. Granulocyte transfusion should be reserved for life-threatening infection; even with transfusion, the results have been disappointing. Chronic mild neutropenia not associated with immunosuppression can be managed expectantly with prompt antimicrobial treatment of soft tissue infections, which usually are caused by *S. aureus* or group A streptococcus.

Frequent courses of antibiotics, including trimethoprim-sulfamethoxazole prophylaxis, and surgical débridement of infections are required in **CGD**. Because *A. fumigatus* can cause serious infection in patients with CGD, moldy hay, decomposing compost, and other nests of fungi must be avoided. The frequency of infection in CGD is lessened by treatment with **recombinant interferon-γ** administered subcutaneously three times a week. Stem cell transplantation (see Chapter 76) may be lifesaving in CGD, LAD-1, and Chédiak-Higashi syndrome.

## PROGNOSIS AND PREVENTION

The prognosis depends on the particular defect. Milder and transient defects in neutrophil numbers have a better prognosis. Prolonged absence of neutrophils or their function has a poor prognosis, especially with the risk of bacterial and fungal sepsis. Treatment with interferon-γ has improved the prognosis of patients with CGD; however, successful stem cell transplantation is the only currently available mode of therapy that can reverse the poor prognosis of severe neutrophil defects. As in other genetic defects, prenatal diagnosis and genetic counseling are possible for all known gene mutations.

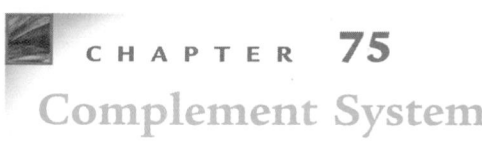

CHAPTER **75**

# Complement System

The **complement system** consists of several plasma and membrane proteins that function in the innate immune response as well as in adaptive immunity by facilitating antibody-mediated immunity. **Complement proteins** can kill pathogens with or without antibody, opsonize pathogens to facilitate their uptake by phagocytes, or mediate inflammation. The complement system can be activated through three pathways—the classic, alternative, or lectin pathways—that involve a cascade-like, sequential activation of complement factors resulting in an amplified response (Fig. 75-1). Disorders of the complement system predispose to recurrent infection, autoimmunity, and angioedema (Table 75-1).

## ETIOLOGY

The three pathways for complement activation are initiated by different mechanisms. The **classic pathway** is activated by antigen-antibody complexes or by C-reactive protein and trypsin-like enzymes. The **alternative pathway** may be activated by C3b generated through classic complement activation or by endotoxin or fungal antigens (zymogen). The **lectin pathway** is initiated by the interaction of mannose-binding lectin with microbial carbohydrate. The three pathways lead to the generation of a C3 convertase, which activates the complement protein C3 and initiates a cascade common to the three pathways, culminating in the formation of a **membrane attack complex (MAC)**, which can lyse pathogens and other target cells (see Fig. 75-1). The MAC is a complex of C5b, C6, C7, C8, and several C9 molecules. The MAC generates pores in the cell membrane, leading to lysis of the cells. The MAC without C9 can form small pores; however, the addition of C9 leads to a large transmembrane pore that enhances lysis of the target cell. C3a and C5a can release histamine from mast cells and basophils, leading to increased vascular permeability and smooth muscle contraction. In addition, C5a has chemotactic activity, attracting phagocytes to the site of complement activation, and it can cause degranulation of phagocytic cells. C3b acts as an opsonin when attached to the surface of a pathogen by binding to phagocytes via complement receptor 1 (CR1). Its degradation product, iC3b, can bind to CR3 on the surface of phagocytes. Activation of the phagocyte leads to ingestion of the C3b-coated or iC3b-coated pathogen.

Activation of the classic pathway by an antigen-antibody complex is initiated by the binding of C1q to the Fc portion of an antibody molecule in the immune complex. C1r autoactivates and cleaves C1s, which cleaves C4 and then C2, forming the C3 convertase, C4b2a. C4b2a is activated by the lectin pathway when lectins, such as mannose-binding protein, bind to sugar residues on the surface of pathogens, and mannose-binding protein–associated proteases cleave C4 and C2. The alternative pathway is always active at a low level and is amplified when active C3 binds to a surface that lacks regulatory proteins. C3b generated from C3 binds to factor B, which is cleaved by factor D to form the alternative pathway C3 convertase, C3bBb. Properdin binds to and stabilizes the C3 convertase (see Fig. 75-1).

The complement system is under tight regulation because it has potent inflammatory activity and the potential to cause significant damage to host cells. The complement cascade is inherently regulated by a short half-life of the sites on C4b and C3b that allow them to bind to cell surfaces and by instability of the C3 convertases, C4b2a and C3bBb. In addition, C1-inhibitor regulates the cascade at an early stage by blocking active sites on C1r, C1s, and the proteases associated with the lectin pathway. Factor I

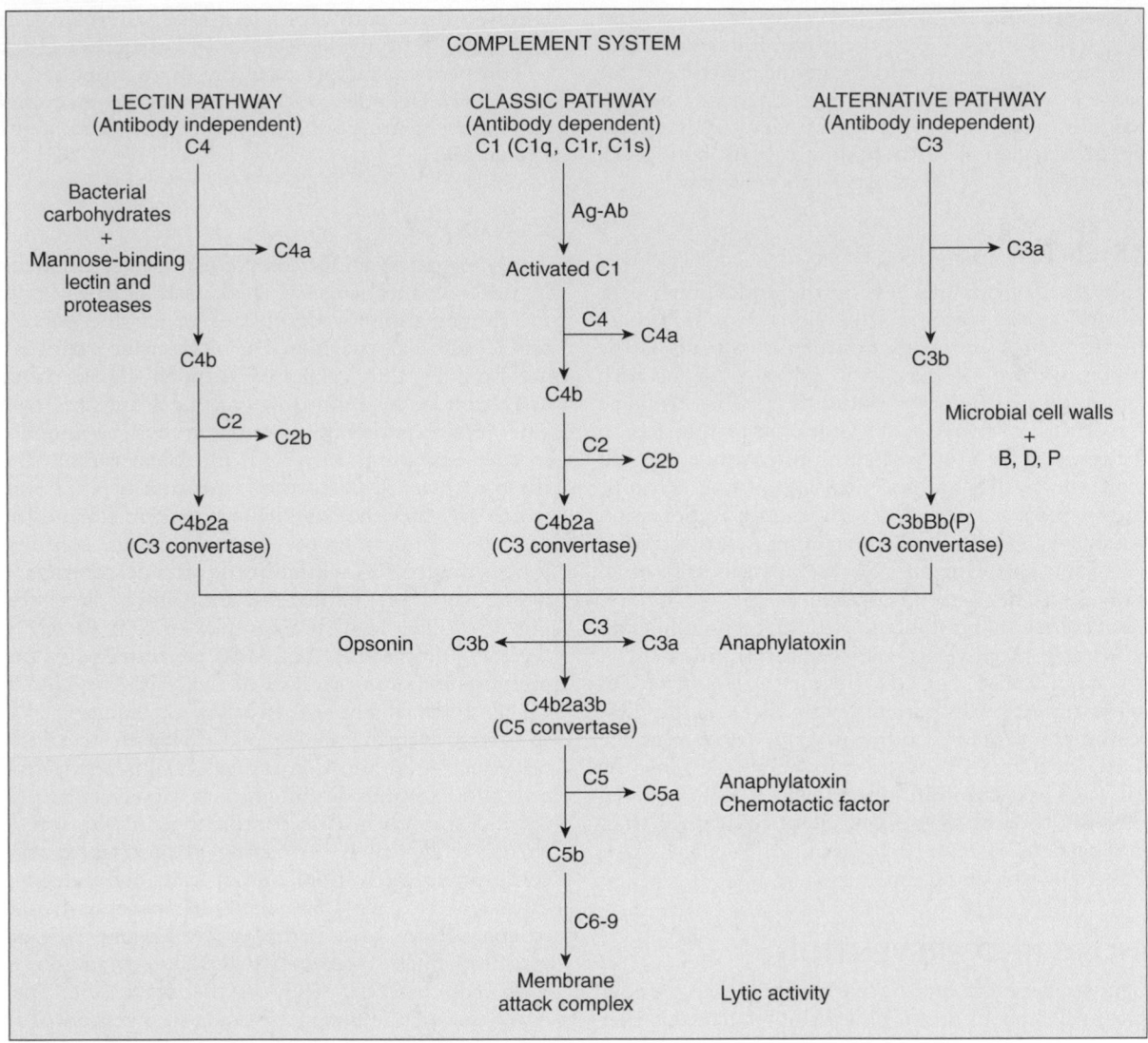

**FIGURE 75-1**

Complement component cascade involving the classic, alternate, and lectin pathways. The initiating events for the pathways differ, but result in production of C3 cleaving enzyme activity, which is the pivotal step as the three pathways converge to the terminal activation sequences. Ag-Ab, antigen-antibody complex; B, factor B; D, factor D (factor B clearing enzyme); P, properdin.

destabilizes C3 convertase complexes and degrades the active fragments. Other inhibitors include membrane proteins, such as decay accelerating factor, CR1, membrane cofactor protein, and plasma proteins such as C4b-binding protein and factor H. Formation of the MAC can be blocked by cell surface CD59, protein S, and other plasma proteins. Deficiency of any of these regulatory proteins can result in an inflammatory response, tissue damage, or excessive complement consumption.

Disorders of complement proteins can result from inherited deficiency or can be secondary to increased consumption. The consequences of decreased complement depend on the affected factor (see Table 75-1). **Deficiencies of early components** of the classic pathway (C1, C2, or C4) are not usually associated with severe infections, although patients with C2 deficiency may present with milder recurrent infections. Patients with C1, C2, or C4 deficiency are susceptible to autoimmune diseases, especially systemic lupus erythematosus. The exact mechanism of this susceptibility is not known but is thought to arise from the role of these early components in clearing immune complexes.

**Deficiency of properdin, C3, or the terminal components** predisposes patients to severe recurrent infections. Deficiency of C3, the major opsonin, due to a genetic defect or secondary to excessive consumption from a deficiency in factor H, factor I, or the presence of C3 nephritic factor predisposes patients to infections, especially with encapsulated organisms. Deficiency of one of the terminal components that compose the MAC predisposes patients to infection with *Neisseria meningitidis*. Complement deficiency may be found in 40% of patients presenting with recurrent neisserial infections. Deficiency of mannose-binding lectin also is associated with an increased frequency of bacterial infections, including sepsis.

Congenital deficiency of C1-inhibitor results in **hereditary angioedema**, characterized by recurrent episodes of nonpruritic angioedema lasting 48 to 72 hours, which occur spontaneously or after minor trauma, stress, or

## TABLE 75-1  Deficiency of Complement and Associated Disease

| Deficient Protein | Associated Disease |
| --- | --- |
| C1q, C1r | SLE, glomerulonephritis; occasional pneumococcal infection |
| C2 | SLE, arthritis, JRA, recurrent infections in some patients, rare glomerulonephritis |
| C3 | Recurrent infections, rare glomerulonephritis, or SLE |
| C4 | SLE-like disease, pyogenic infection |
| C5 | Recurrent meningococcal infections, rare glomerulonephritis, or SLE |
| C6 | Recurrent meningococcal, rare glomerulonephritis, or SLE |
| C7 | Recurrent meningococcal, Raynaud phenomenon |
| C8 | Recurrent infections |
| C9 | Occasional meningococcal infection, autoimmune disease in some patients |
| Properdin | Recurrent infections, meningococcal infection (often fatal) |
| Factor H | Glomerulonephritis, meningococcal infection |
| Factor I | Recurrent infections |
| C4-binding protein | Collagen vascular disease |
| C5a inhibitor | Familial Mediterranean fever |
| C3b receptor | SLE |
| C1 inhibitor | Hereditary angioedema |

JRA, juvenile rheumatoid arthritis; SLE, systemic lupus erythematosus.

anxiety. Angioedema can occur in any tissue. Abdominal edema can cause acute abdominal pain; edema of the upper airway can be life-threatening and may necessitate emergency tracheostomy. The disorder is inherited as an autosomal dominant disease and results from a heterozygous deficiency of C1-inhibitor leading to serum levels less than 30% of normal values. Some mutations (type II hereditary angioedema) result in normal or elevated antigenic levels of C1-inhibitor with defective function. An acquired form of angioedema results from autoantibodies to C1-inhibitor in lymphoid malignancies or autoimmune disorders but is uncommon in childhood. C1-inhibitor is a regulator of Hageman factor (clotting factor XIIa), clotting factor XIa, plasma kallikrein, and plasmin in addition to C1r and C1s. Lack of inhibition of the contact system, Hageman factor and plasma kallikrein, is responsible for the development of angioedema.

## LABORATORY STUDIES

The **CH$_{50}$ test** is a widely available test of classic complement pathway function based on an antibody-dependent hemolytic assay, which measures the serum dilution that results in lysis of 50% of sheep red blood cells. The CH$_{50}$ test depends on the function of all nine complement proteins, C1 through C9, and is the best screen for complement function. The **AP$_{50}$ test**, which measures complement activation using red blood cells from different species (e.g., rabbit) that can activate the alternative pathway, is less widely available than the CH$_{50}$ test. Abnormal results of both tests indicate a deficiency in a terminal component common to both pathways, whereas an abnormal result of one or the other test indicates a deficiency of an early component of the respective pathway. If the CH$_{50}$ or AP$_{50}$ levels are abnormal, individual components can be analyzed in specialized laboratories.

Determination of C1-inhibitor levels and function is needed to diagnose hereditary angioedema. Some functional tests miss rare mutations that allow C1-inhibitor to bind C1s, but not one or more of the other enzymes with which it interacts. Low C1-inhibitor levels or function results in chronically decreased C4 levels and decreased C2 levels during acute attacks. Low C1q levels are found in acquired C1-inhibitor deficiency, which distinguishes it from hereditary angioedema. Tests for autoantibodies to C1-inhibitor and C1q can be performed by enzyme-linked immunosorbent assay.

## TREATMENT

Specific treatment of complement deficiencies with component replacement is not available. Long, frequent courses of antibiotics constitute the primary therapy. Immunization of patients and close contacts with pneumococcal and meningococcal vaccines may be useful, but infections may still occur in immunized complement-deficient patients. Replacement of complement proteins by plasma transfusion has been used in some patients with C2 deficiency or factor H deficiency.

Patients with C1-inhibitor deficiency and frequent episodes of angioedema respond to prophylactic use of an oral attenuated androgen (**stanozolol** or **danazol**), which increases serum concentrations of C1-inhibitor. Adverse effects, including masculinization in females, growth arrest, and hepatitis, limit their use. Care must be taken in using plasma transfusions for angioedema. Prophylactic administration of fresh frozen plasma before surgery can prevent angioedema, but administration during an acute episode may exacerbate the episode. Angioedema of the airway can present as an acute emergency, necessitating tracheostomy because administration of epinephrine, antihistamines, or corticosteroids is ineffective in reversing this type of angioedema. Purified C1-inhibitor is now available and can be used prophylactically (before surgery) and during acute episodes of angioedema. Angiotensin-converting enzyme inhibitors, such as captopril, should be avoided in patients with C1-inhibitor deficiency because they can precipitate episodes of angioedema by inhibiting degradation of kinins that mediate edema formation. Novel therapeutic agents, including a kallikrein inhibitor and a bradykinin receptor 2 antagonist, are being investigated as potential therapy for hereditary angioedema.

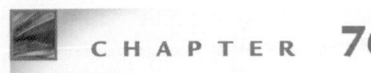

# CHAPTER 76

# Hematopoietic Stem Cell Transplantation

Hematopoietic stem cell transplantation (HSCT) can cure some patients with primary immunodeficiency disease (Table 76-1). It is not available to all patients, however. Use of HSCT is limited to immunodeficiency diseases with T-cell defects, some metabolic storage diseases (see Chapters 55 and 56), malignancies (see Chapter 154), aplastic anemia (see Chapter 150), and a few other disorders. The principle of HSCT is to replace a patient's defective bone marrow stem cells with normal stem cells.

Hematopoietic stem cells reside in the bone marrow and can be obtained from peripheral blood or cord blood. Peripheral blood does not contain a significant proportion of stem cells unless the donor's bone marrow is actively stimulated to generate stem cells. Cord blood is a good source of stem cells and is used for sibling and unrelated HSCT.

**Major histocompatibility complex (MHC) compatibility** is important in the choice of stem cell donor to avoid rejection of the donor cells by the host immune system and to prevent graft-versus-host disease (GVHD) from contaminating mature T cells. The donor stem cells give rise to T cells that develop in the host thymus and need to interact with donor and host antigen-presenting cells. Stem cells from a partially mismatched donor, such as a parent, can give rise to a functioning immune system because the patient shares at least half of the MHC molecules with the donor stem cells. Mature T cells need to be removed

### TABLE 76-1 Immunodeficiency Diseases Curable by Stem Cell Transplantation

Severe combined immunodeficiency (SCID)
  X-linked SCID ($\gamma_c$ deficiency)
  Jak 3 kinase deficiency
  ZAP 70 deficiency and other T-cell activation defects
  RAG1/RAG2 deficiency and other $T^- B^-$ SCID
  Omenn syndrome
  Adenosine deaminase deficiency
  Purine nucleoside phosphorylase deficiency
  Reticular dysgenesis
  Bare lymphocyte syndrome
Wiskott-Aldrich syndrome
X-linked hyper-IgM
X-linked lymphoproliferative syndrome
Cartilage hair hypoplasia
Autoimmune lymphoproliferative syndrome (Fas defect)
Severe congenital neutropenia
Shwachman-Diamond syndrome
Cyclic neutropenia
Chédiak-Higashi syndrome
Leukocyte adhesion deficiency type I
Familial hemophagocytic lymphohistiocytosis

from the bone marrow, however, before transplantation. The reduction in risk of **GVHD** outweighs the disadvantage of a prolonged time of 90 to 120 days before T cells develop in patients with severe combined immunodeficiency (SCID). Patients with other immunodeficiency diseases are at risk for developing **lymphoproliferative disease**, especially associated with Epstein-Barr virus, with T-cell–depleted stem cell transplantation, probably because of the delay in T-cell engraftment. Hematopoietic stem cells can be obtained from MHC-identical siblings (25% chance of a matched sibling), matched unrelated cord blood or bone marrow, or, for patients with SCID, haploidentical bone marrow from a parent (preferred) or a sibling.

MHC molecules are highly polymorphic; typing is performed at the DNA level rather than by serology. Bone marrow and cord blood registries are available worldwide. Searching and identifying a donor can be a lengthy process, especially for some underrepresented ethnic backgrounds. Finding a suitable cord blood donor is faster because the cord blood already has been obtained and stored, whereas bone marrow donors have to be identified, located, and tested. A matched sibling, if available, is the preferred source of hematopoietic stem cells.

Patients with SCID are ideal candidates for HSCT, which is the only option for treatment of SCID at this time. Patients are unlikely to survive beyond 1 to 2 years of age without transplantation, and they have no T-cell function to reject donor cells. Patients with SCID may not need to undergo preconditioning with chemotherapy or irradiation before transplantation. The development of transplantation using T-cell–depleted, haploidentical bone marrow from a parent for SCID has provided almost every patient with SCID a potential donor. The mother is the preferred source for haploidentical bone marrow, if she is able to donate, because some transfer of maternal T cells can occur during pregnancy and these maternal T cells can reject cells obtained from the father. The survival rate after HSCT for SCID is 84% with MHC-identical and 61% with haploidentical bone marrow transplantation. The earlier the patient is transplanted, the better the outcome. Because the outcome of stem cell transplantation as soon after birth as possible is excellent, the risks of in utero transplantation and the inability to observe the fetus for signs of GVHD make it difficult to justify this type of transplantation. In addition, the development of newborn screening for SCID allows initiation of stem cell transplantation as early as possible, providing the best opportunity for a cure.

The decision to treat other patients with primary immunodeficiency diseases is more difficult because HSCT is not always successful. Patients with some, albeit decreased, T-cell function require preconditioning, with the risks that it entails. It is difficult to predict the prognosis of a particular patient because of the variability in clinical course of most primary immunodeficiency diseases, although there is only a small chance of reaching adulthood. The availability of a matched related sibling favors the decision to perform HSCT. Disorders of B cells have not been treated with HSCT because, in many cases, donor B cells do not engraft and patients usually do well with IVIG. If HSCT techniques improve to allow for better B-cell engraftment and the risks of GVHD and preconditioning are reduced, however, treatment of agammaglobulinemia and other immune system diseases with HSCT may be possible.

## COMPLICATIONS

**Rejection** of the grafted cells is the first potential complication of HSCT and depends on the immunocompetence of the patient, the degree of MHC incompatibility, and the number of cells administered. Preconditioning with myeloablative drugs, such as busulfan and cyclophosphamide, can prevent graft rejection but may be complicated by pulmonary toxicity and by veno-occlusive disease of the liver, which results from damage to the hepatic vascular endothelium and can be fatal. Myeloablation results in anemia, leukopenia, and thrombocytopenia, making patients susceptible to infection and bleeding disorders. Neutropenic precautions should be maintained and patients supported with red blood cell and platelet transfusions until the red blood cell, platelet, and neutrophil lineages engraft. Reduced intensity preconditioning has been used recently to prevent graft rejection and decrease the adverse effects of myeloablation. **Lymphoproliferative** disease can develop after T-cell–depleted bone marrow transplantation.

HSCT, in contrast to solid organ transplantation, can be complicated by rejection of the host by mature T cells from the donor. **GVHD** can arise from an MHC-mismatched transplantation or from mismatch in minor histocompatibility antigens that are not tested for before transplantation.

T-cell depletion of haploidentical bone marrow reduces the risk of GVHD. Patients with SCID transplanted with T-cell–depleted haploidentical bone marrow do not usually develop severe GVHD. Acute GVHD begins 6 or more days after transplantation and can result from transfusion of nonirradiated blood products in patients with no T-cell function. **Acute GVHD** presents with fever, skin rash, and severe diarrhea. Patients develop a high, unrelenting fever; a morbilliform maculopapular erythematous rash that is painful and pruritic; hepatosplenomegaly and abnormal liver function tests; and nausea, vomiting, abdominal pain, and watery diarrhea. Acute GVHD is staged from grade 1 to 4 depending on the degree of skin, fever, gastrointestinal, and liver involvement. **Chronic GVHD** results from acute GVHD lasting longer than 100 days and can develop without acute GVHD or after acute GVHD has resolved. Chronic GVHD is characterized by skin lesions (hyperkeratosis, reticular hyperpigmentation, fibrosis, and atrophy with ulceration), limitation of joint movement, interstitial pneumonitis, and immune dysregulation with autoantibody and immune complex formation.

HSCT can be used for any disorder of hematopoiesis such as aplastic anemia, sickle cell disease, and other hemoglobinopathies. It is also used in treatment of malignancy such as leukemia, lymphoma, and solid tumors. In some cases of solid tumor therapy, autologous bone marrow is harvested before high-dose chemotherapy, and then reinfused into the patient to rescue the hematopoietic system.

 **SUGGESTED READING**

Chatila TA, Li N, Garcia-Lloret M, et al: T-cell effector pathways in allergic diseases: transcriptional mechanisms and therapeutic targets, *J Allergy Clin Immunol* 121:812–823, 2008.

Geha RS, Notarangelo LD, Casanova JL, et al: Primary immunodeficiency diseases: an update from the International Union of Immunological Societies Primary Immunodeficiency Diseases Classification Committee, *J Allergy Clin Immunol* 120:776–794, 2007.

Notarangelo LD, Forino C, Mazzolari E: Stem cell transplantation in primary immunodeficiencies, *Curr Opin Allergy Clin Immunol* 6:443–448, 2006.

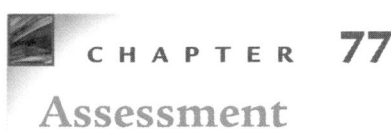

# CHAPTER 77

# Assessment

**Atopy** is a result of a complex interaction between multiple genes and environmental factors. It implies specific IgE-mediated diseases, including allergic rhinitis, asthma, and atopic dermatitis. An **allergen** is an antigen that triggers an IgE response in genetically predisposed individuals.

**Hypersensitivity** disorders of the immune system are classified into four groups based on the mechanism that leads to tissue inflammation (Table 77-1). **Type I reactions** are triggered by the binding of antigen to high-affinity IgE receptors on the surface of tissue mast cells, circulating basophils, or both, causing the release of preformed chemical mediators, such as histamine and tryptase, and newly generated mediators, such as leukotrienes, prostaglandins, and platelet-activating factor, These mediators contribute to the development of allergic symptoms, with anaphylaxis as the most profound symptom. Several hours after the initial response, a **late-phase reaction** may develop with an influx of other inflammatory cells such as basophils, eosinophils, monocytes, lymphocytes, and neutrophils, and their inflammatory mediators. Recruitment of these cells leads to more persistent and chronic symptoms.

**Type II (antibody cytotoxicity) reactions** involve IgM, IgG, or IgA antibodies binding to the cell surface and activating the entire complement pathway resulting in lysis of the cell or release of anaphylatoxins, such as C3a, C4a, and C5a (see Chapter 75). These anaphylatoxins trigger mast cell degranulation, resulting in inflammatory mediator release. The target can be cell surface membrane antigens, such as red blood cells (hemolytic anemia); platelet cell surface molecules (thrombocytopenia); basement membrane molecules in the kidney (Goodpasture syndrome); the alpha chain of the acetylcholine receptor at the neuromuscular junction (myasthenia gravis); and thyroid-stimulating hormone receptor on thyroid cells (Graves' disease).

**Type III (immune complex) reactions** involve the formation of antigen-antibody or immune complexes that enter into the circulation and are deposited in tissues such as blood vessels and filtering organs (liver, spleen, kidney). These complexes initiate tissue injury by activating the complement cascade and recruiting neutrophils that release their toxic mediators. Local reactions caused by the injection of antigen into tissue are called **Arthus reactions**. Administration of large amounts of antigen leads to **serum sickness**, a classic example of a type III reaction. Other type III–mediated reactions include hypersensitivity pneumonitis and some vasculitic syndromes, such as Henoch-Schönlein purpura.

**Type IV (cellular immune–mediated or delayed-hypersensitivity) reactions** involve recognition of antigen by sensitized T cells. Antigen-presenting cells form peptides that are expressed on the cell surface in association with major histocompatibility complex class II molecules. Memory T cells recognize the antigen peptide/major histocompatibility complex class II complexes. Cytokines, such as interferon-$\gamma$, tumor necrosis factor-$\alpha$, and granulocyte-macrophage colony-stimulating factor, are secreted from this interaction, which activates and attracts tissue macrophages. **Contact allergies** (nickel, poison ivy, topical medications) and immunity to tuberculosis are type IV reactions.

## HISTORY

A family history of allergic disease is often present in affected patients. Multiple genes predispose to atopy. If one parent has allergies, the risk that a child will develop allergic disease is 25%. If both parents have allergies, the risk increases to 50% to 70%. Similar allergic diseases tend to occur in families.

## PHYSICAL EXAMINATION

Children with allergic rhinitis exhibit frequent nasal itching and rubbing of the nose with the palm of the hand, the **allergic salute**, which can lead to a transverse nasal crease found across the lower bridge of the nose. **Allergic shiners**, blue-gray to purple discoloration below the lower eyelids that is attributed to venous congestion, are often present in children along with swollen eyelids or conjunctival injection. Dermatologic findings of atopy include hyperlinearity of the palms and soles, white dermatographism, pityriasis alba, prominent creases under the lower eyelids (**Dennie-Morgan folds** or **Dennie lines**), and **keratosis pilaris** (asymptomatic horny follicular papules on the extensor surfaces of the arms).

**TABLE 77-1 Gell and Coombs Classification of Hypersensitivity Disorders**

| Type | Interval Between Exposure and Reaction | Effector Cell | Target or Antigen | Examples of Mediators | Examples |
|---|---|---|---|---|---|
| I—Anaphylactic Immediate Late phase | <30 min 2–12 hr | IgE | Pollens, food, venom, drugs | Histamine, tryptase, leukotrienes, prostaglandins, platelet-activating factor | Anaphylaxis, urticaria, allergic rhinitis, allergic asthma |
| II—Cytotoxic antibody | Variable (minutes to hours) | IgG, IgM, IgA | Red blood cells, platelets | Complement | Rh hemolytic anemia, thrombocytopenia, hemolysis (quinidine), Goodpasture syndrome |
| III—Immune complex reactions | 1–3 weeks after drug exposure | Antigen-antibody/ aggregates | Blood vessels, liver, spleen, kidney, lung | Complement, anaphylatoxin | Serum sickness (cefaclor), hypersensitivity pneumonitis |
| IV—Delayed type | 2–7 days after drug exposure | Lymphocytes | *Mycobacterium tuberculosis,* chemicals | Cytokines (IFN-γ, TNF-α, GM-CSF) | TB skin test reactions, contact dermatitis (neomycin), graft-versus-host disease |

CSF, cerebrospinal fluid; GM-CSF, granulocyte-macrophage colony-stimulating factor; IFN-γ, interferon-γ; TB, tuberculosis; TNF-α, tumor necrosis factor-α.

## COMMON MANIFESTATIONS

Cutaneous manifestations are most common and range from generalized **xerosis** (dry skin) to urticaria to the pruritic, erythematous papules and vesicles of atopic dermatitis. There may be involvement of the upper respiratory tract with allergic rhinitis and the lower respiratory tract with asthma. Allergic disease may involve only the skin or the nose, eyes, lungs, and gastrointestinal tract alone or in combination. It is distinguished by environmental exposure to an inciting trigger and usually a history of previous similar disease or development of symptoms after a suspected trigger. Many patients have more than one allergic symptom.

## INITIAL DIAGNOSTIC EVALUATION

Diagnosis begins with a thorough history with description of all symptoms, exposure to common allergens, and responses to previous therapies. In vivo skin testing and in vitro serum testing are crucial to accurate diagnosis.

## SCREENING TESTS

Atopy is characterized by elevated levels of IgE (Table 77-2) and **eosinophilia** (3% to 10% of white blood cells or an absolute eosinophil count of >250 eosinophils/mm³) with a predominance of Th2 cytokines, including interleukin (IL)-4, IL-5, and IL-13. Extreme eosinophilia suggests a non-allergic disorder such as infections with tissue-invasive parasites, drug reactions, or malignancies (Table 77-3). A classic example of a type IV reaction is the tuberculin skin test. A small amount of purified protein derivative from *Mycobacterium tuberculosis* is injected intradermally (see Chapter 124). In a previously sensitized individual,

a type IV inflammatory reaction develops over the next 24 to 72 hours.

There are two methods for identifying allergen-specific IgE: in vivo skin testing and in vitro serum testing (Table 77-4). **In vivo skin testing** introduces allergen into the skin via a prick/puncture or intradermal injection. The allergen diffuses through the skin to interact with IgE that is bound to mast cells. Cross-linking of IgE causes mast cell degranulation, which results in histamine release; this prompts the development of a **central wheal and erythematous flare**. The wheal and flare are measured 15 to 20 minutes after the allergen has been placed. Properly performed skin tests are the best available method for detecting the presence of allergen-specific IgE.

**In vitro serum testing,** such as the **radioallergosorbent test (RAST)** and enzyme-linked immunosorbent assay, measures levels of antigen-specific IgE. The **CAP-RAST** method uses a newer type of solid phase and shows higher sensitivity, specificity, and reproducibility. These tests are

**TABLE 77-2 Disorders Associated with Elevated Serum Immunoglobulin E**

Allergic disease
Atopic dermatitis (eczema)
Tissue-invasive helminthic infections
Hyperimmunoglobulin-E syndrome
Allergic bronchopulmonary aspergillosis
Wiskott-Aldrich syndrome
Bone marrow transplantation
Hodgkin disease
Bullous pemphigoid
Idiopathic nephrotic syndrome

| TABLE 77-3 Disorders Associated with Eosinophilia |
|---|
| **ALLERGIC DISEASE** |
| Allergic rhinitis |
| Atopic dermatitis |
| Asthma |
| **GASTROINTESTINAL** |
| Eosinophilic gastroenteritis |
| Allergic colitis |
| Inflammatory bowel disease |
| **INFECTIOUS** |
| Tissue-invasive helminthic infections |
| **NEOPLASTIC** |
| Eosinophilic leukemia |
| Hodgkin disease |
| **RESPIRATORY** |
| Eosinophilic pneumonia |
| Allergic bronchopulmonary aspergillosis |
| **SYSTEMIC** |
| Idiopathic hypereosinophilic syndrome |
| Mastocytosis |
| **IATROGENIC** |
| Drug induced |

indicated for patients who have dermatographism or extensive dermatitis; who cannot discontinue medications, such as antihistamines, that interfere with test results; who are very allergic by history, where anaphylaxis is a possible risk; or who are noncompliant for skin testing. The presence of specific IgE antibodies alone is not sufficient for the diagnosis of allergic diseases. Diagnosis must be based on the physician's assessment of the entire clinical picture, including the history and physical examination, the presence of specific IgE antibodies, and the correlation of symptoms to IgE-mediated inflammation.

| TABLE 77-4 Comparison of In Vivo Skin Tests and In Vitro Serum IgE Antibody Immunoassay in Allergic Diagnosis | |
|---|---|
| **In Vivo—Skin Test** | **In Vitro—Serum Immunoassay** |
| Less expensive | No patient risk |
| Greater sensitivity | Patient/physician convenience |
| Wide allergen selection | Not suppressed by antihistamines |
| Results available immediately | Preferable to skin testing for Dermatographism Widespread dermatitis Uncooperative children |

From Skoner DP: Allergic rhinitis: definition, epidemiology, pathophysiology, detection, and diagnosis. *J Allergy Clin Immunol* 108, S2–S8, 2001.

## DIAGNOSTIC IMAGING

Diagnostic imaging has a limited role in the evaluation of allergic disease. Chest radiography is helpful with the differential diagnosis of asthma. Sinus radiography and computed tomography may be useful, but when these images are abnormal, they do not distinguish allergic disease from nonallergic disease.

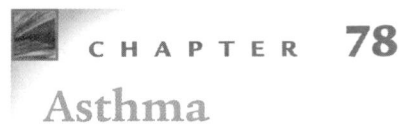

CHAPTER **78**

# Asthma

## ETIOLOGY

Inflammatory cells (mast cells, eosinophils, T lymphocytes, neutrophils), chemical mediators (histamine, leukotrienes, platelet-activating factor, bradykinin), and chemotactic factors (cytokines, eotaxin) mediate the underlying inflammation found in asthmatic airways. Inflammation contributes to **airway hyperresponsiveness**, which is the tendency for the airways to constrict in response to allergens, irritants, viral infections, and exercise. It also results in edema, increased mucus production in the lungs, influx of inflammatory cells into the airway, and epithelial cell denudation. Chronic inflammation can lead to **airway remodeling**, which results from a proliferation of extracellular matrix proteins and vascular hyperplasia and may lead to irreversible structural changes and a progressive loss of pulmonary function.

## EPIDEMIOLOGY

Asthma is the most common chronic disease of childhood in industrialized countries, affecting nearly 6 million children younger than 18 years of age in the United States. The 2003 National Health Interview Survey of the Centers for Disease Control and Prevention yielded a lifetime asthma prevalence of 12.5% and current asthma prevalence of 8.5% in children younger than 18 years of age. Between 1996 and 2004, asthma attack rates and asthma prevalence have stabilized when compared with the previous 12 months.

## CLINICAL MANIFESTATIONS

Children with asthma have symptoms of coughing, wheezing, shortness of breath or rapid breathing, and chest tightness. The history should elicit the frequency, severity, and factors that worsen the child's symptoms. Exacerbating factors include viral infections, exposure to allergens and irritants (smoke, strong odors, fumes), exercise, emotions, and change in weather/humidity. Nighttime symptoms are common. Rhinosinusitis, gastroesophageal reflux, and sensitivity to nonsteroidal anti-inflammatory drugs (especially aspirin) can aggravate asthma. Treatment of these conditions may lessen the frequency and severity of the asthma. Obtaining a family history of allergy and asthma is useful.

During acute episodes, the physical examination may reveal tachypnea, tachycardia, cough, wheezing, and a prolonged expiratory phase. Physical findings may be subtle. Classic wheezing may not be prominent if there is minimal air movement. As the attack progresses, cyanosis, diminished air movement, retractions, agitation, inability to speak, tripod sitting position, diaphoresis, and pulsus paradoxus (decrease in blood pressure with inspiration of >15 mm Hg) may be observed. Physical examination may show evidence of other atopic diseases such as eczema or allergic rhinitis.

## LABORATORY AND IMAGING STUDIES

Objective measurements of pulmonary function (**spirometry**) help establish the diagnosis and treatment of asthma. Spirometry is used to monitor response to treatment, assess degree of reversibility with therapeutic intervention, and measure the severity of an asthma exacerbation. Generally, children older than 5 years of age can perform spirometry maneuvers. Spirometry is preferred to peak flow measures in the diagnosis of asthma because of the variability in predicted peak flow reference values. For younger children who cannot perform spirometry maneuver or peak flow, a therapeutic trial of controller medications helps in the diagnosis of asthma.

**Allergy skin testing** should be included in the evaluation of all children with persistent asthma but not during an exacerbation of wheezing. An allergist offers the special skill of administering and interpreting skin tests to determine immediate hypersensitivity to **aeroallergens** (airborne allergens such as tree and grass pollens, and dust). Positive skin test results correlate strongly with bronchial allergen provocative challenges. In vitro serum tests, such as **radioallergosorbent test (RAST)** and enzyme-linked immunosorbent assay, are generally less sensitive in defining clinically pertinent allergens, are more expensive, and require several days for results compared with several minutes for skin testing (see Table 77-4).

A **chest radiograph** should be performed with the first episode of asthma or with recurrent episodes of undiagnosed cough or wheeze or both to exclude anatomic abnormalities. Repeat chest radiographs are not needed with new episodes unless there is fever, which suggests pneumonia, or localized findings on physical examination.

Two novel forms of monitoring asthma and airway inflammation directly include exhaled **nitric oxide analysis** and quantitative analysis of expectorated sputum for eosinophilia. Currently, both are used mainly in research settings.

## DIFFERENTIAL DIAGNOSIS

Many childhood conditions can cause wheezing and coughing of asthma (Table 78-1) but not all cough and wheeze is asthma. Misdiagnosis delays correcting the underlying cause and exposes children to inappropriate asthma therapy (Table 78-2).

**Allergic bronchopulmonary aspergillosis** is a hypersensitivity type of reaction to antigens of the mold *Aspergillus fumigatus*. It occurs primarily in patients with steroid-dependent asthma and in children with cystic fibrosis.

## TREATMENT

Optimal medical treatment of asthma includes several key components: environmental control; pharmacologic therapy; and patient education, including attainment of self-management skills. Because many children with asthma have coexisting allergies, steps to minimize allergen exposure should be taken (Table 78-3). For all children with asthma, exposures to tobacco and wood smoke and to

---

**TABLE 78-1  Differential Diagnosis of Cough and Wheeze in Infants and Children**

| Upper Respiratory Tract | Middle Respiratory Tract | Lower Respiratory Tract |
|---|---|---|
| Allergic rhinitis | Bronchial stenosis | Asthma |
| Adenoid/tonsillar hypertrophy | Enlarged lymph nodes | Bronchiectasis |
| Foreign body | Epiglottitis | Bronchopulmonary dysplasia |
| Infectious rhinitis | Foreign body | *Chlamydia trachomatis* |
| Sinusitis | Laryngeal webs | Chronic aspiration |
| | Laryngomalacia | Cystic fibrosis |
| | Laryngotracheobronchitis | Foreign body |
| | Mediastinal lymphadenopathy | Gastroesophageal reflux |
| | Pertussis | Hyperventilation syndrome |
| | Toxic inhalation | Obliterative bronchiolitis |
| | Tracheoesophageal fistula | Pulmonary hemosiderosis |
| | Tracheal stenosis | Toxic inhalation, including smoke |
| | Tracheomalacia | Tumor |
| | Tumor | Viral bronchiolitis |
| | Vascular rings | |
| | Vocal cord dysfunction | |

From Lemanske RF Jr, Green CG: Asthma in infancy and childhood. In Middleton E Jr, Reed CE, Ellis EF, et al, editors: Allergy: Principles and Practice, 5th ed, St Louis, 1998, *Mosby–Year Book*, p 878.

### TABLE 78-2 Mnemonic of Causes of Cough in the First Months of Life

**C**—Cystic fibrosis
**R**—Respiratory tract infections
**A**—Aspiration (swallowing dysfunction, gastroesophageal reflux, tracheoesophageal fistula, foreign body)
**D**—Dyskinetic cilia
**L**—Lung and airway malformations (laryngeal webs, laryngotracheomalacia, tracheal stenosis, vascular rings and slings)
**E**—Edema (heart failure, congenital heart disease)

From Schidlow DV: Cough. In Schidlow DV, Smith DS, editors: A Practical Guide to Pediatric Disease, Philadelphia, 1994, *Hanley & Belfus.*

persons with viral infections should be minimized. Asthma medications can be divided into long-term control medications and quick-relief medications.

## Long-Term Control Medications

### Inhaled Corticosteroids

Inhaled corticosteroids are the most effective anti-inflammatory medications for the treatment of chronic, persistent asthma and are the preferred therapy when initiating long-term control therapy. Early intervention with inhaled corticosteroids reduces morbidity but does not alter the natural history of asthma. Regular use reduces airway hyperreactivity, the need for rescue bronchodilator therapy, risk of hospitalization, and risk of death from asthma. Inhaled corticosteroids are available as an inhalation aerosol, dry powder inhaler (DPI), and nebulizer solution.

The potential risks of inhaled corticosteroids are favorably balanced with their benefits. A reduction in growth velocity may occur with poorly controlled asthma or inhaled corticosteroids use. Low-to-medium dose inhaled corticosteroids may decrease growth velocity, although these effects are small (approximately 1 cm in the first year of treatment), generally not progressive, and may be reversible. Potential growth suppression should be monitored by regularly scheduled height measurements. Inhaled corticosteroids do not have clinically significant adverse effects on hypothalamic-pituitary-adrenal axis function, glucose metabolism, or subcapsular cataracts or glaucoma when used at low-to-medium doses in children. Rinsing the mouth after inhalation and using spacers help lessen the local adverse effects of dysphonia and candidiasis and decrease systemic absorption from the gastrointestinal tract. Inhaled corticosteroids should be titrated to the lowest dose needed to maintain control of a child's asthma. For children with severe asthma, higher dose inhaled corticosteroids may be needed to minimize the oral corticosteroid dose.

### TABLE 78-3 Controlling Factors Contributing to Asthma Severity

| Major Indoor Triggers for Asthma | Suggestions for Reducing Exposure |
|---|---|
| Viral upper respiratory tract (RSV, influenza virus) | Limit exposure to viral infections (day care with fewer children) |
| | Annual influenza immunization for children with persistent asthma |
| Tobacco smoke, wood smoke | No smoking around the child or in child's home |
| | Help parents and caregivers quit smoking |
| | Eliminate use of wood stoves and fireplaces |
| Dust mites | Essential actions |
| |    Encase pillow, mattress, and box spring in allergen-impermeable encasement |
| |    Wash bedding in hot water weekly |
| | Desirable actions |
| |    Avoid sleeping or lying on upholstered furniture |
| |    Minimize number of stuffed toys in child's bedroom |
| |    Reduce indoor humidity to <50% |
| |    If possible, remove carpets from bedroom and play areas; if not possible, vacuum frequently |
| Animal dander | Remove the pet from the home or keep outdoors; if removal is not acceptable |
| |    Keep pet out of bedroom |
| |    Use a filter on air ducts in child's room |
| |    Wash pet weekly (the evidence to support this has not been firmly established) |
| Cockroach allergens | Do not leave food or garbage exposed |
| | Use boric acid traps |
| | Reduce indoor humidity to <50% |
| | Fix leaky faucets, pipes |
| Indoor mold | Avoid vaporizers |
| | Reduce indoor humidity to <50% |
| | Fix leaky faucets, pipes |

RSV, respiratory syncytial virus.
From American Academy of Allergy, Asthma and Immunology: Pediatric asthma: promoting best practice. Milwaukee, Wisconsin, 1999, *American Academy of Allergy, Asthma, and Immunology*, p 50.

## Leukotriene Modifiers

Leukotriene modifiers are oral, daily-use, asthma medications. Leukotrienes, synthesized via the arachidonic acid metabolism cascade, are potent mediators of inflammation and smooth muscle bronchoconstriction. Leukotriene modifiers inhibit these biologic effects in the airway. Two classes of leukotriene modifiers include cysteinyl leukotriene receptor antagonists (zafirlukast and montelukast) and leukotriene synthesis inhibitors (zileuton). The leukotriene receptor antagonists have much wider appeal than zileuton. Zafirlukast is approved for children older than 5 years of age and is given twice daily. Montelukast is dosed once daily at night as 4-mg granules or chewable tablets for children 6 months to 5 years, 5-mg chewable tablets for children 6 to 14 years, and 10-mg tablets for adolescents 15 years of age or older. Pediatric studies show the usefulness of leukotriene modifiers in mild asthma and the attenuation of exercise-induced bronchoconstriction. These agents may be helpful as steroid-sparing agents in patients with asthma that is more difficult to control.

## Long-Acting $\beta_2$-Agonists

Long-acting $\beta_2$-agonists, formoterol and salmeterol, have twice-daily dosing and relax airway smooth muscle for 12 hours, but they do not have any significant anti-inflammatory effects. Adding a long-acting bronchodilator to inhaled corticosteroid therapy is more beneficial than doubling the dose of inhaled corticosteroids. Formoterol, available in the DPI form, is approved for use in children older than 5 years of age for maintenance asthma therapy and for prevention of exercise-induced asthma. Formoterol has a rapid onset of action similar to albuterol (15 minutes), whereas salmeterol has onset within 30 minutes. Salmeterol is available in the DPI form and is approved for children 4 years of age or older. A budesonide and formoterol combination product (Symbicort) is available as an inhalation aerosol in two doses, varying by the corticosteroid dosage (80 µg or 160 µg). Each of these strengths contains 4.5 µg of formoterol.

A fluticasone/salmeterol combination product is available either as a DPI (Advair Diskus) or as an inhalation aerosol (Advair HFA). The Advair Diskus is available as 100/50, 250/50, or 500/50, with the dose of corticosteroid listed first (µg) and the dose of salmeterol listed second (µg). The dosing of this medication is usually one puff twice daily. The Advair HFA is available as 45/21, 115/21, or 231/21 dosages and is administered as two inhalations twice daily. Because combination agents administer two medications simultaneously, compliance is generally improved.

## Theophylline

Theophylline was more widely used previously, but because current management is aimed at inflammatory control, its popularity has declined. It is mildly to moderately effective as a bronchodilator and is considered an alternative, add-on treatment to low- and medium-dose inhaled corticosteroids. Theophylline is available in syrup, tablet, and capsule formulations. Serum levels must be monitored and maintained generally between 5 and 15 µg/mL. Levels can be affected by febrile illnesses; diet; and medications, such as macrolide antibiotics, cimetidine, and oral antifungal agents. Adverse effects associated with elevated theophylline levels include nausea, insomnia, headaches, hyperreactivity, and seizures.

## Omalizumab

Omalizumab (Xolair) is a humanized anti-IgE monoclonal antibody that prevents binding of IgE to high-affinity receptors on basophils and mast cells. It is approved for moderate to severe allergic asthma in children 12 years of age and older. Xolair is delivered by subcutaneous injection every 2 to 4 weeks, depending on body weight and pretreatment serum IgE level.

## Quick-Relief Medications

### Short-Acting $\beta_2$-Agonists

Short-acting $\beta_2$-agonists, such as albuterol, levalbuterol, and pirbuterol, are effective bronchodilators that exert their effect by relaxing bronchial smooth muscle within 5 to 10 minutes of administration. They last for 4 to 6 hours. Generally, a short-acting $\beta_2$-agonist is prescribed for acute symptoms and as prophylaxis before allergen exposure and exercise. The inhaled route is preferred because adverse effects—tremor, prolonged tachycardia, and irritability—are fewer. **Overuse** of $\beta_2$-agonists implies inadequate control and that a change in medications may be warranted. The definition of "overuse" depends on the severity of the child's asthma; use of more than one metered dose inhaler canister per month or more than eight puffs per day suggests poor control.

### Anticholinergic Agent

Ipratropium bromide is an anticholinergic bronchodilator that relieves bronchoconstriction, decreases mucus hypersecretion, and counteracts cough-receptor irritability by binding acetylcholine at the muscarinic receptors found in bronchial smooth muscle. It seems to have an additive effect with $\beta_2$-agonists when used for acute asthma exacerbations. Long-term use of anticholinergic medications is not supported by the literature.

### Oral Corticosteroids

Short bursts of oral corticosteroids (3 to 10 days) are administered to children with acute exacerbations. The initial starting dose is 1 to 2 mg/kg/day of prednisone followed by 1 mg/kg/day over the next 2 to 5 days. Oral corticosteroids are available in various liquid or tablet formulations. Prolonged use of oral corticosteroids can result in systemic adverse effects such as hypothalamic-pituitary-adrenal suppression, cushingoid features, weight gain, hypertension, diabetes, cataracts, glaucoma, osteoporosis, and growth suppression. Children with severe asthma may require oral corticosteroids over extended periods. The dose should be tapered as soon as possible to the minimum effective dose, preferably administered on alternate days.

## Approach to Therapy

Current therapy is based on the concept that chronic inflammation is a fundamental feature of asthma and that the processes underlying asthma can vary in intensity over time, requiring treatment to be adjusted accordingly. Based on the 2007 National Asthma Education and Prevention Program guidelines, classification of asthma severity is emphasized for initiation of therapy in patients not currently receiving controller medications. Assessing control is emphasized for monitoring and adjusting therapy. A stepwise approach is used for management of infants, young children 0 to 4 years, children 5 to 11 years (Fig. 78-1), youths 12 years or older, and adults (Fig. 78-2). Medication type, amount, and scheduling are determined by the level of asthma severity or asthma control. Therapy is then increased (**stepped up**) as necessary and decreased (**stepped down**) when possible. A short-acting bronchodilator should be available for all children with asthma. A child with intermittent asthma has asthma symptoms less than two times per week. To determine if a child is having more persistent asthma, the **rule of twos** is helpful: daytime symptoms occurring two or more times per week or nighttime awakening two or more times per month implies a need for daily anti-inflammatory medication.

Inhaled corticosteroids are the preferred initial long-term control therapy for children of all ages (Fig. 78-3). For infants and young children 0 to 4 years of age, daily long-term control therapy is recommended for those who had four or more episodes of wheezing in the previous year that lasted more than 1 day and affected sleep and who have a positive asthma predictive index. For children older than 5 years of age with moderate persistent asthma, combining long-acting bronchodilators with low-to-medium doses of inhaled corticosteroids improves lung function and reduces rescue medication use. For children with severe persistent asthma, a high-dose inhaled corticosteroid and a long-acting bronchodilator are the preferred therapy. The guidelines also recommend that treatment be reevaluated within 2 to 6 weeks of initiating therapy. Once the patient's asthma is under control, control should be assessed on an ongoing basis every 1 to 6 months. The asthma should be well controlled for at least 3 months before stepping down therapy. Note that asthma management guidelines are based on review of the published evidence, not solely on the age recommendations and dosages approved by the U.S. Food and Drug Administration.

## COMPLICATIONS

Most asthma exacerbations can be managed at home successfully. **Status asthmaticus** is an acute exacerbation of asthma that does not respond adequately to therapeutic measures and may require hospitalization. Exacerbations may progress over several days or occur suddenly and can range in severity from mild to life-threatening. Significant respiratory distress, dyspnea, wheezing, cough, and a decrease in peak expiratory flow rates characterize deterioration in asthma control. During severe episodes of wheezing, pulse oximetry is helpful in monitoring oxygenation. In status asthmaticus, arterial blood gases may be necessary for measurement of ventilation. As airway obstruction worsens and chest compliance decreases, carbon dioxide retention can occur. In the face of tachypnea, a *normal* $P_{CO_2}$ (40 mm Hg) indicates impending respiratory arrest.

First-line management of asthma exacerbations includes supplemental oxygen, repetitive or continuous administration of short-acting bronchodilators, and oral or intravenous corticosteroids (Fig. 78-4). Administration of anticholinergic agents (ipratropium) with bronchodilators decreases rates of hospitalization and duration of time in the emergency department. Early administration of oral corticosteroids is important in treating the underlying inflammation. The use of intravenous magnesium sulfate is gaining use in the emergency department in children with severe exacerbations and in children with moderate exacerbations who have clinical deterioration despite treatment with $\beta_2$-agonists, ipratropium, and systemic glucocorticoids. The typical dose is 25 to 75 mg/kg (maximum 2.0 g) intravenously administered over 20 minutes. Epinephrine (intramuscular) or terbutaline (subcutaneous) is rarely used except when severe asthma is associated with anaphylaxis or unresponsive to continuous administration of short-acting bronchodilators.

## PROGNOSIS

For some children, symptoms of wheezing with respiratory infections subside in the preschool years, whereas other children have more persistent asthma symptoms. Prognostic indicators for children younger than 3 years of age who are at risk for asthma include eczema; parental asthma; or two of the following: allergic rhinitis, wheezing with a cold, or eosinophilia of greater than 4%. The strongest predictor for wheezing continuing into persistent asthma is atopy (Table 78-4).

## PREVENTION

Education plays an important role in helping patients and their families adhere to the prescribed therapy and needs to begin at the time of diagnosis. Successful education involves teaching basic asthma facts, explaining the role of medications, teaching environmental control measures, and improving patient skills in the use of spacer devices for metered dose inhalers and peak flow monitoring. Families should have an asthma management plan (Fig. 78-5) for daily care and for exacerbations.

**Peak flow monitoring** is a self-assessment tool that is helpful for children older than 5 years of age. It is advisable for children who are *poor perceivers* of airway obstruction, have moderate to severe asthma, or have a history of severe exacerbations. Peak flow monitoring also can be useful in children who are still learning to recognize asthma symptoms.

To use a peak flow meter, a child should be standing with the indicator placed at the bottom of the scale. The child must inhale deeply, place the device in the mouth, bite down on the mouthpiece, seal the lips around the mouthpiece, and blow out forcefully and rapidly. The indicator moves up the numeric scale. The **peak expiratory flow rate (PEFR)** is the highest number achieved.

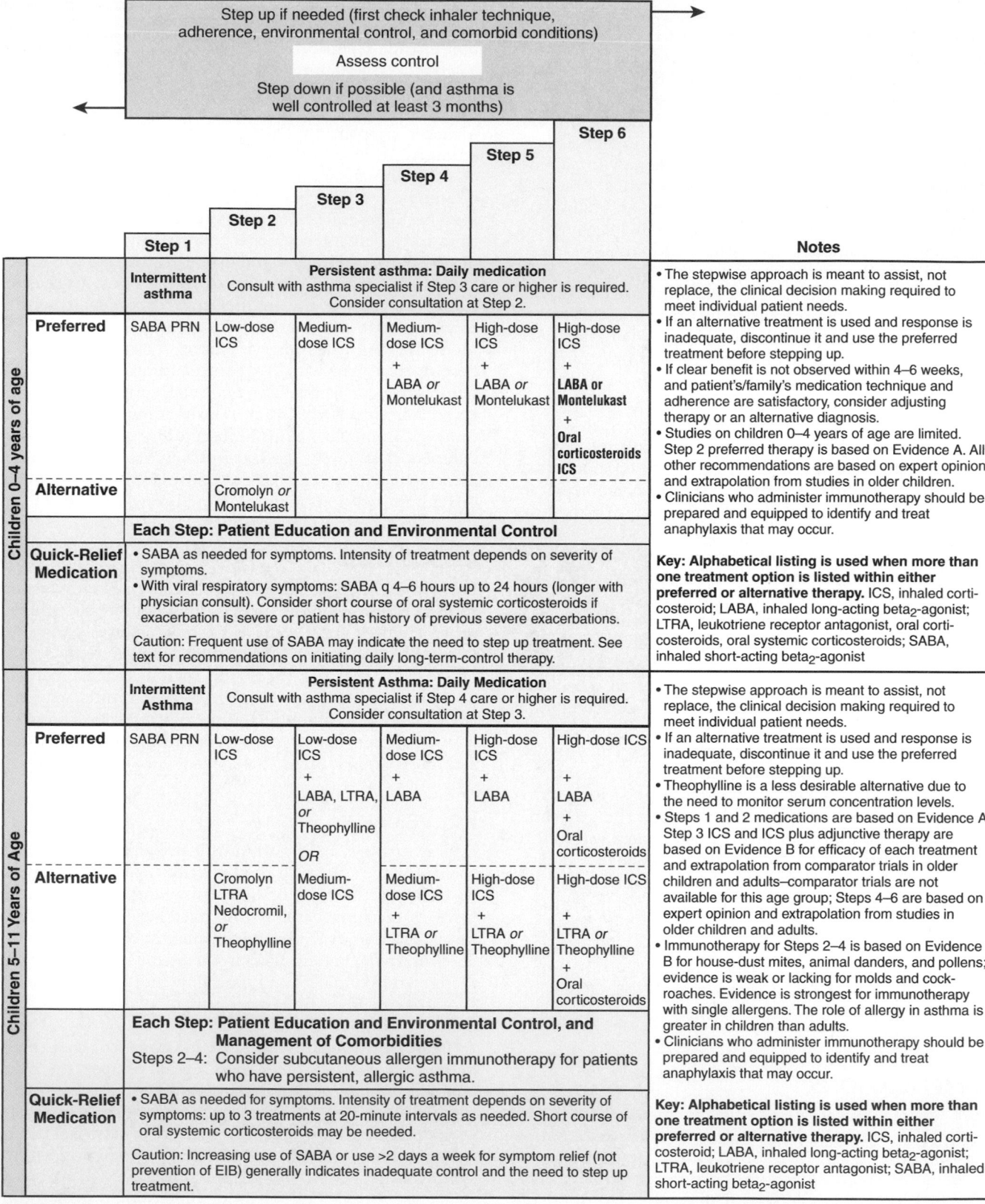

**FIGURE 78-1**

Stepwise long-term approach for managing asthma in children, 0–4 years of age and 5–11 years of age. (From *National Heart Lung Blood Institute, National Asthma Education and Prevention Program:* Expert panel report 3: guidelines for the diagnosis and management of asthma. Summary report 2007, *NIH Publication No. 08-5846,* Bethesda, MD, 2007, U.S. Department of Health and Human Services, p 42, http://www.nhlbi.nih.gov/guidelines/asthma/asthsumm.pdf)

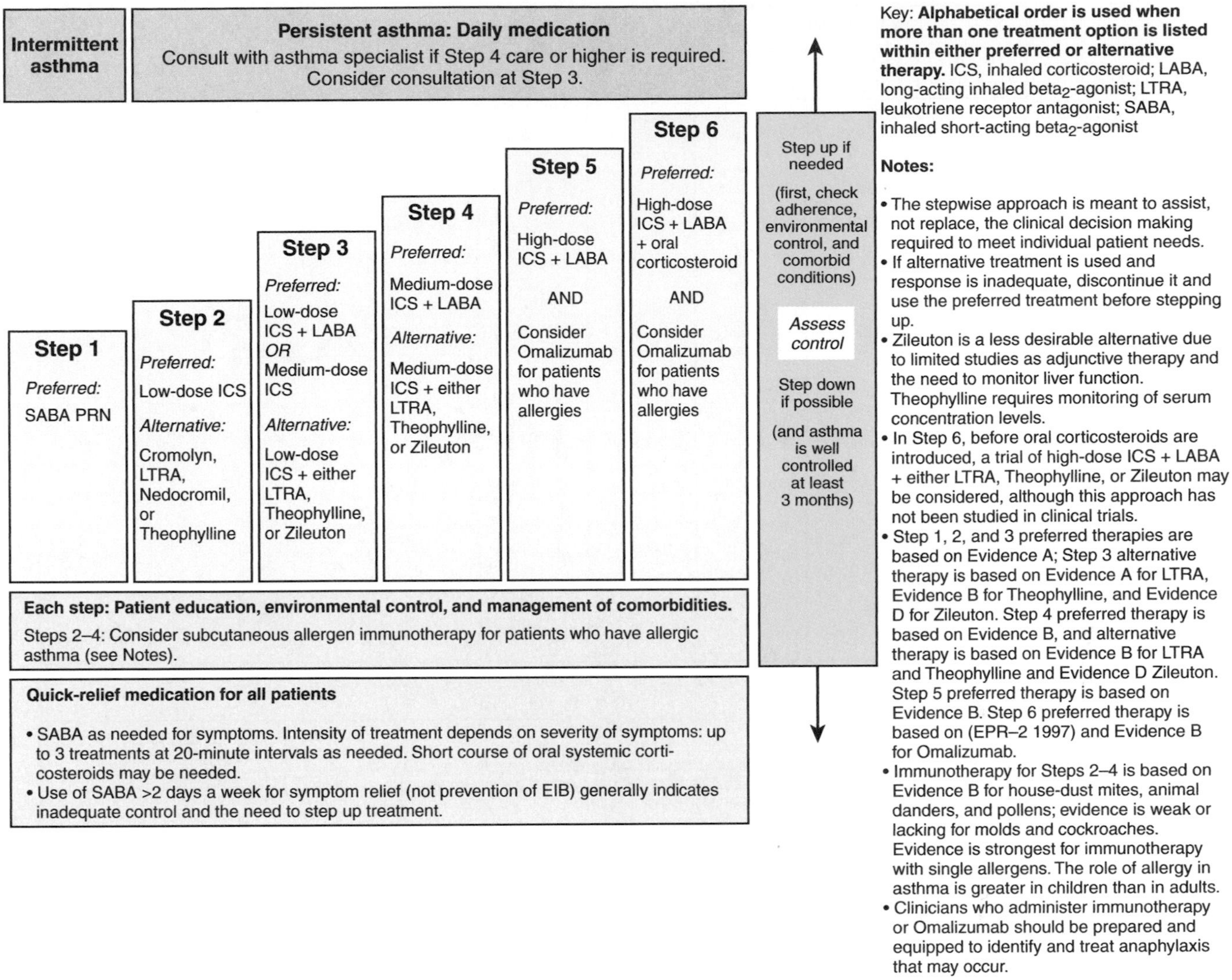

| Intermittent asthma | Persistent asthma: Daily medication<br>Consult with asthma specialist if Step 4 care or higher is required.<br>Consider consultation at Step 3. |
|---|---|

**Step 1**

*Preferred:*

SABA PRN

**Step 2**

*Preferred:*

Low-dose ICS

*Alternative:*

Cromolyn, LTRA, Nedocromil, or Theophylline

**Step 3**

*Preferred:*

Low-dose ICS + LABA OR Medium-dose ICS

*Alternative:*

Low-dose ICS + either LTRA, Theophylline, or Zileuton

**Step 4**

*Preferred:*

Medium-dose ICS + LABA

*Alternative:*

Medium-dose ICS + either LTRA, Theophylline, or Zileuton

**Step 5**

*Preferred:*

High-dose ICS + LABA

AND

Consider Omalizumab for patients who have allergies

**Step 6**

*Preferred:*

High-dose ICS + LABA + oral corticosteroid

AND

Consider Omalizumab for patients who have allergies

**Step up if needed**

(first, check adherence, environmental control, and comorbid conditions)

*Assess control*

**Step down if possible**

(and asthma is well controlled at least 3 months)

**Each step: Patient education, environmental control, and management of comorbidities.**

Steps 2–4: Consider subcutaneous allergen immunotherapy for patients who have allergic asthma (see Notes).

**Quick-relief medication for all patients**

• SABA as needed for symptoms. Intensity of treatment depends on severity of symptoms: up to 3 treatments at 20-minute intervals as needed. Short course of oral systemic corticosteroids may be needed.
• Use of SABA >2 days a week for symptom relief (not prevention of EIB) generally indicates inadequate control and the need to step up treatment.

**Key: Alphabetical order is used when more than one treatment option is listed within either preferred or alternative therapy.** ICS, inhaled corticosteroid; LABA, long-acting inhaled beta$_2$-agonist; LTRA, leukotriene receptor antagonist; SABA, inhaled short-acting beta$_2$-agonist

**Notes:**

• The stepwise approach is meant to assist, not replace, the clinical decision making required to meet individual patient needs.
• If alternative treatment is used and response is inadequate, discontinue it and use the preferred treatment before stepping up.
• Zileuton is a less desirable alternative due to limited studies as adjunctive therapy and the need to monitor liver function. Theophylline requires monitoring of serum concentration levels.
• In Step 6, before oral corticosteroids are introduced, a trial of high-dose ICS + LABA + either LTRA, Theophylline, or Zileuton may be considered, although this approach has not been studied in clinical trials.
• Step 1, 2, and 3 preferred therapies are based on Evidence A; Step 3 alternative therapy is based on Evidence A for LTRA, Evidence B for Theophylline, and Evidence D for Zileuton. Step 4 preferred therapy is based on Evidence B, and alternative therapy is based on Evidence B for LTRA and Theophylline and Evidence D Zileuton. Step 5 preferred therapy is based on Evidence B. Step 6 preferred therapy is based on (EPR–2 1997) and Evidence B for Omalizumab.
• Immunotherapy for Steps 2–4 is based on Evidence B for house-dust mites, animal danders, and pollens; evidence is weak or lacking for molds and cockroaches. Evidence is strongest for immunotherapy with single allergens. The role of allergy in asthma is greater in children than in adults.
• Clinicians who administer immunotherapy or Omalizumab should be prepared and equipped to identify and treat anaphylaxis that may occur.

**FIGURE 78-2**

Stepwise approach for managing asthma in youths 12 years of age or older and adults. (From *National Heart Lung Blood Institute, National Asthma Education and Prevention Program:* Expert panel report 3: guidelines for the diagnosis and management of asthma. Summary report 2007, *NIH Publication No. 08-5846,* Bethesda, MD, 2007, U.S. Department of Health and Human Services, p 45, http://www.nhlbi.nih.gov/guidelines/asthma/asthsumm.pdf)

The test is repeated three times to obtain the best possible effort. Peak flow meters are available as low range ($\leq$300 L/sec) and high range ($\leq$700 L/sec). It is important to provide the appropriate range meter so that accurate measurements can be obtained, and children do not become discouraged because their exhalations barely move the indicator.

A child's personal best is the highest PEFR achieved over a 2-week period when stable. Based on the child's personal best, a **written action plan** can be established, which is divided into three zones, similar to a stoplight. The green zone indicates a PEFR 80% to 100% of the child's personal best value. In this zone, the child is likely asymptomatic and should continue with medications as usual. The yellow zone indicates a PEFR 50% to 80% of the child's personal best value, which generally coincides with more asthma symptoms. Rescue medications, such as albuterol, are added, and a telephone call to the physician may be warranted if the peak flows do not return to the green zone within the next 24 to 48 hours or if asthma symptoms are deteriorating. The red zone indicates a PEFR below 50% and is a medical emergency. Rescue medication should be taken immediately. If the PEFR remains in the red zone or the child has significant airway compromise, a phone call to the physician or emergency care is needed.

A key message for families is that children with asthma should be seen not only when they are ill but also when they are healthy. Regular office visits allow the health care team to review **adherence** to medication and control measures and to determine if doses of medications need adjustment.

| Drug | Low Daily Dose | | | Medium Daily Dose | | | High Daily Dose | | |
|---|---|---|---|---|---|---|---|---|---|
| | Child 0–4 Years of Age | Child 5–11 Years of Age | ≥12 Years of Age and Adults | Child 0–4 Years of Age | Child 5–11 Years of Age | ≥12 Years of Age and Adults | Child 0–4 Years of Age | Child 5–11 Years of Age | ≥12 Years of Age and Adults |
| **Beclomethasone HFA** 40 or 80 µg/puff | NA | 80–160 µg | 80–240 µg | NA | >160–320 µg | >240–480 µg | NA | >320 µg | >480 µg |
| **Budesonide DPI** 90, 180, or 200 µg/inhalation | NA | 180–400 µg | 180–600 µg | NA | >400–800 µg | >600–1,200 µg | NA | >800 µg | >1,200 µg |
| **Budesonide Inhaled** Inhalation suspension for nebulization | 0.25–0.5 mg | 0.5 mg | NA | >0.5–1.0 mg | 1.0 mg | NA | >1.0 mg | 2.0 mg | NA |
| **Flunisolide** 250 µg/puff | NA | 500–750 µg | 500–1,000 µg | NA | 1,000–1,250 µg | >1,000–2,000 µg | NA | >1,250 µg | >2,000 µg |
| **Flunisolide HFA** 80 µg/puff | NA | 160 µg | 320 µg | NA | 320 µg | >320–640 µg | NA | ≥640 µg | >640 µg |
| **Fluticasone** **HFA/MDI:** 44, 110, or 220 µg/puff | 176 µg | 88–176 µg | 88–264 µg | >176–352 µg | >176–352 µg | >264–440 µg | >352 µg | >352 µg | >440 µg |
| **DPI:** 50, 100, or 250 µg/inhalation | NA | 100–200 µg | 100–300 µg | NA | >200–400 µg | >300–500 µg | NA | >400 µg | >500 µg |
| **Mometasone DPI** 200 µg/inhalation | NA | NA | 200 µg | NA | NA | 400 µg | NA | NA | >400 µg |
| **Triamcinolone acetonide** 75 µg/puff | NA | 300–600 µg | 300–750 µg | NA | >600–900 µg | >750–1,500 µg | NA | >900 µg | >1,500 µg |

Key: DPI, dry power inhaler; HFA, hydrofluoroalkane; MDI, metered-dose inhaler; NA, not available (either not approved, no data available, or safety and efficacy not established for this age group)

**Therapeutic Issues:**

• The most important determinant of appropriate dosing is the clinician's judgment of the patient's response to therapy. The clinician must monitor the patient's response on several clinical parameters and adjust the dose accordingly. Once control of asthma is achieved, the dose should be carefully titrated to the minimum dose required to maintain control.

• Preparations are not interchangeable on a µg or per puff basis. This figure presents estimated comparable daily doses. See EPR–3 Full Report 2007 for full discussion.

• Some doses may be outside package labeling, especially in the high-dose range. Budesonide nebulizer suspension is the only inhaler corticosteroid (ICS) with FDA-approved labeling for children <4 years of age.

• For children <4 years of age: The safety and efficacy of ICSs in children <1 year has not been established. Children <4 years of age generally require delivery of ICS (budesonide and fluticasone HFA) through a face mask that should fit snugly over nose and mouth and avoid nebulizing in the eyes. Wash face after each treatment to prevent local corticosteroid side effects. For budesonide, the dose may be administered 1–3 times daily. Budesonide suspension is compatible with Albuterol, Ipratropium, and Levalbuterol nebulizer solutions in the same nebulizer. Use only jet nebulizers, as ultrasonic nebulizers are ineffective for suspensions. For Fluticasone HFA, the dose should be divided 2 times daily; the low dose for children <4 years of age is higher than for children 5–11 years of age due to lower dose delivered with face mask and data on efficacy in young children.

**Potential Adverse Effects of Inhaled Corticosteroids:**

• Cough, dysphonia, oral thrush (candidiasis).

• Spacer or valved holding chamber with non-breath-actuated MDIs and mouthwashing and spitting after inhalation decrease local side effects.

• A number of the ICSs, including Fluticasone, Budesonide, and Mometasone, are metabolized in the gastrointestinal tract and liver by CYP 3A4 isoenzymes. Potent inhibitors of CYP 3A4, such as Ritonavir and Ketoconazole, have the potential for increasing systemic concentrations of these ICSs by increasing oral availability and decreasing systemic clearance. Some cases of clinically significant Cushing syndrome and secondary adrenal insufficiency have been reported.

• In high doses, systemic effects may occur, although studies are not conclusive, and clinical significance of these effects has not been established (e.g., adrenal suppression, osteoporosis, skin thinning, and easy bruising). In low-to-medium doses, suppression of growth velocity has been observed in children, but this effect may be transient, and the clinical significance has not been established.

**FIGURE 78-3**

Estimated comparative daily dosages for inhaled corticosteroids. (Adapted from *National Heart Lung Blood Institute, National Asthma Education and Prevention Program:* Expert panel report 3: guidelines for the diagnosis and management of asthma. Summary report 2007, *NIH Publication No. 08-5846,* Bethesda, MD, 2007, U.S. Department of Health and Human Services, p 49, http://www.nhlbi.nih.gov/guidelines/asthma/asthsumm.pdf)

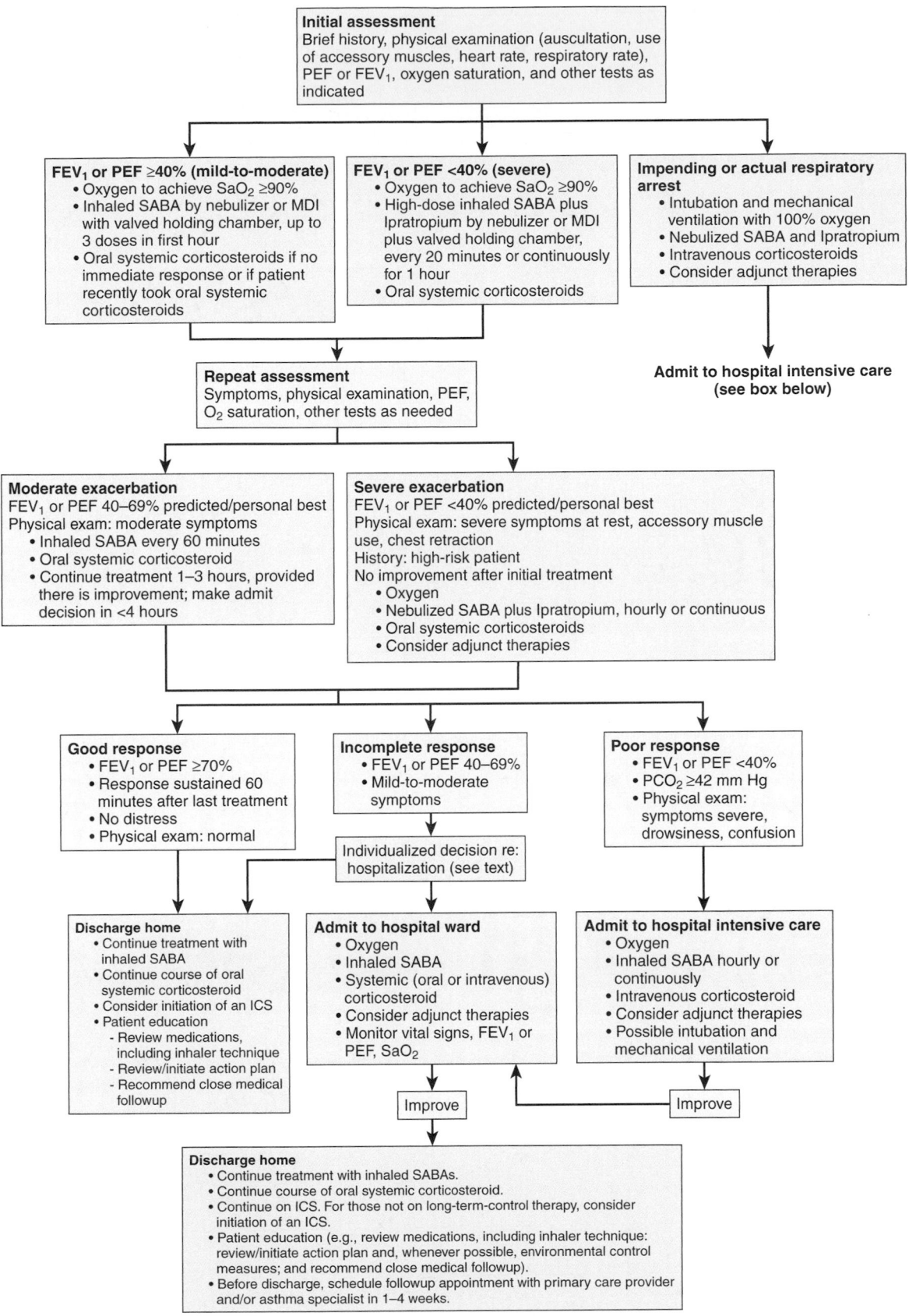

**Initial assessment**
Brief history, physical examination (auscultation, use of accessory muscles, heart rate, respiratory rate), PEF or $FEV_1$, oxygen saturation, and other tests as indicated

**$FEV_1$ or PEF ≥40% (mild-to-moderate)**
- Oxygen to achieve $SaO_2$ ≥90%
- Inhaled SABA by nebulizer or MDI with valved holding chamber, up to 3 doses in first hour
- Oral systemic corticosteroids if no immediate response or if patient recently took oral systemic corticosteroids

**$FEV_1$ or PEF <40% (severe)**
- Oxygen to achieve $SaO_2$ ≥90%
- High-dose inhaled SABA plus Ipratropium by nebulizer or MDI plus valved holding chamber, every 20 minutes or continuously for 1 hour
- Oral systemic corticosteroids

**Impending or actual respiratory arrest**
- Intubation and mechanical ventilation with 100% oxygen
- Nebulized SABA and Ipratropium
- Intravenous corticosteroids
- Consider adjunct therapies

**Admit to hospital intensive care (see box below)**

**Repeat assessment**
Symptoms, physical examination, PEF, $O_2$ saturation, other tests as needed

**Moderate exacerbation**
$FEV_1$ or PEF 40–69% predicted/personal best
Physical exam: moderate symptoms
- Inhaled SABA every 60 minutes
- Oral systemic corticosteroid
- Continue treatment 1–3 hours, provided there is improvement; make admit decision in <4 hours

**Severe exacerbation**
$FEV_1$ or PEF <40% predicted/personal best
Physical exam: severe symptoms at rest, accessory muscle use, chest retraction
History: high-risk patient
No improvement after initial treatment
- Oxygen
- Nebulized SABA plus Ipratropium, hourly or continuous
- Oral systemic corticosteroids
- Consider adjunct therapies

**Good response**
- $FEV_1$ or PEF ≥70%
- Response sustained 60 minutes after last treatment
- No distress
- Physical exam: normal

**Incomplete response**
- $FEV_1$ or PEF 40–69%
- Mild-to-moderate symptoms

**Poor response**
- $FEV_1$ or PEF <40%
- $PCO_2$ ≥42 mm Hg
- Physical exam: symptoms severe, drowsiness, confusion

**Individualized decision re: hospitalization (see text)**

**Discharge home**
- Continue treatment with inhaled SABA
- Continue course of oral systemic corticosteroid
- Consider initiation of an ICS
- Patient education
  - Review medications, including inhaler technique
  - Review/initiate action plan
  - Recommend close medical followup

**Admit to hospital ward**
- Oxygen
- Inhaled SABA
- Systemic (oral or intravenous) corticosteroid
- Consider adjunct therapies
- Monitor vital signs, $FEV_1$ or PEF, $SaO_2$

**Admit to hospital intensive care**
- Oxygen
- Inhaled SABA hourly or continuously
- Intravenous corticosteroid
- Consider adjunct therapies
- Possible intubation and mechanical ventilation

**Improve**

**Improve**

**Discharge home**
- Continue treatment with inhaled SABAs.
- Continue course of oral systemic corticosteroid.
- Continue on ICS. For those not on long-term-control therapy, consider initiation of an ICS.
- Patient education (e.g., review medications, including inhaler technique; review/initiate action plan and, whenever possible, environmental control measures; and recommend close medical followup).
- Before discharge, schedule followup appointment with primary care provider and/or asthma specialist in 1–4 weeks.

Key: $FEV_1$, forced expiratory volume in 1 second; ICS, inhaled corticosteroid; MDI, metered-dose inhaler; $PCO_2$, partial pressure carbon dioxide; PEF, peak expiratory flow; SABA, short-acting beta$_2$-agonist; $SaO_2$, oxygen saturation

**FIGURE 78-4**

Management of asthma exacerbations: emergency department and hospital-based care. (From *National Heart Lung Blood Institute, National Asthma Education and Prevention Program*: Expert panel report 3: guidelines for the diagnosis and management of asthma. Summary report 2007, *NIH Publication No. 08-5846*, Bethesda, MD, 2007, U.S. Department of Health and Human Services, p 55, http://www.nhlbi.nih.gov/guidelines/asthma/asthsumm.pdf)

## Asthma Action Plan

For: _____  Doctor: _____  Date: _____

Doctor's Phone Number _____  Hospital/Emergency Department Phone Number _____

### GREEN ZONE

**Doing Well**
- No cough, wheeze, chest tightness, or shortness of breath during the day or night
- Can do usual activities

**And, if a peak flow meter is used,**

**Peak flow:** more than _____
(80 percent or more of my best peak flow)

My best peak flow is: _____

Take these long-term-control medicines each day (include an anti-inflammatory).

| Medicine | How much to take | When to take it |
|---|---|---|

Identify and avoid and control the things that make your asthma worse, like (list here): _____

Before exercise, if prescribed, take:  □ 2  or  □ 4 puffs  _____  5 to 60 minutes before exercise

### YELLOW ZONE

**Asthma Is Getting Worse**
- Cough, wheeze, chest tightness, or shortness of breath, or
- Waking at night due to asthma, or
- Can do some, but not all, usual activities

-Or-

**Peak flow:** _____ to _____
(50 to 79 percent of my best peak flow)

**First** → **Add: quick-relief medicine—and keep taking your GREEN ZONE medicine.**

_____ □ 2  or  □ 4 puffs, every 20 minutes for up to 1 hour
(short-acting beta₂-agonist) □ Nebulizer, once

If applicable, remove yourself from the thing that made your asthma worse.

If your symptoms (and peak flow, if used) return to GREEN ZONE after 1 hour of above treatment:
- □ Continue monitoring to be sure you stay in the green zone.

-Or-

If your symptoms (and peak flow, if used) do not return to GREEN ZONE after 1 hour of above treatment:

**Second** →

□ Take: _____  □ 2  or  □ 4 puffs  or  □ Nebulizer
(short-acting beta₂-agonist)

□ Add: _____  _____ mg per day. For _____ (3–10) days
(oral corticosteroid)

□ Call the doctor  □ before/ □ within _____ hours after taking the oral corticosteroid.
(phone)

### RED ZONE

**Medical Alert!**
- Very short of breath, or
- Quick-relief medicines have not helped, or
- Cannot do usual activities, or
- Symptoms are same or get worse after 24 hours in Yellow Zone.

-Or-

**Peak flow:** less than _____
(50 percent of my best peak flow)

Take this medicine:

□ _____  □ 4  or  □ 6 puffs  or  □ Nebulizer
(short-acting beta₂-agonist)

□ _____  _____ mg
(oral corticosteroid)

**Then call your doctor NOW.** Go to the hospital or call an ambulance if
- You are still in the red zone after 15 minutes AND
- You have not reached your doctor.

DANGER SIGNS
- Trouble walking and talking due to shortness of breath
- Lips or fingernails are blue

→ ■ Take □ 4  or  □ 6 puffs of your quick-relief medicine **AND**
→ ■ Go to the hospital or call for an ambulance _____ **NOW!**
(phone)

**FIGURE 78-5**

Asthma self-management guideline. (From *National Heart Lung Blood Institute, National Asthma Education and Prevention Program: Expert Panel Report 3: Guidelines for the Diagnosis and Management of Asthma. Summary Report 2007. NIH Publication No. 05-5251.* Bethesda, MD, 2007, U.S. Department of Health and Human Services, p 119. http://www.nhlbi.nih.gov/guidelines/asthma/asthgdln.pdf)

**TABLE 78-4  Risk Factors for Persistent Asthma**

Allergy
  Atopic dermatitis
  Allergic rhinitis
  Elevated total serum IgE levels (first year of life)
  Peripheral blood eosinophilia >4% (2–3 yr of age)
  Food and inhalant allergen sensitization
Gender
  Boys
    Transient wheezing
    Persistent allergy-associated asthma
  Girls
    Asthma associated with obesity and early-onset puberty
    Triad asthma (adulthood)
Parental asthma
Lower respiratory tract infection
  Respiratory syncytial virus, parainfluenza
  Severe bronchiolitis (e.g., requiring hospitalization)
  Pneumonia
Environmental tobacco smoke exposure (including prenatal)

From Liu A, Martinez FD, Taussig LM: Natural history of allergic diseases and asthma. In Leung DYM, Sampson HA, Geha RS, Szefler SJ, editors: Pediatric Allergy: Principles and Practice. St Louis, 2003, *Mosby*, p 15.

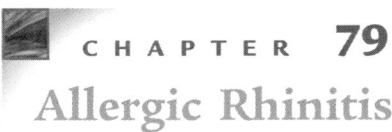

# CHAPTER 79
# Allergic Rhinitis

## ETIOLOGY

**Rhinitis** describes diseases that involve inflammation of the nasal epithelium and is characterized by sneezing, itching, rhinorrhea, and congestion. There are many different causes of rhinitis in children, but approximately half of all cases of rhinitis are caused by allergies.

**Allergic rhinitis**, commonly known as **hay fever**, is caused by a type I, IgE-mediated allergic response. During the early allergic phase, mast cells degranulate and release preformed chemical mediators, such as histamine and tryptase, and newly generated mediators, such as leukotrienes, prostaglandins, and platelet-activating factor. After a quiescent phase in which other cells are recruited, a late phase occurs approximately 4 to 8 hours later. Eosinophils, basophils, CD4 T cells, monocytes, and neutrophils release their chemical mediators, which leads to the development of chronic nasal inflammation.

Allergic rhinitis can be seasonal, perennial, or episodic depending on the particular allergen and the exposure. Some children experience perennial symptoms with seasonal exacerbations. **Seasonal allergic rhinitis** is caused by airborne pollens, which have seasonal patterns. Insect-pollinated plants (flowers, flowering trees) are not a cause of allergic rhinitis. Typically, trees pollinate in the spring, grasses in late spring to summer, and weeds in the summer and fall. The pollen, microscopic in size, can travel airborne hundreds of miles and be inhaled easily into the respiratory tract. **Perennial allergic rhinitis** is primarily caused by indoor allergens, such as house dust mites, animal dander, mold, and cockroaches. **Episodic rhinitis** occurs with intermittent exposure to allergens, such as visiting a friend's home where a pet dwells.

Genetic predisposition and repeated exposure to allergens contribute to the development of allergic rhinitis. It often takes weeks, months, or years to sensitize the immune system to produce sufficient allergen-specific IgE. When an atopic child inhales airborne allergens, these proteins penetrate the nasal mucosal epithelium and interact with allergen-specific IgE on tissue mast cells. Allergic rhinitis is relatively rare in children younger than 6 months of age. If present in infancy, it is caused by foods or household inhalants rather than seasonal pollens. Typically, seasonal allergic rhinitis presents in children older than 3 years of age.

## EPIDEMIOLOGY

Chronic rhinitis is one of the most common disorders encountered in infants and children. Overall, allergic rhinitis is observed in 10% to 25% of the population, with children and adolescents more commonly affected than adults. The prevalence of physician-diagnosed allergic rhinitis may be 40%.

## CLINICAL MANIFESTATIONS

The hallmarks of allergic rhinitis are clear, thin rhinorrhea; nasal congestion; paroxysms of sneezing; and pruritus of the eyes, nose, ears, and palate. Postnasal drip may result in frequent attempts to clear the throat, nocturnal cough, and hoarseness. It is important to correlate the onset, duration, and severity of symptoms with seasonal or perennial exposures, changes in the home or school environment, and exposure to nonspecific irritants, such as tobacco smoke.

The physical examination includes a thorough nasal examination and an evaluation of the eyes, ears, throat, chest, and skin. Physical findings may be subtle. Classic physical findings include pale pink or bluish gray, swollen, boggy nasal turbinates with clear, watery secretions. Frequent nasal itching and rubbing of the nose with the palm of the hand, the **allergic salute**, can lead to a transverse nasal crease found across the lower bridge of the nose. Children may produce clucking sounds by rubbing the soft palate with their tongue. Oropharyngeal examination may reveal lymphoid hyperplasia of the soft palate and posterior pharynx or visible mucus or both. Orthodontic abnormalities may be seen in children with chronic mouth breathing. **Allergic shiners**, dark periorbital swollen areas caused by venous congestion, are often present in children along with swollen eyelids or conjunctival injection. Retracted tympanic membranes from eustachian tube dysfunction or serous otitis media also may be present. Other atopic diseases, such as asthma or eczema, may be present, which helps lead the clinician to the correct diagnosis.

## LABORATORY AND IMAGING STUDIES

Allergy testing can be performed by in vivo skin tests or by in vitro serum tests (radioallergosorbent test [RAST]) to pertinent allergens found in the patient's environment (see Table 77-4). Skin tests (prick/puncture) provide immediate and accurate results. Positive tests correlate strongly with nasal and bronchial allergen provocative challenges. In vitro serum tests are useful for patients with abnormal skin conditions, a tendency for anaphylaxis, or those taking medications that interfere with skin testing. Disadvantages of serum tests include increased cost, inability to obtain immediate results, and reduced sensitivity compared with skin tests. Widespread screening with serum testing without regard to symptoms is not recommended. Measurement of total serum IgE or blood eosinophils generally is not helpful. The presence of eosinophils on the nasal smear suggests a diagnosis of allergy, but eosinophils also can be found in patients with nonallergic rhinitis with eosinophilia. Nasal smear eosinophilia is often predictive of a good clinical response to nasal corticosteroid sprays.

## DIFFERENTIAL DIAGNOSIS

Rhinitis can be divided into allergic and nonallergic rhinitis (Table 79-1). Nonallergic rhinitis describes a group of nasal diseases in which there is no evidence of allergic etiology. It can be divided further into nonanatomic and anatomic etiologies. The most common form of nonallergic rhinitis in children is infectious rhinitis, which may be acute or chronic. Acute infectious rhinitis (the common cold) is caused by viruses, including rhinoviruses and coronaviruses, and typically resolves within 7 to 10 days (see Chapter 102). An average child has three to six common colds per year, with younger children and children attending day care the most affected. Infection is suggested by the presence of sore throat, fever, and poor appetite, especially with a history of exposure to others with colds. Chronic infectious **rhinosinusitis**, or sinusitis, should be suspected if there is mucopurulent nasal discharge with symptoms that persist beyond 10 days (see Chapter 104). Classic signs of acute sinusitis in older children include facial tenderness, tooth pain, headache,

and fever. Classic signs are usually not present in young children who may present with postnasal drainage with cough, throat clearing, halitosis, and rhinorrhea. The character of the nasal secretions with infectious rhinitis varies from purulent to minimal or absent. Coexistence of middle ear disease, such as otitis media or eustachian tube dysfunction, may be additional clues of infection.

**Nonallergic, noninfectious rhinitis** (formerly known as vasomotor rhinitis) can manifest as rhinorrhea and sneezing in children with profuse clear nasal discharge. Exposure to irritants, such as cigarette smoke and dust, and strong fumes and odors, such as perfumes and chlorine in swimming pools, can trigger these nasal symptoms. Nonallergic rhinitis with eosinophilia syndrome is associated with clear nasal discharge and eosinophils on nasal smear and is seen infrequently in children. Cold air (**skier's nose**), hot/spicy food ingestion (**gustatory rhinitis**), and exposure to bright light (**reflex rhinitis**) are examples of physical rhinitis. Treatment with topical ipratropium before exposure may be helpful.

**Rhinitis medicamentosa**, which is due primarily to overuse of topical nasal decongestants such as oxymetazoline, phenylephrine, or cocaine, is not a common condition in younger children. Adolescents or young adults may become dependent on these over-the-counter medications. Treatment requires discontinuation of the offending decongestant spray, topical corticosteroids, and, frequently, a short course of oral corticosteroids.

The most common anatomic problem seen in young children is obstruction secondary to adenoidal hypertrophy, which can be suspected from symptoms such as mouth breathing, snoring, hyponasal speech, and persistent rhinitis with or without chronic otitis media. Infection of the nasopharynx may be secondary to infected hypertrophied adenoid tissue.

**Choanal atresia** is the most common congenital anomaly of the nose and consists of a bony or membranous septum between the nose and pharynx, either unilateral or bilateral. Bilateral choanal atresia classically presents in neonates as cyclic cyanosis because neonates are preferential nose breathers. Airway obstruction and cyanosis are relieved when the mouth is opened to cry and recurs when the calming infant reattempts to breathe through the nose. Some newborns show respiratory difficulty only while

| Allergic | Nonallergic | | Anatomic |
|---|---|---|---|
| | Nonanatomic | | |
| Seasonal | Nonallergic, noninfectious (vasomotor) rhinitis | | Adenoidal hypertrophy |
| Perennial | Infectious rhinosinusitis | | CSF rhinorrhea |
| Episodic | Nonallergic rhinitis with eosinophilia | | Choanal atresia |
| | Physical rhinitis | | Congenital anomalies |
| | Rhinitis medicamentosa | | Foreign body |
| | | | Nasal polyps |
| | | | Septal deviation |
| | | | Tumors |
| | | | Turbinate hypertrophy |

**TABLE 79-1 Classification of the Etiology of Rhinitis in Children**

CSF, cerebrospinal fluid.

feeding. Nearly half of infants with choanal atresia have other congenital anomalies as a part of the **CHARGE association** (**c**oloboma, congenital **h**eart disease, choanal **a**tresia, **r**etardation, **g**enitourinary defects, **e**ar anomalies). Unilateral choanal atresia may go undiagnosed until later in life and presents with symptoms of unilateral nasal obstruction and discharge.

**Nasal polyps** typically appear as bilateral, gray, glistening sacs originating from the ethmoid sinuses and may be associated with clear or purulent nasal discharge. Nasal polyps are rare in children younger than 10 years of age but if present warrant evaluation for an underlying disease process, such as cystic fibrosis or primary ciliary dyskinesia. **Triad asthma** is asthma, aspirin sensitivity, and nasal polyps with chronic or recurrent sinusitis.

**Foreign bodies** are seen more commonly in young children who hide food, small toys, stones, or erasers in their nose. The index of suspicion should be raised by a history of unilateral, purulent nasal discharge, or foul odor. The foreign body can often be seen on examination with a nasal speculum.

Nasal septal deviation in infants can be congenital or the result of birth trauma. In older children, facial trauma from contact sports, automobile or bicycle accidents, or play activities can result in septal deformity. Hypertrophy of the turbinates causing nasal symptoms also can be seen in children. Severe anatomic abnormalities of the septum or turbinates may benefit from surgical intervention.

A rare cause of rhinitis is cerebrospinal fluid rhinorrhea. This condition should be suspected in the presence of unilateral, clear nasal discharge and may occur even in the absence of trauma or recent surgery.

Tumors are extremely rare causes of anatomic obstruction in children and include hemangioma, rhabdomyosarcoma, lymphoma, and olfactory neuroblastoma. Other unusual congenital nasal lesions include dermoid cysts, teratomas, gliomas, and encephaloceles that present as insidious nasal obstruction in children. In adolescent boys, nasal obstruction and severe, recurring nosebleeds may be a sign of **angiofibroma**, a benign tumor.

## TREATMENT

Management of allergic rhinitis is based on disease severity, impact of the disease on the patient, and the ability of the patient to comply with recommendations. Treatment modalities include allergen avoidance, pharmacologic therapy, and immunotherapy. Environmental control and steps to minimize allergen exposure, similar to preventive steps for asthma, should be implemented whenever possible (see Table 78-3).

### Pharmacotherapy

**Intranasal corticosteroids** are the most potent pharmacologic therapy for treatment of allergic and nonallergic rhinitis. These include beclomethasone, budesonide, ciclesonide, flunisolide, fluticasone, mometasone, and triamcinolone. These topical agents work to reduce inflammation, edema, and mucus production. They are effective for symptoms of nasal congestion, rhinorrhea, itching, and sneezing but less helpful for ocular symptoms. Nasal corticosteroid sprays have been used safely in long-term therapy. Deleterious effects on adrenal function or nasal membranes have not been reported when these agents are used appropriately. The most common adverse effects include local irritation, burning, and, sneezing, which occur in 10% of patients. Nasal bleeding from improper technique (spraying the nasal septum) can occur. Rare cases of nasal septal perforation have been reported.

**Antihistamines** are the medications used most frequently to treat allergic rhinitis. They are useful in treating rhinorrhea, sneezing, nasal itching, and ocular itching but are less helpful in treating nasal congestion. **First-generation antihistamines**, such as diphenhydramine and hydroxyzine, easily cross the blood-brain barrier, with sedation as the most common reported adverse effect. Use of first-generation antihistamines in children has an adverse effect on cognitive and academic function. In very young children, a paradoxical stimulatory central nervous system effect, resulting in irritability and restlessness, has been noted. Other adverse effects of first-generation antihistamines include anticholinergic effects, such as blurred vision, urinary retention, dry mouth, tachycardia, and constipation. **Second-generation antihistamines**, such as cetirizine, loratadine, desloratadine, fexofenadine and levocetirizine, are less likely to cross the blood-brain barrier, resulting in less sedation. Cetirizine and loratadine are now over-the-counter medications. Azelastine and olopatadine, topical nasal antihistamine sprays, are approved for children older than 5 years and older than 6 years, respectively.

**Decongestants,** taken orally or intranasally, may be used to relieve nasal congestion. Oral medications, such as pseudoephedrine and phenylephrine, are available either alone or in combination with antihistamines. Adverse effects of oral decongestants include insomnia, nervousness, irritability, tachycardia, tremors, and palpitations. For older children participating in sports, oral decongestant use may be restricted. Topical nasal decongestant sprays are effective for immediate relief of nasal obstruction but should be used for less than 5 to 7 days to prevent rebound nasal congestion (rhinitis medicamentosa).

Topical ipratropium bromide, an anticholinergic nasal spray, is used primarily for nonallergic rhinitis and rhinitis associated with viral upper respiratory infection. Leukotriene modifiers have been studied in the treatment of allergic rhinitis. Montelukast is approved for use in seasonal allergic rhinitis.

### Immunotherapy

If environmental control measures and medication intervention are only partially effective or produce unacceptable adverse effects, immunotherapy may be recommended. The mechanism of action for allergen immunotherapy is complex but includes increased production of an IgG-blocking antibody, decreased production of specific IgE, and alteration of cytokine expression produced in response to an allergen challenge. Immunotherapy is effective for desensitization to pollens, dust mites, and cat and dog proteins. Use in young children may be limited by the need for frequent injections. Immunotherapy must be administered in a physician's office with 20 to 30 minutes of observation after the allergen injection. Anaphylaxis may occur, and the physician must be experienced in the treatment of these severe adverse allergic reactions.

## COMPLICATIONS

Approximately 60% of children with allergic rhinitis have symptoms of reactive airways disease/asthma (see Chapter 78). Chronic allergic inflammation leads to chronic cough from postnasal drip; eustachian tube dysfunction and otitis media; sinusitis; and tonsillar and adenoid hypertrophy, which may lead to obstructive sleep apnea. Children with allergic rhinitis may experience sleep disturbances, limitations of activity, irritability, and mood and cognitive disorders that adversely affect their performance at school and their sense of well-being.

## PROGNOSIS AND PREVENTION

Seasonal allergic rhinitis is a common and prominent condition that may not improve as children grow older. Patients become more adept at self-management. Perennial allergic rhinitis improves with allergen control of indoor allergens.

Removal or avoidance of the offending allergen is advised. The only effective measure for minimizing animal allergens from pets is removal of the pet from the home. Avoidance of pollen and outdoor molds can be accomplished by staying indoors in a controlled environment. Air conditioning and keeping windows and doors closed lower exposure to pollen. High-efficiency particle air (HEPA) filters reduce exposure to allergens (e.g., pet dander, mold spores, or pollen granules). Sealing the mattress, pillow, and covers in allergen-proof encasings is the most effective strategy for reduction of mite allergen. Bed linens and blankets should be washed in hot water (>130 °F) every week.

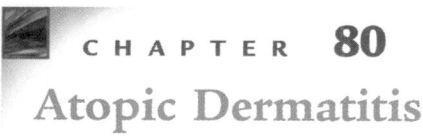

CHAPTER **80**

# Atopic Dermatitis

## ETIOLOGY

Atopic dermatitis is a chronic, pruritic, relapsing inflammatory skin condition. The pathogenesis is multifactorial and involves a complex interplay of factors, including genetic predisposition, immunologic abnormalities, disturbances in skin barrier function, environmental interactions, and infectious triggers. Several genes encoding epidermal or other epithelial structural proteins and genes encoding major elements of the immune system play a major role in atopic dermatitis.

Several immunoregulatory abnormalities have been described in patients with atopic dermatitis. There is an exaggerated cutaneous inflammatory response to environmental triggers, including irritants and allergens. Activated Langerhans cells in the dermis expressing surface-bound IgE stimulate T cells. In acute lesions, activated Th2

lymphocytes infiltrate the dermis. They initiate and maintain local tissue inflammation primarily through interleukin-4 (IL-4) and IL-13, which promote IgE production, and IL-5, which promotes eosinophil differentiation. As the disease progresses from an acute to a chronic phase, there is a switch from Th2 to Th1/Th0 cellular response. Chronic lesions are characterized by increased IL-12 and IL-18.

Patients with atopic dermatitis have **hyperirritable skin**, and many factors can cause the disease to worsen or relapse. Known triggers include anxiety and stress, climate (extremes of temperature and humidity), irritants, allergens, and infections. Approximately 35% to 40% of infants and young children with moderate to severe atopic dermatitis have coexisting food allergies. The more severe the atopic dermatitis and the younger the patient, the more likely a food allergy will be identified as a contributing factor. Egg allergy is the most common cause of food-induced eczematous reactions.

## EPIDEMIOLOGY

The prevalence of atopic dermatitis has increased two- to threefold over the past 30 years. Approximately 15% to 20% of children and 2% to 10% of adults are affected. Atopic dermatitis often starts in early infancy. Approximately 50% of affected children show symptoms in the first year of life, and 80% of these children experience disease onset before 5 years of age. Atopic dermatitis is often the first manifestation of other atopic diseases. Approximately 80% of children with atopic dermatitis develop other allergic diseases, such as asthma or allergic rhinitis. Symptoms of dermatitis often disappear at the onset of respiratory allergy.

## CLINICAL MANIFESTATIONS

The clinical manifestations of atopic dermatitis vary with age. In infants, atopic dermatitis involves the face, scalp, cheeks, and extensor surfaces of the extremities (Fig. 80-1). The diaper area is spared. In older children, the rash localizes to the antecubital and popliteal flexural surfaces, head, and neck. In adolescents and adults, lichenified plaques are seen in the flexural areas (Fig. 80-2) and the head and neck regions. Itching or pruritus has a significant impact on the child and family's quality of life; it is often worse at night, interrupting sleep. Physical examination may show hyperlinearity of the palms and soles, white dermatographism, pityriasis alba, creases under the lower eyelids (**Dennie-Morgan folds or Dennie lines**), and **keratosis pilaris** (asymptomatic horny follicular papules on the extensor surfaces of the arms).

## LABORATORY AND IMAGING STUDIES

The diagnosis of atopic dermatitis is based on clinical features rather than laboratory tests (Table 80-1). Skin biopsy is of little value, but it may be used to exclude other skin diseases that mimic atopic dermatitis. Skin testing or, alternatively, CAP-radioallergosorbent test (RAST) testing, may be helpful in assessing the contribution of food or environmental allergies to disease expression.

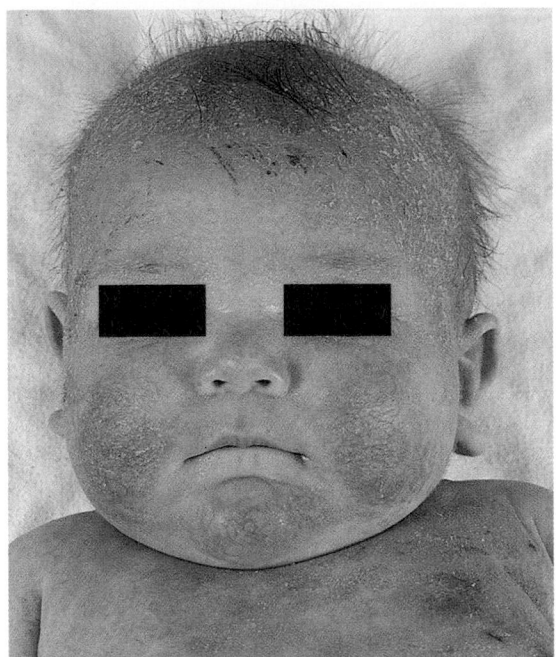

**FIGURE 80-1**

Atopic dermatitis typical cheek involvement. (From Eichenfield LF, Frieden IJ, Esterly NB: Textbook of Neonatal Dermatology, Philadelphia, 2001, *Saunders*, p 242.)

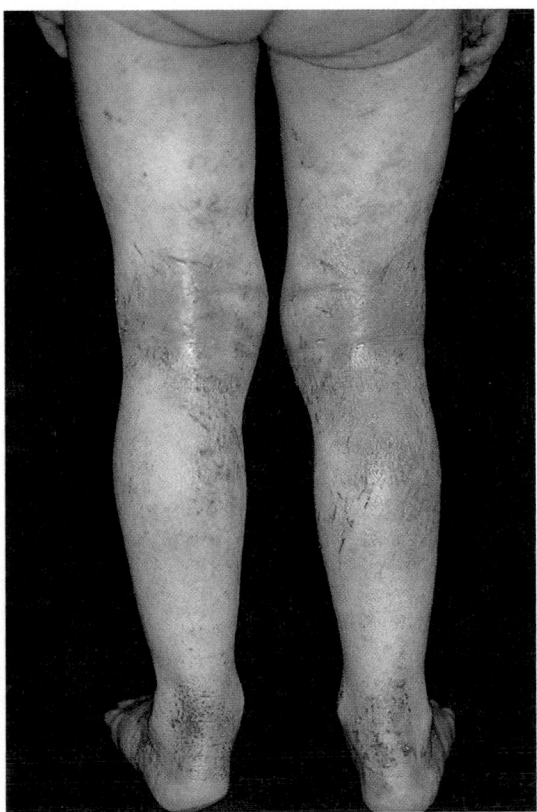

**FIGURE 80-2**

Rubbing and scratching the inflamed flexural areas causes thickened (lichenified) skin. (From Habif T: Clinical Dermatology, 4th ed, Philadelphia, 2004, *Elsevier*.)

| TABLE 80-1 Criteria for the Diagnosis of Atopic Dermatitis |
| --- |
| The diagnosis requires evidence of itchy skin (or parental report of scratching or rubbing) plus three or more of the following: <br> 1. History of involvement of skin creases <br> 2. History of asthma or allergic rhinitis (or history of atopic disease in a first-degree relative if child <4 years) <br> 3. History of generally dry skin in the past year <br> 4. Onset in a child <2 years (criterion not used if child is <4 years) <br> 5. Visible flexural dermatitis (including dermatitis affecting cheeks, forehead, and outer aspects of limbs in children <4 years) |

Modified from Williams HC, et al: Diagnostic criteria for atopic dermatitis. III. Independent hospital validation. *Br J Dermatol* 131:406–416, 1994.

## DIFFERENTIAL DIAGNOSIS

Many conditions share signs and symptoms of atopic dermatitis (Table 80-2). Infants presenting in the first year of life with failure to thrive, recurrent skin or systemic infections, and scaling, erythematous rash should be evaluated for immunodeficiency disorders. Wiskott-Aldrich syndrome is an X-linked recessive syndrome characterized by atopic dermatitis, thrombocytopenia, small-sized platelets, and recurrent infections. Histiocytosis X (Letterer-Siwe disease) is characterized by hemorrhagic or petechial lesions. Scabies is an intensely pruritic skin condition caused by the human scabies mite. The presence of a burrow found in the web spaces of the fingers, the flexor surfaces of the wrists, elbows, axilla, or genitals is pathognomonic. Burrows may be few in number or absent, however.

## TREATMENT

The goals of therapy are to reduce the number and severity of flares and to increase the number of disease-free periods. Successful management involves skin hydration, pharmacologic therapy to reduce pruritus, and identification and avoidance of triggers. Patients with atopic dermatitis have a decrease in skin barrier function and enhanced transepidermal water loss. Daily, lukewarm baths for 15 to 20 minutes followed immediately by the application of fragrance-free emollients to retain moisture are a major component of therapy. Prevention of xerosis is important for control of pruritus and for maintaining the integrity of the epithelial barrier. Emollients should be ointments or creams, such as petrolatum, Aquaphor, Eucerin, or Cetaphil. Lotions are not as effective because they contain water or alcohol and may have a drying effect owing to evaporation. A mild nonsoap cleanser also is recommended.

Topical anti-inflammatory agents, including corticosteroids and immunomodulators, are the cornerstone of therapy for acute flares and prevention of relapses. Topical corticosteroids are used for reducing inflammation and pruritus; they are effective for the acute and chronic phases of the disease. Ointments generally are

**TABLE 80-2 Differential Diagnosis of Atopic Dermatitis**

**CONGENITAL DISORDERS**

Netherton syndrome
Familial keratosis pilaris

**CHRONIC DERMATOSES**

Seborrheic dermatitis
Contact dermatitis (allergic or irritant)
Nummular eczema
Psoriasis
Ichthyoses

**INFECTIONS AND INFESTATIONS**

Scabies
HIV-associated dermatitis
Dermatophytosis

**MALIGNANCIES**

Cutaneous T-cell lymphoma (mycosis fungoides/Sézary syndrome)
Histiocytosis X (Letterer-Siwe disease)

**AUTOIMMUNE DISORDERS**

Dermatitis herpetiformis
Pemphigus foliaceus
Graft-versus-host disease
Dermatomyositis

**IMMUNODEFICIENCIES**

Wiskott-Aldrich syndrome
Severe combined immunodeficiency
Hyper-IgE syndrome

**METABOLIC DISORDERS**

Zinc deficiency
Pyridoxine (vitamin $B_6$) and niacin deficiency
Multiple carboxylase deficiency
Phenylketonuria

From Leung DYM: Atopic dermatitis. In Leung DYM, Sampson HA, Geha RS, Szefler SJ, editors: Pediatric Allergy: Principles and Practice, St Louis, 2003, *Mosby*, p 562.

preferred over creams and lotions because of enhanced potency and skin penetration. Corticosteroids are ranked by potency into seven classes. The least potent corticosteroid that is effective should be used. Higher potency corticosteroids may be necessary to diminish the dermatitis flare but should be used for limited periods. Low-potency, nonfluorinated corticosteroids should be used on the face, intertriginous areas (groin, axilla), and large areas to reduce the risk of adverse effects. Reduced efficacy of topical corticosteroids may be related to disease severity rather than glucocorticoid resistance. Local adverse effects, such as skin atrophy and striae, and systemic adverse effects, such as hypothalamic-pituitary-adrenal axis and growth suppression and hyperglycemia, are related to the

potency, length of use, and extent of medication application. In infants and younger children, the possibility of corticosteroid-induced adverse effects may be greater. When control of inflammatory lesions is achieved, most patients can be managed with emollients and low-potency topical corticosteroids.

The topical immunomodulating drugs, tacrolimus and pimecrolimus, are approved as second-line agents for short-term and intermittent treatment of atopic dermatitis in patients unresponsive to or intolerant of other therapies. They are approved for use in children older than 2 years of age. These agents may be used on all body locations and are especially useful on delicate skin sites, such as the face, neck, and axilla without the adverse effect of cutaneous atrophy seen with topical corticosteroids. These medications have a potential increased cancer risk, and their long-term safety has not been established. Other less serious adverse effects include local burning and the need for sun protection.

Oral corticosteroids are rarely indicated in the treatment of atopic dermatitis. The dramatic improvement seen is frequently associated with a severe rebound flare after the oral corticosteroid has been discontinued. Older sedating antihistamines, such as diphenhydramine and hydroxyzine, are sometimes recommended to help with night-time pruritus.

## COMPLICATIONS

Defective cell-mediated immunity leads to increased susceptibility to many bacterial, viral, and fungal infections of the skin. More than 90% of patients with atopic dermatitis have colonization of lesional skin with *Staphylococcus aureus*, and more than 75% of patients have colonization of uninvolved skin. Colonization and infection by *S. aureus* is associated with disease severity. *S. aureus* secretes exotoxins that act as a superantigen, stimulating T cells and increasing IgE production. Secondarily infected atopic dermatitis often presents as impetiginous, pustular lesions with crusting and honey-colored exudate. Topical antibiotics, such as mupirocin or retapamulin, can be used to treat local areas of infection, or oral antibiotics, such as cephalexin, dicloxacillin, or amoxicillin-clavulanate, can be used for multifocal disease or for infection around the eyes and mouth that is difficult to treat topically. Bacterial cultures may be helpful in patients who do not respond to oral antibiotics or who have infection after multiple antibiotic courses. The incidence of community-acquired methicillin-resistant *S. aureus* is increasing.

Herpes simplex superinfection of affected skin, or **Kaposi varicelliform eruption** or **eczema herpeticum**, results in vesiculopustular lesions that appear in clusters and can become hemorrhagic. Herpes simplex virus infection can be misdiagnosed as bacterial infection and should be considered if skin lesions fail to respond to antibiotics.

In individuals with atopic dermatitis, smallpox vaccination or exposure to a vaccinated individual may lead to **eczema vaccinatum**, a localized vaccinial superinfection of affected skin. Eczema vaccinatum may progress to generalized vaccinia with vaccinial lesions appearing at sites distant from the inoculation. In patients with underlying immunodeficiencies, it may be life-threatening.

Widespread infections with human papillomavirus (warts) and molluscum contagiosum are also common in children with atopic dermatitis.

## PROGNOSIS

Atopic dermatitis is a chronic, relapsing skin disorder that tends to be more severe and prominent in young children. Symptoms become less severe in two thirds of children, with complete remission for approximately 20%. Early-onset disease that is more widespread, concomitant asthma and allergic rhinitis, family history of atopic dermatitis, and elevated serum IgE levels may predict a more persistent course. Patients and families should be taught that a single cause and cure for atopic dermatitis is unlikely but that good control is possible for the majority of affected patients.

## PREVENTION

An important step in the management of atopic dermatitis is to identify and avoid allergens and irritants. Common irritants include soaps, detergents, fragrances, chemicals, smoke, and extremes of temperature and humidity. Wool and synthetic fabrics can be irritating to the skin; 100% cotton fabric is preferred. Sweating is a recognized trigger. Fingernails should be trimmed frequently to minimize excoriations from scratching.

In infants and younger children who do not respond to the usual therapies, identifying and removing a food allergen from the diet may lead to clinical improvement. Food allergy is not a common trigger for older patients. Other environmental exposures, such as dust mites, pet dander, or pollens, can also contribute to the disease state.

C H A P T E R  **81**

# Urticaria, Angioedema, and Anaphylaxis

## ETIOLOGY

**Urticaria**, commonly referred to as **hives**, is swelling of the dermis and one of the most common skin conditions seen in clinical practice. **Angioedema** results from a process similar to urticaria, but the reaction extends below the dermis. Urticaria and angioedema occur in response to release of inflammatory mediators, including histamine, leukotrienes, platelet-activating factor, prostaglandins, and cytokines from mast cells present in the skin. A variety of stimuli can trigger mast cells and basophils to release their chemical mediators. Typically, mast cells degranulate when cross-linking of the membrane-bound IgE occurs. Release of these mediators results in vasodilation, increased vascular leakage, and pruritus. Basophils from the circulatory system also can localize in tissue and release mediators similar to mast cells. Patients with urticaria have elevated histamine content in the skin that is more easily released.

**Anaphylaxis** is mediated by IgE, whereas **anaphylactoid reactions** result from mechanisms that are due to non-immunologic mechanisms. Both reactions are acute, severe, and can be life-threatening due to a massive release of inflammatory mediators. Urticaria, angioedema, and anaphylaxis are best considered as symptoms because they have a variety of causes.

Not all mast cell activation is IgE mediated. Immunologic, nonimmunologic, physical, and chemical stimuli can produce degranulation of mast cells and basophils. **Anaphylatoxins**, C3a and C5a, can cause histamine release in a non–IgE-mediated reaction. Anaphylatoxins are generated in serum sickness (reactions to blood transfusions) (see Chapter 82) and in infectious, neoplastic, and rheumatic diseases. In addition, mast cell degranulation can occur from a direct pharmacologic effect or physical or mechanical activation, such as urticaria after exposure to opiate medications and dermatographism.

Urticaria/angioedema can be classified into three subcategories: acute, chronic, and physical. By definition, **acute urticaria** and **angioedema** are hives and diffuse swelling that last less than 6 weeks. Often, the history is quite helpful in eliciting the cause of the acute reaction (Table 81-1). An IgE mechanism is more commonly found in acute urticaria than in chronic urticaria. **Chronic urticaria** and **angioedema** are characterized by persistence of symptoms beyond 6 weeks (Table 81-2). Some have daily symptoms of hives and swelling, whereas others have intermittent or recurrent episodes. Chronic urticaria can be idiopathic with unknown causal factors. From 35% to 40% of chronic urticaria cases are found to have an autoimmune process due to IgG autoantibodies binding directly to IgE or the IgE receptor. **Physical urticaria** and **angioedema** are characterized by known eliciting external factors that may include pressure, cold, heat, exercise, or exposure to sun or water.

The most common physical urticaria is dermatographism, affecting 2% to 5% of persons. **Dermatographism** means *writing on the skin* and is easily diagnosed by firmly scratching the skin with a blunt point, such as the wooden tip of a cotton swab or tongue depressor. It is characterized by an urticarial reaction localized to the site of skin trauma. It has been suggested that trauma induces an IgE-mediated reaction causing histamine to be released from the mast cells.

**Cholinergic urticaria**, characterized by the appearance of 1- to 3-mm wheals surrounded by large erythematous flares after an increase in core body temperature, occurs commonly in young adults. Lesions may develop during strenuous exercise after a hot bath or emotional stress. The lack of airway symptoms differentiates it from exercise-induced anaphylaxis.

**Cold urticaria** occurs with exposure to cold and may develop within minutes on areas directly exposed to cold or on rewarming of the affected parts. Ingestion of cold drinks may result in lip swelling. Cold urticaria syndromes can be categorized into acquired and familial disorders. Severe reactions resulting in death can occur with swimming or diving into cold water. Patients must never swim alone, avoid total body exposure to cold, and have injectable epinephrine available.

### TABLE 81-1 Etiology of Acute Urticaria

| | |
|---|---|
| Foods | Egg, milk, wheat, peanuts, tree nuts, soy, shellfish, fish, strawberries (direct mast cell degranulation) |
| Medications | Suspect all medications, even over-the-counter or homeopathic medications |
| Insect stings | Hymenoptera (honeybee, yellow jacket, hornets, wasp, fire ants), biting insects (papular urticaria) |
| Infections | Bacterial (group A streptococcus pharyngitis, *Mycoplasma*, sinusitis); viral (hepatitis B, mononucleosis [EBV], coxsackieviruses A and B); parasitic (*Ascaris, Ancylostoma, Echinococcus, Fasciola, Filaria, Schistosoma, Strongyloides, Toxocara, Trichinella*); fungal (dermatophytes, *Candida*) |
| Contact allergy | Latex, pollen, animal saliva, nettle plants, caterpillars |
| Transfusion reactions | Blood, blood products, or IVIG administration |
| Idiopathic | |

EBV, Epstein-Barr virus; IVIG, intravenous immunoglobulin.
From Lasley MV, Kennedy MS, Altman LC: Urticaria and angioedema. In Altman LC, Becker JW, Williams PV, editors: Allergy in Primary Care, Philadelphia, 2000, *Saunders*, p 232.

### TABLE 81-2 Etiology of Chronic Urticaria

| | |
|---|---|
| Idiopathic | 75%–90% of cases |
| | 25%–50% of adult patients have IgG, anti-IgE, and anti-FcεRI (high-affinity IgE receptor alpha chain) autoantibodies |
| Physical | Dermatographism |
| | Cholinergic urticaria |
| | Cold urticaria |
| | Delayed pressure urticaria |
| | Solar urticaria |
| | Vibratory urticaria |
| | Aquagenic urticaria |
| Rheumatologic | Systemic lupus erythematosus |
| | Juvenile rheumatoid arthritis |
| Endocrine | Hyperthyroidism |
| | Hypothyroidism |
| Neoplastic | Lymphoma |
| | Mastocytosis |
| | Leukemia |
| Angioedema | Hereditary angioedema (autosomal dominant inherited deficiency of C1-esterase inhibitor) |
| | Acquired angioedema |
| | Angiotensin-converting enzyme inhibitors |

From Lasley MV, Kennedy MS, Altman LC: Urticaria and angioedema. In Altman LC, Becker JW, Williams PV, editors: Allergy in Primary Care, Philadelphia, 2000, *Saunders*, p 234.

**Hereditary angioedema** is an autosomal dominant disease due to a deficiency of C1 inhibitor. The genetic defect may be caused by spontaneous mutation; approximately 25% of cases occur in patients without any family history. The disease is estimated to affect approximately 10,000 persons in the United States. It is characterized by unpredictable, recurrent attacks of episodic swelling that involves the face, peripheral extremities, genitalia, abdomen, oropharynx, and pharynx. Asphyxiation from laryngeal attacks is a significant cause of mortality. Patients with hereditary angioedema rarely have urticaria associated with angioedema. The majority of patients (85%) have **type 1** disease, which is due to decreased production of C1-esterase inhibitor. A minority of patients (15%) have **type 2** disease, which is due to production of dysfunctional C1-esterase inhibitor. A low C4 level serves as an initial screening test. Patients with reduced C4 should have quantitative and functional levels of C1-esterase inhibitor measured. The U.S. FDA recently approved three products to treat HEA attacks: Berinet (facial or abdominal attacks), Kalbitor® (for children ≥16 years of age), and Cinryze.

**Anaphylactic reactions** are type I, IgE-mediated reactions and result from many causes (Table 81-3). Cross-linking of the IgE molecule with the allergen leads to IgE receptor activation on the mast cell and basophil and release of mediators, including histamine, tryptase, tumor necrosis factor, platelet-activating factor, leukotrienes, prostaglandins, and cytokines. Other cell types involved in the reactions include monocytes, macrophages, eosinophils, neutrophils, and platelets. The mediator release results in the clinical picture of anaphylaxis.

### TABLE 81-3 Common Causes of Anaphylaxis in Children*

| | |
|---|---|
| Foods | Peanuts, tree nuts, milk, eggs, fish, shellfish, seeds, fruits, grains |
| Drugs | Penicillins, cephalosporins, sulfonamides, nonsteroidal anti-inflammatory drugs, opiates, muscle relaxants, vancomycin, dextran, thiamine, vitamin $B_{12}$, insulin, thiopental, local anesthetics |
| Hymenoptera venom | Honeybee, yellow jacket, wasp, hornet, fire ant |
| Latex | |
| Allergen immunotherapy | |
| Exercise | Food-specific exercise, postprandial (non–food-specific) exercise |
| Vaccinations | Tetanus, measles, mumps, influenza |
| Miscellaneous | Radiocontrast media, immunoglobulin, cold temperature, chemotherapeutic agents, blood products, inhalants |
| Idiopathic | |

*In order of frequency.
From Young MC: General treatment of anaphylaxis. In Leung DYM, Sampson HA, Geha RS, Szefler SJ, editors: Pediatric Allergy: Principles and Practice, St Louis, 2003, *Mosby*, p 644.

Anaphylactoid reactions are due to nonimmunologic mechanisms. Mast cells and basophils can be activated by direct, nonspecific stimulation, although the exact underlying mechanism is unknown. Reactions to agents such as opiates and radiocontrast material are classic examples. Complement system activation also can result in mast cell and basophil activation. **Anaphylatoxins**, C3a and C5a, are named because of their ability to trigger mediator release and are generated in serum sickness. The most common cause of this type of reaction is transfusion with blood products. There are other causes of anaphylactoid reactions for which the mechanism has not been clarified.

## EPIDEMIOLOGY

Urticaria and angioedema are common skin conditions affecting 15% to 25% of individuals at some point in their lives. Most cases of urticaria are self-limited, but for some patients, they are chronic. In approximately 50% of patients, urticaria and angioedema occur together. In the remaining 50%, 40% have urticaria alone and 10% have angioedema alone. The incidence of anaphylaxis in children is unknown.

## CLINICAL MANIFESTATIONS

Raised, erythematous lesions with pale centers that are intensely pruritic characterize **urticaria**, commonly called **hives** (Fig. 81-1). The lesions vary in size and can occur anywhere on the body. Typically, urticaria arises suddenly and may resolve within 1 to 2 hours or may persist for 24 hours. **Angioedema** is a similar process that involves the deeper dermis or subcutaneous tissue, with swelling as the principal symptom. Generally, angioedema is not pruritic, may be mildly painful, and persists for longer than

24 hours. In rare cases, it may become life-threatening if swelling affects the upper airway.

The clinical manifestations of **anaphylaxis** and **anaphylactoid** reactions are the same for children and adults. The signs and symptoms vary and can range from mild skin findings to a fatal reaction. Ninety percent of patients present with cutaneous symptoms, including urticaria, angioedema, flushing, and warmth; however, the absence of dermal symptoms does not exclude the diagnosis of anaphylaxis. Other affected organ systems include the respiratory tract (rhinorrhea, oropharyngeal edema, laryngeal edema, hoarseness, stridor, wheezing, dyspnea, and asphyxiation), cardiovascular system (tachycardia, hypotension, shock, syncope, and arrhythmias), gastrointestinal tract (nausea, abdominal pain, crampy diarrhea, and vomiting) and neurologic system (syncope, seizure, dizziness, and a sense of impending doom). The severity of an anaphylactic reaction is often proportionate to the speed of symptom onset.

## LABORATORY AND IMAGING STUDIES

The laboratory evaluation of patients with urticaria and angioedema must be tailored to the clinical situation. Acute urticaria and angioedema do not require specific laboratory evaluation except to document the suspected cause. For patients with chronic urticaria and angioedema, laboratory evaluation should be performed to exclude underlying diseases (Table 81-4). Patients with recurrent angioedema without urticaria should be evaluated for hereditary angioedema (Table 81-5).

Measurement of the mast cell mediators, histamine and tryptase, may be helpful when the diagnosis of anaphylaxis is in question. A tryptase level is a more useful test because histamine is released quickly, has a short half-life, and is often difficult to detect in the serum. Serum tryptase levels peak 1 to 1.5 hours after

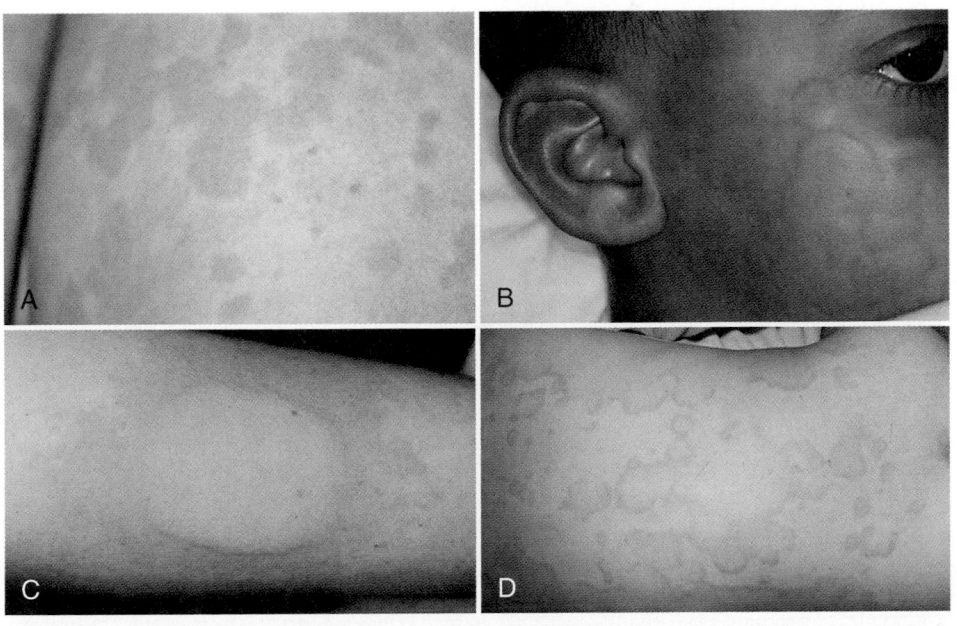

**FIGURE 81-1**

Examples of urticaria. (From Zitelli BJ, Davis HW, editors: Pediatric Physical Diagnosis Electronic Atlas, Philadelphia, 2004, *Mosby*.)

**TABLE 81-4 Suggested Testing for Chronic Urticaria/Angioedema of Unknown Etiology**

| Basic Tests | Discretionary Tests Based on |
|---|---|
| Complete blood count with differential | If vasculitis is suspected |
| Erythrocyte sedimentation rate | Antinuclear antibody |
| Urinalysis | Skin biopsy |
| Liver function tests | $CH_{50}$ |
| Thyroid function and autoantibodies | If liver function tests abnormal |
| Autoimmune chronic urticaria test–anti-FcεR autoantibody | Serology for hepatitis B |

From Zuraw B: Urticaria and angioedema. In Leung DYM, Sampson HA, Geha RS, Szefler SJ, editors: Pediatric Allergy: Principles and Practice, St Louis, 2003, *Mosby*, p 580.

anaphylaxis. Elevated levels may be helpful in establishing the diagnosis, but normal tryptase levels do not rule out the diagnosis. It is best to measure a serum tryptase level 1 to 2 hours after the onset of symptoms. It also can be ordered retrospectively on stored serum that is less than 2 days old.

## DIFFERENTIAL DIAGNOSIS

The diagnosis of urticaria and angioedema is straightforward; finding the etiology may be more difficult. Other dermatologic conditions can mimic urticaria. **Erythema multiforme** has target-shaped, erythematous, macular or papular lesions that may look similar to urticaria, but the lesions are fixed and last for several days. Other dermatologic diseases include dermatitis herpetiformis and bullous pemphigoid, which are quite pruritic, and early on, the lesions may resemble urticaria. Mastocytosis is characterized by mast cell infiltration of various organs, including the skin. Some patients have skin lesions similar in appearance to urticaria rather than the classic urticaria pigmentosa. Urticaria pigmentosa appears as hyperpigmented, red-brown macules, which may coalesce. When these lesions are stroked, they urticate, which is called the **Darier sign**. A rare disorder that should be included in the differential diagnosis of urticaria is **Muckle-Wells syndrome**. It is an autosomal dominant disorder characterized by episodic urticaria presenting in infancy, with sensorineural deafness, amyloidosis, arthralgias, and skeletal abnormalities. Another rare syndrome is **Schnitzler syndrome**, which is characterized by chronic urticaria, macroglobulinemia, bone pain, anemia, fever, fatigue, and weight loss. **Urticarial vasculitis** is a small vessel vasculitis with histologic features of a leukocytoclastic response. The main distinguishing feature is that the lesions last longer than 24 hours, may be tender, and leave behind skin pigmentation. Skin biopsy is required for definitive diagnosis.

The diagnosis of anaphylaxis is usually apparent from the acute and often dramatic onset of multisystem involvement of the skin, respiratory tract, and cardiovascular system. Sudden cardiovascular collapse in the absence of cutaneous symptoms suggests vasovagal collapse, seizure disorder, aspiration, pulmonary embolism, or myocardial infarction. Laryngeal edema, especially with abdominal pain, suggests hereditary angioedema. Many patients with anaphylaxis are initially thought to have septic shock (see Chapter 40).

## TREATMENT

Avoidance of triggering agents is important in management of urticaria and angioedema. The mainstay of pharmacologic treatment is $H_1$ antihistamines. Second-generation $H_1$ antihistamines, such as cetirizine, desloratadine, fexofenadine, levocetirizine, and loratadine, are preferred because they have

**TABLE 81-5 Complement Evaluation of Patients with Recurrent Angioedema**

| Assay | Idiopathic Angioedema | Type I Hereditary Angioedema | Type II Hereditary Angioedema | Acquired C1-Esterase Inhibitor Deficiency | Vasculitis |
|---|---|---|---|---|---|
| C4 | Normal | Low | Low | Low | Low or normal |
| C4d/C4 ratio | Normal | High | High | High | High or normal |
| C1-esterase inhibitor level | Normal | Low | Normal | Low | Normal |
| C1-esterase inhibitor function | Normal | Low | Low | Low | Normal |
| C1q | Normal | Normal | Normal | Low | Low or normal |
| C3 | Normal | Normal | Normal | Normal | Low or normal |

From Zuraw B: Urticaria and angioedema. In Leung DYM, Sampson HA, Geha RS, Szefler SJ, editors: Pediatric Allergy: Principles and Practice, St Louis, 2003, *Mosby*, p 580.

fewer adverse effects. If a second-generation $H_1$ antihistamine, by itself, does not provide adequate relief, the next step is to add a sedating $H_1$ antihistamine at bedtime or $H_2$ antihistamines, such as cimetidine or ranitidine. Tricyclic antidepressants, such as doxepin, exhibit potent activity at both $H_1$ and $H_2$ receptors. Corticosteroids are effective in treating urticaria and angioedema, although adverse effects from long-term use mandate the lowest dose for the shortest time. When urticaria is resistant to treatment, other immunomodulating agents, such as cyclosporine, hydroxychloroquine, methotrexate, cyclophosphamide, and intravenous immunoglobulin, have been used; however, data supporting their use is limited.

Anaphylaxis is a medical emergency; prompt recognition and immediate treatment are crucial (Fig. 81-2). Early administration of intramuscular epinephrine is the mainstay of therapy and should be given at the same time basic measures of cardiopulmonary resuscitation are being performed. If the child is not in a medical setting, emergency medical services should be called. Supplemental oxygen and intravenous fluid should be administered with the child lying in supine position. An airway must be secured; intubation or tracheotomy may be required. Additional pharmacologic therapies, such as corticosteroids, antihistamines, $H_2$-receptor antagonists, and bronchodilators, may be given to improve symptoms. Up to 20% of people with anaphylaxis have **biphasic** or **protracted** anaphylaxis.

A person with **biphasic anaphylaxis** has both an early- and late-phase reaction. The biphasic reaction is a recurrence of anaphylactic symptoms after an initial remission, occurring within 8 to 72 hours after the initial reaction. A person with **protracted anaphylaxis** has signs and symptoms that persist for hours or even days despite treatment, although this is rare.

## PREVENTION

Prevention of urticaria, angioedema, and anaphylaxis focuses on avoidance of known triggers. A referral to an allergy specialist for a thorough history, diagnostic testing, and recommendations for avoidance is suggested for patients following severe reactions or anaphylaxis. Skin testing and serum IgE-specific testing are available for foods, inhalants, insect venoms, drugs (penicillin), vaccines, and latex. Educating the patient and family members about the signs and symptoms of anaphylaxis and using self-administered epinephrine early result in better outcomes. Fatal anaphylaxis has occurred, however, despite timely and appropriate treatment. A **MedicAlert bracelet** with appropriate information should be worn. Medications such as β-blockers, angiotensin-converting enzyme inhibitors, and monoamine oxidase inhibitors should be discontinued because they may exacerbate anaphylaxis or interfere with its treatment.

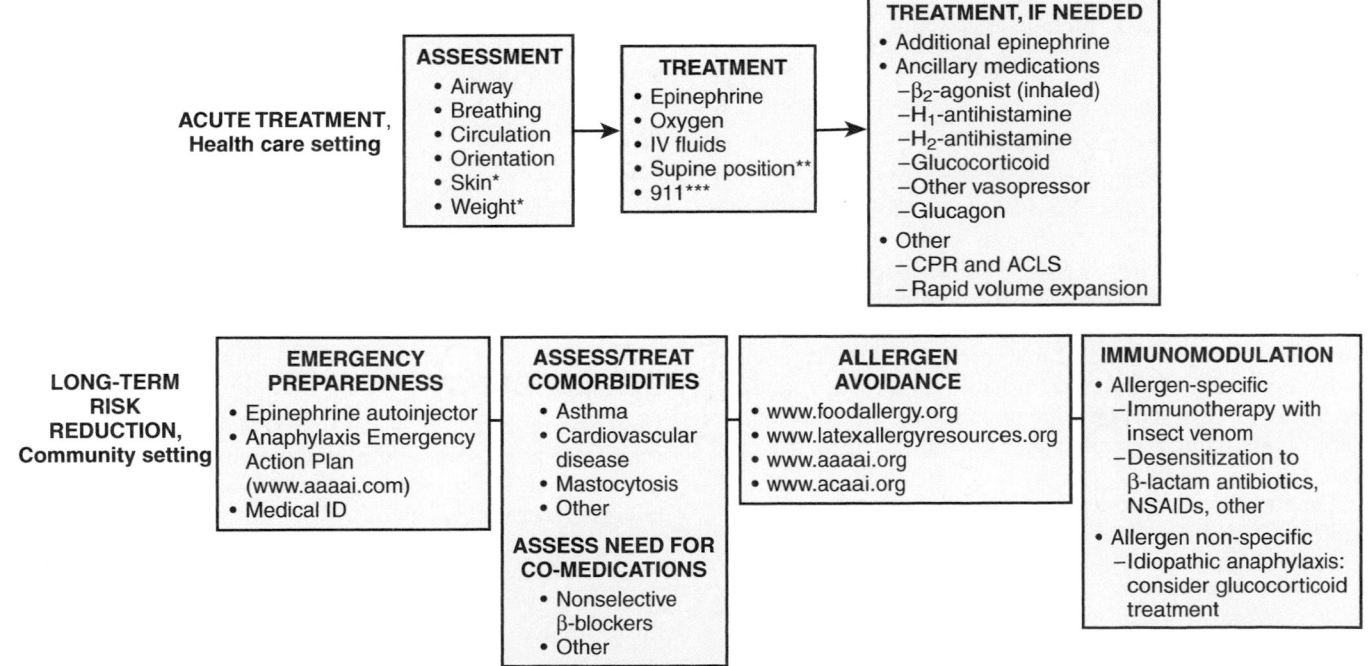

**FIGURE 81-2**

Anaphylaxis management. Summary of anaphylaxis management. Acute treatment is the same regardless of the mechanism or trigger involved in anaphylaxis. In contrast, for long-term risk reduction, avoidance measures and immunomodulation are trigger-specific; currently, immunomodulation is available only for a minority of individuals with anaphylaxis. All at-risk individuals need to have comorbidities and comedications assessed, be taught the importance of emergency preparedness, and be instructed in the use of self-injectable epinephrine.
*The skin should be inspected, and weight estimation is important, especially in infants and children, and also in overweight and obese teens and adults, in order to calculate an optimal dose of epinephrine and other medications needed in treatment and resuscitation.
**Supine position, as tolerated, to prevent empty ventricle syndrome.
***Call 911/emergency medical services for anaphylaxis occurring in community health care facilities such as medical, dental, or infusion clinics, where optimal backup might not be available for resuscitation.
ACLS, advanced cardiac life support; CPR, cardiopulmonary resuscitation; CVS, cardiovascular; GI, gastrointestinal; ID, identification (e.g., bracelet, wallet card); IV, intravenous. (From Simon FER: Anaphylaxis. *J Allergy Clin Immunol* 121:S405, 2008.)

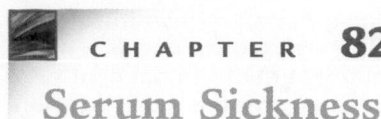

# CHAPTER 82
# Serum Sickness

## ETIOLOGY

Serum sickness is a type III hypersensitivity reaction (see Table 77-1). The patient's immune system recognizes the proteins in the drug or antiserum as foreign and produces antibodies against them. The newly formed antibodies bind with the foreign protein to form antigen-antibody or immune complexes, which may enter the circulation and be deposited in blood vessels and in filtering organs. These complexes cause tissue injury by activating the complement cascade and recruiting neutrophils, resulting in increased capillary permeability, toxic mediator release, and tissue damage.

## EPIDEMIOLOGY

Immune complexes were first described after administration of heterologous serum, such as horse serum for diphtheria. The availability of human-derived biologicals, bioengineered antibodies, and alternative pharmacotherapies has greatly reduced the incidence of serum sickness. Common inciting agents include blood products and foreign proteins, such as antithymocyte globulin and antivenoms. Medications frequently implicated include penicillin, sulfonamides, minocycline, cefaclor, hydantoins, and thiazides.

## CLINICAL MANIFESTATIONS

The symptoms of serum sickness typically occur 7 to 21 days after the administration of drugs, foreign proteins, or infections. Symptom onset may be more rapid (within 1 to 4 days) in previously sensitized individuals. The classic clinical manifestations consist of fever, polyarticular arthralgias, lymphadenopathy, and cutaneous symptoms. Cutaneous lesions vary and may include urticaria, angioedema, erythema multiforme, morbilliform rash, and a palpable purpura or serpiginous rash at the interface of the dorsal and palmar or plantar aspects of the hands and feet.

Carditis, glomerulonephritis, Guillain-Barré syndrome, encephalomyelitis, and peripheral neuritis are rare complications.

## LABORATORY AND IMAGING STUDIES

Laboratory tests may show an elevated erythrocyte sedimentation rate, presence of circulating immune complexes measured by $^{125}$I-C1q binding assay, and depressed complement (C3 and C4) levels. Skin biopsy specimens show immune deposits of IgM, IgA, IgE, or C3. Hematuria or proteinuria or both may be present. The diagnosis is established by history of exposure to an inciting cause, characteristic clinical manifestations, and laboratory testing showing circulating immune complexes and depressed complement levels.

## TREATMENT AND PREVENTION

Serum sickness is self-limited and resolves within 1 to 2 weeks; therefore, treatment is symptomatic relief. Antihistamines may be administered to relieve pruritus. Aspirin and other nonsteroidal anti-inflammatory drugs are given for fever and joint pain, and if necessary, prednisone (1 to 2 mg/kg orally daily) is administered with a tapering dose. Allergy skin testing does not predict the likelihood of serum sickness development.

The primary means of prevention is to avoid exposure to the implicated cause.

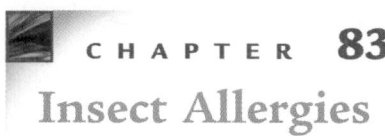

# CHAPTER 83
# Insect Allergies

## ETIOLOGY

Systemic allergic reactions usually result from stinging insects of the order **Hymenoptera**, which include **apids** (honeybee and bumblebee), **vespids** (yellow jacket, wasp, yellow-face and white-face hornets), and **formicids** (fire and harvester ants). Honeybees have a barbed stinger that remains embedded after a sting. Yellow jackets are responsible for most allergic reactions in most parts of the United States, whereas wasps are the most frequent cause of sting reactions in Texas. Fire ants are found in the southeastern and south central United States.

Biting insects rarely cause anaphylaxis. Anaphylaxis has been described, however, after the bites of kissing bug (*Triatoma*), bed bug, blackfly, and deerfly. Large local reactions from biting insects, such as mosquitoes, fleas, and flies, are a more common occurrence. The reaction appears urticarial and is caused by the salivary secretions deposited by the biting insect and does represent an allergic response.

## EPIDEMIOLOGY

Insect sting allergy may develop at any age and typically manifests after several uneventful stings. Although children are stung more frequently than adults, systemic allergic reactions occur in only about 1% of children and 3% of adults. Reactions in adults are generally more severe than in children and can result in death. Large local reactions to insect stings are more common in children, with an estimated incidence of 20% for children and 10% for adults.

## CLINICAL MANIFESTATIONS

The diagnosis of insect sting allergy is dependent on the history of the reaction and the presence of venom-specific IgE. Normal reactions to insect stings, which are observed in 90% of children, include localized pain, swelling, and erythema at the sting site that usually subside within 24 hours. Large local reactions occur in approximately 10% of patients. They are usually late-phase, IgE-mediated

**TABLE 83-1  Classification of Insect Sting Reactions**

| Reaction Type | Characteristics |
|---|---|
| Normal | <2 inches in diameter<br>Transient pain and erythema<br>Duration <24 hr |
| Large local reaction | >2 inches in diameter<br>Swelling contiguous to the site<br>Duration 2–7 days |
| Systemic | |
| Non–life-threatening | Immediate generalized reaction confined to the skin (erythema, urticaria, angioedema) |
| Life-threatening | Immediate generalized reaction not confined to the skin with respiratory (laryngeal edema, bronchospasm) or cardiovascular (hypotension, shock) symptoms |
| Toxic | Follows multiple stings, produced by exogenous vasoactive amines in venom |
| Unusual | Serum sickness, vasculitis, nephrosis, neuritis, encephalitis<br>Symptoms start several days to weeks after the insect sting |

reactions, with large swelling, contiguous to the sting site that develops over 24 to 48 hours and resolves within 2 to 7 days. Virtually all individuals with large local reactions have similar reactions with subsequent stings. Systemic reactions are IgE mediated and occur in 1% of children. They can be mild and non–life-threatening with cutaneous symptoms only or life-threatening with respiratory, cardiovascular, or neurologic symptoms of anaphylaxis (see Chapter 81). Toxic reactions may result if a person receives a large number of stings (50 to 100). Symptoms include malaise, nausea, and emesis resulting from the toxic effects of the venom. Unusual reactions, such as vasculitis, nephrosis, neuritis, serum sickness, and encephalitis, rarely are associated with insect stings (Table 83-1).

## LABORATORY AND IMAGING STUDIES

A positive skin test to Hymenoptera venom extract demonstrates the presence of venom-specific IgE in the context of a positive sting reaction history and helps identify specific insects to which an individual is allergic. Venom-specific IgE antibodies also may be measured by in vitro serum tests (radioallergosorbent test [RAST]). Both testing methods should be considered complementary because neither test alone detects all patients with insect sting allergy. Future reactions correlate more with past individual patterns than the level of sensitivity of venom skin testing or RAST testing.

## DIFFERENTIAL DIAGNOSIS

A history of an immediate systemic reaction is necessary before venom testing and immunotherapy should be considered. Identification of the offending insect is often unreliable. Honeybee stings may be identified by the stinger that remains in place. Vespid stings are usually unprovoked and occur at summer's end when the insects are more aggressive.

## TREATMENT

Local reactions should be treated by cleaning the site, applying cold compresses, and administering oral antihistamines and analgesics. Occasionally, large local reactions may be mistaken for cellulitis. Infection is unlikely if reaction occurs within 24 to 48 hours after a sting. Treatment is with an oral corticosteroid for 4 to 5 days rather than oral antibiotics.

Treatment of systemic reactions is guided by the severity of the reaction, but epinephrine is the cornerstone of therapy and should be administered without delay. Antihistamines may be administered concurrently with epinephrine. Corticosteroids should be given to prevent recurrent or prolonged symptoms. For severe reactions, intravenous fluids and epinephrine, oxygen, and respiratory support in an intensive care unit may be needed. After acute care of a systemic sting reaction, patients should be provided an epinephrine autoinjector, referral to an allergist/immunologist, and instructions on prevention of insect stings.

## COMPLICATIONS

At least 50 to 100 fatalities per year in the United States are attributed to insect sting reactions. Most deaths (80%) occur in adults older than 40 years of age, and only 2% occur in individuals younger than 20 years of age. Approximately one half of deaths occur in persons without any history of a prior sting reaction.

## PROGNOSIS

Successfully avoiding the stinging insect is the most important prognostic factor. More than 85% of adults who complete 5 years of immunotherapy tolerate challenge stings without systemic reactions for 5 to 10 years after completion.

## PREVENTION

Commonsense measures to reduce the chance of accidental sting include exterminating infested areas; not eating or drinking outdoors; wearing long pants and shoes; and avoiding brightly colored clothing, fragrances, or hairspray when outdoors. Common insect repellents are not effective against Hymenoptera.

Current recommendations are to administer **venom immunotherapy** to individuals who have had a systemic life-threatening reaction from an insect sting and have positive venom skin tests or elevated levels of venom-specific IgE. All persons with a history of systemic reactions to insects should be instructed in the use of an epinephrine autoinjector and encouraged to wear a **MedicAlert bracelet.** Children younger than 16 years of age who have only had a cutaneous reaction generally do not require immunotherapy because their prognosis is benign and can be managed with the availability of epinephrine.

CHAPTER **84**

# Adverse Reactions to Foods

## ETIOLOGY AND EPIDEMIOLOGY

An **adverse reaction to food** is a generic description of any untoward reaction after food ingestion, including toxic reactions such as food poisoning and nontoxic reactions, which can be subdivided further into nonimmune and immune reactions. Lactose intolerance is a nonimmune reaction. Food allergy or hypersensitivity reactions encompass immune reactions to food and can be divided further into IgE-mediated reactions, which are typically rapid in onset, and non–IgE-mediated reactions.

**Oral tolerance** is the process of suppression of the immune response to the array of dietary elements ingested daily. **Food allergy or hypersensitivity reactions** are the result of immune reactions to glycoproteins and develop in genetically predisposed individuals. In children, cow's milk, eggs, peanuts, soybean, wheat, tree nuts, fish, and shellfish cause 90% of IgE-mediated reactions. In older children and adults, peanuts, tree nuts, fish, and shellfish account for most reactions. Exposure to the allergenic food protein results in cross-linking of the IgE receptor found on the mast cells and basophils, which become activated and degranulate, releasing numerous potent mediators and cytokines. Non–IgE-mediated reactions typically occur hours to days after the allergen ingestion and are manifest as gastrointestinal symptoms. A cell-mediated immune mechanism may be responsible.

Approximately 6% to 8% of children are affected with food allergy. In adults, this declines to 1% to 2%.

## CLINICAL MANIFESTATIONS

Symptoms of hypersensitivity reactions vary from involvement of the skin, gastrointestinal tract, and respiratory tract to anaphylaxis. Non–IgE-mediated food allergy typically presents during infancy as proctitis/proctocolitis, enteropathy, or enterocolitis (Table 84-1).

| TABLE 84-1 Gastrointestinal Food Allergic Disorders | | | | |
|---|---|---|---|---|
| **Disorder** | **Age Group** | **Characteristics** | **Diagnosis** | **Prognosis/Course** |
| **IGE-MEDIATED** | | | | |
| Acute gastrointestinal hypersensitivity | Any | Onset: minutes to 2 hr Nausea, abdominal pain, emesis, diarrhea Typically in conjunction with cutaneous and/or respiratory symptoms | History, positive PST, and/or serum food-IgE Confirmatory OFC | Variable, food-dependent Milk, soy, egg, and wheat typically outgrown Peanut, tree nuts, seeds, and shellfish typically persist |
| Pollen-food allergy syndrome (oral allergy syndrome) | Any Most common in young adults (50% of birch pollen adults) | Immediate symptoms on contact of raw fruit with oral mucosa Pruritus, tingling, erythema or angioedema of the lips, tongue, oropharynx, throat pruritus/tightness | History, positive PST with raw fruits or vegetables; OFC-positive with raw fruit, negative with cooked | Severity of symptoms may vary with pollen season Symptoms may improve with pollen immunotherapy in subset of patients |
| **IGE- AND/OR NON–IGE-MEDIATED** | | | | |
| Allergic eosinophilic esophagitis | Any, but especially infants, children, adolescents | Children: chronic/intermittent symptoms of gastroesophageal reflux, emesis, dysphagia, abdominal pain, irritability Adults: abdominal pain, dysphagia, food impaction | History, positive PST, and/or food-IgE in 50%, but poor correlation with clinical symptoms Patch testing may be of value Elimination diet and OFC Endoscopy, biopsy provides conclusive diagnosis and response to treatment information | Variable, not well established, improvement with elimination diet within 6–8 wk Elemental diet may be required Often responds to swallowed topical steroids |

**TABLE 84-1 Gastrointestinal Food Allergic Disorders—cont'd**

| Disorder | Age Group | Characteristics | Diagnosis | Prognosis/Course |
|---|---|---|---|---|
| Allergic eosinophilic gastroenteritis | Any | Chronic/intermittent abdominal pain, emesis, irritability, poor appetite, failure to thrive, weight loss, anemia, protein-losing gastroenteropathy | History, positive PST, and/or food-IgE in 50%, but poor correlation with clinical symptoms, elimination diet, and OFC. Endoscopy, biopsy provides conclusive diagnosis and response to treatment information | Variable, not well established, improvement with elimination diet within 6–8 wk. Elemental diet may be required |
| **NON–IGE-MEDIATED** | | | | |
| Allergic proctocolitis | Young infants (<6 mo), frequently breast-fed | Blood-streaked or heme-positive stools, otherwise healthy-appearing | History, prompt response (resolution of gross blood in 48 hr) to allergen elimination. Biopsy conclusive but not necessary in vast majority | Majority able to tolerate milk/soy by 1 yr of age |
| Food protein-induced enterocolitis syndrome | Young infants | Chronic emesis, diarrhea, failure to thrive on chronic exposure. On reexposure following a period of elimination, subacute, repetitive emesis, dehydration (15% shock), diarrhea. Breastfeeding protective | History, response to dietary restriction. OFC | Most resolve in 1–3 yr |
| Dietary protein-induced enteropathy | Young infants | Protracted diarrhea, (steatorrhea), emesis, failure to thrive, anemia in 40% | History, endoscopy, and biopsy. Response to dietary restriction | Most resolve in 1–2 yr |
| Celiac disease (gluten-sensitive enteropathy) | Any | Chronic diarrhea, malabsorption, abdominal distention, flatulence, failure to thrive or weight loss. May be associated with oral ulcers and/or dermatitis herpetiformis | Biopsy diagnostic: villus atrophy. Screening with serum IgA antitissue transglutaminase and antigliadin. Resolution of symptoms with gluten elimination and relapse on oral challenge | Lifelong |

OFC, oral food challenge; PST, prick skin test.
From Adkinson NF Jr, Bochner BS, Busse WW, et al: Middleton's Allergy: Principles and Practice, 7th ed, Philadelphia, 2008, *Mosby*.

## LABORATORY AND IMAGING STUDIES

In acute IgE reactions, skin prick allergy testing and serum testing to foods may help confirm the suspected food allergy.

## DIAGNOSIS

A careful history focuses on symptoms, the time interval from ingestion to onset of symptoms, the quantity of food necessary to evoke the reaction, the most recent reaction, patterns of reactivity, and associated factors such as exercise and medication use. Skin prick testing can be performed to confirm IgE-mediated food allergies. A negative skin test virtually excludes an IgE-mediated reaction (unless the clinical history suggests a severe reaction after an isolated ingestion of the food). A positive skin test indicates sensitization, but does not prove clinical reactivity and must be interpreted based on the history.

An in vitro radioallergosorbent test (RAST) can be obtained for specific allergens. The CAP-RAST is a quantitative measurement of food-specific IgE antibodies and offers improved specificity and reproducibility compared with other RAST methods. These tests provide supplementary information to skin tests. Researchers have tried to determine concentrations of food-specific IgE at which clinical reactions are highly likely to occur (Table 84-2). Patients with CAP-RAST levels greater than 95% of the

| TABLE 84-2 Interpretation of Serum IgE Antibody Concentrations | | |
|---|---|---|
| Food | Food-Specific IgE Antibody Concentrations at or Above Which Clinical Reactions Are Highly Likely (kUa/L) | Positive Predictive Value (%) |
| Egg | 7 | 98 |
| ≤2 yr of age | 2 | 95 |
| Milk | 15 | 95 |
| ≤2 yr of age | 5 | 95 |
| Peanut | 14 | 95–100 |
| Fish | 20 | 100 |
| Soybean | 30 | 73 |
| Wheat | 26 | 74 |
| Tree nuts | ~15 | ~95 |

Adapted from Sampson HA: Food allergy. *J Allergy Clin Immunol* 111: S544, 2003.

predictive value may be considered allergic, and there is no need for an oral food challenge. Monitoring the CAP-RAST level may be helpful in predicting whether a child has outgrown the food allergy. Oral food challenges remain the standard of diagnosis and can be performed to determine if a child can eat the food safely.

## TREATMENT

Currently, management of food allergies consists of educating the patient to avoid ingestion of the responsible allergen and to initiate therapy if ingestion occurs. For mild symptoms limited to the skin only, such as mild itching or hives in the area of allergen contact, oral antihistamines such as diphenhydramine can be administered. If symptoms extend beyond skin, including, but not limited to, difficulty breathing or swallowing, tongue or throat swelling, vomiting, and fainting or symptoms not responding to diphenhydramine within 20 minutes, injectable epinephrine should be administered and immediate medical attention pursued. Types of injectable epinephrine include EpiPen (0.3 mg), EpiPen Jr. (0.15 mg), Twinject (0.3 or 0.15 mg).

## COMPLICATIONS

Anaphylaxis is the most serious complication of allergic food reactions and can result in death (see Chapter 81).

## PROGNOSIS AND PREVENTION

Hypersensitivity to egg, milk, wheat, and soy resolves within the first 5 years of life in approximately 80% of children. Sensitivity to certain foods, such as peanuts, tree nuts, fish, and shellfish, tends to be lifelong. However, 20% of children who manifested peanut allergy younger than 2 years of age may outgrow it.

Avoidance of the suspect food is crucial. Careful reading of food labels is a priority. A **MedicAlert bracelet** with appropriate information should be worn. The Food

Allergy Network (www.foodallergy.org) is a useful educational resource for families and physicians.

Recommendations for prevention of allergic diseases aimed at the *high-risk* newborn who has not manifested atopic disease include (1) breastfeeding for the first 4 to 6 months, or, (2) if supplementing, using a hydrolyzed casein formula (e.g., Alimentum or Nutramigen) or partially hydrolyzed whey formula (e.g., Good Start) for the first 4 to 6 months and delaying introduction of solid foods until 4 to 6 months of age. Other approaches, such as maternal avoidance diets during pregnancy and during lactation, as well as avoidance of allergenic foods for infants beyond 6 months of age, are unproven.

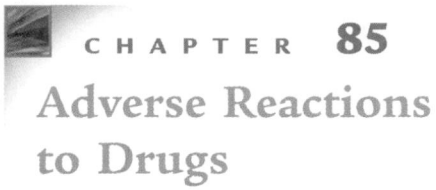

CHAPTER **85**

# Adverse Reactions to Drugs

## ETIOLOGY

An **adverse drug reaction** is defined as an unwanted, negative consequence associated with the use of a drug or biologic agent. Drug reactions can be classified as immunologic or nonimmunologic reactions (Table 85-1). Nearly 75% to 80% of adverse drug reactions are caused by a predictable, nonimmunologic mechanism, and between 5% and 10% of all drug reactions are explained by an immune-mediated mechanism. The remaining drug reactions are caused by an unpredictable mechanism, which may or may not be immune mediated. The **Gell and Coombs classification** can be used to describe some drug-induced allergic reactions (see Table 77-1). Many drug reactions cannot be classified because the exact immune mechanism has not been defined. Most drugs cannot elicit an immune response because of their small size; rather, the drug or a metabolite acts as a hapten and binds to larger molecules, such as tissue or serum proteins, a process called **haptenation**. The multivalent hapten-protein complex forms a new immunogenic epitope that elicits T- and B-lymphocyte responses.

## EPIDEMIOLOGY

Drug reactions to penicillins and cephalosporins are the most common allergic drug reactions encountered in the pediatric population. Approximately 6% to 10% of children are labeled as *penicillin allergic*. Risk factors for drug reactions include previous drug exposure, increasing age (>20 years of age), parenteral or topical administration, higher dose, intermittent repeated exposure, and a genetic predisposition of slow drug metabolism. An atopic background does not predispose an individual to the development of drug reactions but may indicate a greater risk of serious reaction.

**TABLE 85-1 Classification of Adverse Drug Reactions**

| Type | Example |
|------|---------|
| **IMMUNOLOGIC** | |
| Type I reaction (IgE-mediated) | Anaphylaxis from β-lactam antibiotic |
| Type II reaction (cytotoxic) | Hemolytic anemia from penicillin |
| Type III reaction (immune complex) | Serum sickness from antithymocyte globulin |
| Type IV reaction (delayed, cell-mediated) | Contact dermatitis from topical antihistamine |
| Specific T-cell activation | Morbilliform rash from sulfonamides |
| Fas/Fas ligand-induced apoptosis | Stevens-Johnson syndrome; toxic epidermal necrolysis |
| Other | Drug-induced lupus-like syndrome; anticonvulsant hypersensitivity syndrome |
| **NONIMMUNOLOGIC** | |
| *Predictable* | |
| Pharmacologic adverse effect | Dry mouth from antihistamines; tremor from albuterol |
| Secondary pharmacologic adverse effect | Thrush while taking antibiotics; *Clostridium difficile*–associated colitis (pseudomembranous colitis) from clindamycin (and other antibiotics) |
| Drug toxicity | Hepatotoxicity from methotrexate |
| Drug-drug interactions | Torsades de pointes arrhythmia from terfenadine with erythromycin |
| Drug overdose | Hepatic necrosis from acetaminophen |
| *Unpredictable* | |
| Pseudoallergic | Anaphylactoid reaction after radiocontrast media |
| Idiosyncratic | Hemolytic anemia in a patient with G6PD deficiency after primaquine therapy |
| Intolerance | Tinnitus after a single, small dose of aspirin |

G6PD, glucose-6-phosphate dehydrogenase.
Adapted from Riedl MA, Casillas AM: Adverse drug reactions: types and treatment options. *Am Fam Phys* 68:1782, 2003. Copyright ©2003 American Academy of Family Physicians. All rights reserved.

## CLINICAL MANIFESTATIONS

Allergic reactions can be classified into **immediate (anaphylactic) reactions**, which occur within 60 minutes of drug administration; **accelerated reactions**, which begin 1 to 72 hours after drug administration; and **late reactions**, which occur after 72 hours. The most common form of adverse drug reaction is cutaneous. Accelerated reactions are usually dermatologic or serum sickness reactions. Late reactions include desquamating dermatitis, Stevens-Johnson syndrome, toxic epidermal necrolysis, and serum sickness.

## LABORATORY AND IMAGING STUDIES

Skin testing protocols are standardized for penicillin and are well described for other agents, such as local anesthetics, muscle relaxants, vaccines, and insulin. Positive skin testing to such reagents confirms the presence of antigen-specific IgE and supports the diagnosis of a type I hypersensitivity reaction in the appropriate clinical setting.

## DIFFERENTIAL DIAGNOSIS

The broadest experience with managing adverse drug reactions is with penicillin. Penicillin allergy should be evaluated when the individual is well and not in acute need of treatment. Penicillin skin testing is helpful for IgE-mediated reactions because of its negative predictive value; only 1% to 3% of patients with negative skin tests

have a reaction, which is mild, when reexposed to penicillin. Skin testing for penicillin should be performed using the **major determinant, penicilloylpolylysine** (available as Pre-Pen), and **minor determinants**, which include penicillin G, penicilloate, and penilloate. Skin testing to penicillin does not predict non–IgE-mediated reactions. For patients with a history consistent with serum sickness or desquamative-type reactions, skin testing should not be performed, and penicillin should be avoided indefinitely.

The risk of a child, who has reacted positively to penicillin skin testing, suffering an allergic reaction to a cephalosporin antibiotic is less than 2%. It is believed that the first-generation cephalosporins (e.g., cephalexin) are more likely than second-generation (e.g., cefuroxime) or third-generation (cefpodoxime) cephalosporins to be cross-reactive. This is due to the chemical similarity of side chains of the β-lactam ring between penicillin and first-generation cephalosporins.

## TREATMENT

If penicillin skin testing is positive, penicillin should be avoided, and an alternative antibiotic should be used. If there is a definite need for penicillin, **desensitization** can be accomplished by administration of increasing amounts of drug over a short time in a hospital setting. The exact mechanism of desensitization is unclear; however, it is thought to render mast cells unresponsive to the drug. To maintain desensitization, the drug must be given at least twice daily. If the drug is stopped for longer than

48 hours, the patient is no longer *desensitized*, and the same protocol must be repeated before repeated antibiotic use.

For other antibiotics, the relevant allergenic determinants produced by metabolism or degradation are not well defined. Skin testing to the native antibiotic in nonirritating concentrations can be performed. A negative response does not exclude allergy; however, a positive response suggests the presence of IgE-mediated allergy. In the case of a negative skin test response, a graded challenge or test dose may be administered, depending on the clinical history of the reaction. Patients who have experienced Stevens-Johnson syndrome, toxic epidermal necrolysis, or serum sickness should not be challenged.

## COMPLICATIONS

Anaphylaxis is the most serious complication of allergic drug reactions and can result in death (see Chapter 81).

## PROGNOSIS

Most drug reactions do not seem to be allergic in nature. Repeated, intermittent exposure during childhood or early adulthood contributes to an increased incidence of adverse drug reactions in adults.

## PREVENTION

Avoidance of the suspect drug is paramount. A **Medic-Alert bracelet** with appropriate information should be worn. One of the most common concerns in regard to allergic drug reactions is cross-reactivity between penicillin and cephalosporins. In children with a history of penicillin allergy, it is important to determine if they are truly allergic by skin testing to penicillin, using the major and minor determinants. If the penicillin skin test is negative, there is not an increased risk of an allergic reaction to cephalosporins. A positive penicillin skin test leads to an alternate non–cross-reacting antibiotic, a graded challenge to the required cephalosporin under appropriate monitoring, or desensitization to the required cephalosporin.

For children with a history of a cephalosporin allergy who require another cephalosporin, two approaches may be considered: a graded challenge with a cephalosporin that does not share the same side chain determinant, or skin testing with the same or a different cephalosporin. A positive response suggests the presence of IgE-mediated allergy, and the value of a negative test is unknown. Skin testing with cephalosporins has not been standardized or validated.

## SUGGESTED   READING

Bieber T: Atopic dermatitis, *N Engl J Med* 58:483–1494, 2008.

Greer FR, Sicherer SH, Burks AW: Effects of early nutritional interventions on the development of atopic disease in infants and children: the role of maternal dietary restriction, breastfeeding, timing of introduction of complementary foods and hydrolyzed formulas, *Pediatrics* 121:183–191, 2008.

Leung DYM, Sampson HA, Geha RS, et al: Pediatric Allergy: Principles and Practice, St Louis, 2003, *Mosby*.

National Heart Lung and Blood Institute and National Asthma Education and Prevention Program: Expert panel report 3: guidelines for the diagnosis and management of asthma. Full report 2007. *NIH Publication No. 08-4051.* Bethesda, MD, 2007, U.S. Department of Health and Human Services. Available at: http://www.nhlbi.nih.gov/guidelines/asthma/asthgdln.htm.

National Heart Lung Blood Institute and National Asthma Education and Prevention Program: Expert panel report 3: guidelines for the diagnosis and management of asthma. Summary report 2007. *NIH Publication No. 08-5846.* Bethesda, MD, 2007, U.S. Department of Health and Human Services. Available at: http://www.nhlbi.nih.gov/guidelines/asthma/asthsumm.pdf.

Shearer WT, Leung DYM: 2006 Mini-primer on allergic and immunologic diseases, *J Allergy Clin Immunol* 117(2):S429–S493, 2006.

Shearer WT, Leung DYM: Mini-primer on allergic and immunologic diseases, *J Allergy Clin Immunol* 121(2):S263–S425, 2008.

Sicherer SH: Understanding and Managing Your Child's Food Allergies, Baltimore, 2006, *Johns Hopkins University Press.*

Wood RA: Food Allergies for Dummies, Hoboken, 2007, *Wiley Publishing, Inc.*

Williams HC: Atopic dermatitis, *N Engl J Med* 352:2314–2324, 2005.

# RHEUMATIC DISEASES OF CHILDHOOD

Hilary M. Haftel

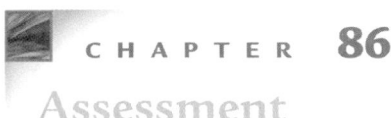

CHAPTER 86

## Assessment

The **rheumatic diseases (collagen vascular or connective tissue diseases)** of childhood are characterized by autoimmunity and inflammation, which may be localized or generalized. The classic rheumatic diseases of children include juvenile rheumatoid arthritis (JRA), systemic lupus erythematosus (SLE), and juvenile dermatomyositis (JDM). Vasculitis is a component of many rheumatic diseases. **Musculoskeletal pain syndromes** are a set of overlapping conditions characterized by poorly localized pain involving the extremities. Scleroderma, Behçet disease, and Sjögren syndrome are rare in childhood. The differential diagnosis of rheumatologic disorders typically includes infections, postinfectious processes, and malignancies (Table 86-1).

## HISTORY

The history identifies symptoms that reflect the source of the inflammation, including whether it is localized or systemic. Symptoms of systemic inflammation tend to be nonspecific. **Fever**, caused by cytokine release, can take many forms. A hectic fever, without periodicity or pattern, is commonly found in vasculitides such as Kawasaki disease but also occurs in children with underlying infection. Certain illnesses, such as systemic-onset JRA, produce a patterned fever with regular temperature spikes once or twice a day. Other rheumatic illnesses cause low-grade fevers. Charting the child's fever pattern, particularly in the absence of antipyretics, is useful. Rashes occur in many forms (see Table 86-1). Other systemic symptoms (malaise, anorexia, weight loss, and fatigue) can vary from mild to debilitating.

Symptoms of localized inflammation vary depending on the involved site. **Arthritis**, or inflammation of the synovium (**synovitis**), leads to joint pain, swelling, and impaired ability to use the affected joint. Morning stiffness or gelling is described. The child may be slow to arise in the morning and may have a limp. Children may refrain from usual activities and athletics. **Enthesitis** is inflammation at the insertion of a ligament to a bone. **Serositis**, inflammation of serosal lining such as pleuritis, pericarditis, or peritonitis, gives rise to chest pain, shortness of breath, or abdominal pain. **Myositis**, inflammation of the muscle, may lead to symptoms of muscle pain, weakness, or difficulty performing tasks of daily living. **Vasculitis**, inflammation of the blood vessels, leads to nonspecific symptoms of rash (petechiae, purpura) and edema when small vessels deep in the papillary dermis are involved; involvement of medium-sized vessels results in a circumscribed tender nodule.

## PHYSICAL EXAMINATION

A thorough history and physical examination is frequently sufficient to narrow the differential diagnosis and elicit the diagnosis. The child's overall appearance, evidence of growth failure or failure to thrive may point to a significant underlying inflammatory disorder. The head and neck examination may show evidence of mucosal ulceration, seen in diseases such as SLE. The eye examination may show pupillary irregularity and synechiae from uveitis or the conjunctivitis of Kawasaki disease. Diffuse lymphadenopathy may be found and is nonspecific. The respiratory and cardiac examinations may show pericardial or pleural friction rubs, indicating serositis. Splenomegaly or hepatomegaly raises suspicion of activation of the reticuloendothelial system that occurs in systemic-onset JRA or SLE.

The joint examination is crucial for the diagnosis of arthritis and may identify evidence of joint swelling, effusion, tenderness, and erythema from increased blood flow. Joint contractures may be seen. The joint lining, or synovium, may be thickened from chronic inflammation. Activation of epiphyseal growth plates in an area of arthritis can lead to localized bony proliferation and limb length discrepancies. Conversely, inflammation at sites of immature growth centers may lead to maldevelopment of bones, such as the carpals or tarsals, resulting in crowding, or the temporomandibular joints, resulting in micrognathia. A rash or evidence of underlying skin disorders, such as skin thickening from scleroderma or sclerodactyly, may be noted. Chronic Raynaud phenomenon may result in nail-fold capillary changes, ulceration, or digital tuft wasting.

**TABLE 86-1  Differential Diagnosis of Pediatric Arthritis Syndromes**

| Characteristic | Systemic Lupus Erythematosus | Juvenile Rheumatoid Arthritis | Rheumatic Fever | Lyme Disease | Leukemia | Gonococcemia | Kawasaki Disease |
|---|---|---|---|---|---|---|---|
| Sex | F > M | Type-dependent | M = F | M = F | M = F | F > M | M = F |
| Age | 10–20 yr | 1–16 yr | 5–15 yr | ≥5–20 yr | 2–10 yr | >12 yr | <5 yr |
| Arthralgia | Yes | Yes | Yes | Yes | Yes | Yes | Yes |
| Morning stiffness | Yes | Yes | No | No | No | Yes | No |
| Rash | Butterfly; discoid | Salmon-pink macules (systemic onset) | Erythema marginatum | Erythema migrans | No | Palms/soles, papulopustules | Diffuse maculopapular (nonspecific), desquamation |
| Monarticular, pauciarticular | Yes | 50% | No | Yes | Yes | Yes | — |
| Polyarticular | Yes | Yes | Yes | No | Yes | No | Yes |
| Small joints | Yes | Yes | No | Rare | Yes | No | Yes |
| Temporomandibular joint | No | Rare | No | Rare | No | No | No |
| Eye disease | Uveitis/retinitis | Iridocyclitis (rare in systemic) | No | Conjunctivitis, keratitis | No | No | Conjunctivitis, uveitis |
| Total WBC count | Decreased | Increased (decreased in macrophage activation syndrome) | Normal to increased | Normal | Increased or neutropenia ± blasts | Increased | Increased |
| ANA | Positive | Positive (50%) | Negative | Negative | Negative | Negative | Negative |
| Rheumatoid factor | Positive | Positive (10%) (polyarticular) | Negative | Negative | Negative | Negative | Negative |
| Other laboratory results | ↓Complement, ↑antibodies to double-stranded DNA | | ↑ASO anti-DNase B | ↑Cryoglobulin, ↑immune complexes | + Bone marrow | + Culture for *Neisseria gonorrhoeae* | Thrombocytosis, ↑immune complexes |
| Erosive arthritis | Rare | Yes | Rare | Rare | No | Yes | No |
| Other clinical manifestations | Proteinuria, serositis | Fever, serositis (systemic onset) | Carditis, nodules, chorea | Carditis, neuropathy, meningitis | Thrombocytopenia | Sexual activity, menses | Fever, lymphadenopathy, swollen hands/feet, mouth lesions |
| Pathogenesis | Autoimmune | Autoimmune | Group A streptococcus | *Borrelia burgdorferi* | Acute lymphoblastic leukemia | *N. gonorrhoeae* | Unknown |
| Treatment | NSAIDs, corticosteroids, hydroxychloroquine, immunosuppressive agents | NSAIDs, etanercept, methotrexate for resistant disease | Penicillin prophylaxis, aspirin, corticosteroids | Penicillin, doxycycline, ceftriaxone | Corticosteroids, chemotherapy | Ceftriaxone | Intravenous immunoglobulin, aspirin |

ANA, antinuclear antibody; ASO, antistreptolysin-O titer; NSAID, nonsteroidal anti-inflammatory drug; WBC, white blood cell.

## COMMON MANIFESTATIONS

The rheumatic diseases of childhood encompass a heterogeneous group of diseases with a shared underlying pathogenesis: disordered functioning of the immune system leading to inflammation directed against native proteins, with secondary increases in numbers of activated lymphocytes; inflammatory cytokines; and circulating antibodies. This antibody production can be nonspecific, or it can be targeted against specific native proteins, leading to subsequent disease manifestations (Table 86-2). Although immune system hyperactivity may be self-limited, the hallmark of most rheumatic diseases of childhood is chronicity, or the perpetuation of the inflammatory process, which can lead to long-term disability.

## INITIAL DIAGNOSTIC EVALUATION

Although rheumatic diseases sometimes present with nonspecific symptoms, especially early in the course, over time a characteristic set of symptoms and physical findings can be elicited. In conjunction with carefully chosen confirmatory laboratory tests, an appropriate differential diagnosis is made, and eventually the correct diagnosis and treatment plan is developed. A correct diagnosis prevents long-term disability.

Most rheumatologic diagnoses are established by clinical findings and fulfillment of classification criteria. Laboratory testing should be judicious and based on a differential diagnosis rather than random screening in search of a diagnosis. Laboratory tests confirm clinical diagnoses rather than develop them.

## SCREENING TESTS

Evidence of an underlying systemic inflammation may be indicated by elevated acute phase reactants, especially the erythrocyte sedimentation rate, but also the white blood cell count, platelet count, and C-reactive protein. The complete blood count may show evidence of a normochromic, normocytic anemia of chronic disease. These laboratory findings are nonspecific for any particular rheumatologic diagnosis. Certain laboratory tests may help confirm a diagnosis, such as autoantibody production in SLE or muscle enzyme elevation in JDM, or identify increased risk for complications, such as uveitis in a patient with JRA with a positive antinuclear antibody.

## DIAGNOSTIC IMAGING

Radiologic studies should focus on areas of concern identified by history or physical examination. Radiography of joints in patients with arthritis on examination may be beneficial, but radiographic abnormalities may lag far behind the clinical examination. Tests with greater sensitivity, such as bone scan, computed tomography scan, and magnetic resonance imaging, may be useful when trying to differentiate between frank synovitis and traumatic soft tissue injury. Magnetic resonance imaging may also be useful to identify evidence of central nervous system involvement with SLE or for evidence of myositis with JDM.

---

#### TABLE 86-2 Manifestations of Autoantibodies

Coombs-positive hemolytic anemia
Immune neutropenia
Immune thrombocytopenia
Thrombosis (anticardiolipin, antiphospholipid, lupus anticoagulant)
Immune lymphopenia
Antimitochondrial (primary biliary cirrhosis, SLE)
Antimicrosomal (chronic active hepatitis, SLE)
Antithyroid (thyroiditis, SLE)
Antineutrophil cytoplasmic antibody (ANCA-cytoplasmic) (Wegener granulomatosis)
ANCA-perinuclear (microscopic polyangiitis)

##### ANTINUCLEAR ANTIBODIES TO SPECIFIC NUCLEAR ANTIGENS AND ASSOCIATED MANIFESTATIONS

Single-stranded DNA (nonspecific, indicates inflammation)
Double-stranded DNA (SLE, renal disease)
DNA-histone (drug-induced SLE)
Sm (Smith) (SLE, renal, CNS)
RNP (ribonucleoprotein) (SLE, Sjögren syndrome, scleroderma, polymyositis, MCTD)
Ro (Robert: SSA) (SLE, neonatal lupus–congenital heart block, Sjögren syndrome)
La (Lane: SSB) (SLE, neonatal lupus (congenital heart block), Sjögren syndrome)
Jo-1 (polymyositis, dermatomyositis)
Scl-70 (scleroderma)
Centromere (CREST syndrome variant of scleroderma)
PM-Scl (scleroderma, UCTD)

ANCA, anti-neutrophil cytoplasmic antibody; CNS, central nervous system; CREST syndrome, calcinosis, Raynaud phenomenon, esophageal dysfunction, sclerodactyly, telangiectasia; MCTD, mixed connective tissue disease; SLE, systemic lupus erythematosus; SSA, Sjögren syndrome antigen A; SSB, Sjögren syndrome antigen B; UCTD, undifferentiated connective tissue disease.
Adapted from Condemi J: The autoimmune diseases. *JAMA* 268:2882–2892, 1992.

---

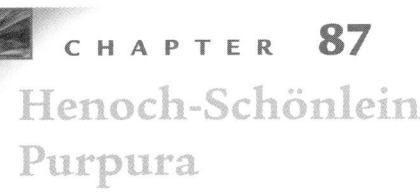

## CHAPTER 87

# Henoch-Schönlein Purpura

## ETIOLOGY

Henoch-Schönlein purpura (HSP) is a vasculitis of unknown etiology characterized by inflammation of small blood vessels with leukocytic infiltration of tissue, hemorrhage, and ischemia. The immune complexes associated with HSP are predominantly composed of IgA, suggesting an allergy-mediated illness, although this is unproven.

## EPIDEMIOLOGY

HSP is the most common systemic vasculitis of childhood and cause of nonthrombocytopenic purpura, with an incidence of 13 per 100,000 children. It occurs primarily in children 3 to 15 years of age, although it has been described in adults. HSP is slightly more common in boys than girls and occurs more frequently in the winter than the summer months.

## CLINICAL MANIFESTATIONS

HSP is characterized by rash, arthritis, and, less frequently, gastrointestinal or renal vasculitis. The hallmark of HSP is **palpable purpura**, caused by small vessel inflammation in the skin leading to extravasation of blood into the surrounding tissues. IgA often is deposited in the lesions. Although the rash can occur anywhere on the body, it is classically found in dependent areas, below the waist on the buttocks and lower extremities (Fig. 87-1). The rash can begin as small macules or urticarial lesions but rapidly progresses to purpura with areas of ecchymosis. The rash also can be accompanied by edema, particularly of the calves and dorsum of the feet, scalp, and scrotum or labia. HSP occasionally is associated with encephalopathy, pancreatitis, and orchitis.

Arthritis occurs in 80% of patients with HSP; it can occur in any joint but tends to affect the lower extremities, most commonly the ankles and knees. The arthritis is acute and can be very painful with refusal to bear weight. Joint swelling can be confused with peripheral edema seen with the rash of HSP.

Gastrointestinal involvement occurs in about one half of affected children and most typically presents as mild to moderate crampy abdominal pain, thought to be due to small vessel involvement of the gastrointestinal tract leading to ischemia. Less commonly, significant abdominal distention, bloody diarrhea, intussusception, or abdominal perforation occurs and requires emergent intervention. Gastrointestinal involvement is typically seen during the acute phase of the illness. It may precede the onset of rash.

One third of children with HSP develop renal involvement, which can be acute or chronic. Although renal involvement is mild in most cases, acute glomerulonephritis manifested by hematuria, hypertension, or acute renal failure can occur. Most cases of glomerulonephritis occur within the first few months of presentation, but rarely patients develop late renal disease, which ultimately can lead to chronic renal disease, including renal failure.

## LABORATORY AND IMAGING STUDIES

Erythrocyte sedimentation rate, C-reactive protein, and white blood cell count are elevated in patients with HSP. The platelet count is the most important test, because HSP is characterized by nonthrombocytopenic purpura with a normal, or even high, platelet count, differentiating HSP from other causes of purpura that are associated with thrombocytopenia such as autoimmune thrombocytopenia, systemic lupus erythematosus, or leukemia. A urinalysis screens for evidence of hematuria. A serum blood urea nitrogen and creatinine should be obtained to evaluate renal function. Testing the stool for blood may identify evidence of gut ischemia. Any question of gut perforation requires radiologic investigation.

## DIFFERENTIAL DIAGNOSIS

The diagnosis of HSP is based on the presence of two of four criteria (Table 87-1), which provides 87.1% sensitivity and 87.7% specificity for the disease. The differential diagnosis includes other systemic vasculitides (Table 87-2) and diseases associated with thrombocytopenic purpura, such as idiopathic thrombocytopenic purpura and leukemia.

## TREATMENT

Therapy for HSP is supportive. A short-term course of nonsteroidal anti-inflammatory drugs can be administered for the acute arthritis. Systemic corticosteroids usually are reserved for children with gastrointestinal disease and provide significant relief of abdominal pain. A typical dosing regimen is prednisone, 1 mg/kg/day for 1 to 2 weeks, followed by a taper schedule. Recurrence of abdominal pain as corticosteroids are weaned may necessitate a longer course of treatment. Acute nephritis typically is treated with corticosteroids but may require more aggressive immunosuppressive therapy.

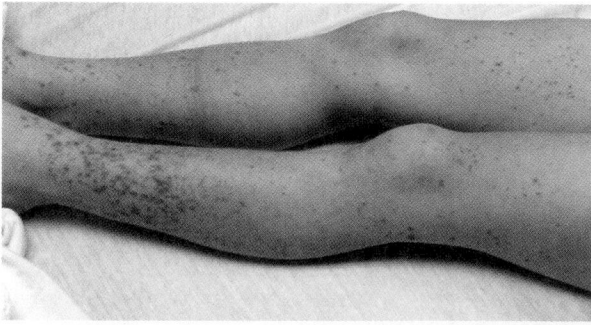

**FIGURE 87-1**

Rash of Henoch-Schönlein purpura on the lower extremities of a child. Note evidence of both purpura and petechiae.

**TABLE 87-1  Criteria for Diagnosis of Henoch-Schönlein Purpura***

| Criteria | Definition |
| --- | --- |
| Palpable purpura | Raised, palpable hemorrhagic skin lesions in the absence of thrombocytopenia |
| Bowel angina | Diffuse abdominal pain or the diagnosis of bowel ischemia |
| Diagnostic biopsy | Histologic changes showing granulocytes in the walls of arterioles or venules |
| Pediatric age group | Age ≤20 years at onset of symptoms |

*The diagnosis of Henoch-Schönlein purpura is based on the presence of two of four criteria.

| TABLE 87-2 Classification of Vasculitides |
| --- |
| **ANTINEUTROPHIL CYTOPLASMIC ANTIBODY–ASSOCIATED VASCULITIS** |
| Wegener granulomatosis |
| Polyarteritis nodosa |
| Churg-Strauss syndrome |
| Microscopic polyangiitis |
| **HYPERSENSITIVITY SYNDROMES** |
| Henoch-Schönlein purpura |
| Serum sickness (e.g., drug-related) |
| Vasculitis associated with infections |
| **CONNECTIVE TISSUE DISEASES** |
| Systemic lupus erythematosus |
| Dermatomyositis |
| Juvenile rheumatoid arthritis |
| **GIANT CELL ARTERITIS** |
| Temporal arteritis |
| Takayasu arteritis |
| **OTHERS** |
| Behçet syndrome |
| Kawasaki disease |
| Hypocomplementemic urticarial vasculitis |

## COMPLICATIONS

Most cases of HSP are monophasic, lasting 3 to 4 weeks and resolving completely. The rash can wax and wane, however, for 1 year after HSP, and parents should be warned regarding possible recurrences. The arthritis of HSP does not leave any permanent joint damage; it does not typically recur. Gastrointestinal involvement can lead to temporary abnormal peristalsis that poses a risk of intussusception, which may be followed by complete obstruction or infarction with bowel perforation. Any child with a recent history of HSP who presents with acute abdominal pain, obstipation, or diarrhea should be evaluated for intussusception. Renal involvement rarely may lead to renal failure.

## PROGNOSIS

The prognosis of HSP is excellent. Most children have complete resolution of the illness without any significant sequelae. Patients with HSP renal disease (elevated blood urea nitrogen, persistent high-grade proteinuria) are at highest risk for long-term complications, such as hypertension or renal insufficiency, particularly if the initial course was marked by significant nephritis. There is a long-term risk of progression to end-stage renal disease in less than 1% of children with HSP. The rare patients who develop end-stage renal disease may require renal transplantation. HSP may recur in the transplanted kidney.

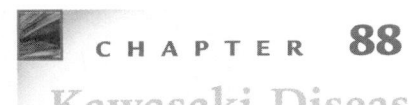

# CHAPTER 88
# Kawasaki Disease

## ETIOLOGY

Kawasaki disease (KD) is a vasculitis of unknown etiology that is characterized by multisystem involvement and inflammation of small to medium-sized arteries with resulting aneurysm formation. Although many causes of KD have been hypothesized, no single underlying etiology has been ascertained.

## EPIDEMIOLOGY

KD is a common vasculitis of childhood that has been described in variable frequency in all parts of the world; the highest frequency is in Japan. Although KD can affect children of all races, it is more common in children of Asian descent. The incidence in the United States is approximately 6 per 100,000 children who are younger than 5 years of age. KD most commonly occurs in children younger than 5 years of age, with a peak between 2 to 3 years, and is rare in children older than 7 years. A seasonal variability has been described with a peak between February and May, but the disease occurs throughout the year.

## CLINICAL MANIFESTATIONS

The clinical course of KD can be divided into three phases, each with its own unique manifestations. Aneurysmal involvement of the coronary arteries is the most important manifestation of KD.

### Acute Phase

The acute phase of KD, which lasts 1 to 2 weeks, is marked by sudden onset of a high, hectic **fever** ($\geq 40\ °C$) without an apparent source. The onset of fever is followed by **conjunctival erythema**; mucosal changes, including dry, **cracked lips** and a **strawberry tongue**; **cervical lymphadenopathy**; and swelling of the hands and feet (Fig. 88-1). Conjunctivitis is bilateral, bulbar, and nonsuppurative. Cervical lymphadenopathy is found in 70% of children and should be greater than 1.5 cm in diameter for the purposes of diagnosis. A rash, which can vary in appearance, occurs in 80% of children with KD and may be particularly accentuated in the inguinal area and on the chest. Extreme irritability is prominent, especially in infants. Abdominal pain and hydrops of the gallbladder, pleocytosis, and arthritis, particularly of medium-sized to large joints, may occur. Carditis in the acute phase may be manifested by tachycardia, shortness of breath, or overt congestive heart failure. **Giant coronary artery aneurysms**, which are rare but occur most commonly in very young children, can appear during this phase.

**FIGURE 88-1**

Facial features of Kawasaki disease with (**A**) morbilliform rash and nonsuppurative conjunctivitis and (**B**) red, chapped lips.

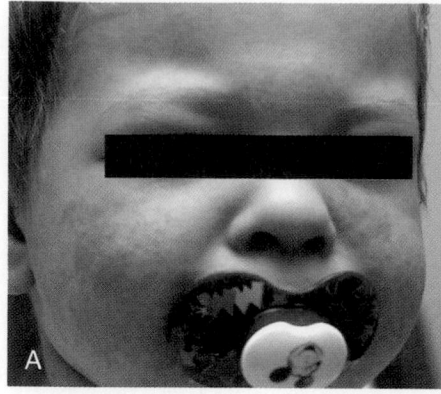 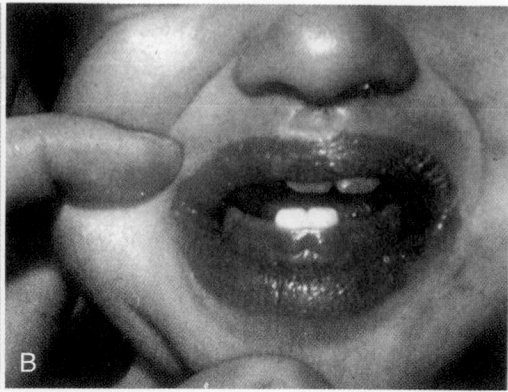

## Subacute Phase

The subacute phase, which lasts until about the fourth week, is characterized by gradual resolution of fever (if untreated) and other symptoms. **Desquamation** of the skin, particularly of the fingers and toes, appears at this point. The platelet count, previously normal or slightly elevated, increases to a significant degree (often >1 million/mm$^3$). This phase heralds the onset of **coronary artery aneurysms**, which may also appear in the convalescent phase, and pose the highest risk of sudden death. Risk factors for development of coronary artery aneurysms include prolonged fever, prolonged elevation of inflammatory parameters such as the erythrocyte sedimentation rate (ESR), age younger than 1 year or older than 6 years, and male gender.

## Convalescent Phase

The convalescent phase begins with the disappearance of clinical symptoms and continues until the ESR returns to normal, usually 6 to 8 weeks after the onset of illness. Beau lines of the fingernails may appear during this phase.

## LABORATORY AND IMAGING STUDIES

It is particularly important to exclude other causes of fever, notably infection. It is appropriate to obtain blood and urine cultures and to perform a chest x-ray. In the acute phase, inflammatory parameters are elevated, including white blood cell count, platelet count, C-reactive protein, and the ESR, which can be profoundly elevated (often >80 mm/hr). A lumbar puncture, if performed to exclude infection, may reveal pleocytosis. Tests of hepatobiliary function may be abnormal. Greatly elevated platelet counts develop during the subacute phase. The development of coronary artery aneurysms is monitored by performing two-dimensional echocardiograms, usually during the acute phase, at 2 to 3 weeks, and at 6 to 8 weeks. More frequent echocardiograms and, potentially, coronary angiography are indicated for patients who develop coronary artery abnormalities.

## DIFFERENTIAL DIAGNOSIS

The diagnosis of KD is based on the presence of fever for more than 5 days without an identifiable source and the presence of four of five other clinical criteria (Table 88-1).

The diagnosis of **incomplete (atypical) KD**, which occurs more commonly in infants, is made when fever is present for at least 5 days even if only two or three clinical criteria are present. The diagnosis of KD should be considered in infants younger than 6 months of age with fever for at least 7 days even if no other criteria are present. Because many of the manifestations of KD are found in other illnesses, many diagnoses must be considered and excluded before the diagnosis of KD can be established (Table 88-2).

## TREATMENT

Intravenous immunoglobulin (IVIG) is the mainstay of therapy for KD, although the mechanism of action is unknown. A single dose of IVIG (2 g/kg over 12 hours) results in rapid defervescence and resolution of clinical illness in most patients and, more importantly, reduces the incidence of coronary artery aneurysms. Aspirin is initially given in **anti-inflammatory doses** (80 to 100 mg/kg/day divided every 6 hours) in the acute phase. Some experts recommend continuing high-dose aspirin until the 14th day and at least 3 days without fever; others recommend only until 48 hours without fever. Aspirin in **antithrombotic**

---

**TABLE 88-1　Criteria for Diagnosis of Kawasaki Disease**

Fever of ≥5 days' duration associated with at least four* of the following five changes:
- Bilateral nonsuppurative conjunctivitis
- One or more changes of the mucous membranes of the upper respiratory tract, including pharyngeal injection, dry fissured lips, injected lips, and "strawberry" tongue
- One or more changes of the extremities, including peripheral erythema, peripheral edema, periungual desquamation, and generalized desquamation
- Polymorphous rash, primarily truncal
- Cervical lymphadenopathy >1.5 cm in diameter

Disease cannot be explained by some other known disease process

---

*A diagnosis of Kawasaki disease can be made if fever and only three changes are present in conjunction with coronary artery disease documented by two-dimensional echocardiography or coronary angiography.

## TABLE 88-2 Differential Diagnosis of Kawasaki Disease

### INFECTIOUS

Scarlet fever
Epstein-Barr virus
Adenovirus
Meningococcemia
Measles
Rubella
Roseola infantum
Staphylococcal toxic shock syndrome
Scalded skin syndrome
Toxoplasmosis
Leptospirosis
Rocky Mountain spotted fever

### INFLAMMATORY

Juvenile rheumatoid arthritis (systemic onset)
Polyarteritis nodosa
Behçet syndrome

### HYPERSENSITIVITY

Drug reaction
Stevens-Johnson syndrome (erythema multiforme)

## TABLE 88-3 Complications of Kawasaki Disease

Coronary artery thrombosis
Peripheral artery aneurysm
Coronary artery aneurysms
Myocardial infarction
Myopericarditis
Congestive heart failure
Hydrops of gallbladder
Aseptic meningitis
Irritability
Arthritis
Sterile pyuria (urethritis)
Thrombocytosis (late)
Diarrhea
Pancreatitis
Peripheral gangrene

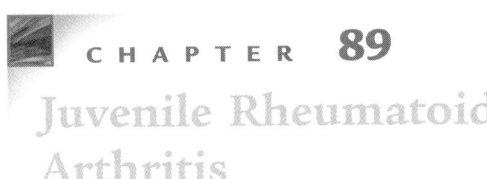

# CHAPTER 89

# Juvenile Rheumatoid Arthritis

doses (3 to 5 mg/kg/day as a single dose) is administered through the subacute and convalescent phases, usually for 6 to 8 weeks, until follow-up echocardiography documents the absence of coronary artery aneurysms.

Approximately 3% to 5% of children with KD initially fail to respond satisfactorily to IVIG therapy. Most of these patients respond to retreatment with IVIG (2 g/kg over 12 hours), but an alternative preparation of IVIG may be required. Corticosteroids or infliximab are rarely used in KD, as opposed to other vasculitides, but may have a role during the acute phase if active carditis is apparent or for children with persistent fever after two doses of IVIG.

## COMPLICATIONS

Most cases resolve without sequelae. Myocardial infarction has been documented, most likely caused by stenosis of a coronary artery at the site of an aneurysm. Coronary artery aneurysms found on autopsy in older children following sudden cardiac death may have been due to past KD. Other complications are listed in Table 88-3.

## PROGNOSIS

IVIG reduces the prevalence of coronary artery disease from 20% to 25% in children treated with aspirin alone to 2% to 4% in children treated with IVIG and aspirin. Other than the risk of persistent coronary artery aneurysms, KD has an excellent prognosis.

## ETIOLOGY

The chronic arthritides of childhood include several types, the most common of which is juvenile rheumatoid arthritis (JRA). The classification of these arthritides is evolving, and newer nomenclature of juvenile idiopathic arthritis (JIA), which includes other types of juvenile arthritis such as enthesitis-related arthritis and psoriatic arthritis, will soon replace the older JRA classification. The etiology of this autoimmune disease is unknown. The common underlying manifestation of this group of illnesses is the presence of chronic **synovitis**, or inflammation of the joint synovium. The synovium becomes thickened and hypervascular with infiltration by lymphocytes, which also can be found in the synovial fluid along with inflammatory cytokines. The inflammation leads to production and release of tissue proteases and collagenases. If left untreated, this can lead to tissue destruction, particularly of the articular cartilage and eventually the underlying bony structures.

## EPIDEMIOLOGY

JRA is the most common chronic rheumatologic disease of childhood, with a prevalence of 1:1000 children. The disease has two peaks, one at 1 to 3 years and one at 8 to 12 years, but it can occur at any age. Girls are affected more commonly than boys, particularly with the pauciarticular form of the illness.

## CLINICAL PRESENTATION

JRA can be divided into three subtypes—pauciarticular, polyarticular, and systemic onset—each with particular disease characteristics (Table 89-1). Although the onset of the arthritis is slow, the actual joint swelling is often noticed by the child or parent acutely, such as after an accident or fall, and can be confused with trauma (although traumatic effusions are rare in children). The child may develop pain and stiffness in the joint that limit use. The child rarely refuses to use the joint at all. Morning stiffness and gelling also can occur in the joint and, if present, can be followed in response to therapy.

On physical examination, signs of inflammation are present, including joint tenderness, erythema, and effusion (Fig. 89-1). Joint range of motion may be limited because of pain, swelling, or contractures from lack of use. In children, because of the presence of an active growth plate, it may be possible to find bony abnormalities of the surrounding bone, causing bony proliferation and localized growth disturbance. In a lower extremity joint, a leg length discrepancy may be appreciable if the arthritis is asymmetric.

All children with chronic arthritis are at risk for chronic **iridocyclitis** or **uveitis**. There is an association between human leukocyte antigens (HLAs) (HLA-DR5, HLA-DR6, and HLA-DR8) and uveitis. The presence of a positive **antinuclear antibody** identifies children with arthritis who are at higher risk for chronic uveitis. Although all children with JRA are at increased risk, the subgroup of children, particularly young girls, with pauciarticular JRA and a positive antinuclear antibody are at highest risk, with an incidence of uveitis of 80%. The uveitis associated with JRA can be asymptomatic until the point of visual loss, making it the primary treatable cause of blindness in children. It is crucial for children with JRA to undergo regular ophthalmologic screening with a slit-lamp examination to identify anterior chamber

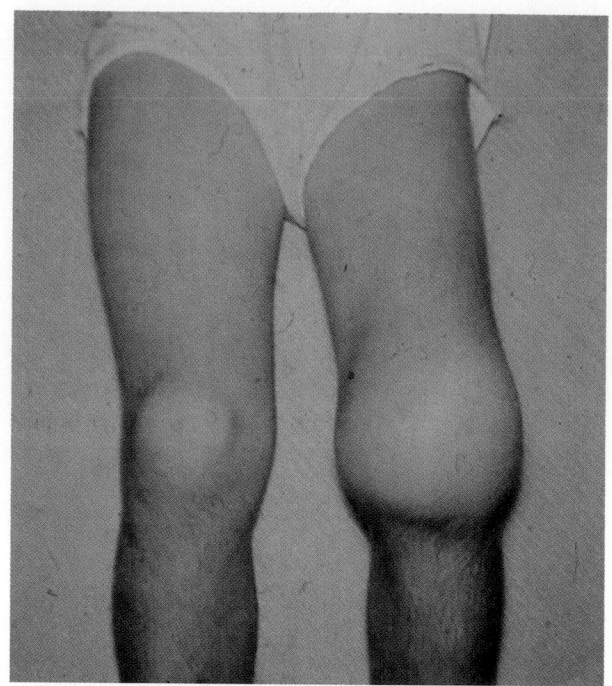

**FIGURE 89-1**

An affected knee in a patient with pauciarticular juvenile rheumatoid arthritis. Note sizeable effusion, bony proliferation, and flexion contracture.

inflammation and to initiate prompt treatment of any active disease.

### Pauciarticular Juvenile Rheumatoid Arthritis

Pauciarticular JRA (or oligoarticular JIA) is defined as the presence of arthritis in fewer than five joints within 6 months of diagnosis. This is the most common form of JRA, accounting for approximately 50% of cases.

---

**TABLE 89-1 Features of Juvenile Rheumatoid Arthritis Subgroups**

| Feature | Pauciarticular | Polyarticular | Systemic Onset |
|---|---|---|---|
| No. joints | <5 | ≥5 | Varies, usually ≥5 |
| Types of joints | Medium to large (also small in extended oligoarthritis) | Small to medium | Small to medium |
| Gender predominance | F > M (especially in younger children) | F > M | F = M |
| Systemic features | None | Some constitutional | Prominent |
| Uveitis | +++ | + | + |
| ANA positivity | ++ | + | − |
| RF positivity | − | + (in older children with early-onset RA) | − |
| Outcomes | Excellent, >90% complete remission | Good, >50% complete remission, some risk of disability | Variable, depends on extent of arthritis |

ANA, antinuclear antibody; RA, rheumatoid arthritis; RF, rheumatoid factor.

Pauciarticular JRA presents in young children, with a peak at 1 to 3 years and another peak at 8 to 12 years. The arthritis is found in medium-sized to large joints; the knee is the most common joint involved, followed by the ankle and the wrist. It is unusual for small joints, such as the fingers or toes, to be involved, although this may occur. Neck and hip involvement also is uncommon. Children with pauciarticular JRA may be otherwise well without any evidence of systemic inflammation (fever, weight loss, or failure to thrive) or have any laboratory evidence of systemic inflammation (elevated white blood cell count or erythrocyte sedimentation rate). A subset of these children later develops polyarticular disease (called extended oligoarthritis in the new JIA classification).

### Polyarticular Juvenile Rheumatoid Arthritis

Polyarticular JRA describes children with arthritis in five or more joints within the first 6 months of diagnosis and accounts for about 40% of cases. Children with polyarticular JRA tend to have symmetric arthritis, which can affect any joint but typically involves the small joints of the hands, feet, ankles, wrists, and knees. The cervical spine can be involved, leading to fusion of the spine over time. In contrast to pauciarticular JRA, children with polyarticular disease can present with evidence of systemic inflammation including malaise, low-grade fever, growth retardation, anemia of chronic disease, and elevated markers of inflammation. Polyarticular JRA can present at any age, although there is a peak in early childhood. There is a second peak in adolescence, but these children differ by the presence of a positive **rheumatoid factor** and most likely represent a subgroup with true adult rheumatoid arthritis; the clinical course and prognosis are similar to the adult entity.

### Systemic-Onset Juvenile Rheumatoid Arthritis

A small subgroup of patients (approximately 10%) with juvenile arthritis do not present with onset of arthritis but rather with preceding **systemic inflammation**. This form of JRA manifests with a typical recurring, spiking fever, usually once or twice per day, which can occur for several weeks to months. This is accompanied by a rash, typically **morbilliform** and **salmon-colored**. The rash may be evanescent and occur only at times of high fever. Rarely, the rash can be urticarial in nature. Internal organ involvement also occurs. Serositis, such as pleuritis and pericarditis, occurs in 50% of children. Pericardial tamponade rarely may occur. Hepatosplenomegaly occurs in 70% of children. Children with systemic-onset JRA appear sick; they have significant constitutional symptoms, including malaise and failure to thrive. Laboratory findings show the inflammation, with elevated erythrocyte sedimentation rate, C-reactive protein, white blood cell count, and platelet counts and anemia. The arthritis of JRA follows the systemic inflammation by 6 weeks to 6 months. The arthritis is typically polyarticular in nature and can be extensive and resistant to treatment, placing these children at highest risk for long-term disability.

## LABORATORY AND IMAGING STUDIES

Most children with pauciarticular JRA have no laboratory abnormalities. Children with polyarticular and systemic-onset disease commonly show elevated acute phase reactants and anemia of chronic disease. In all pediatric patients with joint or bone pain, a complete blood count should be performed to exclude leukemia, which also can present with limb pain (see Chapter 155). All patients with pauciarticular JRA should have an antinuclear antibody test to help identify those at higher risk for uveitis. Older children and adolescents with polyarticular disease should have a rheumatoid factor performed to identify children with early onset adult rheumatoid arthritis.

Diagnostic arthrocentesis may be necessary to exclude suppurative arthritis in children who present with acute onset of monarticular symptoms. The synovial fluid white blood cell count is typically less than 50,000 to 100,000/mm$^3$ and should be predominantly lymphocytes, rather than neutrophils seen with suppurative arthritis. Gram stain and culture should be negative (see Chapter 118).

The most common radiologic finding in the early stages of JRA is a normal bone x-ray. Over time, periarticular osteopenia, resulting from decreased mineralization, is most commonly found. Growth centers may be slow to develop, whereas there may be accelerated maturation of growth plates or evidence of bony proliferation. Erosions of bony articular surfaces may be a late finding. If the cervical spine is involved, fusion of C1–4 may occur, and atlantoaxial subluxation may be demonstrable.

## DIFFERENTIAL DIAGNOSIS

The diagnosis of JRA is established by the presence of arthritis, the duration of the disease for at least 6 weeks, and exclusion of other possible diagnoses. Although a presumptive diagnosis of systemic-onset JRA can be established for a child during the systemic phase, a definitive diagnosis is not possible until arthritis develops. Children must be younger than 16 years of age at time of onset of disease; the diagnosis of JRA does not change when the child becomes an adult. Because there are so many other causes of arthritis, these disorders need to be excluded before providing a definitive diagnosis of JRA (Table 89-2). The acute arthritides can affect the same joints as JRA but have a shorter time course. In particular, JRA can be confused with the spondyloarthropathies, or enthesitis-related arthritidis, which are associated with spinal involvement or inflammation of tendinous insertions. All forms of pediatric arthritides can present with peripheral arthritis before other manifestations and initially may be misclassified (Table 89-3).

## TREATMENT

The treatment of JRA focuses on suppressing inflammation, preserving and maximizing function, preventing deformity, and preventing blindness. Nonsteroidal anti-inflammatory drugs (NSAIDs) are the first choice in the

## TABLE 89-2 Differential Diagnosis of Juvenile Arthritis

### CONNECTIVE TISSUE DISEASES

Juvenile rheumatoid arthritis
Systemic lupus erythematosus
Juvenile dermatomyositis
Scleroderma with arthritis

### SERONEGATIVE SPONDYLOARTHROPATHIES

Seronegative enthesopathy/arthropathy syndrome
Juvenile ankylosing spondylitis
Psoriatic arthritis
Arthritis associated with inflammatory bowel disease

### INFECTIOUS ARTHRITIS

Bacterial arthritis
Viral arthritis
Fungal arthritis
Lyme disease

### REACTIVE ARTHRITIS

Poststreptococcal arthritis
Rheumatic fever
Toxic synovitis
Henoch-Schönlein purpura
Reiter syndrome

### ORTHOPEDIC DISORDERS

Traumatic arthritis
Legg-Calvé-Perthes disease
Slipped capital femoral epiphysis
Osteochondritis dissecans
Chondromalacia patellae

### MUSCULOSKELETAL PAIN SYNDROMES

Growing pains
Hypermobility syndromes
Myofascial pain syndromes/fibromyalgia
Reflex sympathetic dystrophy

### HEMATOLOGIC/ONCOLOGIC DISORDERS

Leukemia
Lymphoma
Sickle cell disease
Thalassemia
Malignant and benign tumors of bone, cartilage, or synovium
Metastatic bone disease

### MISCELLANEOUS

Rickets/metabolic bone disease
Lysosomal storage diseases
Heritable disorders of collagen

treatment of JRA. Naproxen, sulindac, ibuprofen, indomethacin, and others have been used successfully. Aspirin products, the mainstay of arthritis treatment in the past, have been replaced in large part by NSAIDs, not only because of concerns about Reye syndrome but also because of the convenience of twice daily rather than four times daily dosing. Systemic corticosteroid medications, such as prednisone and prednisolone, should be avoided in all but the most extreme circumstances, such as for severe systemic-onset JRA with internal organ involvement or for significant active arthritis leading to inability to ambulate. In this circumstance, the corticosteroids are used as **bridging therapy** until other medications take effect. For patients with a few isolated inflamed joints, intra-articular corticosteroids may be helpful.

Second-line medications, such as hydroxychloroquine and sulfasalazine, have been used in patients whose arthritis is not completely controlled with NSAIDs alone. **Methotrexate**, given either orally or subcutaneously, has become the drug of choice for polyarticular and systemic-onset JRA, which may not respond to baseline agents alone. Methotrexate can cause bone marrow suppression and hepatotoxicity; regular monitoring can minimize these risks. Leflunomide, with a similar adverse effect profile to methotrexate, has also been used. Biologic agents that inhibit tumor necrosis factor-α and block the inflammatory cascade, including **etanercept**, **infliximab**, and **adalimumab,** are effective in the treatment of JRA. The risks of these agents are greater, however, and include serious infection and, possibly, increased risk of malignancy. Anakinra, an interleukin-1 receptor antagonist, is also beneficial in the treatment of systemic-onset JRA.

## COMPLICATIONS

Complications with JRA result primarily from the loss of function of an involved joint secondary to contractures, bony fusion, or loss of joint space. Physical and occupational therapy, professionally and through home programs, are crucial to preserve and maximize function. More serious complications stem from associated uveitis; if left untreated, it can lead to serious visual loss or blindness.

## PROGNOSIS

The prognosis of JRA is excellent, with an overall 85% complete remission rate. Children with pauciarticular JRA uniformly tend to do well, whereas children with polyarticular disease and systemic-onset disease constitute most children with functional disability. Systemic-onset disease, a positive rheumatoid factor, poor response to therapy, and the presence of erosions on x-ray all connote a poorer prognosis. The importance of physical and occupational therapy cannot be overstated because when the disease remits, the physical limitations remain with the patient into adulthood.

**TABLE 89-3  Comparison of Juvenile Rheumatoid Arthritis and Spondyloarthropathies**

| Clinical Manifestations | JRA | JAS | PsA | IBD |
|---|---|---|---|---|
| Gender predominance | F | M | Equal | Equal |
| Peripheral arthritis | +++ | + | ++ | + |
| Back symptoms | − | +++ | + | ++ |
| Family history | − | ++ | ++ | + |
| ANA positivity | ++ | − | − | − |
| HLA-B27 positivity | − | ++ | − | + |
| RF positivity | + (in early-onset JRA) | − | − | − |
| Extra-articular manifestations | Systemic symptoms (systemic-onset JRA) | Enthesopathy | Psoriasis, nail changes | Bowel symptoms |
| Eye disease | Anterior uveitis | Iritis | Posterior uveitis | Anterior uveitis |

ANA, antinuclear antibody; IBD, inflammatory bowel disease; JAS, juvenile ankylosing spondylitis; JRA, juvenile rheumatoid arthritis; PsA, poststreptococcal arthritis; RF, rheumatoid factor.

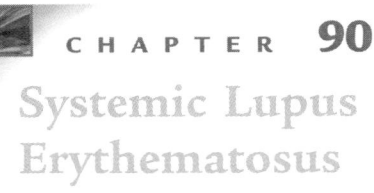

# CHAPTER 90

# Systemic Lupus Erythematosus

## ETIOLOGY

Systemic lupus erythematosus (SLE) is a multisystem disorder of unknown etiology characterized by production of large amounts of **circulating autoantibodies**. This antibody production may be due to loss of T-lymphocyte control on B-lymphocyte activity, leading to hyperactivity of B lymphocytes, which leads to nonspecific and specific antibody and autoantibody production. These antibodies form immune complexes that become trapped in the microvasculature, leading to inflammation and ischemia.

## EPIDEMIOLOGY

Although SLE affects primarily women of childbearing age, approximately 5% of cases present in childhood, mainly around puberty. SLE is rare in children younger than 9 years of age. Although there is a female predominance of this disease in adolescence and adulthood, there is an equal gender distribution in children. The overall prevalence of SLE in the pediatric population is 10 to 25 cases per 100,000 children.

## CLINICAL MANIFESTATIONS

Patients with SLE can present either in an abrupt fashion with fulminant disease or in an indolent manner (Tables 90-1 and 90-2). Nonspecific symptoms are common but can be quite profound and may include significant fatigue and malaise, low-grade fever, and weight loss.

Skin disease can be a prominent finding, occurring in up to 95% of patients. A raised, erythematous rash on the cheeks, called a **malar *butterfly* rash**, is common (Fig. 90-1). This rash also can occur across the bridge of the nose, on the forehead, and on the chin. **Photosensitivity** can be problematic, particularly during the summer months. Both of these rashes improve with appropriate therapy. The rash of **discoid lupus**, by contrast, is an inflammatory process that leads to disruption of the dermal-epidermal junction, resulting in permanent scarring and loss of pigmentation in the affected area. If discoid lupus occurs in the scalp, permanent alopecia ensues because of loss of hair follicles. **Raynaud phenomenon**, although not specific for SLE, and livedo reticularis also can occur.

**Mouth and nasal sores** resulting from mucosal ulceration are a common complaint in patients with SLE and can lead to ulceration and perforation of the nasal septum. Because of reticuloendothelial system stimulation, lymphadenopathy and splenomegaly are common findings in SLE. In particular, axillary lymphadenopathy can be a sensitive indicator of disease activity. Serositis can be seen, with chest pain and pleural or pericardial friction rubs or frank effusion.

Renal involvement is one of the most serious manifestations of SLE and is common in pediatric SLE, occurring in 50% to 70% of children. Renal disease may range from microscopic proteinuria or hematuria to gross hematuria, nephrotic syndrome, and renal failure. Hypertension or the presence of edema suggests lupus renal disease.

Arthralgias and arthritis are common. The arthritis is rarely deforming and typically involves the small joints of the hands; any joint may be involved. Myalgias or frank myositis, with muscle weakness and muscle fatigability, may occur. SLE can affect the central nervous system (CNS), leading to a myriad of symptoms ranging from poor school performance and difficulty concentrating, to seizures, psychosis, and stroke.

## TABLE 90-1  Criteria for Diagnosis of Systemic Lupus Erythematosus*

### PHYSICAL SIGNS

Malar *butterfly* rash
Discoid lupus
Photosensitivity
Oral and nasopharyngeal ulcers
Nonerosive arthritis ($\geq$2 joints with effusion and tenderness)
Pleuritis or pericarditis (serositis)
Seizures or psychosis in absence of metabolic toxins or drugs

### LABORATORY DATA

*Renal Disease (Nephritis)*
    Proteinuria (>500 mg/24 hr) or
    Cellular casts (RBC, granular, or tubular)
*Hematologic Disease*
    Hemolytic anemia with reticulocytosis *or*
    Leukopenia (<4000 on two occasions) *or*
    Lymphopenia (<1500 on two occasions) *or*
    Thrombocytopenia (<100,000/mm$^3$)

### SEROLOGIC DATA

Positive anti-dsDNA *or*
Positive anti-Sm *or*
Evidence of presence of antiphospholipid antibodies
    IgG or IgM anticardiolipin antibodies *or*
    Lupus anticoagulant *or*
    False-positive VDRL for >6 mo
Positive ANA in absence of drugs known to induce lupus

*These are the 1997 revised criteria for diagnosing systemic lupus erythematosus (SLE). A patient must have 4 of the 11 criteria to establish the diagnosis of SLE. These criteria may be present at the same or at different times during the patient's illness. Additional, less specific diagnostic manifestations are noted in Table 90-2.
ANA, antinuclear antibody; RBC, red blood cell; VDRL, Venereal Disease Research Laboratory.

## TABLE 90-2  Additional Manifestations of Systemic Lupus Erythematosus

### SYSTEMIC

Fever
Malaise
Weight loss
Fatigue

### MUSCULOSKELETAL

Myositis, myalgia
Arthralgia

### CUTANEOUS

Raynaud phenomenon
Alopecia
Urticaria-angioedema
Panniculitis
Livedo reticularis

### NEUROPSYCHIATRIC

Personality disorders
Stroke
Peripheral neuropathy
Chorea
Transverse myelitis
Migraine headaches
Depression

### CARDIOPULMONARY

Endocarditis
Myocarditis
Pneumonitis

### OCULAR

Episcleritis
Sicca syndrome
Retinal cytoid bodies

### GASTROINTESTINAL

Pancreatitis
Mesenteric arteritis
Serositis
Hepatomegaly
Hepatitis (chronic lupoid)
Splenomegaly

### RENAL

Nephritis
Nephrosis
Uremia
Hypertension

### REPRODUCTIVE

Repeat spontaneous abortions
Neonatal lupus erythematosus
Congenital heart block

## LABORATORY AND IMAGING STUDIES

Testing for SLE is performed to establish the diagnosis, determine prognosis, and monitor response to therapy. Although nonspecific, a positive **antinuclear antibody** is found in more than 97% of patients with SLE, usually at high titers. Because of its high sensitivity, a negative antinuclear antibody has a high negative predictive value for SLE. The presence of **antibodies to double-stranded DNA** should raise suspicion for SLE because these antibodies are present in most patients with SLE and are found almost exclusively in the disease. Titers of anti–double-stranded DNA antibodies are quantifiable and vary with disease activity. Antibodies directed against Sm (Smith) are specific to SLE but are found in only approximately 30% of persons with SLE, limiting its clinical utility. Antibodies to Ro (SSA) and La (SSB) also can be found in patients with SLE, but they also occur in patients with Sjögren syndrome. Likewise, patients with SLE can have antibodies directed against phospholipids, which also can be seen in other rheumatologic diseases and in primary antiphospholipid syndrome.

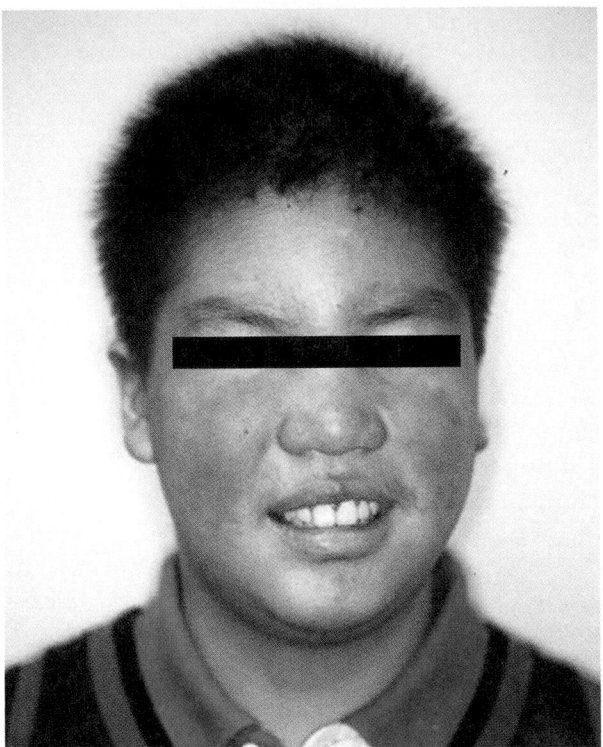

**FIGURE 90-1**

Malar *butterfly* rash on teenage boy with systemic lupus erythematosus. Note erythema on cheeks and chin, sparing the nasolabial folds.

These antibodies lead to an increased risk of arterial and venous thrombosis and can be detected by the presence of anticardiolipin antibodies, a false-positive Venereal Disease Research Laboratory (VDRL) test, or a prolonged activated partial thromboplastin time.

**Hematologic abnormalities** also are prevalent in patients with SLE. Leukopenia, primarily manifest as lymphopenia, is common. Thrombocytopenia and anemia of chronic disease may be found. Rarely, patients with SLE develop Coombs-positive autoimmune hemolytic anemia. Excessive antibody production can lead to polyclonal hypergammopathy with an elevated globulin fraction in the serum. Excessive circulating antibodies and immune complexes also lead to the consumption of complement proteins, with low levels of C3 and C4 and decreased complement function as measured by CH50. Effective therapy returns the low complement levels to normal. This is one way to monitor therapy except in patients with familial deficiency in complement components, which, itself, predisposes to SLE.

Urinalysis may show hematuria and proteinuria, identifying patients with lupus nephritis. Serum blood urea nitrogen and creatinine evaluate renal function. Hypoalbuminemia and hypoproteinemia may be present. Elevation of muscle enzymes may be a clue for the presence of myositis. Elevated cerebrospinal fluid (CSF) protein and an elevated IgG-to-albumin ratio when comparing CSF with serum (IgG index) can indicate antibody production in the CSF and help diagnose SLE affecting the CNS. CNS lupus has a specific pattern on gadolinium-enhanced magnetic resonance imaging.

## DIFFERENTIAL DIAGNOSIS

Because SLE is a multisystem disease, it can be difficult to diagnosis early in the disease course. Suspicion must be high in patients who present with diffuse symptoms, particularly adolescent girls. Many of the clinical manifestations of SLE are found in other inflammatory illnesses and during acute or chronic infection. Criteria have been developed for the diagnosis of SLE (see Table 90-1). The presence of 4 of 11 of these criteria has 98% sensitivity and 97% specificity for SLE.

## TREATMENT

Corticosteroids have been the mainstay of treatment for SLE for decades. Initial use of pulse methylprednisolone and high-dose oral prednisone (up to 2 mg/kg) frequently is required, followed by cautious tapering to minimize recurrence of symptoms. Nonsteroidal anti-inflammatory drugs have been used to treat the arthralgias and arthritis associated with SLE. Hydroxychloroquine is used not only for the treatment of lupus skin disease, such as discoid lupus, but as maintenance therapy. Hydroxychloroquine treatment results in longer periods of wellness between flares of disease as well as decreased numbers of flares.

Corticosteroids and hydroxychloroquine frequently are not sufficient therapies for lupus nephritis or cerebritis. Cyclophosphamide is effective for the worst forms of lupus nephritis, with significant improvements in outcome and decreased rates of progression to renal failure. CNS lupus responds to cyclophosphamide. For patients who are not able to tolerate the tapering of corticosteroids, the use of steroid-sparing agents, such as azathioprine, methotrexate, or mycophenolate mofetil, may be indicated.

Patients with SLE should be counseled to wear sun block and avoid sun exposure as exposure to the sun precipitates flares of the disease. Because of this prohibition, patients benefit from calcium and vitamin D supplementation to reduce the risk of osteoporosis that may result from prolonged corticosteroid use. Early treatment of hyperlipidemia to decrease long-term cardiovascular complications is also indicated.

## COMPLICATIONS

Long-term complications include avascular necrosis secondary to corticosteroid use, infections, and myocardial infarction. Adult patients with SLE develop accelerated atherosclerosis, not only because of prolonged corticosteroid use but also due to the underlying disease. All patients with SLE should be counseled regarding their weight and maintaining an active lifestyle to reduce other cardiac risk factors.

## PROGNOSIS

Outcomes for SLE have improved significantly over the past several decades and depend largely on the organ systems that are involved. Worse prognoses are seen in patients with severe lupus nephritis or cerebritis, with risk of chronic disability or progression to renal failure. With current therapy for the disease and the success of renal transplantation, however, most patients live well into adulthood.

# CHAPTER 91

## Juvenile Dermatomyositis

### ETIOLOGY

The etiology of juvenile dermatomyositis (JDM) is unknown. It is characterized by activation of T and B lymphocytes, leading to vasculitis affecting small vessels of skeletal muscle, with immune complex deposition and subsequent inflammation of blood vessels and muscle. JDM may follow infections, allergic reactions, or sun exposure, but no causal relationship has been shown.

### EPIDEMIOLOGY

JDM is a rare disease, with an incidence of less than 0.1:100,000 children. JDM can occur in all age groups with a peak incidence between 4 to 10 years. The disease is slightly more common in girls than boys.

### CLINICAL MANIFESTATIONS

Dermatomyositis tends to present in a slow, progressive fashion, with insidious onset of fatigue, malaise, and progressive muscle weakness, accompanied by low-grade fevers and rash. Some children present in an acute fashion, however, with rapid onset of severe disease.

The muscle disease of JDM primarily affects the proximal muscles, particularly the hip and shoulder girdles, and the abdominal and neck muscles. Children have difficulty climbing steps, getting out of chairs, and getting off the floor. The patient may have a positive **Gower sign**. In severe cases, the patient is not able to sit up from a supine position or even lift the head off the examination table (see Chapter 182). If muscles of the upper airway and pharynx are involved, the patient's voice will sound nasal and the patient may have difficulty swallowing.

A classic **JDM rash** occurs on the face and across the cheeks but also can be found on the shoulders and back (**shawl sign**). Patients may have **heliotrope discoloration** of the eyelids. Scaly, red plaques (**Gottron papules**) classically are found across the knuckles but can be found on the extensor surfaces of any joint. Patients may have periungual erythema and **dilated nail-fold capillaries**. Less commonly, patients develop cutaneous vasculitis, with inflammation, erythema, and skin breakdown.

At some point, 15% of patients with JDM develop arthritis, commonly affecting small joints, but any joint may be involved. Raynaud phenomenon, hepatomegaly, and splenomegaly may also occur.

### LABORATORY AND IMAGING STUDIES

Many patients with JDM have no evidence of systemic inflammation (normal blood count and erythrocyte sedimentation rate). Evidence of myositis can be identified in 98% of children with active JDM by elevated serum muscle enzymes, including aspartate aminotransferase, alanine aminotransferase, creatine phosphokinase, aldolase, and lactate dehydrogenase. Electromyography and muscle biopsy can document the myositis. Magnetic resonance imaging is a noninvasive means of showing muscle inflammation.

### DIFFERENTIAL DIAGNOSIS

Diagnosis of JDM is based on the presence of documented muscle inflammation in the setting of classic rash (Table 91-1). A small percentage of children have muscle disease without skin manifestations, but polymyositis is sufficiently rare in children that they should have a muscle biopsy to exclude other causes of muscle weakness, such as muscular dystrophy (particularly boys). The differential diagnosis also includes postinfectious myositis and other myopathies (see Chapter 182).

### TREATMENT

Methotrexate, supplemented by short-term use of systemic corticosteroids, is the cornerstone of therapy for JDM. Initial treatment with pulse intravenous methylprednisolone is followed by several months of tapering doses of oral prednisone. Early institution of methotrexate significantly decreases the duration of corticosteroid use and its associated toxicities. In severe or refractory cases, it may be necessary to use cyclosporine or cyclophosphamide. Intravenous immunoglobulin is a useful as adjunctive therapy. Hydroxychloroquine or dapsone has been used for the skin manifestations. These drugs do not significantly affect the muscle disease. Exposure to the sun worsens the cutaneous manifestations and exacerbates the muscle disease; sunlight may lead to flare. Patients should be advised to wear sun block and refrain from prolonged sun exposure. Accordingly, supplementation with calcium and active forms of vitamin D is also indicated.

### COMPLICATIONS

The most serious complication of JDM is the development of **calcinosis**. Dystrophic calcification can occur in the skin and soft tissues in any area of the body; it ranges from mild to extensive (**calcinosis universalis**). Although it is difficult to predict who will develop calcinosis, it occurs more commonly in children with cutaneous vasculitis, prolonged disease activity, or delays in onset of therapy. Patients with JDM who develop vasculitis also are at

---

**TABLE 91-1   Criteria for Diagnosis of Juvenile Dermatomyositis***

Rash typical of dermatomyositis
Symmetric proximal muscle weakness
Elevated muscle enzymes (ALT, AST, LDH, CPK, and aldolase)
EMG abnormalities typical of dermatomyositis (fasciculations, needle insertion irritability, and high-frequency discharges)
Positive muscle biopsy specimen with chronic inflammation

*To make a definitive diagnosis of dermatomyositis, four of five criteria are required.

ALT, alanine aminotransferase; AST, aspartate aminotransferase; CPK, creatine phosphokinase; EMG, electromyography; LDH, lactate dehydrogenase.

risk for gastrointestinal perforation and gastrointestinal bleeding. JDM has been associated with lipoatrophy and insulin resistance, which can progress to type 2 diabetes. Control of insulin resistance frequently leads to improvement in muscle disease in these patients.

## PROGNOSIS

The outcome of JDM depends greatly on the extent of muscle disease and the time between disease onset and initiation of therapy. JDM follows one of three clinical courses: a monophasic course, in which patients are treated and improve without significant sequelae; a chronic recurrent course; and a chronic progressive course marked by poor response to therapy and resulting loss of function. Patients who ultimately develop calcinosis are at risk for chronic loss of mobility depending on the extent of calcium deposition. The association of dermatomyositis with malignancy seen in adults does not occur in children.

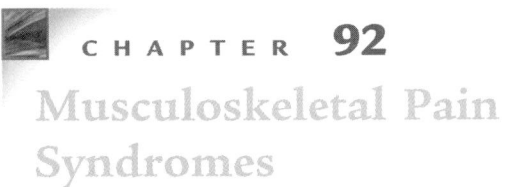

## CHAPTER 92

# Musculoskeletal Pain Syndromes

## GROWING PAINS

**Growing pains**, or benign musculoskeletal pain syndrome, occur in 10% to 20% of school-age children. The peak age range is 3 to 7 years; the syndrome seems to be more common in boys than girls. There is no known etiology, although there seems to be a familial predisposition.

Children with growing pains complain of deep, crampy pain in the calves and thighs. It most typically occurs in the evening or as nocturnal pain that occasionally can waken the child from sleep. Growing pains tend to be more common in children who are extremely active; bouts are exacerbated by increased physical activity. The physical examination is unremarkable, with no evidence of arthritis or muscular tenderness or weakness. Laboratory studies or x-rays, if performed, are normal.

The **diagnosis** of growing pains is based on a typical history and a normal physical examination. **Hypermobility** excludes the diagnosis. It is important to consider leukemia as a cause of nocturnal leg pain in children of this age group, so it is prudent to document a normal complete blood count.

The **treatment** of growing pains consists of reassurance and a regular bedtime ritual of stretching and relaxation. The pain can be relieved by massage. Some patients may benefit from a nighttime dose of acetaminophen or an analgesic dose of a nonsteroidal anti-inflammatory drug (NSAID). Occasionally, nocturnal awakening has been of long duration, leading to disruptive behavior patterns. In these cases, intervention must be aimed at decreasing the secondary gain associated with nighttime parental attention and should focus on sleep hygiene. Other than the negative behavioral patterns that can occur, there are no significant complications. Growing pains are not associated with other illnesses and resolve over time.

## BENIGN HYPERMOBILITY

**Hypermobility syndromes** are disorders of unknown etiology that cause musculoskeletal pain secondary to excessive mobility of joints. These disorders most commonly present in children 3 to 10 years of age. Girls are more commonly affected than boys. There is a familial predisposition to hypermobility syndromes.

Hypermobility can be isolated to a specific joint group or can present as a generalized disorder. Symptoms vary depending on the joints involved. The most consistent symptom is pain, which may occur during the day or night. The discomfort may increase after exertion but rarely interferes with regular physical activity. Children with hypermobility of the ankles or feet may complain of chronic leg or back pain.

Joint hypermobility may be quite marked. Range of motion may be exaggerated with excessive flexion or extension at the metacarpophalangeal joints, wrists, elbows, or knees (genu recurvatum) (Fig. 92-1). There may be excessive pronation of the ankles. Hypermobility of the foot (flat foot; pes planus) is shown by the presence of a longitudinal arch of the foot that disappears with weight bearing and may be associated with a shortened Achilles tendon (see Chapter 200). These findings are rarely associated with tenderness on examination. No laboratory test abnormalities are apparent, and radiographs of affected joints are normal.

The diagnosis of isolated hypermobility is made on the basis of physical examination with demonstration of exaggerated mobility of a joint. Generalized hypermobility is diagnosed by the presence of sufficient criteria (Table 92-1) and the absence of evidence of other underlying disorders. Excessive skin elasticity, easy bruisability, or mitral valve prolapse suggests **Ehlers-Danlos syndrome** or **Marfan syndrome** rather than benign hypermobility.

The **treatment** of hypermobility consists of reassurance and regular stretching, similar to treatment for other benign musculoskeletal disorders. NSAIDs can be administered as needed but do not need to be prescribed on a regular basis. Arch supports can be helpful in children with symptomatic pes planus but are not indicated in the absence of symptoms. Benign hypermobility tends to improve with increasing age and is not associated with long-term complications.

## MYOFASCIAL PAIN SYNDROMES AND FIBROMYALGIA

The myofascial pain syndromes are a group of noninflammatory disorders characterized by diffuse musculoskeletal pain, the presence of multiple **tender points**, fatigue, malaise, and poor sleep patterns. The etiology of these disorders is unknown, although there seems to be a familial predisposition. Although these disorders sometimes follow viral infection or trauma, no causal relationship has been shown. The myofascial pain syndromes are most common in adults but can occur in children (particularly >12 years of age). The syndromes are more common in girls than boys. The prevalence of fibromyalgia in children has been reported to be 6%.

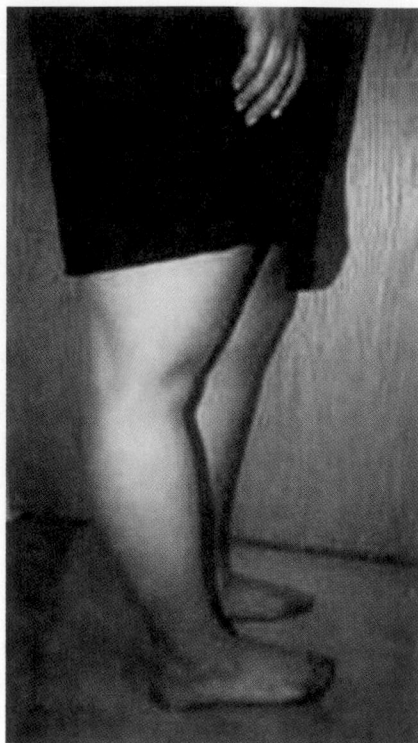

**FIGURE 92-1**

Hyperextension of the knees, an example of hypermobility.

| TABLE 92-1  Criteria for Diagnosis of Benign Hypermobility* | |
|---|---|
| Touch thumb to flexor aspect of the forearm | 1 point each for right and left |
| Extend fifth metacarpophalangeal joint to 90 degrees | 1 point each for right and left |
| >10 degrees hyperextension of elbow | 1 point each for right and left |
| >10 degrees hyperextension of knee | 1 point each for right and left |
| Touch palms to floor with knees straight | 1 point |

*≥6 points defines hypermobility.

Patients with myofascial pain syndromes complain of long-standing diffuse pain in muscles and in the soft tissues around joints that can occur at any time of day, awaken the patient from sleep, and interfere with regular activities. There is frequently a high degree of school absenteeism, despite maintaining adequate school performance. A significant percentage of patients with myofascial pain syndromes exhibit symptoms consistent with depression. An increased incidence of sexual abuse has been reported in children presenting with fibromyalgia.

Physical examination is typically unremarkable with the exception of the presence of specific points that are painful—not just tender—to digital palpation. These points often are located on the neck, back, lateral epicondyles, greater trochanter, and knees. There is no evidence of arthritis or muscular weakness.

Patients with myofascial pain syndromes frequently undergo extensive medical testing because of the concern for underlying inflammatory disease. These tests are invariably normal. Children may have a false-positive antinuclear antibody, which is found in 20% of the normal pediatric population.

The **diagnosis** of myofascial pain syndrome is based on the presence of multiple tender points in the absence of other illness. To fulfill strict criteria for a diagnosis of fibromyalgia, the patient must have a history of diffuse pain for at least 3 months and the presence of 11 of 18 specific tender points on examination. It is important to exclude underlying inflammatory diseases, such as systemic lupus erythematosus, or the postinfectious fatigue that characteristically follows Epstein-Barr virus and influenza virus infection. Mood and conversion disorders also should be considered.

**Treatment** consists of pain control, usually using NSAIDs, physical therapy, relaxation techniques, and education regarding sleep hygiene. Patients may require low doses of medications such as amitriptyline to regulate sleep or gabapentin to reduce pain sensitivity. Education and reassurance are crucial. Because of the disability associated with myofascial pain syndromes, patients and parents frequently believe that the child has a serious underlying condition and may be resistant to reassurance. It should be emphasized that there is no simple cure, and time and perseverance are required.

The long-term outcomes in the myofascial pain syndromes vary. Patients and families who focus on therapy and are positive in their approach tend to have better outcomes. Patients who demand prolonged evaluations, especially from multiple health care providers, may do more poorly. Overall, children with fibromyalgia and myofascial pain syndromes have better prognoses than their adult counterparts.

## SUGGESTED READING

Connelly M, Schanberg L: Latest developments in the assessment and management of chronic musculoskeletal pain syndromes in children, *Curr Opin Rheumatol* 18:496–502, 2006.

Falcini F: Kawasaki disease, *Curr Opin Rheumatol* 18:33–38, 2006.

Feldman BM, Rider LG, Reed AM, et al: Juvenile dermatomyositis and other idiopathic inflammatory myopathies of childhood, *Lancet* 371:2201–2212, 2008.

Gottlieb BS, Ilowite NT: Systemic lupus erythematosus in children and adolescents, *Pediatr Rev* 27:323–330, 2006.

Ravelli A, Martini A: Juvenile idiopathic arthritis, *Lancet* 369:767–778, 2007.

Tizard EJ, Hamilton-Ayres MJJ: Henoch Schönlein purpura, *Arch Dis Child Ed Pract* 93:1–8, 2008.

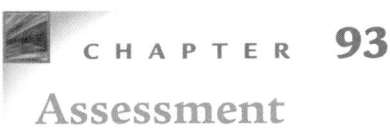

CHAPTER 93

# Assessment

Overlapping clinical symptoms caused by infectious and noninfectious illnesses make the diagnosis of some diseases difficult. Clinicians are concerned that an untreated minor infection may progress to a life-threatening illness, if appropriate treatment is not given. However, unnecessary treatment with antimicrobial agents may lead to a serious problem—emergence of bacteria that are resistant to multiple-antibiotics. Accurate diagnosis of infectious and noninfectious diseases and providing specific treatment only as indicated reduces the unnecessary use of antibiotics. Thus, a thorough assessment of the patient, including a detailed history, complete physical examination, and appropriate diagnostic testing, is critical to making an accurate diagnosis.

## HISTORY

Key elements to include in a complete history are a comprehensive description of symptoms, a detailed environmental history (including sick contacts, travel, and animal exposure), an immunization history, and a determination of the overall health of the patient (Table 93-1). Family history, especially of unexpected deaths of male infants, may suggest familial immunodeficiency (see Chapters 73 through 76). Localization of symptoms to a specific site may narrow diagnostic possibilities (Table 93-2).

## PHYSICAL EXAMINATION

A complete physical examination is essential to identify signs of infection, which may be systemic, such as fever and shock, or focal, including swelling, erythema, tenderness, and limitation of function. Many infectious diseases are associated with characteristic cutaneous signs (see Table 97-1). Accurate otolaryngologic examination is critical for diagnosing upper respiratory tract infections and otitis media, the most common childhood infectious diseases in the United States.

## COMMON MANIFESTATIONS

Respiratory and gastrointestinal infections are the most common illnesses in childhood, reflecting the interface of microbes with the host at these mucosal sites. The host immune response varies with age. Neonates are at risk for different types of infections and have different clinical manifestations than school-age children or adolescents (see Chapters 65 and 66). In addition, the inflammatory response to the infection may be more deleterious than the injury directly attributable to the pathogen. Differentiation between viral and bacterial pathogens is an important determinant for guiding therapy (Table 93-3). However, there is overlap in their clinical presentations.

Some infections present as medical emergencies. Severe gastroenteritis with extreme dehydration or sepsis with hypotension can lead to multiorgan damage and require immediate intervention (see Chapter 40). Infections of the upper airway, such as croup, epiglottitis, retropharyngeal abscess, peritonsillar abscess, or tonsillitis with obstruction can result in airway obstruction and require emergent intubation or, rarely, tracheostomy (see Chapter 135). Fever, headache, vomiting, change in sensorium, and signs of nuchal rigidity suggest acute bacterial meningitis. An emergent lumbar puncture for examination of cerebrospinal fluid, and immediate therapy should be initiated (see Chapter 100).

## DIFFERENTIAL DIAGNOSIS

**Fever** does not always represent infection. Rheumatologic disease, inflammatory bowel disease, Kawasaki disease, poisoning, and malignancy also may present with fever. Importantly, children with overwhelming infection may be afebrile or hypothermic. Common symptoms, such as bone pain or lymphadenopathy that suggest infection, may also be due to leukemia, lymphoma, juvenile rheumatoid arthritis, or Kawasaki disease (see Chapters 88, 89, and 153). Acute mental status changes or focal neurologic impairment could be manifestations of infections (encephalitis, meningitis, or brain abscess) or noninfectious causes (brain or spinal tumors, inflammatory conditions, postinfectious sequelae, or impairment from toxic ingestions or inhalants). Many manifestations of mucosal allergy (rhinitis, diarrhea) may mimic common infectious diseases (see Chapter 77).

Certain infections are more common in specific geographic areas. Parasitic infections are more common in

## TABLE 93-1 Clues from the History for Risk of Infection

Season of year
Age
General health
Weight change
Fever—presence, duration, and pattern
Previous similar symptoms
Previous infections and other illnesses
Previous surgeries, dental procedures
Preceding trauma
Presence of outbreaks or epidemics in the community
Exposures to infected individuals
Exposures to farm or feral animals and pets
Exposures to ticks and mosquitoes
Sexual history, including possibility of sexual abuse
Illicit drug use
Transfusion of blood or blood products
Travel history
Daycare or school attendance
Sources of water and food (e.g., undercooked meat, unpasteurized dairy products)
Home sanitary facilities and hygiene
Pica
Exposure to soil-borne and waterborne organisms (e.g., swimming in brackish water)
Presence of foreign bodies (e.g., indwelling catheters, shunt, grafts)
Immunization history
Current medications

## TABLE 93-3 Differentiating Viral from Bacterial Infections

| Variable | Viral | Bacterial |
|---|---|---|
| Petechiae | Present | Present |
| Purpura | Rare | If severe |
| Leukocytosis | Uncommon* | Common |
| Shift-to-the-left (↑ bands) | Uncommon | Common |
| Neutropenia | Possible | Suggests overwhelming infection |
| ↑ ESR | Unusual* | Common |
| ↑ CRP | Unusual | Common |
| ↑ TNF, IL-1, PAF | Uncommon | Common |
| Meningitis (pleocytosis) | Lymphocytic[†] | Neutrophilic |
| Meningeal signs positive[‡] | Present | Present |

*Adenovirus and herpes simplex may cause leukocytosis and increased ESR; Epstein-Barr virus may cause petechiae and increased ESR.
[†]Early viral (enterovirus, arbovirus) meningitis initially may have a neutrophilic pleocytosis.
[‡]Nuchal rigidity, bulging fontanelle, Kernig sign, Brudzinski sign.
CRP, C-reactive protein; ESR, erythrocyte sedimentation rate; IL, interleukin; PAF, platelet-activating factor; TNF, tumor necrosis factor.

## TABLE 93-2 Localizing Manifestations of Infection

| Site | Localizing Symptoms | Localizing Signs* |
|---|---|---|
| Eye | Eye pain, double vision, photophobia, conjunctival discharge | Periorbital erythema, periorbital edema, drainage, chemosis, limitation of extraocular movements |
| Ear | Ear pain, drainage | Red bulging tympanic membrane, drainage from ear canal |
| Upper respiratory tract | Rhinorrhea, sore throat, cough, drooling, stridor, trismus, sinus pain, tooth pain, hoarse voice | Nasal congestion, pharyngeal erythema, enlarged tonsils with exudate, swollen red epiglottis, regional lymphadenopathy |
| Lower respiratory tract | Cough, chest pain, dyspnea, sputum production, cyanosis | Tachypnea, crackles, wheezing, localized diminished breath sounds, intercostal retractions |
| Gastrointestinal tract | Nausea, vomiting, diarrhea, abdominal pain (focal or diffuse), anorexia, weight loss | Hypoactive or hyperactive bowel sounds, abdominal tenderness (focal or generalized), hematochezia |
| Liver | Anorexia, vomiting, dark urine, light stools | Jaundice, hepatomegaly, hepatic tenderness, bleeding diatheses, coma |
| Genitourinary tract | Dysuria, frequency, urgency, flank or suprapubic pain, vaginal discharge | Costovertebral angle or suprapubic tenderness, cervical motion and adnexal tenderness |
| Central nervous system | Lethargy, irritability, headache, neck stiffness, seizures | Nuchal rigidity, Kernig sign, Brudzinski sign, bulging fontanelle, focal neurologic deficits, altered mental status, coma |
| Cardiovascular | Dyspnea, palpitations, fatigue, exercise intolerance, chest pain | Tachycardia, hypotension, cardiomegaly, hepatomegaly, splenomegaly, crackles, petechiae, Osler nodes, Janeway lesions, Roth spots, new or change in murmur, distended neck veins, pericardial friction rub, muffled heart sounds |
| Musculoskeletal | Limp, bone pain, limited function (pseudoparalysis) | Local swelling, erythema, warmth, limited range of motion, point bone tenderness, joint line tenderness |

*Fever usually accompanies infection as a systemic manifestation.

tropical climates. Diarrhea may be bacterial, viral, or parasitic in the tropics, but in temperate climates parasitic causes of diarrhea, other than giardiasis, are much less likely. Certain fungal infections, such as coccidioidomycosis are common in the southwestern United States, blastomycosis in the upper Midwest, and histoplasmosis in central United States, especially in the states bordering the Mississippi and Ohio Rivers. In other areas, fungal pneumonias are rare except in immunocompromised persons.

Some infections are prone to recurrence, especially if treatment is suboptimal (inadequate antimicrobial or shorter duration). Recurrent, severe, or unusual (opportunistic) infections suggest the possibility of immunodeficiency (see Chapters 72 and 125).

## INITIAL DIAGNOSTIC EVALUATION

The ability to diagnose specific infections accurately begins with an understanding of the epidemiology; risk factors, including exposures; and age-related susceptibility, which reflects the maturity of the immune system. Obtaining a thorough history and physical examination identifies most of these elements (see Tables 93-1 and 93-2).

Antibiotics often are begun before a definitive diagnosis is established, complicating the ability to rely on subsequent cultures for microbiologic diagnosis (see Chapter 95). Although persistent or progressive symptoms despite antibiotic treatment may indicate the need to change the regimen, more frequently this indicates the need to stop all antibiotics to facilitate definitive diagnosis by obtaining appropriate cultures. Antibiotics should not be given before obtaining appropriate cultures unless there is a life-threatening situation (septic shock).

## SCREENING TESTS

Laboratory diagnosis of infection includes examination of bacterial morphology using Gram stain, various culture techniques, molecular microbiologic methods such as polymerase chain reaction, and assessment of the immune response with antibody titers or skin testing. The **acute phase response** is a nonspecific metabolic and inflammatory response to infection, trauma, autoimmune disease, and some malignancies. **Acute phase reactants** such as erythrocyte sedimentation rate and C-reactive protein are commonly elevated during an infection but are not specific for infection and do not identify any specific infection. These tests are often useful to show response to therapy.

A **complete blood count** is frequently obtained for evidence of infection. The initial response to infection, especially in children, is usually a **leukocytosis** (increased number of circulating leukocytes) with an initial neutrophilic response to both bacterial and viral infections. With most viral infections, the initial neutrophilic response is transient and is followed quickly by a characteristic mononuclear response. In general, bacterial infections are associated with greater neutrophil counts than viral infections (see Table 93-3). A **shift-to-the-left** is an increase in the numbers of circulating immature cells of the neutrophil series, including band forms, metamyelocytes, and myelocytes and indicates the rapid release of cells from the bone marrow. It is characteristic of the early

stages of infection and, if sustained, bacterial infections. Transient lymphopenia at the beginning of illness and lasting 24 to 48 hours has been described with many viral infections. **Atypical lymphocytes** are mature T lymphocytes with larger, eccentrically placed, and indented nuclei classically seen with infectious mononucleosis caused by Epstein-Barr virus. Other infections associated with atypical lymphocytosis include cytomegalovirus infection, toxoplasmosis, viral hepatitis, rubella, roseola, mumps, and some drug reactions. **Eosinophilia** is characteristic of allergic diseases but may be seen with tissue-invasive multicellular parasites, such as the migration of the larval stages of parasites through skin, connective tissue, and viscera. High-grade eosinophilia (>30% eosinophils, or a total eosinophil count >3000/μL) frequently occurs during the muscle invasion phase of trichinellosis, the pulmonary phases of ascariasis and hookworm infection (eosinophilic pneumonia), and the hepatic and central nervous system phases of visceral larva migrans.

Other common screening tests include **urinalysis** for urinary tract infections, transaminases for liver function, and **lumbar puncture** for evaluation of the cerebrospinal fluid if there is concern for meningitis or encephalitis (see Chapters 100 and 101). Various tests may help distinguish viral versus bacterial infection, but definitive diagnosis requires identifying the agent by culture or another test, such as polymerase chain reaction.

**Cultures** are the mainstay of diagnosis of many infections. **Blood cultures** are sensitive and specific for bacteremia, which may be primary or secondary to a focal infection (osteomyelitis, gastroenteritis, urinary tract, and endocarditis). Urine cultures are important to confirm urinary tract infection, which may be occult in young infants. Cultures should be obtained with every lumbar puncture, aspiration, or biopsy of other fluid collections or masses. Specific types of cultures (bacterial, fungal, viral, or mycobacterial) are guided by the clinical problem. Tissue culture techniques are used to identify viruses and intracellular bacterial pathogens. **Rapid tests,** such as antigen tests, are useful for preliminary diagnosis and are included in numerous bacterial, viral, fungal, and parasitic antigen detection tests. **Serologic tests**, using enzyme-linked immunosorbent assay or Western blotting, showing an IgM response, high IgG titer, or seroconversion between acute and convalescent sera can be used for diagnosis. **Molecular tests**, such as **polymerase chain reaction** for DNA or RNA, offer the specificity of culture, high sensitivity, and rapid results. When an unusual infection is suspected, a microbiologist should be consulted before samples are obtained.

## DIAGNOSTIC IMAGING

The choice of diagnostic imaging mode should be based on the location of the findings. In the absence of localizing signs and during an acute infection, imaging of the entire body is less productive. **Plain x-rays** are useful initial tests for respiratory tract infections. **Ultrasonography** is a noninvasive, nonirradiating technique well suited to infants and children for imaging solid organs. It also is useful to identify soft tissue abscesses with lymphadenitis and to diagnose suppurative arthritis of the hip. **Computed tomography (CT) (with contrast enhancement)** and **magnetic resonance imaging (MRI) (with gadolinium enhancement)** allow characterization of lesions and precise anatomic localization and are the modalities of choice for the brain. CT shows greater bone detail, and MRI shows greater tissue detail. MRI is especially useful for diagnosis of osteomyelitis, myositis, and necrotizing fasciitis. High-resolution CT is useful for complicated chest infections. Contrast studies (upper gastrointestinal series, barium enema) are used to identify mucosal lesions of the gastrointestinal tract, whereas CT or MRI is preferred for evaluation of appendicitis and intra-abdominal masses. A voiding cystourethrogram (VCUG) may be used to evaluate for vesicoureteral reflux, a predisposing factor for upper urinary tract infections. **Radionuclide scans**, such as technetium-99m for osteomyelitis and dimercaptosuccinic acid (DMSA) for acute pyelonephritis, are often informative.

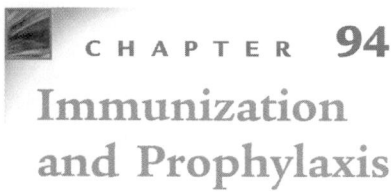

# CHAPTER 94

# Immunization and Prophylaxis

## IMMUNIZATION

Childhood immunization has markedly reduced the impact of major infectious diseases. **Active immunization** induces immunity by vaccination with a **vaccine** or **toxoid** (inactivated toxin). **Passive immunization** includes transplacental transfer of maternal antibodies and the administration of antibody, either as immunoglobulin or monoclonal antibody.

Vaccinations may be with live attenuated viruses (measles, mumps, rubella, varicella, nasal influenza), inactivated or killed viruses (polio, hepatitis A, intramuscular influenza), recombinant products (hepatitis B], human papillomavirus), reassortants (rotavirus), or immunogenic components of bacteria (pertussis, *Haemophilus influenzae* type b, and *Streptococcus pneumoniae*), including toxoids (diphtheria, tetanus). Many purified polysaccharides are T-independent antigens that initiate B-cell proliferation without involvement of CD4 T lymphocytes and are poor immunogens in children younger than 2 years of age. Conjugation of a polysaccharide to a **protein carrier** induces a T-dependent response in infants and creates immunogenic vaccines for *H. influenzae* type b, *S. pneumoniae*, and *Neisseria meningitidis*.

Childhood immunization standards and recommendations in the United States (Figs. 94-1 and 94-2) are formulated by the Advisory Committee on Immunization Practices of the Centers for Disease Control and Prevention (ACIP), the American Academy of Pediatrics (AAP), and the American Academy of Family Physicians (AAFP). In the United States, due to state laws requiring immunization for school entry, approximately 95% of children entering kindergarten are vaccinated for the common infectious diseases. The ACIP recommends that children in the United

States routinely receive vaccines against 16 diseases (see Fig. 94-1). This schedule includes up to 21 injections in four to five visits by 18 months of age. Children and adolescents who are at increased risk for pneumococcal infections should receive the pneumococcal polysaccharide vaccine, as well. Children who are behind in immunization should receive catch-up immunizations as rapidly as feasible. Infants born prematurely, regardless of birth weight, should be vaccinated at the same chronologic age and according to the same schedule as full-term infants and children. The single exception to this practice is providing hepatitis B vaccine for infants weighing less than 2000 g if the mother is hepatitis B virus surface antigen (HB$_s$Ag)–negative at 1 month instead of at birth. Vaccines for adolescents should be given at 11 to 12 years of age. Human papillomavirus vaccine is recommended for all girls at 11 to 12 years of age for the prevention of cervical cancer, precancerous or dysplastic lesions, and genital warts caused by human papillomavirus types 6, 11, 16, and 18. This vaccine may be administered to girls as young as 9 years of age and to women up to 26 years of age. Many colleges and universities require or recommend meningococcal vaccine before matriculation because of the increased risk of meningococcal disease, especially for freshmen living in dormitories.

Vaccines should be administered after obtaining informed consent. The **National Childhood Vaccine Injury Act** requires that all health care providers provide parents or patients with copies of **Vaccine Information Statements** prepared by the Centers for Disease Control and Prevention (http://www.cdc.gov/vaccines/pubs/vis/default.htm) before administering each vaccine dose.

Most vaccines are administered by intramuscular or subcutaneous injection. The preferred sites for administration are the anterolateral aspect of the thigh in infants and the deltoid region in children and adults. Multiple vaccines can be administered simultaneously at anatomically separate sites (different limbs, or separated by >1 in) without diminishing the immune response. Measles, mumps, and rubella (MMR) and varicella vaccines should be administered simultaneously or more than 30 days apart. Administration of blood products and immunoglobulin can diminish response to live virus vaccines if administered before the recommended interval.

**General contraindications** to vaccination include serious allergic reaction (anaphylaxis) after a previous vaccine dose or to a vaccine component, immunocompromised states or pregnancy (live virus vaccines), and moderate or severe acute illness with or without fever. History of anaphylactic-like reactions to eggs is a contraindication to influenza and yellow fever vaccines, which are produced in embryonated chicken eggs. Current preparations of measles and mumps vaccines, which are produced in chick embryo fibroblast tissue culture, do not contain significant amounts of egg proteins and may be administered without testing children with history of egg allergy. Mild acute illness, with or without fever, convalescent phase of illness, recent exposure to infectious diseases, current antimicrobial therapy, breastfeeding, mild to moderate local reaction or low-grade to moderate fever after previous vaccination, and history of penicillin or other nonvaccine allergy or receiving allergen extract immunotherapy are **not contraindications** to immunization.

## Recommended immunization schedule for persons aged 0 through 6 years — United States, 2010

| Vaccine ▼          Age ► | Birth | 1 month | 2 months | 4 months | 6 months | 12 months | 15 months | 18 months | 19–23 months | 2–3 years | 4–6 years |
|---|---|---|---|---|---|---|---|---|---|---|---|
| Hepatitis B[1] | HepB | HepB | | | | HepB | | | | | |
| Rotavirus[2] | | | RV | RV | RV[2] | | | | | | |
| Diphtheria, Tetanus, Pertussis[3] | | | DTaP | DTaP | DTaP | see footnote[3] | DTaP | | | | DTaP |
| *Haemophilus influenzae* type b[4] | | | Hib | Hib | Hib[4] | Hib | | | | | |
| Pneumococcal[5] | | | PCV | PCV | PCV | PCV | | | | PPSV | |
| Inactivated Poliovirus[6] | | | IPV | IPV | | IPV | | | | | IPV |
| Influenza[7] | | | | | | Influenza (Yearly) | | | | | |
| Measles, Mumps, Rubella[8] | | | | | | MMR | | see footnote[8] | | | MMR |
| Varicella[9] | | | | | | Varicella | | see footnote[9] | | | Varicella |
| Hepatitis A[10] | | | | | | HepA (2 doses) | | | | HepA Series | |
| Meningococcal[11] | | | | | | | | | | MCV | |

Range of recommended ages for all children except certain high-risk groups

Range of recommended ages for certain high-risk groups

This schedule includes recommendations in effect as of December 15, 2009. Any dose not administered at the recommended age should be administered at a subsequent visit, when indicated and feasible. The use of a combination vaccine generally is preferred over separate injections of its equivalent component vaccines. Considerations should include provider assessment, patient preference, and the potential for adverse events. Providers should consult the relevant Advisory Committee on Immunization Practices statement for detailed recommendations: http://www.cdc.gov/vaccines/pubs/acip-list.htm. Clinically significant adverse events that follow immunization should be reported to the Vaccine Adverse Event Reporting System (VAERS) at http://www.vaers.hhs.gov or by telephone, 800-822-7967.

1. **Hepatitis B vaccine (HepB).** (Minimum age: birth)
   **At birth:**
   • Administer monovalent HepB to all newborns before hospital discharge.
   • If mother is hepatitis B surface antigen (HBsAg)-positive, administer HepB and 0.5 mL of hepatitis B immune globulin (HBIG) within 12 hours of birth.
   • If mother's HBsAg status is unknown, administer HepB within 12 hours of birth. Determine mother's HBsAg status as soon as possible and, if HBsAg-positive, administer HBIG (no later than age 1 week).
   **After the birth dose:**
   • The HepB series should be completed with either monovalent HepB or a combination vaccine containing HepB. The second dose should be administered at age 1 or 2 months. Monovalent HepB vaccine should be used for doses administered before age 6 weeks. The final dose should be administered no earlier than age 24 weeks.
   • Infants born to HBsAg-positive mothers should be tested for HBsAg and antibody to HBsAg 1 to 2 months after completion of at least 3 doses of the HepB series, at age 9 through 18 months (generally at the next well-child visit).
   • Administration of 4 doses of HepB to infants is permissible when a combination vaccine containing HepB is administered after the birth dose. The fourth dose should be administered no earlier than age 24 weeks.
2. **Rotavirus vaccine (RV).** (Minimum age: 6 weeks)
   • Administer the first dose at age 6 through 14 weeks (maximum age: 14 weeks 6 days). Vaccination should not be initiated for infants aged 15 weeks 0 days or older.
   • The maximum age for the final dose in the series is 8 months 0 days
   • If Rotarix is administered at ages 2 and 4 months, a dose at 6 months is not indicated.
3. **Diphtheria and tetanus toxoids and acellular pertussis vaccine (DTaP).** (Minimum age: 6 weeks)
   • The fourth dose may be administered as early as age 12 months, provided at least 6 months have elapsed since the third dose.
   • Administer the final dose in the series at age 4 through 6 years.
4. ***Haemophilus influenzae* type b conjugate vaccine (Hib).** (Minimum age: 6 weeks)
   • If PRP-OMP (PedvaxHIB or Comvax [HepB-Hib]) is administered at ages 2 and 4 months, a dose at age 6 months is not indicated.
   • TriHiBit (DTaP/Hib) and Hiberix (PRP-T) should not be used for doses at ages 2, 4, or 6 months for the primary series but can be used as the final dose in children aged 12 months through 4 years.
5. **Pneumococcal vaccine.** (Minimum age: 6 weeks for pneumococcal conjugate vaccine [PCV]; 2 years for pneumococcal polysaccharide vaccine [PPSV])
   • PCV is recommended for all children aged younger than 5 years. Administer 1 dose of PCV to all healthy children aged 24 through 59 months who are not completely vaccinated for their age.
   • Administer PPSV 2 or more months after last dose of PCV to children aged 2 years or older with certain underlying medical conditions, including a cochlear implant. See *MMWR* 1997;46(No. RR-8).

6. **Inactivated poliovirus vaccine (IPV)** (Minimum age: 6 weeks)
   • The final dose in the series should be administered on or after the fourth birthday and at least 6 months following the previous dose.
   • If 4 doses are administered prior to age 4 years a fifth dose should be administered at age 4 through 6 years. See *MMWR* 2009;58(30):829–30.
7. **Influenza vaccine (seasonal).** (Minimum age: 6 months for trivalent inactivated influenza vaccine [TIV]; 2 years for live, attenuated influenza vaccine [LAIV])
   • Administer annually to children aged 6 months through 18 years.
   • For healthy children aged 2 through 6 years (i.e., those who do not have underlying medical conditions that predispose them to influenza complications), either LAIV or TIV may be used, except LAIV should not be given to children aged 2 through 4 years who have had wheezing in the past 12 months.
   • Children receiving TIV should receive 0.25 mL if aged 6 through 35 months or 0.5 mL if aged 3 years or older.
   • Administer 2 doses (separated by at least 4 weeks) to children aged younger than 9 years who are receiving influenza vaccine for the first time or who were vaccinated for the first time during the previous influenza season but only received 1 dose.
   • For recommendations for use of influenza A (H1N1) 2009 monovalent vaccine see *MMWR* 2009;58(No. RR-10).
8. **Measles, mumps, and rubella vaccine (MMR).** (Minimum age: 12 months)
   • Administer the second dose routinely at age 4 through 6 years. However, the second dose may be administered before age 4, provided at least 28 days have elapsed since the first dose.
9. **Varicella vaccine.** (Minimum age: 12 months)
   • Administer the second dose routinely at age 4 through 6 years. However, the second dose may be administered before age 4, provided at least 3 months have elapsed since the first dose.
   • For children aged 12 months through 12 years the minimum interval between doses is 3 months. However, if the second dose was administered at least 28 days after the first dose, it can be accepted as valid.
10. **Hepatitis A vaccine (HepA).** (Minimum age: 12 months)
    • Administer to all children aged 1 year (i.e., aged 12 through 23 months). Administer 2 doses at least 6 months apart.
    • Children not fully vaccinated by age 2 years can be vaccinated at subsequent visits
    • HepA also is recommended for older children who live in areas where vaccination programs target older children, who are at increased risk for infection, or for whom immunity against hepatitis A is desired.
11. **Meningococcal vaccine.** (Minimum age: 2 years for meningococcal conjugate vaccine [MCV4] and for meningococcal polysaccharide vaccine [MPSV4])
    • Administer MCV4 to children aged 2 through 10 years with persistent complement component deficiency, anatomic or functional asplenia, and certain other conditions placing tham at high risk.
    • Administer MCV4 to children previously vaccinated with MCV4 or MPSV4 after 3 years if first dose administered at age 2 through 6 years. See *MMWR* 2009; 58:1042–3.

The Recommended Immunization Schedules for Persons Aged 0 through 18 Years are approved by the Advisory Committee on Immunization Practices (http://www.cdc.gov/vaccines/recs/acip), the American Academy of Pediatrics (http://www.aap.org), and the American Academy of Family Physicians (http://www.aafp.org). Department of Health and Human Services • Centers for Disease Control and Prevention

**FIGURE 94-1**

Recommended immunization schedule for persons 0 to 6 years of age, United States (2010). Recommended immunization schedules are approved by the Advisory Committee on Immunization Practices (http://www.cdc.gov/nip/acip), the American Academy of Pediatrics (http://www.aap.org), and the American Academy of Family Physicians (http://www.aafp.org). *(From http://aapredbook.aappublications.org/resources/2010_0-6yrs_Schedule_FINAL.pdf)*

## Recommended immunization schedule for persons aged 7 through 18 years — United States, 2010

| Vaccine ▼      Age ► | 7–10 years | 11–12 years | 13–18 years |
|---|---|---|---|
| Tetanus, Diphtheria, Pertussis[1] | | Tdap | Tdap |
| Human Papillomavirus[2] | see footnote 2 | HPV (3 doses) | HPV series |
| Meningococcal[3] | MCV | MCV | MCV |
| Influenza[4] | Influenza (Yearly) | | |
| Pneumococcal[5] | PPSV | | |
| Hepatitis A[6] | HepA Series | | |
| Hepatitis B[7] | Hep B Series | | |
| Inactivated Poliovirus[8] | IPV Series | | |
| Measles, Mumps, Rubella[9] | MMR Series | | |
| Varicella[10] | Varicella Series | | |

Range of recommended ages for all children except certain high-risk groups

Range of recommended ages for catch-up immunization

Range of recommended ages for certain high-risk groups

This schedule includes recommendations in effect as of December 15, 2009. Any dose not administered at the recommended age should be administered at a subsequent visit, when indicated and feasible. The use of a combination vaccine generally is preferred over separate injections of its equivalent component vaccines. Considerations should include provider assessment, patient preference, and the potential for adverse events. Providers should consult the relevant Advisory Committee on Immunization Practices statement for detailed recommendations: http://www.cdc.gov/vaccines/pubs/acip-list.htm. Clinically significant adverse events that follow immunization should be reported to the Vaccine Adverse Event Reporting System (VAERS) at http://www.vaers.hhs.gov or by telephone, 800-822-7967.

1. **Tetanus and diphtheria toxoids and acellular pertussis vaccine (Tdap).** (Minimum age: 10 years for Boostrix and 11 years for Adacel)
   - Administer at age 11 or 12 years for those who have completed the recommended childhood DTP/DTaP vaccination series and have not received a tetanus and diphtheria toxoid (Td) booster dose.
   - Persons aged 13 through 18 years who have not received Tdap should receive a dose.
   - A 5-year interval from the last Td dose is encouraged when Tdap is used as a booster dose; however, a shorter interval may be used if pertussis immunity is needed.

2. **Human papillomavirus vaccine (HPV).** (Minimum age: 9 years)
   - Two HPV vaccines are licensed: a quadrivalent vaccine (HPV4) for the prevention of cervical, vaginal and vulvar cancers (in females) and genital warts (in females and males), and a bivalent vaccine (HPV2) for the prevention of cervical cancers in females.
   - HPV vaccines are most effective for both males and females when given before exposure to HPV through sexual contact.
   - HPV4 or HPV2 is recommended for the prevention of cervical precancers and cancers in females.
   - HPV4 is recommended for the prevention of cervical, vaginal and vulvar precancers and cancers and genital warts in females.
   - Administer the first dose to females at age 11 or 12 years.
   - Administer the second dose 1 to 2 months after the first dose and the third dose 6 months after the first dose (at least 24 weeks after the first dose).
   - Administer the series to females at age 13 through 18 years if not previously vaccinated.
   - HPV4 may be administered in a 3-dose series to males aged 9 through 18 years to reduce their likelihood of acquiring genital warts.

3. **Meningococcal conjugate vaccine (MCV4).**
   - Administer at age 11 or 12 years, or at age 13 through 18 years if not previously vaccinated.
   - Administer to previously unvaccinated college freshmen living in a dormitory.
   - Administer MCV4 to children aged 2 through 10 years with persistent complement component deficiency, anatomic or functional asplenia, or certain other conditions placing them at high risk.
   - Administer to children previously vaccinated with MCV4 or MPSV4 who remain at increased risk after 3 years (if first dose administered at age 2 through 6 years) or after 5 years (if first dose administered at age 7 years or older). Persons whose only risk factor is living in on-campus housing are not recommended to receive an additional dose. See *MMWR* 2009;58:1042–3.

4. **Influenza vaccine (seasonal).**
   - Administer annually to children aged 6 months through 18 years.
   - For healthy nonpregnant persons aged 7 through 18 years (i.e., those who do not have underlying medical conditions that predispose them to influenza complications), either LAIV or TIV may be used.
   - Administer 2 doses (separated by at least 4 weeks) to children aged younger than 9 years who are receiving influenza vaccine for the first time or who were vaccinated for the first time during the previous influenza season but only received 1 dose.
   - For recommendations for use of influenza A (H1N1) 2009 monovalent vaccine. See *MMWR* 2009;58(No. RR-10)

5. **Pneumococcal polysaccharide vaccine (PPSV).**
   - Administer to children with certain underlying medical conditions, including a cochlear implant. A single revaccination should be administered after 5 years to children with functional or anatomic asplenia or an immunocompromising condition. See *MMWR* 1997;46(No. RR-8).

6. **Hepatitis A vaccine (HepA).**
   - Administer 2 doses at least 6 months apart.
   - HepA is recommended for children aged older than 23 months who live in areas where vaccination programs target older children, who are at increased risk for infection, or for whom immunity against hepatitis A is desired.

7. **Hepatitis B vaccine (HepB).**
   - Administer the 3-dose series to those not previously vaccinated.
   - A 2-dose series (separated by at least 4 months) of adult formulation Recombivax HB is licensed for children aged 11 through 15 years.

8. **Inactivated poliovirus vaccine (IPV).**
   - The final dose in the series should be administered on or after the fourth birthday and at least 6 months following the previous dose.
   - If both OPV and IPV were administered as part of a series, a total of 4 doses should be administered, regardless of the child's current age.

9. **Measles, mumps, and rubella vaccine (MMR).**
   - If not previously vaccinated, administer 2 doses or the second dose for those who have received only 1 dose, with at least 28 days between doses.

10. **Varicella vaccine.**
    - For persons aged 7 through 18 years without evidence of immunity (see *MMWR* 2007;56[No. RR-4]), administer 2 doses if not previously vaccinated or the second dose if only 1 dose has been administered.
    - For persons aged 7 through 12 years, the minimum interval between doses is 3 months. However, if the second dose was administered at least 28 days after the first dose, it can be accepted as valid.
    - For persons aged 13 years and older, the minimum interval between doses is 28 days.

The Recommended Immunization Schedules for Persons Aged 0 through 18 Years are approved by the Advisory Committee on Immunization Practices (http://www.cdc.gov/vaccines/recs/acip), the American Academy of Pediatrics (http://www.aap.org), and the American Academy of Family Physicians (http://www.aafp.org). Department of Health and Human Services ● Centers for Disease Control and Prevention

**FIGURE 94-2**

Recommended immunization schedule for persons 7 to 18 years of age, United States (2010). Recommended immunization schedules are approved by the Advisory Committee on Immunization Practices (http://www.cdc.gov/nip/acip), the American Academy of Pediatrics (http://www.aap.org), and the American Academy of Family Physicians (http://www.aafp.org). (*From http://aapredbook.aappublications.org/resources/2010_7-18yrs_Schedule_FINAL.pdf*)

Severe immunosuppression resulting from congenital immunodeficiency, human immunodeficiency virus (HIV) infection, leukemia, lymphoma, cancer therapy, or a prolonged course of high-dose corticosteroids (>2 mg/kg/day for ≥2 weeks) predisposes to complications and is a contraindication for live virus vaccines. For HIV-infected children who do not have evidence of severe immunosuppression, MMR vaccination is recommended at 12 months of age with a second dose 1 month later rather than waiting until 4 to 6 years of age. Varicella vaccine is contraindicated for persons with cellular immunodeficiency but is recommended for persons with impaired humoral immunity (hypogammaglobulinemia or dysgammaglobulinemia) and at 12 months of age for HIV-infected children without evidence of severe immunosuppression, given as two doses 3 months apart.

The National Childhood Vaccine Injury Act requires that clinically significant adverse events after vaccination be reported to the **Vaccine Adverse Event Reporting System (VAERS)** (http://vaers.hhs.gov or 800-822-7967). Suspected cases of vaccine-preventable diseases should be reported to state or local health departments. The Act also established the **National Vaccine Injury Compensation Program**, a no-fault system in which persons thought to have suffered an injury or death as a result of administration of a covered vaccine can seek compensation.

## PROPHYLAXIS

Prophylaxis may include antibiotics, immunoglobulin or monoclonal antibody, vaccine, or in combination and may be used postexposure, for perinatal exposure, and pre-exposure for persons at increased risk for infection. **Primary prophylaxis** is used to prevent infection before a first occurrence. **Secondary prophylaxis** is used to prevent recurrence after a first episode.

### Meningococcus

Primary prophylaxis to all contacts of index cases of *N. meningitidis* infection should be administered as soon as possible (see Chapter 100). Prophylaxis is recommended for all household contacts, especially young children; child care or nursery school contacts in the previous 7 days; for direct exposure to the index patient's secretions through kissing or sharing of toothbrushes or eating utensils; and for mouth-to-mouth resuscitation or unprotected contact during endotracheal intubation within 7 days before onset of illness. Prophylaxis is also recommended for contacts who frequently sleep or eat in the same dwelling as the index patient or passengers seated directly next to the index case during airline flights lasting longer than 8 hours. Chemoprophylaxis is not recommended for casual contacts with no history of direct exposure to the patient's oral secretions (school or work mate), indirect contact with the index patient, or medical personnel without direct exposure to the patient's oral secretions. Rifampin twice daily for 2 days, ceftriaxone once, and ciprofloxacin once (>18 years of age) are the recommended regimens.

### Tetanus

All postexposure wound treatment begins with immediate, thorough cleansing using soap and water, removal of foreign bodies, and débridement of devitalized tissue. Tetanus prophylaxis after wounds and injuries includes vaccination of persons with incomplete immunization and tetanus immunoglobulin for contaminated wounds (soil, feces, saliva), puncture wounds, avulsions, and wounds resulting from missiles, crushing, burns, and frostbite (Table 94-1).

### Rabies

Rabies immune globulin (RIG) and rabies vaccine are extremely effective for prophylaxis after exposure to rabies but are of no known benefit after symptoms appear. Because rabies is one of the deadliest infections, recognition of potential exposure and prophylaxis are crucial. Any healthy-appearing domestic animal responsible for an apparently unprovoked bite should be observed for 10 days for signs of rabies, without immediate treatment of the victim. Prophylaxis should be administered if the animal is rabid or suspected to be rabid, or if the animal develops signs of rabies while under observation. A captured wild animal should be euthanized (by animal control officials) without a period of observation and its brain examined for evidence of rabies. If the biting animal is not captured, particularly if it is a wild animal of a species known to

---

**TABLE 94-1  Guide to Tetanus Prophylaxis in Routine Wound Management**

| Previous Tetanus Immunization (Doses) | Clean Minor Wounds | | All Other Wounds* | |
|---|---|---|---|---|
| | Tdap or Td[†] | TIG[†,‡] | Tdap or Td | TIG[‡] |
| Uncertain or <3 doses | Yes | No | Yes | Yes |
| ≥3 doses | Yes if ≥10 yr since the last tetanus toxoid–containing vaccine dose | No | Yes if ≥5 yr since the last tetanus toxoid–containing vaccine dose | No |

*Such as, but not limited to, wounds contaminated with dirt, feces, soil, or saliva; puncture wounds; avulsions; and wounds resulting from missiles, crushing, burns, and frostbite.

[†]Tdap is preferred for adolescents who have never received Tdap. Td is preferred to tetanus toxoid for adolescents who received Tdap previously or when Tdap is not available.

[‡]Immune globulin intravenous should be used if TIG is not available.

Tdap, tetanus and diphtheria toxoids, adsorbed (for adolescents >11 yr of age and adults); Td, tetanus-diphtheria toxoid; TIG, tetanus immunoglobulin.

harbor the virus in the region, rabies should be presumed and prophylaxis administered to the victim. Skunks, raccoons, foxes, woodchucks, most other carnivores, and bats are regarded as rabid unless proved negative by testing. Prophylaxis also should be provided following exposure to a bat for persons who might be unaware or unable to relate that a bite or direct contact has occurred, such as a mentally disabled person, a sleeping child, or an unattended infant.

All rabies postexposure management begins with immediate thorough cleansing of the bite using soap and water and, if available, irrigation with a virucidal agent such as povidone-iodine. RIG at a dose of 20 U/kg should be administered, with the full dose of RIG infiltrated subcutaneously into the area around the wound, if possible. Any remaining RIG that cannot be infiltrated into the wound should be administered as an intramuscular injection. Inactivated rabies vaccine should be administered simultaneously as soon as possible, with additional vaccine doses at 3, 7, and 14 days.

# CHAPTER 95
# Anti-infective Therapy

**Empirical or presumptive anti-infective therapy** is based on a clinical diagnosis combined with evidence from the literature and from experience of the probable pathogens causing the infection. **Definitive therapy** depends on microbiologic diagnosis by isolation or other direct evidence of the pathogen. Microbiologic diagnosis permits characterization of the pathogen's anti-infective drug **susceptibilities** and delivery of the appropriate anti-infective agent to the site of infection in sufficient concentration to kill the pathogen or alter it sufficiently to facilitate an effective immune response. Antiviral therapy must include consideration of the intracellular nature of viral replication and, to avoid toxicity to the host's cells, must be targeted to viral-specific proteins, such as the thymidine kinase of herpesviruses or the reverse transcriptase of human immunodeficiency virus (HIV). The choice of antimicrobial therapy depends on the site of infection, probable causative agents, host immunity, and the pathogen's susceptibility to the antimicrobial agent.

Empirical antibiotic therapy usually is initiated after obtaining appropriate laboratory tests, including cultures of appropriate fluids or tissues. In high-risk circumstances, such as neonatal sepsis or bacteremia in immunocompromised persons, empirical therapy includes broad-spectrum antibiotics (see Chapters 96 and 120). Empirical antibiotic therapy may be tailored to specific pathogens based on the clinical diagnosis (e.g., streptococcal pharyngitis) or defined risks (e.g., close exposure to tuberculosis). Definitive therapy is based on culture and antibiotic susceptibility, choosing therapy that minimizes drug toxicity, development of resistant microorganisms, superinfection by fungi, and cost.

Antimicrobial agents are an adjunct to the normal host immune response. Infections associated with a foreign body, such as an intravascular catheter, are difficult to eradicate because of organism-produced biofilms that impair phagocytosis. Similarly, it is difficult for phagocytic cells to eradicate bacteria amid vegetations of fibrin and platelets on infected heart valves. Prolonged therapy with bactericidal antibiotics is required with these infections, and outcomes are not always satisfactory. Foreign body devices may have to be removed if sterilization does not occur promptly. Chronic osteomyelitis, with organisms sequestered in abscesses or poorly perfused bone, as well as other infections in closed spaces with limited perfusion (abscesses) are difficult to cure without surgical drainage, débridement of the infected tissue, and re-establishment of a good vascular supply.

Optimal antimicrobial therapy requires an understanding of the **pharmacokinetic properties** of the drugs being administered to specific patient populations. Immaturity of renal function (premature infants) requires increasing dosing intervals to allow time for drug excretion. The larger volume of distribution of hydrophilic antibiotics and increased renal clearance (e.g., in cystic fibrosis) requires higher doses to achieve therapeutic levels. Weight-based dosage regimens may result in overdoses in obese children due to significantly smaller volumes of distribution for hydrophilic drugs. Determining peak and trough drug levels for antibiotics with lower safety margins (e.g., aminoglycosides and vancomycin) minimizes adverse effects of treatment.

**Oral absorption** and **drug-food interactions** may affect the choice of antimicrobial therapy. The bioavailability of orally administered antibiotics varies depending on the acid stability of the drug; degree of gastric acidity; and whether it is taken with food, antacids, $H_2$ blockers, or other medications. An ileus affects intestinal transit time and may result in unpredictable absorption.

The **site and nature** of the infection may affect the choice of antimicrobials. Aminoglycosides, which are active only against aerobic organisms, have significantly reduced activity in abscesses with low pH and oxygen tension. Infections of the central nervous system or the eye necessitate treatment with antimicrobial agents that penetrate and achieve therapeutic levels in these sites.

**Drug-drug interactions** must be considered when multiple antimicrobial agents are used to treat infection. Use of two or more antimicrobial agents may be justified before the identification of the organism or for the benefit of two drugs with different mechanisms of action. Several drugs are administered in combination (trimethoprim-sulfamethoxazole, amoxicillin-clavulanate, ampicillin-sulbactam, and ticarcillin-clavulanate) because of **synergism** (significantly greater bacterial killing than when either is used alone). The addition of clavulanic acid (a β-lactamase inhibitor with modest antibacterial activity) to amoxicillin broadens its spectrum against gram-negative β-lactamase–producing bacteria such as *Haemophilus influenzae,* gram-positive organisms such as *Staphylococcus aureus,* and anaerobes. The use of a bacteriostatic drug, such as a tetracycline, along with a β-lactam agent, effective only against growing organisms, may result in antibiotic **antagonism**, or less bacterial killing in the presence of both drugs than if either is used alone.

# CHAPTER 96
# Fever without a Focus

Core body temperature is normally maintained within 1° C to 1.5° C in a range of 37° C to 38° C. Normal body temperature is generally considered to be 37° C (98.6° F; range, 97° F to 99.6° F). There is a normal diurnal variation, with maximum temperature in the late afternoon. Rectal temperatures higher than 38° C (>100.4° F) generally are considered abnormal, especially if associated with symptoms.

Normal body temperature is maintained by a complex regulatory system in the anterior hypothalamus. Development of fever begins with release of endogenous pyrogens into the circulation as the result of infection, inflammatory processes, or malignancy. Microbes and microbial toxins act as **exogenous pyrogens** by stimulating release of **endogenous pyrogens**, including cytokines such as interleukin-1, interleukin-6, tumor necrosis factor, and interferons. These cytokines reach the anterior hypothalamus, liberating arachidonic acid, which is metabolized to prostaglandin $E_2$. Elevation of the hypothalamic thermostat occurs via a complex interaction of complement and prostaglandin-$E_2$ production. Antipyretics (acetaminophen, ibuprofen, aspirin) inhibit hypothalamic cyclooxygenase, decreasing production of prostaglandin $E_2$. Aspirin is associated with Reye syndrome in children and is not recommended as an antipyretic. The response to antipyretics does not distinguish bacterial from viral infections.

The **pattern of fever** in children may vary depending on the age of the child and the nature of the illness. Neonates may not have a febrile response and may be hypothermic despite significant infection, whereas older infants and children younger than 5 years of age may have an exaggerated febrile response with temperatures of up to 105° F (40.6° C) in response to either a serious bacterial infection or an otherwise benign viral infection. Fever to this degree is unusual in older children and adolescents and suggests a serious process. The fever pattern does not reliably distinguish fever caused by bacterial, viral, fungal, or parasitic organisms from that resulting from malignancy, autoimmune diseases, or drugs.

Children with fever without a focus present a diagnostic challenge that includes identifying bacteremia and sepsis. **Bacteremia**, a positive blood culture, may be primary or secondary to a focal infection. **Sepsis** is the systemic response to infection that is manifested by hyperthermia or hypothermia, tachycardia, tachypnea, and shock (see Chapter 40). Children with septicemia and signs of central nervous system dysfunction (irritability, lethargy), cardiovascular impairment (cyanosis, poor perfusion), and disseminated intravascular coagulation (petechiae, ecchymosis) are readily recognized as **toxic appearing** or **septic**. Most febrile illness in children may be categorized as follows:

- **Fever of short duration** accompanied by localizing signs and symptoms, in which a diagnosis can often be established by clinical history and physical examination
- **Fever without localizing signs** (**fever without a focus**), frequently occurring in children younger than 3 years of age, in which a history and physical examination fail to establish a cause
- **Fever of unknown origin (FUO)**, defined as fever for longer than 14 days without an identified etiology despite history, physical examination, and routine laboratory tests or after 1 week of hospitalization and evaluation

## FEVER IN INFANTS YOUNGER THAN 3 MONTHS OF AGE

Fever or **temperature instability** in infants younger than 3 months of age is associated with a higher risk of **serious bacterial infections** than in older infants. These younger infants usually exhibit only fever and poor feeding, without localizing signs of infection. Most febrile illnesses in this age group are caused by common viral pathogens, but serious bacterial infections include **bacteremia** (caused by group B streptococcus, *Escherichia coli*, *Listeria monocytogenes* in neonates; and *Streptococcus pneumoniae*, *Haemophilus influenzae*, nontyphoidal *Salmonella*, *Neisseria meningitidis* in 1 to 3-month-old infants), **urinary tract infection (UTI)** (*E. coli*), **pneumonia** (*Staphylococcus aureus*, *S. pneumoniae*, or group B streptococcus), **meningitis** (*S. pneumoniae*, *H. influenzae* type b, group B streptococcus, meningococcus, herpes simplex virus, enteroviruses), **bacterial diarrhea** (*Salmonella*, *Shigella*, *E. coli*), and **osteomyelitis** or **suppurative arthritis (septic arthritis)** (*S. aureus* or group B streptococcus).

Differentiation between viral and bacterial infections in young infants is difficult. Febrile infants younger than 3 months of age who appear ill, especially if follow-up is uncertain, and all febrile infants younger than 4 weeks of age should be admitted to the hospital for empirical antibiotics pending culture results. After blood, urine, and cerebrospinal cultures are obtained, broad-spectrum parenteral antibiotics (cefotaxime and ampicillin or ampicillin and gentamicin) are administered. The choice of antibiotics depends on the pathogens suggested by localizing findings. Well-appearing febrile infants 4 weeks of age and older without an identifiable focus and with certainty of follow-up are at a low risk of developing a serious bacterial infection (0.8% develop bacteremia, and 2% develop a serious localized bacterial infection). Specific criteria identifying these low-risk infants include age older than 1 month, well-appearing without a focus of infection, no history of prematurity or prior antimicrobial therapy, a white blood cell (WBC) count of 5000 to 15,000/μL, urine with less than 10 WBCs/high-power field, stool with less than 5 WBCs/high-power field (obtained for infants with diarrhea), and normal chest x-ray (obtained for infants with respiratory signs). These infants may be followed as outpatients without empirical antibiotic treatment, or, alternatively, may be treated with intramuscular ceftriaxone. Regardless of antibiotic treatment, close follow-up for at least 72 hours, including re-evaluation in 24 hours or immediately with any clinical change, is essential.

# FEVER IN CHILDREN 3 MONTHS TO 3 YEARS OF AGE

A common problem is the evaluation of a febrile but well-appearing child younger than 3 years of age without localizing signs of infection. Although most of these children have self-limited viral infections, some have **occult bacteremia** (bacteremia without identifiable focus) or UTIs, and a few have severe and potentially life-threatening illnesses. It is difficult, even for experienced clinicians, to differentiate patients with bacteremia from those with benign illnesses.

**Observational assessment** is a key part of the evaluation. Descriptions of normal appearance and **alertness** include *child looking at the observer* and *looking around the room*, with eyes that are *shiny* or *bright*. Descriptions that indicate severe impairment include *glassy* and *stares vacantly into space*. Observations such as *sitting, moving arms and legs on table or lap*, and *sits without support* reflect normal motor ability, whereas *no movement in mother's arms* and *lies limply on table* indicate severe impairment. Normal behaviors, such as *vocalizing spontaneously, playing with objects, reaching for objects, smiling*, and *crying with noxious stimuli*, reflect **playfulness**; abnormal behaviors reflect **irritability**. A normal response of the behavior **consolability** of the crying child is *stops crying when held by the parent*, whereas severe impairment is indicated by *continual cry despite being held and comforted*.

Children between 2 months and 3 years of age are at increased risk for infection with organisms with polysaccharide capsules, including *S. pneumoniae, H. influenzae, N. meningitidis*, and nontyphoidal *Salmonella*. Effective phagocytosis of these organisms requires opsonic antibody. Transplacental maternal IgG initially provides immunity to these organisms, but as the IgG gradually dissipates, risk of infection increases. In the United States, use of conjugate *H. influenzae* type b and *S. pneumoniae* vaccines has dramatically reduced the incidence of these infections. Determining the immunization status of the child is essential to evaluate risk of these infections. An approach to evaluation of these children is outlined in Figure 96-1.

Most episodes of fever in children younger than 3 years of age have a demonstrable source of infection that is elicited by history, physical examination, or a simple laboratory test. In this age group, the most commonly identified serious bacterial infection is a UTI. A blood culture to evaluate for occult bacteremia and urinalysis and urine culture to evaluate for a UTI should be performed for all children younger than 3 years of age with fever without localizing signs. Patients with diarrhea should have a stool evaluation for leukocytes. Ill-appearing children should be admitted to the hospital and treated with antibiotics.

Approximately 0.2% of well-appearing febrile children 3 to 36 months of age without localizing signs, who have been vaccinated against *S. pneumoniae* and *H. influenzae*, have occult bacteremia. Risk factors for occult bacteremia include temperature of 102.2° F (39° C) or greater, WBC count of 15,000/mm³ or more, and elevated absolute neutrophil count, band count, erythrocyte sedimentation rate, or C-reactive protein. No combination of demographic (socioeconomic status, race, gender, and age), clinical parameters, or laboratory tests in these children reliably predicts occult bacteremia. Occult bacteremia in otherwise healthy children is usually transient and self-limited but may progress to serious localizing infections. Well-appearing children usually are followed as outpatients without empirical antibiotic treatment or, alternatively, treated with intramuscular ceftriaxone. Regardless of antibiotic treatment, close follow-up for at least 72 hours, including re-evaluation in 24 hours or immediately with any clinical change, is essential. Children with a positive blood culture require immediate re-evaluation, repeat blood culture, consideration for lumbar puncture, and empirical antibiotic treatment.

Children with **sickle cell disease** have impaired splenic function and properdin-dependent opsonization that places them at increased risk for bacteremia, especially during the first 5 years of life. Children with sickle cell disease and fever who appear seriously ill, have a temperature of 104° F (40° C) or greater, or WBC count less than 5000/mm³ or greater than 30,000/mm³ should be hospitalized and treated empirically with antibiotics.

**FIGURE 96-1**

Approach to a child younger than 36 months of age with fever without localizing signs. The specific management varies depending on the age and clinical status of the child.

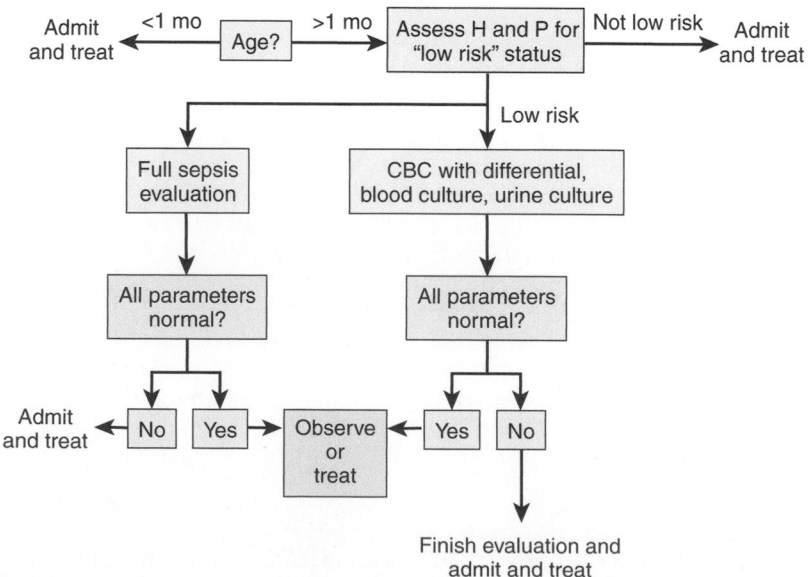

Other children with sickle cell disease and fever should have blood culture, empirical treatment with ceftriaxone, and close outpatient follow-up. Osteomyelitis resulting from *Salmonella* or *S. aureus* is more common in children with sickle cell disease; the blood culture is not always positive in the presence of osteomyelitis.

## FEVER OF UNKNOWN ORIGIN

FUO is defined as temperature greater than 100.4° F (38° C) lasting for more than 14 days without an obvious cause despite a complete history, physical examination, and routine screening laboratory evaluation. Imaging and special diagnostic techniques, including imaging-guided biopsy, have decreased greatly the number of patients with FUO. It is important to distinguish persistent fever from recurrent fever, which usually represents serial acute illnesses.

The initial evaluation of FUO requires a thorough history and physical examination supplemented with a few screening laboratory tests (Fig. 96-2). Additional laboratory and imaging tests are determined by abnormalities on initial evaluation. Important elements of the history include the impact the fever has had on the child's health and activity; weight loss; the use of drugs, medications, or immunosuppressive therapy; history of unusual, severe, or chronic infection suggesting immunodeficiency (see Chapter 72); immunizations; exposure to unprocessed or raw foods; history of pica and exposure to soil-borne or waterborne organisms; exposure to industrial or hobby-related chemicals; blood transfusions; domestic or foreign travel; exposure to animals; exposure to ticks or mosquitoes; ethnic background; recent surgical procedures or dental work; tattooing and body piercing; and sexual activity.

The etiology of most occult infections causing FUO is an unusual presentation of a common disease. Sinusitis, endocarditis, intra-abdominal abscesses (perinephric, intrahepatic, subdiaphragmatic), and central nervous system lesions (tuberculoma, cysticercosis, abscess, toxoplasmosis) may be relatively asymptomatic. Infections are the most common cause of FUO in children, followed by inflammatory diseases, malignancy, and other etiologies (Table 96-1). **Inflammatory diseases** account for approximately 20% of episodes. **Malignancies** are a less common cause of FUO in children than in adults, accounting for about 10% of all episodes. Approximately 15% of children with FUO have no diagnosis. Fever eventually resolves in many of these cases, usually without sequelae, although some may develop definable signs of rheumatic disease over time.

FUO also may be the presentation of an immunodeficiency disease. A history of unusual, severe, or chronic infections suggests immunodeficiency (see Chapter 72) and requires an aggressive evaluation to identify occult infections. Common infections causing FUO in these

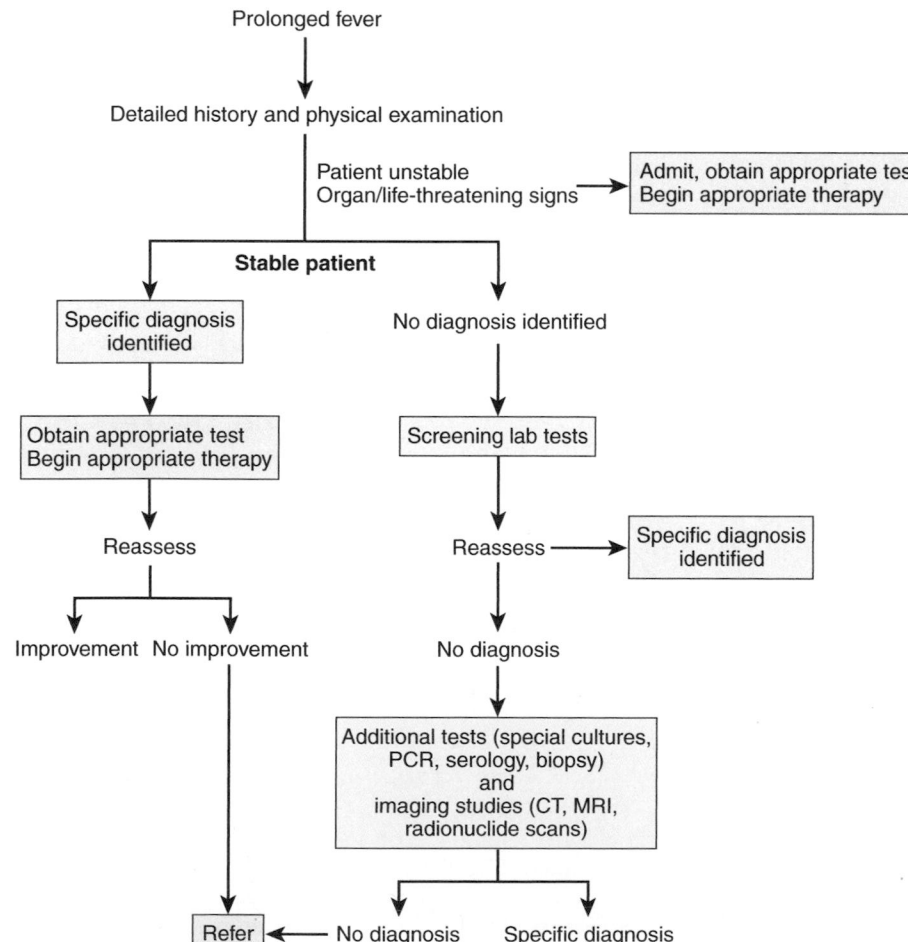

**FIGURE 96-2**

Approach to the evaluation of fever of unknown origin (FUO) in children. Screening laboratory tests include a complete blood count (CBC) and differential white blood cell (WBC) count, platelet count, erythrocyte sedimentation rate, hepatic transaminase levels, urinalysis, bacterial cultures of urine and blood, chest radiograph, and evaluation for rheumatic disease with antinuclear antibody (ANA), rheumatoid factor, and serum complement (C3, C4, $CH_{50}$).

## TABLE 96-1    Causes of Fever of Unknown Origin in Children

### INFECTIONS

*Localized infections*
Abscesses: abdominal, dental, hepatic, pelvic, perinephric, rectal, subphrenic, splenic, periappendiceal, psoas
Cholangitis
Endocarditis
Mastoiditis
Osteomyelitis
Pneumonia
Pyelonephritis
Sinusitis
*Bacterial Diseases*
Brucellosis
*Campylobacter*
Cat-scratch disease (*Bartonella henselae*)
Gonococcemia (chronic)
Leptospirosis
Lyme disease (*Borrelia burgdorferi*)
Meningococcemia (chronic)
Relapsing fever (*Borrelia recurrentis*, other *Borrelia*)
Salmonellosis
*Spirillum minus*
*Streptobacillus moniliformis*
Syphilis
Tuberculosis
Tularemia
*Viral Diseases*
Cytomegalovirus
Hepatitis
HIV (and associated opportunistic infections)
Infectious mononucleosis (Epstein-Barr virus)
*Chlamydial Diseases*
Lymphogranuloma venereum
Psittacosis
*Rickettsial Diseases*
Ehrlichiosis
Q fever
Rocky Mountain spotted fever
*Fungal Diseases*
Blastomycosis (extrapulmonary)
Coccidioidomycosis (disseminated)
Histoplasmosis (disseminated)
*Parasitic Diseases*
Extraintestinal amebiasis
Babesiosis
Giardiasis
Malaria
Toxoplasmosis
Trypanosomiasis
Visceral larva migrans

### INFLAMMATORY DISEASES

Behçet syndrome
Drug fever
Hypersensitivity pneumonitis
Juvenile rheumatoid arthritis (systemic onset, Still disease)
Inflammatory bowel disease (Crohn's disease, ulcerative colitis)
Kawasaki disease
Polyarteritis nodosa
Rheumatic fever
Serum sickness
Systemic lupus erythematosus

### MALIGNANCIES

Atrial myxoma
Ewing sarcoma
Hepatoma
Hodgkin disease
Leukemia
Lymphoma
Neuroblastoma

### MISCELLANEOUS

Anhidrotic ectodermal dysplasia
Deafness, urticaria, amyloidosis syndrome
Diabetes insipidus (central and nephrogenic)
Fabry disease
Familial dysautonomia
Chronic active hepatitis
Granulomatous hepatitis
Hypertriglyceridemia
Ichthyosis
Factitious fever
Hemophagocytic syndromes
Histiocytosis syndromes
Hypothalamic-central fever
Infantile cortical hyperostosis
Pancreatitis
Postoperative (pericardiotomy, craniectomy)
Pulmonary embolism
Sarcoidosis
Spinal cord injury—crisis
Thyrotoxicosis
Central fever

Modified from Powell KR: Fever without a focus. In Kliegman RM, Behrman RE, Jenson HB, et al: Nelson Textbook of Pediatrics, 18th ed, Philadelphia, 2008, *Saunders.*

patients include viral hepatitis, Epstein-Barr virus, cytomegalovirus, *Bartonella henselae,* ehrlichiosis, *Salmonella,* and tuberculosis.

**Factitious fever** or fever produced or feigned intentionally by the patient (**Munchausen syndrome**) or the parent of a child (**Munchausen syndrome by proxy**) is an important consideration, particularly if family members are familiar with health care practices (see Chapter 22). Fever should be recorded in the hospital by a reliable individual who remains with the patient when the temperature is taken. Continuous observation over a long period and repetitive evaluation are essential.

**Screening tests** for FUO include complete blood count with WBC and differential count, platelet count, erythrocyte sedimentation rate, C-reactive protein, hepatic transaminase levels, urinalysis, cultures of urine and blood, chest radiograph, and evaluation for rheumatic disease with antinuclear antibody, rheumatoid factor, and serum complement (C3, C4, CH$_{50}$). Additional tests for FUO that may include throat culture, stool culture, tuberculin skin test with controls, HIV antibody, Epstein-Barr virus antibody profile, and *B. henselae* antibody. Consultation with infectious disease, immunology, rheumatic disease, or oncology specialists should be considered. Further tests may include lumbar puncture for cerebrospinal fluid analysis and culture; computed tomography or magnetic resonance imaging of the chest, abdomen, and head; radionuclide scans; and bone marrow biopsy for cytology and culture.

# CHAPTER 97
# Infections Characterized by Fever and Rash

Rashes are a common manifestation of many infections. The characteristic distribution and appearance provide important clues to the diagnosis (Table 97-1).

## MEASLES (RUBEOLA)

### Etiology

Measles (rubeola) is caused by a single-stranded RNA paramyxovirus with one antigenic type. Humans are the only natural host. Measles virus infects the upper respiratory tract and regional lymph nodes and is spread systemically during a brief, low-titer primary viremia. A secondary viremia occurs within 5 to 7 days as virus-infected monocytes spread the virus to the respiratory tract, skin, and other organs. Virus is present in respiratory secretions, blood, and urine of infected individuals. Measles virus is transmitted by large droplets from the upper respiratory tract and requires close contact. The virus is stable at room temperature for 1 to 2 days. Infected persons are contagious from 1 to 2 days before onset of symptoms (about 5 days before onset of rash) to 4 days after the appearance of the rash.

### Epidemiology

Measles is endemic in regions of the world where measles vaccination is not available and is responsible for about 1 million deaths per year. Since 2000, there typically have been fewer than 100 cases reported annually in the United States, although outbreaks occur. Infections of nonimmigrant children during outbreaks may occur as a result of age (too young to be vaccinated) or low immunization rates. Most young infants are protected by transplacental antibody, but infants become susceptible toward the end of the first year of life.

### Clinical Manifestations

Measles infection is divided into four phases: incubation, prodromal (catarrhal), exanthematous (rash), and recovery. The incubation period is 8 to 12 days from exposure to the onset of symptoms and 14 days from exposure to the onset of rash. The manifestations of the 3-day prodromal period are cough, coryza, conjunctivitis, and the pathognomonic **Koplik spots** (gray-white, sand grain–sized dots on the buccal mucosa opposite the lower molars) that last 12 to 24 hours. The conjunctiva may reveal a characteristic transverse line of inflammation along the eyelid margin (**Stimson line**). The classic symptoms of cough, coryza, and conjunctivitis occur during the secondary viremia of the exanthematous phase, which often is accompanied by high fever (40° C to 40.5° C [104° F to 105° F]). The macular rash begins on the head (often above the hairline) and spreads over most of the body in 24 hours in a cephalad to caudal pattern. Areas of the rash often are confluent. The rash fades in the same pattern. The severity of the illness is related to the extent of the rash. It may be petechial or hemorrhagic (**black measles**). As the rash fades, it undergoes brownish discoloration and desquamation.

Cervical lymphadenitis, splenomegaly, and mesenteric lymphadenopathy with abdominal pain may be noted with the rash. Otitis media, pneumonia, and diarrhea are more common in infants. Liver involvement is more common in adults.

The term **modified measles** describes mild cases of measles occurring in persons with partial protection against measles. Modified measles occurs in persons vaccinated before 12 months of age or with coadministration of immune serum globulin, in infants with disease modified by transplacental antibody, or in persons receiving immunoglobulin.

### Laboratory and Imaging Studies

Routine laboratory findings are nonspecific and do not aid in diagnosis. Leukopenia is characteristic. In patients with acute encephalitis, the cerebrospinal fluid reveals an increased protein, a lymphocytic pleocytosis, and normal glucose levels. Measles virus culture is not generally available. Serologic testing for IgM antibodies, which appear within 1 to 2 days of the rash and persist for 1 to 2 months, confirms the clinical diagnosis. Chest x-rays may show interstitial or perihilar infiltrates but may indicate measles pneumonia or bacterial superinfection. Suspected cases should immediately be reported to the local or state health department.

### Differential Diagnosis

The constellation of fever, rash, cough, and conjunctivitis is diagnostic for measles. Koplik spots are pathognomonic but are not always present at the time the rash is most pronounced. Confirmation is by identification of multinucleated giant cells in nasal mucosal smears and diagnostic antibody increases in acute and convalescent serum. The rash must be differentiated from rubella, roseola, enteroviral or adenoviral infection, infectious mononucleosis, toxoplasmosis, meningococcemia, scarlet fever, rickettsial disease, Kawasaki syndrome, serum sickness, and drug rash.

**TABLE 97-1 Differential Diagnosis of Fever and Rash**

| Lesion | Pathogen or Disease |
| --- | --- |
| **MACULAR OR MACULOPAPULAR RASH** | |
| Viruses | Adenovirus |
| | Measles |
| | Rubella |
| | Roseola (HHV-6 or HHV-7) |
| | Erythema infectiosum (fifth disease, parvovirus B19) |
| | Epstein-Barr virus |
| | Echoviruses |
| | HBV (papular acrodermatitis or Gianotti-Crosti syndrome) |
| | HIV |
| Bacteria | Erythema marginatum (rheumatic fever) |
| | Scarlet fever (group A streptococcus) |
| | Erysipelas (group A streptococcus) |
| | *Arcanobacterium haemolyticum* |
| | Secondary syphilis |
| | Leptospirosis |
| | *Pseudomonas* |
| | Meningococcal infection (early) |
| | *Salmonella typhi* (typhoid fever) |
| | Lyme disease (erythema migrans) |
| | *Mycoplasma pneumoniae* |
| Rickettsiae | Rocky Mountain spotted fever (early) |
| | Typhus (scrub, endemic) |
| | Ehrlichiosis |
| Other | Kawasaki disease |
| | Rheumatoid arthritis |
| | Drug reaction |
| **DIFFUSE ERYTHRODERMA** | |
| Bacteria | Scarlet fever (group A streptococcus) |
| | Staphylococcal scalded skin syndrome |
| | Toxic shock syndrome (*Staphylococcus aureus*) |
| Fungi | *Candida albicans* |
| Other | Kawasaki syndrome |
| **URTICARIAL RASH** | |
| Viruses | Epstein-Barr virus |
| | HBV |
| | HIV |
| Bacteria | *M. pneumoniae* |
| | Group A streptococcus |
| Other | Drug reaction |
| **VESICULAR, BULLOUS, PUSTULAR** | |
| Viruses | Herpes simplex viruses |
| | Varicella-zoster virus |
| | Coxsackievirus |
| Bacteria | Staphylococcal scalded skin syndrome |
| | Staphylococcal bullous impetigo |
| | Group A streptococcal crusted impetigo |
| Rickettsiae | Rickettsialpox |
| Other | Toxic epidermal necrolysis |
| | Erythema multiforme (Stevens-Johnson syndrome) |
| **PETECHIAL-PURPURIC** | |
| Viruses | Adenovirus |
| | Atypical measles |
| | Congenital rubella |

**TABLE 97-1  Differential Diagnosis of Fever and Rash—cont'd**

| Lesion | Pathogen or Disease |
|---|---|
| | Congenital cytomegalovirus |
| | Enterovirus |
| | Papular-purpuric gloves and socks (parvovirus B19) |
| | HIV |
| | Hemorrhagic fever viruses |
| Bacteria | Sepsis (meningococcal, gonococcal, pneumococcal, *Haemophilus influenzae* type b) |
| | Infective endocarditis |
| | Ecthyma gangrenosum (*Pseudomonas aeruginosa*) |
| Rickettsiae | Rocky Mountain spotted fever |
| | Epidemic typhus |
| | Ehrlichiosis |
| Fungi | Necrotic eschar (*Aspergillus*, *Mucor*) |
| Other | Vasculitis |
| | Thrombocytopenia |
| | Henoch-Schönlein purpura |
| | Malaria |
| **ERYTHEMA NODOSUM** | |
| Viruses | Epstein-Barr virus |
| | HBV |
| Bacteria | Group A streptococcus |
| | *Mycobacterium tuberculosis* |
| | *Yersinia* |
| | Cat-scratch disease (*Bartonella henselae*) |
| Fungi | Coccidioidomycosis |
| | Histoplasmosis |
| Other | Sarcoidosis |
| | Inflammatory bowel disease |
| | Estrogen-containing oral contraceptives |
| | Systemic lupus erythematosus |
| | Behçet disease |

HBV, hepatitis B virus; HHV, human herpesvirus.

## Treatment

Routine supportive care includes maintaining adequate hydration and antipyretics. High-dose vitamin A supplementation improves the outcome of malnourished infants with measles and should be considered for persons at high risk for severe complications, including hospitalized infants 6 months to 2 years of age as well as immunodeficient children. The World Health Organization and United Nations and International Children's Emergency Fund recommend routine administration of vitamin A therapy in areas with known vitamin A deficiency or a measles case fatality rate of greater than 1%.

## Complications and Prognosis

Otitis media is the most common complication of measles infection. Interstitial (measles) pneumonia or pneumonia may result from secondary bacterial infection with *Streptococcus pneumoniae*, *Staphylococcus aureus*, or group A streptococcus. Persons with impaired cell-mediated immunity may develop **giant cell (Hecht) pneumonia**, which is usually fatal. Anergy associated with measles may activate latent tuberculosis. Myocarditis and mesenteric lymphadenitis are infrequent complications.

Encephalomyelitis occurs in 1 to 2 per 1000 cases and usually occurs 2 to 5 days after the onset of the rash. Early encephalitis probably is caused by direct viral infection of brain tissue, whereas later onset encephalitis is a demyelinating and probably an immunopathologic phenomenon. **Subacute sclerosing panencephalitis** is a late neurologic complication of slow measles infection that is characterized by progressive behavioral and intellectual deterioration and eventual death. It occurs in approximately 1 in every 1 million cases of measles, an average of 8 to 10 years after measles. There is no effective treatment.

Deaths most frequently result from bronchopneumonia or encephalitis, with much higher risk in persons with malignancy or human immunodeficiency virus (HIV) infection. Deaths in adolescents and adults usually result from subacute sclerosing panencephalitis. Other forms of measles encephalitis in immunocompetent persons are associated with a mortality rate of approximately 15%, with 20% to 30% of survivors having serious neurologic sequelae.

## Prevention

Live measles vaccine prevents infection and is recommended as measles, mumps, and rubella (MMR) for children at 12 to 15 months and 4 to 6 years of age. The MMRV (MMR combined with varicella vaccine) is an alternative vaccine for children 12 months to 12 years of age, provided there are no contraindications. The second dose of MMR is not a booster dose but significantly reduces the primary vaccine failure rate, which is less than 5%. Contraindications to measles vaccine include immunocompromised states resulting from congenital immunodeficiency, severe HIV infection, leukemia, lymphoma, cancer therapy, or an immunosuppressive course of corticosteroids (>2 mg/kg/day for >14 days); pregnancy; or recent administration of immunoglobulin (3 to 11 months, depending on dose). MMR vaccination is recommended for all HIV-infected persons without evidence of severe immunosuppression (low age-specific total CD4 T-lymphocyte count or a low CD4 T-lymphocyte count as a percentage of total lymphocytes), children with cancer in remission who have not received chemotherapy in the previous 3 months, and children who have not received immunosuppressive corticosteroids in the previous month. Susceptible household contacts with a chronic disease or who are immunocompromised when exposed to measles should receive **postexposure prophylaxis** with measles vaccine, within 72 hours of exposure, or immunoglobulin within 6 days of exposure.

## RUBELLA (GERMAN OR 3-DAY MEASLES)

### Etiology

Rubella, also known as **German measles** or **3-day measles**, is caused by a single-stranded RNA virus with a glycolipid envelope, which is a member of the togavirus family. Humans are the only natural host. Rubella virus invades the respiratory epithelium and disseminates via a primary viremia. After replication in the reticuloendothelial system, a secondary viremia ensues, and virus can be isolated from peripheral blood monocytes, cerebrospinal fluid, and urine.

Infection **in utero** results in significant morbidity from **congenital rubella syndrome** (see Chapter 66). Maternal infection during the first trimester results in fetal infection and generalized vasculitis in more than 90% of cases. Rubella virus is most contagious from 2 days before until 5 to 7 days after onset of the rash, although virus may be present in nasopharyngeal secretions from 7 days before until 14 days after the rash. Infants with congenital rubella may shed virus in nasopharyngeal secretions and urine for longer than 12 months after birth and may transmit the virus to susceptible contacts.

### Epidemiology

In unvaccinated populations, rubella usually occurs in the spring, with epidemics occurring in cycles of every 6 to 9 years. Subclinical cases outnumber clinically apparent cases by a ratio of 2:1. Fewer than 20 cases of rubella occur annually in the United States. Outbreaks of rubella in nonvaccinated groups occasionally occur in adults in workplaces, prisons, colleges, and health care centers from internationally imported cases. Transplacental antibody is protective during the first 6 months of life.

### Clinical Manifestations

The incubation period for postnatal rubella is 14 to 23 days. The mild catarrhal symptoms of the prodromal phase of rubella may go unnoticed. The characteristic signs of rubella are retroauricular, posterior cervical, and posterior occipital lymphadenopathy accompanied by an erythematous, maculopapular, discrete rash. The rash begins on the face and spreads to the body and lasts for 3 days. The rash is less prominent than with measles. Rose-colored spots on the soft palate, known as **Forchheimer spots**, develop in 20% of patients and may appear before the rash. Other manifestations of rubella include mild pharyngitis, conjunctivitis, anorexia, headache, malaise, and low-grade fever. Polyarthritis, usually of the hands, may occur, especially among adult females, but usually resolves without sequelae. Paresthesias and tendinitis may occur.

### Laboratory and Imaging Studies

Routine laboratory findings in cases of rubella are nonspecific and generally do not aid in diagnosis. The white blood cell count usually is normal or low, and thrombocytopenia rarely occurs. Diagnosis is confirmed by serologic testing for IgM antibodies or by a fourfold or greater increase in specific IgG antibodies in paired acute and convalescent sera. Cases of suspected congenital rubella syndrome and postnatal rubella infection should be reported to the local and state health department.

### Differential Diagnosis

The rash must be differentiated from measles, roseola, enteroviral or adenoviral infection, infectious mononucleosis, toxoplasmosis, scarlet fever, rickettsial disease, Kawasaki syndrome, serum sickness, and drug rash.

### Treatment

There is no specific therapy for rubella. Routine supportive care includes maintaining adequate hydration and antipyretics.

### Complications and Prognosis

Complications of rubella are rare. Rubella infection during pregnancy may result in **congenital rubella syndrome** with intrauterine growth retardation, cataracts, deafness, neurologic deficits, and a patent ductus arteriosus (see Chapter 66). The prognosis for rubella is excellent. Deaths rarely occur with rubella encephalitis.

### Prevention

Live rubella vaccine prevents infection and is recommended as MMR for children at 12 to 15 months and at 4 to 6 years of age. After vaccination, rubella virus is shed from the nasopharynx for several weeks, but it is not communicable. Pregnant women who are susceptible to rubella should be immunized after delivery. In children, rubella vaccine rarely is associated with adverse effects, but in postpubertal females, it causes arthralgias in 25% of vaccinees and acute arthritis-like symptoms in 10% of vaccinees. These symptoms typically develop 1 to 3 weeks after vaccination and last 1 to 3 days.

**Contraindications** to rubella vaccine include immuno-compromised states resulting from congenital immunodeficiency, HIV infection, leukemia, lymphoma, cancer therapy, or an immunosuppressive course of corticosteroids (>2 mg/kg/day for >14 days); pregnancy; or recent administration of immunoglobulin (3 to 11 months, depending on dose). Vaccine virus has been recovered from fetal tissues, although no cases of congenital rubella syndrome have been identified among infants born to women inadvertently vaccinated against rubella in pregnancy. Nevertheless, women are cautioned to avoid pregnancy after receipt of rubella-containing vaccine for 28 days. All pregnant women should have prenatal serologic testing to determine their immune status to rubella, and susceptible mothers should be vaccinated after delivery and before hospital discharge.

Susceptible, nonpregnant persons exposed to rubella should receive rubella vaccination. Immunoglobulin should be administered to susceptible, pregnant women exposed to rubella.

# ROSEOLA INFANTUM (EXANTHEM SUBITUM)

## Etiology

**Roseola infantum (exanthem subitum, sixth disease)** is caused primarily by human herpesvirus type 6 (HHV-6), and by HHV-7 in 10% to 30% of cases. HHV-6 and HHV-7 are large, enveloped double-stranded DNA viruses that are members of the herpesvirus family. They infect mature mononuclear cells and cause a relatively prolonged (3 to 5 days) viremia during primary infection. They can be detected in the saliva of healthy adults, which suggests, as with other herpesviruses, the development of lifelong latent infection and intermittent shedding of virus.

## Epidemiology

Transplacental antibody protects most infants until 6 months of age. The incidence of infection increases as maternally derived antibody levels decline. By 12 months of age, approximately 60% to 90% of children have antibodies to HHV-6, and essentially all children are seropositive by 2 to 3 years of age. The virus is likely acquired from asymptomatic adults who periodically shed these viruses. HHV-6 is a major cause of acute febrile illnesses in infants and may be responsible for 20% of visits to the emergency department for children 6 to 18 months of age.

## Clinical Manifestations

Roseola is characterized by high fever (often >40° C) with an abrupt onset that lasts 3 to 5 days. A maculopapular, rose-colored rash erupts coincident with defervescence, although it may be present earlier. The rash usually lasts 1 to 3 days but may fade rapidly and is not present in all infants with HHV-6 infection. Upper respiratory symptoms, nasal congestion, erythematous tympanic membranes, and cough may occur. Gastrointestinal symptoms are described. Most children with roseola are irritable and appear toxic. Roseola is associated with approximately one third of febrile seizures. Roseola caused by HHV-6 and HHV-7 is clinically indistinguishable, although HHV-6–associated roseola typically occurs in younger infants. Reactivation of HHV-6 following bone marrow transplantation may result in bone marrow suppression.

## Laboratory and Imaging Studies

Routine laboratory findings are nonspecific and do not aid in diagnosis. Encephalitis with roseola is characterized by pleocytosis (30 to 200 cells/mm$^3$) with mononuclear cell predominance, elevated protein concentration, and normal glucose concentration. Serologic testing showing a fourfold rise in acute and convalescent sera or documenting HHV-6 DNA by polymerase chain reaction in the cerebrospinal fluid is diagnostic.

## Differential Diagnosis

The pattern of high fever for 3 to 5 days without significant physical findings followed by onset of rash with defervescence of fever is characteristic. Many febrile illnesses may be easily confused with roseola during the pre-eruptive stage. Serious infections must be excluded, although most children are alert, behave normally, and continue with their usual daily activities.

## Treatment

There is no specific therapy for roseola. Routine supportive care includes maintaining adequate hydration and antipyretics.

## Complications and Prognosis

The prognosis for roseola is excellent. A few deaths have been attributed to HHV-6, usually in cases complicated by encephalitis or virus-associated **hemophagocytosis syndrome**.

## Prevention

There are no guidelines for prevention of roseola.

# ERYTHEMA INFECTIOSUM (FIFTH DISEASE)

## Etiology

**Erythema infectiosum (fifth disease)** is caused by the human parvovirus B19, a single-stranded DNA virus producing a benign viral exanthem in healthy children. The affinity of this virus to red blood cell progenitor cells makes it an important cause of aplastic crisis in patients with hemolytic anemias, including sickle cell disease, spherocytosis, and thalassemia. Parvovirus B19 also causes fetal anemia and hydrops fetalis after primary infection during pregnancy. The cell receptor for parvovirus B19 is the **erythrocyte P antigen**, a glycolipid present on erythroid cells. The virus replicates in actively dividing erythroid stem cells, leading to cell death that results in erythroid aplasia and anemia.

## Epidemiology

Erythema infectiosum is common. Parvovirus B19 seroprevalence is only 2% to 9% in children younger than 5 years of age, but it increases to 15% to 35% in children 5 to 18 years and 30% to 60% in adults. Community epidemics usually occur in the spring. The virus is transmitted by respiratory secretions and by blood product transfusions.

## Clinical Manifestations

The incubation period is typically 4 to 14 days and rarely may last 21 days. Parvovirus B19 infections usually begin with a mild, nonspecific illness characterized by fever, malaise, myalgias, and headache. In some cases, the characteristic rash appears 7 to 10 days later. Erythema infectiosum is manifested by rash, low-grade or no fever, and occasionally pharyngitis and mild conjunctivitis. The rash appears in three stages. The initial stage is typically a **"slapped cheek" rash** with circumoral pallor. An erythematous symmetrical, maculopapular, truncal rash appears 1 to 4 days later, then fades as central clearing takes place, giving a distinctive **lacy, reticulated rash** that lasts 2 to 40 days (mean, 11 days). This rash may be pruritic, does not desquamate, and may recur with exercise, bathing, rubbing, or stress. Adolescents and adults may experience myalgia, significant arthralgia or arthritis, headache, pharyngitis, coryza, and gastrointestinal upset.

Children with shortened erythrocyte life span (e.g., sickle cell disease) may develop a **transient aplastic crisis** characterized by ineffective erythroid production (see Chapter 150). Most children with parvovirus B19–induced transient aplastic crisis have multiple symptoms, including fever, lethargy, malaise, pallor, headache, gastrointestinal symptoms, and respiratory symptoms. The reticulocyte count is extremely low or zero, and the hemoglobin level is lower than usual for the patient. Transient neutropenia and thrombocytopenia also commonly occur.

Persistent parvovirus B19 infection may develop in children with immunodeficiency, causing severe anemia resulting from pure red blood cell aplasia. These children do not display the typical manifestations of erythema infectiosum.

## Laboratory and Imaging Studies

Many abnormalities occur with parvovirus infection, including reticulocytopenia lasting 7 to 10 days, mild anemia, thrombocytopenia, lymphopenia, and neutropenia. Parvovirus B19 can be detected by polymerase chain reaction and by electron microscopy of erythroid precursors in the bone marrow. Serologic tests showing antibody response to parvovirus, especially the presence of specific IgM antibody to parvovirus, are diagnostic.

## Differential Diagnosis

The diagnosis of erythema infectiosum in children is established on the basis of the clinical findings of typical facial rash with absent or mild prodromal symptoms, followed by a reticulated rash over the body that waxes and wanes. The differential diagnosis includes measles, rubella, scarlet fever, enteroviral or adenoviral infection, infectious mononucleosis, scarlet fever, Kawasaki disease, systemic lupus erythematosus, serum sickness, and drug reaction.

## Treatment

There is no specific therapy. Routine supportive care includes maintaining adequate hydration and antipyretics. Transfusions may be required for transient aplastic crisis. Intrauterine transfusion has been performed for hydrops fetalis associated with fetal parvovirus B19 infection. Intravenous immunoglobulin may be used for immunocompromised persons with severe anemia.

## Complications and Prognosis

The prognosis for erythema infectiosum is excellent. Fatalities associated with transient aplastic crisis are rare. Parvovirus B19 is not teratogenic, but in utero infection of fetal erythroid cells may result in fetal heart failure, hydrops fetalis, and fetal death. Of the approximately 50% of women of childbearing age susceptible to parvovirus B19 infection, 30% of exposed women develop infection, with 25% of exposed fetuses becoming infected and 10% of these culminating in fetal death.

## Prevention

The greatest risk is to pregnant women. Effective control measures are limited. Exclusion of affected children from school is not recommended, because children generally are not infectious by the time the rash is present. Good handwashing and hygiene are practical measures that should help reduce transmission.

# VARICELLA-ZOSTER VIRUS INFECTION (CHICKENPOX AND ZOSTER)

## Etiology

Chickenpox and zoster are caused by varicella-zoster virus (VZV), an enveloped, icosahedral, double-stranded DNA virus that is a member of the herpesvirus family. Humans are the only natural host. **Chickenpox (varicella)** is the manifestation of primary infection. VZV infects susceptible individuals via the conjunctivae or respiratory tract and replicates in the nasopharynx and upper respiratory tract.

It disseminates by a primary viremia and infects regional lymph nodes, the liver, the spleen, and other organs. A secondary viremia follows, resulting in a cutaneous infection with the typical vesicular rash. After resolution of chickenpox, the virus persists in latent infection in the dorsal root ganglia cells. **Zoster (shingles)** is the manifestation of reactivated latent infection of endogenous VZV. Chickenpox is highly communicable in susceptible individuals, with a secondary attack rate of more than 90%. The period of communicability ranges from 2 days before to 7 days after the onset of the rash, when all lesions are crusted.

## Epidemiology

In the prevaccine era, the peak age of occurrence was 5 to 10 years, with peak seasonal infection in late winter and spring. Transmission is by direct contact, droplet, and air. **Zoster** is a recurrence of latent VZV. Only 5% of cases of zoster occur in children younger than 15 years of age. The overall incidence of zoster (215 cases per 100,000 person-years) results in a cumulative lifetime incidence of approximately 10% to 20%, with 75% of cases occurring after 45 years of age. The incidence of zoster is increased in immunocompromised persons.

## Clinical Manifestations

The incubation period of varicella is generally 14 to 16 days, with a range of 11 to 20 days after contact. Prodromal symptoms of fever, malaise, and anorexia may precede the rash by 1 day. The characteristic rash appears initially as small red papules that rapidly progress to nonumbilicated, oval, "teardrop" vesicles on an erythematous base. The fluid progresses from clear to cloudy, and the vesicles ulcerate, crust, and heal. New crops appear for 3 to 4 days, usually beginning on the trunk followed by the head, the face, and, less commonly, the extremities. There may be a total of 100 to 500 lesions, with all forms of lesions being present at the same time. Pruritus is universal and marked. Lesions may be present on mucous membranes. Lymphadenopathy may be generalized. The severity of the rash varies, as do systemic signs and fever, which generally abate after 3 to 4 days.

The pre-eruption phase of **zoster** includes intense localized and constant pain and tenderness **(acute neuritis)** along a dermatome, accompanied by malaise and fever. In several days, the eruption of papules, which quickly vesiculate, occurs in the dermatome or in two adjacent dermatomes. Groups of lesions occur for 1 to 7 days and then progress to crusting and healing. Thoracic and lumbar regions are typically involved. Lesions generally are unilateral and are accompanied by regional lymphadenopathy. In one third of patients, a few vesicles occur outside the primary dermatome. Any branch of cranial nerve V may be involved, which also may cause corneal and intraoral lesions. Involvement of cranial nerve VII may result in facial paralysis and ear canal vesicles (**Ramsay Hunt syndrome**). Ophthalmic zoster may be associated with ipsilateral cerebral angiitis and stroke. Immunocompromised persons may have unusually severe, painful herpes zoster that involves cutaneous and, rarely, visceral dissemination (to liver, lungs, and central nervous system). **Postherpetic neuralgia**, defined as pain persisting longer than 1 month, is uncommon in children.

## Laboratory and Imaging Studies

Laboratory testing confirmation for diagnosis is usually unnecessary. Vesicles exhibit polymorphonuclear leukocytes. Cytology and electron microscopy of vesicular fluid or scrapings may reveal intranuclear inclusions, giant cells, and virus particles. VZV is fastidious and difficult to culture. Cytology consistent with either HSV or VZV in the presence of a negative culture suggests VZV. Detection of varicella-specific antigen in vesicular fluid by immunofluorescence using monoclonal antibodies or demonstration of a fourfold antibody increase of acute and convalescent sera are diagnostic.

## Differential Diagnosis

The diagnosis of varicella and zoster is based on the distinctive characteristics of the rash. **Eczema herpeticum**, or **Kaposi varicelliform eruption**, is a localized, vesicular eruption caused by HSV that develops on skin affected by underlying eczema or trauma. The differentiation between zoster and HSV infection may be difficult because HSV may cause eruption that appears to be in a dermatomal distribution. Coxsackievirus A infection has a vesiculopustular appearance, but lesions are usually localized to the extremities and oropharynx. A previously healthy patient with more than one recurrence probably has HSV infection, which can be confirmed by viral culture.

## Treatment

Symptomatic therapy of varicella includes nonaspirin antipyretics, cool baths, and careful hygiene. Early therapy with antivirals in immunocompromised persons is effective in preventing severe complications, including pneumonia, encephalitis, and death from varicella. Early administration of acyclovir, famciclovir, or valacyclovir for chickenpox may decrease the incidence of varicella pneumonia and is recommended for nonpregnant persons older than 13 years of age and children older than 12 months of age with chronic cutaneous or pulmonary disease; receiving short-course, intermittent, or aerosolized corticosteroids; or receiving long-term salicylate therapy. The dose of acyclovir for VZV infections is much higher than for HSV. Routine oral administration of acyclovir is not recommended in otherwise healthy children with chickenpox because of marginal therapeutic benefit, the lack of difference in complications, and the cost of acyclovir treatment.

Antiviral treatment of zoster accelerates cutaneous healing, hastens the resolution of acute neuritis, and reduces the risk of postherpetic neuralgia. Oral famciclovir and valacyclovir have much greater oral bioavailability than acyclovir and are recommended for treatment of zoster in adults. Acyclovir is recommended for children and is an alternative therapy for adults. The necessity of concomitant oral corticosteroids for zoster is controversial.

## Complications and Prognosis

Secondary infection of skin lesions by streptococci or staphylococci is the most common complication. These infections may be mild, resembling impetigo, or life-threatening with toxic shock syndrome or necrotizing fasciitis. Pneumonia is uncommon in healthy children but occurs in 15% to 20% of healthy adults and immunocompromised persons. Myocarditis, pericarditis, orchitis, hepatitis, ulcerative gastritis, glomerulonephritis, and arthritis may complicate varicella. Reye syndrome may follow varicella; thus, aspirin use is contraindicated during varicella infection.

Neurologic complications frequently include postinfectious encephalitis, cerebellar ataxia, nystagmus, and tremor. Less common neurologic complications include Guillain-Barré syndrome, transverse myelitis, cranial nerve palsies, optic neuritis, and hypothalamic syndrome.

Primary varicella can be a fatal disease in immunocompromised persons as a result of visceral dissemination, encephalitis, and pneumonitis. The mortality rate approaches 15% in children with leukemia who do not receive prophylaxis or therapy for varicella (see Chapter 66).

A severe form of neonatal varicella may develop in newborns of mothers with varicella (but not shingles) occurring 5 days before or 2 days after delivery. The fetus is exposed to a large inoculum of virus but is born before the maternal antibody response develops. These infants should be treated as soon as possible with varicella-zoster immunoglobulin (VZIG) to attempt to prevent or ameliorate the infection.

Primary varicella usually resolves spontaneously. The mortality rate is much higher for persons older than 20 years of age and for immunocompromised persons. Zoster usually is self-limited, especially in children. Advanced age and severity of pain at presentation and at 1 month are predictors of prolonged pain. Scarring is more common with zoster because of involvement of the deeper layers of the skin.

## Prevention

Children with chickenpox should not return to school until all vesicles have crusted. A hospitalized child with chickenpox should be isolated in a negative-pressure room to prevent transmission.

A live attenuated varicella vaccine—two doses for all children—is recommended. The first dose should be administered at age 12 to 15 months and the second dose at 4 to 6 years. Varicella vaccine is 85% effective in preventing any disease and 97% effective in preventing moderately severe and severe disease. Transmission of vaccine virus from a healthy vaccinee is rare but possible.

Passive immunity can be provided by VZIG, which is indicated within 96 hours of exposure for susceptible individuals at increased risk for severe illness. Administration of VZIG does not eliminate the possibility of disease in recipients and prolongs the incubation period up to 28 days.

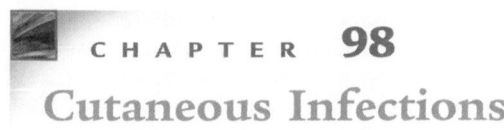

## CHAPTER 98

# Cutaneous Infections

## SUPERFICIAL BACTERIAL INFECTIONS

### Impetigo

**Nonbullous or crusted impetigo** is caused most often by *Staphylococcus aureus* and occasionally by group A streptococcus. It begins as a single erythematous papulovesicle that progresses to one or many **honey-colored, crusted lesions** weeping serous drainage. **Bullous impetigo** accounts for approximately 10% of all impetigo. The skin lesions are thin-walled (0.5 to 3 cm) bullae with erythematous margins resembling second-degree burns and are associated with *S. aureus* phage type 71. Impetigo most frequently occurs on the face, around the nares and mouth, and on the extremities. Fever is uncommon. The diagnosis usually is established by the clinical appearance alone, without the need for culture.

Recommended treatment for nonbullous impetigo is topical 2% mupirocin or oral antistaphylococcal antibiotics. Extensive or disseminated lesions, bullous impetigo, lesions around the eyes, or lesions otherwise are not amenable to topical therapy are best treated with oral antibiotics. Streptococcal impetigo is associated with increased risk of poststreptococcal glomerulonephritis but not acute rheumatic fever (see Chapter 163). Antibiotic treatment for streptococcal impetigo does not decrease the risk of poststreptococcal glomerulonephritis but is recommended to decrease possible spread of nephritogenic strains to close contacts. Children with impetigo should remain out of school or day care until 24 hours of antibiotic therapy has been completed.

### Cellulitis

**Cellulitis** is infection involving the subcutaneous tissues and the dermis and is usually caused by *S. aureus or* group A streptococcus. Cellulitis typically presents with indurated, warm, and erythematous macules with indistinct borders that expand rapidly. Additional manifestations commonly include fever, lymphangitis, regional lymphadenitis, and less often bacteremia, which may lead to secondary foci and sepsis. **Erysipelas** is a superficial variant of cellulitis usually caused by group A streptococcus that involves only the dermis. The rapidly advancing lesions are tender, bright red in appearance, and have sharp margins with an *orange peel* quality. Blood cultures are recommended. Empirical antibiotic treatment for cellulitis is recommended with a first-generation cephalosporin unless the rate of *S. aureus* methicillin-resistance is high. Hospitalization and initial intravenous antibiotic treatment is recommended for erysipelas and cellulitis of the face, hands, feet, or perineum or with lymphangitis. Many patients may be managed with oral antibiotics with close outpatient follow-up.

**Ecthyma** usually is caused by group A streptococcus and may complicate impetigo. Initially, it is characterized by a lesion with a rim of erythematous induration surrounding an eschar, which, if removed, reveals a shallow ulcer. **Ecthyma gangrenosum** is a serious skin infection that occurs in immunocompromised persons due to hematogenous spread of septic emboli to the skin. It classically is caused by *Pseudomonas aeruginosa*, other gram-negative organisms, or occasionally *Aspergillus*. The lesions begin as purple macules that undergo central necrosis to become exquisitely tender, deep, punched-out ulcers 2 to 3 cm in diameter with a dark necrotic base, raised red edges, and sometimes a yellowish green exudate. Fever usually is present.

**Necrotizing fasciitis** is the most extensive form of cellulitis and involves deeper subcutaneous tissues and fascial planes. It may progress to **myonecrosis** of the underlying muscle. It usually is caused by *S. aureus* and group A streptococcus alone or in combination with anaerobic organisms, such as *Clostridium perfringens*. Risk factors include underlying immunodeficiency, recent surgery or trauma, and varicella infection. Lesions progress rapidly with raised or sharply demarcated margins. Subcutaneous gas formation confirms anaerobic infection. Necrotizing fasciitis is a surgical emergency that is associated with systemic toxicity and shock. Early consultation with an experienced surgeon is recommended. Adjunctive tests such as magnetic resonance imaging can confirm the presence of gas in tissues. Treatment includes surgical débridement of all necrotic tissues and intravenous antibiotics, such as clindamycin plus cefotaxime or ceftriaxone, with or without an aminoglycoside.

## Folliculitis

**Folliculitis** refers to small, dome-shaped pustules or erythematous papules located in the hair follicle predominantly caused by *S. aureus,* with superficial, limited inflammatory reaction in the surrounding tissue. A **furuncle (boil)** is a deeper infection of the hair follicle that manifests as nodules with intense surrounding inflammatory reaction. These occur most frequently on the neck, trunk, axillae, and buttocks. A **carbuncle** represents the deepest and most complicated of hair follicle infections and is characterized by multiseptate, loculated abscesses that frequently require incisional drainage. Superficial folliculitis can be treated with topical therapy, such as an antibacterial chlorhexidine wash or an antibacterial lotion or solution such as clindamycin 1%, applied twice a day for 7 to 10 days. Oral antibiotics are necessary for unresponsive or persistent cases, with widespread involvement, or for furuncles or carbuncles. Furuncles and carbuncles may need incision and drainage.

*P. aeruginosa* folliculitis **(hot tub folliculitis)** is associated with hot tubs. It presents as pruritic papules; pustules; or deeper, purple-red nodules that are predominantly on areas of skin that were covered by a swimsuit. Folliculitis develops 8 to 48 hours after exposure, usually without associated systemic symptoms. It usually resolves in 1 to 2 weeks without treatment.

## Perianal Dermatitis

**Perianal dermatitis** (perianal streptococcal disease) is caused by group A streptococcus and is characterized by well-demarcated, tender perianal erythema extending 2 cm from the anus. Manifestations include anal pruritus and painful defecation, sometimes with blood-streaked stools. The differential diagnosis includes diaper dermatitis, candidiasis, pinworm infection, and simple anal fissures. Treatment is oral penicillin V or erythromycin.

## SUPERFICIAL FUNGAL INFECTIONS

Cutaneous fungal infections are common in children (Table 98-1). The estimated lifetime risk of developing a **dermatophytosis** is 10% to 20%. The diagnosis usually is established by visual inspection and may be confirmed by potassium hydroxide (KOH) examination or fungal culture of skin scrapings from the margins of the lesion. **Recommended treatment** of tinea corporis, tinea pedis, and tinea cruris is with a topical antifungal cream (e.g., miconazole, clotrimazole, ketoconazole, tolnaftate) for about 2 weeks or for 1 week after resolution. The diagnosis of **onychomycosis** always should be confirmed by KOH examination and fungal culture. Recommended treatment is terbinafine or itraconazole for at least 12 weeks.

## SUPERFICIAL VIRAL INFECTIONS

### Herpes Simplex Virus

Primary herpetic infections can occur after inoculation of the virus at any mucocutaneous site. Herpes simplex virus (HSV) type 1 is common in children and classically infects skin and mucous membranes above the waist. Cutaneous HSV type 2 may present as part of neonatal HSV infection (see Chapter 65) but otherwise is rare in childhood and classically infects the genitalia as a sexually transmitted infection (see Chapter 116).

**Herpes gingivostomatitis** is a primary HSV infection involving the gingivae and the vermilion border of the lips. Herpes labialis **(cold sores or fever blisters)** is limited to the vermilion border involving skin and mucous membranes. Clinical manifestations of primary HSV gingivostomatitis include typical oropharyngeal vesicular lesions with high fever, malaise, stinging mouth pain, drooling, fetid breath, and cervical lymphadenopathy. After primary infection, HSV establishes latency in the trigeminal ganglion. About 20% to 40% of adults experience recurrent oral episodes of HSV labialis throughout life.

Herpetic skin lesions are quite painful and characteristically begin as erythematous papules that quickly progress to the characteristically grouped, 2- to 4-mm, fluid-filled vesicles on an erythematous base. Removal of the vesicle roof reveals a small, sharply demarcated ulcer with a *punched-out* appearance. The characteristic grouped vesicles distinguish HSV from chickenpox (see Chapter 97). Within several days, the vesicles become pustular, rupture, become crusted and may appear as impetigo. They gradually heal. Scarring is uncommon, but there may be residual hyperpigmentation. After primary infection, the virus remains latent in the dorsal root ganglia. Recurrences occur

**TABLE 98-1  Superficial Fungal Infections**

| Name | Etiology | Manifestations | Diagnosis | Therapy |
|------|----------|----------------|-----------|---------|
| **DERMATOPHYTES** | | | | |
| Tinea capitis (ringworm) | *Microsporum audouinii, Trichophyton tonsurans, Microsporum canis* | Prepubertal infection of scalp, hair-shafts; *black dot* alopecia; *T. tonsurans* common in blacks | *M. audouinii* fluorescence: blue-green with Wood lamp*; +KOH, culture | Griseofulvin; terbinafine, itraconazole |
| Kerion | Inflammatory reaction to tinea capitis | Swollen, boggy, crusted, purulent, tender mass with lymphadenopathy; secondary distal *id* reaction common | As above | As above, plus steroids for *id* reactions |
| Tinea corporis (ringworm) | *M. canis, Trichophyton rubrum,* others | Slightly pruritic ringlike, erythematous papules, plaques with scaling and slow outward expansion of the border; check cat or dog for *M. canis* | +KOH, culture; *M. canis* fluorescence: blue-green with Wood lamp; differential diagnosis: granuloma annulare, pityriasis rosea, nummular eczema, psoriasis | Topical miconazole, clotrimazole, terbinafine, econazole, ketoconazole, or tolnaftate |
| Tinea cruris (jock itch) | *Epidermophyton floccosum, Trichophyton mentagrophytes, T. rubrum* | Symmetrical, pruritic, scrotal sparing, scaling plaques | +KOH, culture; differential diagnosis: erythrasma (*Corynebacterium minutissimum*) | See Tinea corporis, Therapy; wear loose cotton underwear |
| Tinea pedis (athlete's foot) | *T. rubrum, T. mentagrophytes* | Moccasin or interdigital distribution, dry scales, interdigital maceration with secondary bacterial infection | +KOH, culture; differential diagnosis: *C. minutissimum* erythrasma | Medications as above; wear cotton socks |
| Tinea unguium (onychomycosis) | *T. mentagrophytes, T. rubrum, Candida albicans* | Uncommon before puberty; peeling of distal nail plate; thickening, splitting of nails | +KOH, culture | Oral terbinafine or itraconazole |
| Tinea versicolor | *Malassezia furfur* | Tropical climates, steroids or immunosuppressive drugs; uncommon before puberty; chest, back, arms; oval hypopigmented or hyperpigmented in blacks, red-brown in whites; scaling patches | +KOH; orange-gold fluorescence with Wood lamp; differential diagnosis: pityriasis alba | Topical selenium sulfide, oral ketoconazole |
| **YEAST** | | | | |
| Candidiasis | *Candida albicans* | Diaper area, intense erythematous plaques or pustules, isolated or confluent | +KOH, culture | Topical nystatin; oral nystatin treats concomitant oral thrush |

*Wood lamp examination uses an ultraviolet source in a completely darkened room. *Trichophyton* usually has no fluorescence.
KOH, potassium hydroxide.

in roughly the same location and may be preceded by prodromal symptoms of tingling or burning but without fever and lymphadenopathy.

Viral paronychia **(herpetic whitlow)** is a painful, localized infection of a digit, usually of the distal pulp space, with erythematous and occasionally vesiculopustular eruption. It occurs in children who suck their thumbs and bite their nails and especially in children with herpetic gingivostomatitis. **Herpes gladiatorum** occurs in wrestlers and rugby players who acquire cutaneous herpes from close body contact with the cutaneous infections of other players. Cutaneous HSV infection in persons with an underlying skin disorder, often atopic dermatitis, can result in **eczema herpeticum (Kaposi varicelliform eruption)**, which is a disseminated cutaneous infection. There may be hundreds of herpetic vesicles over the body, usually concentrated in the areas of skin affected by the underlying disorder.

Treatment with oral valacyclovir or famciclovir may shorten duration of disease for primary and recurrent infection. Topical antiviral therapy, with penciclovir cream, is effective only for recurrent gingivostomatitis and must be started with the first symptoms. Infants, persons with eczema, and persons with immunodeficiency are at increased risk for disseminated and severe HSV disease and should receive intravenous acyclovir therapy.

## Human Papillomaviruses (Warts)

Warts are caused by the human papillomaviruses (HPVs), which are nonenveloped, double-stranded DNA viruses that infect keratinocytes of the skin and mucous membranes. More than 100 serotypes of HPV have been identified, with different serotypes accounting for the variation in location and clinical presentation of warts. There are 15 to 20 **oncogenic (high-risk)** types, including 16, 18, 31, 33, 35, 39, 45, 51, 52, and 58. HPV types 16 and 18 are associated with 70% of cases of cervical cancer as well as vulvar and vaginal cancers. Common **nononcogenic (low-risk)** types include 1, 2, 3, 6, 10, 11, 40, 42, 43, 44, and 54. Regardless of the infecting serotype, all warts are associated with hyperplasia of the epidermal cells.

Warts occur at all ages. **Common warts (verruca vulgaris),** associated with HPV types 1 and 2, are the most common form (71%). They occur frequently in school-age children, with a prevalence of 4% to 20%. They are transmitted by direct contact or by fomites and have an incubation period of approximately 1 month before clinical presentation. The common wart is a painless, well-circumscribed, small (2- to 5-mm) papule with a papillated or verrucous surface typically distributed on the fingers, toes, elbows, and knees. They also may be found on the nose, ears, and lips. **Filiform warts** are verrucous, exophytic, 2-mm papules that have a narrow or pedunculated base. **Flat warts (verruca plana)** are associated with HPV types 3 and 10 and are multiple, flat-topped 2- to 4-mm papules clustered on the dorsal surface of the hands, on the soles of the feet (**plantar warts**), or on the face. Plantar warts may be painful because of the effect of pressure and friction on the lesions. **Genital warts (condylomata acuminata)** are associated the HPV types 6 and 11 (90%). They are flesh-colored, hyperpigmented, or erythematous lesions that are filiform, fungating, or plaquelike in appearance and involve multiple sites on the vulva, vagina, penis, or perineum. Genital warts are the most common sexually transmitted infection, with 1 million new cases each year.

Warts typically are self-limited and resolve spontaneously over years without specific treatment. Treatment options are available for common and flat warts as well as condylomata acuminata. Topical application of preparations containing salicylic acid to common and flat warts results in a cure of approximately 75% patients. Alternative therapies include cryotherapy with liquid nitrogen and electrodesiccation. Treatment of anogenital warts is complex, and specific treatment guidelines (www.cdc.gov/std/hpv/default.htm) may include topical podophyllotoxin or imiquimod. Additional treatment methods include laser ablation and immunotherapy with intralesional interferon; immunotherapy may result in significant toxicities.

The most serious consequence of HPV infection is cervical, vulvar, and vaginal cancers. A quadrivalent, recombinant HPV vaccine against HPV types 6, 11, 31, and 33 is recommended for all girls at 11 to 12 years of age. It may be given to girls as young as 9 and to women 26 years of age or younger. It is given as a three-dose regimen at 0, 2, and 6 months. The vaccine has 98% to 100% efficacy in preventing the precancerous dysplasia that precedes cervical cancer.

## Molluscum Contagiosum

Molluscum contagiosum virus, a poxvirus that replicates in host epithelial cells, produces discrete, small (2 to 4 mm), pearly flesh-colored or pink, nontender, dome-shaped papules with central umbilication. Papules occur most commonly in intertriginous regions, such as the axillae, groin, and neck. They rarely occur on the face or in the periocular region. The infection typically affects toddlers and young children and is acquired through direct contact with an infected individual. Spread occurs by autoinoculation. Infection with molluscum contagiosum may be complicated by a surrounding dermatitis. Severely immunocompromised persons or persons with extensive atopic dermatitis often have widespread lesions.

Diagnosis is made clinically by the appearance of the rash. Lesions are self-limited, resolving over months to years, and usually no specific treatment is recommended. Available treatment options are limited to destructive modalities, such as cryotherapy with topical liquid nitrogen, vesicant therapy with topical 0.9% cantharidin, or removal by curettage and should be reserved for extensive disease.

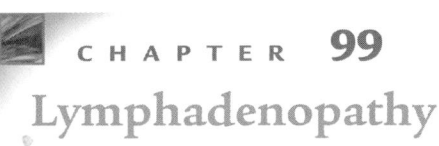

CHAPTER **99**

# Lymphadenopathy

## ETIOLOGY

Lymphoid tissue steadily enlarges until puberty, after which it undergoes progressive atrophy throughout life. Lymph nodes are most prominent in children 4 to 8 years of age. Normal lymph node size is 10 mm in diameter, with the exceptions of 15 mm for inguinal nodes, 5 mm for epitrochlear nodes, and 2 mm for supraclavicular nodes, which are usually undetectable. **Lymphadenopathy** is enlargement of lymph nodes and occurs in response to a wide variety of infectious, inflammatory, and malignant processes. **Generalized lymphadenopathy** is enlargement of two or more noncontiguous lymph node groups, whereas **regional lymphadenopathy** involves only one lymph node group.

**Lymphadenitis** is acute or chronic inflammation of lymph nodes. Acute lymphadenitis usually results when bacteria and toxins from a site of acute inflammation are carried via lymph to regional nodes. Numerous infections cause lymphadenopathy, and lymphadenitis (Tables 99-1 and 99-2). Causes of inguinal regional lymphadenopathy also include sexually transmitted infections (see Chapter 116). **Lymphocutaneous syndromes** are regional lymphadenitis associated with a characteristic skin lesion at the site of inoculation. **Lymphangitis** is an inflammation of subcutaneous lymphatic channels that presents as an acute bacterial infection, usually caused by *Staphylococcus aureus* and group A streptococcus.

Cervical lymphadenitis is the most common regional lymphadenitis among children and is associated most commonly with pharyngitis caused by group A streptococcus (see Chapter 103), respiratory viruses, and Epstein-Barr virus (EBV). Other common infectious causes of cervical lymphadenitis include *Bartonella henselae* (cat-scratch disease) and nontuberculous mycobacteria.

EBV is the primary cause of **infectious mononucleosis**, a clinical syndrome characterized by fever, fatigue and malaise, cervical or generalized lymphadenopathy, tonsillitis, and pharyngitis. EBV, a member of the herpesvirus family, infects B lymphocytes and is spread by salivary secretions. After primary infection, EBV is maintained latently in multiple episomes in the cell nucleus of resting B lymphocytes and establishes lifelong infection that remains clinically inapparent. Most persons

### TABLE 99-1 Infectious Causes of Generalized Lymphadenopathy

#### VIRAL

Epstein-Barr virus (infectious mononucleosis)
Cytomegalovirus (infectious mononucleosis–like syndrome)
HIV (acute retroviral syndrome)
Hepatitis B virus
Hepatitis C virus
Varicella
Adenoviruses
Rubeola (measles)
Rubella

#### BACTERIAL

Endocarditis
*Brucella* (brucellosis)
*Leptospira interrogans* (leptospirosis)
*Streptobacillus moniliformis* (bacillary rat-bite fever)
*Mycobacterium tuberculosis* (tuberculosis)
*Treponema pallidum* (secondary syphilis)

#### FUNGAL

*Coccidioides immitis* (coccidioidomycosis)
*Histoplasma capsulatum* (histoplasmosis)

#### PROTOZOAL

*Toxoplasma gondii* (toxoplasmosis)

### TABLE 99-2 Infectious Causes of Regional Lymphadenopathy

#### NONVENEREAL ORIGIN

*Staphylococcus aureus*
Group A streptococcus
Group B streptococcus (in infants)
*Bartonella henselae* (cat-scratch disease)
*Yersinia pestis* (plague)
*Francisella tularensis* (glandular tularemia)
*Mycobacterium tuberculosis*
Nontuberculous mycobacteria
*Sporothrix schenckii* (sporotrichosis)
Epstein-Barr virus
*Toxoplasma gondii*

#### SEXUALLY TRANSMITTED INFECTIONS (PRIMARILY INGUINAL LYMPHADENOPATHY)

*Neisseria gonorrhoeae* (gonorrhea)
*Treponema pallidum* (syphilis)
Herpes simplex virus
*Haemophilus ducreyi* (chancroid)
*Chlamydia trachomatis* serovars $L_{1-3}$ (lymphogranuloma venereum)

#### LYMPHOCUTANEOUS SYNDROMES

*Bacillus anthracis* (anthrax)
*F. tularensis* (ulceroglandular tularemia)
*B. henselae* (cat-scratch disease)
*Pasteurella multocida* (dog or cat bite)
*Spirillum minus* (spirillary rat-bite fever)
*Y. pestis* (plague)
*Nocardia* (nocardiosis)
Cutaneous diphtheria (*Corynebacterium diphtheriae*)
Cutaneous coccidioidomycosis (*Coccidioides immitis*)
Cutaneous histoplasmosis (*Histoplasma capsulatum*)
Cutaneous sporotrichosis (*S. schenckii*)

shed EBV intermittently, with approximately 20% of healthy individuals shedding EBV at any given time. Cytomegalovirus (CMV), *Toxoplasma gondii*, adenoviruses, hepatitis B virus, hepatitis C virus, and initial human immunodeficiency virus (HIV) infection, known as **acute retroviral syndrome**, can cause an infectious mononucleosis–like syndrome with lymphadenopathy.

The cause of **cat-scratch disease** is *B. henselae*, a small, pleomorphic, gram-negative bacillus that stains with Warthin-Starry silver stain. *B. henselae* does not seem to cause disease in cats despite bacteremia. *B. henselae* is transmitted to humans by bites and scratches, which may be minor. *B. henselae* also causes bacillary angiomatosis and peliosis hepatis in persons with HIV infection (see Chapter 125).

**Nontuberculous mycobacteria** are ubiquitous in soil, vegetation, dust, and water. *Mycobacterium* species commonly causing lymphadenitis in children include *M. avium* complex, *M. scrofulaceum*, and *M. kansasii*. *M. tuberculosis* is an important but uncommon cause of cervical lymphadenitis.

## EPIDEMIOLOGY

Acute cervical lymphadenitis as a complication of group A streptococcal infection parallels the incidence of streptococcal pharyngitis (see Chapter 103). Many cases are caused by S. aureus. EBV and CMV are ubiquitous, with most infections occurring in young children, who may often be asymptomatic or only mildly symptomatic. Risk factors for other specific causes of lymphadenopathy may be indicated by past medical and surgical history; preceding trauma; exposure to animals; contact with persons infected with tuberculosis; sexual history; travel history; food and ingestion history, especially of undercooked meat or unpasteurized dairy products; and current medications.

## CLINICAL MANIFESTATIONS

The exact location and detailed measurement of the size, shape, characteristics, and number of involved nodes should be noted, including their consistency, mobility, tenderness, warmth, fluctuant nature, firmness, and adherence to adjacent tissues. Important findings include presence or absence of dental disease, oropharyngeal or skin lesions, ocular disease, other nodal enlargement, and any other signs of systemic illness, including hepatosplenomegaly and skin lesions.

Acute cervical lymphadenopathy associated with pharyngitis is characterized by small and rubbery lymph nodes in the anterior cervical chain with minimal to moderate tenderness. Suppurative cervical lymphadenitis, frequently caused by S. aureus or group A streptococcus, shows erythema and warmth of the overlying skin with moderate to exquisite tenderness.

The characteristic triad of EBV infectious mononucleosis is fever, pharyngitis, and lymphadenopathy. The pharynx shows enlarged tonsils and exudate and sometimes an enanthem with pharyngeal petechiae. Lymphadenopathy is most prominent in the anterior and posterior cervical and submandibular lymph nodes and less commonly involves axillary and inguinal lymph nodes. Other findings include splenomegaly in 50% of cases, hepatomegaly in 10% to 20%, and maculopapular or urticarial rash in 5% to 15%. A diffuse, erythematous rash develops in approximately 80% of patients with infectious mononucleosis treated with oral ampicillin, known as **ampicillin rash**. Compared with EBV infection, infectious mononucleosis–like illness caused by CMV has minimal pharyngitis and often more prominent splenomegaly; it often presents only with fever. The most common manifestation of toxoplasmosis is asymptomatic cervical lymphadenopathy, but approximately 10% of cases of acquired toxoplasmosis develop chronic posterior cervical lymphadenopathy and fatigue, usually without significant fever.

Cat-scratch disease typically presents with a cutaneous papule or conjunctival granuloma followed by lymphadenopathy localized to the draining regional nodes. The nodes are tender, with suppuration in approximately 10% of cases. Lymphadenopathy may persist 1 to 4 months. Less common features of cat-scratch disease include erythema nodosum, osteolytic lesions, encephalitis, oculoglandular (Parinaud) syndrome, hepatic or splenic granulomas, endocarditis, polyneuritis, and transverse myelitis.

Lymphadenitis caused by nontuberculous mycobacteria usually is unilateral in the cervical, submandibular, or preauricular nodes. The nodes usually are relatively painless and firm initially, but over time they gradually soften, then rupture and drain. The local reaction is circumscribed, and although the skin overlying the node may develop a violaceous discoloration, it is not warm to the touch. Fever and systemic symptoms are minimal or absent.

## LABORATORY AND IMAGING STUDIES

Initial laboratory tests of regional lymphadenopathy include a complete blood count and an erythrocyte sedimentation rate. Infectious mononucleosis is characterized by a lymphocytosis with **atypical lymphocytes**. Thrombocytopenia and elevated hepatic enzymes are common with EBV disease.

Cultures of infected skin lesions and tonsillar exudates should be obtained. Isolation of group A streptococcus from the oropharynx suggests, but does not confirm, streptococcal cervical lymphadenitis. A blood culture should be obtained from children with systemic signs and symptoms of bacteremia.

Serologic testing for EBV and for B. henselae (cat-scratch disease) should be obtained if there are appropriate findings. The most reliable test for diagnosis of acute EBV infection is the IgM anti–viral capsid antigen (Fig. 99-1). Heterophil antibody also is diagnostic but this test is not reliably positive in children younger than 4 years of age with infectious mononucleosis.

Extended diagnostic workup for lymphadenopathy is guided by the specific risk factors in the history and physical examination findings. Chest radiograph, throat culture, antistreptolysin O titer, and serologic tests for CMV, toxoplasmosis, syphilis, tularemia, Brucella, histoplasmosis, and coccidioidomycosis may be indicated. Genital tract evaluation and specimens should be obtained with regional inguinal lymphadenopathy (see Chapter 116). Intradermal skin testing for tuberculosis can be performed using the standard (5 tuberculin units) Mantoux test, which may also be positive with atypical mycobacterial infection.

Aspiration is indicated for acutely inflamed, fluctuant cervical lymph nodes, especially if they are larger than 3 cm in diameter and not responding to antibiotic treatment. Ultrasound or computed tomography may be useful in establishing the extent of lymphadenopathy and defining whether the mass is solid, cystic, or suppurative with formation of an abscess. Pus from fluctuant lesions should be examined by Gram stain and acid-fast stain and cultured for aerobic and anaerobic bacteria and mycobacteria. Biopsy should be performed if lymphoma is suspected because of firm, matted, nontender nodes and other systemic findings.

If the diagnosis remains uncertain and the lymphadenopathy persists despite empirical antibiotic therapy for presumed S. aureus and group A streptococcus, excisional biopsy of the entire node should be performed if possible. This is curative for nontuberculous mycobacterial lymphadenitis. Biopsy material should be submitted for histopathology as well as Gram, acid-fast, Giemsa, periodic

**FIGURE 99-1**

The development of antibodies to various Epstein-Barr virus antigens in patients with infectious mononucleosis. The titers are geometric mean values expressed as reciprocals of the serum dilution. The IgM response to viral capsid antigen (VCA) is divided because of the significant differences noted according to age of the patient. (From Jenson HB, Ench Y: Epstein-Barr virus. In Rose NR, Hamilton RG, Detrick B: Manual of Clinical Laboratory Immunology, ed 7, Washington DC, 2006, *American Society for Microbiology Press*, p. 640.)

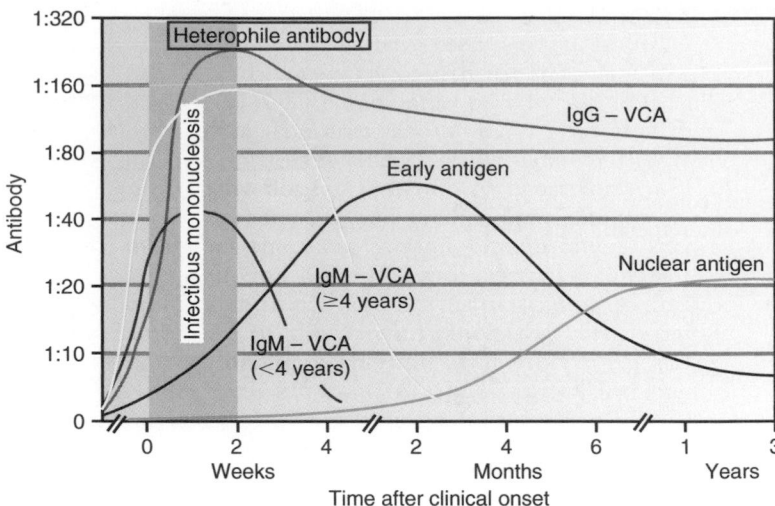

acid–Schiff, Warthin-Starry silver (*B. henselae*), and methenamine silver stains. Cultures for aerobic and anaerobic bacteria, mycobacteria, and fungi should be performed.

## DIFFERENTIAL DIAGNOSIS

Noninfectious causes of cervical lymphadenopathy include congenital and acquired cysts, Kawasaki disease, sarcoidosis, benign neoplasms, and malignancies. The differential diagnosis for generalized lymphadenopathy includes juvenile idiopathic arthritis; systemic lupus erythematosus; and serum sickness and other adverse drug reactions, especially with phenytoin and other antiepileptic medications, allopurinol, isoniazid, antithyroid medications, and pyrimethamine. Leukemia, lymphoma, and occasionally neuroblastoma may have lymph nodes that are usually painless, not inflamed, matted, and firm in consistency (see Chapters 155 and 156). A syndrome of **periodic fever, aphthous stomatitis, pharyngitis, and adenitis** is an occasional cause of recurrent fever and cervical lymphadenitis (see Chapter 103).

## TREATMENT

Management of lymphadenopathy and lymphadenitis depends on the age of the patient, associated findings, size and location of the nodes, and severity of the acute systemic symptoms. In children, most cases of cervical lymphadenopathy, without other signs of acute inflammation, require no specific therapy and usually regress within 2 to 3 weeks. Progression to lymphadenitis or development of generalized lymphadenopathy requires further evaluation.

The specific treatment of cervical lymphadenitis depends on the underlying etiology. The most common causes of acute suppurative cervical lymphadenitis are *S. aureus* and group A streptococcus. Empirical treatment includes a penicillinase-resistant penicillin or first-generation cephalosporin. For patients with hypersensitivity to β-lactam antibiotics, or if community-acquired methicillin-resistant *S. aureus* is suspected, clindamycin is appropriate. Response to empirical antibiotic therapy for suppurative cervical lymphadenitis obviates the need for

further evaluation. Absence of a clinical response within 48 to 72 hours is an indication for further laboratory evaluation and possible excisional biopsy and culture.

There is no specific treatment for infectious mononucleosis. Cat-scratch disease usually does not require treatment because the lymphadenopathy resolves in 2 to 4 months without sequelae. Aspiration is indicated for suppurative nodes. Azithromycin may hasten resolution and reduces node size at 30 days but there is no benefit of treatment at 90 days. The recommended treatment of cervical lymphadenitis caused by nontuberculous mycobacteria is complete surgical excision. Antimycobacterial drugs are necessary only if there is recurrence or inability to excise the infected nodes completely, or if *M. tuberculosis* is identified, which requires 6 months of antituberculous chemotherapy (see Chapter 124). Localized cutaneous or lymphocutaneous sporotrichosis is treated with oral itraconazole.

## COMPLICATIONS AND PROGNOSIS

Most acute infections caused by *S. aureus* and group A streptococcus respond to treatment and have an excellent prognosis. Complications such as abscess formation, cellulitis, and bacteremia may occur. Abscess formation is treated with incision and drainage in conjunction with appropriate antibiotic therapy.

Infectious mononucleosis usually resolves in 2 to 4 weeks, but fatigue and malaise may wax and wane for several weeks to months. EBV also is associated with numerous complications during the acute illness. Neurologic complications include seizures, aseptic meningitis syndrome, Bell palsy, transverse myelitis, encephalitis, and Guillain-Barré syndrome. Hematologic complications include Coombs-positive hemolytic anemia, antibody-mediated thrombocytopenia, hemophagocytic syndrome, and, rarely, aplastic anemia. Corticosteroids have been used for respiratory compromise resulting from tonsillar hypertrophy, which responds rapidly, and for thrombocytopenia, hemolytic anemia, and neurologic complications. Splenic rupture is very rare. **X-linked lymphoproliferative disease,** which results from a mutation of the *SH2D1A* gene located in the Xq25 region, manifests as fulminant infectious mononucleosis with primary EBV infection and progresses to malignant lymphoproliferative disease or dysgammaglobulinemia.

EBV infection, as with other herpesviruses, persists for life, but no symptoms are attributed to intermittent reactivation. EBV is causally associated with nasopharyngeal carcinoma; Burkitt lymphoma; Hodgkin disease; leiomyosarcoma in immunocompromised persons; and EBV lymphoproliferative disease, especially in post-transplant patients and in those with acquired immunodeficiency syndrome (AIDS).

Lymphadenitis caused by nontuberculous mycobacteria has an excellent prognosis. Surgical excision of cervical lymphadenitis caused by nontuberculous mycobacteria is curative in greater than 97% of cases.

## PREVENTION

The incidence of suppurative regional lymphadenitis reflects the incidence of predisposing conditions, such as dental disease, streptococcal pharyngitis, otitis media, impetigo, and other infections involving the face and scalp. There are no guidelines to prevent lymphadenitis caused by nontuberculous mycobacteria.

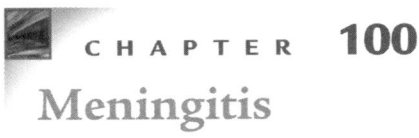

# CHAPTER 100

# Meningitis

## ETIOLOGY

**Meningitis**, inflammation of the leptomeninges, can be caused by bacteria, viruses, or, rarely, fungi. The term **aseptic meningitis** refers principally to viral meningitis, but a similar picture may be seen with other infectious organisms (Lyme disease, syphilis, tuberculosis), parameningeal infections (brain abscess, epidural abscess, venous sinus empyema), chemical exposure (nonsteroidal anti-inflammatory drugs, intravenous immunoglobulin), autoimmune disorders, and many other diseases.

The organisms commonly causing bacterial meningitis (Table 100-1) before the availability of current conjugate vaccines were *Haemophilus influenzae*, *Streptococcus pneumoniae*, and *Neisseria meningitidis*. In the United States, the rate of *H. influenzae* type b meningitis has declined to less than 5% of its previous rate, and the rate of *S. pneumoniae* disease has declined substantially after the introduction of targeted vaccines. The bacteria causing neonatal meningitis are the same as the bacteria that cause neonatal sepsis (see Chapter 65). Staphylococcal meningitis occurs primarily in patients who have had neurosurgery or experience penetrating head trauma.

**Partially treated meningitis** refers to bacterial meningitis complicated by oral antibiotic treatment before the lumbar puncture, which may result in negative cerebrospinal fluid (CSF) cultures, although other CSF findings suggestive of bacterial infection persist. The etiology can be confirmed by antigen detection in the CSF and urine.

**TABLE 100-1 Bacterial Causes of Meningitis**

| Age | Most Common | Less Common |
|---|---|---|
| Neonatal | Group B streptococcus | *Listeria monocytogenes* |
| | *Escherichia coli* | Coagulase-negative staphylococci |
| | *Klebsiella* | *Enterococcus faecalis* |
| | *Enterobacter* | *Citrobacter diversus* |
| | | *Salmonella* |
| | | *Pseudomonas aeruginosa* |
| | | *Haemophilus influenzae* types a, b, c, d, e, f, and nontypable |
| >1 mo | *Streptococcus pneumoniae* | *H. influenzae* type b |
| | *Neisseria meningitidis* | Group A streptococcus |
| | | Gram-negative bacilli |
| | | *L. monocytogenes* |

Viral meningitis is caused principally by enteroviruses, including coxsackieviruses, echoviruses, and, in unvaccinated individuals, polioviruses. Fecal excretion and transmission are continuous and persist for several weeks. Enteroviruses and arboviruses (St. Louis, LaCrosse, West Nile, California encephalitis viruses) are the principal causes of meningoencephalitis (see Chapter 101). Other viruses that cause meningitis include herpes simplex virus, Epstein-Barr virus, cytomegalovirus, lymphocytic choriomeningitis virus, and human immunodeficiency virus (HIV). Mumps virus is a common cause of viral meningitis in unvaccinated children. Uncommon causes of meningitis include *Borrelia burgdorferi* (Lyme disease), *Bartonella henselae* (cat-scratch disease), *Mycobacterium tuberculosis*, *Toxoplasma*, fungi (*Cryptococcus*, *Histoplasma*, and *Coccidioides*), and parasites (*Angiostrongylus cantonensis*, *Naegleria fowleri*, and *Acanthamoeba*).

## EPIDEMIOLOGY

The incidence of bacterial meningitis is highest among children younger than 1 year of age. Extremely high rates are found in Native Americans, Alaskan Natives, and Australian aboriginals, suggesting that genetic factors play a role in susceptibility. Other risk factors include acquired or congenital immunodeficiencies, hemoglobinopathies such as sickle cell disease, functional or anatomic asplenia, and crowding such as occurs in some households, day care centers, or college and military dormitories. A CSF leak resulting from congenital anomaly or following a basilar skull fracture increases the risk of meningitis, especially that caused by *S. pneumoniae*.

Enteroviruses cause meningitis with peaks during summer and fall. These infections are more prevalent among low socioeconomic groups, young children, and immunocompromised persons. The prevalence of arboviral meningitis is determined by geographic distribution and seasonal activity of the arthropod (mosquito) vectors. In the United States, most arboviral infections occur during the summer and fall.

## CLINICAL MANIFESTATIONS

Preceding upper respiratory tract symptoms are common. Rapid onset is typical of *S. pneumoniae* and *N. meningitidis*. Indications of meningeal inflammation include headache, irritability, nausea, nuchal rigidity, lethargy, photophobia, and vomiting. Fever usually is present. Kernig and Brudzinski signs of meningeal irritation are often positive in children older than 12 months of age. In young infants, signs of meningeal inflammation may be minimal with only irritability, restlessness, depressed mental status, and poor feeding. Focal neurologic signs, seizures, arthralgia, myalgia, petechial or purpuric lesions, sepsis, shock, and coma may occur. Increased intracranial pressure is reflected in complaints of headache, diplopia, and vomiting. A bulging fontanelle may be present in infants. Ptosis, sixth nerve palsy, anisocoria, bradycardia with hypertension, and apnea are signs of increased intracranial pressure with brain herniation. Papilledema is uncommon, unless there is occlusion of the venous sinuses, subdural empyema, or brain abscess.

## LABORATORY AND IMAGING STUDIES

If bacterial meningitis is suspected, a lumbar puncture should be performed unless there is evidence of cardiovascular instability or of increased intracranial pressure, other than a bulging fontanelle (because of the risk of herniation). Routine CSF examination includes a white blood cell count, differential, protein and glucose levels, and Gram stain (Table 100-2). CSF should be cultured for

| TABLE 100-2 Cerebrospinal Fluid (CSF) Findings in Various Central Nervous System Disorders | | | | | |
|---|---|---|---|---|---|
| Condition | Pressure | Leukocytes (/μL) | Protein (mg/dL) | Glucose (mg/dL) | Comments |
| Normal | 50–180 mm H₂O | <4; 60%–70% lymphocytes, 30%–40% monocytes, 1%–3% neutrophils | 20–45 | >50% of serum glucose | |
| Acute bacterial meningitis | Usually elevated | 100–60,000+; usually a few thousand; PMNs predominate | 100–500 | Usually <40 or <40% of glucose | Organisms may be seen on Gram stain and recovered by culture |
| Partially treated bacterial meningitis | Normal or elevated | 1–10,000; PMNs usual but mononuclear cells may predominate if pretreated for extended period | >100 | Depressed or normal | Organisms may be seen; pretreatment may render CSF sterile in pneumococcal and meningococcal disease, but antigen may be detected |
| Tuberculous meningitis | Usually elevated; may be low because of CSF block in advanced stages | 10–500; PMNs early but lymphocytes and monocytes predominate later | 100–500; may be higher in presence of CSF block | Usually <50; decreases with time if treatment not provided | Acid-fast organisms may be seen on smear; organisms can be recovered in culture or by PCR; PPD, chest x-ray positive |
| Fungal | Usually elevated | 25–500; PMNs early; mononuclear cells predominate later | 20–500 | Usually <50; decreases with time if treatment not provided | Budding yeast may be seen; organisms may be recovered in culture; India ink preparation may be positive and antigen usually positive in cryptococcal disease |
| Viral meningitis or meningoencephalitis | Normal or slightly elevated | PMNs early; mononuclear cells predominate later; rarely more than 1000 cells except in eastern equine | <200 | Generally normal; may be depressed to 40 in some viral diseases (in 15%–20% of mumps) | Enteroviruses may be recovered from CSF by appropriate viral cultures or detected by PCR; HSV detected by PCR |
| Abscess (parameningeal infection) | Normal or elevated | 0–100 PMNs unless rupture into CSF | 20–200 | Normal | Profile may be completely normal |

HSV, herpes simplex virus; PCR, polymerase chain reaction; PMNs, polymorphonuclear leukocytes; PPD, purified protein derivative of tuberculin.

bacteria and, when appropriate, fungi, viruses, and myco-bacteria. The polymerase chain reaction test is used to diagnose enteroviruses and herpes simplex virus; it is more sensitive and more rapid than viral culture. Leukocytosis is common on the complete blood count. Blood cultures are positive in 90% of cases of bacterial meningitis. An electroencephalogram may confirm an encephalitis component (see Chapter 101).

## DIFFERENTIAL DIAGNOSIS

Many disorders may show signs of meningeal irritation and increased intracranial pressure, including the infectious causes of meningitis, encephalitis, hemorrhage, rheumatic diseases, and malignancies. Seizures are associated with meningitis, encephalitis, and intracranial abscess or can be the sequelae of brain edema, cerebral infarction or hemorrhage, or vasculitis.

## TREATMENT

Treatment of bacterial meningitis focuses on sterilization of the CSF by antibiotics (Table 100-3) and maintenance of adequate cerebral and systemic perfusion. Because of increasing resistance of S. pneumoniae to both penicillin and cephalosporins, cefotaxime (or ceftriaxone) *plus* vancomycin should be administered until antibiotic susceptibility testing is available. Cefotaxime or ceftriaxone are adequate to treat N. meningitidis and H. influenzae types a through f. For infants younger than 2 months of age, ampicillin is added to cover the possibility of Listeria monocytogenes and Escherichia coli. Duration of treatment is 10 to 14 days for S. pneumoniae, 5 to 7 days for N. meningitidis, and 7 to 10 days for H. influenzae.

Dexamethasone therapy (0.6 to 0.8 mg/kg daily in two to three divided doses for 2 days), as **adjunctive therapy** initiated just before or concurrently with the first dose of antibiotics, significantly diminishes the incidence of hearing loss and neurologic deficits resulting from H. influenzae meningitis. In addition, it improves outcomes in both children and adults with pneumococcal meningitis.

Supportive therapy involves treatment of dehydration, shock, disseminated intravascular coagulation, syndrome of inappropriate antidiuretic hormone (SIADH) secretion, seizures, increased intracranial pressure, apnea, arrhythmias, and coma. Adequate cerebral perfusion must be maintained in the presence of cerebral edema.

## COMPLICATIONS AND PROGNOSIS

SIADH secretion may complicate meningitis and necessitates monitoring of urine output and fluid administration. Computed tomography or magnetic resonance imaging commonly detects subdural effusions with S. pneumoniae and H. influenzae meningitis. Most effusions are sterile and asymptomatic, and they do not necessitate drainage unless associated with increased intracranial pressure or focal neurologic signs. Persistent fever is common during treatment, but it also may be related to infective or immune complex-mediated pericardial or joint effusions, thrombophlebitis, drug fever, or nosocomial infection. A repeat lumbar puncture is not indicated for fever in the absence of other signs of persistent central nervous system infection.

Even with appropriate antibiotic therapy, the mortality rate for bacterial meningitis in children is significant: 25% for S. pneumoniae, 15% for N. meningitidis, and 8% for H. influenzae. Of survivors, 35% have sequelae, particularly after pneumococcal infection, including deafness, seizures, learning disabilities, blindness, paresis, ataxia, or hydrocephalus. All patients with meningitis should have hearing evaluation before discharge and at follow-up. Poor prognosis is associated with young age, long duration of illness before effective antibiotic therapy, seizures, coma at presentation, shock, low or absent CSF white blood cell count in the presence of visible bacteria on Gram stain of the CSF, and immunocompromised status.

Rarely, **relapse** may occur 3 to 14 days after treatment, possibly from parameningeal foci or resistant organisms. **Recurrence** may indicate an underlying immunologic or anatomic defect that predisposes the patient to meningitis.

## PREVENTION

Routine **immunizations** against H. influenzae and S. pneumoniae are recommended for children beginning at 2 months of age. Vaccines against N. meningitidis are recommended for young adolescents, college freshmen, military personnel, and travelers to highly endemic areas (see Chapter 94). **Chemoprophylaxis** is recommended for close contacts of persons with N. meningitidis infection plus the index case as well as for close contacts of persons with H. influenzae disease and the index case. Treatment with rifampin, ciprofloxacin, or ceftriaxone is recommended.

### TABLE 100-3  Initial Antimicrobial Therapy by Age for Presumed Bacterial Meningitis

| Age | Recommended Treatment | Alternative Treatments |
|---|---|---|
| Newborns (0–28 days) | Cefotaxime or ceftriaxone plus ampicillin with or without gentamicin | Gentamicin plus ampicillin Ceftazidime plus ampicillin |
| Infants and toddlers (1 mo–4 yr) | Ceftriaxone or cefotaxime plus vancomycin | Cefotaxime or ceftriaxone plus rifampin |
| Children and adolescents (5–13 yr) and adults | Ceftriaxone or cefotaxime plus vancomycin | Cefepime or ceftazidime plus vancomycin |

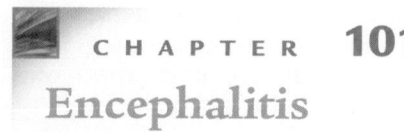

# CHAPTER 101

# Encephalitis

## ETIOLOGY

**Encephalitis** is an inflammatory process of the brain parenchyma leading to cerebral dysfunction. It is usually an acute process but may be a postinfectious encephalomyelitis, a chronic degenerative disease, or a slow viral infection. Encephalitis may be diffuse or localized. Organisms cause encephalitis by one of two mechanisms: (1) direct infection of the brain parenchyma or (2) an apparent immune-mediated response in the central nervous system that usually begins several days after the appearance of extraneural manifestations of the infection.

Viruses are the principal causes of acute infectious encephalitis (Table 101-1). The most common viral causes of encephalitis in the United States are the arboviruses, enteroviruses, and herpesviruses. Human immunodeficiency virus (HIV) is an important cause of subacute encephalitis in children and adolescents and may present as an acute febrile

**TABLE 101-1  Viral Causes of Acute Encephalitis**

| Acute | Frequency* |
|---|---|
| Adenoviruses | Infrequent |
| Arboviruses | Frequent |
| *In North America* | |
| Eastern equine encephalitis | |
| Western equine encephalitis | |
| St. Louis encephalitis | |
| California encephalitis | |
| West Nile encephalitis | |
| Colorado tick fever | |
| *Outside North America* | |
| Venezuelan equine encephalitis | |
| Japanese encephalitis | |
| Tick-borne encephalitis | |
| Murray Valley encephalitis | |
| Enteroviruses | Infrequent |
| Herpesviruses | |
| Herpes simplex viruses | Frequent |
| Epstein-Barr virus | Infrequent |
| Cytomegalovirus (congenital) | Rare |
| Varicella-zoster virus | Infrequent |
| Human herpesvirus-6 | Infrequent |
| Human herpesvirus-7 | Rare |
| Influenza viruses | Infrequent |
| Lymphocytic choriomeningitis virus | Infrequent |
| Measles virus (native or vaccine) | Infrequent |
| Mumps virus (native or vaccine) | Frequent |
| Rabies virus | Frequent |
| Rubella virus | Infrequent |

*Frequency of occurrence of encephalitis as a component of infection.
Adapted from Cherry JD, Shields WD: Encephalitis and meningoencephalitis. In Feigin RD, Cherry JD, Demmler GJ, et al: Textbook of Pediatric Infectious Diseases, 5th ed, Philadelphia, 2004, *Saunders*.

illness but more commonly is insidious in onset (see Chapter 125). Other causes of subacute encephalitis include measles, slow viruses (e.g., JC virus), and prion-associated diseases (e.g., Creutzfeldt-Jakob disease). Encephalitis also may result from metabolic, toxic, and neoplastic disorders.

**Acute disseminated encephalomyelitis (ADEM)** is the abrupt development of multiple neurologic signs related to an inflammatory, demyelinating disorder of the brain and spinal cord. ADEM follows childhood viral infections such as measles and chickenpox or vaccinations and resembles multiple sclerosis clinically.

## EPIDEMIOLOGY

Arboviral and enteroviral encephalitides characteristically appear in clusters or epidemics that occur from midsummer to early fall, although sporadic cases of enteroviral encephalitis occur throughout the year. Herpesviruses and other infectious agents account for additional sporadic cases throughout the year.

Arboviruses tend to be limited to certain geographic areas, reflecting the reservoir and mosquito vector. St. Louis encephalitis virus is present throughout the United States in birds. California encephalitis virus, common in the Midwest, is carried by rodents and spread by mosquitoes. Eastern equine encephalitis virus is limited to the East Coast in birds. Western equine encephalitis virus is present throughout the Midwest and West in birds. West Nile virus infection occurs worldwide and causes outbreaks of summer encephalitis in North America. The principal vector for West Nile virus is the *Culex pipiens* mosquito, but the organism can be isolated in nature from a wide variety of *Culex* and *Aedes* species. A broad range of birds serves as the major reservoir for West Nile virus.

## CLINICAL MANIFESTATIONS

Acute infectious encephalitis usually is preceded by a prodrome of several days of nonspecific symptoms such as cough, sore throat, fever, headache, and abdominal complaints followed by the characteristic symptoms of progressive lethargy, behavioral changes, and neurologic deficits. Seizures are common at presentation. Children with encephalitis also may have a maculopapular rash and severe complications such as fulminant coma, transverse myelitis, anterior horn cell disease, or peripheral neuropathy.

West Nile encephalitis produces a broad spectrum of illness from asymptomatic infection to death. Severity of disease increases with advancing age. Most children are asymptomatic. Typical symptoms include mild, nonspecific extraneurologic illness characterized by fever, rash, arthralgias, lymphadenopathy, gastrointestinal complaints, and conjunctivitis.

## LABORATORY AND IMAGING STUDIES

The diagnosis of viral encephalitis is supported by examination of the cerebrospinal fluid (CSF), which typically shows a lymphocytic pleocytosis, slight elevation in protein content, and normal glucose level. The CSF occasionally may be normal. Extreme elevations of protein and reductions of glucose suggest tuberculosis, cryptococcal infection, or meningeal carcinomatosis. The electroencephalogram (EEG) is the definitive test and shows diffuse, slow wave activity, although focal changes may be present. Neuroimaging studies may be normal or may show diffuse cerebral swelling of the parenchyma or focal abnormalities. A temporal lobe focus on EEG or brain imaging is the characteristic feature of herpes simplex virus (HSV) infection.

Serologic studies should be obtained for arboviruses (including West Nile virus), Epstein-Barr virus, *Mycoplasma pneumoniae*, cat-scratch disease, and Lyme disease. Additional serologic testing for less common pathogens should be performed as indicated by the travel, social, or medical history. In addition to serologic testing, viral cultures of CSF and stool and a nasopharyngeal swab should be obtained. In most cases of viral encephalitis, the virus is difficult to isolate from the CSF. Polymerase chain reaction tests for HSV, enteroviruses, West Nile virus, and other viruses are available and should be sent if no specific cause is found. Even with extensive testing and the use of polymerase chain reaction assays, the cause of encephalitis remains undetermined in one third of cases.

Brain biopsy is seldom performed but may be useful in patients with focal neurologic findings. It may be appropriate for patients with severe encephalopathy who show no clinical improvement if the diagnosis remains obscure. Rabies encephalitis and prion-related diseases (Creutzfeldt-Jakob disease and kuru) may be routinely diagnosed by culture or pathologic examination of brain biopsy tissue. Brain biopsy may be helpful to identify arbovirus and enterovirus infections, tuberculosis, fungal infections, and noninfectious illnesses, particularly primary central nervous system vasculopathies and malignancies.

## DIFFERENTIAL DIAGNOSIS

The diagnosis is established presumptively by the presence of characteristic neurologic signs, typical epidemiology findings, and evidence of infection by CSF analysis, EEG, and brain imaging techniques. Encephalitis may result from infections with bacteria, *Mycoplasma, Rickettsia,* fungi, and parasites and from many noninfectious diseases, including metabolic diseases (encephalopathy) such as Reye syndrome, hypoglycemia, collagen vascular disorders, drugs, hypertension, and malignancies.

## TREATMENT

With the exception of HSV, varicella-zoster virus, cytomegalovirus, and HIV, there is no specific therapy for viral encephalitis. Management is supportive and frequently requires intensive care unit admission to facilitate aggressive therapy for seizures, timely detection of electrolyte abnormalities, and, when necessary, airway monitoring and protection or reduction of increased intracranial pressure and maintenance of adequate cerebral perfusion pressure.

Intravenous acyclovir is the treatment of choice for HSV and varicella-zoster virus infections. Cytomegalovirus infection is treated with ganciclovir. HIV infections may be treated with a combination of antiretroviral agents. *M. pneumoniae* infections may be treated with doxycycline, erythromycin, azithromycin, or clarithromycin, although the clinical value of treating encephalitis associated with mycoplasmal disease is uncertain.

ADEM has been treated with high-dose intravenous corticosteroids, but it is unclear whether the improved outcome with corticosteroids reflects milder cases recognized by magnetic resonance imaging, fewer cases of ADEM caused by measles (which causes severe ADEM), or improved supportive care.

## COMPLICATIONS AND PROGNOSIS

Among survivors, symptoms usually resolve over several days to 2 to 3 weeks. Although most patients with epidemic forms of infectious encephalitis (St. Louis, California, West Nile and enterovirus infections) in the United States recover without sequelae, severe cases leading to death or substantial neurologic sequelae can occur with virtually any of these neurotropic viruses. About two thirds of patients recover fully before being discharged from the hospital. The remainder show clinically significant residua, including paresis or spasticity, cognitive impairment, weakness, ataxia, and recurrent seizures. Most patients with neurologic sequelae of infectious encephalitis at the time of hospital discharge gradually recover some or all of their function. The overall mortality for infectious encephalitis is approximately 5%.

Disease caused by HSV, Eastern equine encephalitis, or *M. pneumoniae* is associated with a worse prognosis. The prognosis may be worse for encephalitis in children younger than 1 year of age or with coma. Rabies is, with very rare exceptions, fatal.

Relapses of ADEM occur in 14%, usually within 1 year with the same or new clinical signs. Recurrences of ADEM may represent onset of multiple sclerosis in childhood.

## PREVENTION

The best prevention for arboviral encephalitis is to avoid mosquito-borne or tick-borne exposures and to remove ticks carefully (see Chapter 122). There are no vaccines in use in the United States for prevention of arboviral infection or for enteroviruses except for poliomyelitis. There are no specific preventive measures for HSV encephalitis except for cesarean section for mothers with active genital lesions (see Chapter 65). Rabies can be prevented by preexposure or postexposure vaccination. Influenza encephalitis can be prevented by use of influenza vaccination. Reye syndrome can be prevented by avoiding use of aspirin or aspirin-containing compounds for children with fever as well as use of varicella and influenza vaccines.

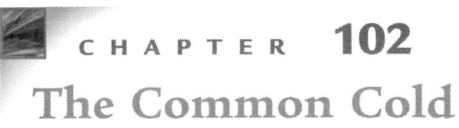

# CHAPTER 102
# The Common Cold

## ETIOLOGY

The common cold is a viral infection with prominent symptoms of rhinorrhea and nasal obstruction, absent or mild fever, and no systemic manifestations. It is often referred to as **rhinitis** but usually involves the sinus mucosa and is more correctly termed **rhinosinusitis**.

The viruses primarily associated with colds are rhinoviruses and, less commonly, coronaviruses. Other viruses that cause common cold symptoms include respiratory syncytial virus and, less commonly, influenza, parainfluenza, and adenoviruses. Viral infection of nasal epithelium causes an acute inflammatory response with mucosal infiltration by inflammatory cells and release of cytokines. The inflammatory response is partly responsible for many of the symptoms.

## EPIDEMIOLOGY

Colds occur throughout the year with peak incidence from early fall through late spring, reflecting the seasonal prevalence of viral pathogens and confined habitation during colder months. Young children have an average of 6 to 7 colds each year, and 10% to 15% of children have at least 12 colds each year. The annual number of colds decreases with age, to 2 to 3 colds each year by adulthood. Children in out-of-home day care during the first year of life have 50% more colds than children cared for only at home. This difference diminishes during subsequent years in day care.

## CLINICAL MANIFESTATIONS

Common cold symptoms typically develop 1 to 3 days after viral infection and include nasal obstruction, rhinorrhea, sore or *scratchy* throat, and occasional nonproductive cough. Colds usually persist about 1 week, although 10% last 2 weeks. There is often a change in the color or consistency of nasal secretions, which is not indicative of sinusitis or bacterial superinfection. Examination of the nasal mucosa may reveal swollen, erythematous nasal turbinates.

## LABORATORY AND IMAGING STUDIES

Laboratory studies often are not helpful. A **nasal smear** for eosinophils may be useful in the evaluation for allergic rhinitis (see Chapter 79).

## DIFFERENTIAL DIAGNOSIS

The differential diagnosis of the common cold includes allergic rhinitis, foreign body (especially with unilateral nasal discharge), sinusitis, pertussis, and streptococcal nasopharyngitis. Allergic rhinitis is characterized by absence of fever, eosinophils in the nasal discharge, and other manifestations, such as allergic shiners, nasal polyps, a transverse crease on the nasal bridge, and pale, edematous, nasal turbinate mucosa. Rare causes of rhinorrhea are choanal atresia or stenosis, cerebrospinal fluid fistula, diphtheria, tumor, congenital syphilis (with *snuffles*), nasopharyngeal malignancy, and Wegener granulomatosis.

## TREATMENT

There is no specific therapy for the common cold. Antibacterial therapy is not beneficial. Management consists of symptomatic therapies. Antihistamines, decongestants, and combination antihistamine–decongestants are not recommended for children younger than 6 years of age because of adverse effects and lack of benefits. Fever infrequently is associated with an uncomplicated common cold and antipyretic treatment is usually unnecessary, although acetaminophen may reduce symptoms of sore throat. Cough suppressants and expectorants have not been shown to be beneficial. Vitamin C and inhalation of warm, humidified air are no more effective than placebo. The benefit of zinc lozenges or sprays has been inconsistent.

## COMPLICATIONS AND PROGNOSIS

Otitis media is the most common complication and occurs in 5% to 20% of children with a cold (see Chapter 105). Other complications include bacterial sinusitis, which should be considered if rhinorrhea or daytime cough persists without improvement for at least 10 to 14 days or if severe signs of sinus involvement develop, such as fever, facial pain, or facial swelling (see Chapter 104). Colds may lead to exacerbation of asthma and may result in inappropriate antibiotic treatment.

## PREVENTION

There are no proven methods for prevention of colds other than good handwashing and avoiding contact with infected persons. No significant effect of vitamin C or echinacea for prevention of the common cold has been confirmed.

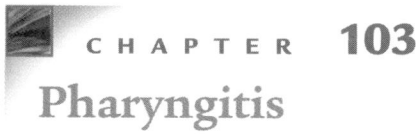

CHAPTER **103**

# Pharyngitis

## ETIOLOGY

Many infectious agents can cause pharyngitis (Table 103-1). Group A streptococci (*Streptococcus pyogenes*) are gram-positive, nonmotile cocci that are facultative anaerobes. On sheep blood agar, the colonies are small (1 to 2 mm in diameter) and have a surrounding zone of β (clear) hemolysis. Other bacterial organisms less often associated with pharyngitis include group C streptococcus (also β-hemolytic), *Arcanobacterium haemolyticum* (β-hemolytic, gram-positive rod), and *Francisella tularensis* (gram-negative coccobacillus and cause of tularemia). *Chlamydophila pneumoniae*, strain TWAR, is associated with lower respiratory disease but also causes sore throat. *Mycoplasma pneumoniae* is associated with atypical pneumonia and may cause mild pharyngitis without distinguishing clinical manifestations. Other bacteria, including *Staphylococcus aureus*, *Haemophilus influenzae*, and *Streptococcus pneumoniae* are cultured frequently from the throats of children with pharyngitis, but their role in causing pharyngitis is unclear.

Many viruses cause acute pharyngitis. Some viruses, such as adenoviruses, are more likely than others to cause pharyngitis as a prominent symptom, whereas other viruses, such as rhinoviruses, are more likely to cause pharyngitis as a minor part of an illness that primarily features other symptoms, such as rhinorrhea or cough. Epstein-Barr virus, enteroviruses (herpangina), herpes simplex virus, and primary human immunodeficiency virus (HIV) infection also produce pharyngitis.

**TABLE 103-1 Major Microbial Causes of Acute Pharyngitis**

| Agent | Syndrome or Disease | Estimated Proportion of All Pharyngitis (%) |
|---|---|---|
| **BACTERIAL** | | |
| Group A streptococcus (*Streptococcus pyogenes*) | Pharyngitis, tonsillitis | 15–30 |
| Group C streptococcus | Pharyngitis, tonsillitis | 1–5 |
| *Arcanobacterium haemolyticum* | Pharyngitis | 0.5–3 |
| Other (e.g., *Corynebacterium diphtheriae*) | Pharyngitis, laryngitis | <5 |
| **VIRAL** | | |
| Rhinoviruses (>100 types) | Common cold | 20 |
| Coronaviruses (>4 types) | Common cold | ≥5 |
| Adenoviruses (types 3, 4, 7, 14, 21) | Pharyngoconjunctival fever, acute respiratory disease | 5 |
| Herpes simplex viruses (types 1 and 2) | Gingivitis, stomatitis, pharyngitis | 4 |
| Parainfluenza viruses (types 1–4) | Common cold, croup | 2 |
| Influenza viruses (types A and B) | Influenza | 2 |
| Epstein-Barr virus | Mononucleosis | Unknown |
| **UNKNOWN** | | 40 |

Adapted from Hayden GF, Hendley JO, Gwaltney JM Jr: Management of the ambulatory patient with a sore throat. *Curr Clin Top Infect Dis* 1988;9:62–75.

## EPIDEMIOLOGY

Sore throat is the primary symptom in approximately one third of upper respiratory tract illnesses. Streptococcal pharyngitis is relatively uncommon before 2 to 3 years of age, but the incidence increases in young school-age children and then declines in late adolescence and adulthood. Streptococcal pharyngitis occurs throughout the year in temperate climates, with a peak during the winter and spring. The illness often spreads to siblings and classmates. Viral infections generally spread via close contact with an infected person and peak during winter and spring.

## CLINICAL MANIFESTATIONS

Pharyngeal inflammation causes cough, sore throat, dysphagia, and fever. If involvement of the tonsils is prominent, the term **tonsillitis** or **tonsillopharyngitis** is often used.

The onset of streptococcal pharyngitis is often rapid and associated with prominent sore throat and moderate to high fever. Headache, nausea, vomiting, and abdominal pain are frequent. In a typical, florid case, the pharynx is distinctly red. The tonsils are enlarged and covered with a yellow, blood-tinged exudate. There may be petechiae or *doughnut-shaped* lesions on the soft palate and posterior pharynx. The uvula may be red, stippled, and swollen. Anterior cervical lymph nodes are enlarged and tender to touch. Many children, however, present with only mild pharyngeal erythema without tonsillar exudate or cervical lymphadenitis. The diagnosis of streptococcal pharyngitis cannot be made on clinical features alone.

In addition to sore throat and fever, some patients exhibit the stigmata of **scarlet fever**: circumoral pallor, strawberry tongue, and a fine diffuse erythematous macular-papular rash that has the feeling of goose flesh. The tongue initially has a white coating, but red and edematous lingual papillae later project through this coating, producing a **white strawberry tongue**. When the white coating peels off, the resulting **red strawberry tongue** is beefy red with prominent papillae. Patients infected with *A. haemolyticum* may present with similar findings.

Compared with classic streptococcal pharyngitis, the onset of viral pharyngitis is typically more gradual, and symptoms more often include rhinorrhea, cough, and diarrhea. Many upper respiratory tract infections present with symptoms of rhinorrhea and nasal obstruction, whereas systemic symptoms and signs, such as myalgia and fever, are absent or mild.

**Gingivostomatitis** is characteristic of herpes simplex virus-1 (see Chapter 65). **Herpangina** is an enteroviral infection with sudden onset of high fever, vomiting, headache, malaise, myalgia, backache, conjunctivitis, poor intake, drooling, sore throat, and dysphagia. The oral lesions of herpangina may be nonspecific, but classically there are one or more small, tender, papular, or pinpoint vesicular lesions on an erythematous base scattered over the soft palate, uvula, and tongue. These vesicles enlarge from 1 to 2 mm to 3 to 4 mm over 3 to 4 days, rupture, and produce small, punched-out ulcers that persist for several days.

## Mononucleosis

▶ SEE CHAPTER 99

## LABORATORY EVALUATION

The principal challenge is to distinguish pharyngitis caused by group A streptococcus from pharyngitis caused by nonstreptococcal (usually viral) organisms. A rapid streptococcal antigen test, a throat culture, or both are often performed to improve diagnostic precision and to identify children most likely to benefit from antibiotic therapy of streptococcal disease.

Many rapid diagnostic techniques for streptococcal pharyngitis are available with excellent specificity of 95% to 99%. The sensitivity of these rapid tests varies, however, and negative rapid tests should be confirmed by throat culture.

Throat culture is the diagnostic *gold standard* for establishing the presence of streptococcal pharyngitis. False-positive cultures can occur if other organisms are incorrectly identified as group A streptococcus. As many as 20% of positive cultures in children during winter months reflect **streptococcal carriers** and not acute pharyngitis.

The predictive values of white blood cell count and differential, erythrocyte sedimentation rate, and C-reactive protein are not sufficient to distinguish streptococcal from nonstreptococcal pharyngitis, and these tests are not routinely recommended. The white blood cell count in patients with infectious mononucleosis usually shows a predominance of atypical lymphocytes.

## DIFFERENTIAL DIAGNOSIS

The differential diagnosis of infectious pharyngitis includes other local infections of the oral cavity, retropharyngeal abscesses (*S. aureus,* streptococci, anaerobes), diphtheria (if unimmunized), peritonsillar abscesses (with quinsy sore throat or unilateral tonsil swelling caused by streptococci, anaerobes, or, rarely, *S. aureus*), and epiglottitis. In addition, neutropenic mucositis (leukemia, aplastic anemia), thrush (candidiasis secondary to T-cell immune deficiency), autoimmune ulceration (systemic lupus erythematosus, Behçet disease), and Kawasaki disease may cause pharyngitis. Pharyngitis is often a prominent feature of Epstein-Barr virus–associated mononucleosis (see Chapter 99).

**Vincent infection** or **trench mouth** is a fulminant form of **acute necrotizing ulcerative gingivitis** with synergistic infection with certain spirochetal organisms, notably *Treponema vincentii*, with anaerobic *Selenomonas* and *Fusobacterium*. **Vincent angina** refers to a virulent form of anaerobic pharyngitis wherein gray pseudomembranes are found on the tonsils, accounting for the synonym **false diphtheria**.

**Noma**, also known as **cancrum oris** or **gangrenous stomatitis**, typically begins as a focal gingival lesion and rapidly progresses to gangrene and consequent destruction of bone, teeth, and soft tissues. Mortality rates of 70% to 90% occur in the absence of prompt surgical intervention. Noma has been associated with infection by *Borrelia vincentii* and *Fusobacterium nucleatum* and seems to be related to severe malnutrition or to immunodeficiency states.

**Ludwig angina** is a mixed anaerobic bacterial cellulitis of the submandibular and sublingual regions. Although often applied to any infection of the sublingual or submandibular region, the term originally was reserved for a rapidly spreading bilateral cellulitis of the sublingual and submandibular spaces. It typically is due to spreading from a periapical abscess of the second or third mandibular molar. It also has been associated with tongue piercing. A propensity for rapid spread, glottic and lingual swelling, and consequent airway obstruction makes prompt intervention imperative.

A syndrome of **periodic fever, aphthous stomatitis, pharyngitis, and cervical adenitis (PFAPA)** is a rare cause of recurrent fever in children. Recurring nonspecific pharyngitis is accompanied by fever and painful solitary vesicular lesions in the mouth. The fevers begin at a young age (usually <5 years). Episodes last approximately 5 days, with a mean of 28 days between episodes. Episodes are shorter with oral prednisone and unresponsive to nonsteroidal anti-inflammatory drugs or antibiotics. The syndrome resolves in some but persist in other children. Long-term sequelae do not develop.

## TREATMENT

Even if untreated, most episodes of streptococcal pharyngitis resolve uneventfully over a few days. Early antimicrobial therapy accelerates clinical recovery by only 12 to 24 hours. The major benefit of antimicrobial therapy is prevention of acute rheumatic fever (see Chapter 146). Because the latent (incubation) period of acute rheumatic fever is relatively long (1 to 3 weeks), treatment instituted within 9 days of illness is virtually 100% successful in preventing rheumatic fever. Treatment begun more than 9 days after the onset of illness, although less than 100% successful, has some preventive value. Antibiotic therapy should be started promptly in children with a positive rapid test for group A streptococcus, scarlet fever, symptomatic pharyngitis whose sibling has documented streptococcal pharyngitis, a past history of rheumatic fever or a recent family history of rheumatic fever, or symptomatic pharyngitis who are living in an area experiencing an epidemic of acute rheumatic fever or poststreptococcal glomerulonephritis.

A variety of antimicrobial agents can be used to treat streptococcal pharyngitis (Table 103-2). Cephalosporins have superior pharyngeal bacterial eradication rates compared with penicillin. One proposed explanation is that staphylococci or anaerobes in the pharynx produce β-lactamase, which inactivates penicillin and reduces its efficacy. Another possible explanation is that cephalosporins are more effective in eradicating streptococcal carriage.

---

**TABLE 103-2  Antimicrobial Treatment of Group A Streptococcal Pharyngitis**

Penicillin
Oral penicillin V (2–3 times daily for 10 days) 10 mg/kg/dose, maximum dose 250 mg/dose
*or*
Intramuscular benzathine penicillin G (single dose)
For children ≤27 kg: 600,000 U
For larger children and adults: 1.2 million U
*For persons allergic to β-lactams*
Erythromycin
Erythromycin ethyl succinate: 40–50 mg/kg/day (max 1 g/day) in 3–4 doses for 10 days
Erythromycin estolate: 20–40 mg/kg/day in 2–4 doses (max 1 g/day) for 10 days
*Alternative therapies:*
Cephalexin 20 mg/kg (max 500 mg/dose) orally every 12 hours for 10 days
Azithromycin, children: 12 mg/kg orally once daily for 5 days (to maximum adult dose); adults: 500 mg orally on day 1, then 250 mg orally on days 2–5

Children with recurrent throat culture episodes of group A streptococcal pharyngitis pose a particular problem. An alternative antibiotic may be chosen to treat β-lactamase producing flora, which may be responsible for the recurrences. Either amoxicillin-clavulanate or clindamycin is an effective regimen for eliminating streptococcal carriage.

Specific antiviral therapy is unavailable for most cases of viral pharyngitis. Patients with primary herpetic gingivostomatitis benefit from early treatment with oral acyclovir.

## COMPLICATIONS AND PROGNOSIS

Pharyngitis caused by streptococci or respiratory viruses usually resolves completely. The complications of group A streptococcal pharyngitis include local suppurative complications, such as parapharyngeal abscess and other infections of the deep fascial spaces of the neck, and nonsuppurative complications, such as acute rheumatic fever and acute postinfectious glomerulonephritis. Viral respiratory tract infections, including infections caused by influenza A, adenoviruses, parainfluenza type 3, and rhinoviruses, may predispose to bacterial middle ear infections.

## PREVENTION

Antimicrobial prophylaxis with daily oral penicillin V prevents recurrent streptococcal infections and is recommended only to prevent recurrences of rheumatic fever.

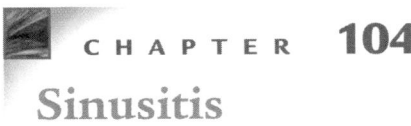

# CHAPTER 104
# Sinusitis

## ETIOLOGY

**Sinusitis** is a suppurative infection of the paranasal sinuses and often complicates the common cold and allergic rhinitis. The maxillary and ethmoid sinuses are present at birth, but only the ethmoidal sinuses are pneumatized. The maxillary sinuses become pneumatized at 4 years of age. Frontal sinuses begin to develop at 7 years of age and are not completely developed until adolescence. The sphenoid sinuses are present by 5 years of age. The ostia draining the sinuses are narrow (1 to 3 mm) and drain into the middle meatus in the **ostiomeatal complex**. The mucociliary system maintains the sinuses as normally sterile.

Obstruction to mucociliary flow, such as mucosal edema resulting from the common cold, impedes sinus drainage and predisposes to bacterial proliferation. In 90% of children with acute sinusitis, the bacterial causes are *Streptococcus pneumoniae*, nontypable *Haemophilus influenzae, Moraxella catarrhalis, Staphylococcus aureus,* and group A streptococcus. Anaerobes emerge as important pathogens in subacute and chronic sinusitis. Indwelling nasogastric and nasotracheal tubes predispose to nosocomial sinusitis, which may be caused by gram-negative bacteria (*Klebsiella* and *Pseudomonas*). Antibiotic therapy predisposes to infection with antibiotic-resistant organisms. Sinusitis in neutropenic and immunocompromised persons may be caused by *Aspergillus* and the Zygomycetes (e.g., *Mucor, Rhizopus*).

## EPIDEMIOLOGY

The true incidence of sinusitis is unknown. The common cold is the major predisposing factor for developing sinusitis at all ages. Other risk factors include cystic fibrosis, immunodeficiency, human immunodeficiency virus (HIV) infection, nasogastric or nasotracheal intubation, immotile cilia syndrome, nasal polyps, and nasal foreign body. Sinusitis also is a frequent problem in immunocompromised children after organ transplantation.

## CLINICAL MANIFESTATIONS

Clinical manifestations most commonly include persistent, mucopurulent, unilateral or bilateral rhinorrhea, nasal stuffiness, and cough, especially at night. Less common symptoms include a nasal quality to the voice, halitosis, facial swelling, facial tenderness and pain, and headache. Sinusitis may exacerbate asthma.

## LABORATORY AND IMAGING STUDIES

Culture of the nasal mucosa is not useful. Sinus aspirate culture is the most accurate diagnostic method but is not practical or necessary. Transillumination may show evidence of fluid, but this is difficult to perform in children and is not reliable.

Plain x-ray and computed tomography may reveal sinus clouding, mucosal thickening, or an air-fluid level. Abnormal radiographic findings do not differentiate infection from allergic disease; computed tomography and magnetic resonance imaging often show abnormalities, including air-fluid levels, in the sinuses of asymptomatic persons. Conversely, normal radiographs have high negative predictive value for bacterial sinusitis.

## DIFFERENTIAL DIAGNOSIS

The diagnosis usually is based on history and physical findings for longer than 10 to 14 days without improvement or increased severity of symptoms compared with the common cold.

## TREATMENT

Amoxicillin administered for 7 days after resolution of symptoms is recommended for treatment of uncomplicated sinusitis. Alternative antibiotics for penicillin-allergic patients include cefuroxime axetil, cefpodoxime, clarithromycin, and azithromycin. For children at increased risk for resistant bacteria (antibiotic treatment in the preceding 1 to 3 months, day care attendance, age <2 years), and for children who fail to respond to initial therapy with amoxicillin within 72 hours, high-dose amoxicillin-clavulanate (80 to 90 mg/kg/day of amoxicillin and 6.4 mg/kg/day of clavulanate) is recommended. Failure to respond to this regimen necessitates referral to an otolaryngologist.

## COMPLICATIONS AND PROGNOSIS

Complications include orbital cellulitis, epidural or subdural empyema, brain abscess, dural sinus thrombosis, osteomyelitis of the outer or inner table of the frontal sinus (**Pott's puffy tumor**), and meningitis. These all should be managed with sinus drainage and broad-spectrum parenteral antibiotics. Sinusitis also may exacerbate bronchoconstriction in asthmatic patients.

**Orbital cellulitis** is a serious complication of sinusitis that follows bacterial spread into the orbit through the wall of the infected sinus. It typically begins as ethmoid sinusitis and spreads through the lamina papyracea, a thin, bony plate that separates the medial orbit and the ethmoid sinus. Orbital involvement can lead to subperiosteal abscess, ophthalmoplegia, cavernous sinus thrombosis, and vision loss. Manifestations of orbital cellulitis include orbital pain, proptosis, chemosis, ophthalmoplegia and limited extraocular muscle motion, diplopia, and reduced visual acuity. Infection of the orbit must be differentiated from that of the preseptal (anterior to the palpebral fascia) or periorbital space. **Preseptal (periorbital) cellulitis** usually occurs in children younger than 3 years of age; these children do not have proptosis or ophthalmoplegia. Periorbital cellulitis is associated with a skin lesion or trauma and usually is caused by *S. aureus* or group A streptococcus.

The diagnosis of orbital cellulitis is confirmed by a computed tomography scan of the orbit, which determines the extent of orbital infection and the need for surgical drainage. Disorders to be considered in the differential diagnosis are zygomycosis (mucormycosis), aspergillosis, rhabdomyosarcoma, neuroblastoma, Wegener granulomatosis, inflammatory pseudotumor of the orbit, and trichinosis. Therapy for orbital cellulitis involves broad-spectrum parenteral antibiotics, such as oxacillin and ceftriaxone.

More than half of children with acute bacterial sinusitis recover without any antimicrobial therapy. Fever and nasal discharge should improve dramatically within 48 hours of initiating treatment. Persistent symptoms suggest another etiology.

## PREVENTION

The best means of prevention are good handwashing to minimize acquisition of colds and management of allergic rhinitis.

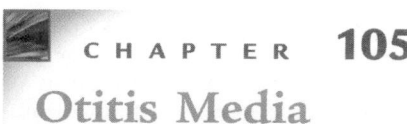

CHAPTER    **105**

# Otitis Media

## ETIOLOGY

**Otitis media (OM)** is a suppurative infection of the middle ear cavity. Bacteria gain access to the middle ear when the normal patency of the eustachian tube is blocked by upper airway infection or hypertrophied adenoids. Air trapped in the middle ear is resorbed, creating negative pressure in this cavity and facilitating reflux of nasopharyngeal bacteria. Obstructed flow of secretions from the middle ear to the pharynx combined with bacterial reflux leads to infected middle ear effusion.

Both bacteria and viruses can cause OM. The common bacterial pathogens are *Streptococcus pneumoniae*, nontypable *Haemophilus influenzae*, *Moraxella catarrhalis*, and, less frequently, group A streptococcus. *S. pneumoniae* that is **relatively resistant** to penicillin (minimal inhibitory concentration 0.1 to 1 µg/mL) or **highly resistant** to penicillin (minimal inhibitory concentration ≥2 µg/mL) is isolated with increasing frequency from young children, particularly those who attend day care or have received antibiotics recently. Viruses, including rhinoviruses, influenza, and respiratory syncytial virus, are recovered alone or as copathogens in 20% to 25% of patients.

## EPIDEMIOLOGY

Diseases of the middle ear account for approximately one third of office visits to pediatricians. The peak incidence of acute OM is between 6 to 15 months of life. By the first birthday, 62% of children experience at least one episode. Few first episodes occur after 18 months of age. OM is more common in boys and in patients of lower socioeconomic status. There is increased incidence of OM in Native Americans and Alaskan Natives and in certain high-risk populations, such as children with human immunodeficiency virus (HIV), cleft palate, and trisomy 21. In most of the United States, OM is a seasonal disease with a distinct peak in January and February, which corresponds to the rhinovirus, respiratory syncytial virus, and influenza seasons. It is less common from July to September. The major risk factors for acute OM are young age, bottle-feeding as opposed to breastfeeding, drinking a bottle in bed, parental history of ear infection, presence of a sibling in the home (especially a sibling with a history of ear infection), sharing a room with a sibling, passive exposure to tobacco smoke, and increased exposure to infectious agents (day care).

As defined by the presence of six or more acute OM episodes in the first 6 years of life, at least 12% of children in the general population have **recurrent OM** and would be considered **otitis-prone**. Craniofacial anomalies and immunodeficiencies often are associated with recurrent OM; most children with recurrent acute OM are otherwise healthy.

## CLINICAL MANIFESTATIONS

In infants, the most frequent symptoms of acute OM are nonspecific and include fever, irritability, and poor feeding. In older children and adolescents, acute OM usually is associated with fever and **otalgia** (acute ear pain). Acute OM also may present with **otorrhea** (ear drainage) after spontaneous rupture of the tympanic membrane. Signs of a common cold, which predisposes to acute OM, are often present (see Chapter 102). A bulging tympanic membrane, air fluid level, or visualization of purulent material by otoscopy are reliable signs of infection (Table 105-1).

## LABORATORY AND IMAGING STUDIES

Routine laboratory studies, including complete blood count and erythrocyte sedimentation rate, are not useful in the evaluation of OM. **Tympanometry** provides objective acoustic measurements of the tympanic membrane–middle

**TABLE 105-1 Definition of Acute Otitis Media (AOM)**

A diagnosis of AOM requires
  History of acute onset of signs and symptoms
  Presence of middle ear effusion
  Signs and symptoms of middle ear inflammation
The definition of AOM includes all of the following:
  Recent, usually abrupt, onset of signs and symptoms of middle ear inflammation and middle ear effusion
  The presence of middle ear effusion that is indicated by any of the following:
    Bulging of the tympanic membrane
    Limited or absent mobility of the tympanic membrane
    Air-fluid level behind the tympanic membrane
    Otorrhea
  Signs or symptoms of middle ear inflammation as indicated by either
    Distinct erythema of the tympanic membrane or
    Distinct otalgia (discomfort clearly referable to the ear that results in interference with or precludes normal activity or sleep)

ear system by reflection or absorption of sound energy from the external ear duct as pressure in the duct is varied. Measurements of the resulting **tympanogram** correlate well with the presence or absence of middle ear effusion.

Instruments using **acoustic reflectometry** are available for office and home use. Use of reflectometry as a screening test for acute OM should be followed by examination with pneumatic otoscopy when abnormal reflectometry is identified.

Bacteria recovered from the nasopharynx do not correlate with bacteria isolated by tympanocentesis. Tympanocentesis and middle ear exudate culture are not always necessary, but they are required for accurate identification of bacterial pathogens and may be useful in neonates, immunocompromised patients, and patients not responding to therapy.

## DIFFERENTIAL DIAGNOSIS

Examination of the ears is essential for diagnosis and should be part of the physical examination of any child with fever. The hallmark of OM is the presence of effusion in the middle ear cavity (see Table 105-1). The presence of an effusion does not define its nature or potentially infectious etiology, but it does define the need for appropriate diagnosis and therapy.

**Pneumatic otoscopy**, using an attachment to a hermetically sealed otoscope, allows evaluation of ventilation of the middle ear and is a standard for clinical diagnosis. The tympanic membrane of the normal, air-filled middle ear has much greater compliance than if the middle ear is fluid-filled. With acute OM, the tympanic membrane is characterized by **hyperemia**, or red color rather than the normal pearly gray color, but it can be pink, white, or yellow with a full to bulging position and with poor or absent mobility to negative and positive pressure. The light reflex is lost, and the middle ear structures are obscured and difficult to distinguish. A hole in the tympanic membrane or purulent drainage confirms perforation. Occasionally, bullae are present on the lateral aspect of the tympanic membrane, which characteristically are associated with severe ear pain.

The major difficulty is differentiation of acute OM from **OM with effusion**, which also is referred to as **chronic OM**. Acute OM is accompanied by signs of acute illness, such as fever, pain, and upper respiratory tract inflammation. OM with effusion is the presence of effusion without any of the other signs and symptoms.

## TREATMENT

Recommendations for treatment are based on certainty of diagnosis and severity of illness. A certain diagnosis can be made if there is rapid onset, signs of middle ear effusion, and signs and symptoms of middle ear inflammation. The recommended first-line therapy for most children with a certain diagnosis of acute OM or those with an uncertain diagnosis but who are younger than 2 years of age or have fever greater than 39 ° C or otalgia is amoxicillin (80 to 90 mg/kg/day in two divided doses). Children with an uncertain diagnosis who are older than 2 years of age may be observed if appropriate follow-up can be arranged. Failure of initial therapy with amoxicillin at 3 days suggests infection with β-lactamase–producing *H. influenzae* or *M. catarrhalis* or resistant *S. pneumoniae*. Recommended next-step treatments include high-dose amoxicillin-clavulanate (amoxicillin 80 to 90 mg/kg/day), cefuroxime axetil, cefdinir, or ceftriaxone (50 mg/kg intramuscularly in daily doses for 1 to 3 days). Intramuscular ceftriaxone is especially appropriate for children younger than 3 years of age with vomiting that precludes oral treatment. Tympanocentesis may be required for patients who are difficult to treat or who do not respond to therapy. Acetaminophen and ibuprofen are recommended for fever. Decongestants or antihistamines are not effective.

## COMPLICATIONS AND PROGNOSIS

The complications of OM are chronic effusion, hearing loss, cholesteatoma (masslike keratinized epithelial growth), petrositis, intracranial extension (brain abscess, subdural empyema, or venous thrombosis), and mastoiditis. **Acute mastoiditis** is a suppurative complication of OM with inflammation and potential destruction of the mastoid air spaces. The disease progresses from a periostitis to an osteitis with mastoid abscess formation. Posterior auricular tenderness, swelling, and erythema, in addition to the signs of OM, are present. The pinna is displaced downward and outward. Radiographs or computed tomography scan of the mastoid reveals clouding of the air cells, demineralization, or bone destruction. Treatment includes systemic antibiotics and drainage if the disease has progressed to abscess formation.

**OM with effusion** is the most frequent sequela of acute OM and occurs most frequently in the first 2 years of life. **Persistent middle ear effusion** may last for many weeks or months in some children but usually resolves by 3 months following infection. Evaluating young children for this condition is part of all well-child examinations.

Conductive hearing loss should be assumed to be present with persistent middle ear effusion; the loss is mild to moderate and often is transient or fluctuating. **Glue ear** is used to describe the presence of a viscous, gluelike effusion that is produced when the chronically inflamed middle ear mucosa produces an excess of mucus that, because of absence of the normal clearance of the middle ear cavity, is retained for prolonged periods.

Normal tympanograms after 1 month of treatment obviate the need for further follow-up. In children at developmental risk or with frequent episodes of recurrent acute OM, 3 months of persistent effusion with significant bilateral hearing loss is a reasonable indicator of need for intervention with insertion of pressure equalization tubes.

## PREVENTION

Parents should be encouraged to continue exclusive breastfeeding as long as possible and should be cautioned about the risks of *bottle-propping* and of children taking a bottle to bed. The home should be a smoke-free environment.

Children identified at high-risk for recurrent acute OM are candidates for prolonged courses of antimicrobial prophylaxis, which can reduce recurrences significantly. Amoxicillin (20 to 30 mg/kg/day) or sulfisoxazole (50 mg/kg/day) given once daily at bedtime for 3 to 6 months or longer is used for prophylaxis.

The conjugate *S. pneumoniae* vaccine reduces pneumococcal OM caused by vaccine serotypes by 50%, all pneumococcal OM by 33%, and all OM by 6%. Annual immunization against influenza virus may be helpful in high-risk children.

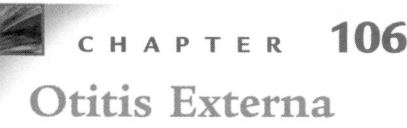

CHAPTER **106**

# Otitis Externa

## ETIOLOGY

Otitis externa, also known as **swimmer's ear**, is defined by inflammation and exudation in the external auditory canal in the absence of other disorders, such as otitis media or mastoiditis. It results from the interaction of host, environmental, and microbial factors.

The most common bacterial pathogen is *Pseudomonas aeruginosa*, especially in association with swimming in pools or lakes. Otitis externa develops in approximately 20% of children with **tympanostomy tubes**, associated with *Staphylococcus aureus, Streptococcus pneumoniae, Moraxella catarrhalis, Proteus, Klebsiella*, and occasionally anaerobes. Coagulase-negative staphylococci and *Corynebacterium* are isolated frequently from cultures of the external canal but represent normal flora. **Malignant otitis externa** is caused by *P. aeruginosa* in immunocompromised persons and adults with diabetes.

## EPIDEMIOLOGY

Otitis externa is a frequent complaint in summer, in contrast to otitis media, which occurs primarily in colder seasons in association with viral upper respiratory tract infections. Cleaning of the auditory canal, swimming, and, in particular, diving disrupt the integrity of the cutaneous lining of the ear canal and local defenses, predisposing to otitis externa.

## CLINICAL MANIFESTATIONS

Pain, tenderness, and aural discharge are the characteristic clinical findings of otitis externa. Fever is notably absent, and hearing is unaffected. Tenderness with movement of the pinnae, especially the tragus, and with chewing is particularly characteristic. This is not present in otitis media and is a valuable diagnostic criterion. Inspection usually reveals that the lining of the auditory canal is inflamed with mild to severe erythema and edema. Scant to copious discharge from the auditory canal may obscure the tympanic membrane. The most common symptoms of **malignant otitis externa** are similar, but facial nerve palsy occasionally occurs. The most common physical findings are swelling and granulation tissue in the canal, usually with a discharge from the external auditory canal.

## LABORATORY AND IMAGING STUDIES

The diagnosis of uncomplicated otitis externa usually is established solely on the basis of the clinical symptoms and physical examination findings without the need for additional laboratory or microbiologic evaluation. In malignant otitis externa, an elevated erythrocyte sedimentation rate is a constant finding. Cultures are required to identify the etiologic agent, which is usually *P. aeruginosa*, and the antimicrobial susceptibility.

## DIFFERENTIAL DIAGNOSIS

**Otitis media with tympanic perforation** and discharge into the auditory canal may be confused with otitis externa, particularly when it is difficult to clear the discharge. Pain on movement of the pinnae or tragus, which is typical of otitis externa, is not present. Local and systemic signs of mastoiditis indicate a process more extensive than otitis externa. **Malignancies** presenting in the auditory canal are rare in children but may present with discharge, unusual pain, or hearing loss.

## TREATMENT

Local therapy with acetic acid preparations (2%) designed to restore the acid pH of the auditory canal is usually effective. It may be necessary to remove the aural exudate with a swab or with suction to permit instillation of the solution. The predisposing activity, such as swimming or diving, should be avoided until the inflammation has resolved.

The most widely used topical otic preparations contain a combination of an aminoglycoside with a topical corticosteroid. Topical quinolone antibiotic drops (ciprofloxacin, ofloxacin) are more popular despite the cost. They are active against *S. aureus* and most gram-negative bacteria, including *P. aeruginosa*. None of these antibiotics has any antifungal activity.

Otic solutions containing corticosteroids are used frequently to reduce local inflammation. Solutions that combine antibiotics and corticosteroids are a reasonable choice in severe cases and when therapy with acetic acid preparations has not been effective. Treatment with topical otic analgesics and cerumenolytics is usually unnecessary. It is important with any topical therapy to remove purulent discharge from the external auditory canal so the treatment will work effectively.

Fungi such as *Aspergillus, Candida,* and dermatophytes occasionally are isolated from the external ear. It may be difficult to determine whether they represent normal flora or are the cause of inflammation. In most cases, local therapy and restoration of normal pH as recommended for bacterial otitis externa are sufficient.

**Tympanostomy tube otorrhea** is best treated with quinolone otic drugs, considered less likely to be ototoxic.

**Malignant otitis externa** is treated by parenteral antimicrobials with activity against *P. aeruginosa,* such as an expanded-spectrum penicillin (mezlocillin, piperacillin-tazobactam) or a cephalosporin with activity against *P. aeruginosa* (ceftazidime, cefepime) plus an aminoglycoside.

## COMPLICATIONS AND PROGNOSIS

Acute otitis externa usually resolves promptly without complications within 1 to 2 days of initiating treatment. Persistent pain, especially if severe or if accompanied by other symptoms, such as fever, should prompt re-evaluation for other conditions.

Complications of malignant otitis externa include invasion of the bones of the base of the skull, which may cause cranial nerve palsies. A mortality of 15% to 20% occurs in adults with malignant otitis media. Relapses within the first year after treatment are common.

## PREVENTION

Overly vigorous cleaning of an asymptomatic auditory canal should be avoided. Drying the auditory canals with acetic acid (2%), Burow solution, or diluted isopropyl alcohol (rubbing alcohol) after swimming may be used prophylactically to help prevent the maceration that facilitates bacterial invasion. Often underwater gear, such as earplugs or diving equipment, must be avoided to prevent recurrent disease. There is no role for prophylactic otic antibiotics.

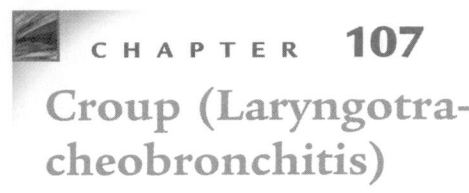

CHAPTER **107**

# Croup (Laryngotracheobronchitis)

## ETIOLOGY AND EPIDEMIOLOGY

Croup, or laryngotracheobronchitis, is the most common infection of the middle respiratory tract (Table 107-1). The most common causes of croup are parainfluenza viruses (types 1, 2, and 3) and respiratory syncytial virus. Laryngotracheal airway inflammation disproportionately affects children because a small decrease in diameter secondary to mucosal edema and inflammation exponentially increases airway resistance and significantly increases the work of breathing. During inspiration, the walls of the subglottic space are drawn together, aggravating the obstruction and producing the stridor characteristic of croup. Croup is most common in children 6 months to 3 years of age, with a peak in fall and early winter. It typically follows a common cold. Symptomatic reinfection is common, yet reinfections are usually mild.

## CLINICAL MANIFESTATIONS

The manifestations of croup are a harsh cough described as **barking** or **brassy**, hoarseness, inspiratory stridor, low-grade fever, and respiratory distress that may develop slowly or quickly. **Stridor** is a harsh, high-pitched respiratory sound produced by turbulent airflow. It is usually inspiratory, but it may be biphasic and is a sign of upper airway obstruction (Table 107-2). Signs of upper airway obstruction, such as labored breathing and marked suprasternal, intercostal, and subcostal retractions, may be evident on examination (see Chapter 135). Wheezing may be present if there is associated lower airway involvement.

## LABORATORY AND IMAGING STUDIES

Anteroposterior radiographs of the neck often, but not always, show the diagnostic subglottic narrowing of croup known as the **steeple sign** (Fig. 107-1). Routine laboratory studies are not useful in establishing the diagnosis. Leukocytosis is uncommon and suggests epiglottitis or bacterial tracheitis. Many rapid tests (polymerase chain reaction or antigen) are available for parainfluenza viruses and respiratory syncytial virus and other less common viral causes of croup, such as influenza and adenoviruses.

## DIFFERENTIAL DIAGNOSIS

The diagnosis of croup usually is established by clinical manifestations. Stridor in infants younger than 4 months of age or persistence of symptoms for longer than 1 week indicates an increased probability of another lesion (subglottic stenosis or hemangioma) and the need for direct laryngoscopy (see Chapter 135).

**TABLE 107-1  Clinical Features of Laryngotracheal Respiratory Tract Infections**

| Feature | Viral Laryngotracheobronchitis | Epiglottitis | Bacterial Tracheitis | Spasmodic Croup |
|---|---|---|---|---|
| Viral prodromal illness | ++ | − | + | + |
| Mean age | 6–36 mo (60% <24 mo) | 3–4 yr (25% <2 yr) | 4–5 yr | 6–36 mo (60% <24 mo) |
| Onset of illness | Gradual (2–3 days) | Acute (6–24 hr) | Acute (1–2 days) | Sudden (at night) |
| Fever | ± | + | + | − |
| Toxicity | − | + | ++ | − |
| Quality of stridor | Harsh | Mild | Harsh | Harsh |
| Drooling, neck hyperextension | − | ++ | + | − |
| Cough | ++ | − | ++ | ++ |
| Sore throat | ± | ++ | ± | − |
| Positive blood culture | − | + | ± | − |
| Leukocytosis | − | + | + | − |
| Recurrence | + | − | − | ++ |
| Hospitalization and endotracheal intubation | Rare | Frequent | Frequent | Rare |

+, frequently present; −, absent; ±, may or may not be present; ++, present and usually pronounced.
From Bell LM: Middle respiratory tract infections. In Jenson HB, Baltimore RS: Pediatric Infectious Diseases: Principles and Practice, 2nd ed, Philadelphia, 2002, *Saunders*, p 772.

**TABLE 107-2  Differential Diagnosis of Stridor**

| Infectious | Mechanical | Other |
|---|---|---|
| Acute laryngotracheobronchitis (croup) | Foreign body aspiration | Hypocalcemia |
| Epiglottitis | Spasmodic croup | Vocal cord paralysis |
| Pharyngitis | Laryngomalacia | |
| Parapharyngeal abscess | Congenital subglottic stenosis | |
| Bacterial tracheitis | Extrinsic compression (goiter, cyst, hemangioma, mediastinal mass) | |
| Laryngeal papillomatosis | Vascular ring | |
| | Angioedema | |

Table 107-2 provides the differential diagnosis of stridor in children. **Epiglottitis** is a medical emergency because of the risk of sudden airway obstruction. This illness is now rare and usually caused by group A streptococcal or *Staphylococcus aureus* infections. The patients typically have a preference for sitting, often with the head held forward, the mouth open, and the jaw thrust forward (**sniffing position**). Lateral radiograph reveals thickened and bulging epiglottis (**thumb sign**) and swelling of the aryepiglottic folds. The diagnosis is confirmed by direct observation of the inflamed and swollen supraglottic structures and swollen, cherry-red epiglottitis, which should be performed only in the operating room with a competent surgeon and anesthesiologist prepared to place an endotracheal tube or perform a tracheostomy if needed. Epiglottitis requires endotracheal intubation to maintain the airway and antibiotic therapy. Clinical recovery is rapid, and most children can be extubated safely within 48 to 72 hours.

**Bacterial tracheitis** is a rare but serious superinfection of the trachea that may follow viral croup and is most commonly caused by *S. aureus*. **Spasmodic croup** describes sudden onset of croup symptoms, usually at night, but without a significant upper respiratory tract prodrome. These episodes may be recurrent and severe but usually are of short duration. Spasmodic croup has a milder course than viral croup and responds to relatively simple therapies, such as exposure to cool or humidified air. The etiology is not well understood and may be allergic.

## TREATMENT

Oral or intramuscular dexamethasone for children with mild, moderate, or severe croup reduces symptoms, the need for hospitalization, and shortens hospital stays. Dexamethasone phosphate (0.6 to 1 mg/kg) may be given once intramuscularly or dexamethasone (0.6 to 1 mg/kg) once orally. Alternatively, prednisolone (2 mg/kg per day) may be given orally in two to three divided doses. For significant airway compromise, administration of aerosolized racemic (D- and L-) or L-epinephrine reduces

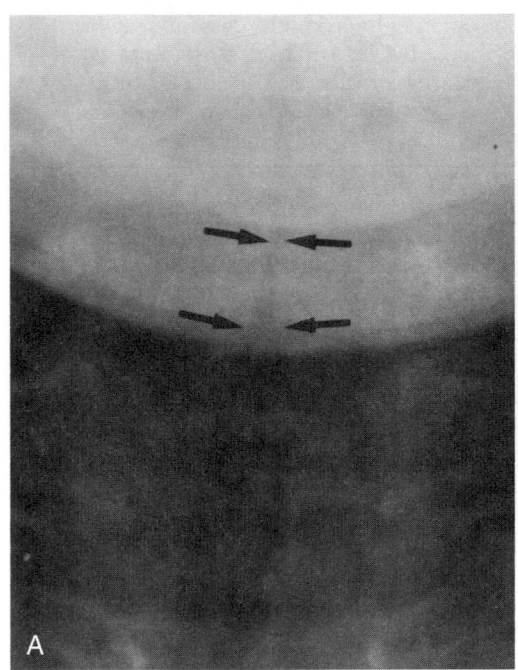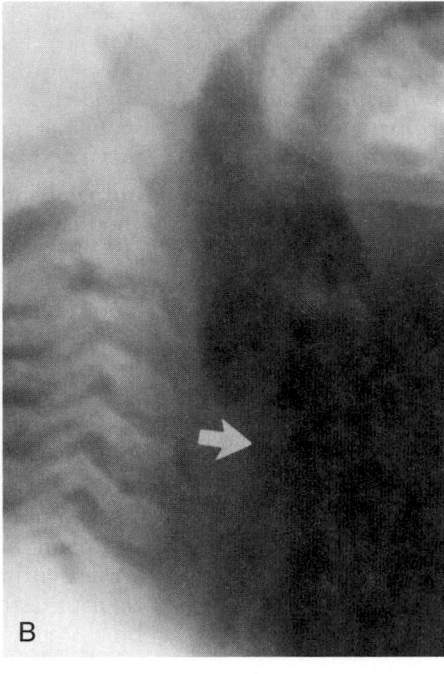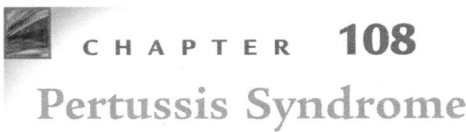

**FIGURE 107-1**

Croup (laryngotracheobronchitis). **A,** Posteroanterior view of the upper airway shows the so-called steeple sign, the tapered narrowing of the immediate subglottic airway (*arrows*). **B,** Lateral view of the upper airway shows good delineation of the supraglottic anatomy. The subglottic trachea is hazy and poorly defined (*arrow*) because of the inflammatory edema that has obliterated the sharp undersurface of the vocal cords and extends down the trachea in a diminishing manner. (From Bell LM: Middle respiratory tract infections. In Jenson HB, Baltimore RS: Pediatric Infectious Diseases: Principles and Practice, 2nd ed, Philadelphia, 2002, *Saunders*, p 774.)

subglottic edema by adrenergic vasoconstriction, temporarily producing marked clinical improvement. The peak effect is within 10 to 30 minutes and fades within 60 to 90 minutes. A rebound effect may occur, with worsening of symptoms as the effect of the drug dissipates. Aerosol treatment may need to be repeated every 20 minutes (for no more than 1 to 2 hours) in severe cases.

Children should be kept as calm as possible to minimize forceful inspiration. One useful calming method is for a child with croup to sit in the parent's lap. Sedatives should be used cautiously and only in the intensive care unit. Cool mist administered by face mask may help prevent drying of the secretions around the larynx.

Hospitalization is often required for children with stridor at rest. Children receiving aerosol treatment should be hospitalized or observed for at least 2 to 3 hours because of the risk of rebound airway obstruction. Subsidence of symptoms may indicate improvement or fatigue and impending respiratory failure.

## COMPLICATIONS AND PROGNOSIS

The most common complication of croup is viral pneumonia, which occurs in 1% to 2% of children with croup. Parainfluenza virus pneumonia and secondary bacterial pneumonia are more common in immunocompromised persons.

The prognosis for croup is excellent. Illness usually lasts approximately 5 days. As children grow, they become less susceptible to the airway effects of viral infections of the middle respiratory tract.

## PREVENTION

There is no vaccine for parainfluenza.

## CHAPTER 108

# Pertussis Syndrome

## ETIOLOGY

The pertussis syndrome includes disease caused by *Bordetella pertussis* and certain other infectious agents. Classic pertussis, **whooping cough syndrome**, is caused by *B. pertussis,* a gram-negative pleomorphic bacillus with fastidious growth requirements. Some cases of pertussis syndrome are caused by other organisms, including *Bordetella parapertussis,* which causes a similar but milder illness that is not affected by *B. pertussis* vaccination. *B. pertussis* and *B. parapertussis* infect only humans and are transmitted person to person by coughing. Adenoviruses have been associated with pertussis syndrome.

## EPIDEMIOLOGY

The mean incubation period is 6 days. Patients are most contagious during the earliest stage. The annual rate of pertussis was approximately 100 to 200 cases per 100,000 population in the prevaccination era, and presently it may be higher in developing countries. In the United States, the incidence of pertussis has increased steadily since the 1980s with more than 15,000 cases reported in 2006. The peak age incidence of pertussis in the United States is less than 4 months of age—among infants too young to be completely immunized and most likely to have the complications of pneumonia and severe infection that are associated with a high mortality rate. Infections in adolescents have also been rising, likely due to waning immunity from previous vaccines.

When vaccination rates are low, pertussis rates increase. In the United Kingdom, there was a steady decline in the incidence of pertussis until the late 1970s, when the incidence increased dramatically as the rate of vaccination declined. These data, a similar episode in Japan at about the same time, and the decline in the incidence of cases when vaccines were first tested are major events indicating the efficacy of vaccination.

## CLINICAL MANIFESTATIONS

Classic pertussis is the syndrome seen in children between 1 and 10 years of age. The progression of the disease is divided into catarrhal, paroxysmal, and convalescent stages. The **catarrhal stage** is marked by nonspecific signs (injection, increased nasal secretions, and low-grade fever) lasting 1 to 2 weeks. The **paroxysmal stage** is the most distinctive stage of pertussis and lasts 2 to 4 weeks. Coughing occurs in **paroxysms** during expiration, causing young children to lose their breath. This pattern of coughing is needed to dislodge plugs of necrotic bronchial epithelial tissues and thick mucus. The forceful inhalation against a narrowed glottis that follows this paroxysm of cough produces the characteristic **whoop**. Post-tussive emesis is common. The **convalescent stage** is marked by gradual resolution of symptoms over 1 to 2 weeks. Coughing becomes less severe, and the paroxysms and whoops slowly disappear. Although the disease typically lasts 6 to 8 weeks, residual cough may persist for months, especially with physical stress or respiratory irritants.

Infants may not display the classic pertussis syndrome. The first sign in the neonate may be episodes of apnea. Young infants are unlikely to have the classic whoop, more likely to have central nervous system (CNS) damage as a result of hypoxia, and more likely to have secondary bacterial pneumonia. Adolescents and adults with pertussis usually present with a prolonged bronchitic illness with persistent, nonproductive cough that often begins as a nonspecific upper respiratory tract infection. Generally adolescents and adults do not have a whoop with the cough, although they may have severe paroxysms. The cough may persist many weeks to months.

## LABORATORY AND IMAGING STUDIES

The diagnosis depends on isolation of *B. pertussis* and detection of antigens or nucleic acids from the organism. Culture on specialized media is usually accomplished during the early phases of illness on specimens from nasopharyngeal swabs or aspirates. Polymerase chain reaction (PCR) and nucleic acid detection are sensitive and specific tests that are available in clinical laboratories. Direct fluorescent antibody staining to detect the organism is technically difficult, is dependent on the skills of the technologist, and has low sensitivity (~60%). Available serologic tests are not useful for diagnosis of acute infection.

In classic *B. pertussis*–associated pertussis, **lymphocytosis** is present in 75% to 85% of patients, although in young infants the rate is much lower. The white blood cell (WBC) count may increase from 20,000 cells/mm$^3$ to more than 50,000 cells/mm$^3$, consisting primarily of mature lymphocytes.

It is not unusual for physical and radiographic signs of segmental lung atelectasis to develop during pertussis, especially during the paroxysmal stage. Perihilar infiltrates are common and are similar to what is seen in viral pneumonia.

## DIFFERENTIAL DIAGNOSIS

For a young child with classic pertussis syndrome, the diagnosis based on the pattern of illness is quite accurate. The paroxysmal stage is the most distinctive part of the syndrome. Respiratory viruses such as respiratory syncytial virus (RSV), parainfluenza virus, and *Chlamydophila pneumoniae* can produce bronchitic illnesses among infants. In older children and young adults, *Mycoplasma pneumoniae* may produce a prolonged bronchitic illness that is not distinguished easily from pertussis in this age group.

## TREATMENT

Erythromycin, clarithromycin, or azithromycin are recommended for children under 1 month of age. Azithromycin should be used in neonates due to the association of erythromycin treatment and the development of pyloric stenosis. Early treatment eradicates nasopharyngeal carriage of organisms within 3 to 4 days and lessens the severity of symptoms. Treatment is not effective in the paroxysmal stage. TMP-SMZ (trimethoprim and sulfamethoxazole) may be beneficial as an alternative, but this remains unproved.

## COMPLICATIONS AND PROGNOSIS

Major complications are most common among infants and young children and include hypoxia, apnea, pneumonia, seizures, encephalopathy, and malnutrition. The most frequent complication is pneumonia caused by *B. pertussis* itself or resulting from secondary bacterial infection from *Streptococcus pneumoniae, Haemophilus influenzae*, and *Staphylococcus aureus*. Atelectasis may develop secondary to mucous plugs. The force of the paroxysm may produce pneumomediastinum, pneumothorax, or interstitial or subcutaneous emphysema; epistaxis; hernias; and retinal and subconjunctival hemorrhages. Otitis media and sinusitis may occur.

Most children do well with complete healing of the respiratory epithelium and have normal pulmonary function after recovery. Young children can die from pertussis and are more likely to be hospitalized than older children. Most permanent disability is a result of encephalopathy.

## PREVENTION

Active immunity is induced with acellular pertussis components given in combination with the tetanus and diphtheria toxoids (DTaP). The acellular pertussis vaccines contain two to –five antigens of *B. pertussis* including pertussis toxin, pertactin, filamentous hemagglutinin, and fimbrial agglutinogens, FIM-2 and FIM-3. DTaP vaccine is recommended at 2, 4, 6, and 15 to 18 months, with a booster at 4 to 6 years, and has an efficacy of 70% to 90%.

Tdap vaccine is recommended for all adolescents at 11 to 12 years of age and is preferred to using tetanus and diphtheria for subsequent boosters every 10 years.

Macrolides are effective in preventing secondary cases in contacts exposed to pertussis. Close contacts under 7 years of age who have received only four doses of vaccine should receive a booster dose of DTaP (unless a booster dose has been given within the preceding 3 years) and a macrolide antibiotic for 10 to 14 days. Close contacts 7 years of age and older should receive prophylactic macrolide antibiotic for 10 to 14 days and Tdap, although the effectiveness of this strategy has not yet been determined.

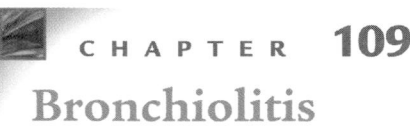

# CHAPTER 109
# Bronchiolitis

## ETIOLOGY

**Bronchiolitis** is the term used for first-time wheezing with a viral respiratory infection. The distinctive element of acute bronchiolitis is respiratory tract inflammation with airway obstruction resulting from swelling of small bronchioles leading to inadequate expiratory airflow. Most severe cases of bronchiolitis occur among infants, probably as a consequence of smaller airways and an immature immune system. Bronchiolitis is potentially life-threatening.

Respiratory syncytial virus (RSV) is the primary cause of bronchiolitis, followed in frequency by human metapneumovirus, parainfluenza viruses, influenza viruses, adenoviruses, rhinoviruses, and, infrequently, *Mycoplasma pneumoniae*. Viral bronchiolitis is extremely contagious and is spread by contact with infected respiratory secretions. Although coughing produces aerosols, hand carriage of contaminated secretions is the most frequent mode of transmission.

## EPIDEMIOLOGY

Bronchiolitis is the leading cause of hospitalization of infants. Approximately 50% of children experience bronchiolitis during the first 2 years of life, with a peak age at 2 to 6 months. The incidence falls rapidly between the ages of 1 and 5 years, after which bronchiolitis is uncommon. It is estimated that only 10% of healthy children with bronchiolitis and wheezing require hospitalization. Children with chronic lung disease such as bronchopulmonary dysplasia, hemodynamically significant congenital heart disease, neuromuscular weakness, or immunodeficiency are at increased risk of severe, potentially fatal disease. Children acquire infection after exposure to infected family members, who typically have symptoms of an upper respiratory tract infection, or from infected children in day care. In the United States, annual peaks are usually in the late winter months from December through March. Boys are affected more commonly than girls in a ratio of 1.5:1.

## CLINICAL MANIFESTATIONS

Bronchiolitis caused by RSV has an incubation period of 4 to 6 days. Bronchiolitis classically presents as a progressive respiratory illness that is similar to the common cold in its early phase with cough, coryza, and rhinorrhea. It progresses over 3 to 7 days to noisy, raspy breathing and audible wheezing. There is usually a low-grade fever accompanied by irritability, which may reflect the increased work of breathing. In contrast to the classic progression of disease, young infants infected with RSV may not have a prodrome and may have apnea as the first sign of infection.

Physical signs of bronchiolar obstruction include prolongation of the expiratory phase of breathing, intercostal retractions of the lower ribs, suprasternal retractions, and air trapping with hyperexpansion of the lungs. During the wheezing phase of the illness, percussion of the chest usually reveals only hyperresonance, but auscultation usually reveals diffuse wheezes and crackles throughout the breathing cycle. With more severe disease, grunting and cyanosis may be present.

## LABORATORY AND IMAGING STUDIES

Routine laboratory tests lack specificity for diagnosing bronchiolitis and are not required to confirm the diagnosis. A mild leukocytosis of 12,000 to 16,000 cells/μL is encountered frequently but is not specific. It is important to assess oxygenation in severe cases of bronchiolitis. **Pulse oximetry** is generally adequate for monitoring oxygen saturation. Frequent, regular assessments and cardiorespiratory monitoring of infants are necessary because respiratory failure may develop precipitously in very tired infants even though blood gas values taken before rapid decompensation are not alarming.

Antigen tests (usually by immunofluorescence or ELISA [enzyme-linked immunosorbent assay]) of nasopharyngeal secretions for RSV, parainfluenza viruses, influenza viruses, and adenoviruses are the most sensitive tests to confirm the infection. Rapid viral diagnosis also is performed by polymerase chain reaction (PCR). Identifying the viral agent is helpful for cohorting children with the same infection.

The chest radiograph frequently shows signs of hyperexpansion of the lungs, including increased lung radiolucency and flattened or depressed diaphragms. Areas of increased density may represent either viral pneumonia or localized atelectasis.

## DIFFERENTIAL DIAGNOSIS

The major difficulty in the diagnosis of bronchiolitis is to differentiate other diseases associated with wheezing. It may be impossible to differentiate asthma from bronchiolitis by physical examination, but age of presentation, presence of fever, and no history (personal or family) of asthma are the major differential factors. Bronchiolitis occurs primarily in the first year of life and is accompanied by fever, whereas asthma usually presents in older children with previous wheezing episodes that usually are not accompanied by fever unless a respiratory tract infection is the trigger for the asthma attack.

Wheezing also may be due to a foreign body in the airway, congenital airway obstructive lesion, cystic fibrosis, exacerbation of bronchopulmonary dysplasia, viral or bacterial pneumonia, and other lower respiratory tract diseases (see Chapter 78). **Cardiogenic asthma**, which can be confused with bronchiolitis in infants, is wheezing associated with pulmonary congestion secondary to left-sided heart failure.

Wheezing associated with gastroesophageal reflux is likely to be chronic or recurrent, and the patient may have a history of frequent emesis. Cystic fibrosis is associated with poor growth, chronic diarrhea, and a positive family history. A focal area on radiography that does not inflate or deflate suggests a **foreign body**.

## TREATMENT

Treatment of bronchiolitis consists of supportive therapy, including respiratory monitoring, control of fever, good hydration, upper airway suctioning, and oxygen administration. Supplemental oxygen by nasal cannula is often necessary, with intubation and ventilatory assistance for respiratory failure or apnea.

Indications for hospitalization include young age (<6 months old), moderate to marked respiratory distress, hypoxemia ($Po_2 < 60$ mm Hg or oxygen saturation <92% on room air), apnea, inability to tolerate oral feeding, and lack of appropriate care available at home. Hospitalization of high-risk children with bronchiolitis should be considered. Bronchodilators and corticosteroids have not been shown to be effective treatment of bronchiolitis.

## COMPLICATIONS AND PROGNOSIS

Most hospitalized children show marked improvement in 2 to 5 days with supportive treatment alone. The course of the wheezing phase varies, however. There may be tachypnea and hypoxia after admission, progressing to respiratory failure requiring assisted ventilation. Apnea is a major concern for very young infants with bronchiolitis.

Most cases of bronchiolitis resolve completely, although minor abnormalities of pulmonary function and bronchial hyperreactivity may persist for several years. Recurrence is common but tends to be mild and should be assessed and treated similarly to the first episode. The incidence of asthma seems to be higher for children hospitalized for bronchiolitis as infants, but it is unclear whether this is causal or if children prone to asthma are more likely to be hospitalized with bronchiolitis. There is a 1% to 2% mortality rate, highest among infants with preexisting cardiopulmonary or immunologic impairment.

## PREVENTION

Monthly injections of **palivizumab**, an RSV-specific monoclonal antibody, initiated just before the onset of the RSV season confers some protection from severe RSV disease. Palivizumab is indicated for some infants under 2 years old with chronic lung disease (bronchopulmonary dysplasia), very low birth weight infants, and infants with hemodynamically significant cyanotic and acyanotic congenital heart disease. Immunization with influenza vaccine in children above 6 month of age may prevent influenza-associated disease.

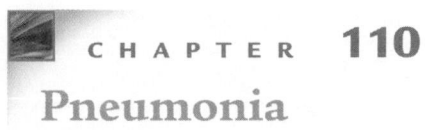

CHAPTER **110**

# Pneumonia

## ETIOLOGY

**Pneumonia** is an infection of the lower respiratory tract that involves the airways and parenchyma with consolidation of the alveolar spaces. The term **lower respiratory tract infection** is often used to encompass bronchitis, bronchiolitis (see Chapter 109), or pneumonia or any combination of the three. **Pneumonitis** is a general term for lung inflammation that may or may not be associated with consolidation. **Lobar pneumonia** describes pneumonia localized to one or more lobes of the lung. **Atypical pneumonia** describes patterns other than lobar pneumonia. **Bronchopneumonia** refers to inflammation of the lung that is centered in the bronchioles and leads to the production of a mucopurulent exudate that obstructs some of these small airways and causes patchy consolidation of the adjacent lobules. **Interstitial pneumonitis** refers to inflammation of the interstitium, which is composed of the walls of the alveoli, the alveolar sacs and ducts, and the bronchioles. Interstitial pneumonitis is characteristic of acute viral infections but also may be a chronic process.

Defects in host defenses increase the risk of pneumonia. Lower airways and secretions are sterile as a result of a multicomponent cleansing system. Airway contaminants are caught in the mucus secreted by the goblet cells. Cilia on epithelial surfaces, composing the **ciliary elevator system**, beat synchronously to move particles upward toward the central airways and into the throat, where they are swallowed or expectorated. Polymorphonuclear neutrophils from the blood and tissue macrophages ingest and kill microorganisms. IgA secreted into the upper airway fluid protects against invasive infections and facilitates viral neutralization.

Infectious agents that commonly cause community-acquired pneumonia vary by age (Table 110-1). Most common causes are respiratory syncytial virus (RSV) in infants (see Chapter 109), respiratory viruses (RSV, parainfluenza viruses, influenza viruses, adenoviruses) in children younger than 5 years old, and *Mycoplasma pneumoniae* in children older than age 5. *Streptococcus pneumoniae* occurs in children of any age, outside the neonatal period. *M. pneumoniae* and *Chlamydophila pneumoniae* are principal causes of **atypical pneumonia**.

Additional agents occasionally or rarely cause pneumonia. **Severe acute respiratory syndrome (SARS)** is due to SARS-associated coronavirus (SARS-CoV). **Avian influenza**, also known as **bird flu**, is a highly contagious viral disease of poultry and other birds that is caused by **influenza A (H5N1)**. There were outbreaks among humans in South East Asia in 1997 and 2003–2004 with high mortality rates. **Hantavirus cardiopulmonary syndrome** is caused by Sin Nombre virus, which is carried by *Peromyscus maniculatus* (the deer mouse) and transmitted to humans by aerosolized rodent excreta. Legionnaires' disease caused by *Legionella pneumophila* is a rare cause of pneumonia in children.

**TABLE 110-1 Etiologic Agents and Empirical Antimicrobial Therapy for Pneumonia in Patients without History of Recent Antibiotic Therapy**

| Age Group | Common Pathogens* (in order of frequency) | Outpatients[†] (7–10 days total duration of treatment) | Patients Requiring Hospitalization[‡] (10–14 days total duration of treatment) | Patients Requiring Intensive Care*[‡] (10–14 days total duration of treatment) |
|---|---|---|---|---|
| Neonates (up to 1 month of age) | Group B streptococci, *Escherichia coli*, other gram-negative bacilli, *Streptococcus pneumoniae*, *Haemophilus influenzae* (type b,[§] nontypable) | Outpatient management not recommended | Ampicillin *plus* cefotaxime or an aminoglycoside *plus* an antistaphylococcal agent if *Staphylococcus aureus* is suspected | Ampicillin *plus* cefotaxime or an aminoglycoside *plus* an antistaphylococcal agent if *S. aureus* is suspected |
| 1 to 3 months Febrile pneumonia | Respiratory syncytial virus, other respiratory viruses (parainfluenza viruses, influenzaviruses, adenoviruses), *S. pneumoniae*, *H. influenzae* (type b,[§] nontypable) | Initial outpatient management not recommended | Cefuroxime or cefotaxime or ceftriaxone *plus* nafcillin or oxacillin | Cefotaxime or ceftriaxone *plus* nafcillin or oxacillin |
| Afebrile pneumonia | *Chlamydia trachomatis*, *Mycoplasma hominis*, *Ureaplasma urealyticum*, cytomegalovirus | Erythromycin, azithromycin, or clarithromycin with close follow-up | Erythromycin, azithromycin, or clarithromycin | Erythromycin, azithromycin, or clarithromycin *plus* cefotaxime or ceftriaxone *plus* nafcillin or oxacillin |
| 3 to 12 months | Respiratory syncytial virus, other respiratory viruses (parainfluenza viruses, influenzaviruses, adenoviruses), *S. pneumoniae*, *H. influenzae* (type b,[§] nontypable), *C. trachomatis*, *Mycoplasma pneumoniae*, group A streptococci | Amoxicillin, erythromycin, azithromycin, or clarithromycin | Ampicillin or cefuroxime | Cefuroxime or ceftriaxone *plus* erythromycin or clarithromycin |
| 12 to 60 months | Respiratory viruses (parainfluenza viruses, influenzaviruses, adenoviruses), *S. pneumoniae*, *H. influenzae* (type b,[§] nontypable), *M. pneumoniae*, *Chlamydophila pneumoniae*, *S. aureus*, group A streptococci | Amoxicillin, erythromycin, azithromycin, or clarithromycin | Ampicillin or cefuroxime | Cefuroxime or ceftriaxone *plus* erythromycin, azithromycin, or clarithromycin |
| 5 to 18 years | *M. pneumoniae*, *S. pneumoniae*, *C. pneumoniae*, *H. influenzae* (type b,[§] nontypable), | Erythromycin, azithromycin, or clarithromycin | Erythromycin, azithromycin, or clarithromycin with or without cefuroxime or ampicillin | Cefuroxime or ceftriaxone *plus* erythromycin or clarithromycin |

*Continued*

**TABLE 110-1 Etiologic Agents and Empirical Antimicrobial Therapy for Pneumonia in Patients without History of Recent Antibiotic Therapy—cont'd**

| Age Group | Common Pathogens* (in order of frequency) | Outpatients[†] (7–10 days total duration of treatment) | Patients Requiring Hospitalization[‡] (10–14 days total duration of treatment) | Patients Requiring Intensive Care*[‡] (10–14 days total duration of treatment) |
|---|---|---|---|---|
| | influenzaviruses, adenoviruses, other respiratory viruses | | | |
| ≥18 years[¶] | *M. pneumoniae, S. pneumoniae, C. pneumoniae, H. influenzae* (type b,[§] nontypable), influenzaviruses, adenoviruses, *Legionella pneumophila* | Erythromycin, azithromycin, clarithromycin, doxycycline, moxifloxacin, gatifloxacin, levofloxacin, or gemifloxacin | Moxifloxacin, gatifloxacin, levofloxacin, or gemifloxacin *or* Azithromycin or clarithromycin *plus* cefotaxime, ceftriaxone, or ampicillin-sulbactam | Cefotaxime, ceftriaxone, or ampicillin-sulbactam *plus either* azithromycin or clarithromycin *or* moxifloxacin, gatifloxacin, levofloxacin, or gemifloxacin |

*Severe pneumonia, from *S. pneumoniae, S. aureus,* group A streptococci, *H. influenzae* type b, or *M. pneumoniae,* requiring admission to an intensive care unit. Antipseudomonal agents should be added if *Pseudomonas* is suspected.

[†]Oral administration.

[‡]Intravenous administration for inpatients except for the macrolides (erythromycin, azithromycin, and clarithromycin), which are given orally.

[§]*H. influenzae* type b infection is uncommon with universal *H. influenzae* type b immunization.

[¶]Fluoroquinolones are contraindicated for children, adolescents younger than 18 years of age, and pregnant and lactating women. Tetracyclines are not recommended for children younger than 9 years.

*Chlamydia trachomatis* and less commonly *Mycoplasma hominis, Ureaplasma urealyticum,* and cytomegalovirus (CMV) cause a similar respiratory syndrome in infants 1 to 3 months of age with subacute onset of an **afebrile pneumonia** with cough and hyperinflation as the predominant signs. These infections are difficult to diagnose and to distinguish from each other. In adults, these organisms are carried primarily as part of the genital mucosal flora. Women who harbor these agents may transmit them perinatally to newborns.

Causes of pneumonia in immunocompromised persons include gram-negative enteric bacteria, mycobacteria (*M. avium* complex), fungi (aspergillosis, histoplasmosis), viruses (CMV), and *Pneumocystis jirovecii (carinii).* Pneumonia in patients with cystic fibrosis usually is caused by *Staphylococcus aureus* in infancy and *Pseudomonas aeruginosa* or *Burkholderia cepacia* in older patients.

## EPIDEMIOLOGY

Immunizations have had a great impact on the incidence of pneumonia caused by pertussis, diphtheria, measles, *Haemophilus influenzae,* and *S. pneumoniae.* Where used, bacille Calmette-Guérin (BCG) for tuberculosis also has had a significant impact. More than 4 million deaths each year in developing countries are due to acute respiratory tract infections. Risk factors for lower respiratory tract infections include gastroesophageal reflux, neurologic impairment (aspiration), immunocompromised states, anatomic abnormalities of the respiratory tract, residence in residential care facilities for handicapped children, and hospitalization, especially in an intensive care unit (ICU) or requiring invasive procedures.

## CLINICAL MANIFESTATIONS

Age is a determinant in the clinical manifestations of pneumonia. Neonates may have fever only with subtle or absent physical findings of pneumonia (see Chapter 65). The typical clinical patterns of viral and bacterial pneumonias usually differ between older infants and children, although the distinction is not always clear for a particular patient. Fever, chills, tachypnea, cough, malaise, pleuritic chest pain, retractions, and apprehension, because of difficulty breathing or shortness of breath, are common in older infants and children.

Viral pneumonias are associated more often with cough, wheezing, or stridor; fever is less prominent than with bacterial pneumonia. Bacterial pneumonias typically are associated with higher fever, chills, cough, dyspnea, and auscultatory findings of lung consolidation. Atypical pneumonia in young infants is characterized by tachypnea, cough, crackles on auscultation, and often concomitant chlamydial conjunctivitis. Other signs of respiratory distress include flaring of the alae of the nose, intercostal and subcostal retractions, and grunting. All significant pneumonias have localized crackles and decreased breath sounds; a pleural effusion may cause dullness to percussion.

## LABORATORY AND IMAGING STUDIES

Bacterial flora of the upper respiratory tract is not an accurate reflection of the causes of lower respiratory tract infection, and good quality sputum is rarely obtainable from children. In otherwise healthy children without life-threatening disease, invasive procedures to obtain lower respiratory tissue or secretions usually are not indicated. Serologic tests are not useful for the most common causes of bacterial pneumonia.

The white blood cell (WBC) count with viral pneumonias is often normal or mildly elevated, with a predominance of lymphocytes, whereas with bacterial pneumonias the WBC count is elevated (>20,000/mm$^3$) with a predominance of neutrophils. Mild eosinophilia is characteristic of infant *C. trachomatis* pneumonia. Blood cultures should be performed to attempt to diagnose a bacterial cause of pneumonia. Blood cultures are positive in 10% to 20% of bacterial pneumonia and are considered to be confirmatory of the cause of pneumonia if positive for a recognized respiratory pathogen. Urinary antigen tests are especially useful for *L. pneumophila* (Legionnaires' disease).

Relatively accurate for the diagnosis of viral respiratory pneumonia are cultures or rapid viral antigen detection of upper respiratory secretions, but neither rules out concomitant bacterial pneumonia. *M. pneumoniae* should be suspected if cold agglutinins are present in peripheral blood samples; this may be confirmed by *Mycoplasma* IgM or more specifically polymerase chain reaction (PCR). CMV and enterovirus can be cultured from the nasopharynx, urine, or bronchoalveolar lavage fluid. The diagnosis of *M. tuberculosis* is established by tuberculin skin test, blood interferon assays, and analysis of sputum or gastric aspirates by culture, antigen detection, or PCR.

The need to establish an etiologic diagnosis of pneumonia is greater for patients who are ill enough to require hospitalization, immunocompromised patients, patients with recurrent pneumonia, or patients with pneumonia unresponsive to empirical therapy. For these patients, bronchoscopy with bronchoalveolar lavage and brush mucosal biopsy, needle aspiration of the lung, and open lung biopsy are methods of obtaining material for microbiologic diagnosis.

When there is effusion or empyema, performing a thoracentesis to obtain pleural fluid can be diagnostic and therapeutic. Evaluation differentiates between empyema and a sterile parapneumonic effusion caused by irritation of the pleura contiguous with the pneumonia. Gram stain and culture may lead to microbiologic diagnosis. The pleural fluid should be cultured for bacteria, mycobacteria, fungi, and viruses. If the fluid is grossly purulent, removal reduces the patient's toxicity and associated discomfort and may facilitate more rapid recovery. If the accumulation is large and impairs the ability of the lung to expand, removal of the fluid improves pulmonary mechanics and gas exchange.

Frontal and lateral radiographs are required to localize the diseased segments and to visualize adequately infiltrates behind the heart or the diaphragmatic leaflets. There are characteristic radiographic findings of pneumonia, although there is much overlap that precludes definitive diagnosis by radiography alone. Bacterial pneumonia characteristically shows lobar consolidation, or a round pneumonia, with pleural effusion in 10% to 30% of cases (Fig. 110-1). Viral pneumonia characteristically shows diffuse, streaky infiltrates of bronchopneumonia (Fig. 110-2). Atypical pneumonia, such as with *M. pneumoniae* and *C. pneumoniae*, shows increased interstitial markings or bronchopneumonia (Fig. 110-3). The chest radiograph

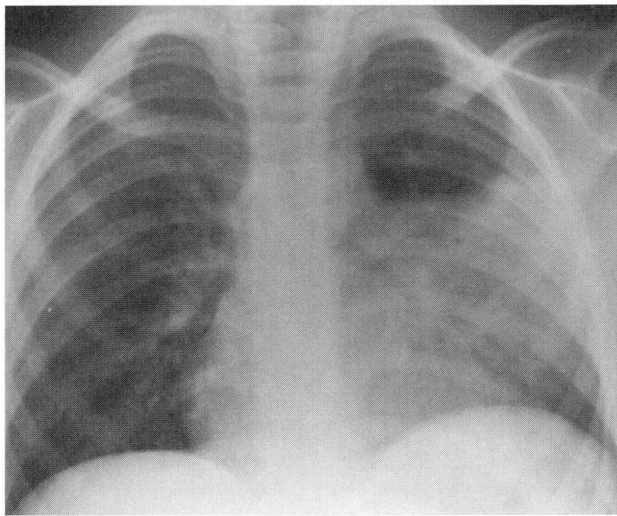

**FIGURE 110-1**

**Acute lobar pneumonia of the lingula in a 6-year-old child with high fever, cough, and chest pain.** Frontal chest radiograph shows airspace consolidation, which obliterates the silhouette of the heart border on the left. The left hemidiaphragm is mildly elevated as a result of splinting. (From Markowitz RI: Diagnostic imaging. In Jenson HB, Baltimore RS [eds]: Pediatric Infectious Diseases: Principles and Practice, 2nd ed. Philadelphia, *WB Saunders*, 2002, p 133.)

may be normal in early pneumonia, with appearance of an infiltrate during the treatment phase of the disease when edema fluid is greater. Hilar lymphadenopathy is uncommon with bacterial pneumonia, but may be a sign of tuberculosis, histoplasmosis, or an underlying

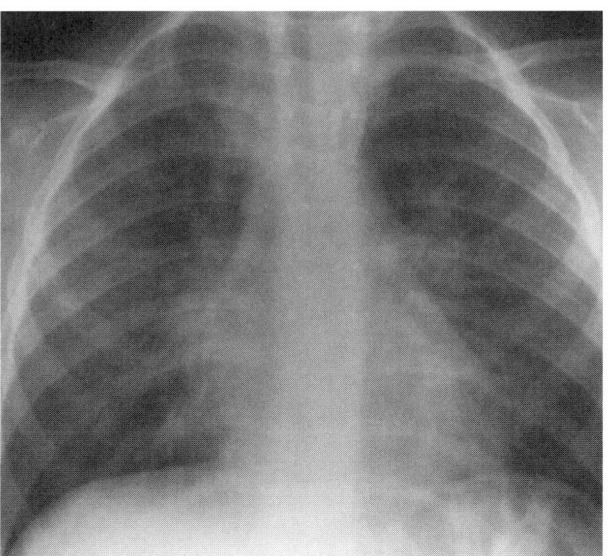

**FIGURE 110-2**

**Diffuse viral bronchopneumonia in a 12-year-old boy with cough, fever, and wheezing.** Frontal chest radiograph shows bilateral, perihilar, peribronchial thickening and shaggy infiltrate. Focal airspace disease representing consolidation or atelectasis is present in the medial portion of the right upper lobe. The findings are typical of bronchopneumonia. (From Markowitz RI: Diagnostic imaging. In Jenson HB, Baltimore RS [eds]: Pediatric Infectious Diseases: Principles and Practice, 2nd ed. Philadelphia, *WB Saunders*, 2002, p 132.)

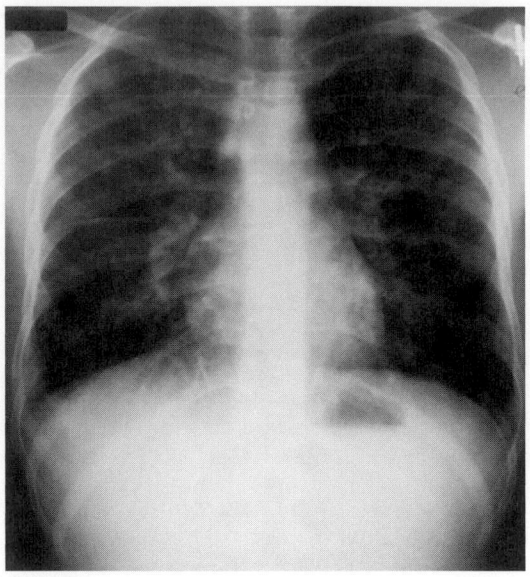

**FIGURE 110-3**

*Mycoplasma pneumoniae* infection (atypical pneumonia) in a 14-year-old boy with malaise, dry cough, and mild shortness of breath for 1 week. Frontal chest radiograph shows a diffuse pattern of increased interstitial markings, including Kerley lines. The heart is normal, and there are no focal infiltrates. Cold agglutinins were markedly elevated, and the patient responded to erythromycin. This radiographic pattern of reticulonodular interstitial disease is observed in 25% to 30% of patients with pneumonia caused by *Mycoplasma pneumoniae*. (From Baltimore RS: Pneumonia. In Jenson HB, Baltimore RS [eds]: Pediatric Infectious Diseases: Principles and Practice, 2nd ed. Philadelphia, *WB Saunders*, 2002, p 808.)

| TABLE 110-2 Differential Diagnosis of Recurrent Pneumonia |
| --- |
| **HEREDITARY DISORDERS** |
| Cystic fibrosis |
| Sickle cell disease |
| **DISORDERS OF IMMUNITY** |
| AIDS |
| Bruton agammaglobulinemia |
| Selective IgG subclass deficiencies |
| Common variable immunodeficiency syndrome |
| Severe combined immunodeficiency syndrome |
| **DISORDERS OF LEUKOCYTES** |
| Chronic granulomatous disease |
| Hyperimmunoglobulin E syndrome (Job syndrome) |
| Leukocyte adhesion defect |
| **DISORDERS OF CILIA** |
| Immotile cilia syndrome |
| Kartagener syndrome |
| **ANATOMIC DISORDERS** |
| Sequestration |
| Lobar emphysema |
| Esophageal reflux |
| Foreign body |
| Tracheoesophageal fistula (H type) |
| Gastroesophageal reflux |
| Bronchiectasis |
| Aspiration (oropharyngeal incoordination) |

malignant neoplasm. Decubitus views or ultrasound should be used to assess size of pleural effusions and whether they are freely mobile. Computed tomography (CT) is used to evaluate serious disease, pleural abscesses, bronchiectasis, and delineating effusions. Unusual etiologies or recurrent pneumonias require special considerations (Table 110-2). Lung abscesses, pneumatoceles, and empyema all require special management.

## DIFFERENTIAL DIAGNOSIS

Complete physical examination is important to identify other foci of disease or associated findings that may suggest an etiology. Mucosal congestion and inflammation of the upper airway suggest a viral infection. Tachypnea can be caused by airway inflammation resulting in obstruction or by pneumonia resulting in inadequate gas exchange and hypoxia. Generalized or peripheral cyanosis indicates hypoxia with severe diffuse or multilobular pneumonia or a large pleural effusion. With a young infant, apneic spells may be the first sign of pneumonia.

Asymmetry or shallow breathing may be due to splinting from pain. Low diaphragms by percussion indicate air trapping, which is common in asthma, but also frequently accompanies viral lower respiratory infections. Poor diaphragmatic excursion may indicate hyperexpanded lungs or an inability for expansion because a large consolidation is causing poor lung compliance. Hyperexpansion may push the diaphragm and liver downward. Dullness to percussion may be due to lobar or segmental infiltrates or pleural fluid. Auscultation may be normal in early or very focal pneumonia, but the presence of localized crackles, rhonchi, and wheezes may help one to detect and locate pneumonia. Distant breath sounds may indicate a large, poorly ventilated area of consolidation or pleural fluid.

The various types of pneumonia—lobar pneumonia, bronchopneumonia, interstitial and alveolar pneumonias—need to be differentiated on the basis of radiologic or pathologic diagnosis. Pneumonia must be differentiated from other acute lung diseases, including lung edema caused by heart failure, allergic pneumonitis, and aspiration, and autoimmune diseases, such as rheumatoid disease and systemic lupus erythematosus. Radiographically, pneumonia must be differentiated from lung trauma and contusion, hemorrhage, foreign body obstruction, and irritation from subdiaphragmatic inflammation.

## TREATMENT

Therapy for pneumonia includes supportive and specific treatment and depends on the degree of illness, complications, and knowledge of the infectious agent likely causing the pneumonia. Age, severity of the illness, complications noted on the chest radiograph, degree of respiratory distress, and ability of the family to care for the child and to assess the progression of the symptoms all must be taken into consideration in the choice of ambulatory treatment over hospitalization (Table 110-3). Most cases of pneumonia in healthy children can be managed on an outpatient basis.

Although viruses cause most community-acquired pneumonias in young children, in most situations experts recommend empirical antibiotic treatment for the most probable treatable causes (see Table 110-1). Exceptional situations include lack of response to empirical therapy, unusually severe presentations, nosocomial pneumonia, and immunocompromised children susceptible to infections with opportunistic pathogens (Table 110-4). In contrast to pneumococcal meningitis, presumed pneumococcal pneumonia can be treated with high-dose cephalosporin therapy even with high-level penicillin resistance. Vancomycin can be used if the isolate shows high-level resistance and the patient is severely ill. For infants 4 to 18 weeks old with afebrile pneumonia most likely caused by *C. trachomatis,* a macrolide is the recommended treatment.

## COMPLICATIONS AND PROGNOSIS

Bacterial pneumonias frequently cause inflammatory fluid to collect in the adjacent pleural space, causing a **parapneumonic effusion** or, if grossly purulent, an **empyema**. Small effusions may not require any special therapy. Large effusions may restrict breathing and require drainage. Air dissection within lung tissue results in a **pneumatocele**, or air pocket. Scarring of the airways and lung tissue may leave dilated bronchi, resulting in **bronchiectasis** and increased risk for recurrent infection.

Pneumonia that causes necrosis of lung tissue may evolve into a **lung abscess**. Lung abscess is an uncommon problem in children and usually is caused by aspiration or infection behind an obstructed bronchus. The most

### TABLE 110-4 Antimicrobial Therapy for Pneumonia Caused by Specific Pathogens*

| Pathogen | Recommended Treatment | Alternative Treatment |
|---|---|---|
| *Streptococcus pneumoniae*[†] | Ceftriaxone, cefotaxime, penicillin G, or penicillin V | Cefuroxime axetil, erythromycin, clindamycin, or vancomycin |
| Group A streptococci | Penicillin G | Cefuroxime, cefuroxime axetil, or erythromycin |
| Group B streptococci | Penicillin G | |
| *Haemophilus influenzae* type b | Ceftriaxone, cefotaxime, ampicillin-sulbactam, or ampicillin | Cefuroxime, cefuroxime axetil |
| *Mycoplasma pneumoniae* | Erythromycin, azithromycin, or clarithromycin | Doxycycline (in patients older than 9 years of age)[‡] Fluoroquinolone (in patients older than 18 years) |
| Gram-negative aerobic bacilli (except *P. aeruginosa*) | Cefotaxime (or ceftriaxone) with or without an aminoglycoside | Piperacillin-tazobactam plus an aminoglycoside[§] |
| *P. aeruginosa* | Ceftazidime with or without an aminoglycoside[§] | Piperacillin-tazobactam plus an aminoglycoside[§] |
| *Staphylococcus aureus* | Nafcillin, cephazolin, clindamycin (for MRSA) | Vancomycin (for MRSA) |
| *Chlamydophila pneumoniae* | Erythromycin, azithromycin, or clarithromycin | Doxycycline (in patients older than 9 years of age)[‡] Fluoroquinolone (in patients older than 18 years) |
| *Chlamydia trachomatis* (afebrile pneumonia in infants) | Erythromycin, azithromycin, or clarithromycin | |
| Herpes simplex virus | Acyclovir | |

*Oral outpatient therapy may be used for mild illness. Intravenous inpatient therapy should be used for moderate to severe illness.
[†]Antibiotic should be chosen on the basis of antibiotic susceptibility of the isolate or susceptibility of the prevalent isolates in the community.
[‡]Appropriate fluoroquinolones include moxifloxacin, gatifloxacin, levofloxacin, and gemifloxacin. Fluoroquinolones are contraindicated for children, adolescents younger than 18 years of age, and pregnant and lactating women. Tetracyclines are not recommended for children younger than 9 years.
[§]Aminoglycoside dosing should be guided by serum antibiotic concentrations after a steady state has been reached.
MRSA, methicillin-resistant *Staphylococcus aureus*; TMP-SMX, trimethoprim-sulfamethoxazole.

commonly involved sites are the posterior segments of the upper lobes and the superior segments of the lower lobes, where aspirated material drains when the child is recumbent. Anaerobic bacteria usually predominate, along with various streptococci, *Escherichia coli, Klebsiella pneumoniae, Pseudomonas aeruginosa,* and *Staphylococcus aureus.* Chest radiograph or CT scan reveals a cavitary lesion, often with an air-fluid level, surrounded by parenchymal inflammation. If the cavity communicates with the bronchi, organisms may be isolated from sputum. Diagnostic bronchoscopy may be indicated to exclude a foreign body and obtain microbiologic specimens. Lung abscesses usually respond to appropriate antimicrobial therapy with clindamycin, penicillin G, or ampicillin-sulbactam.

Most children recover from pneumonia rapidly and completely, although radiographic abnormalities may take 6 to 8 weeks to return to normal. In a few children, pneumonia may persist longer than 1 month or may be recurrent. In such cases, the possibility of underlying disease must be investigated further, such as with tuberculin skin test, sweat chloride determination for cystic fibrosis, serum immunoglobulin and IgG subclass determinations, bronchoscopy to identify anatomic abnormalities or foreign body, and barium swallow for gastroesophageal reflux.

Severe adenovirus pneumonia may result in **bronchiolitis obliterans**, a subacute inflammatory process in which the small airways are replaced by scar tissue, resulting in a reduction in lung volume and lung compliance. **Unilateral hyperlucent lung**, or **Swyer-James syndrome**, is a focal sequela of severe necrotizing pneumonia in which all or part of a lung has increased translucency radiographically and has been linked to adenovirus type 21.

## PREVENTION

Annual influenza vaccine is recommended for all children 6 to 18 years of age (see Chapter 94). Children 6 months to 5 years of age are at higher risk for influenza complications. Trivalent inactivated vaccine or the live, attenuated influenza vaccine can be used for persons 2 to 49 years of age. Some trivalent vaccines are licensed for use beginning at 6 months of age. Universal childhood vaccination with conjugate vaccines for *H influenzae* type b and *S. pneumoniae* have greatly diminished the incidence of these pneumonias. The severity of RSV infections can be reduced by use of palivizumab in high-risk patients (see Chapter 109).

Reducing the duration of mechanical ventilation and administering antibiotics judiciously reduces the incidence of ventilator-associated pneumonias. The head of the bed should be raised to 30 to 45 degrees for intubated patients to minimize risk of aspiration, and all suctioning equipment and saline should be sterile. Hand washing before and after every patient contact and use of gloves for invasive procedures are important measures to prevent nosocomial transmission of infections. Hospital staff with respiratory illnesses or who are carriers of certain organisms, such as methicillin-resistant *S. aureus,* should comply with infection control policies to prevent transfer of organisms to patients. Treating sources of aerosols, such as air coolers, can prevent *Legionella* pneumonia.

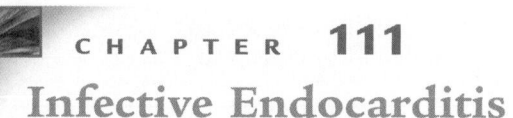

## CHAPTER 111

# Infective Endocarditis

## ETIOLOGY

**Infective endocarditis** is an infection on the endothelial surface of the heart, including the heart valves. The management of infections on the endothelial surfaces of blood vessels is very similar. Infectious endothelial lesions, called **vegetations**, usually occur on the valve leaflets and are composed of microorganisms trapped in a fibrin mesh that extends into the bloodstream. Because antibiotics must reach the organisms by passive diffusion through the fibrin mesh, high doses of bactericidal antibiotics are required for an extended period of treatment.

Many microorganisms have been reported to cause endocarditis, although there are only a few principal causes in children (Table 111-1). Viridans streptococci are the principal causes in children with congenital heart diseases without previous surgery. *Staphylococcus aureus* and coagulase-negative staphylococci are important causes of endocarditis, especially following cardiac surgery and in the presence of prosthetic cardiac and endovascular materials.

## EPIDEMIOLOGY

Infective endocarditis among children is primarily a complication of congenital heart disease and cardiac surgery. High-risk cardiac lesions include tetralogy of Fallot, ventricular septal defect, aortic stenosis, aortic regurgitation, patent ductus arteriosus, and transposition of the great vessels. The risk is increased after dental and oral procedures or instrumentation or surgical procedures of the respiratory tract, genitourinary tract, or gastrointestinal tract. Rheumatic heart disease is a risk factor but is now uncommon. Neonatal endocarditis is associated with the use of central vascular catheters and surgery in neonates. Endocarditis is a sporadic disease with no geographic predisposition and little gender or socioeconomic predisposition in children. In adults, there is a male preponderance and association with social and behavioral factors, such as intravenous (IV) drug abuse and atherosclerotic heart disease.

## CLINICAL MANIFESTATIONS

The most common early symptoms of infective endocarditis are nonspecific and include fever, malaise, and weight loss. Tachycardia and a new or changed heart murmur are common findings. The subtle and nonspecific findings underscore the need to obtain blood cultures if endocarditis is suspected, especially for children with congenital heart disease and for unexplained illness after dental or surgical procedures. Endocarditis is usually a **subacute**, slowly progressive process, but **acute endocarditis** is often due to *S. aureus* and may resemble sepsis. Heart failure, splenomegaly, petechiae, and embolic phenomena (Osler nodes, Roth spots, Janeway lesions, and splinter hemorrhages) may be present.

## TABLE 111-1 Pathogens Causing Infective Endocarditis in Children

### BACTERIA

Viridans streptococci (the most common causative organism at all ages)*
*Staphylococcus aureus*\*
*Enterococcus*\*
Coagulase-negative staphylococci
Hemolytic streptococci: groups A, B (in neonates and elderly), C, G, D
*Streptococcus pneumoniae*
Gram-negative enteric bacilli
HACEK organisms (i.e., *Haemophilus aphrophilus, Actinobacillus actinomycetemcomitans, Cardiobacterium hominis, Eikenella corrodens,* and *Kingella kingae*)

### FUNGI

*Candida albicans*
Non-albicans *Candida*
*Aspergillus*
*Cryptococcus neoformans*

### OTHERS

*Coxiella burnetii* (Q fever)
*Chlamydia*
Agent (?) of culture-negative endocarditis

\*Most common causes of infective endocarditis in children.

## LABORATORY STUDIES AND IMAGING

The key to diagnosis is confirming continuous bacteremia or fungemia by culturing the blood. Multiple blood cultures are performed before initiating antibiotic therapy. Three separate venipunctures for blood culture achieve near-maximal sensitivity (about 95%) among patients who have not been treated recently with antibiotics. Patients who have been treated with antibiotics recently or who are currently receiving antibiotics should have additional serial cultures performed. Despite adequate blood culture techniques, the microbiologic diagnosis is not confirmed in 10% to 15% of cases, known as **culture-negative endocarditis**.

Erythrocyte sedimentation rate (ESR) and C-reactive protein (CRP) are often elevated. Leukocytosis, anemia, and hematuria are common laboratory findings. A positive rheumatoid factor may also be seen.

Echocardiography visualizes endocardial and valvular vegetations measuring 2 mm or greater. Transesophageal echocardiography is more sensitive than transthoracic echocardiography for adolescents and adults and for patients with prosthetic valves, but is often unnecessary in children.

## DIFFERENTIAL DIAGNOSIS

Infective endocarditis must be differentiated from other causes of bacteremia or other cardiac conditions using the **Modified Duke Criteria** for categorizing the strength of the endocarditis diagnosis (Table 111-2). Noninfectious causes of endocardial vegetations must be excluded, such as sterile clots and vegetations associated with rheumatoid disease and lupus erythematosus. Prolonged bacteremia can be caused by infectious endothelial foci outside the heart, often associated with congenital malformations, vascular trauma, an infected venous thrombosis, and previous vascular surgery.

## TABLE 111-2 Modified Duke Clinical Criteria for Diagnosis of Infective Endocarditis

### DEFINITE INFECTIVE ENDOCARDITIS

*Histopathologic Criteria*
Microorganisms shown by culture or histopathologic examination in a vegetation, emboli, intracardiac abscess *or*
Active endocardial lesions on pathologic examination
*Clinical Criteria—*
*Two major criteria or one major and three minor criteria or five minor criteria)*
*Major Criteria*
Positive blood cultures
    Two or more separate cultures positive with typical organisms for infective endocarditis
    Two or more positive cultures of blood drawn more than 12 hours apart or 4 positive blood cultures irrespective of timing of obtaining specimen
    A positive blood culture for *Coxiella burnetii* or positive IgG titer >1:800
Evidence of endocardial involvement
    Positive findings on echocardiogram (vegetation on valve or supporting structure, abscess, new valvular regurgitation)
*Minor Criteria*
Predisposition—predisposing heart condition *or* injection drug use
Fever—temperature >38° C (>100.4° F)
Vascular phenomena (major arterial emboli, septic pulmonary infarcts, mycotic aneurysm, intracranial hemorrhage, conjunctival hemorrhages, Janeway lesions)
Immunologic phenomena (glomerulonephritis, Osler nodes, Roth spots, rheumatoid factor)
Microbiologic evidence (positive blood culture result, but not meeting major criteria, *or* serologic evidence of active infection with organism consistent with infective endocarditis)

### POSSIBLE INFECTIVE ENDOCARDITIS

*Clinical Criteria*
One major and one minor criteria *or* three minor criteria

### REJECTED

Firm alternative diagnosis for manifestations of endocarditis *or*
Resolution of manifestations of endocarditis with antibiotic therapy for ≤4 days *or*
No pathologic evidence of endocarditis at surgery or autopsy after antibiotic therapy of ≥4 days *or* does not meet criteria for possible endocarditis

Adapted from Tissières P, Gervaix A, Beghetti M, et al: Value and limitations of the van Reyn, Duke, and modified Duke criteria for the diagnosis of infective endocarditis in children. *Pediatrics* 112: e467–e471, 2003.

## TREATMENT

Severely ill patients must be stabilized with supportive therapies for cardiac failure, pulmonary edema, and low cardiac output (see Chapter 145). Multiple blood cultures should be obtained before initiating antibiotic therapy after which empirical antibiotic therapy may be started for acutely ill persons. With subacute disease, awaiting results of blood cultures to confirm the diagnosis is recommended to direct therapy according to the susceptibility of the isolate. Antibiotic treatment typically requires treatment with bactericidal antibiotics for 4 to 8 weeks. Infective carditis from suspectible viridans streptococci can be treated with monotherapy penicillin G for 4 weeks. A 2-week regimen of penicillin G plus an aminoglycoside is effective in adults. Surgery is indicated if medical treatment is unsuccessful, with persistent bacteremia, an unusual, difficult to treat pathogen (fungal endocarditis), valve annulus or myocardial abscess, rupture of a valve leaflet, valvular insufficiency with acute or refractory heart failure, recurrent serious embolic complications, or refractory prosthetic valve disease.

## COMPLICATIONS AND PROGNOSIS

The major complications of infective endocarditis are direct damage to the heart and heart valves and distant complications secondary to sterile and **septic emboli** from vegetations. Damage to the heart and heart valves may include regurgitation with vegetations or actual defects in the leaflets resulting from embolization of the leaflet tissue, abscess of the valve ring, or myocardial abscess. These complications should be monitored by physical examination and echocardiography. Cerebral abscesses or aneurysms can cause a strokelike picture. Splenic abscesses can cause fatal bleeding.

The outcome of infective endocarditis caused by the most common organisms is often good. The cure rate is greater than 90% in uncomplicated endocarditis caused by viridans streptococci on a natural valve, 75% to 90% for *Enterococcus* endocarditis treated by a synergistic combination of antibiotics, and 60% to 75% for *S. aureus* endocarditis with an acute, severe presentation. The prognosis for endocarditis caused by gram-negative bacilli and rarer organisms is poor. Fungal endocarditis has the poorest prognosis, with a cure rate of about 50% even with valve replacement.

## PREVENTION

Patients at high risk for infective endocarditis include those with prosthetic cardiac valves or prior infective endocarditis; children who have unrepaired cyanotic congenital heart disease, are within 6 months of repair using prosthetic material, or have residual defects at or near a site of prosthetic material; or transplant patients who develop valvular lesions. In these high-risk patients, prophylactic antibiotics are required before and during all dental procedures that involve manipulation of gingival tissue or the periapical region as well as invasive procedures of the respiratory tract, infected skin, or muscle. In most cases, oral amoxicillin 50 mg/kg (maximum dose, 2 g) taken 30 to 60 minutes before the procedure is the recommended regimen. Clindamycin or azithromycin are alternative regimens indicated for most patients allergic to β-lactams. Prolonged or continuous antibiotic prophylaxis is not recommended.

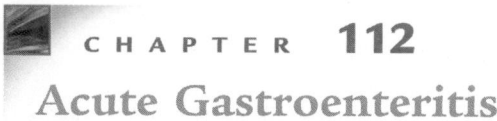

CHAPTER **112**

# Acute Gastroenteritis

## ETIOLOGY AND EPIDEMIOLOGY

**Acute enteritis** or **acute gastroenteritis** refers to **diarrhea**, which is abnormally frequent and liquidity of fecal discharges. Diarrhea is caused by different infectious or inflammatory processes in the intestine that directly affect enterocyte secretory and absorptive functions (Table 112-1). Some of these processes act by increasing cyclic adenosine monophosphate (AMP) levels (*Vibrio cholerae, Escherichia coli* heat-labile toxin, vasoactive intestinal peptide–producing tumors). Other processes (*Shigella* toxin, congenital chloridorrhea) cause secretory diarrhea by affecting ion channels or by unknown mechanisms. Enteritis has many viral, bacterial, and parasitic causes (Table 112-2).

Diarrhea is a leading cause of morbidity and a common disease in children in the United States In the developing world, it is a major cause of childhood fatality. The epidemiology of gastroenteritis depends on the specific organisms. Some organisms are spread person to person, others are spread via contaminated food or water, and some are spread from animal to human. Many organisms spread by multiple routes. The ability of an organism to infect relates to the mode of spread, ability to colonize the gastrointestinal tract, and minimum number of organisms required to cause disease.

Viral causes of gastroenteritis in children include rotaviruses, caliciviruses (including the noroviruses), astroviruses, and enteric adenoviruses (serotypes 40 and 41). Rotavirus invades the epithelium and damages villi of the upper small intestine and, in severe cases, involves the entire small bowel and colon. Rotavirus is the most frequent cause of diarrhea during the winter months. Vomiting may last 3 to 4 days, and diarrhea may last 7 to 10 days. Dehydration is common in younger children. Primary infection with rotavirus may cause moderate to severe disease in infancy but is less severe later in life.

**Typhoid fever** is caused by *Salmonella typhi* and, occasionally, *Salmonella paratyphi*. Worldwide, there are an estimated 16 million cases of typhoid fever annually, resulting in 600,000 deaths. The typhoid bacillus infects humans only. These infections are distinguished by prolonged fever and extraintestinal manifestations despite inconsistent presence of diarrhea. In the United States, approximately 400 cases of typhoid fever occur each year. Most occur in travelers returning from other countries. The incubation period of typhoid fever is usually 7 to 14 days (range 3–60 days). Infected persons without symptoms, or **chronic carriers**, serve as reservoirs and sources of continuous spread. Carriers often have cholelithiasis.

**TABLE 112-1  Mechanisms of Diarrhea**

| Primary Mechanism | Defect | Stool Examination | Examples | Comments |
|---|---|---|---|---|
| Secretory | Decreased absorption, increased secretion: electrolyte transport | Watery, normal osmolality; osmoles = 2 × (Na$^+$ + K$^+$) | Cholera, toxigenic *Escherichia coli*; carcinoid, VIP, neuroblastoma, congenital chloride diarrhea, *Clostridium difficile*, cryptosporidiosis (in AIDS) | Persists during fasting; bile salt malabsorption also may increase intestinal water secretion; no stool leukocytes |
| Osmotic | Maldigestion, transport defects, ingestion of unabsorbable solute | Watery, acidic, + reducing substances; increased osmolality; osmoles > 2 × (Na$^+$ + K$^+$) | Lactase deficiency, glucose-galactose malabsorption, lactulose, laxative abuse | Stops with fasting, increased breath hydrogen with carbohydrate malabsorption, no stool leukocytes |
| Motility | | | | |
| Increased motility | Decreased transit time | Loose to normal-appearing stool, stimulated by gastrocolic reflex | Irritable bowel syndrome, thyrotoxicosis, postvagotomy dumping syndrome | Infection also may contribute to increased motility |
| Decreased motility | Defect in neuromuscular unit(s); stasis (bacterial overgrowth) | Loose to normal-appearing stool | Pseudo-obstruction, blind loop | Possible bacterial overgrowth |
| Mucosal invasion | Inflammation, decreased mucosal surface area and/or colonic reabsorption, increased motility | Blood and increased WBCs in stool | Celiac disease, *Salmonella* infection, shigellosis, amebiasis, yersiniosis, *Campylobacter* infection, rotavirus enteritis | Dysentery (blood, mucus, and WBCs) |

VIP, vasoactive intestinal peptide; WBCs, white blood cells.

From Wyllie R: Major symptoms and signs of digestive tract disorders. In Kliegman RM, Behrman RE, Jenson HB Stanton BF (eds): Nelson Textbook of Pediatrics, 18th ed. Philadelphia, *WB Saunders*, 2007, Table 303-7, p 152.

**Nontyphoidal *Salmonella*** produce diarrhea by invading the intestinal mucosa. The organisms are transmitted through contact with infected animals (chickens, pet iguanas, other reptiles, turtles) or from contaminated food products, such as dairy products, eggs, and poultry. A large inoculum, of 1000 to 10 billion organisms, is required because *Salmonella* are killed by gastric acidity. The incubation period for gastroenteritis ranges from 6 to 72 hours, but usually is less than 24 hours. Chronic carriage may develop.

*Shigella dysenteriae* may cause disease by producing **Shiga toxin**, either alone or combined with tissue invasion. The incubation period is 1 to 7 days. Infected adults may shed organisms for 1 month. Infection is spread by person-to-person contact or by the ingestion of contaminated food with 10 to 100 organisms. The colon is selectively affected. High fever and seizures may occur in addition to diarrhea.

Only certain strains of *E. coli* produce diarrhea. *E. coli* strains associated with enteritis are classified by the mechanism of diarrhea: enteropathogenic (EPEC), enterotoxigenic (ETEC), enteroinvasive (EIEC), enterohemorrhagic (EHEC), or enteroaggregative (EAEC). EPEC is responsible for many of the epidemics of diarrhea in newborn nurseries and in day care centers. ETEC strains produce **heat-labile (cholera-like) enterotoxin**, **heat-stable enterotoxin**, or both. ETEC causes 40% to 60% of cases of **traveler's diarrhea**. EPEC and ETEC adhere to the epithelial cells in the upper small intestine and produce disease by liberating toxins that induce intestinal secretion and limit absorption. EIEC invades the colonic mucosa, producing widespread mucosal damage with acute inflammation, similar to *Shigella*. EHEC, especially the *E. coli* O157:H7 strain, produce a **Shiga-like toxin** that is responsible for a hemorrhagic colitis and most cases of **hemolytic uremic syndrome (HUS)**, which is a syndrome of microangiopathic hemolytic anemia, thrombocytopenia, and renal failure (see Chapter 164). EHEC is associated with contaminated food, including unpasteurized fruit juices and especially undercooked beef. EHEC is associated with a self-limited form of gastroenteritis, usually with bloody diarrhea, but production of this toxin blocks host cell protein synthesis and affects vascular endothelial cells and glomeruli, resulting in the clinical manifestations of HUS.

**TABLE 112-2 Common Pathogenic Organisms Causing Diarrhea and Their Virulence Mechanisms**

| Organisms | Pathogenic Mechanism(s) |
|---|---|
| **VIRUSES** | |
| Rotaviruses | Damage to microvilli |
| Caliciviruses | Mucosal lesion |
| Astroviruses | Mucosal lesion |
| Enteric adenoviruses (serotypes 40 and 41) | Mucosal lesion |
| **BACTERIA** | |
| *Campylobacter jejuni* | Invasion, enterotoxin |
| *Clostridium difficile* | Cytotoxin, enterotoxin |
| *Escherichia coli* | |
|   Enteropathogenic (EPEC) | Adherence, effacement |
|   Enterotoxigenic (ETEC) (traveler's diarrhea) | Enterotoxins (heat-stable or heat-labile) |
|   Enteroinvasive (EIEC) | Invasion of mucosa |
|   Enterohemorrhagic (EHEC) (includes O157: H7 causing HUS) | Adherence, effacement, cytotoxin |
|   Enteroaggregative (EAEC) | Adherence, mucosal damage |
| *Salmonella* | Invasion, enterotoxin |
| *Shigella* | Invasion, enterotoxin, cytotoxin |
| *Vibrio cholerae* | Enterotoxin |
| *Vibrio parahaemolyticus* | Invasion, cytotoxin |
| *Yersinia enterocolitica* | Invasion, enterotoxin |
| **PARASITES** | |
| *Entamoeba histolytica* | Invasion, enzyme and cytotoxin production; cyst resistant to physical destruction |
| *Giardia lamblia* | Adheres to mucosa; cyst resistant to physical destruction |
| Spore-forming intestinal protozoa | Adherence, inflammation |
|   *Cryptosporidium parvum* | |
|   *Isospora belli* | |
|   *Cyclospora cayetanensis* | |
|   Microsporidia (*Enterocytozoon bieneusi, Encephalitozoon intestinalis*) | |

HUS, hemolytic uremic syndrome.

*Campylobacter jejuni* is spread by person-to-person contact and by contaminated water and food, especially poultry, raw milk, and cheese. The organism invades the mucosa of the jejunum, ileum, and colon. *Yersinia enterocolitica* is transmitted by pets and contaminated food, especially chitterlings. Infants and young children characteristically have a diarrheal disease whereas older children usually have acute lesions of the terminal ileum or acute mesenteric lymphadenitis mimicking appendicitis or Crohn disease. Postinfectious arthritis, rash, and spondylopathy may develop.

*Clostridium difficile* causes **C. difficile–associated diarrhea**, or **antibiotic-associated diarrhea**, secondary to its toxin. The organism produces spores that spread from person to person. *C. difficile*–associated diarrhea may follow exposure to any antibiotic.

*Entamoeba histolytica* (amebiasis), *Giardia lamblia,* and *Cryptosporidium parvum* are important enteric parasites found in North America. Amebiasis occurs in warmer climates, whereas giardiasis is endemic throughout the United States and is common among infants in day care centers. *E. histolytica* infects the colon; amebae may pass through the bowel wall and invade the liver, lung, and brain. Diarrhea is of acute onset, is bloody, and contains leukocytes. *G. lamblia* is transmitted through ingestion of cysts, either from contact with an infected individual or from food or freshwater or well water contaminated with infected feces. The organism adheres to the microvilli of the duodenal and jejunal epithelium. *Cryptosporidium* causes mild, watery diarrhea in immunocompetent persons that resolves without treatment. It produces severe, prolonged diarrhea in persons with acquired immunodeficiency syndrome (AIDS) (see Chapter 125).

## CLINICAL MANIFESTATIONS

Gastroenteritis may be accompanied by systemic findings, such as fever, lethargy, and abdominal pain.

Viral diarrhea is characterized by watery stools, with no blood or mucus. Vomiting may be present, and dehydration may be prominent. Fever, when present, is low grade. **Typhoid fever** is characterized by bacteremia and fever that usually precede the final enteric phase. Fever, headache, and abdominal pain worsen over 48 to 72 hours with nausea, decreased appetite, and constipation over the first week. If untreated, the disease persists for 2 to 3 weeks marked by significant weight loss and occasionally hematochezia or melena. Bowel perforation is a common complication in adults, but is rare in children. **Dysentery** is enteritis involving the colon and rectum, with blood and mucus, possibly foul smelling, and fever. *Shigella* is the prototype cause of dysentery, which must be differentiated from infection with EIEC, EHEC, *E. histolytica* (**amebic dysentery**), *C. jejuni, Y. enterocolitica,* and nontyphoidal *Salmonella*. Gastrointestinal bleeding and blood loss may be significant. **Enterotoxigenic disease** is caused by agents that produce enterotoxins, such as *V. cholerae* and ETEC. Fever is absent or low grade. Diarrhea usually involves the ileum with watery stools without blood or mucus and usually lasts 3 to 4 days with four to five loose stools per day. Insidious onset of progressive anorexia, nausea, gaseousness, abdominal distention, watery diarrhea, secondary lactose intolerance, and weight loss is characteristic of giardiasis.

A chief consideration in management of a child with diarrhea is to assess the degree of dehydration as evident from clinical signs and symptoms, ongoing losses, and daily requirements (see Chapter 33). The degree of dehydration dictates the urgency of the situation and the volume of fluid needed for rehydration. Mild to moderate dehydration usually can be treated with oral rehydration; severe dehydration usually requires intravenous (IV) rehydration and may require ICU admission.

## LABORATORY AND IMAGING STUDIES

Initial laboratory evaluation of moderate to severe diarrhea includes electrolytes, blood urea nitrogen (BUN), creatinine, and urinalysis for specific gravity as an indicator of hydration. Stool specimens should be examined for mucus, blood, and leukocytes, which indicate colitis in response to bacteria that diffusely invade the colonic mucosa such as *Shigella, Salmonella, C. jejuni,* and invasive *E. coli.* Patients infected with Shiga toxin–producing *E. coli* and *E. histolytica* generally have minimal fecal leukocytes.

A rapid diagnostic test for rotavirus in stool should be performed, especially during the winter. Bacterial stool cultures are recommended for patients with fever, profuse diarrhea, and dehydration or if HUS is suspected. If the stool test result is negative for blood and leukocytes, and there is no history to suggest contaminated food ingestion, a viral etiology is most likely. Stool evaluation for parasitic agents should be considered for acute dysenteric illness, especially in returning travelers, and in protracted cases of diarrhea in which no bacterial agent is identified. The diagnosis of *E. histolytica* is based on identification of the organism in the stool. Serologic tests are useful for diagnosis of extraintestinal amebiasis, including amebic hepatic abscess. Giardiasis can be diagnosed by identifying trophozoites or cysts in stool; less often a duodenal aspirate or biopsy of the duodenum or upper jejunum is needed. *Giardia* is excreted intermittently; three specimens are required. If stool tests are nondiagnostic, the duodenal fluid may be examined using the Entero-Test, a nylon string affixed to a gelatin capsule, which is swallowed. After several hours, the string is withdrawn and duodenal contents are examined for *G. lamblia* trophozoites.

Positive blood cultures are uncommon with bacterial enteritis except for *S. typhi* (typhoid fever), nontyphoidal *Salmonella,* and *E. coli* enteritis in very young infants. In typhoid fever, blood cultures are positive early in the disease, whereas stool cultures become positive only after the secondary bacteremia.

## DIFFERENTIAL DIAGNOSIS

Diarrhea can be caused by infection, toxins, gastrointestinal allergy (including allergy to milk or its components), malabsorption defects, inflammatory bowel disease, celiac disease, or any injury to enterocytes. Specific infections are differentiated from each other by the use of stool cultures and enzyme-linked immunosorbent assay (ELISA) or polymerase chain reaction (PCR) tests, when necessary. Acute enteritis may mimic other acute diseases, such as intussusception and acute appendicitis, which are best identified by diagnostic imaging. Many noninfectious causes of diarrhea produce chronic diarrhea, with persistence for more than 14 days. Persistent or chronic diarrhea may require tests for malabsorption or invasive studies, including endoscopy and small bowel biopsy (see Chapter 129).

**Common-source diarrhea** usually is associated with ingestion of contaminated food. In the United States, the most common bacterial food-borne causes (in order of frequency) are nontyphoidal *Salmonella, Campylobacter, Shigella, E. coli* O157:H7, *Yersinia, Listeria monocytogenes,* and *V. cholerae.* The most common parasitic food-borne causes are *Cryptosporidium parvum* and *Cyclospora cayetanensis.*

Common-source diarrhea also includes ingestion of preformed enterotoxins produced by bacteria, such as *S. aureus* and *Bacillus cereus,* which multiply in contaminated foods, and nonbacterial toxins such as from fish, shellfish, and mushrooms. After a short incubation period, vomiting and cramps are prominent symptoms, and diarrhea may or may not be present. Heavy metals that leach into canned food or drinks causing gastric irritation and emetic syndromes may mimic symptoms of acute infectious enteritis.

## TREATMENT

Most infectious causes of diarrhea in children are self-limited. Management of viral and most bacterial causes of diarrhea is primarily supportive and consists of correcting dehydration and ongoing fluid and electrolyte deficits and managing secondary complications resulting from mucosal injury.

Hyponatremia is common; hypernatremia is less common. Metabolic acidosis results from losses of bicarbonate in stool, lactic acidosis results from shock, and phosphate retention results from transient prerenal-renal insufficiency. Traditionally, therapy for 24 hours with oral rehydration solutions alone is effective for viral diarrhea. Therapy for severe fluid and electrolyte losses involves IV hydration. Less severe degrees of dehydration (<10%) in the absence of excessive vomiting or shock may be managed with oral rehydration solutions containing glucose and electrolytes. Ondansetron may be administered to reduce emesis when persistent.

Antibiotic therapy is necessary only for patients with *S. typhi* (typhoid fever) and sepsis or bacteremia with signs of systemic toxicity, those with metastatic foci, or infants younger than 3 months with nontyphoidal salmonella. Antibiotic treatment of *Shigella* produces a bacteriologic cure in 80% of patients after 48 hours, reducing the spread of the disease. Many *Shigella sonnei* isolates, the predominant strain affecting children, are resistant to amoxicillin and trimethoprim-sulfamethoxazole (TMP-SMZ). Recommended treatment for children is an oral third-generation cephalosporin or a fluoroquinolone for patients 18 years and older.

Treatment of *C. difficile* includes discontinuation of the antibiotic and, if diarrhea is severe, oral metronidazole or vancomycin. *E. histolytica* dysentery is treated with metronidazole followed by a luminal agent, such as iodoquinol. The treatment of *G. lamblia* is with albendazole, metronidazole, furazolidone, or quinacrine. Nitazoxanide can be used in children younger than 12 months of age for the treatment of *Cryptosporidium.*

## COMPLICATIONS AND PROGNOSIS

The major complication of gastroenteritis is dehydration and the cardiovascular compromise that can occur with severe hypovolemia. Seizures may occur with high fever, especially with *Shigella.* Intestinal abscesses can form with *Shigella* and *Salmonella* infections, especially typhoid fever, leading to intestinal perforation, a life-threatening complication. Severe vomiting associated with gastroenteritis can cause esophageal tears or aspiration.

Deaths resulting from diarrhea reflect the principal problem of disruption of fluid and electrolyte homeostasis, which leads to dehydration, electrolyte imbalance, vascular instability, and shock. In the United States, approximately 75 to 150 deaths occur annually from diarrheal disease, primarily in children under 1 year of age. These deaths occur in a seasonal pattern between October and February, concurrent with the rotavirus season.

At least 10% of patients who have typhoid fever shed *S. typhi* for about 3 months, and 4% become chronic carriers. The risk of becoming a chronic carrier is low in children. Ciprofloxacin is recommended for adult carriers with persistent *Salmonella* excretion.

## PREVENTION

The most important means of preventing childhood diarrhea is the provision of clean, uncontaminated water and proper hygiene in growing, collecting, and preparing foods. Good hygienic measures, especially good hand washing with soap and water, are the best means of controlling person-to-person spread of most organisms causing gastroenteritis. Similarly, poultry products should be considered potentially contaminated with *Salmonella* and should be handled and cooked appropriately.

Immunization against rotavirus infection is recommended for all children beginning at 6 weeks of age, with the first dose by 14 weeks 6 days and the last dose by 8 months (see Chapter 94). Two typhoid vaccines are licensed in the United States: an oral live attenuated vaccine (Ty21a) for children 6 years and older, and a capsular polysaccharide vaccine (ViCPS) for intramuscular (IM) administration for persons 2 years and older. These are not recommended for travelers to endemic areas of developing countries or for household contacts of *S. typhi* chronic carriers.

Families should be aware of the risk of acquiring salmonellosis from household reptile pets. Transmission of *Salmonella* from reptiles can be prevented by thorough hand washing with soap and water after handling reptiles or reptile cages. Children under 5 years of age and immunocompromised persons should avoid contact with reptiles. Pet reptiles should not roam freely in the home or living areas and should be kept out of kitchens and food preparation areas to prevent contamination.

The risk for traveler's diarrhea, caused primarily by ETEC, may be minimized by avoiding uncooked food and untreated drinking water. Prophylaxis with bismuth subsalicylate (Pepto-Bismol) for adults (2 oz or 2 tablets orally four times a day) may be effective for prevention but is not recommended for children. Symptomatic self-treatment for mild diarrhea with loperamide (Imodium) and WHO **oral rehydration solution (ORS)** is recommended for children at least 6 years of age and adults. Self-treatment of moderate diarrhea and fever with a fluoroquinolone is recommended in adults at least 18 years old. Prompt medical evaluation is indicated for disease persisting more than 3 days, bloody stools, fever above 102°F or chills, persistent vomiting, or moderate to severe dehydration, especially in children.

*Lactobacillus acidophilus* is a **probiotic** and reduces the incidence of community-acquired and antibiotic-associated diarrhea in children treated with oral antibiotics for other infectious diseases.

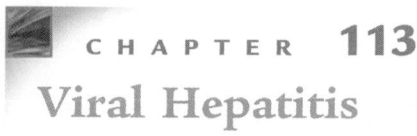

CHAPTER **113**

# Viral Hepatitis

## ETIOLOGY

There are six primary hepatotropic viruses:

Hepatitis A virus (HAV)
Hepatitis B virus (HBV)
Hepatitis C virus (HCV)
Hepatitis D virus (HDV)
Hepatitis E virus (HEV)
Hepatitis G virus (HGV)

They differ in their virologic characteristics, transmission, severity, likelihood of persistence, and subsequent risk of hepatocellular carcinoma (Table 113-1). HDV, also known as the **delta agent**, is a defective virus that requires HBV for spread and causes either coinfection with HBV or superinfection in chronic HBsAg (hepatitis B surface antigen) carriers. HBV, HCV, and HDV infections can result in chronic hepatitis, or a chronic carrier state, which facilitates spread. The causes of 10% to 15% of cases of acute hepatitis are unknown.

## EPIDEMIOLOGY

HAV causes approximately half of all cases of viral hepatitis in the United States. Among U.S. children, approximately 70% to 80% of all new cases of viral hepatitis are caused by HAV, 5% to 30% by HBV, and 5% to 15% by HCV. The major risk factors for HBV and HCV are injectable drug use, frequent exposure to blood products, and maternal infection. HEV occurs following travel to endemic areas outside the United States. HGV is prevalent in HIV-infected persons. HBV and HCV cause chronic infection, which may lead to cirrhosis and is a significant risk factor for hepatocellular carcinoma and represents a persistent risk of transmission.

## CLINICAL MANIFESTATIONS

There is considerable overlap in the characteristic clinical courses of HAV, HBV, and HCV (Fig. 113-1). The **preicteric phase**, which lasts approximately 1 week, is characterized by headache, anorexia, malaise, abdominal discomfort, nausea, and vomiting and usually precedes the onset of clinically detectable disease. Infants with perinatal HBV may have immune complexes accompanied by urticaria and arthritis before the onset of icterus. Jaundice and tender hepatomegaly are the most common physical findings and are characteristic of the **icteric phase**. Prodromal symptoms, particularly in children, may abate during the icteric phase. Asymptomatic or mild, nonspecific illness without icterus is common with HAV, HBV, and HCV, especially in young children. Hepatitic enzymes may increase 15- to 20-fold. Resolution of the hyperbilirubinemia and normalization of the transaminases may take 6 to 8 weeks.

**TABLE 113-1 Characteristics of Agents Causing Acute Viral Hepatitis**

| Feature | Hepatitis Viruses | | | | | | |
| --- | --- | --- | --- | --- | --- | --- | --- |
| | HAV* | HBV | HCV† | HDV | HEV‡ | HGV | TTV, SEN-V |
| Viral structure | 27-nm ssRNA virus | 42-nm dsDNA virus | 30- to 60-nm ssRNA virus | 36-nm circular ssRNA hybrid particle with HBsAg coat | 27-34 nm ssRNA virus | 50- to 100-nm ssRNA virus | 30- to 50-nm ssDNA virus |
| Family | Picornavirus | Hepadnavirus | Flavivirus | Satellite Similar to HBV | Flavivirus | Flavivirus | Circovirus |
| Transmission | Fecal-oral, rarely parenteral | Transfusion, sexual, inoculation, perinatal | Parenteral, transfusion, perinatal | | Fecal-oral (endemic and epidemic) | Parenteral, transfusion | Parenteral, perinatal |
| Incubation period | 15-30 days | 60-180 days | 30-60 days | Co-infection with HBV | 35-60 days | Unknown | Unknown |
| Serum markers | Anti-HAV | HBsAg, HBcAg, HBeAg, anti-HBs, anti-HBc | Anti-HCV (IgG, IgM), RIBA, PCR assay for HCV RNA | Anti-HDV, RNA | Anti-HEV | RNA by RT-PCR assay | |
| Fulminant liver failure | Rare | <1% unless co-infection with HDV | Uncommon | 2-20% | 20% | Probably no | |
| Persistent infection | No | 5-10% (90% with perinatal infection) | 85% | 2-70% | No | Persistent infection common; chronic disease rare | |
| Increased risk of hepatocellular carcinoma | No | Yes | Yes | No | No | Unknown | |
| Prophylaxis | Vaccine: immune serum globulin | Vaccine: hepatitis B immunoglobulin (HBIG) | | | | | |

*I.e., enterovirus 72.

†Formerly post-transfusion non-A, non-B virus.

‡Formerly enteral non-A, non-B virus.

dsDNA, double-stranded DNA; HAV, hepatitis A virus; HBV, hepatitis B virus; HCV, hepatitis C virus; HDV, hepatitis D virus; HEV, hepatitis E virus; HGV, hepatitis G virus; PCR, polymerase chain reaction; RIBA, recombinant immunoblot assay; RT-PCR, reverse transcriptase–polymerase chain reaction; ssDNA/ssRNA, single-stranded DNA/RNA; TTV, transfusion-transmitted virus.

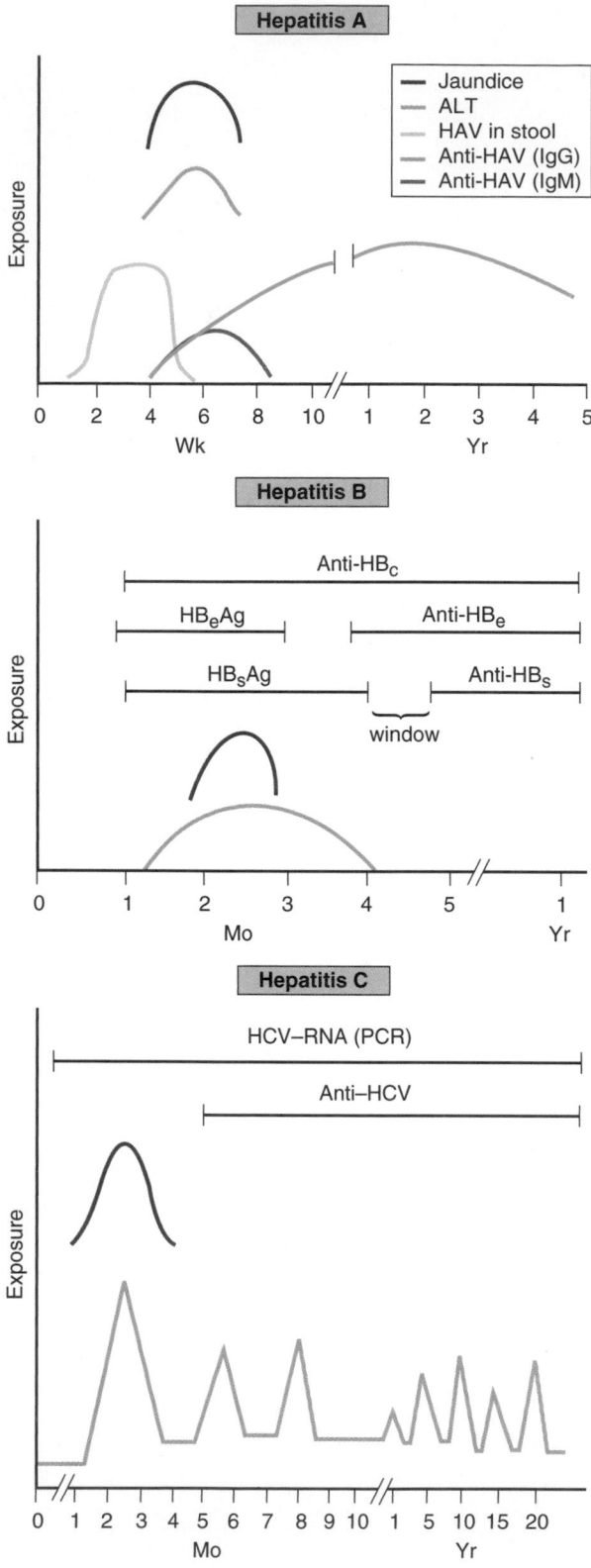

**FIGURE 113-1**

**Clinical course and laboratory findings associated with hepatitis A, hepatitis B, and hepatitis C.** ALT, alanine aminotransferase; HAV, hepatitis A virus; anti-HBc, antibody to hepatitis B core antigen; HBeAg, hepatitis B early antigen; anti-HBe, antibody to hepatitis B early antigen; HBsAg, hepatitis B surface antigen; anti-HBs, antibody to hepatitis B surface antigen; HCV, hepatitis C virus; PCR, polymerase chain reaction.

## LABORATORY AND IMAGING STUDIES

Alanine aminotransferase and aspartate aminotransferase levels are elevated and generally reflect the degree of parenchymal inflammation. Alkaline phosphatase, 5α-nucleotidase, and total and direct (conjugated) bilirubin levels indicate the degree of cholestasis, which results from hepatocellular and bile duct damage. The prothrombin time is a good predictor of severe hepatocellular injury and progression to fulminant hepatic failure (see Chapter 130).

The diagnosis of viral hepatitis is confirmed by serologic testing (see Table 113-1 and Fig. 113-1). The presence of IgM-specific antibody to HAV with low or absent IgG antibody to HAV is presumptive evidence of HAV. There is no chronic carrier state of HAV. The presence of HBsAg signifies acute or chronic infection with HBV. Antigenemia appears early in the illness and is usually transient, but is characteristic of chronic infection. Maternal HBsAg status always should be determined when HBV infection is diagnosed in children younger than 1 year of age because of the likelihood of vertical transmission. Hepatitis B early antigen (HBeAg) appears in the serum with acute HBV. The continued presence of HBsAg and HBeAg in the absence of antibody to e antigen (anti-HBe) indicates high risk of transmissibility that is associated with ongoing viral replication. Clearance of HBsAg from the serum precedes a variable **window period** followed by the emergence of the antibody to surface antigen (anti-HBs), which indicates development of lifelong immunity and is also a marker of immunization. Antibody to core antigen (anti-HBc) is a useful marker for recognizing HBV infection during the window phase (when HBsAg has disappeared, but before the appearance of anti-HBs). Anti-HBe is useful in predicting a low degree of infectivity during the carrier state. Seroconversion after HCV infection may occur 6 months after infection. A positive result of HCV enzyme-linked immunosorbent assay (ELISA) should be confirmed with the more specific recombinant immunoblot assay, which detects antibodies to multiple HCV antigens. Detection of HCV RNA by polymerase chain reaction (PCR) is a sensitive marker for active infection, and results of this test may be positive 3 days after inoculation.

## DIFFERENTIAL DIAGNOSIS

Many other viruses may cause hepatitis as part of systemic infection including Epstein-Barr virus (EBV), cytomegalovirus (CMV), varicella zoster virus (VZV) (chickenpox), herpes simplex virus, and adenoviruses. Bacterial infections that may cause hepatitis include *Escherichia coli* sepsis and leptospirosis. Patients with cholecystitis, cholangitis, and choledocholithiasis may present with acute symptoms and jaundice. Other causes of acute liver disease in childhood include drugs (isoniazid, phenytoin, valproic acid, carbamazepine, oral contraceptives, acetaminophen), toxins (ethanol, poisonous mushroom), Wilson disease, metabolic disease (galactosemia, tyrosinemia), $\alpha_1$-antitrypsin deficiency, tumor, shock, anoxia, and graft-versus-host disease (see Chapter 130).

## TREATMENT

The treatment of acute hepatitis is largely supportive and involves rest, hydration, and adequate dietary intake. Hospitalization is indicated for persons with severe vomiting and dehydration, a prolonged prothrombin time, or signs of hepatic encephalopathy. When the diagnosis of viral hepatitis is established, attention should be directed toward preventing its spread to close contacts. For HAV, hygienic measures include hand washing and careful disposal of excreta, contaminated diapers or clothing, needles, and other blood-contaminated items.

Chronic HBV infection may be treated with interferon alfa-2b or lamivudine, and HCV may be treated with interferon alfa alone or usually in combination with oral ribavirin. Most experience with these treatment regimens is in adults. The decision to treat is based on the patient's current age, age at HBV acquisition, development of viral mutations during therapy, and stage of viral infection. Transmission of HBV by vertical transmission or infection early in life often results in chronic HBV infection in an immune tolerant phase, in which interferon usually is not effective.

## COMPLICATIONS AND PROGNOSIS

A protracted or relapsing course may develop in 10% to 15% of cases of HAV in adults, lasting up to 6 months with an undulating course before eventual clinical resolution. **Fulminant hepatitis** with encephalopathy, gastrointestinal bleeding from esophageal varices or coagulopathy, and profound jaundice is uncommon, but is associated with a high mortality rate.

Most cases of acute viral hepatitis resolve without specific therapy, with less than 0.1% of cases progressing to fulminant hepatic necrosis. HAV and HEV cause only acute infection. HBV, HCV, and HDV may persist as chronic infection with chronic inflammation, fibrosis, and cirrhosis and the associated risk of hepatocellular carcinoma.

From 5% to 10% of adults with HBV develop persistent infection, defined by persistence of HBsAg in the blood for more than 6 months, compared with 90% of children who acquire HBV by perinatal transmission. Chronic HBsAg carriers are usually HBeAg-negative and have no clinical, biochemical, or serologic evidence of active hepatitis, unless there is superinfection with HDV. Approximately 10% to 15% of HBsAg carriers eventually clear HBsAg.

Approximately 85% of persons infected with HCV remain chronically infected, which is characterized by fluctuating transaminase levels (see Fig. 113-1). There is poor correlation of symptoms with ongoing liver damage. Approximately 20% of persons with chronic infection develop cirrhosis, and approximately 25% of those develop hepatocellular carcinoma. Human immunodeficiency virus (HIV) infection and ethanol use increase the risk of HCV progression.

## PREVENTION

Good hygienic practices significantly reduce the risk of fecal-oral transmission of HAV. Screening blood donors for evidence of hepatitis significantly reduces the risk of blood-borne transmission. Specific postexposure measures are recommended to prevent secondary cases in susceptible persons.

HAV vaccine is recommended for routine immunization of all children beginning at 12 months, and for unvaccinated older children in areas with targeted vaccination programs. Unvaccinated household and sexual contacts of persons with HAV should receive postexposure prophylaxis as soon as possible and within 2 weeks of the last exposure. A single dose of HAV vaccine at the age-appropriate dose is preferred for persons 12 months to 40 years of age. Immunoglobulin (0.02 mL/kg) given intramuscularly is preferred for children under 12 months of age, persons over 40 years of age, and immunocompromised persons. Unvaccinated travelers to endemic regions should receive a single dose of HAV vaccine administered at any time before departure.

HBV vaccine is recommended for routine immunization of all infants beginning at birth and for all children and adolescents through 18 years of age who have not been immunized previously (see Fig. 94-1). It also is recommended as a pre-exposure vaccination for older children and adults at increased risk of exposure to HBV including persons undergoing hemodialysis, recipients of clotting factor concentrates, residents and staff of institutions for developmentally disabled persons, men who have sex with men, injectable drug users, inmates of juvenile detention and other correctional facilities, and health care workers. HBV vaccine already has shown effectiveness in reducing the incidence of hepatocellular carcinoma in high-risk populations. Routine prenatal screening for HBsAg is recommended for all pregnant women in the United States. Infants born to HBsAg-positive mothers should receive HBV vaccine and hepatitis B immunoglobulin (HBIG) (0.5 mL) within 12 hours of birth, with subsequent vaccine doses at 1 month and 6 months of age followed by testing for HBsAg and anti-HBs at 9 to 15 months of age. Infants born to mothers whose HBsAg status is unknown should receive vaccine within 12 hours of birth. If maternal testing is positive for HBsAg, the infant should receive HBIG as soon as possible (no later than 1 week of age). The combination of HBIG and vaccination is 99% effective in preventing vertical transmission of HBV. Vaccination alone without HBIG may prevent 75% of cases of perinatal HBV transmission and approximately 95% of cases of symptomatic childhood HBV infection.

Postexposure prophylaxis of unvaccinated persons using HBIG and vaccine is recommended following needle stick injuries with blood from an HBsAg-positive patient and for household members with intimate contact, including sex partners.

# CHAPTER 114

# Urinary Tract Infection

## ETIOLOGY

Urinary tract infections (UTIs) include **cystitis** (infection localized to the bladder), **pyelonephritis** (infection of the renal parenchyma, calyces, and renal pelvis), and **renal abscess**, which may be intrarenal or perinephric. The urinary tract and urine are normally sterile. *Escherichia coli*, ascending from bowel flora, accounts for 90% of first infections and 75% of recurrent infections. Over 90% of nephritogenic *E. coli* possess P fimbriae that binds to uroepithelial cells and P blood group antigens, which are glycolipids containing the disaccharide α-D-galactopyranosyl-(1,4)-β-D-galactopyranose (Gal-Gal). Individuals with high-level expression of P1 blood group antigen are predisposed to pyelonephritis and bacteremia, as well as recurrent UTIs. Other bacteria commonly causing infection include *Klebsiella, Proteus, Enterococcus,* and *Pseudomonas. Staphylococcus saprophyticus* is associated with UTI in some children and in sexually active adolescent girls. *S. saprophyticus, Chlamydia trachomatis,* and *E. coli* are the chief causes of the **acute urethral syndrome**, or **postcoital urethritis**, which typically occurs 12 to 72 hours after sexual intercourse.

## EPIDEMIOLOGY

Approximately 8% of girls and 2% of boys have a UTI by 11 years of age. The lifetime incidence of UTI in females is about 30% compared to only 1% in males. Approximately 75% of infants younger than 3 months of age with bacteriuria are male compared with only 10% between 3 and 8 months of age. After 12 months of age, UTI in healthy children usually is seen in girls.

A short urethra predisposes girls to UTI. Uncircumcised male infants are at 5- to 12-fold increased risk for UTI compared with circumcised male infants. Obstruction to urine flow and urinary stasis is the major risk factor and may result from anatomic abnormalities, nephrolithiasis, renal tumor, indwelling urinary catheter, ureteropelvic junction obstruction, megaureter, extrinsic compression, and pregnancy. Vesicoureteral reflux, whether primary (70% of cases) or secondary to urinary tract obstruction, predisposes to chronic infection and renal scarring. Scarring also may develop in the absence of reflux.

## CLINICAL MANIFESTATIONS

The symptoms and signs of UTI vary markedly with age. Few have high positive predictive values in neonates, with failure to thrive, feeding problems, and fever the most consistent symptoms. Direct hyperbilirubinemia may develop secondary to gram-negative endotoxin. Infants 1 month to 2 years old may present with feeding problems, failure to thrive, diarrhea, vomiting, or unexplained fever. The symptoms may masquerade as gastrointestinal illness with *colic*, irritability, and screaming periods. At 2 years of age, children begin to show the classic signs of UTI such as urgency, dysuria, frequency, and abdominal or back pain. The presence of UTI should be suspected in all infants and young children with unexplained fever and in patients of all ages with fever and congenital anomalies of the urinary tract.

## LABORATORY AND IMAGING STUDIES

The diagnosis of UTI requires a culture of the urine. Urine samples for urinalysis should be examined promptly (within 20 minutes) or refrigerated until cultured. Urine obtained by midstream, clean-catch technique (for older children and adolescents) is considered significant with bacterial growth of a single organism of more than 100,000 colony-forming units (CFU)/mL and has a 95% positive correlation with positive culture by suprapubic aspiration. Urine obtained by catheterization is considered significant with bacterial growth of more than 10,000 CFU/mL. Urine obtained by suprapubic aspiration is considered significant with bacterial growth of more than 1000 CFU/mL. Suprapubic percutaneous aspiration of the bladder may be performed in young infants if they have not voided for 1 to 3 hours. Perineal bags for urine collection are prone to contamination and are not recommended for urine collection for culture.

For infants and young children with unexplained fever who require immediate antibiotic therapy, a urine specimen should be obtained by catheterization. For infants and young children with unexplained fever who do not require antibiotic treatment, a urine specimen should be obtained by catheterization or alternatively by the most convenient method with a repeat urine collection by catheterization, or suprapubic aspiration in young infants, if the urinalysis suggests a UTI.

Urinalysis showing **pyuria** (leukocyturia of >10 white blood cells [WBCs]/mm$^3$) suggests infection, but also is consistent with urethritis, vaginitis, nephrolithiasis, glomerulonephritis, and interstitial nephritis. Urinary dipstick tests that combine both the leukocyte esterase and nitrite have sensitivity of 88% and specificity of 93% for detecting a UTI. Either test used alone has poor sensitivity. The presence of numerous motile bacteria in freshly voided, uncentrifuged urine from symptomatic infants and children has a 94% correlation with a positive culture by suprapubic aspiration. The presence of even scant bacteria has an 82% correlation with a positive culture by suprapubic aspiration.

Ultrasonography, voiding cystourethrogram (VCUG), radionuclide cystography, renal nucleotide scans, and computed tomography (CT) or magnetic resonance imaging (MRI) can be used for anatomic and functional assessment of the urinary tract. Ultrasound provides limited information about renal scarring and is performed to exclude an anatomic abnormality. VCUG is the best imaging study for determining the presence or absence of vesicoureteral reflux, which is ranked from grade I (ureter only) to grade V (complete gross dilation of the ureter and obliteration of caliceal and pelvic anatomy) (see Chapter 167). A technetium-99m DMSA scan can identify acute pyelonephritis and is most useful to define renal scarring as a late effect of UTI.

## DIFFERENTIAL DIAGNOSIS

The diagnosis of a UTI is confirmed by a positive urine culture, although this does not distinguish between upper tract and lower tract infection. Localization of a UTI is important because upper UTI is associated more frequently with bacteremia and with anatomic abnormalities than is uncomplicated cystitis. The clinical manifestations of UTI do not reliably distinguish the site of infection in neonates, infants, and toddlers. Fever and abdominal pain may occur with either lower or upper UTI, although high fever, costovertebral tenderness, high erythrocyte sedimentation rate (ESR), leukocytosis, and bacteremia each suggest upper tract involvement. Indirect findings such as WBC casts, inability to concentrate urine maximally, presence of antibody-coated bacteria detected by immunofluorescence, and $\beta_2$-microglobulin excretion are of limited value in localizing the site of the UTI to the upper tract. DMSA scan is sensitive for detecting acute pyelonephritis.

The manifestations of UTI overlap with signs of sepsis seen in young children and with enteritis, appendicitis, mesenteric lymphadenitis, and pneumonia in older children. Dysuria may indicate pinworm infection, hypersensitivity to soaps or detergents, vaginitis, or sexual abuse and infection.

## TREATMENT

Empirical therapy should be initiated for symptomatic children and for all children with a urine culture confirming UTI. For an older child who does not appear ill but with a positive urine culture, antibiotic therapy should be initiated either parenterally or orally. For a child with suspected UTI who appears toxic, appears dehydrated, or is unable to retain oral fluids, initial antibiotic therapy should be administered parenterally, and hospitalization should be considered.

Neonates with UTI are treated for 10 to 14 days with parenteral antibiotics because of the higher rate of bacteremia. Older children with acute cystitis are treated for 7 to 14 days with an oral antibiotic. Increasing bacterial resistance has limited the usefulness of some antibiotics such as amoxicillin. Trimethoprim-sulfamethoxazole (TMP-SMZ) is used frequently, although resistance to this drug also is increasing. Oral third-generation cephalosporins such as cefixime and cefpodoxime are effective but more expensive. Children with high fever or other manifestations of acute pyelonephritis often are hospitalized for initial treatment with parenteral antibiotics. Patients with systemic toxicity such as chills and high fever should be hospitalized and treated with intravenous (IV) cefotaxime and gentamicin or another aminoglycoside. When the patient has improved and is afebrile, oral therapy with an agent to which the cultured organism is susceptible is administered to complete 7 to 14 days of total therapy.

The degree of toxicity, dehydration, and ability to retain oral intake of fluids should be assessed carefully. Restoring or maintaining adequate hydration, including correction of electrolyte abnormalities that are often associated with vomiting or poor oral intake, is important.

Infants and children who do not show the expected clinical response within 2 days of starting antimicrobial therapy should be re-evaluated, have another urine specimen obtained for culture, and undergo ultrasound promptly and either VCUG or radionuclide cystography, which should be performed at the earliest convenient time.

## COMPLICATIONS AND PROGNOSIS

Bacteremia occurs in 2% to 5% of episodes of pyelonephritis and is more likely in infants than in older children. Focal renal abscesses are an uncommon complication.

The relapse rate of UTI is approximately 25% to 40%. Most relapses occur within 2 to 3 weeks of treatment. Follow-up urine cultures should be obtained 1 to 2 weeks after completing therapy to document sterility of the urine. Prophylactic antibiotics should be administered until the VCUG has been completed and the presence of reflux is known. TMP-SMZ (2 mg/kg TMP, 10 mg/kg SMZ) and nitrofurantoin (1 to 2 mg/kg) given once daily at bedtime are recommended as prophylactic agents, which, in contrast to amoxicillin and cephalosporins, are associated with low rates of developing antibiotic resistance. Clinical follow-up for at least 2 to 3 years is prudent, with repeat urine culture as indicated. Some experts recommend that follow-up urine cultures after recurrent cystitis or pyelonephritis are obtained monthly for 3 months, at 3-month intervals for 6 months, then yearly for 2 to 3 years.

Grade 1 to 3 reflux resolves at a rate of about 13% per year for the first 5 years, then at a rate of 3.5% per year. Grade 4 to 5 reflux resolves at a rate of about 5% per year. Bilateral reflux resolves more slowly than unilateral reflux (see Chapter 167).

## PREVENTION

Primary prevention is achieved by promoting good perineal hygiene and managing underlying risk factors for UTI, such as chronic constipation, encopresis, and daytime and nighttime urinary incontinence. Secondary prevention of UTI with antibiotic prophylaxis given once daily is directed toward preventing recurrent infections, although the impact of secondary prophylaxis to prevent renal scarring is unknown. Acidification of the urine with cranberry juice is not recommended as the sole means of preventing UTI in children at high risk.

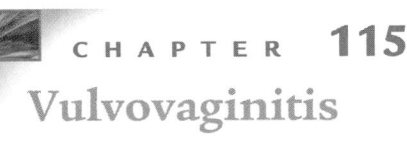

CHAPTER 115

# Vulvovaginitis

## ETIOLOGY

**Vulvovaginitis**, which is inflammation of the vulva or the vagina or both, is the most common gynecologic problem in children. Low prepubertal levels of estrogen result in thin, atrophic vaginal epithelium that is susceptible to bacterial invasion. At puberty, estrogen increases, and the pH of the vagina becomes more acidic. There are several specific causes of vulvovaginitis (Table 115-1) including sexually transmitted infections (STIs) such as *Trichomonas vaginalis* and herpes simplex virus (HSV) (see Chapter 116). **Nonspecific vaginitis** results from overgrowth of normal aerobic vaginal flora that is associated with poor hygiene. **Bacterial vaginosis** is caused by *Gardnerella vaginalis*, which interacts synergistically with vaginal anaerobes, including *Bacteroides, Mobiluncus,* and *Peptostreptococcus.*

## TABLE 115-1 Characteristics of Vulvovaginitis

| Etiologic Condition/Disorder | Presentation | Diagnosis | Treatment |
|---|---|---|---|
| Physiologic vaginal discharge (physiologic leukorrhea) | Minimal, clear, thin discharge without pruritus or inflammation; occurs soon after birth and again at 6–12 months before menarche | No pathogenic organisms on culture | Reassurance |
| Nonspecific vaginitis | Vaginal discharge, dysuria, itching; fecal soiling of underwear | Evidence of poor hygiene; no pathogenic organisms on culture | Improved hygiene, sitz baths |
| Bacterial vaginosis | Often asymptomatic; possible thin vaginal discharge with a "fishy" odor | At least 3 of the following 4 criteria: (1) thin, homogeneous vaginal discharge; (2) vaginal pH $\geq$4.5; (3) a fishy odor of volatile amines on the addition of a drop of 10% potassium hydroxide to a drop of vaginal discharge (the whiff test); and (4) the presence of clue cells on a saline wet mount of vaginal discharge (*Gardnerella vaginalis* and anaerobes) | Metronidazole, clindamycin |
| Candidiasis | Itching, dysuria, white "cottage cheese" vaginal discharge | *Candida* on saline wet mount of vaginal discharge | Topical antifungal (e.g., butoconazole, clotrimazole, miconazole, nystatin, fluconazole) |
| Enterobiasis (pinworms) | Perineal pruritus (nocturnal); gastrointestinal symptoms; variable vulvovaginal contamination from feces | Adult worms in stool or eggs on perianal skin | Mebendazole or albendazole |
| Giardiasis | Asymptomatic fecal contaminant, vaginal discharge, diarrhea, malabsorption syndrome | Protozoal flagellate (cyst or trophozoites) in feces | Metronidazole or albendazole |
| Molluscum contagiosum | Vulvar lesions, nodules with papule; white core of curd-like material | Isolation of poxvirus | Dermal curettage of umbilicated area |
| *Phthirus pubis* infection (pediculosis pubis) | Pruritus, excoriation, sky-blue macules; inner thigh or lower abdomen | Nits on hair shafts, lice on skin or clothing | 1% permethrin |
| *Sarcoptes scabiei* infection (scabies) | Nocturnal pruritus, pruritic vesicles, pustules in runs | Mites; ova black, dots of feces (microscopic) | 5% permethrin |
| *Shigella* infection | Bloody vaginal discharge; fever, malaise, fecal contamination, diarrhea; blood and mucus in stool, abdominal cramps | Stools: white blood cells and red blood cells, positive for *Shigella* | Oral third-generation cephalosporin |
| *Staphylococcus, Streptococcus* infection | Vaginal discharge, possibly bloody; spread from primary lesion | | First-generation cephalosporin or dicloxacillin |
| Foreign body | Foul-smelling vaginal discharge, sometimes bloody | Foreign body on physical examination | Removal of foreign body |

## EPIDEMIOLOGY

Nonspecific vaginitis is the most common cause of vulvovaginitis in young girls. *G. vaginalis* is often present as part of the normal vaginal flora in preadolescent girls, but is more common in girls who are sexually active. *Candida* is much less common in preadolescent girls than in women.

## CLINICAL MANIFESTATIONS

The primary symptoms of vulvovaginitis are vaginal discharge, erythema, and pruritus. A thin, gray, homogeneous discharge with a *fishy* odor suggests bacterial vaginosis. A white *cottage cheese* discharge suggests *Candida*. Bloody discharge suggests group A streptococcus or *Shigella*. Foul-smelling discharge suggests a foreign body.

## LABORATORY AND IMAGING STUDIES

Wet mount microscopic examination, prepared by mixing vaginal secretions with normal saline solution, and culture may be used to confirm a specific diagnosis (see Table 115-1). **Clue cells** are vaginal epithelial cells that are covered with *G. vaginalis* and have a granular appearance. Vaginal cultures for *G. vaginalis* are not useful. *Candida* may be identified by saline wet mount or by culture.

## DIFFERENTIAL DIAGNOSIS

Noninfectious causes of vulvovaginitis include physical agents (foreign body, sand), chemical agents (bubble bath, soap, detergent), and vulvar skin disease (atopic dermatitis, seborrhea, psoriasis). Physiologic vaginal discharge or **physiologic leukorrhea** of desquamated vaginal cells and mucus occurs normally in girls soon after birth, with discharge lasting for about 1 week, and again at 6 to 12 months before menarche. There is minimal, clear, thin discharge without pruritus or inflammation. No treatment is necessary.

## TREATMENT

The treatment of vulvovaginitis depends on the etiology (see Table 115-1). Treatment of nonspecific vaginitis includes improving perineal hygiene and sitz baths two to three times a day as needed. The recommended treatment for bacterial vaginosis is oral metronidazole. Imidazole creams and vaginal tablets and suppositories all are effective for the treatment of acute vulvovaginal candidiasis. Douching or vaginal irrigation is not beneficial and is not recommended.

## COMPLICATIONS AND PROGNOSIS

Complications are rare. The prognosis is excellent.

## PREVENTION

There are no recognized prophylactic measures for bacterial vaginosis or nonspecific vaginitis. Douching reduces normal vaginal flora, which are protective against pathogenic organisms, and is not protective.

## CHAPTER 116
# Sexually Transmitted Infections

Adolescents have the highest rates of sexually transmitted infections (STIs). Biologic agents, such as *Chlamydia trachomatis*, may predispose adolescents to certain STIs. Compared with adults, sexually active adolescents are more likely to believe that they will not contract an STI, more likely to come into contact with an infected sexual partner, less likely to receive health care when an STI develops, and less likely to be compliant with treatment for an STI.

Although numerous organisms cause STIs, the diseases can be grouped by the characteristic clinical presentation. **Urethritis** and **endocervicitis** (Table 116-1) are characteristic of *Neisseria gonorrhoeae* and *C. trachomatis* and are the most common STIs. More than 70% of genital chlamydial infections in women are asymptomatic. **Genital ulcers** (Table 116-2) are characteristic of syphilis (*Treponema pallidum*), genital herpes simplex virus (HSV) infections, chancroid (*Haemophilus ducreyi*), and granuloma inguinale, also known as donovanosis (*Calymmatobacterium granulomatis*). **Vaginal discharge** (Table 116-3) is a symptom of trichomoniasis (*Trichomonas vaginalis*) and is part of the spectrum of vulvovaginitis (see Chapter 115), which is not always associated with sexual activity. Human papillomavirus (HPV) cause **condylomata acuminata,** or **genital warts** (Table 116-4) and are the major risk factor for cervical, vulvar, and vaginal cancers.

STIs are associated with significant physiologic and psychological morbidity. Early diagnosis and treatment are important for preventing medical complications and infertility. All STIs are preventable; primary prevention of STIs should be a goal for all health care providers for adolescents. Diagnosis of an STI necessitates evaluation or treatment for concomitant STIs and notification and treatment of sexual partners.

Many infections that are not traditionally considered STIs are sexually transmissible including those caused by human immunodeficiency virus (HIV), human T cell leukemia viruses types I and II, cytomegalovirus (CMV), Epstein-Barr virus (EBV), human herpes virus (HHV-6, HHV-7), hepatitis B virus (HBV), molluscum contagiosum virus, and *Sarcoptes scabiei*. The presence of any STI suggests behavior that increases risk for HIV (see Chapter 125), and HIV counseling and testing should be provided to all adolescents with STIs. Acquisition of gonorrhea, syphilis, HSV-2, and trichomoniasis in prepubertal children beyond the neonatal period indicates sexual contact and signifies the need to investigate for possible sexual abuse (see Chapter 22). The association of vulvovaginitis and genital HPV infection, which may result from skin or genital HPV types, with sexual abuse is less certain.

**TABLE 116-1 Features of Sexually Transmitted Infections Caused by *Chlamydia trachomatis* and *Neisseria gonorrhoeae*\***

| Feature | C. trachomatis | N. gonorrhoeae |
|---|---|---|
| Incubation period | 5–12 days | 3–14 days |
| Possible presentations | Pharyngitis, conjunctivitis (including neonatal conjunctivitis), disseminated disease (arthritis, dermatitis, endocarditis, meningitis) | |
| | *Female* | *Male* |
| | Asymptomatic | Asymptomatic |
| | Urethritis | Urethritis |
| | Skenitis/bartholinitis | Epididymo-orchitis |
| | PID | Proctitis |
| Signs/symptoms of common syndromes | | |
| Urethritis | *Female* | *Male* |
| | Dysuria, frequency | Penile discharge |
| | >10 PMNs/hpf | >10 PMNs/hpf |
| Mucopurulent cervicitis | Cervical erythema, friability, with thick creamy discharge | |
| | >10 PMNs/hpf | |
| | Mild cervical tenderness | |
| | Gram-negative intracellular diplococci | |
| Pelvic inflammatory disease | Onset of symptoms day 3–10 of menstrual cycle | |
| | Lower abdominal pain (95%) | |
| | Adnexal tenderness, mass (95%) | |
| | Pain on cervical motion (95%) | |
| | Fever (35%) | |
| | Mucopurulent cervical discharge (variable) | |
| | Menstrual irregularities (variable) | |
| | Nausea, vomiting (variable) | |
| | Weakness, syncope, dizziness (variable) | |
| | Perihepatitis (5%) | |
| Diagnostic tests | NAAT, culture (using Thayer-Martin selective media) | NAAT |
| Treatment | Cefixime *or* ceftriaxone *plus* doxycycline *or* azithromycin | |

Co-infection is common, and clinical presentations have significant overlap.

NAAT, nucleic acid amplification test; PID, pelvic inflammatory disease; PMN, polymorphonuclear cells

## PELVIC INFLAMMATORY DISEASE

Direct extension of *N. gonorrhoeae*, often in combination with *C. trachomatis*, to the endometrium, fallopian tubes, and peritoneum causes **pelvic inflammatory disease**. Complications of pelvic inflammatory disease include tubo-ovarian abscess and perihepatitis (**Fitz-Hugh–Curtis syndrome**), which is inflammation of the capsule of the liver. A major sequela of pelvic inflammatory disease is infertility. The differential diagnosis of pelvic inflammatory disease includes ectopic pregnancy, septic abortion, ovarian cyst torsion or rupture, UTI, appendicitis, mesenteric lymphadenitis, and inflammatory bowel disease. Pelvic ultrasound may detect thickened adnexal structures and is the imaging study of choice for other possible diagnoses. Clinical criteria for diagnosis of pelvic inflammatory disease are lower abdominal tenderness, uterine/adnexal tenderness, and cervical motion tenderness. Additional criteria that support the diagnosis are fever, mucopurulent vaginal discharge, elevated white blood cell (WBC) count (in 45%), elevated erythrocyte sedimentation rate (ESR) (in 65%) or C-reactive protein (CRP), and documented infection with *N. gonorrhoeae* or *C. trachomatis*. Adolescents should be hospitalized for treatment if there is uncertainty about the diagnosis; pregnancy; no clinical response to oral therapy with 72 hours; inability to adhere to or tolerate oral therapy; a tubo-ovarian abscess; or severe illness with high fever, nausea, and vomiting. The recommended parenteral treatment is cefotetan or cefoxitin, plus doxycycline orally. The recommended oral treatment of pelvic inflammatory disease for younger persons is ceftriaxone in a single dose, plus doxycycline orally, for 14 days, with or without metronidazole for 14 days. Follow-up examination should be performed within 72 hours, with hospitalization for parenteral therapy if there has not been clinical improvement.

## GONORRHEA (*Neisseria gonorrhoeae*)

*N. gonorrhoeae*, a gram-negative coccus, is often seen as diplococci. Gonorrhea is a common STI among adolescents. The greatest increase in incidence is in the 15- to 19-year-old age group, especially among girls. The organism causes infection at the site of acquisition, which commonly results in mucopurulent cervicitis and urethritis (see Table 116-1). **Disseminated gonococcal infections**

**TABLE 116–2 Features of Sexually Transmitted Infections Characterized by Genital Ulcers**

| | Syphilis | Genital Herpes | Chancroid | Granuloma Inguinale (Donovanosis) |
|---|---|---|---|---|
| Agent | *Treponema pallidum* | HSV-1, HSV-2 | *Haemophilus ducreyi* | *Calymmatobacterium granulomatis* |
| Incubation | 10–90 days | 4–14 days | 3–10 days | 8–80 days |
| Systemic findings | Fever, rash, malaise, anorexia, arthralgia, lymphadenopathy | Headache, fever, malaise, myalgia in one third of cases | None | Local spread only |
| Inguinal lymphadenopathy | Late, bilateral, nontender, no suppuration | Early, bilateral, tender, no suppuration | Early, rapid, tender, and unilateral; suppuration likely | Lymphatic obstruction |
| Primary lesion | Papule | Vesicle | Papule to pustule | Papule |
| Ulcer characteristics | | | | |
|   Number | ≥1 | Multiple | ≤3 | ≥1, may coalesce |
|   Edges | Distinct | Reddened, ragged | Ragged, undermined | Rolled, distinct |
|   Depth | Shallow | Shallow | Deep | Raised |
|   Base | Red, smooth | Red, smooth | Necrotic | Beefy red, clean |
|   Secretion | Serous | Serous | Pus, blood | None |
|   Induration | Firm | None | None | Firm |
|   Pain | None | Usual | Often | None |
| Diagnosis | | | | |
|   Serology | VDRL *or* RPR<br><br>MHA-TP *or* FTA-ABS | Seroconversion (primary infection only) | None | None |
|   Isolation | No in vitro test; rabbit inoculation | Culture | Aspirate of node, swab of ulcer on selective medium | None |
|   Microscopic | Dark-field examination | Pap smear; Tzanck smear; direct FA staining | Gram-negative pleomorphic rods | Staining of ulcer biopsy material for Donovan bodies |
| Treatment | *Early:* Benzathine penicillin G (2.4 million U IM) once<br><br>*Late (>1 yr duration):* Benzathine penicillin G (2.4 million U IM) weekly × 3 doses | Acyclovir *or* famciclovir *or* valacyclovir | Aspirate fluctuant nodes<br><br>Incision and drainage of buboes >5 cm<br><br>Azithromycin *or* ciprofloxacin *or* erythromycin | Doxycycline *or* TMP-SMZ |

FTA-ABS, fluorescent treponemal antibody–absorption; HSV, herpes simplex virus; MHA-TP, microhemagglutination assay–*Treponema pallidum*; RPR, rapid plasma reagin; TMP-SMZ, trimethoprim-sulfamethoxazole; VDRL, Venereal Disease Research Laboratory.

can occur with hematogenous spread and results in petechial or pustular acral skin lesions, asymmetrical arthralgia, tenosynovitis or septic arthritis, and occasionally endocarditis or meningitis. Perinatal transmission of maternal infection can lead to neonatal sepsis and meningitis (see Chapter 65) and ophthalmia neonatorum (see Chapter 119).

Treatment regimens should be effective against *N. gonorrhoeae* and *C. trachomatis* because of the high frequency of concomitant infection. Increasing rates of resistance to fluoroquinolones limit treatment options. A single dose of intramuscular (IM) ceftriaxone (125 mg) or oral cefixime (400 mg) is recommended for uncomplicated gonococcal infections of the cervix, urethra, and

**TABLE 116-3 Features of Sexually Transmitted Infections Characterized by Vaginal Discharge**

| Feature | Physiologic Leukorrhea (Normal) | Trichomoniasis | Bacterial Vaginosis (*Gardnerella vaginalis–* Associated Vaginitis) |
|---|---|---|---|
| Agent | Normal flora | *Trichomonas vaginalis* | *G. vaginalis* and anaerobes |
| Incubation | — | 3–28 days | Not necessarily sexually transmitted |
| Predominant symptoms | | | |
| Pruritus | None | Mild to moderate | None to mild |
| Discharge | Minimal | Moderate to severe | Mild to moderate |
| Pain | None | Mild | Uncommon |
| Vulvar inflammation | None | Common | Uncommon |
| Characteristics of discharge | | | |
| Amount | Small | Profuse | Moderate |
| Color | Clear, milky | Yellow-green or gray | Gray |
| Consistency | Flocculent | Frothy | Homogeneous |
| Viscosity | Thin | Thin | Thin |
| Foul odor | None | None | Yes |
| Odor with KOH | None | Possible | Characteristic fishy odor (amine) |
| pH | <4.5 | ≥5.0 | >4.5 |
| Diagnosis | | | |
| Saline drop | Squamous and few WBCs | Motile flagellates, slightly larger than WBCs, and WBCs | Squamous cells studded with bacteria ("clue cells") and WBCs |
| Gram stain | Gram-positive and gram-negative rods and cocci | *Trichomonas* killed | Predominance of gram-negative rods |
| Culture | Mixed flora with *Lactobacillus* predominant | Culture generally not indicated; antigen detection and antibody tests available | Culture not useful |
| Treatment | Reassurance | Metronidazole | Metronidazole or clindamycin |

KOH, potassium hydroxide; WBCs, white blood cells.

rectum. Hospitalization and treatment with ceftriaxone are recommended for disseminated gonococcal infections. For all gonococcal infections, azithromycin or doxycycline also is administered unless chlamydial infection is excluded. Sexual partners should be notified and treated.

## CHLAMYDIA INFECTION (*Chlamydia trachomatis*)

Chlamydiae are obligate intracellular bacteria with a biphasic life cycle, existing as relatively inert elementary bodies in their extracellular form and as **reticulate bodies** when phagocytosed and replicating within a phagosome. Reticulate bodies divide by binary fission and, after 48 to 72 hours, reorganize into elementary bodies that are released from the cell. *Chlamydia* infects nonciliated squamo-columnar cells and the transitional epithelial cells that line the mucosa of the urethra, cervix, rectum, and conjunctiva.

*C. trachomatis* serovars D through K cause urethritis, cervicitis, pelvic inflammatory disease, inclusion conjunctivitis in newborns, and infant pneumonia. *C. trachomatis* serovars L1–3 cause lymphogranuloma venereum, an infrequent STI characterized by unilateral, painful inguinal lymphadenitis. *C. trachomatis* serovars A, B, Ba, and C produce trachoma (hyperendemic blinding), which eventually leads to blindness from extensive local scarring.

*Chlamydia* is the most frequently diagnosed bacterial STI in adolescents and accounts for most cases of **nongonococcal urethritis and cervicitis** (see Table 116-1). There is a 5:1 female-to-male ratio. Males often have dysuria and a mucopurulent discharge, although approximately 25% may be asymptomatic. Women are more often asymptomatic (approximately 70%) or may have minimal symptoms including dysuria, mild abdominal pain, or vaginal discharge. Prepubertal girls may have vaginitis. At least 30% of persons with gonococcal cervicitis, urethritis, proctitis, or epididymitis have a concomitant *C. trachomatis* infection.

*Chlamydia* infection usually is diagnosed by detection of bacterial nucleic acids (PCR tests, using ligase chain reaction and transcription-mediated amplification) of cervical, urethral, and early morning first-voided urine specimens. Amplification tests have supplanted less sensitive culture and ELISA (enzyme-linked immunosorbent assay) tests.

**TABLE 116-4 Features of Sexually Transmitted Infections Characterized by Nonulcerative External Genital Symptoms**

| Feature | Genital Warts | Vulvovaginal Candidiasis | Pediculosis Pubis (Crabs) |
|---|---|---|---|
| Agent | Human papillomavirus | *Candida albicans* | *Phthirus pubis* |
| Incubation/transmission | 30–90 days | Uncommon sexual transmission | 5–10 days |
| Presenting complaints | Genital warts are seen or felt | Vulvar itching or discharge | Pubic itching; live organisms may be seen; sexual partner has "crabs" |
| Signs | Firm, gray-to-pink, single or multiple, fimbriated, painless excrescences on vulva, introitus, vagina cervix, perineum, anus | Inflammation of vulva, with thick, white, "cottage cheese" discharge, pH < 5; friable mucosa that easily bleeds | Eggs (nits) at base of pubic hairs, lice may be visible; excoriated, red skin secondary to infestation |
| Clinical associations | Cervical neoplasia, dysplasia | Oral contraceptives, diabetes, antibiotics | — |
| Diagnosis | Clinical appearance; most infections asymptomatic; acetowhite changes on colposcopy; enlarged cells with perinuclear halo and hyperchromatic nuclei | KOH (10%): pseudohyphae; Gram stain: gram-positive pseudohyphae; Nickerson or Sabouraud medium for culture | History and clinical appearance |
| Treatment | *Patient-applied therapies*: Podofilox solution or gel *or* Imiquimod cream *Provider-applied therapies*: cryotherapy with liquid nitrogen or cryoprobe *or* topical podophyllin resin *or* trichloroacetic acid or dichloroacetic acid *or* surgical removal | *Intravaginal agents*: butoconazole *or* clotrimazole *or* miconazole *or* nystatin *or* tioconazole *or* terconazole *Oral agent*: fluconazole | Permethrin 1% cream *or* lindane 1% shampoo *or* pyrethrin with piperonyl butoxide |

KOH, potassium hydroxide.

Because of false positive results, only culture should be used for medicolegal purposes to confirm *C. trachomatis* infection in cases of suspected sexual abuse.

Treatment regimens should be effective against *C. trachomatis* and *N. gonorrhoeae* because of the high frequency of concomitant infection. A single oral dose of azithromycin (1 g) or doxycycline for 7 days is recommended, which can be combined with a single oral dose of cefixime (400 mg) to treat concomitant gonorrhea infection. Sexual partners should be notified and treated.

## SYPHILIS (*Treponema pallidum*)

Syphilis is caused by *T. pallidum*, a long, slender, coiled spirochete. It cannot be cultivated routinely in vitro but can be observed by dark-field microscopy. Untreated infection progresses through several clinical stages (see Table 116-2). **Primary syphilis** is manifested as a single, painless genital ulcer, or **chancre**, usually on the genitalia, that appears 3 to 6 weeks after inoculation. **Secondary syphilis** follows 6 to 8 weeks later and is manifested as fever, generalized lymphadenopathy, and a disseminated maculopapular rash that also is present on the palms and soles. Plaquelike skin lesions, **condylomata lata**, and mucous membrane lesions occur and are infectious. **Tertiary syphilis** is a slowly progressive disease that involves the cardiovascular, neurologic, and musculoskeletal systems and is not seen in children. **Latent syphilis** is asymptomatic infection that is detected by serologic testing. Early latent syphilis indicates acquisition within

the preceding year; all other cases of latent syphilis are either late latent syphilis or designated latent syphilis of unknown duration. Infection can be passed from pregnant women and infect their infants resulting in **congenital syphilis** (see Chapter 66).

The diagnosis of syphilis is based on serologic testing. **Nontreponemal antibody tests**, the **Venereal Disease Research Laboratory (VDRL)** test, and the **rapid plasma reagin (RPR)** test are screening tests and can be quantified as titers increase with increasing duration of infection and decrease in response to therapy. A nonquantitative VDRL test can be performed on cerebrospinal fluid (CSF), but is insensitive. Rheumatic disease and other infectious diseases may cause false positive results. Confirmatory, specific **treponemal antibody tests**, the **microhemagglutination assay–T. pallidum** and **fluorescent treponemal antibody-absorption**, are more specific and are used to confirm the diagnosis of syphilis. These tests usually remain positive for life even if the infection is treated and cured. Dark-field examination of chancres, mucous membranes, or cutaneous lesions may reveal motile organisms.

The treatment of choice for all stages of syphilis is penicillin G. Primary syphilis, secondary syphilis, and early latent syphilis is treated with a single IM dose of benzathine penicillin G. Tertiary, late latent, and latent syphilis of unknown duration is treated with three doses at 1-week intervals. Neurosyphilis is treated with intravenous (IV) aqueous crystalline penicillin G for 10 to 14 days. A systemic, febrile **Jarisch-Herxheimer reaction** occurs in 15% to 20% of syphilitic patients treated with penicillin.

## HERPES SIMPLEX VIRUS INFECTION

HSV-1 and HSV-2 are large, double-stranded DNA viruses of the herpesvirus family that have a linear genome contained within an icosahedral capsid. There is significant DNA homology between types 1 and 2. The virus initially infects mucosal surfaces and enters cutaneous neurons where it migrates along the axons to the sensory ganglia. As viral replication occurs in the ganglia, infectious virus moves along the axon to infect and destroy epithelial cells. Infection may disseminate to other organs in immunocompromised patients. Virus latency is maintained in the ganglia where it undergoes periodic reactivation and replication triggered by undefined events. Although either virus can be found in any site, nongenital type 1 (HSV-1) more commonly occurs above the waist (central nervous system, eyes, mouth), and genital type 2 (HSV-2) more commonly involves genitalia and skin below the waist. Reinfection can occur with exposure to the other type or even a second strain of the same type.

**Primary genital herpes** is characterized by painful, multiple, grouped vesicles or ulcerative and crusted external genital lesions on an erythematous base (see Table 116-2). In females, the cervix also is involved. Symptoms may include regional lymphadenopathy, discharge, and dysuria. Primary illness lasts 10 to 20 days with recurrences in 50% to 80% of patients. **Secondary, recurrent, or reactivation eruptions** are not as dramatic and are not associated with systemic symptoms. In primary infection, viral shedding lasts 10 to 14 days, and vesicles and ulcers resolve in 16 to 20 days. In recurrent disease, often with several episodes annually, virus shedding lasts for less than 7 days, and vesicles resolve in 8 to 10 days. Many persons experience five to eight recurrences per year. Some primary and many secondary lesions are asymptomatic.

Viral cultures are the most reliable method of diagnosis and show cytopathic effect in 2 to 5 days. The diagnosis is suggested by a **Tzanck smear** or Papanicolaou smear showing characteristic multinucleated giant cells with intranuclear inclusions. Latency develops as the virus becomes dormant in the sacral nerve ganglion. Serologic testing is useful only for primary infection, to show seroconversion between acute and convalescent sera. There is much overlap between types 1 and 2 in serologic tests for HSV. Titers are not helpful in guiding management of recurrences.

Oral acyclovir, famciclovir, and valacyclovir are effective treatments in reducing the severity and duration of symptoms in primary cases, and may reduce recurrences. Once-daily suppressive therapy reduces the frequency of genital herpes recurrences by 70% to 80% among patients who have frequent recurrences (>6 recurrences per year). Local hygiene and sitz baths may relieve some discomfort. The use of condoms provides some protection against sexual transmission of HSV.

## TRICHOMONIASIS (*Trichomonas vaginalis*)

Trichomoniasis is caused by the protozoan *T. vaginalis* and often is associated with other STIs such as gonorrhea and *Chlamydia* infection. Infected males either are asymptomatic or have nongonococcal urethritis. Infected females have vaginitis with thin, malodorous, frothy yellow-green discharge, vulvar irritation, and cervical "strawberry hemorrhages" (see Table 116-3). The diagnosis is based on visualization of motile, flagellated protozoans in the urine or in a saline wet mount, which has a sensitivity of only 60% to 70%. Culture is the most sensitive method of diagnosis. Single-dose treatment of both sexual partners with oral metronidazole (2 g) is recommended.

## GENITAL WARTS (HUMAN PAPILLOMAVIRUSES)

HPV infections, the cause of genital warts (**condylomata acuminata**), may be the most common STI with an estimated prevalence of 20 million active infections and over 6 million new infections each year, mostly in 15- to 24-year-olds. Most HPV infections are asymptomatic or subclinical. HPV types 6 and 11 cause 90% of genital warts and are nononcogenic. HPV types 16 and 18 are associated with 70% of cases of cervical cancer. HPV types 31, 33, and 35 are also ongogenic.

Genital warts can occur on the squamous epithelium or mucous membranes of the genital and perineal structures of females and males (see Table 116-4). Genital warts are usually multiple, firm, gray-to-pink excrescences. Untreated genital warts may remain unchanged, increase in size or number, or resolve spontaneously. They can become tender if macerated or secondarily infected. The diagnosis usually is established by appearance without biopsy. The differential diagnosis of genital warts includes condylomata lata (secondary syphilis) and tumors.

The goal of treatment is removal of symptomatic warts to induce wart-free periods. On cornified skin, patient-applied therapies include podofilox solution or gel or imiquimod cream. Provider-applied therapies include cryotherapy with liquid nitrogen or cryoprobe, topical podophyllin resin, and trichloroacetic acid or dichloroacetic acid, all of which can be applied until the lesions regress. An alternative is surgical removal. Intralesional interferon and laser surgery also have been effective. Factors that may influence selection of treatment include wart number, size, anatomic sites, wart morphology, patient preference, cost of treatment, convenience, adverse effects, and provider experience. Recurrences after treatment are common and are commonly asymptomatic.

## PUBIC LICE (*Phthirus pubis*)

Pubic lice, or pediculosis pubis, are caused by infestation with *Phthirus pubis*, the **pubic crab louse**. The louse is predominantly sexually transmitted and lives out its life cycle on pubic hair, where it causes characteristic, intense pruritus (see Table 116-4). Erythematous papules and **egg cases (nits)** are not seen before puberty. Treatment consists of education regarding personal and environmental hygiene and the application of an appropriate pediculicide, such as permethrin 1% cream, lindane 1% shampoo, or pyrethrins with piperonyl butoxide. Bedding and clothing should be decontaminated (machine washed and machine dried using the heat cycle or dry cleaned) or removed from body contact for at least 72 hours.

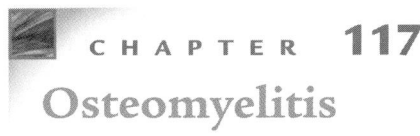

CHAPTER 117

# Osteomyelitis

## ETIOLOGY

Syndromes of pediatric osteomyelitis include acute **hematogenous osteomyelitis**, which is accompanied by bacteremia; **subacute osteomyelitis**, which usually follows local inoculation by penetrating trauma and is not associated with systemic symptoms; and **chronic osteomyelitis**, which results from an untreated or inadequately treated bone infection. In children beyond the newborn period and without hemoglobinopathies, bone infections occur almost exclusively in the metaphysis. Sluggish blood flow through tortuous vascular loops unique to this site in long bones is a possible explanation for this phenomenon. Preceding nonpenetrating trauma often is reported and may lead to local bone injury that predisposes to infection. Bone infections in children with sickle cell disease occur in the diaphyseal portion of the long bones, probably as a consequence of antecedent focal infarction. In children younger than 1 year of age, capillaries perforate the epiphyseal growth plate, permitting spread of infection across the epiphysis which can lead to suppurative arthritis (Fig. 117-1A). In older children, the infection is contained in the metaphysis because the vessels no longer cross the epiphyseal plate (see Fig. 117-1B).

*Staphylococcus aureus* is responsible for most culture-positive skeletal infections (Table 117-1). Group B streptococcus and *S. aureus* are major causes in neonates. Sickle cell disease and other hemoglobinopathies predispose to osteomyelitis caused by *Salmonella* and *S. aureus*. *Pasteurella*

### TABLE 117-1 Pathogenic Organisms Identified in Culture-Positive Acute Osteomyelitis in Children Beyond the Neonatal Period

| Organism | Frequency (%) |
|---|---|
| *Staphylococcus aureus* | 25–60 |
| *Haemophilus influenzae* type b | 4–12 |
| *Streptococcus pneumoniae* | 2–5 |
| Group A streptococci | 2–4 |
| *Mycobacterium tuberculosis* | <1 |
| *Neisseria meningitidis* | <1 |
| *Salmonella** | <1 |
| None identified | 10–15 |

*Especially in persons with hemoglobinopathies.

*multocida* osteomyelitis may follow cat or dog bites. The use of polymerase chain reaction testing reveals that a significant percentage of culture negative osteomyelitis is due to *Kingella kingae*. Conjugate vaccine has reduced greatly the incidence of *Haemophilus influenzae* infections; similar reductions of *Streptococcus pneumoniae* infections are anticipated with the conjugate pneumococcal vaccine.

Subacute focal bone infections caused by *Pseudomonas aeruginosa* and *S. aureus* usually occur in ambulatory persons who sustain **puncture wounds** of the foot. *Pseudomonas* **chondritis** is associated strongly with puncture wounds through sneakers, which harbor *Pseudomonas* in the foam insole. *S. aureus* is the most common cause of chronic osteomyelitis. **Multifocal recurrent osteomyelitis** is a poorly understood syndrome characterized by recurrent episodes of fever, bone pain, and radiographic findings of osteomyelitis; no pathogen has been confirmed as the cause of this syndrome.

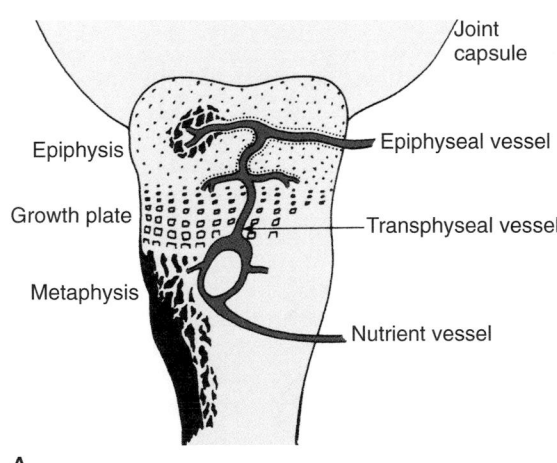

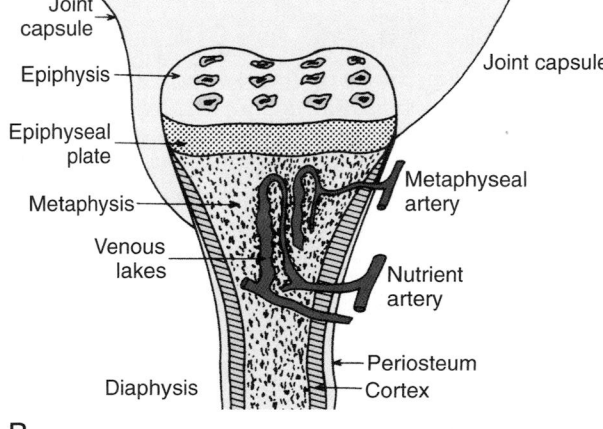

**FIGURE 117-1**

**A,** Major structures of the bone of an infant before maturation of the epiphyseal growth plate. Note the transphyseal vessel, which connects the vascular supply of the epiphysis and metaphysis, facilitating spread of infection between these two areas. **B,** Major structures of the bone of a child. Joint capsule *A* inserts below the epiphyseal growth plate, as in the hip, elbow, ankle, and shoulder. Rupture of a metaphyseal abscess in these bones is likely to produce pyarthrosis. Joint capsule *B* inserts at the epiphyseal growth plate, as in other tubular bones. Rupture of a metaphyseal abscess in these bones is likely to lead to a subperiosteal abscess, but seldom to an associated pyarthrosis. (From Gutman LT: Acute, subacute, and chronic osteomyelitis and pyogenic arthritis in children. *Curr Prob Pediatr* 15:1–72, 1985.)

## EPIDEMIOLOGY

Osteomyelitis may occur at any age but is most common in children 3 to 12 years of age and affects boys twice as frequently as girls. Hematogenous osteomyelitis is the most common form in infants and children. Osteomyelitis from penetrating trauma or peripheral vascular disease is more common in adults. Osteomyelitis from penetrating injuries of the foot is more common in summer months when children are outdoors and exploring.

## CLINICAL MANIFESTATIONS

The most common presenting complaints are focal pain, exquisite point tenderness over the bone, warmth, erythema, swelling, and decreased use of the affected extremity. Fever, anorexia, irritability, and lethargy may accompany the focal findings. Weight bearing and active and passive motion are refused, which mimics paralysis (**pseudoparalysis**). Muscle spasm may make the extremity difficult to examine. The adjacent joint space may be involved in young children (see Chapter 118).

Usually only one bone is involved. The femur, tibia, or humerus is affected in two thirds of patients. Infections of the bones of the hands or feet account for an additional 15% of cases. Flat bone infections, including the pelvis, account for approximately 10% of cases. Vertebral osteomyelitis is notable for an insidious onset, vague symptoms, backache, occasional spinal cord compression, and usually little associated fever or systemic toxicity. Patients with osteomyelitis of the pelvis may present with fever, limp, and vague abdominal, hip, groin, or thigh pain.

## LABORATORY AND IMAGING STUDIES

The presence of leukocytosis is inconsistent. Blood cultures are important but are negative in many cases. Elevated acute phase reactants, erythrocyte sedimentation rate (ESR) and C-reactive protein (CRP), are sensitive but nonspecific findings of osteomyelitis. Serial determinations of ESR and CRP are helpful in monitoring the course of the illness and response to treatment. Direct subperiosteal or metaphyseal needle aspiration is the definitive procedure for establishing the diagnosis. Identification of bacteria in aspirated material by Gram stain can establish the diagnosis within hours of clinical presentation. Surgical drainage may be needed after bone aspiration.

Plain radiographs are a useful initial study (Fig. 117-2). The earliest radiographic finding of acute systemic osteomyelitis, at about 9 days, is **loss of the periosteal fat line**. **Periosteal elevation** and **periosteal destruction** are later findings. **Brodie abscess** is a subacute intraosseous abscess that does not drain into the subperiosteal space and is classically located in the distal tibia. **Sequestra**, portions of avascular bone that have separated from adjacent bone, frequently are covered with a thickened sheath, or **involucrum**, both of which are hallmarks of chronic osteomyelitis.

Radionuclide scanning for osteomyelitis has largely been supplanted by magnetic resonance imaging (MRI), which is sensitive to the inflammatory changes in the marrow even during the earliest stages of osteomyelitis.

Technetium-99m bone scans are useful for identifying multifocal disease. Gallium-67 scans are often positive if the technetium-99m bone scan is negative.

## DIFFERENTIAL DIAGNOSIS

Osteomyelitis must be differentiated from infectious arthritis (see Chapter 118), cellulitis, fasciitis, diskitis, trauma, juvenile rheumatoid arthritis, and malignancy.

## TREATMENT

Initial antibiotic therapy for osteomyelitis is based on the likely organism for the age of the child, Gram stain of bone aspirate, and associated diseases (Table 117-2). Initial therapy includes an antibiotic that targets *S. aureus* such as oxacillin, nafcillin, or clindamycin. Vancomycin should be used if methicillin-resistant *S. aureus* is suspected. For patients with sickle cell disease, initial therapy should include an antibiotic with activity against *Salmonella*.

There is usually a response to intravenous (IV) antibiotics within 48 hours. Lack of improvement after 48 hours indicates that surgical drainage may be necessary or that an unusual pathogen may be present. Surgical drainage is indicated if **sequestrum** is present, the disease is chronic or atypical, the hip joint is involved, or spinal cord compression is present. Antibiotics are administered for a minimum of 4 to 6 weeks. After initial inpatient treatment and a good clinical response, including decreases in CRP or ESR, home therapy with IV antibiotics or oral antibiotics may be considered if adherence can be ensured.

## COMPLICATIONS AND PROGNOSIS

Complications of acute osteomyelitis are uncommon and usually arise because of inadequate or delayed therapy or due to concominant bacteremia. Young children are more likely to have spread of infection across the epiphysis, leading to suppurative arthritis (see Chapter 118). Vascular insufficiency, which affects delivery of antibiotics, and trauma are associated with higher rates of complications.

Hematogenous osteomyelitis has an excellent prognosis if treated promptly and if surgical drainage is performed when appropriate. The poorest outcome is in neonates and in infants with involvement of the hip or shoulder joints (see Chapter 118). Approximately 4% of acute infections recur despite adequate therapy, and approximately 25% of these fail to respond to extensive surgical débridement and prolonged antimicrobial therapy, ultimately resulting in bone loss, sinus tract formation, and occasionally amputation. Sequelae related to retarded growth are most common with neonatal osteomyelitis.

## PREVENTION

There are no effective means to prevent hematogenous *S. aureus* osteomyelitis. Universal immunization of infants with conjugate Hib (*Haemophilus influenzae* type b) vaccine has practically eliminated serious bacterial infections from this organism, including bone and joint infections. Because the serotypes of *S. pneumoniae* causing joint infections are represented in the conjugate pneumococcal

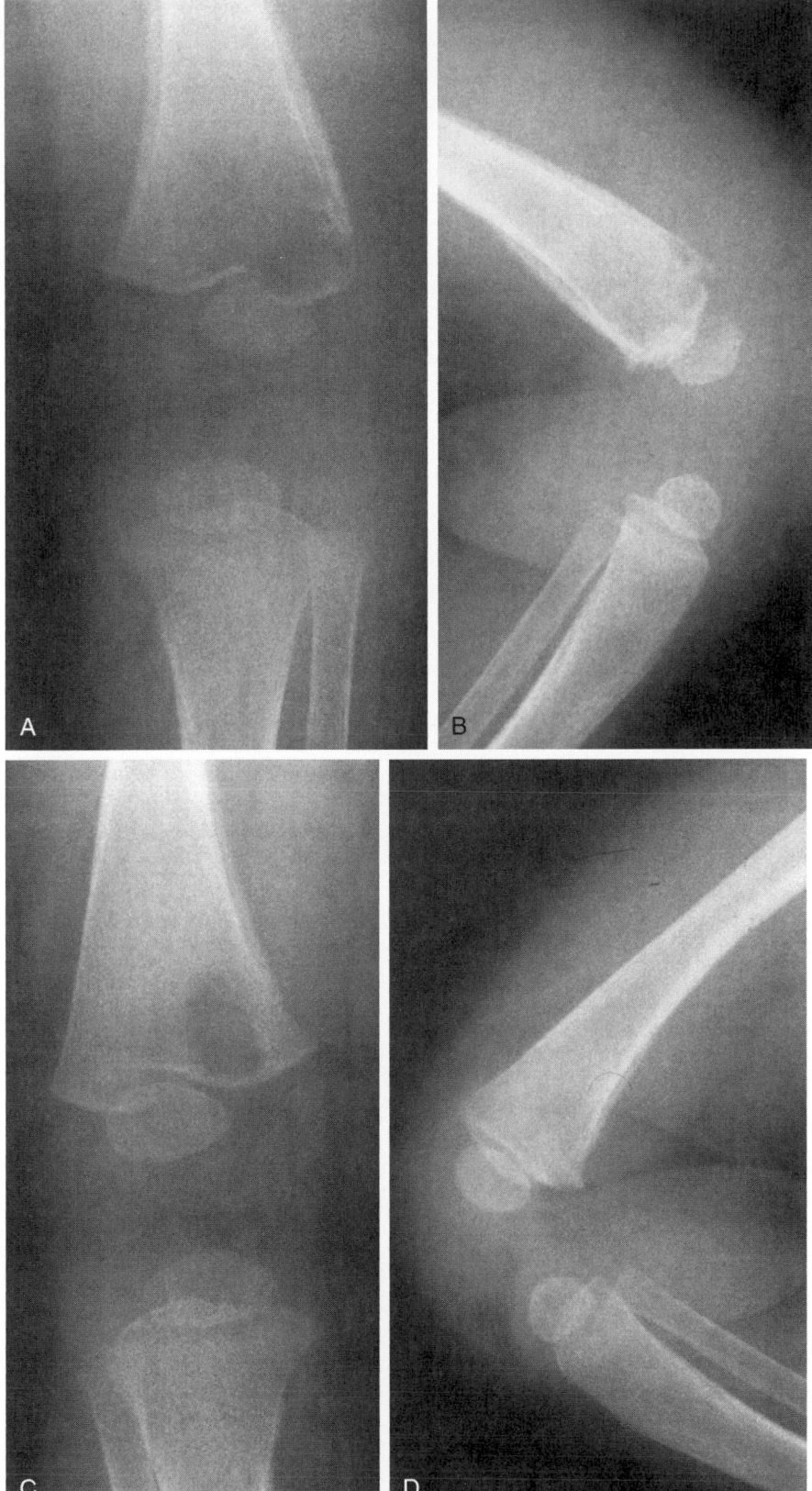

**FIGURE 117-2**

**Multifocal acute osteomyelitis in a 3-week-old infant with multiple joint swelling and generalized malaise.** Frontal (**A**) and lateral (**B**) radiographs of the left knee show focal destruction of the distal femoral metaphysis with periosteal reaction and generalized soft tissue swelling. Frontal (**C**) and lateral (**D**) views of the right knee show an area of focal bone destruction at the distal femoral metaphysis with periosteal reaction and medial soft tissue swelling. Needle aspiration of multiple sites revealed *Staphylococcus aureus*. (From Moffett KS, Aronoff SC: Osteomyelitis. In Jenson HB, Baltimore RS [eds]: Pediatric Infectious Diseases: Principles and Practice, 2nd ed. Philadelphia, *WB Saunders*, 2002, p 1038.)

**TABLE 117-2 Recommended Antibiotic Therapy for Osteomyelitis in Children**

| Common Pathogen | Recommended Treatment* |
|---|---|
| **ACUTE HEMATOGENOUS OSTEOMYELITIS** | |
| *Staphylococcus aureus* | |
| Methicillin-sensitive | Nafcillin (or oxacillin) *or* cephazolin |
| Methicillin-resistant | Clindamycin *or* vancomycin *or* linezolid |
| *Streptococcus pneumoniae* | Penicillin G *or* ceftriaxone/cefotaxime *or* vancomycin |
| *Streptococcus pyogenes* (group A streptococci) | Penicillin G |
| **SUBACUTE FOCAL OSTEOMYELITIS** | |
| *Pseudomonas aeruginosa* | Ceftazidime *or* piperacillin-tazobactam *plus* an aminoglycoside |
| *Kingella kingae* | Penicillin G *or* oxacillin |

*Optimal specific therapy is based on susceptibilities of the organism that is isolated.

vaccine, the incidence of pneumococcal osteomyelitis should decrease with widespread immunization.

Children with puncture wounds to the foot should receive prompt irrigation, cleansing, débridement, removal of any visible foreign body or debris, and tetanus prophylaxis. The value of oral prophylactic antibiotics for preventing osteomyelitis after penetrating injury is uncertain.

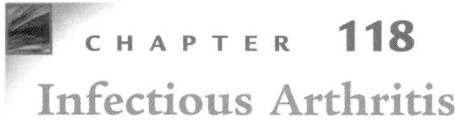

# CHAPTER 118

# Infectious Arthritis

## ETIOLOGY

Infectious arthritis, or **suppurative** or **septic arthritis**, is a serious bacterial infection of the joint space that results from hematogenous dissemination of bacteria in children. Infectious arthritis less often results from contiguous spread of infection from surrounding soft tissues or direct inoculation into the joint (penetrating trauma). Spread of osteomyelitis is common and occurs with rupture into the joint space via transphyseal vessels to the epiphysis or rupture of a metaphyseal abscess in the joint where the joint capsule inserts below the epiphysis (see Fig. 117-1A). The bacteria causing infectious arthritis are similar to bacteria causing osteomyelitis (Table 118-1). Lyme disease also may cause arthritis as part of the late disease (see Chapter 122).

The arthritis of **disseminated gonococcal infections** includes both reactive and suppurative forms of arthritis in early and late gonococcal disease, respectively. With untreated genital infection, gonococcemia may occur with fever and a polyarticular, symmetrical arthritis and rash, known as the **arthritis-dermatitis syndrome**. Bacterial cultures of the synovium are sterile at this stage despite a relatively high prevalence of bacteremia. Monarticular arthritis of large, weight-bearing joints develops days to weeks later. Cultures of affected synovial fluid at this stage often yield the pathogen.

**Reactive arthritis** is immune-mediated synovial inflammation that follows a bacterial or viral infection,

especially *Yersinia* and other enteric infections. Reactive arthritis of the hip joints in children 3 to 6 years of age is known as **toxic synovitis** or **transient synovitis** of the hip (see Chapter 199).

## EPIDEMIOLOGY

Infectious arthritis occurs most commonly in children younger than 5 years of age and adolescents.

**TABLE 118-1 Pathogenic Organisms Causing Arthritis in Children**

| Common | Uncommon |
|---|---|
| **YOUNG INFANTS (<2 MONTHS)** | |
| Group B streptococci | *Neisseria gonorrhoeae* |
| *Staphylococcus aureus* | *Candida* |
| *Escherichia coli* | |
| *Klebsiella pneumoniae* | |
| **OLDER INFANTS AND CHILDREN (2 MONTHS TO MATURITY)** | |
| *Streptococcus pneumoniae* | Anaerobic bacteria |
| *S. aureus* | *Pseudomonas aeruginosa* |
| *Haemophilus influenzae* type b* | Group A streptococci |
| *Kingella kingae* | Enterobacteriaceae organisms |
| *N. gonorrhoeae* | *Mycobacterium tuberculosis* |
| *Borrelia burgdorferi* (Lyme disease) | |
| **REACTIVE ARTHRITIS** | |
| *Yersinia enterocolitica* | |
| *Campylobacter jejuni* | |
| *Shigella flexneri* | |
| *Salmonella* | |
| Group A streptococci | |
| *Neisseria meningitidis* | |
| *Coccidioides immitis* | |
| Rubella virus | |

*The incidence of invasive infections caused by *H. influenzae* type b has diminished greatly with universal childhood Hib vaccination.

## CLINICAL MANIFESTATIONS

The typical features of suppurative arthritis include erythema, warmth, swelling, and tenderness over the affected joint with a palpable effusion and decreased range of movement. The onset may be sudden or insidious with symptoms noted only when the joint is moved, such as during a diaper change, or if parents become aware of decreased voluntary movement of a joint or limb. Toddlers may exhibit a limp. In septic arthritis of the hip, the lower limb may be preferentially held in external rotation and flexion to minimize pain from pressure on the joint capsule. Similarly, the knee and elbow joints usually are held in flexion. The joints of the lower extremity are most often involved: the knees (40%), the hips (20%), and the ankles (14%). Small joints, such as those of the hand, usually are involved after penetrating trauma or closed fist injuries.

Minor genital tract symptoms that have been ignored may precede development of the early arthritis-dermatitis syndrome associated with disseminated gonococcal infection. A history of febrile illness antedating the development of monarticular arthritis characterizes late gonococcal arthritis.

Reactive arthritis is typically symmetrical, polyarticular, and usually involves the large joints, especially the hips. Patients may have had a preceding episode of gastroenteritis or urethritis. Urethritis may appear with the arthritis.

## LABORATORY AND IMAGING STUDIES

Leukocytosis and an elevated erythrocyte sedimentation rate (ESR) and C-reactive protein (CRP) are common. Arthrocentesis and analysis of the effusion is the test of choice for rapid diagnosis of infectious arthritis (Table 118-2). Adolescents with acute infectious arthritis should have urethral, cervical, rectal, and pharyngeal examination and cultures or nucleic acid amplification tests performed for *Neisseria gonorrhoeae*.

Blood or joint cultures are positive in 70% to 85% of cases. Joint fluid that exhibits the characteristics of pyogenic infection may not reveal bacterial pathogens in 30% of patients, even in the absence of preceding antibiotic therapy, because of the bacteriostatic effects of synovial fluid. Gram stain, acid-fast stain, and potassium hydroxide (KOH) preparation for fungi should be performed and are often informative even if the cultures are negative.

Plain radiographs typically add little information to the physical findings. Radiographs may show swelling of the joint capsule, a widened joint space, and displacement of adjacent normal fat lines. Radionuclide scans are of limited use, although technetium-99m bone scans may be helpful to exclude concurrent bone infection, either adjacent or distant from the infected joint. Ultrasound is especially useful for identifying joint effusions and is the diagnostic procedure of choice for evaluation of suppurative infections of the hip. Magnetic resonance imaging (MRI) is useful in distinguishing joint infections from cellulitis or deep abscesses.

## DIFFERENTIAL DIAGNOSIS

The differential diagnosis of infectious arthritis in infants, children, and adolescents includes other infectious diseases, rheumatoid disorders, rheumatic fever, and trauma. Suppurative arthritis must be distinguished from Lyme disease, osteomyelitis, suppurative bursitis, fasciitis, myositis, cellulitis, and soft tissue abscesses. Psoas muscle abscess often presents with fever and pain on hip flexion and rotation. Juvenile rheumatoid arthritis, Kawasaki syndrome, Schönlein-Henoch purpura, other rheumatoid disorders, and Crohn disease must be differentiated from infectious arthritis. In most of these diseases, the presence of symmetrical or multiple joint involvment often excludes infectious arthritis. **Suppurative bursitis** with *Staphylococcus aureus* occurs most often in older boys and men and is usually a consequence of trauma or, less commonly, a complication of bacteremia.

## TREATMENT

Initial antibiotic therapy for infectious arthritis is based on the likely organism for the age of the child and the Gram stain of joint fluid. Suppurative arthritis of the hip joint, especially, or shoulder joint necessitates prompt surgical drainage. With insertion of the joint capsule below the epiphysis in these ball-and-socket joints, increased pressure in the joint space can affect adversely the vascular supply to the head of the femur or humerus, leading to ischemic injury and necrosis. Infections of the knee may be treated with repeated arthrocenteses in addition to appropriate parenteral antibiotics.

Several antimicrobial agents provide adequate antibiotic levels in joint spaces (Table 118-3). Initial therapy for neonates should include antibiotics, such as nafcillin and cefotaxime, with activity against *S. aureus,* group B streptococcus, and aerobic gram-negative rods. Initial therapy for children 3 months to 5 years old should include antibiotics with activity against *S. aureus.* Addition of appropriate antibiotics should be considered if the child is unimmunized against *Haemophilus influenzae.* Confirmed methicillin-susceptible *S. aureus* infections are treated with nafcillin or oxacillin, and methicillin-resistant *S. aureus* infections are treated with vancomycin, or clindamycin if susceptible.

The duration of therapy depends on clinical resolution of fever and pain and decline of the ESR and CRP. Infection with virulent organisms, such as *S. aureus,* usually necessitates treatment for at least 21 days. Treatment may be changed to oral antibiotics if adherence can be ensured. Oral agents with excellent activity against *S. aureus* that are often used to complete therapy include cephalexin, amoxicillin-clavulanate, dicloxacillin, clindamycin, and ciprofloxacin (for patients ≥18 years).

## COMPLICATIONS AND PROGNOSIS

The major complications of neonatal, childhood, and gonococcal arthritis are loss of joint function resulting from damage to the articular surface. The highest incidence of these complications occurs with hip infections, presumably as a result of ischemic injury to the head of the femur. As a result, prompt open drainage of infected hip joints and often shoulder joints is critical. The high incidence of concurrent suppurative arthritis with adjacent osteomyelitis in neonates places the epiphyseal growth plate at high risk for growth abnormalities.

The prognosis for the common forms of infectious arthritis encountered in infants and children is excellent.

## TABLE 118-2 Synovial Fluid Findings in Various Joint Diseases

| Condition | Appearance | WBC Count (mm³/L) | PMNs (%) | Mucin Clot | Synovial Fluid–Blood Glucose Difference (mg/dL) | Comments |
|---|---|---|---|---|---|---|
| Normal | Clear, yellow | 0–200 (200)* | <10 | Good | No difference | — |
| Trauma | Clear, turbid, or hemorrhagic | 50–4000 (600) | <30 | Good | No difference | Common in hemophilia |
| Systemic lupus erythematosus | Clear or slightly turbid | 0–9000 (3,000) | <20 | Good to fair | No difference | LE cell positive, complement decreased |
| Rheumatoid arthritis, reactive arthritis (Reiter syndrome, inflammatory bowel disease) | Turbid | 250–80,000 (19,000) | >70 | Poor | 30 | Decreased complement |
| Infectious | | | | | | |
| Pyogenic infection | Turbid | 10,000–250,000 (80,000) | >90 | Poor | 50–90 | Positive culture result, positive Gram stain |
| Tuberculosis | Turbid | 2500–100,000 (20,000) | >60 | Poor | 40–70 | Positive results on culture, PPD testing, and acid-fast stain |
| Lyme arthritis | Turbid | 500–100,000 (20,000) | >60 | Poor | 70 | History of tick bite or erythema migrans |

LE, lupus erythematosus; PMN, polymorphonuclear cell; PPD, purified protein derivative of tuberculin; WBC, white blood cell.
*Average in parentheses.

**TABLE 118-3 Recommended Antibiotic Therapy for Infectious Arthritis in Children**

| Age Group | Common Pathogens | Recommended Treatment |
|---|---|---|
| Infants (younger than 2 months of age) | Group B streptococci | Ampicillin *plus* aminoglycoside |
| | *Escherichia coli* | Cefotaxime (*or* ceftriaxone) *plus* aminoglycoside |
| | *Klebsiella pneumoniae* | Cefotaxime (*or* ceftriaxone) *plus* aminoglycoside |
| | *Staphylococcus aureus* | Nafcillin (*or* oxacillin), vancomycin |
| Older infants and children | *S. aureus* | Nafcillin (*or* oxacillin), vancomycin |
| | *Streptococcus pneumoniae* | Penicillin G *or* cefotaxime (*or* ceftriaxone) *or* vancomycin (based on susceptibilities) |
| | Group A streptococci | Penicillin G |
| | *Kingella kingae* | Penicillin G *or* nafcillin (*or* oxacillin) |
| | *Haemophilus influenzae* type b* | Cefuroxime (*or* cefotaxime *or* ceftriaxone) |
| | *Neisseria gonorrhoeae*: disseminated gonococcal infection | Ceftriaxone |

*The incidence of invasive infections caused by *H. influenzae* type b has diminished greatly with universal childhood Hib vaccination.

The poorest outcome is for infectious arthritis of the hip or shoulder. Neonates with osteomyelitis have an approximately 40% to 50% likelihood of growth disturbances with loss of longitudinal bone growth and ultimate limb shortening.

## PREVENTION

There are no effective means to prevent hematogenous *S. aureus* arthritis. Universal immunization of infants with conjugate Hib (*Haemophilus influenzae* type b) vaccine has practically eliminated serious bacterial infections from this organism, including bone and joint infections. Because the serotypes of *Streptococcus pneumoniae* causing joint infections are represented in the conjugate pneumococcal vaccine, the incidence of pneumococcal joint infections should decrease with widespread immunization.

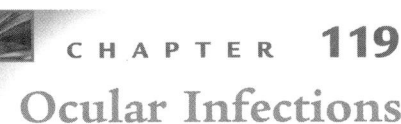

CHAPTER **119**

# Ocular Infections

## ETIOLOGY

**Acute conjunctivitis** is usually a bacterial or viral infection of the eye characterized by a rapid onset of symptoms that persists for a few days. The most common causes of bacterial conjunctivitis are nontypable *Haemophilus influenzae*, *Streptococcus pneumoniae*, and *Mycoplasma catarrhalis* (Table 119-1). Other causes include *Neisseria gonorrhoeae* and *Pseudomonas aeruginosa*, which is associated with extended-wear soft contact lenses. Viral conjunctivitis most commonly is caused by adenoviruses, which cause **epidemic keratoconjunctivitis**, and less frequently by coxsackieviruses and other enteroviruses. **Keratitis**, or inflammation of the cornea, is not commonly associated with conjunctivitis but occurs with *N. gonorrhoeae*, herpes simplex virus (HSV), and adenovirus infections.

Neonatal conjunctivitis, or **ophthalmia neonatorum**, is purulent conjunctivitis during the first 10 days of life, usually acquired during birth. The common causes of neonatal conjunctivitis, in order of decreasing prevalence, are: silver nitrate if used for gonococcal prophylaxis, *Chlamydia trachomatis*, common bacterial causes of conjunctivitis, *Escherichia coli*, other gram-negative enteric bacilli, and *N. gonorrhoeae*. Neonatal conjunctivitis also can occur as a part of perinatal HSV infection.

## EPIDEMIOLOGY

Conjunctivitis is common in young children, especially if they come in contact with other children with conjunctivitis. Predisposing factors for bacterial infection include nasolacrimal duct obstruction, sinus disease, ear infection, and allergic children who rub their eyes frequently. Conjunctivitis occurs in 1% to 12% of neonates. A mild to moderate chemical conjunctivitis commonly is present from 24 to 48 hours of age in most newborns who receive ophthalmic silver nitrate as gonococcal prophylaxis. Neonatal acquisition of *C. trachomatis* occurs in approximately 50% of infants born vaginally to infected mothers. In infants with perinatal acquisition of *C. trachomatis*, the risk of chlamydial conjunctivitis, also called **inclusion conjunctivitis**, is 25% to 50%.

## CLINICAL MANIFESTATIONS

Symptoms include redness, discharge, matted eyelids, and mild photophobia. Physical examination findings include chemosis, injection of the conjunctiva, and edema of the eyelids. Corneal involvement suggests gonococcal or herpetic infection. Herpetic corneal lesions appear as dendritic or ameboid ulcers or, more commonly, in recurrent infection, as a deep keratitis. Unilateral conjunctivitis with ipsilateral otitis media is often caused by nontypable *H. influenzae*.

The timing and manifestations of neonatal conjunctivitis are helpful in identifying the cause (Table 119-2). *N. gonorrhoeae* causes severe conjunctivitis with profuse purulent discharge. Chlamydial conjunctivitis usually occurs in the second week of life but may appear 3 days to 6 weeks after delivery. There is mild to moderate inflammation with purulent discharge issuing from one or both eyes.

**TABLE 119-1  Manifestations of Acute Conjunctivitis in Children**

| Feature | Clinical Characteristics | |
| --- | --- | --- |
| | Bacterial | Viral |
| Common pathogens | *Haemophilus influenzae* (usually nontypable) *Streptococcus pneumoniae* *Moraxella catarrhalis* | Adenoviruses types 8, 19 Enteroviruses Herpes simplex virus |
| Incubation | 24–72 hours | 1–14 days |
| Symptoms | | |
| Photophobia | Mild | Moderate to severe |
| Blurred vision | Common with discharge | If keratitis is present |
| Foreign body sensation | Unusual | Yes |
| Signs | | |
| Discharge | Purulent discharge | Mucoid/serous discharge |
| Palpebral reaction | Papillary response | Follicular response |
| Preauricular lymph node | Unusual for acute (<10%) | More common (20%) |
| Chemosis | Moderate | Mild |
| Hemorrhagic conjunctivae | Occasionally with *Streptococcus* or *Haemophilus* | Frequent with enteroviruses |
| Treatment (topical) | Polymyxin B–trimethoprim *or* sulfacetamide 10% *or* erythromycin | Adenovirus: self-limited Herpes simplex virus: trifluridine 1% solution *or* vidarabine 3% ointment; ophthalmologic consultation |
| End of contagious period | 24 hours after start of effective treatment | 7 days after onset of symptoms |

## LABORATORY AND IMAGING STUDIES

Cultures are not routinely obtained because bacterial conjunctivitis is usually self-limited or responds quickly to antibiotic treatment. If gonococcal conjunctivitis is suspected, especially in neonates, Gram stain and culture must be obtained. In these infants, further testing of blood or other sites of infection should be cultured. Additional testing for chlamydia, human immunodeficiency virus (HIV), and syphilis should be performed as well.

## DIFFERENTIAL DIAGNOSIS

Distinguishing bacterial from viral conjunctivitis by presentation and appearance is difficult (see Table 119-1). Vesicular lid lesions, if present, suggest the diagnosis of HSV. **Hyperpurulent conjunctivitis** characterized by reaccumulation of purulent discharge within minutes is characteristic of *N. gonorrhea* infection. The differential diagnosis is delineated in Table 119-3.

**Blepharitis** is associated with staphylococcal infections, seborrhea, and meibomian gland dysfunction. The child complains of photophobia, burning, irritation, and a foreign body sensation that causes the child to rub the eyes. Eyelid hygiene with an **eyelid scrub** routine is the initial step in treatment.

**Hordeola** are acute suppurative nodular inflammatory lesions of the eyelids associated with pain and redness. **External hordeola** or **styes** occur on the anterior eyelid, in the Zeis glands, or in the lash follicles and usually are caused by staphylococci. **Internal hordeola** occur in the meibomian glands and may be infected with staphylococci or may be sterile. If the meibomian gland becomes obstructed, the gland secretions accumulate, and a

**chalazion** develops. Hordeola usually respond spontaneously to local treatment measures, but may recur.

**Dacryocystitis** is an infection or inflammation of the lacrimal sac, which is usually obstructed, and is most commonly caused by *Staphylococcus aureus* or coagulase-negative staphylococci. A mucopurulent discharge can be expressed with gentle pressure on the nasolacrimal sac. Treatment usually requires probing of the nasolacrimal system to establish communication.

**Endophthalmitis** is an emergent, sight-threatening infection that usually follows trauma, surgery, or hematogenous spread from a distant focus. Causative organisms include coagulase-negative staphylococci, *S. aureus, S. pneumoniae, Bacillus cereus,* and *Candida albicans.* Examination is difficult because of severe blepharospasm and extreme photophobia. A hypopyon and haze may be visible on examination.

## TREATMENT

The lids should be treated as needed with warm compresses to remove accumulated discharge. Acute bacterial conjunctivitis is frequently self-limited, but topical antibiotics hasten resolution. Antibiotics are instilled between the eyelids four times a day until the discharge and chemosis subside. Recommended treatment includes topical ciprofloxacin solution, sulfacetamide 10% solution trimethoprim-polymyxin B solution, and erythromycin ointment. Gonococcal conjunctivitis in adults is treated with a single intramuscular (IM) dose of ceftriaxone (1 g) plus azithromycin (to treat possible concominant chlamydial infection).

The treatment of ophthalmia neonatorum depends on the cause (see Table 119-2). Gonococcal ophthalmia neonatorum is treated with a single dose of ceftriaxone (25–50 mg/kg intravenous [IV] or IM; maximum dose

**TABLE 119-2 Clinical Manifestations and Treatment of Neonatal Conjunctivitis**

| Etiologic Agent | % of Cases | Discharge and External Examination | Typical Age at Onset | Diagnosis | Associated Manifestations | Treatment |
|---|---|---|---|---|---|---|
| Chemical: silver nitrate | Variable (1%), depending on use of silver nitrate | Watery discharge | 1–3 days | No organisms on smear or culture | None | None |
| Neisseria gonorrhoeae | <1% | Copious, purulent discharge; swelling of lids and conjunctivae; corneal involvement common; risk for perforation and corneal scar | 1–7 days | Gram stain (gram-negative intracellular diplococci); culture on chocolate agar. Culture other sites including blood and CSF | May be associated with severe disseminated gonococcal infection | Ceftriaxone. Hospitalize patient |
| Bacterial: Staphylococcus, Streptococcus, Pseudomonas, E. coli | 30–50% | Purulent moderate discharge; mild lid and conjunctival swelling; corneal involvement with risk for perforation | 2–7 days | Gram stain; culture on blood agar | | Topical therapy |
| Chlamydia trachomatis (inclusion conjunctivitis) | 2–40% | Scant discharge; mild swelling; hyperemia; follicular response; late corneal staining | 4–19 days | Test of discharge with a DIF test or PCR assay | May presage C. trachomatis pneumonia (at 3 weeks–3 months of age) | Erythromycin (oral) |
| HSV | <1% | Clear or serosanguineous discharge; lid swelling; keratitis with cloudy cornea; dendrite formation | 3 days– 3 weeks | Viral culture; DIF test | May be associated with disseminated perinatal HSV infection | Acyclovir (intravenous) for systemic involvement |

CSF, cerebrospinal fluid; DIF, direct immunofluorescence; HSV, herpes simplex virus; PCR, polymerase chain reaction.

**TABLE 119-3 Differential Diagnosis of Ocular Infections**

| Condition | Etiologic Agents | Signs and Symptoms | Treatment |
|---|---|---|---|
| Bacterial conjunctivitis | *Haemophilus influenzae, Haemophilus aegyptius, Streptococcus pneumoniae, Neisseria gonorrhoeae* | Mucopurulent unilateral or bilateral discharge, normal vision, photophobia, conjunctival injection and edema (chemosis); gritty sensation | Topical antibiotics, parenteral ceftriaxone for gonococcus |
| Viral conjunctivitis | Adenovirus, echovirus, coxsackievirus | Same as for bacterial infection; may be hemorrhagic, unilateral | Self-limited |
| Neonatal conjunctivitis | *Chlamydia trachomatis*, gonococcus, chemical (silver nitrate), *Staphylococcus aureus* | Palpebral conjunctival follicle or papillae; same as for bacterial infection | Ceftriaxone for gonococcus and oral erythromycin for *C. trachomatis* |
| Allergic conjunctivitis | Seasonal pollens or allergen exposure | Itching, incidence of bilateral chemosis (edema) greater than that of erythema, tarsal papillae | Antihistamines, steroids, cromolyn |
| Keratitis | Herpes simplex, adenovirus, *S. pneumoniae, S. aureus, Pseudomonas, Acanthamoeba*, chemicals | Severe pain, corneal swelling, clouding, limbus erythema, hypopyon, cataracts; contact lens history with amebic infection | Specific antibiotics for bacterial/fungal infections; keratoplasty, acyclovir for herpes |
| Endophthalmitis | *S. aureus, S. pneumoniae, Candida albicans*, associated surgery or trauma | Acute onset, pain, loss of vision, swelling, chemosis, redness; hypopyon and vitreous haze | Antibiotics |
| Anterior uveitis (iridocyclitis) | JRA, Reiter syndrome, sarcoidosis, Behçet disease, inflammatory bowel disease | Unilateral/bilateral; erythema, ciliary flush, irregular pupil, iris adhesions; pain, photophobia, small pupil, poor vision | Topical steroids, plus therapy for primary disease |
| Posterior uveitis (choroiditis) | Toxoplasmosis, histoplasmosis, *Toxocara canis* | No signs of erythema, decreased vision | Specific therapy for pathogen |
| Episcleritis/scleritis | Idiopathic autoimmune disease (e.g., SLE, Schönlein-Henoch purpura) | Localized pain, intense erythema, unilateral; blood vessels bigger than in conjunctivitis; scleritis may cause globe perforation | Episcleritis is self-limiting; topical steroids for fast relief |
| Foreign body | Occupational or other exposure | Unilateral, red, gritty feeling; visible or microscopic size | Irrigation, removal; check for ulceration |
| Blepharitis | *S. aureus, Staphylococcus epidermidis*, seborrheic, blocked lacrimal duct; rarely molluscum contagiosum, *Phthirus pubis, Pediculus capitis* | Bilateral, irritation, itching, hyperemia, crusting, affecting lid margins | Topical antibiotics, warm compresses |
| Dacryocystitis | Obstructed lacrimal sac: *S. aureus, H. influenzae, S. pneumoniae* | Pain, tenderness, erythema and exudate in areas of lacrimal sac (inferomedial to inner canthus); tearing (epiphora); possible orbital cellulitis | Systemic, topical antibiotics; surgical drainage |
| Dacryoadenitis | *S. aureus, S. pneumoniae*, CMV, measles, EBV, enteroviruses; trauma, sarcoidosis, leukemia | Pain, tenderness, edema, erythema over gland area (upper temporal lid); fever, leukocytosis | Systemic antibiotics; drainage of orbital abscesses |
| Orbital cellulitis (postseptal cellulitis) | Paranasal sinusitis: *H. influenzae, S. aureus, S. pneumoniae*, other streptococci Trauma: *S. aureus* Fungi: *Aspergillus, Mucor* if immunodeficient | Rhinorrhea, chemosis, vision loss, painful extraocular motion, proptosis, ophthalmoplegia, fever, lid edema, leukocytosis | Systemic antibiotics, drainage of orbital abscesses |
| Periorbital cellulitis (preseptal cellulitis) | Trauma: *S. aureus*, other streptococci Bacteremia: pneumococcus, streptococci, *H. influenzae* | Cutaneous erythema, warmth, normal vision, minimal involvement of orbit; fever, leukocytosis, toxic appearance | Systemic antibiotics |

CMV, cytomegalovirus; EBV, Epstein-Barr virus; JRA, juvenile rheumatoid arthritis; SLE, systemic lupus erythematosus.

125 mg). These infants should be hospitalized. Antibiotic treatment also is recommended for newborns to mothers with untreated gonorrhea. The mother and infant should be tested for chlamydial infection. Chlamydial conjunctivitis is treated with oral erythromycin for 14 days, partly to reduce the risk of subsequent chlamydial pneumonia.

## COMPLICATIONS AND PROGNOSIS

The prognosis for bacterial and viral conjunctivitis is excellent. The major complication is keratitis, which can lead to ulcerations and perforation. This complication is uncommon except with *N. gonorrhoeae* infection. Complications of neonatal conjunctivitis are uncommon except with *N. gonorrhoeae* and HSV infections. Chlamydial conjunctivitis may progress in infants to chlamydial pneumonia, which typically develops from 4 to 12 weeks of age (see Chapter 110).

## PREVENTION

Careful hand washing is important to prevent spread of conjunctivitis. Bacterial conjunctivitis is considered contagious for 24 hours after initiating effective treatment. Children may return to school, but treatment measures must be continued until there is complete clinical resolution.

All infants should receive prophylaxis for gonococcal ophthalmia neonatorum. Silver nitrate 1% is used frequently but usually causes a chemical conjunctivitis. Alternative methods are equally effective and less irritating and include a single application of erythromycin 0.5% ointment or tetracycline 1% ointment. Prophylaxis is administered to all newborns, whether delivered vaginally or by cesarean section, as soon as possible after delivery.

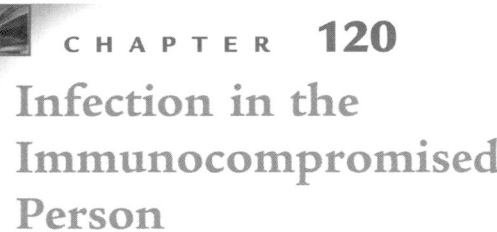

CHAPTER **120**

# Infection in the Immunocompromised Person

## ETIOLOGY

Many diseases or their treatments adversely affect the immune system, including genetic immunodeficiencies, human immunodeficiency virus (HIV) infection and acquired immunodeficiency syndrome (AIDS), cancer, stem cell and organ transplantation, and immunosuppressive drugs used to treat cancer, autoimmune diseases, and transplant patients. These patients are at significant risk of life-threatening infections from invasive **endogenous infection** from bacterial or fungal flora of the oropharynx and gastrointestinal tract, acquisition of **exogenous infection** from infected persons, and reactivation of latent virus until marrow and immune function recover (Table 120-1).

Episodes of fever and **neutropenia**, defined as an **absolute neutrophil count** of less than 500/mm$^3$ neutrophils and bands, are especially common in cancer and transplant patients. The evaluation of fever in immunocompromised persons differs from that in immunocompetent hosts. The types of infections often can be predicted by which component of the immune system is abnormal. The use of corticosteroids and potent immunosuppressive drugs that impair the activation of T cells increases the risk for pathogens that normally are controlled by T cell–mediated responses, such as *Pneumocystis jirovecii* and *Toxoplasma gondii*, and intracellular pathogens, such as *Salmonella, Listeria,* and *Mycobacterium*.

Bacteria cause most infections in immunocompromised persons (see Table 120-1). *Staphylococcus aureus, Escherichia coli, Pseudomonas aeruginosa, Klebsiella pneumoniae,* and coagulase-negative staphylococci are the most commonly identified bacterial pathogens. Central indwelling catheters often are associated with coagulase-negative staphylococci, *Staphylococcus aureus,* and less frequently gram-negative bacteria, *Enterococcus,* and *Candida*.

Fungal pathogens account for approximately 10% of all infections associated with childhood cancer. *Candida* causes 60% of all fungal infections, with *Aspergillus* the second most common pathogen. Besides cancer-associated or therapy-associated cellular immunity defects, risk factors for fungal infections include oropharyngeal and gastrointestinal mucositis facilitating systemic fungal invasion, presence of long-term indwelling intravascular catheters, and broad-spectrum antibacterial therapy that promotes fungal colonization as a precursor to infection.

Infections with *P. jirovecii* and *T. gondii* represent reactivation of quiescent infection facilitated by cancer-associated or therapy-associated cellular immunodeficiency. *P. jirovecii* primarily causes pneumonitis in patients with leukemia, lymphoma, or HIV or on long-term corticosteroids, but it also can cause extrapulmonary disease (sinusitis, otitis media).

Viral opportunistic infections in patients with cancer usually represent symptomatic reactivation from latency facilitated by cancer-associated or therapy-associated cellular immunodeficiency. Herpes simplex virus (HSV) can cause severe and prolonged mucocutaneous infection or disseminated disease. Cytomegalovirus (CMV) can cause focal disease in immunocompromised persons, especially in stem cell transplant patients. Manifestations of CMV disease include hepatitis, pneumonitis, esophagitis, and enteritis with ulcerations of the gastrointestinal mucosa. Varicella zoster virus (VZV) can cause serious primary infection in susceptible persons, often with accompanying encephalitis, hepatitis, or, most ominously, pneumonitis. Zoster also can reactivate during chemotherapy and may cause disseminated zoster.

## EPIDEMIOLOGY

Chemotherapeutic agents target rapidly dividing cells, especially myeloproliferative cells, which causes myelosuppression. Children receiving allogeneic transplants are at greater risk for infection than children receiving autologous transplants. Prolonged time to hematologic engraftment is a significant risk factor for infection in these patients. Children receiving stem cell or organ transplants have significantly greater immunosuppression as a consequence of the myeloablative conditioning regimens. Foreign bodies (shunts, central venous catheters) interfere with cutaneous barriers against infection and together with neutropenia or immunosuppression increase the risk of bacterial or fungal infections (see Chapter 121).

## TABLE 120-1 Pathogens of Importance in Patients with Cancer

| Bacteria | Fungi | Protozoa | Viruses |
|---|---|---|---|
| *Bacteroides fragilis* | *Aspergillus* | *Cryptosporidium parvum* | Adenoviruses |
| *Campylobacter* | *Blastoschizomyces capitatus* | *Cyclospora cayetanensis* | Cytomegalovirus |
| *Clostridium difficile* | *Candida* | *Enterocytozoon bieneusi* | Echoviruses |
| *Clostridium septicum,* | *Chrysosporium* | *Giardia lamblia* | Hepatitis A virus |
| *Clostridium perfringens* | *Cryptococcus neoformans* | *Isospora belli* | Herpes simplex viruses |
| *Comamonas acidovorans* | *Cunninghamella bertholletiae* | *Leisbmania donovani* | Influenza viruses |
| *Enterobater cloacae* | *Fusarium proliferatum, Fusarium solani* | *Septata intestinalis* | Parvovirus B19 |
| *Enterrococcus* | *Geotrichum candidium* | | Human metapneumovirus |
| *Escherichia coli* | *Hansenula anomala* | | Respiratory syncytial virus |
| *Haemophilus influenzae* | *Malassezia furfur* | | Varicella-zoster virus |
| *Klebsiella pneumoniae* | *Scopulariopsis* | | |
| *Listeria monocytogenes* | *Trichosporon beigelii* | | |
| *Moraxella catarrbalis* | | | |
| *Mycobacterium avium* complex | | | |
| *Mycobacterium chelonae* | | | |
| *Mycobacterium haemophilum* | | | |
| *Nocardia asteroides* | | | |
| *Pediococcus acidilactici* | | | |
| *Propionibacterium granulosum* | | | |
| *Pseudomonas aeruginosa* | | | |
| *Pseudomonas pseudomallei* | | | |
| Coagulase-negative staphylococci | | | |
| *Staphylococcus aureus* | | | |
| *Vibrio vulnificus* | | | |

The relative rate of infection in patients with cancer at admission or during hospitalization is 10% to 15%. The most frequently infected sites, in descending order, are the respiratory tract, the bloodstream, surgical wounds, and the urinary tract.

## CLINICAL MANIFESTATIONS

Fever is the most common and sometimes the only presenting symptom of serious infection in cancer and transplant patients. The presence of fever with neutropenia, even in the absence of other signs or symptoms, demands prompt evaluation because of the potential for life-threatening infection. Despite being immunocompromised, these patients develop fever with infection as well as the typical signs and symptoms associated with infections. All symptoms and signs should be evaluated thoroughly, in addition to the evaluation necessitated because of fever in the presence of underlying immunodeficiency.

## LABORATORY TESTS AND IMAGING

Assessing fever and neutropenia in immunocompromised persons requires blood cultures for bacterial and fungal pathogens obtained by peripheral venipuncture and from all lumens of any indwelling vascular catheters. A complete blood count (CBC) with differential, C-reactive protein (CRP), complete chemistry panel, culture of urine and gram staining/culture of potential sites of specific infection found during history and physical should be performed. Antigen tests, especially for serum cryptococcal antigen, should be considered. Chest radiographs are important to assess for the presence of pulmonary infiltrates. Specialized imaging studies, such as computed tomography (CT) or magnetic

resonance imaging (MRI), can be useful in selected cases, such as with suspected sinusitis or intra-abdominal infection, or to further delineate the location and extent of abnormalities seen on plain radiographs.

In the absence of neutrophils to contain and induce localized signs of inflammation, it often is difficult to determine the source of infection by physical examination. Chest findings may be absent despite significant infection and revealed only by chest radiograph. Sinus infection with bacteria, *Aspergillus,* or Zygomycetes is common in neutropenic hosts and may be detected only on CT scan.

## DIFFERENTIAL DIAGNOSIS

Initially, the patient should have a complete physical examination, including careful scrutiny of the oropharynx, nares, external auditory canals, skin and axilla, groin, perineum, and rectal area. The exit site and subcutaneous tunnel of any indwelling vascular catheter should be examined closely for erythema and palpated for tenderness and expression of purulent material. Perirectal abscess is a potentially serious infection in neutropenic hosts, with tenderness and erythema that may be the only clues to infection. Any presumptive infection identified during the evaluation should direct appropriate cultures and tailor anti-infective therapy.

## TREATMENT

Treatment should be provided as appropriate for focal infections identified by physical examination or diagnostic imaging. Select *low-risk* patients may be managed as outpatients. Empirical treatment of fever and neutropenia without an identified source should include an extended-spectrum penicillin or cephalosporin with activity against gram-negative bacilli, including *P. aeruginosa*, sometimes in combination with an aminoglycoside (Fig. 120-1). If the patient has an indwelling vascular catheter, vancomycin should be added because of the increasing prevalence of methicillin-resistant *S. aureus*, but can be discontinued if *S. aureus* is not cultured after 48 to 72 hours. Specific antibiotic regimens should be guided by local antibiotic resistance patterns at each institution.

If no microbiologic cause is isolated, empirical broad-spectrum antibiotics are continued as long as the patient remains neutropenic, regardless of whether the fever resolves (see Fig. 120-2). Antibiotic therapy should be modified as indicated by new findings or if the patient's

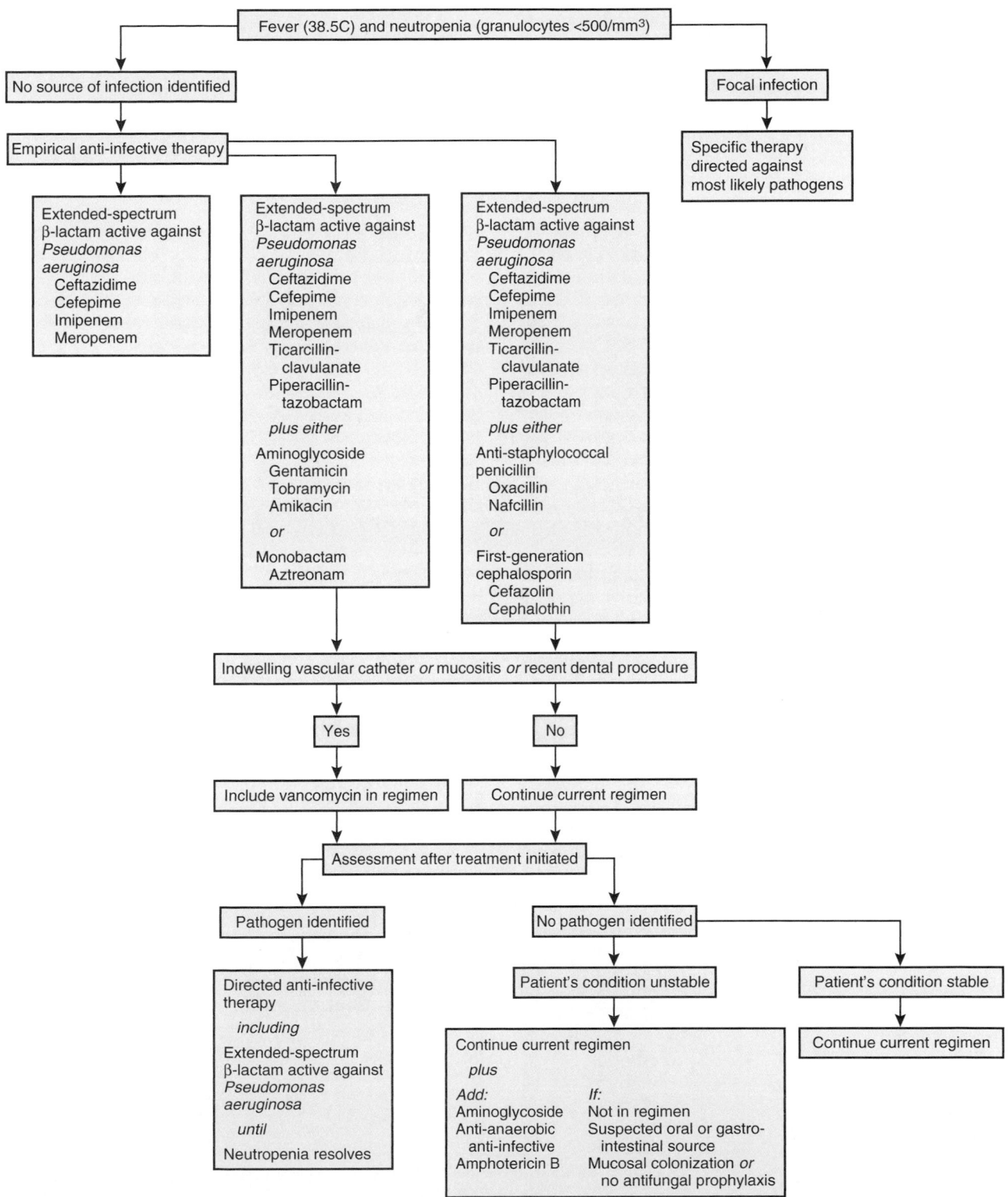

**FIGURE 120-1**

**Initial management of fever and neutropenia without an identified source in cancer and transplant patients.** (From Conrad DA: Patients with cancer. In Jenson HB, Baltimore RS [eds]: Pediatric Infectious Diseases: Principles and Practice, 2nd ed. Philadelphia, *WB Saunders*, 2002, p 1161.)

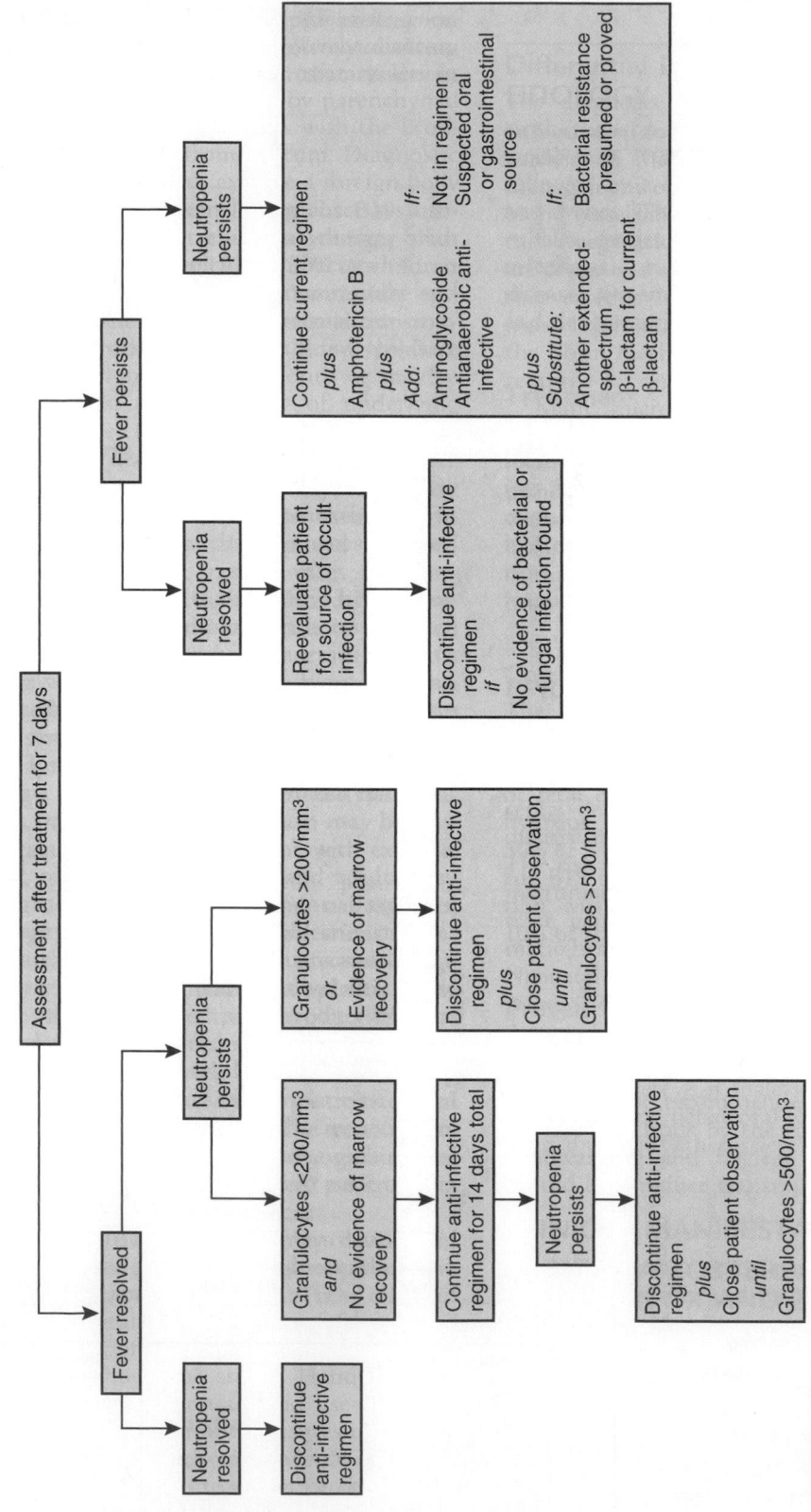

**FIGURE 120–2**

Continuing management of possible infection after 7 days of fever without an identified source in cancer and transplant patients. (From Conrad DA: Patients with cancer. In Jenson HB, Baltimore RS [eds]: Pediatric Infectious Diseases: Principles and Practice, 2nd ed. Philadelphia, WB Saunders, 2002, p 1165.)

clinical status deteriorates. Further investigation for fungal infection and empirical treatment with amphotericin B or another antifungal agent is instituted in patients who have neutropenia and persistent fever without a focus despite broad-spectrum antibacterial therapy for 5 days (Fig. 120-2).

The use of recombinant granulocyte colony-stimulating factor (G-CSF) or granulocyte-macrophage colony-stimulating factor (GM-CSF) stimulates neutrophil production by the bone marrow, reduces the duration and severity of neutropenia, and decreases the risk of infection. Some chemotherapeutic protocols for the treatment of solid tumors that result in prolonged neutropenia incorporate hematopoietic cytokine therapy as part of the treatment protocol.

## PREVENTION

Current guidelines discourage the use of broad-spectrum prophylactic antibiotics to prevent fever and neutropenia because of lack of efficacy and concerns about development of antibiotic resistance. Administration of trimethoprim-sulfamethoxazole (TMP-SMZ) to prevent *P. jirovecii* infection is routine for patients with leukemia or lymphoma and for many patients undergoing intensive chemotherapy for solid tumors. Prophylaxis generally is begun with initiation of anticancer therapy and continued until 6 months after chemotherapy has been completed. In select populations, such as patients undergoing hematopoetic stem cell transplant, prophylactic antifungals such as fluconazole are beneficial.

Immunocompromised susceptible persons exposed to chickenpox within 2 days before the onset of rash until 5 days after the onset of rash in the index case should receive varicella zoster immune globulin (VZIG). Modified infection after VZIG may not result in protective immunity, and persons who receive VZIG prophylaxis should be considered to still be at risk with any subsequent exposures.

# CHAPTER 121

# Infections Associated with Medical Devices

Infections are a common and important complication of medical devices and are a major part of **health care–associated infections** (formerly known as **nosocomial infections**).

## VASCULAR DEVICE INFECTIONS

**Vascular catheters** are inserted in most inpatients and used in many outpatients. The use of catheters for long-term access to the bloodstream has been an important advance for the care of persons who require parenteral nutrition, chemotherapy, or extended parenteral antibiotic therapy. The major complication of catheters is infection.

Short, peripheral intravenous (IV) catheters used for short-term access in stable patients are associated with a low rate of infection, especially in children. **Peripherally inserted central catheters** are commonly used for short-term venous access. **Central catheters** are commonly placed for extended venous access, such as for chemotherapy, using tunneled silicone elastomer catheters (**Broviac or Hickman catheters**) which are surgically inserted into a central vein, passed through a subcutaneous tunnel before exiting the skin, and anchored by a subcutaneous cuff. Contamination of the catheter hub or any connection of the IV tubing is common and is a major predisposition to catheter-associated infection. Totally implanted venous access systems (Port-a-Cath, Infuse-a-Port) have a silicone elastomer catheter tunneled beneath the skin to a reservoir implanted in a subcutaneous pocket. Implanted catheters or ports decrease, but do not eliminate, the opportunity for microbial entry at the skin site.

Catheter-related thrombosis and catheter-related infection can develop separately or together. Ultrasound or radiographs can identify thrombi but infection can be identified only by culture. **Thrombophlebitis** is inflammation with thrombosis. **Septic thrombophlebitis** is thrombosis with organisms embedded in the clot. **Catheter-related bloodstream infection** implies isolation of the same organism from a catheter and from peripheral blood of a patient with clinical symptoms of bacteremia and no other apparent source of infection. Confirmation requires quantitative colony counts of both samples, which is not routinely performed. Possible sources of the bacteremia include the infusate, contamination via tubing and catheter connections, or established infection, which may or may not be clinically apparent. Infection may appear as an **exit site infection** limited to the insertion site or may extend along the catheter tunnel of buried catheters to cause a **tunnel infection**.

Many microorganisms cause catheter-related infections, most commonly *Staphylococcus aureus,* coagulase-negative staphylococci, *Enterococcus,* and *Candida* (Table 121-1). Gram-positive cocci, primarily staphylococci, cause more than 50% of central venous catheter associated bacteremias and exit site infections. Other skin flora, diphtheroids, and *Bacillus* are often involved. Gram-negative organisms cause 25% to 40% of infections. Polymicrobial infections of central venous catheters are common. Fungal catheter infections, usually *Candida albicans,* are most common among persons receiving broad-spectrum antibiotics or parenteral nutrition.

The rates of bloodstream infection of peripheral venous catheters are from 0 to 2 per 1000 catheter-days and for central catheters from less than 2 to 30 per 1000 catheter-days. Risk factors for infection include prematurity, burns and skin disorders that adversely affect the skin integrity, neutropenia, and other immunodeficiencies (see Chapter 120). Infection rates are lower for tunneled and implanted catheters. Catheters inserted in emergency settings are more likely to be infected than catheters placed electively.

**TABLE 121-1 Organisms Causing Catheter-Related Infections**

| Classification of Pathogen | Common | Uncommon |
|---|---|---|
| Gram-positive organisms | Coagulase-negative staphylococci, *Staphylococcus aureus*, *Enterococcus* | Diphtheroids, *Bacillus*, *Micrococcus* |
| Gram-negative organisms | *Escherichia coli*, *Klebsiella*, *Pseudomonas aeruginosa* | *Acinetobacter*, *Enterobacter*, *Neisseria* |
| Fungi | *Candida albicans* | *Malassezia furfur*, *Candida parapsilosis*, *Candida glabrata*, *Candida tropicalis* |
| Miscellaneous | | Nontuberculous mycobacteria |

Clinical signs of catheter-associated bacteremia or fungemia range from mild fever to overwhelming sepsis. Infection at the site of central catheter entrance is manifested as a localized cellulitis with warmth, tenderness, swelling, erythema, and discharge. Tunnel infection is manifested by similar findings along the tunnel route. Peripheral phlebitis or catheter-related infection is classically manifested as a warm, erythematous, tender palpable cord originating at the IV catheter site, but may be subclinical or manifested only by fever without signs of local inflammation.

The treatment of catheter-related infection depends on the site of the infection and the pathogen involved. Catheters that are no longer necessary should be removed if infection is suspected. Catheter-associated bacteremia can be treated with simple catheter removal, removal plus antibiotics, or, in a stable patient, an attempt of antibiotic therapy alone (see Fig. 121-1). Infection with organisms of low virulence may be manifested by fever alone, and removal of the catheter frequently is followed by prompt defervescence and complete resolution of infection. Initial therapy should include antibiotics active against gram-negative organisms such as a broad-spectrum cephalosporin, and against *S. aureus* and coagulase-negative

staphylococci such as oxacillin, nafcillin, or vancomycin. Antibiotic regimens should be tailored to the specific organism identified. Eradication of infection can be accomplished without removal of the central line in 89% of uncomplicated bacteremic infections, 94% of exit site infections, and 25% of tunnel infections. If the patient is not critically ill and the pathogen is likely to be susceptible to antibiotic therapy, a trial of antibiotics is given through the infected catheter. The total duration of therapy depends on the pathogen and the duration of positive cultures and is usually 10 to 14 days after sterilization of the bloodstream. Catheter removal is indicated with sepsis, septic thrombophlebitis, clinical deterioration despite appropriate therapy, persistently positive blood culture results after 48 to 72 hours of appropriate antimicrobial therapy, embolic lesions, or fungal infection because of poor response to antifungal therapy alone (Fig. 121-1). Infection of the pocket around an implanted port is unlikely to respond to antibiotics, and removal of the foreign body is usually necessary.

**Antibiotic-lock** is a method of sterilizing intravascular catheters by using high concentrations of antibiotics infused into the portion of the catheter between the hub and the vessel entry. The solution is allowed to dwell within the catheter segment for several hours. It also may be useful for treatment of catheter-associated infections and for prevention of infection.

Aseptic technique is essential during catheter insertion. Catheters that are placed during emergency situations should be replaced as soon as medically feasible. Care of indwelling catheters involves meticulous attention to sterile technique whenever the system is entered. The number and use of stopcocks should be minimized. Care of the catheter entry site commonly involves a topical antibiotic or disinfectant. Catheters that are no longer necessary should be removed.

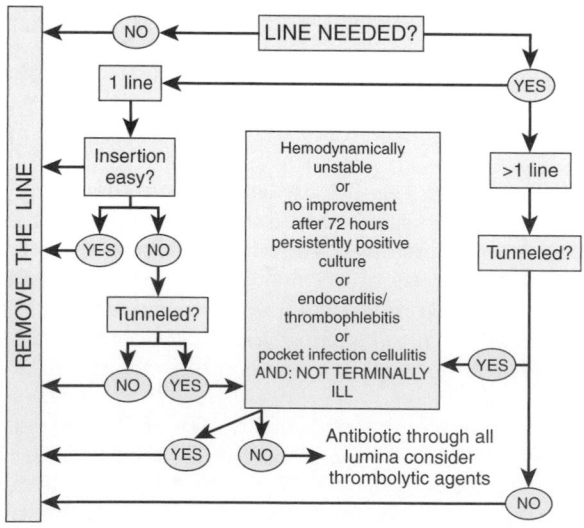

**FIGURE 121-1**

Management of central venous catheter infection. (From De Paw BE, Verwij PE: Infections in patients with hematologic malignancies. In Mandell GL, Bennett JE, Dolin R [eds]: Principles and Practice of Infectious Diseases, 6th ed. Philadelphia, *Churchill Livingstone*, 2005, Fig. 307-1 p 3434.)

## VENTILATOR-ASSOCIATED PNEUMONIA

Intubation of the airway provides direct access to the lungs and bypasses normal host defenses. Organisms enter the lungs directly through the lumen of the tube or by descending around the tube, which may result in ventilator-associated pneumonia. Contaminated respiratory equipment, humidification systems, or condensate introduces bacteria directly into lower airways. The continuously open upper airway increases the risk of aspiration of oropharyngeal flora and reflux of gastric contents and interferes with clearance of the airway by coughing because an effective cough requires a closed glottis. Suctioning of the upper respiratory tract or mouth requires clean technique but does not require aseptic technique. Suction catheters that reach the lower airways must be sterile and usually are designed for single use.

## URINARY CATHETERS

The most important risk factors for urinary tract infections (UTIs) are the presence of catheters, instrumentation, and anatomic abnormalities (see Chapter 114). Organisms enter the bladder through the catheter by instillation of contaminated irrigation fluids, backflow of contaminated urine from the drainage bag, or ascent of bacteria around the meatus along the outside of the catheter. Indwelling catheters facilitate direct access to the bladder and should have a closed drainage system. After simple, straight catheterization, the incidence of UTI is 1% to 2%. Organisms that cause catheter-associated UTIs include fecal flora, such as gram-negative enteric bacilli, most commonly *Escherichia coli*, and *Enterococcus*. With concomitant antibiotic treatment, resistant organisms predominate, and fungi emerge as pathogens.

The most important aspect of prevention is to minimize the duration and use of catheterization. Intermittent catheterization is preferred over indwelling catheter drainage whenever feasible. Insertion of catheters must be performed with aseptic technique, and the drainage system must remain closed at all times, with sterile technique used whenever the system is entered. Drainage bags always should be dependent to avoid backflow of urine into the bladder.

## PERITONEAL DIALYSIS–ASSOCIATED INFECTIONS

Indwelling catheters used for peritoneal dialysis may be complicated by exit site infection, tunnel infection, and peritonitis. The usual route of infection is from the skin surface along the tunnel and into the peritoneum. The most common pathogens are skin flora, including *Staphylococcus;* organisms that contaminate water, such as *Pseudomonas* and *Acinetobacter;* enteric flora, such as *E. coli* and *Klebsiella;* and fungi, such as *C. albicans*. Peritonitis may present with fever, vague abdominal pain, and cloudy dialysate. The diagnosis is established on clinical manifestations and confirmed by culture of the dialysate. Prevention of infection requires careful planning of the location of the exit site to minimize contamination, aseptic insertion of the catheter, meticulous care of the catheter site, securing of the catheter to avoid tension and motion, and aseptic technique during dialysis.

## CENTRAL NERVOUS SYSTEM SHUNTS

Important risk factors of health care–associated central nervous system (CNS) infections are surgery, ventriculoperitoneal shunts, and cerebrospinal fluid (CSF) leaks. Infection of ventriculoperitoneal shunts results from contamination of the system at the time of placement or from hematogenous seeding. Externalized ventricular drains and subdural bolts allow direct access of skin flora to the CSF. For these devices, the rates of infection increase with the duration of catheterization, especially beyond 5 days.

The most common pathogens causing shunt infections are coagulase-negative staphylococci and *S. aureus*. After skull fracture or cranial surgery, a CSF leak may facilitate ascending infection, especially with *Streptococcus pneumoniae*, which frequently colonizes the nasopharynx. Patients with shunt infections may present with only fever and headache, or may present with typical signs and symptoms of meningitis (see Chapter 100). Infections caused by coagulase-negative staphylococci typically present with insidious onset of fever, malaise, headache, and vomiting. Empiric therapy is with vancomycin, with additional antibiotics if gram-negative bacteria are suspected.

Antibiotics frequently are used perioperatively during placement of shunts and other neurosurgical procedures. There is no proof that antibiotics decrease infection rates in these clean procedures. External ventricular drains should be maintained as closed systems with aseptic technique and removed as soon as possible. Drainage bags always should be dependent to avoid backflow.

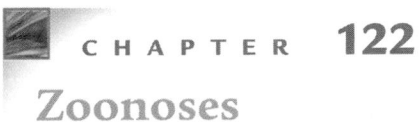

CHAPTER **122**

# Zoonoses

**Zoonoses** are infections that are transmitted in nature between vertebrate animals and humans. Many zoonotic pathogens are maintained in nature by means of an **enzootic cycle**, in which mammalian hosts and arthropod vectors reinfect each other. Humans frequently are only incidentally infected. Of the more than 150 different human zoonotic diseases that have been described, Lyme disease (*Borrelia burgdorferi*) accounts for 90% of reported vector-borne infections in the United States. Other common pathogens include *Rickettsia rickettsii* (Rocky Mountain spotted fever), ehrlichiosis (*Ehrlichia chaffeensis*), West Nile virus, and anaplasmosis (*Anaplasma phagocytophilum*). The epidemiology of zoonoses is related to the geographic distribution of the hosts and, if vector-borne, the distribution and seasonal life cycle of the vector (Table 122-1).

Many zoonoses are spread by ticks including Lyme disease, Rocky Mountain spotted fever, ehrlichiosis, tularemia, tick typhus, and babesiosis. Mosquitoes transmit the arboviral encephalitides (see Chapter 101), dengue fever, malaria, and yellow fever. Preventive measures to avoid tick-borne and mosquito-borne diseases include using insect repellants that contain **DEET** (*N,N*-diethyl-*m*-toluamide) on skin and insect repellants that contain **permethrin** on clothing; avoiding tick-infested habitats (thick scrub oak, briar, poison ivy sites); avoiding excretory products of wild animals; wearing shoes or boots and not sandals; completely covering the arms and legs, with trousers tucked into shoes or socks to prevent ticks from crawling under clothing; wearing light-colored clothing to facilitate detection of crawling ticks; conducting thorough inspections of the body and of pets after returning from the outdoors; and removing ticks promptly.

**TABLE 122-1  Major Zoonotic and Vector-Borne Infections***

| Disease | Causative Agent | Common Animal Reservoirs | Vector(s)/Mode(s) of Transmission | Geographic Distribution |
|---|---|---|---|---|
| **BACTERIAL DISEASES** | | | | |
| Anthrax | Bacillus anthracis | Cattle, goats, sheep, swine, cats, wild animals | Aerosol inhalation of spores in hides and other animal by-products, direct contact | Worldwide; rare in United States |
| Brucellosis | Brucella | Cattle, sheep, goats, swine, horses, dogs | Aerosol inhalation, direct contact, ingestion of contaminated goat cheese and milk | Worldwide |
| Campylobacteriosis | Campylobacter jejuni | Rodents, dogs (puppies), cats, fowl (chickens), swine | Direct contact, ingestion of contaminated food or water | Worldwide |
| Cat-scratch disease | Bartonella henselae | Cats, dogs | Bites and scratches | United States |
| Erysipeloid | Erysipelothrix rhusiopathiae | Sheep, swine, turkeys, ducks, fish | Direct contact | Worldwide |
| Listeriosis | Listeria monocytogenes | Cattle, fowl, goats, sheep | Ingestion of contaminated food, unpasteurized cheese and dairy products | Worldwide |
| Plague | Yersinia pestis | Wild and domestic rodents, cats, dogs | Direct contact, flea bite | New Mexico, Arizona, Utah, Colorado, California |
| Rat-bite fever (bacillary fever) | Streptobacillus moniliformis | Mice, rats, hamsters | Bites, ingestion of contaminated food or water | Japan, Asia; rare in United States |
| Salmonellosis | Nontyphoidal Salmonella | Fowl, dogs, cats, reptiles, amphibians | Direct contact, ingestion of contaminated food or water | Worldwide |
| Tularemia | Francisella tularensis | Rabbits, squirrels, dogs, cats | Aerosol inhalation, direct contact, ingestion of contaminated meat, tick bite, deerfly bite | California, Utah, Arkansas, Oklahoma |
| Yersiniosis | Yersinia enterocolitica, Yersinia pseudotuberculosis | Rodents, cattle, goats, sheep, swine, fowl, dogs | Direct contact, ingestion of contaminated food or water | Worldwide |
| Wound infection, bacteremia | Pasteurella multocida, Capnocytophaga canimorsus | Cats, dogs, rodents | Direct contact, bites and scratches | Worldwide |
| **MYCOBACTERIAL DISEASES** | | | | |
| Wound infection | Mycobacterium marinum, Mycobacterium fortuitum, Mycobacterium kansasii | Fish, aquarium | Direct contact, scratches | Worldwide |
| **SPIROCHETAL DISEASES** | | | | |
| Leptospirosis | Leptospira interrogans | Dogs, rodents, livestock | Direct contact, contact with water or soil contaminated by urine of infected animals | Worldwide |

**TABLE 122-1  Major Zoonotic and Vector-Borne Infections*—cont'd**

| Disease | Causative Agent | Common Animal Reservoirs | Vector(s)/Mode(s) of Transmission | Geographic Distribution |
|---|---|---|---|---|
| Lyme disease | *Borrelia burgdorferi* | Deer, rodents | Tick bite (*Ixodes scapularis, Ixodes pacificus*) | Northeast and Midwest United States, California |
| Rat-bite fever (Haverhill fever) | *Spirillum minus* | Mice, rats, hamsters | Bites, ingestion of contaminated food or water | Japan, Asia; rare in United States |
| Relapsing fever | *Borrelia* | Rodents, fleas | Louse bite, flea bite, transplacental transmission | Western and southern United States |
| Southern tick-associated rash illness | *Borrelia lonestari* | Deer, rodents | Tick bite (*I. scapularis*) | Southeastern and south-central United States |

**RICKETTSIAL DISEASES**

*Spotted Fever Group*

| Disease | Causative Agent | Common Animal Reservoirs | Vector(s)/Mode(s) of Transmission | Geographic Distribution |
|---|---|---|---|---|
| Rocky Mountain spotted fever | *Rickettsia rickettsii* | Dogs, rodents | Tick bite (*Dermacentor variabilis*, the American dog tick; *Dermacentor andersoni*, the wood tick; *Rhipicephalus sanguineus*, the brown dog tick; *Amblyomma cajennense*) | Western hemisphere |
| Mediterranean spotted fever (boutonneuse fever) | *Rickettsia conorii* | Dogs, rodents | Tick bite | Africa, Mediterranean region, India, Middle East |
| African tick-bite fever | *Rickettsia africae* | Cattle, goats (?) | Tick bite | Sub-Saharan Africa, Caribbean |
| Rickettsialpox | *Rickettsia akari* | Mice | Mite bite | North America, Russia, Ukraine, Adriatic region, Korea, South Africa |
| Murine typhus–like illness | *Rickettsia felis* | Opossums, cats, dogs | Flea bite | Western hemisphere, Europe |

*Typhus Group*

| Disease | Causative Agent | Common Animal Reservoirs | Vector(s)/Mode(s) of Transmission | Geographic Distribution |
|---|---|---|---|---|
| Murine typhus | *Rickettsia typhi* | Rats | Rat flea or cat flea feces | Worldwide |
| Epidemic typhus | *Rickettsia prowazekii* | Humans | Louse feces | Africa, South America, Central America, Mexico, Asia |
| Brill-Zinsser disease (recrudescent typhus) | *R. prowazekii* | Humans | Reactivation of latent infection | Potentially worldwide; United States, Canada, Eastern Europe |
| Flying squirrel (sylvatic) typhus | *R. prowazekii* | Flying squirrels | Lice or fleas of flying squirrel | United States |

*Scrub Typhus*

| Disease | Causative Agent | Common Animal Reservoirs | Vector(s)/Mode(s) of Transmission | Geographic Distribution |
|---|---|---|---|---|
| Scrub typhus | *Orientia tsutsugamushi* | Rodents (?) | Chigger bite | Southern Asia, Japan, Indonesia, Australia, Korea, Asiatic Russia, India, China |

*Continued*

### TABLE 122-1 Major Zoonotic and Vector-Borne Infections*—cont'd

| Disease | Causative Agent | Common Animal Reservoirs | Vector(s)/Mode(s) of Transmission | Geographic Distribution |
|---|---|---|---|---|
| *Ehrlichiosis and Anaplasmosis* | | | | |
| Human monocytic ehrlichiosis | *Ehrlichia chaffeensis* | Deer, dogs | Tick bite (*Amblyomma americanum*) | United States, Europe, Africa |
| Anaplasmosis (human granulocytic ehrlichiosis) | *Anaplasma phagocytophilum* | Rodents, deer, ruminants | Tick bite (*I. scapularis*) | United States, Europe |
| Human ewingii ehrlichiosis | *Ehrlichia ewingii* | Dogs | Tick bite | United States |
| Sennetsu ehrlichiosis | *Neorickettsia sennetsu* | Unknown | Ingestion of helminth-contaminated fish (?) | Japan, Malaysia |
| *Q Fever* | | | | |
| Q fever | *Coxiella burnetii* | Cattle, sheep, goats, cats, rabbits | Inhalation of infected aerosols, ingestion of contaminated dairy products, tick bite (?) | Worldwide |
| **VIRAL DISEASES** | | | | |
| Colorado tick fever | Orbivirus | Rodents, ticks | Aerosol inhalation, tick bite, blood transfusion, ingestion of contaminated food | Rocky Mountains, Pacific Northwest, western Canada |
| Dengue fever | Dengue viruses (types 1–4) | Humans | Mosquito bite (*Aedes aegypti, Aedes albopictus*) | Tropical areas of the Caribbean, the Americas, and Asia |
| Hantavirus cardiopulmonary syndrome | Hantavirus | Rodents, mice, cats | Aerosol inhalation | Southwestern United States |
| Herpesvirus B infection | Herpesvirus B | Old World primates (rhesus, *Macaca cynomolgus*) | Animal bite | Africa, Asia (and primate centers worldwide) |
| Lymphocytic choriomeningitis | Lymphocytic choriomeningitis virus | Rodents, hamsters, mice | Aerosol inhalation, direct contact, bite | Worldwide |
| Rabies | Rabies virus | Dogs, skunks, bats, raccoons, foxes, cats | Bites and scratches | Worldwide |
| Vesicular stomatitis | Vesicular stomatitis virus | Horses, cattle, swine | Direct contact | Americas |
| **PROTOZOAN DISEASES** | | | | |
| African trypanosomiasis | | | | |
| East African sleeping sickness | *Trypanosoma brucei rhodesiense* | Wild and domestic animals | Insect bite (tsetse fly) | East Africa |
| West African sleeping sickness | *Trypanosoma brucei gambiense* | Wild and domestic animals | Insect bite (tsetse fly) | West Africa |
| American trypanosomiasis (Chagas disease) | *Trypanosoma cruzi* | Wild and domestic animals | Insect bite (reduviid bug); contact with fecal material of reduviid bug | South America, Central America, South Texas |
| Babesiosis | *Babesia* | Cattle, wild and domestic rodents | Tick bite (*I. scapularis*), blood transfusion | Worldwide |

**TABLE 122-1  Major Zoonotic and Vector-Borne Infections*—cont'd**

| Disease | Causative Agent | Common Animal Reservoirs | Vector(s)/Mode(s) of Transmission | Geographic Distribution |
|---|---|---|---|---|
| Leishmaniasis, mucocutaneous and cutaneous | *Leishmania* | Domestic and wild dogs | Sandfly bite | Tropics |
| Leishmaniasis, visceral | *Leishmania donovani* complex | Domestic and wild dogs | Sandfly bite | Tropics |
| Malaria | *Plasmodium* | Humans | Mosquito bite (*Anopheles*) | Usually imported to the United States, Southern California |
| Toxoplasmosis | *Toxoplasma gondii* | Cats, livestock, pigs | Ingestion of oocysts in fecally contaminated material or ingestion of tissue cysts in undercooked meat | Worldwide |

*Many helminths are also zoonotic (see Tables 123-2, 123-3, and 123-4).
Adapted from Christenson JC: Epidemiology of infectious diseases. In Jenson HB, Baltimore RS (eds): Pediatric Infectious Diseases: Principles and Practice, 2nd ed. Philadelphia, *WB Saunders*, 2002, pp 18–20.

Ticks are best removed using blunt forceps or tweezers to grasp the tick as close to the skin as possible to pull the tick steadily outward. Squeezing, twisting, or crushing the tick should be avoided because the tick's bloated abdomen can act like a syringe if squeezed. Transmission of infection seems to be most efficient after 30 to 36 hours of nymphal tick attachment for human granulocytic ehrlichiosis, after 36 to 48 hours for *B. burgdorferi*, and after 56 to 60 hours for *Babesia*. Prophylactic antimicrobial therapy after a tick bite or exposure is not recommended.

## LYME DISEASE (*Borrelia burgdorferi*)

### Etiology

Lyme disease is a tick-borne infection caused by the spirochete, *B. burgdorferi*. The vector in the eastern and midwestern United States is *Ixodes scapularis*, the **black-legged tick** that is commonly known as the **deer tick**. The vector on the Pacific Coast is *Ixodes pacificus*, the **western black-legged tick**. Ticks usually become infected by feeding on the white-footed mouse (*Peromyscus leucopus*), which is a natural reservoir for *B. burgdorferi*. The larvae are dormant over winter and emerge the following spring in the nymphal stage, which is the stage of the tick that is most likely to transmit the infection to humans.

### Epidemiology

Over 20,000 cases are reported annually in the United States, with 95% of cases reported from New England and the eastern parts of the Middle Atlantic states and the upper Midwest; with a small endemic focus along the Pacific coast (Fig. 122-1). In Europe, most cases occur in Scandinavian countries and central Europe. Because exposure to ticks is more common in warm months, Lyme disease is noted predominantly in summer. The incidence is highest among children 5 to 10 years old, at almost twice the incidence among adolescents and adults.

### Clinical Manifestations

The clinical manifestations are divided into early and late stages. Early infection may be localized or disseminated. **Early localized disease** develops 7 to 14 days after a tick bite as the site forms an erythematous papule that expands to form a red, raised border, often with central clearing. The lesion, **erythema migrans**, harbors *B. burgdorferi* and may be 15 cm wide, pruritic, or painful. Systemic manifestations may include malaise, lethargy, fever, headache, arthralgias, stiff neck, myalgias, and lymphadenopathy. The skin lesions and early manifestations resolve without treatment over 2 to 4 weeks. Not all patients with Lyme disease recall a tick bite or develop erythema migrans.

Approximately 20% of patients develop **early disseminated disease** with multiple secondary skin lesions, aseptic meningitis, pseudotumor, papilledema, cranioneuropathies including Bell palsy, polyradiculitis, peripheral neuropathy, mononeuritis multiplex, or transverse myelitis. Carditis with various degrees of heart block rarely may develop during this stage. Neurologic manifestations usually resolve by 3 months, but may recur or become chronic.

**Late disease** begins weeks to months after infection. Arthritis is the usual manifestation and may develop in 50% to 60% of untreated patients. The male-female ratio is 7:1. The knee is involved in greater than 90% of cases, but any joint may be affected. Symptoms may resolve over 1 to 2 weeks, but often recur in other joints. If untreated, most cases resolve, but chronic erosive arthritis persists in 10% of patients as the episodes increase in duration and severity. Cardiac abnormalities occur in approximately 10% of untreated patients. **Neuroborreliosis**, the late manifestations of Lyme disease involving the central nervous system (CNS), is rarely reported in children.

Reported Cases of Lyme Disease - United States, 2008

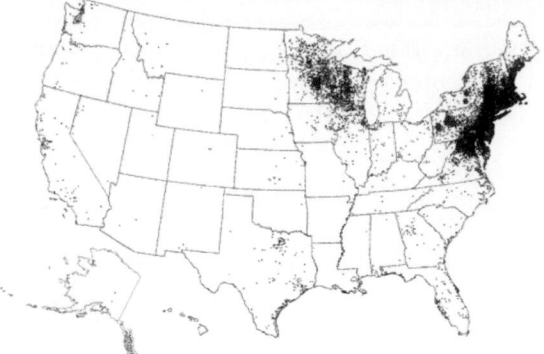

1 dot placed randomly within county of residence for each confirmed case

**FIGURE 122-1**

The geographic distribution of 28,921 confirmed cases of Lyme disease in the United States in 2008. The risk for acquiring Lyme disease varies by the distribution of *Ixodes scapularis* and *Ixodes pacificus*, the proportion of infected ticks for each species at each stage of the tick's life cycle, and the presence of grassy or wooded locations favored by white-tailed deer. (From Centers for Disease Control and Prevention: Lyme Disease—United States, 2008, available from the CDC website: *www.cdc.gov/ncidod/dvbid/Lyme/ld_Incidence.htm.*)

## Laboratory and Imaging Studies

Antibody tests during early, localized Lyme disease may be negative and are not useful. The diagnosis of late disease is confirmed by serologic tests specific for *B. burgdorferi*. The sensitivity and specificity of serologic tests for Lyme disease vary substantially. A positive enzyme-linked immunosorbent assay (ELISA) or immunofluorescence assay result must be confirmed by immunoblot showing antibodies against at least either two to three (for IgM) or five (for IgG) proteins of *B. burgdorferi* (at least one of which is one of the more specific, low-molecular-weight, outer-surface proteins).

In late disease, the erythrocyte sedimentation rate (ESR) is elevated and complement may be reduced. The joint fluid shows an inflammatory response with total white blood cell (WBC) count of 25,000 to 125,000 cells/mm$^3$, often with a polymorphonuclear predominance (see Table 118-1). The rheumatoid factor and antinuclear antibody are negative, but the Venereal Disease Research Laboratory (VDRL) test may be falsely positive. With CNS involvement, the cerebrospinal fluid (CSF) shows a lymphocytic pleocytosis with normal glucose and slightly elevated protein.

## Differential Diagnosis

A history of a tick bite and the classic rash are helpful, but are not always present. Erythema migrans of early, localized disease may be confused with nummular eczema, tinea corporis, granuloma annulare, an insect bite, or cellulitis. **Southern tick-associated rash illness**, which is similar to erythema migrans, has been described in southeastern and south-central states and is associated with the bite of *Amblyomma americanum*, the lone star tick. A spirochete that has been named *Borrelia lonestari* has been detected by DNA analysis, but has not yet been cultured.

During early, disseminated Lyme disease, multiple lesions may appear as erythema multiforme or urticaria. The aseptic meningitis is similar to viral meningitis, and the seventh nerve palsy is indistinguishable from herpetic or idiopathic Bell palsy. Lyme carditis is similar to viral myocarditis. Monarticular or pauciarticular arthritis of late Lyme disease may mimic suppurative arthritis, juvenile idiopathic arthritis, or rheumatic fever (see Chapter 89). The differential diagnosis of neuroborreliosis includes degenerative neurologic illness, encephalitis, and depression.

## Treatment

Early, localized disease and early, disseminated disease, including facial nerve palsy (or other cranial nerve palsy) and carditis with first-degree or second-degree heart block, is treated with doxycycline or amoxicillin for 14 to 21 days. Early disease with carditis with third-degree heart block or meningitis and late neurologic disease (other than facial nerve or other cranial nerve palsy) are treated with intravenous (IV) or intramuscular (IM) ceftriaxone or IV penicillin G for 14 to 28 days. Arthritis is treated with doxycycline (for children >9 years of age) or amoxicillin for 28 days. If there is recurrence, treatment should be with a repeated oral regimen or with the regimen for late neurologic disease.

## Complications and Prognosis

Carditis, especially conduction disturbances, and arthritis are the major complications of Lyme disease. Even untreated, most cases eventually resolve without sequelae.

Lyme disease is readily treatable and curable. The long-term prognosis is excellent for early and late disease. Early treatment may prevent progression to carditis and meningitis. Recurrences of arthritis are rare after recommended treatment. A community-based study of children with Lyme disease found no evidence of impairment 4 to 11 years later.

## Prevention

Measures to minimize exposure to tick-borne diseases are the most reasonable means of preventing Lyme disease. Postexposure prophylaxis is not routinely recommended because the overall risk of acquiring Lyme disease after a tick bite is only 1% to 2% even in endemic areas, and treatment of the infection, if it develops, is highly effective. Nymphal stage ticks must feed for 36 to 48 hours, and adult ticks must feed for 48 to 72 hours before the risk of transmission of *B. burgdorferi* from infected ticks becomes substantial. In hyperendemic regions, prophylaxis of adults with doxycycline, 200 mg as a single dose, within 72 hours of a nymphal tick bite is effective in preventing Lyme disease.

# ROCKY MOUNTAIN SPOTTED FEVER (*Rickettsia rickettsii*)

## Etiology

The cause of Rocky Mountain spotted fever is *R. rickettsii,* gram-negative coccobacillary organisms that resemble bacteria but have incomplete cell walls and require an intracellular site for replication. The organism invades and proliferates within the endothelial cells of blood vessels causing vasculitis and resulting in increased vascular permeability, edema, and, eventually, decreased vascular volume, altered tissue perfusion, and widespread organ failure. Many tick species are capable of transmitting *R. rickettsii.* The principal ticks are the **American dog tick** (*Dermacentor variabilis*) in the eastern United States and Canada, the **wood tick** (*Dermacentor andersoni*) in the western United States and Canada, the **brown dog tick** (*Rhipicephalus sanguineus*) in Mexico, and *Amblyomma cajennense* in Central and South America.

## Epidemiology

Rocky Mountain spotted fever is the most common rickettsial illness in the United States, occurring primarily in the eastern coastal, southeastern, and western states. Most cases occur from May to October after outdoor activity in wooded areas, with peak incidence among children 1 to 14 years of age. Approximately 40% of infected persons are unable to recall a tick bite.

## Clinical Manifestations

The incubation period of Rocky Mountain spotted fever is 2 to 14 days, with an average of 7 days. The onset is nonspecific with headache, malaise, and fever. A pale, rose-red macular or maculopapular rash appears in 90% of cases. The rash begins peripherally and spreads to involve the entire body, including palms and soles. The early rash blanches on pressure and is accentuated by warmth. It progresses over hours or days to a petechial and purpuric eruption that appears first on the feet and ankles, then the wrists and hands, and progresses centripetally to the trunk and head. Myalgias, especially of the lower extremities, and intractable headaches are common. Severe cases progress with splenomegaly, myocarditis, renal impairment, pneumonitis, and shock.

## Laboratory and Imaging Studies

Thrombocytopenia (usually <100,000 cells/mm$^3$), anemia, hyponatremia, and elevated hepatic transaminase levels are common laboratory findings. Organisms can be detected in skin biopsy specimens by fluorescent antibodies, although this test is not widely available. Serologic testing is used to confirm the diagnosis, although treatment is begun before confirmation.

## Differential Diagnosis

The differential diagnosis includes meningococcemia, bacterial sepsis, toxic shock syndrome, leptospirosis, ehrlichiosis, measles, enteroviruses, infectious mononucleosis, collagen vascular diseases, Schönlein-Henoch purpura, and idiopathic thrombocytopenic purpura. The diagnosis of Rocky Mountain spotted fever should be suspected with fever and petechial rash, especially with a history of a tick bite or outdoor activities during spring and summer in endemic regions. Fever, headache, and myalgias lasting more than 1 week in patients in endemic areas indicate Rocky Mountain spotted fever. Delayed diagnosis and late treatment usually result from atypical initial symptoms and late appearance of the rash.

## Treatment

Therapy for suspected Rocky Mountain spotted fever should not be postponed pending results of diagnostic tests. Doxycycline is the drug of choice, even for young children despite the theoretical risk of dental staining in children younger than 9 years of age. Fluoroquinolones also are active against *R. rickettsii* and may be an alternative treatment for adults.

## Complications and Prognosis

In severe infections, capillary leakage results in noncardiogenic pulmonary edema (acute respiratory distress syndrome), hypotension, disseminated intravascular coagulation, circulatory collapse, and multiple organ failure including encephalitis, myocarditis, hepatitis, and renal failure.

Untreated illness may persist for 3 weeks before progressing to multisystem involvement. The mortality rate is 25% without treatment, which is reduced to 3.4% with treatment. Permanent sequelae are common after severe disease.

## Prevention

Preventive measures to avoid tick-borne infections and careful removal of ticks are recommended.

# EHRLICHIOSIS (*Ehrlichia chaffeensis*) AND ANAPLASMOSIS (*Anaplasma phagocytophilum*)

## Etiology

The term **ehrlichiosis** often is used to refer to all forms of infection with *Ehrlichia.* **Human monocytic ehrlichiosis** is caused by *E. chaffeensis,* which infects predominantly monocytic cells and is transmitted by the tick *A. americanum.* **Human anaplasmosis**, formerly named **granulocytic ehrlichiosis**, is caused by *A. phagocytophilum* and is transmitted by the tick *I. scapularis.* Disease caused by *Ehrlichia ewingii* has been identified by various names, including **ehrlichiosis ewingii**.

## Epidemiology

Ehrlichiosis occurs commonly in the United States. Human monocytic ehrlichiosis occurs in broad areas across the southeastern, south central, and mid-Atlantic United States in a distribution that parallels that of Rocky Mountain spotted fever. Anaplasmosis is the most frequently recognized ehrlichiosis and is found mostly in the northeastern and upper midwestern United States, but infections have now been identified in northern California, the mid-Atlantic states, and broadly across Europe.

## Clinical Manifestations

Human monocytic ehrlichiosis, anaplasmosis, and ehrlichiosis ewingii cause similar acute febrile illness characterized by fever, malaise, headache, myalgias, anorexia, and nausea, but often without a rash. In contrast to adult patients, nearly two thirds of children with human monocytic ehrlichiosis present with a macular or maculo-papular rash, although petechial lesions may occur. Symptoms usually last for 4 to 12 days.

## Laboratory and Imaging Studies

Characteristic laboratory findings include leukopenia, lymphocytopenia, thrombocytopenia, anemia, and elevated hepatic transaminases. Morulae are found infrequently in circulating monocytes of persons with human monocytic ehrlichiosis, but are found in 40% of circulating neutrophils in 20% to 60% of persons with anaplasmosis (Fig. 122-2). Seroconversion or fourfold rise in antibody titer confirms the diagnosis.

## Differential Diagnosis

Ehrlichiosis is clinically similar to other arthropod-borne infections, including Rocky Mountain spotted fever, tularemia, babesiosis, early Lyme disease, murine typhus, relapsing fever, and Colorado tick fever. The differential diagnosis also includes infectious mononucleosis, Kawasaki disease, endocarditis, viral infections, hepatitis, leptospirosis, Q fever, collagen vascular diseases, and leukemia.

## Treatment

As with Rocky Mountain spotted fever, therapy for suspected ehrlichiosis should not be postponed pending results of diagnostic tests. Ehrlichiosis and anaplasmosis are treated with tetracyclines, primarily doxycycline.

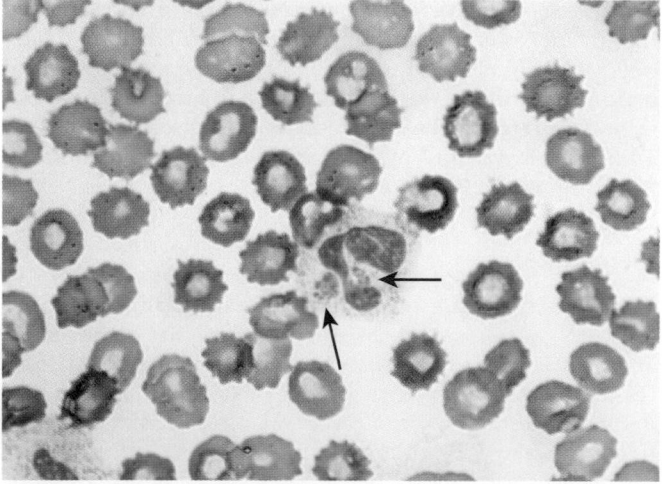

**FIGURE 122-2**

A morula (*arrowhead*) containing *Anaplasma phagocytophilum* in a neutrophil. *Ehrlichia chaffeensis* and *A. phagocytophilum* have similar morphologies but are serologically and genetically distinct. (Wright stain, original magnification ×1200.) (From Walker DH, Dumler JS: *Ehrlichia chaffeensis* (human monocytotropic ehrlichiosis), *Anaplasma phagocytophilum* (human granulocytotropic anaplasmosis), and other ehrlichieae. In Mandell GL, Bennett JE, Dolin R [eds]: Principles and Practice of Infectious Diseases, 6th ed. Philadelphia, *Churchill Livingstone*, 2005; Fig. 190-2, p 2315.)

## Complications and Prognosis

Severe pulmonary involvement with acute respiratory distress syndrome has been reported in several cases. Other reported severe complications include meningoencephalitis and myocarditis. Most patients improve within 48 hours.

## Prevention

Preventive measures to avoid tick-borne infections and careful removal of ticks are recommended.

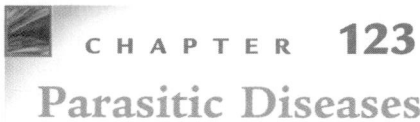

CHAPTER **123**

# Parasitic Diseases

## PROTOZOAL DISEASES

Protozoa are the simplest organisms of the animal kingdom. They are unicellular, and most are free living, but some have a commensal or parasitic existence. Protozoal diseases include malaria, toxoplasmosis, babesiosis, and the intestinal protozoal diseases, amebiasis, cryptosporidiosis, and giardiasis.

## Malaria

### Etiology

Malaria is caused by obligate intracellular protozoa of the genus *Plasmodium*, including *P. falciparum*, *P. malariae*, *P. ovale*, and *P. vivax*. *Plasmodium* has a complex life cycle that enables survival in different cellular environments in the human host and in the mosquito vector. There are two major phases in the life cycle, an **asexual phase (schizogony)** in humans and a **sexual phase (sporogony)** in mosquitoes. The **erythrocytic phase** of *Plasmodium* asexual development begins when the merozoites released from exoerythrocytic schizonts in the liver penetrate erythrocytes. When inside the erythrocyte, the parasite transforms into the **ring form**, which enlarges to become a **trophozoite**. These latter two forms can be identified with Giemsa stain on blood smear, which is the primary means of confirming the diagnosis of malaria.

The parasites usually are transmitted to humans by female *Anopheles* mosquitoes. Malaria also can be transmitted through blood transfusion, via contaminated needles, and transplacentally to a fetus.

### Epidemiology

Malaria is a worldwide problem with transmission in more than 100 countries with a combined population of more than 1.6 billion people. Malaria is an important cause of fever and morbidity in the tropical world. The principal areas of transmission are sub-Saharan Africa, southern Asia, South East Asia, Mexico, Haiti, the Dominican Republic, Central and South America, Papua New Guinea, and the Solomon Islands. Approximately 1000 to 2000 imported cases are recognized annually in the United States, with most cases occurring among infected foreign civilians from endemic areas who travel to the United States and among U.S. citizens who travel to endemic areas without appropriate chemoprophylaxis.

## Clinical Manifestations

The clinical manifestations of malaria range from asymptomatic infection to fulminant illness and death depending on the virulence of the infecting malaria species and the host immune response. The incubation period ranges from 6 to 30 days depending on the *Plasmodium* species (Table 123-1). The most characteristic clinical feature of malaria, which is seldom noted with other infectious diseases, is **febrile paroxysms** alternating with periods of fatigue but otherwise relative wellness. The classic symptoms of the febrile paroxysms of malaria include high fever, rigors, sweats, and headache. Paroxysms coincide with the rupture of schizonts that occur every 48 hours

with *P. vivax* and *P. ovale* (**tertian periodicity**) and every 72 hours with *P. malariae* (**quartan periodicity**).

**Short-term relapse** describes the recurrence of symptoms after a primary attack that is due to the survival of erythrocyte forms in the bloodstream. **Long-term relapse** describes the renewal of symptoms long after the primary attack, usually due to release of merozoites from an exoerythrocytic source in the liver. Long-term relapse occurs with *P. vivax* and *P. ovale* because of persistence in the liver and with *P. malariae* because of persistence in the erythrocyte.

## Laboratory and Imaging Studies

The diagnosis of malaria is established by identification of organisms on stained smears of peripheral blood. In nonimmune persons, symptoms typically occur 1 to 2 days before parasites are detectable on blood smear. Although *P. falciparum* is most likely to be identified from blood during a febrile paroxysm, the timing of the smears is less

**TABLE 123-1 Characteristics of *Plasmodium* Species Causing Malaria**

| Characteristic | P. falciparum | P. vivax | P. ovale | P. malariae |
|---|---|---|---|---|
| Exoerythrocytic cycle | 5.5–7 days | 6–8 days | 9 days | 12–16 days |
| Erythrocytic cycle | 48 hours | 42–48 hours | 49–50 hours | 72 hours |
| Prepatent period | 9–10 days | 11–13 days | 10–14 days | 15 days |
| Usual incubation period (range) | 12 days (9–14 days) | 13 days (12–17 days; may be longer) | 17 days (16–18 days; may be longer) | 28 days (18–40 days; may be longer) |
| Merozoites per hepatic schizont | 30,000 | 10,000 | 15,000 | 2000 |
| Erythrocyte preference | Young erythrocytes, but can infect all | Reticulocytes | Reticulocytes | Older erythrocytes |
| Usual parasite load (% erythrocytes infected) | ≥1–5 | 1–2 | 1–2 | 1–2 |
| Secondary exoerythrocytic cycle (hypnozoites) and relapses | Absent | Present | Present | Absent |
| Duration of untreated infection | 1–2 years | 1.5–4 years (includes liver stage) | 1.5–4 years (includes liver stage) | 3–50 years |
| Severity of primary attack | Severe in nonimmune forms; subpatent patients—**a medical emergency**—failure to recognize and treat can lead to death | Mild to severe—danger of splenic rupture, relapse related to persistence of latent exoerythrocytic forms | Mild—danger of splenic rupture, relapse related to persistence of latent exoerythrocytic forms | Can be chronic in subclinical and subpatent forms; can cause nephritis in children |
| Usual periodicity of febrile attacks | None | 48 hours | 48 hours | 72 hours |
| Duration of febrile paroxysm | 16–36 hours (may be longer) | 8–12 hours | 8–12 hours | 8–10 hours |

Adapted from Strickland GT: Malaria. In Strickland GT (ed): Hunter's Tropical Medicine, 7th ed. Philadelphia, *WB Saunders*, 1991, p 589.

important than obtaining smears several times each day over 3 successive days. Both thick and thin blood smears should be examined. The concentration of erythrocytes on a **thick smear** is approximately 20 to 40 times greater than on a **thin smear**. Thick smears are used to scan large numbers of erythrocytes quickly. Thin smears allow for positive identification of the malaria species and determination of the percentage of infected erythrocytes, which also is useful in following the response to therapy.

## Differential Diagnosis

The most important aspect of diagnosis of malaria in children is to consider the possibility of malaria in any child who has fever, chills, splenomegaly, anemia, or decreased level of consciousness with a history of recent travel or residence in an endemic area, regardless of the use of chemoprophylaxis. The differential diagnosis is broad and includes many infectious diseases, such as tuberculosis, typhoid fever, brucellosis, relapsing fever, infective endocarditis, influenza, poliomyelitis, yellow fever, trypanosomiasis, kala-azar, and amebic liver abscess.

## Treatment

Oral chloroquine is the recommended treatment except for chloroquine-resistant *P. falciparum*. Quinine sulfate plus tetracycline, quinine plus pyrimethamine-sulfadoxine, or mefloquine are used for chloroquine-resistant malaria. Patients with malaria usually require hospitalization and may require intensive care unit (ICU) admission. Quinidine gluconate is used for parenteral treatment.

## Complications and Prognosis

Cerebral malaria is a complication of *P. falciparum* infection and a frequent cause of death (20–40% of cases), especially among children and nonimmune adults. Similar to other complications, cerebral malaria is more likely to occur among patients with intense parasitemia ($\geq$5%). Other complications include splenic rupture, renal failure, severe hemolysis (**blackwater fever**), pulmonary edema, hypoglycemia, thrombocytopenia, and **algid malaria** (sepsis syndrome with vascular collapse).

Death may occur with any of the malarial species, but is most frequent with complicated *P. falciparum* malaria. The likelihood of death is increased in children with preexisting health problems, such as measles, intestinal parasites, schistosomiasis, anemia, and malnutrition. Death is much more common in developing countries.

## Prevention

There are two components of malaria prevention: reduction of exposure to infected mosquitoes and chemoprophylaxis. Mosquito protection is necessary because no prophylactic regimen can guarantee protection in every instance because of the widespread development of resistant organisms.

**Chemoprophylaxis** is necessary for all visitors to and residents of the tropics who have not lived there since infancy. Children of nonimmune women should have chemoprophylaxis from birth. Children of women from endemic areas have passive immunity until 3 to 6 months of age, after which they are increasingly likely to acquire malaria. Chemoprophylaxis should be started 1 to 2 weeks before a person enters the endemic area except for doxycycline, which can be started 1 to 2 days before, and should continue for at least 4 weeks after the person leaves. In the few remaining areas of the world that are free of chloroquine-resistant malaria strains, chloroquine is given once per week. In areas where chloroquine-resistant *P. falciparum* exists, mefloquine is recommended for all ages. Travelers to South East Asia, especially to the Thai-Cambodian and Thai-Myanmar (Burma) border areas, the Amazon basin, and some countries in Africa should take atovaquone-proguanil or doxycycline. Mefloquine should not be used for self-treatment because of the frequency of serious adverse effects at treatment doses. There have been several reports of mefloquine and pyrimethamine-sulfadoxine resistance.

## Toxoplasmosis

Toxoplasmosis is a zoonosis caused by *Toxoplasma gondii*, an intracellular protozoan parasite. Infection is acquired by infectious oocysts, such as those excreted by newly infected cats, which play an important role in amplifying the organism in nature, or from ingesting cysts in contaminated, undercooked meat. Less commonly, transmission occurs transplacentally during acute infection of pregnant women. In the United States, the incidence of congenital infection is 1 to 2 per 1000 live births.

Acquired toxoplasmosis is usually asymptomatic. Symptomatic infection is typically a heterophile-negative mononucleosis syndrome that includes lymphadenopathy, fever, and hepatosplenomegaly. Disseminated infection, including myocarditis, pneumonia, and central nervous system (CNS) toxoplasmosis, is more common among immunocompromised persons, especially persons with acquired immunodeficiency syndrome (AIDS). Among women infected during pregnancy, 40% to 60% give birth to an infected infant. The later in pregnancy that infection occurs, the more likely it is that the fetus will be infected, but the less severe the illness (see Chapter 66). Serologic diagnosis can be established by a fourfold increase in antibody titer or seroconversion, a positive IgM antibody titer, or positive polymerase chain reaction (PCR) for *T. gondii* in peripheral white blood cells (WBCs), cerebrospinal fluid (CSF), serum, or amniotic fluid.

Treatment includes pyrimethamine and sulfadiazine, which act synergistically against *Toxoplasma*. Because these compounds are folic acid inhibitors, they are used in conjunction with folinic acid. Spiramycin, which is not licensed in the United States, also is used in therapy of pregnant women with toxoplasmosis. Corticosteroids are reserved for patients with acute CNS or ocular infection.

Ingesting only well-cooked meat and avoiding cats or soil in areas where cats defecate are prudent measures for pregnant or immunocompromised persons. Administration of spiramycin to infected pregnant women has been associated with lower risks of congenital infection in their offspring.

# HELMINTHIASES

Helminths are divided into three groups: roundworms, or nematodes, and two groups of flatworms, the trematodes (flukes) and the cestodes (tapeworms).

## Hookworm Infections

Hookworm infection is caused by several species of hookworms, with *Ancylostoma duodenale* and *Necator americanus* being the most important (Table 123-2). There are more than 9 million humans worldwide infected with hookworms. *Ancyclostoma duodenale* is the predominant species in Europe, the Mediterranean region, northern Asia, and the west coast of South America. *N. americanus* predominates in the Western hemisphere, sub-Saharan Africa, South East Asia, and the Pacific Islands. Optimal soil conditions and fecal contamination are found in many agrarian tropical countries and in the southeastern United States. Infection typically occurs in young children, especially during the first decade of life. The larvae are found in warm, damp soil and infect humans by penetrating the skin. They migrate to the lungs, ascend the trachea, are swallowed, and reside in the intestine. The worms mature and attach to the intestinal wall, where they suck blood and shed eggs.

Infections are usually asymptomatic. Intense pruritus (**ground itch**) occurs at the site of larval penetration, usually the soles of the feet or between the toes, and may include papules and vesicles. Migration of larvae through the lungs usually is asymptomatic. Symptoms of abdominal pain, anorexia, indigestion, fullness, and diarrhea occur with hookworm infestation. The major manifestation of infection is anemia. Examination of fresh stool for hookworm eggs is diagnostic. Therapy includes anthelmintic treatment with albendazole, mebendazole, or pyrantel pamoate and treatment for anemia. Eradication depends on sanitation of the patient's environment and chemotherapy.

## Ascariasis

Ascariasis is caused by *Ascaris lumbricoides,* a large nematode. It is the most prevalent helminthiasis, affecting 1 billion people (see Table 123-2). After humans ingest the eggs, larvae are released and penetrate the intestine, migrate to the lungs, ascend the trachea, and are swallowed. On entering the intestines again, they mature and produce eggs that are excreted in the stool and are deposited in the soil, where they survive for prolonged periods.

**TABLE 123-2 Major Pediatric Syndromes Caused by Parasitic Nematodes**

| Syndrome | Etiologic Agent | Transmission | Treatment |
|---|---|---|---|
| Hookworm iron deficiency | *Ancylostoma duodenale* | Larval ingestion and penetration | Albendazole *or* mebendazole *or* pyrantel pamoate |
| | *Necator americanus* | Larval penetration | |
| Cutaneous larva migrans | *Ancylostoma braziliense* (a zoonotic hookworm) | Larval penetration (and failure to migrate) | Albendazole *or* ivermectin *or* thiabendazole topically |
| Infant ancylostomiasis | *A. duodenale* | Perinatal (?) | Albendazole *or* mebendazole *or* pyrantel pamoate |
| *Trichuris* dysentery or colitis | *Trichuris trichiura* | Egg ingestion | Mebendazole *or* albendazole *or* pyrantel pamoate and oxantel pamoate |
| Intestinal ascariasis | *Ascaris lumbricoides* | Ingestion of *Ascaris* eggs | Albendazole *or* mebendazole *or* pyrantel pamoate |
| Neonatal ascariasis | | Transplacental | |
| Visceral larva migrans | *Toxocara canis* | Egg ingestion | Albendazole *or* mebendazole |
| Ocular larva migrans | *Toxocara cati* *Baylisascaris procyonis* | | |
| Diarrhea, malabsorption (celiac-like) | *Strongyloides stercoralis* | Larval penetration | Ivermectin *or* thiabendazole |
| Swollen belly syndrome | *Strongyloides fuelleborni* | Perinatal | Ivermectin *or* thiabendazole |
| Pinworm | *Enterobius vermicularis* | Ingestion of embryonated eggs | Albendazole *or* mebendazole *or* pyrantel pamoate |
| Trichinellosis | *Trichinella spiralis* | Ingestion of infected undercooked meat | Mebendazole *or* albendazole *plus* corticosteroids for severe symptoms |
| Abdominal angiostrongyliasis | *Angiostrongylus costaricensis* | Ingestion of contaminated food | Mebendazole *or* thiabendazole |
| Eosinophilic meningitis | *Angiostrongylus cantonensis* (rat lungworm) | Ingestion of undercooked contaminated seafood | Mebendazole |

Manifestations may be the result of migration of the larvae to other sites of the body or the presence of adult worms in the intestine. **Pulmonary ascariasis** occurs as the larvae migrate through the lung, producing cough, blood-stained sputum, eosinophilia, and transient infiltrates on chest x-ray films. Adult larvae in the small intestine may cause abdominal pain and distention. Intestinal obstruction from adult worms rarely occurs. Migration of worms into the bile duct may rarely cause acute biliary obstruction. Examination of fresh stool for characteristic eggs is diagnostic. Effective control depends on adequate sanitary treatment and disposal of infected human feces.

## Visceral Larva Migrans

Visceral larva migrans is a systemic nematodiasis caused by ingestion of the eggs of the dog tapeworm, *Toxocara canis*, or, less commonly, the cat tapeworm, *Toxocara cati*, or the raccoon tapeworm, *Baylisascaris procyonis* (see Table 123-2). These organisms also cause **ocular larva migrans**.

Visceral larva migrans is most common in young children with pica who have dogs or cats as pets. Ocular toxocariasis occurs in older children. The eggs of these roundworms are produced by adult worms residing in the dog and cat intestine. Ingested eggs hatch into larvae that penetrate the gastrointestinal tract and migrate to the liver, lung, eye, CNS, and heart, where they die and calcify.

Symptoms of visceral larva migrans are the result of the number of migrating worms and the associated immune response. Light infections are often asymptomatic. Symptoms include fever, cough, wheezing, and seizures. Physical findings may include hepatomegaly, crackles, rash, and lymphadenopathy. Visual symptoms may include decreased acuity, strabismus, periorbital edema, or blindness. Eye examination may reveal granulomatous lesions near the macula or disc. Ocular larva migrans is characterized by isolated, unilateral ocular disease and no systemic findings. Larvae probably enter the anterior vitreous of the eye from a peripheral branch of the retinal artery and elicit granulomas in the posterior and peripheral poles that cause vision loss.

Eosinophilia and hypergammaglobulinemia associated with elevated isohemagglutinin levels suggest the diagnosis, which is confirmed by serology (ELISA [enzyme-linked immunosorbent assay]) or, less commonly, by biopsy. This is usually a self-limited illness. In severe disease, albendazole or mebendazole is used. Deworming puppies and kittens, major excreters of eggs, decreases the risk of infection.

## Enterobiasis (Pinworm)

Pinworm is caused by *Enterobius vermicularis*, a nematode that is distributed worldwide. Enterobiasis affects individuals at all socioeconomic levels, especially children. Crowded living conditions predispose to infection. Humans ingest the eggs carried on hands, present in house dust or on bedclothes. The eggs hatch in the stomach, and the larvae migrate to the cecum and mature. At night, the females migrate to the perianal area to lay their eggs, which are viable for 2 days.

The most common symptoms are nocturnal anal pruritus (**pruritus ani**) and sleeplessness, presumably resulting from the migratory female worms. Vaginitis and salpingitis may develop secondary to aberrant worm migration. The eggs are detected by microscopically examining adhesive cellophane tape pressed against the anus in the morning to collect eggs. Less commonly, a worm may be seen in the perianal region. Treatment is with albendazole (400 mg), mebendazole (100 mg), or pyrantel pamoate (11 mg/kg, maximum 1 g) each given as a single oral dose and repeated in 2 weeks.

## Schistosomiasis

Schistosomiasis (bilharziasis) is caused by flukes that parasitize the bloodstream, including *Schistosoma haematobium*, *Schistosoma mansoni*, *Schistosoma japonicum*, and, rarely, *Schistosoma intercalatum* and *Schistosoma mekongi* (Table 123-3). Schistosomiasis affects more than 2 million people, mainly children and young adults with a peak age range of 10 to 20 years. Humans are infected by cercariae in contaminated water that emerge in an infectious form from snails and penetrate intact skin. Each adult worm migrates to specific sites: *S. haematobium* to the **bladder plexus** and *S. intercalatum* and *S. mekongi* to the **mesenteric vessels**. The eggs are deposited by the adult flukes in urine (*S. haematobium*) or stool (*S. mansoni* and *S. japonicum*). *S. haematobium* is prevalent in Africa and the Middle East; *S. mansoni* in Africa, the Middle East, the Caribbean, and South America; *S. japonicum* in China, the Philippines, and Indonesia; *S. mekongi* in the Far East; and *S. intercalatum* in West Africa.

The manifestations of schistosomiasis result from eggs that are trapped at the site of deposition or at metastatic locations. Within 3 to 12 weeks of infection, while the worms are maturing, a syndrome of fever, malaise, cough, abdominal pain, and rash can occur. This syndrome is followed by a resultant inflammatory response that leads to further symptoms. **Katayama fever** is an acute condition, with fever, weight loss, hepatosplenomegaly, and eosinophilia. Eggs may be found in the urine (*S. haematobium*) or stool (*S. mansoni* and *S. japonicum*) of infected individuals. Sanitary measures, molluscacides, and therapy for infected individuals may help control the illness.

## Echinococcosis

Echinococcosis includes **hydatid or unilocular cyst disease**, caused by *Echinococcus granulosus* (the **minute dog tapeworm**) or *Echinococcus vogeli*, and **alveolar cyst disease**, caused by *Echinococcus multilocularis* (Table 123-4). Dogs become infected with tapeworms by eating infected sheep or cattle viscera and excrete eggs in their stools. Humans acquire echinococcosis by ingesting eggs and become an intermediate host. The eggs hatch in the intestinal tract, and the larva (**oncospheres**) penetrate the mucosa and enter the circulation to pass to the liver and other visceral organs, forming cysts 2 cm in diameter.

*E. granulosus* has a worldwide distribution and is endemic in sheep-raising and cattle-raising areas of Australia, South

| TABLE 123-3 Major Pediatric Syndromes Caused by Parasitic Trematodes | | | |
|---|---|---|---|
| **Syndrome** | **Etiologic Agent** | **Transmission** | **Treatment** |
| Schistosomiases | | Freshwater contact with penetration through the skin | |
| Intestinal or hepatic schistosomiasis | *Schistosoma mansoni* | | Praziquantel *or* oxamniquine |
| | *Schistosoma japonicum* | | Praziquantel |
| | *Schistosoma mekongi* | | Praziquantel |
| Urinary schistosomiasis | *Schistosoma haematobium* | | Praziquantel |
| Parasitoses due to other trematodes | | Ingestion of raw or inadequately cooked foods | |
| Clonorchiasis | *Clonorchis sinensis* (Chinese liver fluke) | | Praziquantel *or* albendazole |
| Fascioliasis | *Fasciola hepatica* (sheep liver fluke) | | Triclabendazole *or* bithionol |
| Fasciolopsiasis | *Fasciolopsis buski* | | Praziquantel |
| Heterophyiasis | *Heterophyes heterophyes* | | Praziquantel |
| Metagonimiasis | *Metagonimus yokogawai* | | Praziquantel |
| Metorchiasis | *Metorchis conjunctus* (North American liver fluke) | | Praziquantel |
| Nanophyetiasis | *Nanophyetus salmincola* (salmon fluke) | | Praziquantel |
| Opisthorchiasis | *Opisthorchis viverrini* (Southeast Asian liver fluke) | | Praziquantel |
| Paragonimiasis | *Paragonimus westermani, P. miyazaki, P. mexicanus, P. kellicotti, P. uterobilateralis, P. skjabini, P. hueitungensis, P. heterotrema, P. africanus* (lung flukes) | | Praziquantel *or* bithionol |

| TABLE 123-4 Major Pediatric Syndromes Caused by Parasitic Cestodes | | | |
|---|---|---|---|
| **Syndrome** | **Etiologic Agent** | **Transmission** | **Treatment** |
| Echinococcosis | | Ingestion of *Echinococcus* eggs | |
| Unilocular echinococcosis | *Echinococcus granulosus* | | Surgical resection *plus* albendazole |
| | *Echinococcus granulosus* var. *canadensis* | | Expectant observation |
| Alveolar echinococcosis | *Echinococcus multilocularis* | | Surgical resection is only reliable means of treatment; some reports suggest adjunct use of albendazole or mebendazole |
| Neurocysticercosis | Larval stage of *Taenia solium* (cysticerci) | Ingestion of infected raw/ undercooked pork | Albendazole *or* praziquantel |
| Adult tapeworm infections | *T. solium* (pork tapeworm) | Ingestion of contaminated raw/ undercooked pork | Praziquantel |
| | *Hymenolepis diminuta* | Fecal-oral transmission | Praziquantel |
| | *Hymenolepis nana* | Fecal-oral transmission | Praziquantel |

America, South Africa, the former Soviet Union, and the Mediterranean region. The prevalence is highest in children. Symptoms caused by *E. granulosus* result from space-occupying cysts. Pulmonary cysts may cause hemoptysis, cough, dyspnea, and respiratory distress. Brain cysts appear as tumors; liver cysts cause problems as they compress and obstruct blood flow. Ultrasonography identifies cystic lesions, and the diagnosis is confirmed by serologic testing. Large or asymptomatic granulosa cysts are removed surgically. Treatment with albendazole has shown some benefit.

## Neurocysticercosis

Neurocysticercosis is caused by infection with the larval stages (**cysticerci**) of the **pork tapeworm**, *Taenia solium*, and is the most frequent helminthic infection of the CNS (see Table 123-4). Human cysticercosis is a biologic "dead end" infection. Humans are infected after consuming cysticerci in raw or undercooked larva-containing pork. *T. solium* is endemic in Asia, Africa, and Central and South America.

Cysts typically enlarge slowly, causing no or minimal symptoms for years or decades until the organism begins to die. The cyst then begins to swell, and leakage of antigen incites an inflammatory response, resulting in the presenting signs of focal or generalized seizures and calcified cerebral cysts identified by computed tomography (CT) or magnetic resonance imaging (MRI). The CSF shows lymphocytic or eosinophilic pleocytosis. The diagnosis is confirmed by serologic testing. Neurocysticercosis is treated with albendazole or praziquantel, corticosteroids for concomitant cerebral inflammation from cyst death, and anticonvulsant drugs.

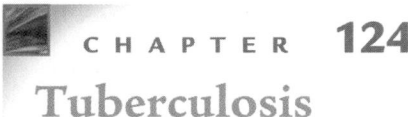

CHAPTER **124**

# Tuberculosis

## ETIOLOGY

The agent of human tuberculosis is *Mycobacterium tuberculosis*. The **tubercle bacilli** are pleomorphic, weakly gram-positive curved rods 2 to 4 μm long. Mycobacteria are **acid fast**, which is the capacity to form stable mycolate complexes with arylmethane dyes. The term **acid-fast bacilli** is practically synonymous with mycobacteria. Mycobacteria grow slowly and culture from clinical specimens on solid synthetic media usually takes 3 to 6 weeks. Drug-susceptibility testing requires an additional 4 weeks. Growth can be detected in 1 to 3 weeks in selective liquid media using radiolabeled nutrients. Polymerase chain reaction (PCR) of clinical specimens allows rapid diagnosis in many laboratories.

## EPIDEMIOLOGY

Susceptibility to infection with *M. tuberculosis* disease depends on the likelihood of exposure to an individual with infectious tuberculosis and the ability of the person's immune system to control the initial infection and keep it latent. An estimated 10 to 15 million persons in the United States have latent tuberculosis infection. Without treatment, tuberculosis *disease* develops in 5% to 10% of immunologically normal adults with tuberculosis *infection* at some time during their lives. An estimated 8 million new cases of tuberculosis occur each year among adults worldwide, and 3 million deaths are attributed to the disease annually. In developing countries, 1.3 million new cases of the disease occur in children under 15 years of age, and 450,000 children die each year of tuberculosis. Most children with tuberculosis infection and disease acquire *M. tuberculosis* from an infectious adult.

Transmission of *M. tuberculosis* is from person to person, usually by **respiratory droplets** that become airborne when the ill individual coughs, sneezes, laughs, sighs, or breathes. Infected droplets dry and become **droplet nuclei**, which may remain suspended in the air for hours, long after the infectious person has left the environment. Only particles less than 10 μm in diameter can reach the alveoli and establish infection.

Several patient-related factors are associated with an increased chance of transmission. Of these, a positive acid-fast smear of the sputum most closely correlates with infectivity. Children with primary pulmonary tuberculosis disease rarely, if ever, infect other children or adults. Tubercle bacilli are relatively sparse in the endobronchial secretions of children with primary pulmonary tuberculosis, and a significant cough is usually lacking. When young children cough, they rarely produce sputum, lacking the tussive force necessary to project and suspend infectious particles of the requisite size. Hospitalized children with suspected pulmonary tuberculosis are placed in respiratory isolation initially. Most infectious patients become noninfectious within 2 weeks of starting effective treatment, and many become noninfectious within several days.

In North America, tuberculosis rates are highest in foreign-born persons from high-prevalence countries, residents of prisons, residents of nursing homes, homeless persons, users of illegal drugs, persons who are poor and medically indigent, health care workers, and children exposed to adults in high-risk groups. Among U.S. urban dwellers with tuberculosis, persons with acquired immunodeficiency syndrome (AIDS) and racial minorities are overrepresented. Most children are infected with *M. tuberculosis* from household contacts, but outbreaks of childhood tuberculosis centered in elementary and high schools, nursery schools, family day care homes, churches, school buses, and stores still occur. A high-risk adult working in the area has been the source of the outbreak in most cases.

## CLINICAL MANIFESTATIONS

**Tuberculosis infection** describes the asymptomatic stage of infection with *M. tuberculosis*, also termed **latent tuberculosis**. The tuberculin skin test (TST) is positive but the chest radiograph is normal and there are no signs or symptoms of illness. **Tuberculosis disease** occurs when there are clinical signs and symptoms or an abnormal chest radiograph. The term *tuberculosis* usually refers to the disease. The interval between latent tuberculosis and the onset of disease may be several weeks or many decades in adults. In young children, tuberculosis usually develops as an immediate complication of the primary infection, and the distinction between infection and disease may be less obvious.

**Primary pulmonary tuberculosis** in older infants and children is usually an asymptomatic infection. Often the disease is manifested by a positive TST with minimal abnormalities on the chest radiograph, such as an infiltrate with hilar lymphadenopathy or **Ghon complex**. Malaise, low-grade fever, erythema nodosum, or symptoms resulting from lymph node enlargement may occur after the development of delayed hypersensitivity.

**Progressive primary disease** is characterized by a primary pneumonia that develops shortly after initial infection. Progression to pulmonary disease or disseminated miliary disease, or progression of central nervous system (CNS) granulomas to meningitis occurs most commonly in the first year of life. Hilar lymphadenopathy may compress the bronchi or trachea.

**Tuberculous pleural effusion**, which may accompany primary infection, generally represents the immune response to the organisms and most commonly occurs in older children or adolescents. Pleurocentesis reveals lymphocytes and an increased protein level, but the pleural fluid usually does not contain bacilli. A pleural biopsy may be necessary to obtain tissue to confirm the diagnosis by showing the expected granuloma formation and acid-fast organisms.

**Reactivation pulmonary tuberculosis**, common in adolescents and typical in adults with tuberculosis, usually is confined to apical segments of upper lobes or superior segments of lower lobes. There is usually little lymphadenopathy and no extrathoracic infection because of established hypersensitivity. This is a manifestation of a secondary expansion of infection at a site seeded years previously during primary infection. Advanced disease is associated with cavitation and endobronchial spread of bacilli. Symptoms include fever, night sweats, malaise, and weight loss. A productive cough and hemoptysis often herald cavitation and bronchial erosion.

**Tuberculous pericarditis** usually occurs when organisms from the lung or pleura spread to the contiguous surfaces of the pericardium. Accumulation of fluid with lymphocytic infiltration occurs in the pericardial space. Persistent inflammation may result in a cellular immune response with rupture of granulomas into the pericardial space and the development of constrictive pericarditis. In addition to antimycobacterial therapy, tuberculous pericarditis is managed with corticosteroids to decrease inflammation.

**Lymphadenopathy** is common in primary pulmonary disease. The most common extrathoracic sites of lymphadenitis are the cervical, supraclavicular, and submandibular areas (**scrofula**). Enlargement may cause compression of adjacent structures. **Miliary tuberculosis** refers to widespread hematogenous dissemination to multiple organs. The lesions are of roughly the same size as a millet seed, from which the name *miliary* is derived. Miliary tuberculosis is characterized by fever, general malaise, weight loss, lymphadenopathy, night sweats, and hepatosplenomegaly. Diffuse bilateral pneumonitis is common, and meningitis may be present. The chest radiograph reveals bilateral miliary infiltrates, showing overwhelming infection. The TST may be nonreactive as a result of **anergy**. Liver or bone marrow biopsy is useful for the diagnosis.

**Tuberculous meningitis** most commonly occurs in children under 5 years old and often within 6 months of primary infection. Tubercle bacilli that seed the meninges during the primary infection replicate, triggering an inflammatory response. This condition may have an insidious onset, initially characterized by low-grade fever, headache, and subtle personality change. Progression of the infection results in basilar meningitis with impingement of the cranial nerves and is manifested by meningeal irritation and eventually increased intracranial pressure, deterioration of mental status, and coma. Computed tomography (CT) scans show hydrocephalus, edema, periventricular lucencies, and infarctions. CSF analysis reveals pleocytosis (50–500 leukocytes/mm$^3$), which early in the course of disease may be either lymphocytes or polymorphonuclear leukocytes. Glucose is low, and protein is significantly elevated. Acid-fast bacilli are not detected frequently in the cerebrospinal fluid (CSF) by either routine or fluorescent staining procedures. Although culture is the standard for diagnosis, PCR for *M. tuberculosis* is useful to confirm meningitis. Treatment regimens for tuberculous meningitis generally include four antituberculosis drugs and corticosteroids.

**Skeletal tuberculosis** results from either hematogenous seeding or direct extension from a **caseous lymph node**. This is usually a chronic disease with an insidious onset that may be mistaken for chronic osteomyelitis caused by *Staphylococcus aureus*. Radiographs reveal cortical destruction. Biopsy and culture are essential for proper diagnosis. Tuberculosis of the spine, **Pott's disease**, is the most common skeletal site followed by the hip and the fingers and toes (**dactylitis**).

Other forms of tuberculosis include **abdominal tuberculosis** that occurs from swallowing infected material. This is a relatively uncommon complication in developed nations where dairy herds are inspected for bovine tuberculosis. **Tuberculous peritonitis** is associated with abdominal tuberculosis and presents as fever, anorexia, ascites, and abdominal pain. **Urogenital tuberculosis** is a late reactivation complication and is rare in children. Symptomatic illness presents as dysuria, frequency, urgency, hematuria, and *sterile* pyuria.

## LABORATORY AND IMAGING STUDIES

### Tuberculin Skin Test

The TST response to tuberculin antigen is a manifestation of a T cell–mediated delayed hypersensitivity and is the most important diagnostic tool for tuberculosis. It is usually positive 2 to 6 weeks after onset of infection (occasionally 3 months) and at the time of symptomatic illness. The **Mantoux test**, an intradermal injection of 5 TU (tuberculin units) (**intermediate test strength**) of Tween-stabilized purified tuberculous antigen (**purified protein derivative standard [PPD-S]**) usually on the volar surface of the forearm, is the standard for screening high-risk populations and for diagnosis ill patients or contacts. False negative responses may occur early in the illness, with use of inactivated antigen (as a result of poor storage practice or inadequate administration), or as a result of immunosuppression (secondary to underlying illness, AIDS, malnutrition, or overwhelming tuberculosis). Tests with questionable results should be repeated after several weeks of therapy and adequate nutrition. Because of poor nutrition, a high proportion of internationally adopted children arriving in the United States have an initial false positive tuberculin skin test. All internationally adopted children with an initially negative tuberculin skin test should have a repeat tuberculin skin test after 3 months in the United States.

The only TST that should be used in ordinary practice is the 5-TU test (Mantoux test). It is interpreted based on the host status and size of induration (Table 124-1). Only persons at high risk should be offered a Mantoux test (Table 124-2). When persons at low risk are given the TST, the positive predictive value of a positive test decreases, and persons with active tuberculosis (mainly those with asymptomatic infection with atypical mycobacteria) are subjected to unnecessary treatment.

A whole blood test of interferon-gamma (INF-$\gamma$) (Quanitferon gold), a cytokine elaborated by lymphocytes in response to tuberculosis antigens, is currently the recommended diagnostic test for persons older than 5 years of age in the United States. It has similar sensitivity as the TST but improved specificity as it is unaffected by prior bacille Calmette-Guérin (BCG) vaccination or exposure to nontuberculous mycobacterial antigens.

## Culture

The ultimate diagnostic confirmation relies on culture of the organism, a process that usually is more successful with tissue, such as pleura or pericardial membrane from biopsy rather than only pleural or pericardial fluid. Sputum is an excellent source for diagnosis in adults but is difficult to obtain in young children. Induced sputum or gastric fluid obtained via an indwelling nasogastric tube with samples taken before or immediately on waking contains swallowed sputum and provides appropriate samples in young children. Large volumes of fluid (CSF, pericardial fluid) yield a higher rate of recovery of organisms, but slow growth of the mycobacteria makes culture less helpful in very ill children. When the organism is grown, drug susceptibilities should be determined because of the increasing incidence of resistant organisms.

Antigen detection and DNA probes have expedited diagnosis, especially with CNS disease.

## Diagnostic Imaging

Because many cases of pulmonary tuberculosis in children are clinically relatively silent, radiography is a cornerstone for the diagnosis of disease. The initial parenchymal inflammation is not visible radiographically. A localized, nonspecific infiltrate with an overlying pleural reaction may be seen, however. This lesion usually resolves within 1 to 2 weeks. All lobar segments of the lung are at equal risk of being the focus of the initial infection. In 25% of cases, two or more lobes of the lungs are involved, although disease usually occurs at only one site. Spread of infection to regional lymph nodes occurs early.

The hallmark of childhood pulmonary tuberculosis is the relatively large size and importance of the hilar lymphadenitis compared with the less significant size of the initial parenchymal focus, together historically referred to as the **Ghon complex** (with or without calcification of the lymph nodes). Hilar lymphadenopathy is inevitably present with childhood tuberculosis but it may not be detected on a plain radiograph if calcification is not present. Partial bronchial obstruction caused by external compression from the enlarging nodes can cause air trapping, hyperinflation, and lobar emphysema. Occasionally, children have a picture of lobar pneumonia without impressive hilar lymphadenopathy. If the infection is progressively destructive, liquefaction of the lung parenchyma leads to formation of a thin-walled primary tuberculous cavity. Adolescents with pulmonary tuberculosis may develop segmental lesions with hilar lymphadenopathy or the apical infiltrates, with or without cavitation, that are typical of adult reactivation tuberculosis.

| **TABLE 124-1** Criteria for Positive Tuberculin Skin Test Results in Clinically Defined Pediatric Populations* | |
|---|---|
| **Positive Result** | **Population(s)** |
| *Induration* ≥5 mm | Children in close contact with persons with known or suspected contagious tuberculosis disease |
| | Children suspected to have tuberculosis disease |
| |     Findings on chest radiograph consistent with active or previously active tuberculosis |
| |     Clinical evidence of tuberculosis disease[†] |
| | Children receiving immunosuppressive therapy[‡] or with immunosuppressive conditions, including HIV infection |
| *Induration* ≥10 mm | Children at increased risk for disseminated disease |
| |     Children <4 years of age |
| |     Children with other medical conditions, including Hodgkin disease, lymphoma, diabetes mellitus, chronic renal failure, and malnutrition |
| | Children with increased exposure to tuberculosis disease |
| |     Children born, or whose parents were born, in high-prevalence regions of the world |
| |     Children frequently exposed to adults who are HIV-infected, homeless, users of illicit drugs, residents of nursing homes, incarcerated or institutionalized, or migrant farm workers |
| |     Children who travel to high-prevalence regions of the world |
| *Induration* ≥15 mm | Children ≥4 years of age without any risk factors |

*These criteria apply regardless of previous bacille Calmette-Guérin immunization. Erythema at tuberculin skin test site does not indicate a positive test result. Tuberculin reactions should be read at 48 to 72 hours after placement.

[†]Evidence by physical examination or laboratory assessment that would include tuberculosis in the working differential diagnosis (e.g., meningitis).

[‡]Including immunosuppressive doses of corticosteroids.

---

**TABLE 124-2 Tuberculin Skin Test (TST) Recommendations for Infants, Children, and Adolescents[a]**

**Children for Whom Immediate TST or IGRA is Indicated:[b]**

- Contacts of people with confirmed or suspected contagious tuberculosis (contact investigation)
- Children with radiographic or clinical findings suggesting tuberculosis disease
- Children immigrating from countries with endemic infection (e.g., Asia, Middle East, Africa, Latin America, countries of the former Soviet Union), including international adoptees
- Children with travel histories to countries with endemic infection and substantial contact with indigenous people from such countries

**Children Who Should Have Annual TST or IGRA:[c]**

- Children infected with HIV infection (TST only)
- Incarcerated adolescents

**Children at Increased Risk of Progression of LTBI to Tuberculosis Disease:**

Children with other medical conditions, including diabetes mellitus, chronic renal failure, malnutrition, and congenital or acquired immunodeficiencies deserve special consideration. Without recent exposure, these people are not at increased risk of acquiring tuberculosis infection. Underlying immune deficiencies associated with these conditions theoretically would enhance the possibility for progression to severe disease. Initial histories of potential exposure to tuberculosis should be included for all of these patients. If these histories or local epidemiologic factors suggest a possibility of exposure, immediate and periodic TST or IGRA should be considered. **An initial TST or IGRA should be performed before initiation of immunosuppressive therapy, including prolonged steroid administration, use of tumor necrosis factor–alpha antagonists, or other immunosuppressive therapy in any child requiring these treatments.**

Recommendations from American Academy of Pediatrics. Tuberculosis. In: Pickering LK, Baker CJ, Kimberlin DW, Long SS, eds. Red Book: 2009 Report of the Committee on Infectious Diseases. 28th ed. Elk Grove Village, IL: *American Academy of Pediatrics*; 2009: page 684.

HIV, human immunodeficiency virus; IGRA, interferon-gamma release assay; LTBI, latent tuberculosis infection.

[a]Bacille Calmette-Guérin immunization is not a contraindication to a TST.

[b]Beginning as early as 3 months of age.

[c]If the child is well, the TST or IGRA should be delayed for up to 10 weeks after return.

---

Radiographic studies aid greatly in the diagnosis of **extrapulmonary tuberculosis** in children. Plain radiographs, CT, and magnetic resonance imaging (MRI) of the tuberculous spine usually show collapse and destruction of the vertebral body with narrowing of the involved disk spaces. Radiographic findings in bone and joint tuberculosis range from mild joint effusions and small lytic lesions to massive destruction of the bone.

In tuberculosis of the CNS, CT or MRI of the brains of patients with tuberculous meningitis may be normal during early stages of the infection. As disease progresses, basilar enhancement and communicating hydrocephalus with signs of cerebral edema or early focal ischemia are the most common findings. In children with renal tuberculosis, intravenous (IV) pyelograms may reveal mass lesions, dilation of the proximal ureters, multiple small filling defects, and hydronephrosis if ureteral stricture is present.

## DIFFERENTIAL DIAGNOSIS

The differential diagnosis of tuberculosis includes a multitude of diagnoses because tuberculosis may affect any organ and in early disease the symptoms and signs may be nonspecific. In pulmonary disease, tuberculosis may appear similar to pneumonia, malignancy, and any systemic disease in which generalized lymphadenopathy occurs. The diagnosis of tuberculosis should be suspected if the TST is positive or if there is history of tuberculosis in a close contact.

The differential diagnosis of tuberculous lymphadenopathy includes infections caused by atypical mycobacteria, cat-scratch disease, fungal infection, viral or bacterial disease, toxoplasmosis, sarcoidosis, drug reactions, and malignancy. The diagnosis may be confirmed by fine needle aspiration but may necessitate excisional biopsy accompanied by appropriate histologic and microbiologic studies.

## TREATMENT

The treatment of tuberculosis is affected by the presence of naturally occurring drug-resistant organisms in large bacterial populations, even before therapy is initiated, and the fact that mycobacteria replicate slowly and can remain dormant in the body for prolonged periods. Although a population of bacilli as a whole may be considered drug susceptible, a subpopulation of drug-resistant organisms occurs at fairly predictable frequencies of $10^5$ to $10^7$, depending on the drug. Cavities may contain $10^9$ tubercle bacilli with thousands of organisms resistant to any one drug, but only rare organisms that are resistant to multiple drugs. The chance that an organism is naturally resistant to two drugs is on the order of $10^{11}$ to $10^{13}$. Because populations of this number rarely occur in patients, organisms naturally resistant to two drugs are essentially nonexistent.

For patients with large populations of bacilli, such as adults with cavities or extensive infiltrates, at least two antituberculosis drugs must be given. For patients with tuberculosis infection but no disease, the bacterial population is small and a single drug, such as isoniazid, can be given. Therapy for latent infection is aimed at eradicating the presumably small inoculum of organisms sequestered within macrophages and suppressed by normal T cell activity. To prevent reactivation of these latent bacilli, therapy with a single agent (usually isoniazid for 9 months) is suggested. Children with primary pulmonary tuberculosis and patients with extrapulmonary tuberculosis have medium-sized populations in which significant numbers of drug-resistant organisms may or may not be present. In general, these patients are treated with at least two drugs (Table 124-3) for a prolonged course, typically 9 to 12 months, depending on the type of disease. Isoniazid and rifampin are bactericidal for *M. tuberculosis* and are effective against all populations of mycobacteria. Along with pyrazinamide, they form the backbone of the antimicrobial treatment of tuberculosis. Other drugs are used in special circumstances, such as tuberculous meningitis and antibiotic-resistant tuberculosis. Ethambutol, ethionamide, streptomycin, and cycloserine are bacteriostatic and are used with bactericidal antituberculosis agents to prevent emergence of resistance.

A 9-month regimen of isoniazid and rifampin cures greater than 98% of cases of drug-susceptible pulmonary tuberculosis. After daily administration for the first 1 to 2 months, both drugs can be given daily or twice weekly for the remaining 7 to 8 months, with equivalent results and low rates of adverse reactions. The addition of pyrazinamide for the first 2 months of the regimen reduces the total duration of treatment to 6 months and has similar efficacy. **Noncompliance**, or **nonadherence**, is a major problem in tuberculosis control because of the long-term nature of treatment and the sometimes difficult social circumstances of the patients. As treatment regimens become shorter, adherence assumes an even greater importance. Improvement in compliance occurs with **directly observed therapy**, which means that the health care worker is physically present when the medications are administered, and is the standard of care in most settings.

## COMPLICATIONS AND PROGNOSIS

Tuberculosis of the spine may result in angulation or **gibbus** formation that requires surgical correction after the infection is cured. With extrapulmonary tuberculosis, the major problem is often delayed recognition of the cause of disease and delayed initiation of treatment. Most childhood tuberculous meningitis occurs in developing countries, where the prognosis is poor.

**TABLE 124-3 Recommended Treatment Regimens for Drug-Susceptible Tuberculosis in Infants, Children, and Adolescents**

| Infection or Disease Category | Regimen | Comments |
|---|---|---|
| Latent tuberculosis infection (positive TST result, no disease) | | |
| Isoniazid-susceptible | 9 months of isoniazid, once a day | If daily therapy is not possible, DOT twice a week can be used for 9 months. |
| Isoniazid-resistant | 6 months of rifampin, once a day | |
| Isoniazid-rifampin-resistant | Consult a tuberculosis specialist. | |
| Pulmonary and extrapulmonary (except meningitis) | 2 months of isoniazid, rifampin, and pyrazinamide daily, followed by 4 months of isoniazid and rifampin twice weekly under DOT | If possible drug resistance is a concern, another drug (ethambutol or an aminoglycoside) is added to the initial three-drug therapy until drug susceptibilities are determined. DOT is highly desirable. If hilar lymphadenopathy only, a 6-month course of isoniazid and rifampin is sufficient. Drugs can be given 2 or 3 times per week under DOT in the initial phase if nonadherence is likely. |
| Meningitis | 2 months of isoniazid, rifampin, pyrazinamide, and an aminoglycoside or ethionamide, once a day, followed by 7–10 months of isoniazid and rifampin, once a day or twice a week (9–12 months total) | A fourth drug, usually an aminoglycoside, is given with initial therapy until drug susceptibility is known. For patients who may have acquired tuberculosis in geographic areas where resistance to streptomycin is common, capreomycin, kanamycin, or amikacin may be used instead of streptomycin. |

Recommendations from Pickering LK, Baker CJ, Long SS, et al: Red Book: 2006 Report of the Committee on Infectious Diseases, 27th ed. Elk Grove Village, IL, *American Academy of Pediatrics*, 2006, p 686.
DOT, directly observed therapy; TST, tuberculin skin test.

In general, the prognosis of tuberculosis in infants, children, and adolescents is excellent with early recognition and effective chemotherapy. In most children with pulmonary tuberculosis, the disease completely resolves, and ultimately radiographic findings are normal. The prognosis for children with bone and joint tuberculosis and tuberculous meningitis depends directly on the stage of disease at the time antituberculosis medications are started.

## PREVENTION

Tuberculosis control programs involve case finding and treatment, which interrupts secondary transmission of infection from close contacts. Infected close contacts are identified by positive TST reactions and can be started on appropriate treatment to prevent transmission.

Prevention of transmission in health care settings involves appropriate physical ventilation of the air around the source case. Offices, clinics, and hospital rooms used by adults with possible tuberculosis should have adequate ventilation, with air exhausted to the outside (**negative-pressure ventilation**). Health care providers should have annual TSTs.

The only available vaccine against tuberculosis is the **BCG (bacille Calmette-Guérin) vaccine**. The original vaccine organism was a strain of *Mycobacterium bovis* attenuated by subculture every 3 weeks for 13 years. The preferred route of administration is intradermal injection with a syringe and needle because this is the only method that permits accurate measurement of an individual dose. The official recommendation of the World Health Organization is a single dose administered during infancy. In the United Kingdom, a single dose is administered during adolescence following a negative TST. In many countries, the first dose is given in infancy and then one or more additional vaccinations are given during childhood. In some countries, repeat vaccination is universal; in others, it is based either on tuberculin negativity or on the absence of a typical scar. This vaccine is not routinely used in the United States. Some studies show BCG to provide 80% to 90% protection from tuberculosis, and other studies show no protective efficacy at all. Many infants who receive BCG vaccine never have a positive TST reaction. When a reaction does occur, the induration size is usually less than 10 mm, and the reaction wanes after several years.

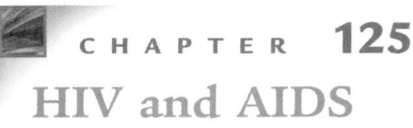

## CHAPTER 125

# HIV and AIDS

## ETIOLOGY

The cause of AIDS (acquired immunodeficiency syndrome) is HIV (human immunodrficiency virus), a single-stranded RNA virus of the retrovirus family that produces a **reverse transcriptase** enabling the viral RNA to act as a template for DNA transcription and integration into the host genome. HIV-1 causes 99% of all human cases. HIV-2,

which is less virulent, causes 1% to 9% of cases in parts of Africa and is very rare in the United States.

HIV infects human **helper T cells (CD4 cells)** and cells of monocyte-macrophage lineage via interaction of viral protein gp120 with the CD4 molecule and chemokines (CXCR4 and CCR5) that serve as coreceptors, facilitating membrane fusion and cell entry. Because helper T cells are important for delayed hypersensitivity, T cell–dependent B cell antibody production, and T cell–mediated lymphokine activation of macrophages, their destruction produces a profound combined (B and T cell) immunodeficiency. A lack of T cell regulation and unrestrained antigenic stimulation result in polyclonal hypergammaglobulinemia with nonspecific and ineffective globulins. Other cells bearing CD4, such as microglia, astrocytes, oligodendroglia, and placental tissues also may be infected with HIV.

HIV infection is a continuously progressive process with a variable period of clinical latency before development of AIDS-defining conditions. All untreated patients have evidence of ongoing viral replication and progressive CD4 lymphocyte depletion. There are no overt manifestations of immunodeficiency until CD4 cell numbers decline to critical threshold levels. Quantitation of the viral load has become an important parameter in management.

**Horizontal transmission** of HIV is by sexual contact (vaginal, anal, or orogenital), percutaneous contact (from contaminated needles or other sharp objects), or mucous membrane exposure to contaminated blood or body fluid. Transmission by contaminated blood and blood products has been eliminated in developed countries, but still occurs in developing countries. **Vertical transmission** of HIV from mother to infant may occur transplacentally in utero, during birth, or by breastfeeding. Risk factors for perinatal transmission include prematurity, rupture of membranes more than 4 hours, and high maternal circulating levels of HIV at delivery. Perinatal transmission can be decreased from approximately 25% to less than 8% with antiretroviral treatment of the mother before and during delivery and postnatal treatment of the infant. Breastfeeding by HIV-infected mothers increases the risk of vertical transmission by 30% to 50%. In untreated infants, the mean incubation interval for development of an AIDS-defining condition after vertical transmission is 5 months (range, 1 to 24 months) compared with an incubation period after horizontal transmission of generally 7 to 10 years.

## EPIDEMIOLOGY

Worldwide, as of 2007, approximately 35 million persons have been infected with HIV, including 2.5 million children. More than 25 million persons have died of AIDS, with 80% of the deaths in Africa. An estimated 2.5 million persons worldwide acquired HIV in 2007. In areas of Africa and Asia, infection rates of 40% are largely the result of heterosexual transmission. There are more than 900,000 persons who have been diagnosed with AIDS in the United States, including 9300 children less than 13 years of age. In 2006, approximately 435,000 people were living with HIV/AIDS including approximately 6000 children who were infected perinatally. There were an estimated 56,300 new HIV infections in the United States in 2006.

Vertical transmission accounts for more than 90% of all cases of AIDS in children in the United States. Currently, approximately 100 to 200 infants are born with HIV infection each year in the United States. The effectiveness of perinatal prophylaxis has reduced dramatically the numbers of new cases of pediatric AIDS in the United States and developed countries. Most pediatric cases now occur in adolescents who engage in unprotected sexual activities.

## CLINICAL MANIFESTATIONS

In adolescents and adults, primary infection results in the **acute retroviral syndrome** that develops after an incubation period of 2 to 6 weeks and consists of fever, malaise, weight loss, pharyngitis, lymphadenopathy, and often a maculopapular rash. The risk of opportunistic infections and other AIDS-defining conditions is related to the depletion of CD4 T cells. A combination of CD4 cell count and percentage and clinical manifestations is used to classify HIV infection in children (Tables 125-1, 125-2). Initial symptoms with vertical transmission vary and may include failure to thrive, neurodevelopmental delay, lymphadenopathy, hepatosplenomegaly, chronic or recurrent diarrhea, interstitial pneumonia, or oral thrush. These findings may be subtle and remarkable only by their persistence. Manifestations that are more common in children than adults with HIV infection include recurrent bacterial infections, lymphoid hyperplasia, chronic parotid swelling, lymphocytic interstitial pneumonitis, and earlier onset of progressive neurologic deterioration. Pulmonary manifestations of HIV infection are common and include *Pneumocystis jirovecii* pneumonia, which can present early in infancy as a primary pneumonia characterized by hypoxia, tachypnea, retractions, elevated serum lactate dehydrogenase, and fever.

In the United States, most pregnant women are screened and, if indicated, treated for HIV infection. Infants born to HIV-infected mothers receive prophylaxis and are prospectively tested for infection. The diagnosis of HIV infection in most infants born in the United States is confirmed before development of clinical signs of infection.

## LABORATORY AND IMAGING STUDIES

HIV infection can be diagnosed definitively by 1 month of age and in virtually all infected infants by 6 months of age using viral diagnostic assays (RNA polymerase chain reaction [PCR], DNA PCR, or virus culture). Maternal antibodies may be detectable until 12 to 15 months of age, and a positive serologic test is not considered diagnostic until 18 months of age.

HIV DNA PCR is the preferred virologic method for diagnosing HIV infection during infancy and identifies 38% of infected infants at 48 hours and 96% at 28 days. Diagnostic viral testing should be performed by 48 hours of age, at 1 to 2 months of age, and at 3 to 6 months of age. An additional test at 14 days of age is often performed because the diagnostic sensitivity increases rapidly by 2 weeks of age. HIV RNA PCR has 25% to 40% sensitivity during the first weeks of life, increasing to 90% to 100% by 2 to 3 months of age. However, a negative HIV RNA PCR cannot be used to exclude infection and, thus, is not recommended as first-line testing. HIV culture is complicated and not routinely performed.

HIV infection of an exposed infant is confirmed if virologic tests are positive on two separate occasions. HIV infection can be reasonably excluded in nonbreastfed infants with at least two virologic tests performed at older than 1 month of age, with one test being performed after 4 months of age, or at least two negative antibody tests performed after 6 months of age, with an interval of at least 1 month between the tests. Loss of HIV antibody combined with negative HIV DNA PCR confirms absence of HIV infection. Persistence of a positive HIV antibody test after 18 months of age indicates HIV infection.

## DIFFERENTIAL DIAGNOSIS

The differential diagnosis of AIDS in infants includes primary immunodeficiency syndromes and intrauterine infections with cytomegalovirus (CMV) and syphilis. Prominence of individual symptoms, such as diarrhea, may suggest other etiologies.

---

**TABLE 125-1  1994 Revised HIV Pediatric Classification System: Immune Categories**

| Immune Category | Laboratory Criteria | | | | | |
|---|---|---|---|---|---|---|
| | <12 months | | 1–5 years | | 6–12 years | |
| | CD4$^+$ Cells/mm$^3$ | % Total Lymphocytes | CD4$^+$ Cells/mm$^3$ | % Total Lymphocytes | CD4$^+$ Cells/mm$^3$ | % Total Lymphocytes |
| Category 1 (no suppression) | ≥1500 | ≥25 | ≥1000 | ≥25 | ≥500 | ≥25 |
| Category 2 (moderate suppression) | 750–1499 | 15–24 | 500–999 | 15–24 | 200–499 | 15–24 |
| Category 3 (severe suppression) | <750 | <15 | <500 | <15 | <200 | <15 |

From Centers for Disease Control and Prevention: 1994 revised classification system for human immunodeficiency virus infection in children less than 13 years of age. *MMWR* 43(RR-12):1–10, 1994.

## TABLE 125-2  1994 Revised HIV Pediatric Classification System: Clinical Categories

*Category N: Not Symptomatic*
Children who have no signs or symptoms considered to be the result of HIV infection or who have only one of the conditions listed in category A

*Category A: Mildly Symptomatic*
Children with two or more of the following conditions, but none of the conditions listed in categories B and C:
  Lymphadenopathy (nodal tissue enlargement of $\geq$0.5 cm palpable at more than two sites; bilateral = one site)
  Hepatomegaly
  Splenomegaly
  Dermatitis
  Parotitis
  Recurrent or persistent upper respiratory infection, sinusitis, or otitis media

*Category B: Moderately Symptomatic*
Children who have symptomatic conditions, other than those listed for category A or category C, that are attributed to HIV infection. Examples of
  conditions in clinical category B include, but are not limited to, the following:
  Anemia (<8 g/dL), neutropenia (<1000/mm$^3$), or thrombocytopenia (<100,000/mm$^3$) persisting $\geq$30 days
  Bacterial meningitis, pneumonia, or sepsis (single episode)
  Candidiasis, oropharyngeal (i.e., thrush) persisting for >2 months in children younger than 6 months of age
  Cardiomyopathy
  Cytomegalovirus infection with onset before the age of 1 month
  Diarrhea, recurrent or chronic
  Hepatitis
  HSV stomatitis, recurrent (i.e., >2 episodes within 1 year)
  HSV bronchitis, pneumonitis, or esophagitis with onset before the age of 1 month
  Herpes zoster (i.e., shingles) involving at least 2 distinct episodes or >1 dermatome
  Leiomyosarcoma
  LIP or pulmonary lymphoid hyperplasia complex
  Nephropathy
  Nocardiosis
  Fever lasting >1 month
  Varicella, disseminated (i.e., complicated chickenpox)

*Category C: Severely Symptomatic*
Serious bacterial infections, multiple or recurrent (i.e., any combination of at least two culture-confirmed infections within a 2-year period), of the
  following types: septicemia, pneumonia, meningitis, bone or joint infection, or abscess of an internal organ or body cavity (excluding otitis media,
  superficial skin or mucosal abscesses, and indwelling catheter-related infections)
  Candidiasis, esophageal or pulmonary (bronchi, trachea, lungs)
  Coccidioidomycosis, disseminated (at site other than or in addition to lungs or cervical or hilar lymph nodes)
  Cryptococcosis, extrapulmonary
  Cryptosporidiosis or isosporiasis with diarrhea persisting >1 month
  Cytomegalovirus disease with onset of symptoms before the age of 1 month (other than liver, spleen, or lymph nodes)
  Encephalopathy (at least one progressive deficit present for at least 2 months in the absence of a concurrent illness): (a) failure to attain or loss of
    developmental milestones/intellectual ability, verified by standard scale or tests; (b) impaired brain growth or acquired microcephaly; (c)
    acquired symmetrical motor deficit manifested by two or more of the following: paresis, pathologic reflexes, ataxia, or gait disturbance
  Herpes simplex virus infection (mucocutaneous ulcer persisting for >1 month; bronchitis, pneumonitis, or esophagitis affecting a child younger
    than 1 month of age
  Histoplasmosis, disseminated (other than or in addition to lungs or cervical or hilar lymph nodes)
  Kaposi sarcoma
  Lymphoma (primary tumor, in brain; Burkitt's lymphoma; immunoblastic or large cell lymphoma of B cell or unknown immunologic phenotype)
  *Mycobacterium tuberculosis*, disseminated or extrapulmonary
  *Mycobacterium*, other species or unidentified species, disseminated (other than or in addition to lungs, skin, or cervical or hilar lymph nodes)
  *Mycobacterium avium* complex or *Mycobacterium kansasii*, disseminated (other than or in addition to lungs, skin, or cervical or hilar lymph nodes)
  *Pneumocystis jirovecii (carinii)* pneumonia
  Progressive multifocal leukoencephalopathy
  *Salmonella* (nontyphoid) septicemia, recurrent
  Toxoplasmosis of the brain with onset before the age of 1 month
  Wasting syndrome in the absence of a concurrent illness could explain the following findings: (a) persistent weight loss >10% of baseline *or*
    (b) downward crossing of at least two percentile lines on the weight-for-age chart *or* (c) below the 5th percentile on the weight-for-height chart
    on two consecutive measurements, $\geq$30 days apart, *plus* (1) chronic diarrhea (i.e., 2 or more loose stools per day for >30 days) *or* (2) documented
    fever (for $\geq$30 days, intermittent or constant)

HIV, human immunodeficiency virus infection; HSV, herpes simplex virus; LIP, lymphoid interstitial pneumonia.
From the Working Group on Antiretroviral Therapy and Medical Management of HIV-Infected Children: Guidelines for the Use of Antiretroviral
Agents in Pediatric HIV Infection. Department of Health and Human Services. February 23, 2009. Available at *http://aidsinfo.nih.gov/contentfiles/
PediatricGuidelines.pdf.* Updated from Centers for Disease Control and Prevention: 1994 revised classification system for human immunodeficiency
virus infection in children less than 13 years of age. *MMWR* 43(RR-12):1–10, 1994.

# TREATMENT

Management of HIV infection in children and adolescents is rapidly evolving and becoming increasingly complex. It should be directed by a specialist in the treatment of HIV infection. Therapy is initiated based on the severity of HIV disease, as indicated by AIDS-defining conditions, and the risk of disease progression, as indicated by CD4 cell count and plasma HIV RNA level (Table 125-3). Initiation of antiretroviral therapy while the patient is still asymptomatic may preserve immune function and prevent clinical progression, but incurs the adverse effects of therapy and may facilitate emergence of drug-resistant virus. Because the risk of HIV progression is fourfold to sixfold greater in infants and very young children, treatment recommendations for children are more aggressive than for adults. All age groups show rapid increases in risk as CD4 cell percentage declines to less than 15%.

Initiation of therapy (Table 125-4) is recommended for infants less than 12 months of age regardless of symptoms of HIV disease or HIV RNA level. Initiation of therapy is recommended for all children 1 to 5 years of age with AIDS or significant HIV-related symptoms or CD4 below 25% (clinical category C or most clinical category B) regardless of symptoms or HIV RNA level. For children older than 5 years with AIDS or significant HIV-related symptoms, CD4 count below 350/mm$^3$ should be treated. Indications for treatment of adolescents and adults include CD4 cell count less than 200 to 350/mm$^3$ or plasma HIV RNA levels above 55,000 copies/mL.

Combination therapy with **highly active antiretroviral therapy (HAART)** is recommended based on the risk of disease progression as determined by CD4 percentage or count and plasma HIV RNA copy number; the potential benefits and risks of therapy; and the ability of the caregiver to adhere to administration of the therapeutic regimen. Antiretroviral regimens include nucleoside analog or nucleoside reverse transcriptase inhibitors, non-nucleoside reverse transcriptase inhibitors, protease inhibitors, and fusion inhibitors (see Table 125-4). Effective combination therapy significantly reduces viral loads and leads to the amelioration of clinical symptoms and opportunistic infections. Combination therapy with dual nucleoside reverse transcriptase inhibitors (zidovudine-lamivudine, zidovudine-didanosine, or stavudine-lamivudine) and a protease inhibitor is a common initial regimen for children.

The ability of HIV to develop resistance to antiretroviral agents rapidly and the development of cross-resistance to several classes of agents simultaneously are major problems. Determination of HIV RNA, CD4 cell count and HIV phenotype and genotype is essential for monitoring and modifying antiretroviral treatment.

Routine immunizations are recommended to prevent vaccine-preventable infections, but may result in suboptimal immune responses. In addition to heptavalent pneumococcal conjugate vaccine, 23-valent pneumococcal polysaccharide vaccine is recommended for HIV-infected children at 2 years of age, and adolescents and adults with CD4 counts at or above 200/mm$^3$. Because of the risk of fatal measles in children with AIDS, children without severe immunosuppression should receive their first dose of MMR at 12 months of age and may receive the booster as soon as 4 weeks later. Varicella zoster virus (VZV) vaccine should be given only to asymptomatic, nonimmunosuppressed

---

**TABLE 125-3 Indications for Initiation of Antiretroviral Therapy in Children Infected with HIV**

| Age | Criteria | Recommendation |
|---|---|---|
| <12 months | ● Regardless of clinical symptoms, immune status, or viral load | Treat |
| 1<5 years | ● AIDS or significant HIV-related symptoms[1] | Treat |
| | ● CD4 <25%, regardless of symptoms or HIV RNA level[2] | Treat |
| | ● Asymptomatic or mild symptoms[3] *and* | Consider |
| | ○ CD4 ≥25% *and* | |
| | ○ HIV RNA ≥100,000 copies/mL | |
| | ● Asymptomatic or mild symptoms[3] *and* | Defer[4] |
| | ○ CD4 ≥25% *and* | |
| | ○ HIV RNA <100,000 copies/mL | |
| ≥5 years | ● AIDS or significant HIV-related symptoms[1] | Treat |
| | ● CD4 <350 cells/mm$^{3,5}$ | Treat |
| | ● Asymptomatic or mild symptoms[3] *and* | Consider |
| | ○ CD4 ≥350 cells/mm$^3$ *and* | |
| | ○ HIV RNA ≥100,000 copies/mL | |
| | ● Asymptomatic or mild symptoms[3] *and* | Defer[4] |
| | ○ CD4 ≥350 cells/mm$^3$ *and* | |
| | ○ HIV RNA <100,000 copies/mL | |

[1]CDC clinical categories C and B (except for the following category B conditions: single episode of serious bacterial infection or lymphoid interstitial pneumonitis)
[2]The data supporting this recommendation are stronger for those with CD4 percentage <20% than for those with CD4 percentage of 20% to 24%.
[3]CDC clinical category A or N or the following category B conditions: single episode of serious bacterial infection or lymphoid interstitial pneumonitis.
[4]Clinical and laboratory data should be re-evaluated every 3 to 4 months.
[5]The data supporting this recommendation are stronger for those with CD4 count <200 than for those with CD4 counts of 200 to 350 cells/mm$^3$.

CHAPTER 125 ● HIV and AIDS 461

**TABLE 125-4 Recommended Antiretroviral Regimens for Initial Therapy for HIV Infection in Children**

A combination antiretroviral regimen in treatment-naïve children generally contains one NNRTI plus a two-NRTI backbone or one PI plus a two-NRTI backbone. A three-NRTI regimen consisting of zidovudine, abacavir, and lamivudine is recommended only if a PI or NNRTI regimen cannot be used. Regimens should be individualized based on advantages and disadvantages of each combination.

**Non-Nucleoside Reverse Transcriptase Inhibitor-Based Regimens**

| | |
|---|---|
| Preferred Regimen | Children ≥3 years old: Two NRTIs *plus* efavirenz[1] |
| | Children <3 years old or who can't swallow capsules: Two NRTIs *plus* nevirapine[1] |
| Alternative | Two NRTIs *plus* nevirapin[1] (children ≥3 years old) |

**Protease Inhibitor-Based Regimens**

| | |
|---|---|
| Preferred Regimen | Two NRTIs *plus* lopinavir/ritonavir |
| Alternative (listed alphabetically) | Two NRTIs *plus* atazanavir *plus* low-dose ritonavir (children ≥6 years old) |
| | Two NRTIs *plus* fosamprenavir *plus* low-dose ritonavir (children ≥6 years old) |
| | Two NRTIs *plus* nelfinavir (children ≥2 years old) |

**Use in Special Circumstances**

| | |
|---|---|
| | Two NRTIs *plus* atazanavir unboosted (for treatment-naïve adolescents ≥13 years of age and >39 kg) |
| | Two NRTIs *plus* fosamprenavir unboosted (children ≥2 years old ) |
| | Zidovudine *plus* lamivudine *plus* abacavir |

**2-NRTI Backbone Options (For Use in Combination with Additional Drugs) (Alphabetical Ordering)**

| | |
|---|---|
| Preferred | Abacavir *plus* (lamivudine *or* emtricitabine) |
| | Didanosine *plus* emtricitabine |
| | Tenofovir *plus* (lamivudine *or* emtricitabine) (for Tanner stage 4 *or* postpubertal adolescents only) |
| | Zidovudine *plus* (lamivudine *or* emtricitabine) |
| Alternative | Abacavir *plus* zidovudine |
| | Zidovudine *plus* didanosine |
| Use in Special Circumstances | Stavudine *plus* (lamivudine *or* emtricitabine) |

**Insufficent Data to Recommend for Initial Therapy**

| | |
|---|---|
| | Low-dose ritonavir-boosted PI regimens, with exceptions of lopinavir/ritonavir (any age), atazanavir/ritonavir in children ≥6 years old, and fosamprenavir/ritonavir in children ≥6 years old[2] |
| | Dual (full-dose) PI regimens |
| | NRTI *plus* NNRTI *plus* PI |
| | Tenofovir-containing regimens in children in Tanner stage 1 to 3 |
| | Unboosted atazanavir-containing regimens in children <13 years of age and/or <39 kg |
| | Tipranavir- or darumavir-containing regimens |
| | Etravirine-containing regimens |
| | Enfuvirtide (T-20)-containing regimens |
| | Maraviroc-containing regimens |
| | Raltegravir-containing regimens |

[1]Efavirenz is currently available only in capsule form and should only be used in children ≥3 years old with weight ≥10 kg; nevirapine would be the preferred NNRTI for children age <3 years old or who require a liquid formulation. Unless adequate contraception can be assured, efavirenz-based therapy is not recommended for adolescent females who are sexually active and may become pregnant.

[2]With the exception of lopinavir/ritonavir, atazanavir/ritonavir in children ≥6 years old, and fosamprenavir in combination with low-dose ritonavir in children ≥6 years old, use of other boosted PIs as a component of initial therapy is not recommended, although such regimens have utility as secondary treatment regimens for children who have failed initial therapy.

children beginning at 12 months of age as two doses of vaccine at least 3 months apart. Inactivated split influenza virus vaccine should be administered annually to all HIV-infected children at or after 6 months of age. HIV-infected children exposed to varicella or measles should receive varicella zoster immune globulin (VZIG) or immunoglobulin prophylaxis.

## COMPLICATIONS

The approach to the numerous opportunistic infections in HIV-infected patients involves treatment and prophylaxis for infections likely to occur as CD4 cells are depleted. With potent antiretroviral therapy and immune reconstitution, routine prophylaxis for common opportunistic infections depends on the child's age and CD4 count. Infants born to HIV-infected mothers receive prophylaxis for *P. jirovecii* pneumonia with TMP-SMZ (trimethoprim-sulfamethoxazole) beginning at 4 to 6 weeks of age and continued for the first year of life or discontinued if HIV infection is subsequently excluded. TMP-SMZ prophylaxis for *P. jirovecii* pneumonia for older children and adolescents is provided if CD4 cell counts are less than 200/mm$^3$ or there is history of oropharyngeal candidiasis. Clarithromycin prophylaxis for *Mycobacterium avium*-complex infection is provided if CD4 cell counts are below 50/mm$^3$. *P. jirovecii* pneumonia is treated with high-dose TMP-SMZ and corticosteroids. Oral and gastrointestinal candidiasis is common in children and usually responds to imidazole therapy. VZV infection may be severe and should be treated with acyclovir or other antivirals. Recurrent herpes simplex virus (HSV) infections also may require long-term antiviral prophylaxis. Other common infections in HIV-infected patients include toxoplasmosis, CMV, Epstein-Barr virus (EBV) infection, salmonellosis, and tuberculosis.

Children and adults with HIV are prone to malignancies, especially non-Hodgkin lymphomas, with the gastrointestinal tract being the most common site. Leiomyosarcomas are the second most common tumors among HIV-infected children. Kaposi sarcoma, caused by HHV-8, is distinctly rare in children with HIV. It was once common among adults with AIDS and is now infrequent with HAART.

## PROGNOSIS

The availability of HAART has improved the prognosis for HIV and AIDS dramatically. Children with opportunistic infections, especially *P. jirovecii* pneumonia, encephalopathy, or wasting syndrome have the poorest prognosis, with 75% dying before 3 years of age.

## PREVENTION

Identification of HIV-infected women before or during pregnancy is crucial to providing optimal therapy for infected women and their infants and to preventing perinatal transmission. Prenatal HIV counseling and testing with consent should be provided for all pregnant women in the United States. Women who use illicit drugs during pregnancy pose special concerns because they are least likely to obtain prenatal care.

The rate of vertical transmission is reduced to less than 8% by chemoprophylaxis with a regimen of zidovudine to the mother (100 mg five times/24 hours orally) started by 4 weeks gestation, continued during delivery (2 mg/kg loading dose intravenously followed by 1 mg/kg/hour intravenously), and then administered to the newborn for the first 6 weeks of life (2 mg/kg every 6 hours orally). Other regimens incorporating single-dose nevirapine for infants have been shown to be similarly effective and are used in developing countries. Currently, combination drug regimens tailored to whether the mother has previously received HIV therapy are recommended. Scheduled cesarean section at 38 weeks to prevent vertical transmission is recommended for women with HIV RNA levels greater than 1000 copies/mL, but it is unclear if cesarean section is beneficial if viral load is less than 1000 copies/mL or when membranes have already ruptured.

Preventing HIV infection in adults decreases the incidence of infection in children. Adult prevention results from behavior changes such as "safe sex" practices, decrease in intravenous drug use, and needle exchange programs. Prevention of pediatric AIDS includes avoidance of pregnancy and breastfeeding (in developed countries) in high-risk women. Screening of blood donors has almost eliminated the risk of HIV transmission from blood products. HIV infection almost never is transmitted in a casual or nonsexual household setting.

## SUGGESTED READING

Feigin RD, Cherry J, Demmler GJ, et al: Textbook of Pediatric Infectious Diseases, 6th ed, Philadelphia, 2009, *WB Saunders.*

Isaacs D: Evidence-based Pediatric Infectious Disease, Malden, MA, 2007, *Blackwell Publishing.*

Kliegman RB, Behrman RE, Jenson HB, et al: Nelson Textbook of Pediatrics, 18th ed, Philadelphia, 2007, *WB Saunders.*

Long SS, Pickering LK, Prober CG: Principles and Practice of Pediatric Infectious Diseases, 3rd ed, Philadelphia, 2008, *Churchill Livingstone.*

Mandell GL, Bennett JE, Dolin R: Principles and Practice of Infectious Diseases, 6th ed, Philadelphia, 2005, *Churchill Livingstone.*

Pickering LK, Baker CJ, Long SS, et al: Red Book: 2006 Report of the Committee on Infectious Diseases, 27th ed, Elk Grove Village, IL, 2006, *American Academy of Pediatrics.*

Plotkin SA, Orenstein WA, Offit PA: Vaccines, 5th ed, Philadelphia, 2008, *WB Saunders.*

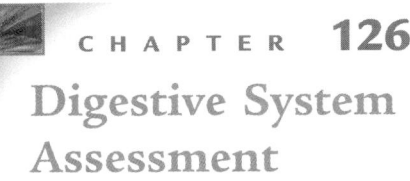

CHAPTER 126

# Digestive System Assessment

Children commonly present with symptoms originating in the digestive tract. The pediatrician needs to be able to evaluate a child's symptoms quickly using knowledge, careful history, physical examination, and appropriate diagnostic tests.

## HISTORY

Younger children may not be able to describe symptoms accurately, so reports of caregivers are important. Proper assessment of the history before moving on to physical examination and diagnostic testing helps narrow the possibilities and allows a focused examination and precise use of diagnostic studies.

Onset and progression of the major symptom should be characterized. Changes in symptoms, triggers that aggravate or alleviate the symptom and associated symptoms (e.g., fever, weight loss), and exposures to others (through travel or environmental exposure) should be identified.

Next, the pediatrician should ask about the child's current status, what investigations have been performed, and whether therapies have been used. Important issues include the frequency and duration of symptoms and their the relationship to meals and defecation and impact on activities (school attendance). If medications have been used, therapeutic effect should be determined. Finally, the initial visit should include a thorough review of systems, family history, social history, and past medical history.

## PHYSICAL EXAMINATION

Children with gastrointestinal (GI) complaints need a full general examination and a thorough abdominal examination. Extraintestinal disorders may produce GI manifestations (e.g., emesis and group A streptococcal pharyngitis;

abdominal pain and lower lobe pneumonia). A careful external inspection should evaluate for abdominal distention, bruising or discoloration, abnormal veins, jaundice, surgical scars, and ostomies. Abnormalities of intensity and pitch of bowel sounds should be determined. Palpation should assess for tenderness, noting location, facial expression, guarding, and rebound tenderness. The liver and spleen should be examined, measuring enlargement with a tape measure and noting abnormal firmness or contour. Assessment for the presence of palpable feces and mass lesions should occur. A rectal examination needs to be done when it is indicated. Children with history suggesting constipation, GI bleeding, abdominal pain, chronic diarrhea, and suspicion of inflammatory bowel disease (IBD) may have important findings on rectal examination. The rectal examination includes external inspection for fissures, skin tags, abscesses, and fistulous openings. Digital rectal examination should include assessment of anal sphincter tone, anal canal size and elasticity, tenderness, extrinsic masses, presence of fecal impaction, and caliber of the rectum. Stool obtained on the glove should be tested for occult blood.

## SCREENING TESTS

After the history and physical examination, laboratory testing may guide the diagnosis or treatment. Careful selection of tests minimizes cost, discomfort, and risk to the patient.

A complete blood count may provide evidence of inflammation (white blood cell [WBC] and platelet count), poor nutrition or bleeding (hemoglobin, red blood cell volume, reticulocyte count), and infection (WBC number and differential, presence of toxic granulation). Serum electrolytes, blood urea nitrogen (BUN), and creatinine help define hydration status. Tests of liver function include total and direct bilirubin, alanine aminotransferase, aspartate aminotransferase, and γ-glutamyltransferase or alkaline phosphatase for more specific evidence of bile duct injury. Hepatic synthetic function can be assessed by coagulation factor levels, coagulation times, and albumin level. Pancreatic enzyme tests (amylase, lipase, trypsinogen) provide evidence of pancreatic injury or inflammation. Tests also are available for specific conditions, such as celiac disease, viral hepatitis, $\alpha_1$-antitrypsin deficiency,

463

Wilson disease, ulcerative colitis (UC), Crohn's disease (CD), and metabolic conditions. Urinalysis can be helpful in gauging dehydration and assessing effects of digestive system disease on the urinary tract.

## DIAGNOSTIC IMAGING

### Radiology

Plain abdominal radiographs and barium studies have great utility. There is usually no reason to start with computed tomography (CT) or magnetic resonance imaging (MRI) for evaluation of most symptoms. In choosing an imaging study, consultation with a radiologist is often advisable, not only to discuss the best imaging method, but to decide what variants of the technique should be used and how to prepare the patient for the study. In some cases, it is important for the patient to be fasting (ultrasound examination of the gallbladder). An intravenous (IV) catheter may be needed for contrast agent or radionuclide administration, or a preparatory enema may be required.

It is not necessary to obtain a plain abdominal x-ray to document excessive retained stool in a child whose history is consistent with constipation and encopresis. Examination alone can confirm the presence of a fecal mass in the left lower quadrant. Rectal examination can disclose fecal impaction. Similarly, if a simple barium upper GI series is planned to diagnose small bowel Crohn's disease, a CT scan may not be needed, unless there are other concerns, such as abscess or lymphoma.

### Endoscopy

Endoscopy permits the direct visualization of the interior of the gut. Modern equipment includes **video endoscopes** with high-quality electronic optics. Endoscopes are small and flexible, and may be used even in very small infants. The design of endoscopes permits a great deal of control of tip movement, illumination, image acquisition, and endoscope advancement through the gut. Endoscopes also allow for suction of intestinal contents and air and water insufflation; they have a separate channel for introducing instruments, such as biopsy forceps, snares, foreign body retrievers, electrocoagulators, injection needles, and other specialized tools. **Wireless capsule endoscopy** (Fig. 126-1) extends the diagnostic capabilities of endoscopy, enabling visualization of lesions beyond the reach of conventional endoscopes.

## COMMON MANIFESTATIONS OF GASTROINTESTINAL DISORDERS

### Abdominal Pain

#### General Considerations

Abdominal pain can result from injury to the intra-abdominal organs, injury to overlying somatic structures in the abdominal wall, or extra-abdominal diseases. **Visceral pain** results when nerves within the gut detect injury. Visceral sensation is transmitted by nonmyelinated fibers and is vague, dull, slow in onset, and poorly localized.

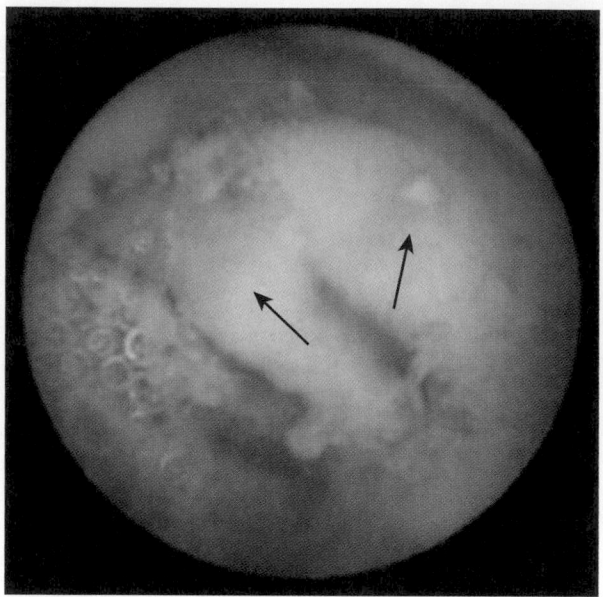

**FIGURE 126-1**

**Wireless capsule endoscopy:** Aphthous ulcers (*arrows*) in jejunum diagnostic of Crohn's disease in patient with negative findings on upper endoscopy and colonoscopy.

A variety of stimuli, including normal peristalsis and various chemical and osmotic states, activate these fibers to some degree, allowing some sensation of normal activity. Regardless of the stimulus, visceral pain is perceived when a threshold of intensity or duration is crossed. Lower degrees of activation may result in perception of non-painful or perhaps vaguely uncomfortable sensations, whereas more intensive stimulation of these fibers results in pain. Overactive sensation may be the basis of some kinds of abdominal pain, such as functional abdominal pain.

In contrast to visceral pain, **somatic pain** results when overlying body structures are injured. Somatic structures include the parietal peritoneum, fascia, muscles, and skin of the abdominal wall. In contrast to the vague, poorly localized pain emanating from visceral injury, somatic nociceptive fibers are myelinated and are capable of rapid transmission of well-localized painful stimuli. When intra-abdominal processes extend to cause inflammation or injury to the parietal peritoneum or abdominal wall structures, poorly localized visceral pain becomes well-localized somatic pain. In acute appendicitis, visceral nociceptive fibers are activated initially, yielding poorly localized discomfort in the midabdomen. When the inflammatory process extends to involve the overlying parietal peritoneum, the pain becomes severe and localizes to the right lower quadrant. This is called **somatoparietal pain**.

**Referred pain** is a painful sensation in a body region distant from the true source of pain. The physiologic cause is the activation of spinal cord somatic sensory cell bodies by intense signaling from visceral afferent nerves, located at the same level of the spinal cord. The location of referred pain is predictable based on the locus of visceral injury. Stomach pain is referred to the epigastric and retrosternal regions. Liver and pancreas pain is referred to the epigastric region. Gallbladder pain often is referred to the region below the right scapula. Splenic pain is referred to the left shoulder. Somatic pathways stimulated by small bowel visceral afferents affect the periumbilical area. Colonic injury results in infraumbilical referred pain.

## Acute Abdominal Pain

### Distinguishing Features

Acute abdominal pain can signal the presence of a dangerous intra-abdominal process, such as appendicitis or bowel obstruction, or may originate from extraintestinal sources, such as lower lobe pneumonia or urinary tract infection or stone. Not all episodes of acute abdominal pain require emergency intervention. Appendicitis must be ruled out as quickly as possible. Only a few children presenting with acute abdominal pain actually have a surgical emergency. These surgical cases must be separated from cases that can be managed conservatively (see Tables 126-2 and 126-3).

### Diagnostic Evaluation

Important clues to the diagnosis can be determined by history and physical examination (Tables 126-1 to 126-3). The **onset of pain** can provide clues. Events that occur abruptly (e.g., passage of a stone, perforation of a viscus, or infarction) result in a sudden onset. Gradual onset of pain is common with infectious or inflammatory causes (e.g., appendicitis, IBD).

A standard group of laboratory tests usually is performed for abdominal pain (see Table 126-1). After an abdominal x-ray series is obtained, further imaging studies may be warranted. CT can visualize the appendix if appendicitis is suspected. If the initial evaluation suggests intussusception, a barium or pneumatic (air) enema may be the first choice to diagnose and treat this condition with hydrostatic reduction (see Chapter 129).

**TABLE 126-1  Diagnostic Approach to Acute Abdominal Pain**

| HISTORY | |
| --- | --- |
| Onset | Sudden or gradual, prior episodes, association with meals, history of injury |
| Nature | Sharp versus dull, colicky or constant, burning |
| Location | Epigastric, periumbilical, generalized, right or left lower quadrant, change in location over time |
| Fever | Presence suggests appendicitis or other infection |
| Extraintestinal symptoms | Cough, dyspnea, dysuria, urinary frequency, flank pain |
| Course of symptoms | Worsening or improving, change in nature or location of pain |

| PHYSICAL EXAMINATION | |
| --- | --- |
| General | Growth and nutrition, general appearance, hydration, degree of discomfort, body position |
| Abdominal | Tenderness, distention, bowel sounds, rigidity, guarding, mass |
| Genitalia | Testicular torsion, hernia, pelvic inflammatory disease, ectopic pregnancy |
| Surrounding structures | Breath sounds, rales, rhonchi, wheezing, flank tenderness, tenderness of abdominal wall structures, ribs, costochondral joints |
| Rectal examination | Perianal lesions, stricture, tenderness, fecal impaction, blood |

| LABORATORY | |
| --- | --- |
| CBC, C-reactive protein, ESR | Evidence of infection or inflammation |
| AST, ALT, GGT, bilirubin | Biliary or liver disease |
| Amylase, lipase | Pancreatitis |
| Urinalysis | Urinary tract infection, bleeding due to stone, trauma, or obstruction |
| Pregnancy test (older females) | Ectopic pregnancy |

| RADIOLOGY | |
| --- | --- |
| Plain flat and upright abdominal films | Bowel obstruction, appendiceal fecalith, free intraperitoneal air, kidney stones |
| CT scan | Rule out abscess, appendicitis, Crohn disease, pancreatitis, gallstones, kidney stones |
| Barium enema | Intussusception, malrotation |
| Ultrasound | Gallstones, appendicitis, intussusception, pancreatitis, kidney stones, ovarian/tube diseases |

| ENDOSCOPY | |
| --- | --- |
| Upper endoscopy | Suspected peptic ulcer or esophagitis |

ALT, alanine aminotransferase; AST, aspartate aminotransferase; CBC, complete blood count, ESR, erythrocyte sedimentation rate; GGT, γ-glutamyltransferase.
Adapted from Andreoli TE, Carpenter CJ, Plum F, et al: Cecil Essentials of Medicine. Philadelphia, *WB Saunders*, 1986.

## TABLE 126-2  Differential Diagnosis of Acute Abdominal Pain

### TRAUMATIC

Duodenal hematoma
Ruptured spleen
Perforated viscus

### FUNCTIONAL

Constipation*
Irritable bowel syndrome*
Dysmenorrhea*
Mittelschmerz (ovulation)*
Infantile colic*

### INFECTIOUS

Appendicitis*
Viral or bacterial gastroenteritis/mesenteric adenitis*
Abscess
Spontaneous bacterial peritonitis
Pelvic inflammatory disease
Cholecystitis
Urinary tract infection*
Pneumonia (lower lobes)
Bacterial typhlitis
Hepatitis

### GENITAL

Testicular torsion
Ovarian torsion
Ectopic pregnancy

### GENETIC

Sickle cell crisis*
Familial Mediterranean fever
Porphyria

### METABOLIC

Diabetic ketoacidosis

### INFLAMMATORY

Inflammatory bowel disease
Vasculitis
Henoch-Schönlein purpura*
Pancreatitis

### OBSTRUCTIVE

Intussusception*
Malrotation with volvulus
Ileus*
Incarcerated hernia
Postoperative adhesion
Meconium ileus equivalent (cystic fibrosis)
Duplication cyst, congenital stricture

### BILIARY

Gallstone
Gallbladder hydrops
Biliary dyskinesia

### PEPTIC

Gastric or duodenal ulcer
Gastritis*
Esophagitis

### RENAL

Kidney stone
Hydronephrosis

*Common.

## Differential Diagnosis (Table 126-2)

Acute pain requires an urgent evaluation to rule out surgical emergencies. In young children, malrotation, incarcerated hernia, congenital anomalies, and intussusception are common concerns. In older children and teenagers, appendicitis is more common. An acute surgical abdomen is characterized by signs of peritonitis, including tenderness, abdominal wall rigidity, guarding, and absent or diminished bowel sounds. Helpful characteristics of onset, location, referral, and quality of pain are noted in Table 126-3.

## Functional Abdominal Pain and Irritable Bowel Syndrome

Recurrent abdominal pain is a common problem, affecting more than 10% of all children. The peak incidence occurs between ages 7 and 12 years. The differential diagnosis of recurrent abdominal pain is fairly extensive (Table 126-4). However, most children with this condition do not have a serious (or identifiable) underlying illness causing the pain.

## Differential Diagnosis

Children with **functional abdominal pain** characteristically have pain almost daily. The pain is not associated with meals or relieved by defecation, and is often associated with a tendency toward anxiety and perfectionism. Symptoms often result from stress at school or in novel social situations. The pain often is worst in the morning and prevents or delays them from attending school. **Irritable bowel syndrome (IBS)** is a subset of functional abdominal pain, characterized by onset of pain at the time of a change in stool frequency or consistency, a stool pattern fluctuating between diarrhea and constipation, and relief of pain with defecation. Symptoms in IBS are linked to gut motility. Pain is commonly accompanied in both groups of children by school avoidance, secondary gains, anxiety about imagined causes, lack of coping skills, and disordered peer relationships.

## Distinguishing Features

One needs to distinguish between functional pain/IBS and more serious underlying disorders. **Warning signs** for underlying illness are listed in Table 126-5. If any

**TABLE 126-3  Distinguishing Features of Abdominal Pain in Children**

| Disease | Onset | Location | Referral | Quality | Comments |
|---|---|---|---|---|---|
| Functional: irritable bowel syndrome | Recurrent | Periumbilical, splenic and hepatic flexures | None | Dull, crampy, intermittent; duration 2 hr | Family stress, school phobia, diarrhea and constipation; hypersensitive to pain from distention |
| Esophageal reflux | Recurrent, after meals, at bedtime | Substernal | Chest | Burning | Sour taste in mouth; Sandifer syndrome |
| Duodenal ulcer | Recurrent, before meals, at night | Epigastric | Back | Severe burning, gnawing | Relieved by food, milk, antacids; family history important; GI bleeding |
| Pancreatitis | Acute | Epigastric-hypogastric | Back | Constant, sharp, boring | Nausea, emesis, marked tenderness |
| Intestinal obstruction | Acute or gradual | Periumbilical-lower abdomen | Back | Alternating cramping (colic) and painless periods | Distention, obstipation, bilious emesis, increased bowel sounds |
| Appendicitis | Acute | Periumbilical or epigastric; localizes to right lower quadrant | Back or pelvis if retrocecal | Sharp, steady | Nausea, emesis, local tenderness, ± fever, avoids motion |
| Meckel diverticulum | Recurrent | Periumbilical-lower abdomen | None | Sharp | Hematochezia; painless unless intussusception, diverticulitis, or perforation |
| Inflammatory bowel disease | Recurrent | Depends on site of involvement | | Dull cramping, tenesmus | Fever, weight loss, ± hematochezia |
| Intussusception | Acute | Periumbilical-lower abdomen | None | Cramping, with painless periods | Guarded position with knees pulled up, currant jelly stools, lethargy |
| Lactose intolerance | Recurrent with milk products | Lower abdomen | None | Cramping | Distention, gaseousness, diarrhea |
| Urolithiasis | Acute, sudden | Back | Groin | Severe, colicky pain | Hematuria |
| Pyelonephritis | Acute, sudden | Back | None | Dull to sharp | Fever, costochondral tenderness, dysuria, urinary frequency, emesis |
| Cholecystitis and cholelithiasis | Acute | Right upper quadrant | Right shoulder | Severe, colicky pain | Hemolysis ± jaundice, nausea, emesis |

GI, gastrointestinal.
Adapted from Andreoli TE, Carpenter CJ, Plum F, et al: Cecil Essentials of Medicine. Philadelphia, *WB Saunders*, 1986.

warning signs are present, further investigation is necessary. Even if the warning signs are absent, some laboratory evaluation is warranted. A judicious laboratory evaluation after a careful history and complete physical examination can assure parents and physicians that no serious illness is being missed. The initial evaluation recommended in Table 126-6 is a sensible approach, avoiding unnecessary testing and providing ample sensitivity for most serious underlying disorders. A 3-day trial of a lactose-free diet can rule out lactose intolerance. If tests are normal and no warning signs are present, testing should be stopped. If there are warning signs, progression of symptoms, or laboratory abnormalities that suggest a specific diagnosis, additional investigation may be warranted. For example, if antacids consistently relieve pain, an upper GI endoscopy to look for peptic disease may be considered. If the child is losing weight, a barium upper GI series with a small bowel follow-through or CT can be performed to look for

**TABLE 126-4 Differential Diagnosis of Recurrent Abdominal Pain**

Functional abdominal pain*
Irritable bowel syndrome*
Chronic pancreatitis
Gallstones
Peptic disease
    Duodenal ulcer
    Gastric ulcer
    Esophagitis
Lactose intolerance*
Fructose malabsorption
Inflammatory bowel disease*
    Crohn disease
    Ulcerative colitis
Constipation*
Obstructive uropathy
Congenital intestinal malformation
    Malrotation
    Duplication cyst
    Stricture or web
Celiac disease*

*Common.

**TABLE 126-5 Warning Signs of Underlying Illness in Recurrent Abdominal Pain**

Vomiting
Abnormal screening laboratory study
Fever
Bilious emesis
Growth failure
Pain awakening child from sleep
Weight loss
Location away from periumbilical region
Blood in stools or emesis
Delayed puberty

evidence of inflammatory bowel disease. Celiac disease (see Chapter 129) also should be considered and diagnosed by antibody testing and endoscopic duodenal biopsy.

### Treatment

A child who is repeatedly kept home from school because of pain receives attention for his symptoms, is excused from responsibilities, and withdraws from full social functioning. This situation tends to both increase anxiety and provide positive reinforcement for being ill. To break the cycle of pain and disability, the child with functional pain must be assisted in returning to normal activities immediately. The child should not be sent home from school with stomachaches; rather, the child may be allowed to take a short break from class until the cramping abates. It is useful to inform the child and the parents that the pain is likely to be worse on the day the child returns to school, because anxiety worsens dysmotility and enhances pain perception. Sometimes, medications can be helpful. **Fiber supplements** are useful to manage symptoms of IBS. In difficult and persistent cases, amitriptyline or a selective serotonin reuptake inhibitor may be helpful. When significant anxiety or social dysfunction persists, a mental health professional should be consulted.

## Vomiting

**Vomiting** is a coordinated, sequential series of events that leads to forceful oral emptying of gastric contents. It is a common problem in children and has many causes. Vomiting should be distinguished from **regurgitation** of stomach contents, also known as gastroesophageal reflux (GER), chalasia, or *spitting up*. Although the end result of vomiting and regurgitation is similar, they have completely different characteristics. Vomiting is usually preceded by nausea, followed by forceful gagging and retching. Regurgitation, on the other hand, is effortless and not preceded by nausea.

**TABLE 126-6 Suggested Evaluation of Recurrent Abdominal Pain**

| Initial Evaluation | Follow-up Evaluation* |
|---|---|
| Complete history and physical examination | CT scan of the abdomen and pelvis with oral, rectal, and intravenous contrast |
| Ask about "warning signs" (see Table 126-5) | |
| Determine degree of functional impairment (e.g., missing school) | Celiac disease serology—endomysial antibody or tissue transglutaminase antibody |
| CBC | Barium upper GI series with small bowel follow-through |
| ESR | Endoscopy of the esophagus, stomach, and duodenum |
| Amylase, lipase | Colonoscopy |
| Urinalysis | |
| Abdominal ultrasound—examine liver, bile ducts, gallbladder, pancreas, kidneys, ureters | |
| Trial of 3-day lactose-free diet | |

*Consider using one or more of these to investigate warning signs, abnormal laboratory tests, or specific or persistent symptoms.
CBC, complete blood count; CT, computed tomography; ESR, erythrocyte sedimentation rate; GI, gastrointestinal.

## Differential Diagnosis

In neonates with true vomiting, congenital obstructive lesions should be considered. Allergic reactions to formula also are common in the first 2 months of life. **Infantile GER** ("spitting up") occurs in most infants and can be large in volume, but is effortless and these infants do not appear ill. **Pyloric stenosis** occurs in the first month of life and is characterized by steadily worsening, forceful vomiting which occurs immediately after feedings. Prior to vomiting a distended stomach, often with visible peristaltic waves is often seen. Pyloric stenosis is more common in male infants, and there may be a positive family history. Other obstructive lesions, such as intestinal duplication cysts, atresias, webs, and midgut malrotation must be ruled out. **Metabolic disorders** (organic acidemias, galactosemia, urea cycle defects, etc.) can cause vomiting in infants. In older children with acute vomiting, viral illnesses are common. Other infections, especially streptococcal pharyngitis, urinary tract infections, and otitis media, commonly result in vomiting. When vomiting is chronic, central nervous system (CNS) causes (increased intracranial pressure, migraine) must be considered. When abdominal pain or bilious emesis accompanies vomiting, evaluation for bowel obstruction, peptic disorders, and appendicitis must be immediately initiated.

## Distinguishing Features

Physicians caring for children see hundreds of patients with viral gastroenteritis for every one with a less common diagnosis. It is important to be alert for unusual features that suggest another diagnosis (Table 126-7). Viral gastroenteritis usually is not associated with severe abdominal pain or headache and does not recur at frequent intervals.

## Assessment

**Physical examination** should include assessment of the child's hydration status, including examination of capillary refill, moistness of mucous membranes, and skin turgor (see Chapter 38). The chest should be auscultated for evidence of pulmonary involvement. The abdomen must be examined carefully for distention, organomegaly, bowel sounds, tenderness, and guarding. A rectal examination and testing stool for occult blood should be performed.

**TABLE 126-7  Differential Diagnosis of Vomiting by Historical Features**

| Potential Diagnosis | Historical Clues |
| --- | --- |
| Viral gastroenteritis | Fever, diarrhea, sudden onset, absence of pain |
| Gastroesophageal reflux | Effortless, not preceded by nausea, chronic |
| Hepatitis | Jaundice, history of exposure |
| Extragastrointestinal infections | |
|   Otitis media | Fever, ear pain |
|   Urinary tract infection | Dysuria, unusual urine odor, frequency, incontinence |
|   Pneumonia | Cough, fever, chest discomfort |
| Allergic | |
|   Milk or soy protein intolerance (infants) | Associated with particular formula or food, blood in stools |
|   Other food allergy (older children) | |
| Peptic ulcer or gastritis | Epigastric pain, blood or coffee-ground material in emesis, pain relieved by acid blockade |
| Appendicitis | Fever, abdominal pain migrating to the right lower quadrant, tenderness |
| Anatomic obstruction | |
|   Intestinal atresia | Neonate, usually bilious, polyhydramnios |
|   Midgut malrotation | Pain, bilious vomiting, gastrointestinal bleeding, shock |
|   Intussusception | Colicky pain, lethargy, vomiting, currant jelly stools, mass occasionally |
|   Duplication cysts | Colic, mass |
|   Pyloric stenosis | Nonbilious vomiting, postprandial, <4 mo old, hunger |
| Bacterial gastroenteritis | Fever, often with bloody diarrhea |
| Central nervous system | |
|   Hydrocephalus | Large head, altered mental status |
|   Meningitis | Fever, stiff neck |
|   Migraine syndrome | Attacks scattered in time, relieved by sleep; headache |
|   Cyclic vomiting syndrome | Similar to migraine, usually no headache |
|   Brain tumor | Morning vomiting, accelerating over time, headache, diplopia |
| Motion sickness | Associated with travel in vehicle |
| Labyrinthitis | Vertigo |
| Metabolic disease | Presentation early in life, worsens when catabolic or with exposure to substrate |
| Pregnancy | Morning, sexually active, cessation of menses |
| Drug reaction or side effect | Associated with increased dose or new medication |
| Cancer chemotherapy | Temporally related to administration of chemotherapeutic drugs |

**Laboratory evaluation** of vomiting should include serum electrolytes, tests of renal function, complete blood count, amylase, lipase, and liver function tests. Additional testing may be required immediately when history and examination suggest a specific etiology. Ultrasound is useful to look for pyloric stenosis, gallstones, renal stones, hydronephrosis, biliary obstruction, pancreatitis, appendicitis, malrotation, intussusception, and other anatomic abnormalities. CT may be indicated to rule out appendicitis or to observe structures that cannot be visualized well by ultrasound. Barium studies can show obstructive or inflammatory lesions of the gut and can be therapeutic, as in the use of contrast enemas for intussusception (see Chapter 129).

## Treatment

**Treatment** of vomiting needs to address the consequences and causes of the vomiting. Dehydration must be treated with fluid resuscitation. This can be accomplished in most cases with oral fluid-electrolyte solutions, but IV fluids are commonly required. Electrolyte imbalances should be corrected by appropriate choice of fluids. Underlying causes should be treated when possible.

The use of **antiemetic medications** is controversial. These drugs should not be prescribed until the etiology of the vomiting is known and then only for severe symptoms. Phenothiazines, such as prochlorperazine, may be useful for reducing symptoms in food poisoning and motion sickness. Their side effect profile must be considered carefully, and the dose prescribed should be conservative. Anticholinergics, such as scopolamine, and antihistamines, such as dimenhydrinate, are useful for the prophylaxis and treatment of motion sickness. Drugs that block serotonin 5-HT$_3$ receptors, such as ondansetron and granisetron, are used for viral gastroenteritis, and can improve tolerance of oral rehydration therapy. They are clearly helpful for chemotherapy-induced vomiting, often combined with dexamethasone. No antiemetic should be used in patients with surgical emergencies or when a specific treatment of the underlying condition is possible. Correction of dehydration, ketosis, and acidosis by oral or intravenous rehydration is helpful to reduce vomiting in most patients with viral gastroenteritis.

## Acute and Chronic Diarrhea

Parents use the word *diarrhea* to describe loose or watery stools, excessively frequent stools, or stools that are large in volume. Constipation with overflow incontinence can be mislabeled as diarrhea. A more exact definition is excessive daily stool liquid volume (>10 mL stool/kg body weight/day).

Diarrhea is a major cause of childhood morbidity and fatality worldwide. Deaths from diarrhea are rare in developed countries, but are common elsewhere. **Acute diarrhea** is a major problem when it occurs with malnutrition or in the absence of basic medical care (see Chapter 30). In North America, most acute diarrhea is viral, is self-limited, and requires no diagnostic testing or specific intervention. Bacterial agents tend to cause more severe illness and typically are seen in outbreaks or in regions with poor public sanitation. Bacterial enteritis should be suspected when there is **dysentery** (bloody diarrhea with fever) and whenever severe symptoms are present. These infections can be diagnosed by stool culture or other assays for specific pathogens. **Chronic diarrhea** lasts more than 2 weeks and has a wide range of possible causes, including more difficult to diagnose serious and benign conditions.

## Differential Diagnosis

Diarrhea may be classified by etiology or by physiologic mechanisms (secretory or osmotic). Etiologic agents include viruses, bacteria or their toxins, chemicals, parasites, malabsorbed substances, and inflammation (Table 126-8). **Secretory diarrhea** occurs when the intestinal mucosa directly secretes fluid and electrolytes into the stool. Secretion may be the result of inflammation, as in inflammatory bowel disease, or a chemical stimulus. Cholera is a secretory diarrhea stimulated by the enterotoxin of *Vibrio cholerae* which causes increased levels of cyclic adenosine monophosphate (cAMP) within enterocytes, leading to secretion into the small bowel lumen. Secretion also is stimulated by mediators of inflammation and by various hormones, such as vasoactive intestinal peptide secreted by a neuroendocrine tumor.

**Osmotic diarrhea** occurs after malabsorption of an ingested substance, which "pulls" water into the bowel lumen. A classic example is the diarrhea of lactose intolerance. Osmotic diarrhea also can result from maldigestion, such as that seen with pancreatic insufficiency, or with malabsorption caused by intestinal injury. Certain nonabsorbable laxatives, such as polyethylene glycol and milk of magnesia, also cause osmotic diarrhea. Fermentation of malabsorbed substances (e.g., lactose) often occurs, resulting in gas, cramps, and acidic stools. The most common non infectious cause of loose stools in early childhood is **functional diarrhea**, commonly known as **toddler's diarrhea**. This condition is defined by frequent watery stools in the setting of normal growth and weight gain. It is caused by excessive intake of carbohydrate-containing sweet liquids, overwhelming the absorptive capacity of the intestine. Diarrhea typically improves tremendously when the child's beverage intake is reduced or changed.

## Distinguishing Features

Stools are isosmotic—that is, they have the same osmolarity as body fluids. This is true even in osmotic diarrhea, because of the relatively free exchange of water across the intestinal mucosa. Osmoles present in the stool are a mixture of electrolytes and other osmotically active solutes. To determine whether the diarrhea is osmotic or secretory, the **osmotic gap** may be calculated:

$$\text{Osmotic gap} = 290 - 2([Na^+] + [K^+])$$

The formula for the osmotic gap assumes that the stool is isosmotic (an osmolarity of 290 mOsm/L). Stool sodium and potassium are measured, added together, and multiplied by 2 to account for their associated anions. This result is subtracted from 290. Secretory diarrhea is characterized by an osmotic gap of less than 50 because most of the dissolved substances in the stool are electrolytes.

## TABLE 126-8 Differential Diagnosis of Diarrhea

| Type/Frequency | Infant | Child | Adolescent |
|---|---|---|---|
| **ACUTE** | | | |
| Common | Gastroenteritis* | Gastroenteritis* | Gastroenteritis* |
| | Systemic infection | Food poisoning | Food poisoning |
| | Antibiotic-associated | Systemic infection | Antibiotic-associated |
| | Overfeeding | Antibiotic-associated | |
| Rare | Primary disaccharidase deficiency | Toxic ingestion | Hyperthyroidism |
| | Hirschsprung toxic colitis | | |
| | Adrenogenital syndrome | | |
| **CHRONIC** | | | |
| Common | Postinfectious secondary lactase deficiency | Postinfectious secondary lactase deficiency | Irritable bowel syndrome |
| | Cow's milk/soy protein intolerance | Irritable bowel syndrome | Inflammatory bowel disease |
| | Chronic nonspecific diarrhea of infancy (toddler's diarrhea) | Celiac disease | Lactose intolerance |
| | Celiac disease | Lactose intolerance | Giardiasis |
| | Cystic fibrosis | Giardiasis | Laxative abuse (anorexia nervosa) |
| | AIDS enteropathy | Inflammatory bowel disease | |
| Rare | Primary immune defects | AIDS enteropathy | AIDS enteropathy |
| | Familial villous atrophy | Acquired immune defects | Secretory tumors |
| | Secretory tumors | Secretory tumor | Primary bowel tumor |
| | Congenital chloridorrhea | Pseudo-obstruction | |
| | Acrodermatitis enteropathica | Factitious | |
| | Lymphangiectasia | | |
| | Abetalipoproteinemia | | |
| | Eosinophilic gastroenteritis | | |
| | Short bowel syndrome | | |
| | Intractable diarrhea syndrome | | |
| | Autoimmune enteropathy | | |
| | Factitious | | |

*Gastroenteritis includes viral (rotavirus, norovirus, astrovirus) and bacterial (*Salmonella, Shigella, Escherichia coli, Clostridium difficile, Yersinia, Campylobacter*, other) agents.
AIDS, acquired immunodeficiency syndrome.

A number significantly higher than 50 defines osmotic diarrhea and indicates that malabsorbed substances other than electrolytes account for fecal osmolarity.

Another way to differentiate between osmotic and secretory diarrhea is to stop all oral feedings and observe whether the diarrhea stops. It must be done only in a hospitalized patient receiving IV fluids to prevent dehydration. If the diarrhea stops completely, the patient has osmotic diarrhea. A child with secretory diarrhea continues to have stool output. Neither method for classifying diarrhea works perfectly, as most diarrheal illnesses are a mixture of secretory and osmotic components. Viral enteritis damages the intestinal lining, causing malabsorption and osmotic diarrhea. The associated inflammation results in release of mediators that cause excessive secretion. A child with viral enteritis may have decreased stool volume while not receiving oral feedings (NPO), but the secretory component persists until the inflammation resolves.

The **history** should include the onset of diarrhea, number and character of stools, estimates of stool volume, and presence of other symptoms, such as blood in the stool, fever, and weight loss. Recent travel should be documented, dietary factors should be investigated, and a list of medications recently used should be obtained. Factors that seem to worsen or improve the diarrhea should be determined. **Physical examination** should be thorough, including evaluation for abdominal distention, tenderness, bowel sound characteristics, presence of blood, and evidence of dehydration or shock.

**Laboratory testing** includes stool culture and complete blood count if bacterial enteritis is suspected. If diarrhea occurs after a course of antibiotics, a *Clostridium difficile* toxin assay should be ordered. If stools are oily or fatty, fecal fat content should be checked. Tests for specific diagnoses should be sent when appropriate, such as serum antibody tests for celiac disease or colonoscopy for suspected inflammatory bowel disease. A trial of lactose restriction for several days is helpful to rule out lactose intolerance.

## Constipation and Encopresis

Constipation is a common problem in childhood, accounting for a significant proportion of clinic visits. When a child is thought to be constipated, the parents may be concerned about straining with defecation, hard stool consistency, large stool size, decreased stool frequency, fear of passing stools, or any combination of these. Physicians define **constipation** as *two or fewer stools per week or passage of hard, pellet-like stools for at least 2 weeks*. A common pattern of constipation is **functional constipation**, which is characterized by two or fewer stools per week, voluntary withholding of stool and infrequent passage of large diameter, often painful, stools. Children with functional fecal retention often exhibit *retentive posturing* (standing or sitting with legs extended and stiff or crossed legs) and have associated fecal incontinence caused by leakage of retained stool (**encopresis**).

### Differential Diagnosis

Young children are vulnerable to **functional constipation**. Functional constipation commonly occurs during toilet training, when the child is unwilling to defecate on the toilet. Retained stool becomes harder and larger over time, leading to painful defecation. This aggravates voluntary withholding of stool, with perpetuation of the constipation.

**Hirschsprung disease** is characterized by delayed meconium passage in newborns, abdominal distention, vomiting, occasional fever, and foul-smelling stools. This condition is caused by failure of ganglion cells to migrate into the distal bowel, resulting in spasm and functional obstruction of the aganglionic segment. Only about 6% of infants with Hirschsprung disease pass meconium in the first 24 hours of life compared with 95% of normal infants. Most affected babies rapidly become ill with symptoms of enterocolitis or obstruction. Affected older children do not pass large-caliber stools because of rectal spasm. They do not have encopresis. When evaluating a 3-year-old with fear of defecation, large stools, fecal soiling, and no history of neonatal constipation, Hirschsprung disease is not a likely diagnosis. Other causes of constipation include spinal cord abnormalities, hypothyroidism, drugs, cystic fibrosis, and anorectal malformations (Table 126-9). A variety of systemic disorders affecting metabolism or

**TABLE 126-9 Common Causes of Constipation and Characteristic Features**

| Cause of Constipation | Clinical Features |
|---|---|
| Hirschsprung disease | *History:* Failure to pass stool in first 24 hr, abdominal distention, vomiting, symptoms of enterocolitis (fever, foul-smelling diarrhea, megacolon); not associated with large-caliber stools or encopresis<br>*Physical examination:* Snug anal sphincter, empty, contracted rectum; may have explosive release of stool as examiner's finger is withdrawn<br>*Laboratory:* Absence of ganglion cells on rectal suction biopsy specimen, absent relaxation of the internal sphincter, "transition zone" from narrow distal bowel to dilated proximal bowel on barium enema |
| Functional constipation | *History:* No history of significant neonatal constipation, onset at potty training, large-caliber stools, retentive posturing; may have encopresis<br>*Physical examination:* Normal or reduced sphincter tone, dilated rectal vault, fecal impaction, soiled underwear, palpable fecal mass in left lower quadrant<br>*Laboratory:* No abnormalities, barium enema would show dilated distal bowel |
| Anorectal and colonic malformations<br>  Anal stenosis<br>  Anteriorly displaced anus<br>  Imperforate anus<br>  Colonic stricture | *History:* Constipation from birth due to abnormal anatomy<br>*Physical examination:* Anorectal abnormalities are shown easily on physical examination; anteriorly displaced anus is found chiefly in females, with a normal-appearing anus located close to the posterior fourchette of the vagina<br>*Laboratory:* Barium enema shows the anomaly |
| Multisystem disease<br>  Muscular dystrophy<br>  Cystic fibrosis<br>  Diabetes mellitus<br>  Developmental delay | *History:* Presence of other symptoms or prior diagnosis<br>*Physical examination:* Specific abnormalities may be present that directly relate to the underlying diagnosis<br>*Laboratory:* Tests directed at suspected disorder confirm the diagnosis |
| Spinal cord abnormalities<br>  Meningomyelocele<br>  Tethered cord<br>  Sacral teratoma or lipoma | *History:* History of swelling or exposed neural tissue in the lower back, history of urinary incontinence<br>*Physical examination:* Lax sphincter tone due to impaired innervation, visible or palpable abnormality of lower back usually (but not always) present<br>*Laboratory:* Bony abnormalities often present on plain x-ray; MRI of spinal cord reveals characteristic abnormalities |
| Drugs<br>  Narcotics<br>  Psychotropics | *History:* Recent use of drugs known to cause constipation<br>*Physical examination:* Features suggest functional constipation<br>*Laboratory:* No specific tests available |

MRI, magnetic resonance imaging.

muscle function can result in constipation. Children with **developmental disabilities** have a great propensity for constipation because of diminished capacity to cooperate with toileting, reduced effort or control of pelvic floor muscles during defecation, and diminished perception of the need to pass stool.

## Distinguishing Features

Congenital malformations usually cause symptoms from birth. Functional constipation is overwhelmingly the most common diagnosis in older patients. Constipation in older children often begins after starting school, when free and private access to toilets may be restricted. Use of some drugs, especially opiates and some psychotropic medications, also is associated with constipation.

For a few specific causes of constipation, directed diagnostic testing can make the diagnosis. Hirschsprung disease can be suggested by findings on barium enema: a narrowed aganglionic distal bowel and dilated proximal bowel. Rectal suction biopsy confirms the absence of

ganglion cells in the rectal submucosal plexus, with hypertrophy of nerve fibers. Lack of internal anal sphincter relaxation can be shown by anorectal manometry in Hirschsprung disease. Hypothyroidism is diagnosed by thyroid function testing. Anorectal malformations are easily detected by rectal examination. Cystic fibrosis (meconium ileus) is diagnosed by sweat chloride determination or *CFTR* gene mutation analysis (see Chapter 137). Most children with constipation have functional constipation and do not have any laboratory abnormality. Examination reveals normal or reduced anal sphincter tone (owing to stretching by passage of large stools). Fecal impaction is usually present, but a large caliber, empty rectum may be found if a stool has just been passed.

## Evaluation and Treatment of Functional Constipation

In most cases of constipation, the history is consistent with functional constipation—absence of neonatal constipation, active fecal retention, and infrequent, large stools

**TABLE 126-10  Causes and Distinguishing Characteristics of Gastrointestinal Bleeding**

| Age | Type of Bleeding | Characteristics |
|---|---|---|
| **NEWBORN** | | |
| Ingested maternal blood* | Hematemesis or rectal, large amount | Apt test indicates adult hemoglobin is present |
| Peptic disease | Hematemesis, amount varies | Blood found in stomach on lavage |
| Coagulopathy | Hematemesis or rectal, bruising, other sites | History of home birth (no vitamin K) |
| Allergic colitis* | Streaks of bloody mucus in stool | Eosinophils in feces and in rectal mucosa |
| Necrotizing enterocolitis | Rectal | Sick infant with tender and distended abdomen |
| Duplication cyst | Hematemesis | Cystic mass in abdomen on imaging study |
| Volvulus | Hematemesis, hematochezia | Acute tender distended abdomen |
| **INFANCY TO 2 YEARS** | | |
| Peptic disease | Usually hematemesis, rectal possible | Epigastric pain, coffee-ground emesis |
| Esophageal varices | Hematemesis | History or evidence of liver disease |
| Intussusception* | Rectal bleeding | Crampy pain, distention, mass |
| Meckel diverticulum* | Rectal | Massive, bright red bleeding; no pain |
| Bacterial enteritis* | Rectal | Bloody diarrhea, fever |
| NSAID injury | Usually hematemesis, rectal possible | Epigastric pain, coffee-ground emesis |
| **>2 YEARS** | | |
| Peptic disease | See above | See above |
| Esophageal varices | See above | See above |
| NSAID injury* | See above | See above |
| Inflammatory bowel disease | Usually rectal | Crampy pain, poor weight gain, diarrhea |
| Bacterial enteritis* | Rectal | Fever, bloody stools |
| Pseudomembranous colitis | Rectal | History of antibiotic use, bloody diarrhea |
| Juvenile polyp | Rectal | Painless, bright red blood in stool; not massive |
| Meckel diverticulum* | See above | See above |
| Nodular lymphoid hyperplasia | Rectal | Streaks of blood in stool, no other symptoms |
| Mallory-Weiss syndrome* | Hematemesis | Bright red or coffee-ground, follows retching |
| Hemolytic uremic syndrome | Rectal | Thrombocytopenia, anemia, uremia, diarrhea |

*Common.
NSAID, nonsteroidal anti-inflammatory drug.

with soiling. In these patients, no testing is necessary other than a good physical examination. A prolonged course of stool softener therapy is needed in these children to alleviate fear of defecation. The child should be asked to sit on the toilet for a few minutes on awakening in the morning and immediately after meals, when the colon is most active and it is easiest to pass a stool. Use of a positive reinforcement system for taking medication and sitting on the toilet is a helpful for younger children. The stool softener chosen should be non–habit forming, safe, and palatable. Polyethylene glycol (PEG) and milk of magnesia are the most commonly used agents. PEG, which is tasteless and minimally absorbed, has become the preferred stool-softening laxative for most situations.

## Gastrointestinal Bleeding

GI tract bleeding can be an emergency when large volume bleeding is present, but the presence of small amounts of blood in stool or vomitus is also sufficient to cause concern. Evaluation of bleeding should include confirmation that blood truly is present, estimation of the amount of bleeding, stabilization of vital signs, localization of the source of bleeding, and appropriate treatment of the underlying cause. When bleeding is massive, it is crucial that the patient receive adequate resuscitation with fluid and blood products before moving ahead with diagnostic testing.

## Differential Diagnosis

In newborns, blood in vomitus or stool may be maternal blood swallowed during delivery or during breastfeeding. Blood-streaked stools are particularly associated with allergic colitis or necrotizing enterocolitis in this age group, but small streaks of bright red blood also can be seen in the diaper of infants with an anal fissure or milk allergy. Coagulopathy, peptic disease, and arteriovenous malformations can cause upper or lower GI tract bleeding in neonates.

In infants up to 2 years of age, peptic disease or nonsteroidal anti-inflammatory drug (NSAID)–induced gastric injury causes hematemesis; esophageal varices also occur in this age group with portal hypertension caused by conditions such as biliary atresia. After this age, peptic disease and esophageal varices continue to be common causes of hematemesis. Rectal bleeding in older children is likely to be caused by a juvenile polyp, IBD, Meckel's diverticulum, or nodular lymphoid hyperplasia. The presence of diarrhea and mucus in the stool particularly suggests IBD or bacterial dysentery. When rectal bleeding is massive and painless, Meckel's diverticulum is a common cause. The bleeding caused by polyps or lymphoid hyperplasia can be significant, but seldom is profuse enough to result in changes in pulse or blood pressure (Table 126-10).

## Distinguishing Features

Red substances in foods or beverages occasionally can be mistaken for blood. A test for occult blood is worth performing whenever the diagnosis is in doubt.

Blood may not be coming from the GI tract. The clinician should ask about cough, look in the mouth and nostrils, and examine the lungs carefully to exclude these sources of hematemesis. Blood in the toilet or diaper may be coming from the urinary tract, vagina, or even a severe diaper rash. If the bleeding is GI, the clinician needs to determine whether it is originating high in the GI tract or distal to the ligament of Treitz. Vomited blood is always proximal. Rectal bleeding may be coming from anywhere in the gut. When dark clots or melena are seen mixed with stool, a higher location is suspected, whereas bright red blood on the surface of stool probably is coming from lower in the colon. When upper GI tract bleeding is suspected, a nasogastric tube may be placed and gastric contents aspirated for evidence of recent bleeding in the proximal gut.

The location and hemodynamic significance of the bleeding can also be assessed by history and examination. The parents should be asked to quantify the bleeding. Details of associated symptoms should be sought. The vital signs should be evaluated and assessment for orthostatic changes performed when bleeding volume is large. Pulses, capillary refill, and pallor of the mucous membranes should be assessed. Laboratory assessment and imaging studies should be ordered as indicated (Table 126-11).

---

### TABLE 126-11 Evaluation of Gastrointestinal Bleeding

#### LABORATORY INVESTIGATION

*All Patients*
CBC and platelet count
Coagulation tests: prothrombin time, partial thromboplastin time
Liver function tests: AST, ALT, GGT, bilirubin
Occult blood test of stool or vomitus
Blood type and crossmatch
*Evaluation of Bloody Diarrhea*
Stool culture, *Clostridium difficile* toxin
Sigmoidoscopy or colonoscopy—rule out inflammatory bowel disease
Barium enema or CT with contrast
*Evaluation of Rectal Bleeding with Formed Stools*
External and digital rectal examination
Sigmoidoscopy or colonoscopy—rule out fissures, polyps
Meckel scan—rule out Meckel diverticulum
Mesenteric arteriogram or capsule endoscopy—rule out arteriovenous malformation

#### INITIAL RADIOLOGIC EVALUATION

*All Patients*
Abdominal x-ray series

#### EVALUATION OF HEMATEMESIS

Upper endoscopy
Barium upper GI series if endoscopy not available
*Evaluation of Bleeding with Pain and Vomiting (Bowel Obstruction)*
Abdominal x-ray series
Pneumatic or contrast enema—rule out intussusception
Upper GI series or ultrasound—rule out malrotation, volvulus

ALT, alanine aminotransferase; AST, aspartate aminotransferase; CBC, complete blood count; GGT, γ-glutamyltransferase; GI, gastrointestinal.

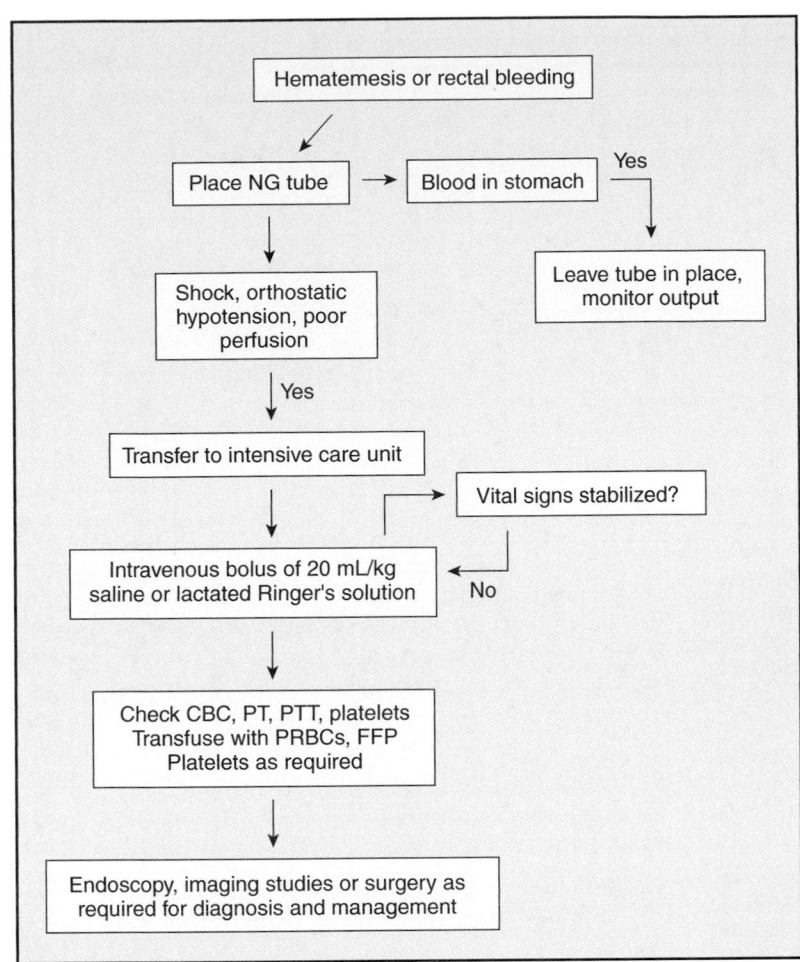

FIGURE 126-2

**Initial management of gastrointestinal bleeding.** CBC, complete blood count; FFP, fresh frozen plasma; NG, nasogastric; PRBCs, packed red blood cells; PT, prothrombin time; PTT, partial thromboplastin time.

## Treatment

Treatment of GI bleeding should begin with an initial assessment, rapid stabilization of shock, if present, and a logical sequence of diagnostic tests. When a treatable cause is identified, specific therapy should be started. In many cases, the amount of blood is small, and no resuscitation is required. For children with large volume bleeds, the **ABCs** of resuscitation (check airway, breathing, and circulation) should be addressed first (see Chapters 38 and 40). Oxygen should be administered and the airway protected with an endotracheal tube if massive hematemesis is present. Two large bore IV lines are needed to restore adequate circulation with fluid boluses or transfuse with packed red blood cells as required. Frequent reassessment is needed (Fig. 126-2).

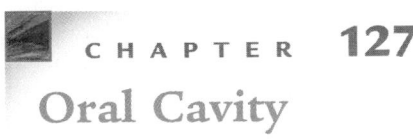

CHAPTER **127**

# Oral Cavity

The oral cavity is a complex structure including the lips, gums, tongue, teeth, and surrounding structures involved in the functions of chewing and swallowing. The health of oral tissues has a significant impact on the ability to take adequate nourishment and to protect the airway from aspiration. Systemic disorders may have manifestations in the oral cavity that are readily detectable on examination.

## EFFECTS OF SYSTEMIC DISEASE ON THE ORAL CAVITY

Medications taken for a variety of conditions may cause oral abnormalities. Drugs with anticholinergic properties diminish saliva production and increase the risk of dental caries and parotitis. Tetracyclines taken before the eruption of the permanent teeth stain the enamel. Excessive fluoride in vitamin preparations or in drinking water can result in mottled teeth. Gingival hypertrophy may be caused by cyclosporine, phenytoin, and calcium channel blockers.

Gastroesophageal reflux (GER) can lead to substantial enamel erosion and caries. Neonatal hyperbilirubinemia can result in discoloration of the deciduous teeth. Renal failure is associated with mottled enamel of the permanent teeth. Congenital syphilis causes marked abnormalities in the shape of teeth, especially incisors and molars. Crohn's disease is associated with oral ulcers. Abnormal pigmentation of the lips and buccal mucosa is seen with Peutz-Jeghers syndrome and Addison disease. Candidiasis is seen commonly with immunodeficiency disorders and diabetes. Leukemic infiltrates result in gum hyperplasia and bleeding; treatment of neoplastic conditions can cause severe mucositis. Some tumors, including lymphoma, may present as mass lesions of the buccal cavity.

| | Primary, Age (mo) | | Permanent, Age (yr) | |
|---|---|---|---|---|
| **Tooth Type** | Upper | Lower | Upper | Lower |
| Central incisor | 6 ± 2 | 7 ± 2 | 7–8 | 6–7 |
| Lateral incisor | 9 ± 2 | 7 ± 2 | 8–9 | 7–8 |
| Cuspids | 18 ± 2 | 16 ± 2 | 11–12 | 9–10 |
| First bicuspids | — | — | **10–11** | **10–12** |
| Second bicuspids | — | — | **10–12** | **11–12** |
| First molars | 14 ± 4 | 12 ± 4 | 6–7 | 6–7 |
| Second molars | 24 ± 4 | 20 ± 4 | 12–13 | 11–13 |
| Third molars | — | — | 17–21 | 17–21 |

**TABLE 127-1 Time of Eruption of the Primary and Permanent Teeth**

Osteogenesis imperfecta is associated with abnormal dentin and risk of caries. Children with ectodermal dysplasias commonly have malformed or missing teeth. Pierre Robin syndrome is associated with micrognathia and cleft palate. Disorders resulting in facial dysmorphism can have a profound effect on dental occlusion and mandibular function. Examples include mandibulofacial dysostosis, Crouzon syndrome, conditions associated with dwarfism, and others.

## DECIDUOUS AND PRIMARY TEETH

Most infants are born without teeth. *Natal teeth* are present at birth, are usually supernumerary, and may be poorly attached. No treatment is usually necessary, but removal by a dentist is sometimes needed if they are causing difficulties with feeding or injuries to the tongue. Table 127-1 presents the ages when normal **deciduous teeth** are acquired. The lower central incisors are the first to erupt, followed by the upper central incisors, lateral incisors, first molars, and bicuspids. **Delayed eruption** may occur in association with hypopituitarism, hypothyroidism, osteopetrosis, Gaucher disease, Down syndrome, cleidocranial dysplasia, and rickets. Deciduous teeth begin to be replaced by the permanent teeth around age 6 years. The sequence of replacement is similar to that of the appearance of deciduous teeth.

## DENTAL CARIES

### Etiology

Dental caries, commonly referred to as "cavities," occur as a result of interactions between the tooth enamel, dietary carbohydrates, and oral flora. There is increased susceptibility if the enamel is abnormal or hypoplastic. Bacteria (*Streptococcus mutans*) that can adhere to and colonize the teeth, survive at low pH, and produce acids during fermentation of carbohydrates cause dental caries. The diet has a significant role. A classic example is "bottle mouth," or **baby bottle caries**. This condition results from allowing an infant to have a bottle in the mouth for prolonged periods, especially during sleep, and with sweet beverages or milk in the bottle. This practice allows bacteria to have continuous substrate for acid production and can result in destruction of multiple teeth, especially the upper incisors. Sticky sweet foods, such as candy, have the same effect.

### Epidemiology and Treatment

Risk of caries is associated with lack of dental care and poor socioeconomic status and predictably is greatest in developing countries. Baby bottle caries is seen in 50% to 70% of low-income infants. Treatment of caries involves dental restorative surgery. The carious portion is removed and filled with silver amalgam or plastic. When not properly treated, dental decay results in inflammation and infection of the dental pulp and surrounding alveolar bone, which can lead to abscess and facial space infections.

### Prevention

Avoiding inappropriate use of bottles and excessive sweets is a common-sense remedy for baby bottle caries. Oral hygiene offers some protection, but young children (<8 years of age) do not have the ability to brush their own teeth adequately; brushing should be done by the parents. Fluoride supplementation of community water supplies to a concentration of 1 ppm is highly effective in reducing dental caries. Home water supplies, such as from a well, should have the fluoride content tested before prescribing supplements. Excessive supplementation causes fluorosis, a largely cosmetic defect of chalky white marks and brown stains on the teeth. Finally, occlusal sealants applied by a dentist after the eruption of the secondary molars can reduce the cavity rate by about 50%.

## CLEFT LIP AND PALATE

### Epidemiology

Cleft lip and palate occur separately or together and affect approximately 1 in 700 infants. Clefting is more common in Asians (1:500) and least common in African Americans (1:2500). It occurs with two possible patterns: isolated soft tissue cleft palate or cleft lip with or without associated clefts of the hard palate. Isolated cleft palate is associated with a higher risk of other congenital malformations. The combined cleft lip/palate type has a male predominance.

### Etiology

Cleft lip is due to hypoplasia of the mesenchymal tissues with subsequent failure of fusion. There is a strong genetic component; the risk is highest in children with affected first-degree relatives. Monozygotic twins are affected with only 60% concordance, suggesting other nongenomic factors. Environmental factors during gestation also increase risk, including drugs (phenytoin, valproic acid, thalidomide), maternal alcohol and tobacco use, dioxins and other herbicides, and possibly high altitude. Chromosomal and nonchromosomal syndromes are associated with clefting, as are specific genes in some families.

### Clinical Manifestations and Treatment

Cleft lip can be unilateral or bilateral and associated with cleft palate and defects of the alveolar ridge and dentition. When present, palatal defects allow direct communication between the nasal and oral cavities, creating problems with speech and feeding. Feeding infants with clefts requires the use of squeeze-bottles, special nipples, nipples with attached shields to seal the palate, or even gastrostomy in severe cases. Surgical closure of the cleft lip is usually done by 3 months of age. Closure of the palate follows, usually before 1 year of age. Cosmetic results are often good but depend on the severity of the defect.

### Complications

Speech is nasal as a result of the cleft palate. Surgical treatment is effective, but sometimes does not restore palatal function completely. Speech therapy or occasionally the use of a speech-assisting appliance may help. Frequent episodes of otitis media are common, as are defects of teeth and the alveolar ridge.

## THRUSH

### Epidemiology

Oropharyngeal *Candida albicans* infection, or thrush, is common in healthy neonates. The organism may be acquired in the birth canal or from the environment. Persistent infection is common in breastfed infants as a result of colonization or infection of the mother's nipples. Thrush in healthy, older patients can occur but suggests a possible immunodeficiency, except after recent broad-spectrum antibiotic use or when found in diabetics.

### Clinical Manifestations

Thrush is easily visible as white plaques, often with a *fuzzy* appearance, on oral mucous membranes. When scraped with a tongue depressor, the plaques are difficult to remove, and the underlying mucosa is inflamed and friable. Clinical diagnosis is usually adequate, but may be confirmed by fungal culture or potassium hydroxide smear. Oropharyngeal candidiasis is sometimes painful (especially if associated with esophagitis) and can interfere with feeding.

### Treatment

Thrush is treated with topical nystatin or an azole antifungal agent such as fluconazole. When the mother's nipples are infected and painful, consideration should be given to treating her at the same time. Because thrush is commonly self-limited in newborns, withholding therapy in asymptomatic infants and treating only persistent or severe cases is a reasonable approach.

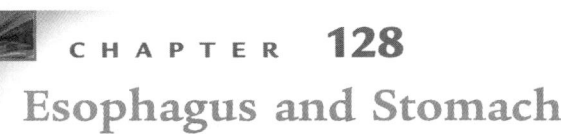

## CHAPTER 128
# Esophagus and Stomach

## GASTROESOPHAGEAL REFLUX

### Etiology and Epidemiology

Gastroesophageal reflux (GER) is defined as the effortless retrograde movement of gastric contents into the esophagus. In infancy, GER is not always an abnormality. **Physiologic GER** (*spitting up*) is normal in infants younger than 8 to 12 months of age. Nearly half of all infants are reported to spit up at 2 months of age. Infants who regurgitate stomach contents meet the criteria for physiologic GER, so long as they maintain adequate nutrition and have no signs of respiratory complications or esophagitis. Factors involved in causing infantile GER include liquid diet; horizontal body position; short, narrow esophagus; small, noncompliant stomach; frequent, relatively large volume feedings; and an immature lower esophageal sphincter (LES). As infants grow, they spend more time upright, eat more solid foods, develop a longer and larger diameter esophagus, have a larger and more compliant stomach, and experience lower caloric needs per unit of body weight. Most infants stop spitting up by 9 to 12 months of age.

### Clinical Manifestations

The presence of GER is easy to observe in an infant who spits up. In older children, the refluxate is usually kept down by reswallowing, but GER may be suspected by associated symptoms, such as heartburn, cough, dysphagia (trouble swallowing), wheezing, aspiration pneumonia, hoarse voice, failure to thrive, and recurrent otitis media or sinusitis. In severe cases of esophagitis, there may be laboratory evidence of anemia and hypoalbuminemia secondary to esophageal bleeding and inflammation.

**Pathologic GER** is diagnosed after 18 months of age or if there are complications, such as esophagitis, respiratory symptoms, or failure to thrive in younger infants. In older children, normal protective mechanisms against GER include antegrade esophageal motility, tonic contraction of the LES, and the geometry of the gastroesophageal junction. Abnormalities that cause GER in older children and adults include reduced tone of the LES, transient relaxations of the LES, esophagitis (which impairs esophageal motility), increased intra-abdominal pressure, cough, respiratory difficulty (asthma or cystic fibrosis), and hiatal hernia. When esophagitis develops as a result of acid reflux, esophageal motility and LES function are impaired further, creating a cycle of reflux and esophageal injury.

## Laboratory and Imaging Studies

A clinical diagnosis is often sufficient in children with classic effortless regurgitation and no complications. Diagnostic studies are indicated if there are persistent symptoms or complications or if other symptoms suggest the possibility of GER. A child with recurrent pneumonia, chronic cough, or apneic spells without overt emesis may have occult GER. A **barium upper gastrointestinal series** helps to rule out gastric outlet obstruction, malrotation, or other anatomic contributors to GER. Because of the brief nature of the examination, a negative barium study does *not* rule out GER. Another study, a **24-hour esophageal pH probe monitoring**, uses a pH electrode placed transnasally into the distal esophagus, with continuous recording of esophageal pH. Data typically are gathered for 24 hours, following which the number and temporal pattern of acid reflux events are analyzed. A similar test, which does not require the presence of acid in the stomach, is **esophageal impedance monitoring**, which records the migration of electrolyte-rich gastric fluid in the esophagus. **Endoscopy** is useful to rule out esophagitis, esophageal stricture, and anatomic abnormalities.

## Treatment

In otherwise healthy young infants, no treatment is necessary. For infants with complications of GER, pharmacologic therapy with a proton-pump inhibitor should be offered (Table 128-1). Lesser benefits are obtained with $H_2$ receptor antagonists. Prokinetic drugs, such as metoclopramide, are occasionally helpful by enhancing gastric emptying and increasing LES tone, but are seldom very effective. When severe symptoms persist despite medication, or if life-threatening aspiration is present, surgical intervention may be required. Fundoplication procedures, such as the Nissen operation, enhance the antireflux anatomy of the LES. In children with a severe neurologic defect who cannot tolerate oral or gastric tube feedings, placement of a feeding jejunostomy can be considered as an alternative to fundoplication.

## ESOPHAGEAL ATRESIA AND TRACHEOESOPHAGEAL FISTULA

### Etiology and Epidemiology

The esophagus and trachea develop in close proximity to each other during weeks 4 to 6 of fetal life. Defects in the mesenchyme separating the two structures result in a tracheoesophageal fistula (TEF), often in association with other anomalies (involving the kidneys, heart, spine, or limbs). This defect occurs in about 1:3000 live births. TEF is not thought to be a genetic defect because concordance between monozygotic twins is poor.

### Clinical Manifestations

The most common forms of TEF occur with esophageal atresia; the **H-type** TEF without atresia is uncommon, as is esophageal atresia without TEF (Fig. 128-1). Associated defects include the **VACTERL** association—**v**ertebral anomalies (70%), **a**nal atresia (imperforate anus) (50%), **c**ardiac anomalies (30%), **TE**F (70%), **r**enal anomalies (50%), and **l**imb anomalies (polydactyly, forearm defects, absent thumbs, syndactyly) (70%). A single artery umbilical cord is often noted. Infants with esophageal atresia have a history of polyhydramnios, exhibit drooling, and have mucus and saliva bubbling from the nose and mouth. Patients with TEF are vulnerable to aspiration pneumonia. When TEF is suspected, the first feeding should be delayed until a diagnostic study is performed.

### TABLE 128-1 Treatment of Gastroesophageal Reflux

| Therapy | Comments |
|---|---|
| **CONSERVATIVE MANAGEMENT** | |
| Towel on caregiver's shoulder | Cheap, effective; useful only for physiologic reflux |
| Thickened feedings | Reduces number of episodes, enhances nutrition |
| Smaller, more frequent feedings | Can be of some help; be careful not to *underfeed* child |
| Avoidance of tobacco smoke and alcohol | Always a good idea; may help control reflux symptoms |
| Abstaining from caffeine | Inexpensive, offers some benefit |
| Positional therapy—upright in seat, elevate head of crib or bed | Prone positioning with head up is helpful, but *not* for young infants due to risk of SIDS |
| **MEDICAL THERAPY** | |
| Proton pump inhibitor | Effective medical therapy for heartburn and esophagitis |
| Histamine $H_2$ receptor antagonist | Reduces heartburn, less effective for healing esophagitis |
| Metoclopramide | Enhances stomach emptying and LES tone |
| | Benefit often minimal |
| **SURGICAL THERAPY** | |
| Nissen or other fundoplication procedure | For life-threatening or medically unresponsive cases |
| Feeding jejunostomy | Useful in child requiring tube feeds—delivering feeds downstream eliminates GERD |

GERD, gastroesophageal reflux disease; LES, lower esophageal sphincter; SIDS, sudden infant death syndrome.

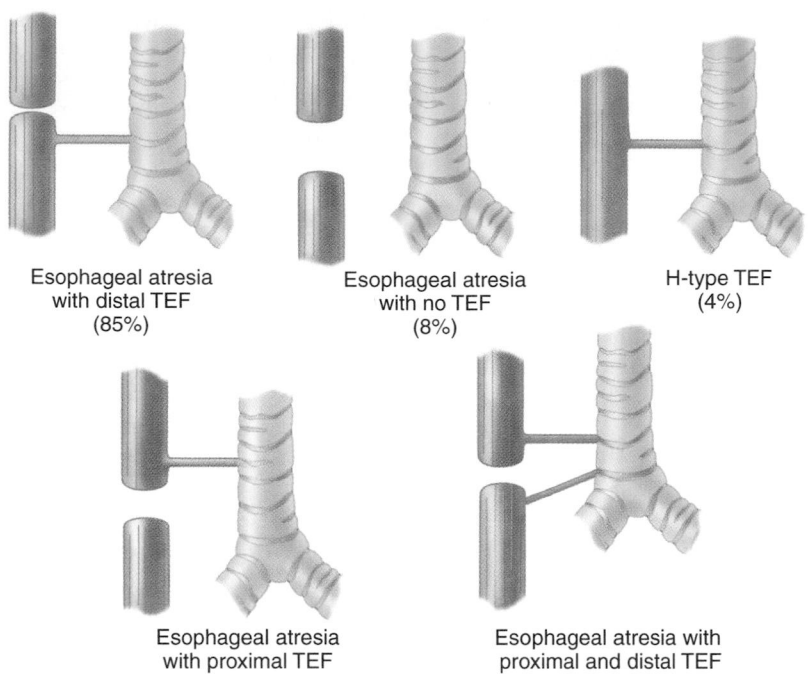

Esophageal atresia
with distal TEF
(85%)

Esophageal atresia
with no TEF
(8%)

H-type TEF
(4%)

Esophageal atresia
with proximal TEF
(2%)

Esophageal atresia with
proximal and distal TEF
(1%)

## Laboratory and Imaging Studies

The simplest test for TEF is to attempt gently to place a nasogastric tube via the mouth into the stomach. The passage of the tube is blocked at the level of the atresia. Confirmation is by chest x-ray with the tube coiled in the esophageal pouch. Air can be injected through the tube to outline the atretic pouch. Barium should not be used because of extreme risk of aspiration, but a tiny amount of dilute water-soluble contrast agent can be given carefully.

## Treatment and Prognosis

The treatment of TEF is surgical. A thoracotomy provides access to the mediastinum via extrapleural dissection. The fistula is divided and ligated. The esophageal ends are approximated and anastomosed. In some cases, primary anastomosis cannot be performed because of a long gap between the proximal and distal portions of the esophagus. Various techniques have been described to deal with this problem, including pulling up the stomach, elongating the esophagus by myotomy, using intestinal segments to span the gap, and delaying the anastomosis and providing continuous suction to the upper pouch, allowing for growth.

## Complications

The surgically reconstructed esophagus is not normal and is prone to poor motility, GER, anastomotic stricture, recurrent fistula, and leakage. The tracheal cartilage is also malformed; tracheomalacia (a soft trachea that collapses easily) is common.

# ESOPHAGEAL FOREIGN BODIES

## Etiology and Epidemiology

Young children often place nonfood items in their mouths. When these items are swallowed, they may become lodged in the upper esophagus at the thoracic inlet. The most common objects are coins. Smaller objects may pass harmlessly into the stomach, where they rarely cause symptoms. Other common esophageal foreign bodies include food items, small toys or toy parts, disc batteries, and other small household items. Children with a prior history of esophageal atresia or with poor motility secondary to GER are more prone to food impactions, which seldom occur in the normal esophagus.

## Clinical Manifestations

Some children are asymptomatic, but most exhibit some degree of drooling, food refusal, or chest discomfort. Older children usually can point to the region of the chest where they feel the object to be lodged. Respiratory symptoms tend to be minimal, but cough may be present, especially when the esophagus is completely blocked by a large object, such as a piece of meat, which presses on the trachea.

## Diagnosis

Plain chest and abdominal radiographs should be taken when foreign body ingestion is suspected. Metallic objects are easily visualized. A plastic object often can be seen on x-ray if the child is given a small amount of dilute contrast material to drink, although endoscopy is probably safer and more definitive.

## Treatment

Endoscopy is ultimately necessary in most cases to remove an esophageal foreign body. Various devices can be used to remove the object, depending on its size, shape, and location. Coins usually are grasped and removed with a special-purpose forceps. Nets, baskets, and snares also are available. Whenever objects that may threaten the airway are being recovered, endoscopy should be performed with endotracheal intubation and under general anesthesia.

## Complications

Sharp objects may lacerate or perforate the esophagus; smooth objects present for a long time also may result in perforation. Corrosive objects, such as zinc-containing pennies and disc batteries, can cause considerable local tissue injury and esophageal perforation.

# CAUSTIC INJURIES AND PILL ULCERS

## Etiology and Epidemiology

In adolescents, caustic ingestion injuries are usually the result of suicide attempts. In toddlers, the accidental ingestion of household cleaning products is common. Typical injurious agents include drain cleaners, toilet bowl cleaners, dishwasher detergents, and powerful bleaching agents. Childproof lids for commercial products offer some protection, but have not eliminated the problem. Lye-based drain cleaners, especially liquid products, cause the worst injuries because they are swallowed easily and liquefy tissue rapidly. Solid-phase products are less likely to cause esophageal injury during accidental exposures because they burn the tongue and often are expelled before swallowing. Less caustic agents, such as bleach and detergents, cause less serious injury. **Pill ulcers** occur when certain medications (tetracyclines and nonsteroidal anti-inflammatory drugs) are swallowed without sufficient liquids, allowing prolonged direct contact of the pill with the esophageal mucosa.

## Clinical Manifestations

Caustic burns cause immediate and severe mouth pain. The child cries out, drools, spits, and usually drops the container immediately. Burns of the lips and tongue are visible almost immediately. These burns indicate the possibility of esophageal involvement, although esophageal injury can occur in the absence of oral burns. Symptoms may not be present; further evaluation by endoscopy usually is indicated with any significant history of caustic ingestion. Pill injury causes severe chest pain and often prominent odynophagia (painful swallowing) and dysphagia.

## Laboratory and Imaging Studies

A chest x-ray should be obtained to rule out aspiration and to inspect for mediastinal air. The child should be admitted to the hospital and given intravenous fluids until endoscopy. The true extent of burns may not be endoscopically apparent immediately, but delayed endoscopy can increase the risk of perforation. Most endoscopists perform the initial endoscopy soon after injury, when the patient has been stabilized. The extent of injury and severity of the burn should be carefully determined. Risk of subsequent esophageal strictures is related to the degree of burn and whether the injury is circumferential.

## Treatment

A nasogastric tube can be placed at the time of the initial endoscopy to provide a route for feeding and to stent the esophagus. Systemic steroid use does not reduce the risk of stricture. Broad-spectrum antibiotics should be prescribed if infection is suspected.

## Complications

Esophageal strictures, if they occur, usually develop within 1 to 2 months and are treated with balloon dilation. The risk of perforation during dilation is significant. When esophageal destruction is severe, surgical reconstruction of the esophagus using stomach or intestine may be necessary.

# PYLORIC STENOSIS

## Etiology and Epidemiology

Pyloric stenosis is an acquired condition caused by hypertrophy of the pyloric muscle, resulting in gastric outlet constriction. It occurs in 6 to 8 per 1000 live births and has a 5:1 male predominance. It is more common in first-born children.

## Clinical Manifestations

Infants with pyloric stenosis typically begin vomiting during the first month of life, but onset of symptoms may be delayed. The emesis becomes increasingly more frequent and forceful as time passes. Vomiting in pyloric stenosis differs from spitting up because of its extremely forceful and often projectile nature. The vomited material does not contain bile because the gastric outlet obstruction is proximal to the duodenum. This feature differentiates pyloric stenosis from most other obstructive lesions of early childhood. Affected infants are ravenously hungry early in the course of the illness, but become more lethargic with increasing malnutrition and dehydration. The stomach becomes massively enlarged with retained food and secretions, and gastric **peristaltic waves** are often visible in the left upper quadrant. A hypertrophied pylorus (the *olive*) may be palpable. As the illness progresses, very little of each feeding is able to pass through the pylorus, and the child becomes progressively thinner and more dehydrated.

## Laboratory and Imaging Studies

Repetitive vomiting of purely gastric contents results in loss of hydrochloric acid; the classic laboratory finding is a **hypochloremic metabolic alkalosis** with elevated blood urea nitrogen (BUN) secondary to dehydration.

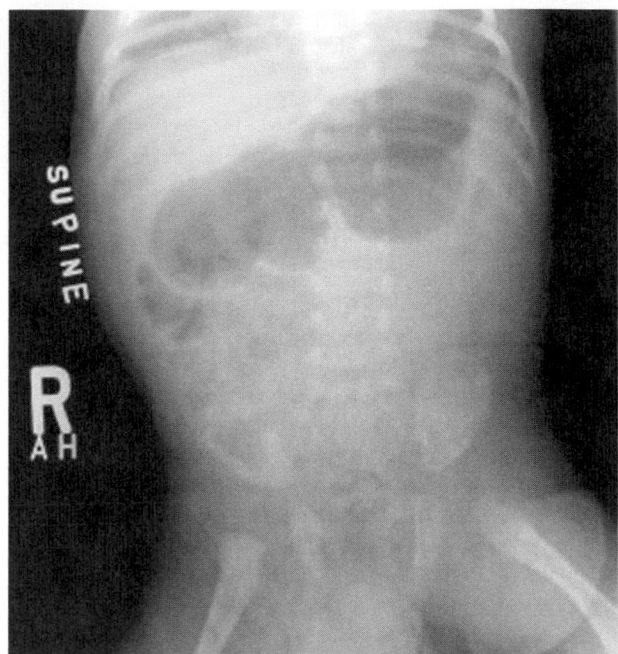

**FIGURE 128-2**

**Pyloric stenosis.** Note the huge, gas-filled stomach extending across the midline, with minimal air in the intestine downstream. *(Courtesy of Warren Bishop, MD.)*

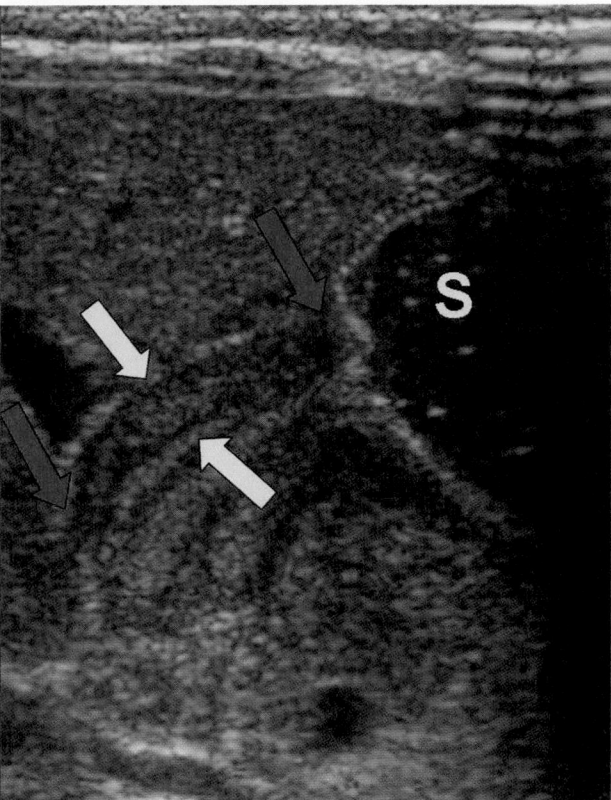

**FIGURE 128-3**

**Ultrasound image of infant with pyloric stenosis.** Large, fluid-filled stomach (*S*) is seen at right, with an elongated, thickened pylorus. The length of the pylorus is marked by the *red arrows*; the wall thickness is marked by the *yellow arrows*.

Jaundice with unconjugated hyperbilirubinemia also is common. Plain abdominal x-rays typically show a huge stomach and diminished or absent gas in the intestine (Fig. 128-2). Ultrasonography of the pylorus is the preferred study, showing elongation and thickening of the pylorus (Fig. 128-3). A barium upper gastrointestinal series, which is seldom necessary, shows a **string sign** caused by barium filling the elongated, constricted pyloric channel.

### Treatment

Treatment of pyloric stenosis includes intravenous fluid and electrolyte resuscitation followed by surgical pyloromyotomy. Before surgery, dehydration and hypochloremic alkalosis must be corrected, generally with an initial normal saline fluid bolus followed by infusions of half-normal saline containing 5% dextrose. Potassium chloride is added to the solution after urine output is observed. For pyloromyotomy, a small incision is made, and the pyloric muscle is incised longitudinally to release the constriction. Care is taken not to cut into the mucosa itself.

## PEPTIC DISEASE

### Etiology and Epidemiology

Acid-related injury can occur in the esophagus, stomach, or duodenum. Table 128-2 lists risk factors for **peptic ulcer disease** in children. *Helicobacter pylori* is responsible for more than half of ulcers in the stomach and the duodenum in adults. *H. pylori* plays a significant but lesser role in childhood ulcer disease. Risk factors for acquisition of

*H. pylori* are low socioeconomic status and poor sanitation, with the highest incidence in developing countries. GER (see Chapter 128) allows acidic gastric contents to injure the esophagus, resulting in **esophagitis**. Esophagitis is characterized by retrosternal and epigastric burning pain and is best diagnosed by endoscopy. It can range from minimal, with only erythema and microscopic inflammation on biopsy, to superficial erosions and finally to frank ulceration.

**TABLE 128-2  Risk Factors for Peptic Ulcer Disease**

*Helicobacter pylori* infection
Drugs
  NSAIDs, including aspirin
  Tobacco use
  Bisphosphonates
  Alcohol
  Potassium supplements
Family history
Sepsis
Head trauma
Burn injury
Hypotension

NSAIDs, nonsteroidal anti-inflammatory drugs.

## Clinical Manifestations

Typical symptoms are listed in Table 128-3. The presence of burning epigastric and retrosternal pain strongly suggests esophagitis. With duodenal ulcers, pain typically occurs several hours after meals and often awakens patients at night. Eating tends to relieve the pain. Gastric ulcers differ in that pain may be aggravated by eating, resulting in weight loss. Gastrointestinal bleeding from either can occur. Most patients report significant symptom relief with antacids or acid blockers.

## Laboratory and Imaging Studies

Whenever pain is localized to the upper abdomen or the retrosternal region, upper gastrointestinal endoscopy is indicated, although a short course of empiric therapy using a proton-pump inhibitor may be considered, with endoscopy reserved for nonresponders. The possibilities of inflammatory bowel disease, an anatomic abnormality such as malrotation, pancreatitis, and biliary disease should each be ruled out by appropriate testing when suspected (see Chapter 126 and Table 128-3 for recommended studies). Testing for *H. pylori* should be performed by biopsy during every endoscopy.

## Treatment

If *H. pylori* is present in association with ulcers, it should be treated with a multidrug regimen, such as omeprazole-clarithromycin-metronidazole, omeprazole-amoxicillin-clarithromycin, or omeprazole-amoxicillin-metronidazole, given twice daily for 1 to 2 weeks. Other proton-pump inhibitors may be substituted for omeprazole. Tetracycline is useful in adults, but should be avoided in children. In the absence of *H. pylori*, esophagitis and peptic ulcer disease are treated with a proton-pump inhibitor, which yields higher rates of healing than $H_2$ receptor antagonists. Gastric and duodenal ulcers heal in 4 to 8 weeks. Esophagitis requires 4 to 5 months of proton-pump inhibitor treatment for optimal healing.

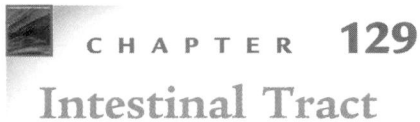

**CHAPTER 129**

# Intestinal Tract

## MIDGUT MALROTATION

### Etiology and Epidemiology

During early fetal life, the midgut is attached to the yolk sac and loops outward into the umbilical cord. Beginning at around 10 weeks' gestation, the bowel reenters the abdomen and rotates counterclockwise around the superior mesenteric artery until the cecum arrives in the right lower quadrant. The duodenum rotates behind the artery and terminates at the **ligament of Treitz** in the left upper quadrant. The base of the mesentery becomes fixed along a broad attachment posteriorly, running from the cecum to the ligament of Treitz (Fig. 129-1A). When rotation is incomplete or otherwise abnormal, **malrotation** is present. Incomplete rotation occurs when the cecum stops near the right upper quadrant, and the duodenum fails to move behind the mesenteric artery; this results in an extremely narrow mesenteric root (see Fig. 129-1B) that makes the child susceptible to midgut **volvulus** (Fig. 129-2). It is common for abnormal mesenteric attachments (Ladd bands) to extend from the cecum across the duodenum, causing partial obstruction.

### Clinical Manifestations

About 60% of children with malrotation present with bilious vomiting during the first month of life; the remaining 40% present later in infancy or childhood. The emesis initially may be due to obstruction by Ladd bands without volvulus. When midgut volvulus occurs, the venous drainage of the gut is impaired, and congestion results in ischemia, pain, tenderness, and often bloody emesis and stools. The bowel eventually becomes necrotic, causing peritonitis and sepsis. Physicians caring for children must be alert to the possibility of malrotation in patients with vomiting and fussiness or abdominal pain.

---

**TABLE 128-3  Peptic Disorders, Symptoms, and Clinical Investigation**

| Syndrome and Associated Symptoms | Clinical Investigation |
| --- | --- |
| **ESOPHAGITIS** | |
| Retrosternal and epigastric location | Endoscopy |
| Burning pain | Therapeutic trial of acid-blocker therapy |
| Sensation of regurgitation | pH probe study |
| Dysphagia, odynophagia | |
| **NONULCER DYSPEPSIA** | |
| Upper abdominal location | Endoscopy |
| Fullness | Therapeutic trial of acid-blocker therapy |
| Bloating | Upper GI series to ligament of Treitz: rule out malrotation |
| Nausea | CBC, ESR, amylase, lipase, abdominal ultrasound |
| **PEPTIC ULCER DISEASE** | |
| Alarm symptoms | Endoscopy—mandatory with alarm symptoms |
| Weight loss | |
| Hematemesis | Test for *Helicobacter pylori* |
| Melena, heme-positive stools | CBC, ESR, amylase, lipase, abdominal ultrasound |
| Chronic vomiting | Same as for esophagitis and nonulcer dyspepsia |
| Microcytic anemia | |
| Nocturnal pain | |
| Other symptoms | |

CBC, complete blood count; ESR, erythrocyte sedimentation rate; GI, gastrointestinal.

## Laboratory and Imaging Studies

Plain abdominal x-rays show evidence of obstruction. Abdominal ultrasound may demonstrate malrotation. An upper gastrointestinal (GI) series must be done and reveals absence of the normal *C-loop* of the duodenum, with the jejunum on the right side of the abdomen. When doubt exists about the normalcy of the duodenal course, the contrast material can be followed until it reaches the cecum. High placement of the cecum on follow-through (or by contrast enema) confirms the diagnosis. Laboratory studies are nonspecific, showing evidence of dehydration, electrolyte loss, or evidence of sepsis. A decreasing platelet count is a common indicator of bowel ischemia.

## Treatment

Treatment is surgical. The bowel is untwisted. Ladd bands and other abnormal membranous attachments are divided. The mesentery is spread out and flattened against the posterior abdominal wall by moving the cecum to the left side of the abdomen. Sutures may be used to hold the bowel in position, but postoperative adhesions tend to hold the mesentery in place, resulting in a broad attachment and eliminating the risk of recurrent volvulus. Necrotic bowel is resected which may result in short gut syndrome.

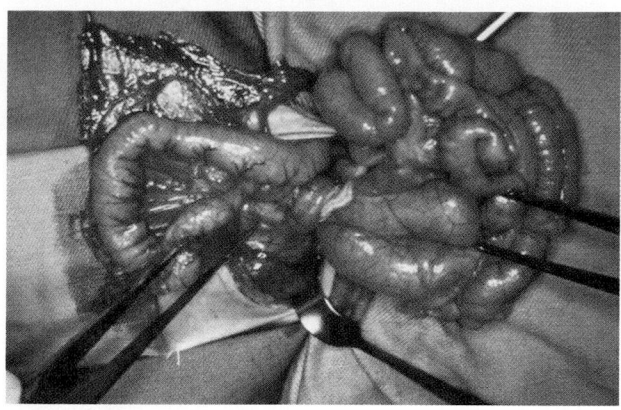

**FIGURE 129-2**

**Malrotation with volvulus.** Midgut is twisted around the mesentery, with an area of darker, ischemic intestine visible. *(Courtesy of Robert Soper, MD.)*

## INTESTINAL ATRESIA

### Etiology and Epidemiology

Congenital partial or complete blockage of the intestine is a developmental defect that occurs in about 1:1500 live births. Atresia occurs in several forms (Fig. 129-3). One or more segments of bowel may be missing completely,

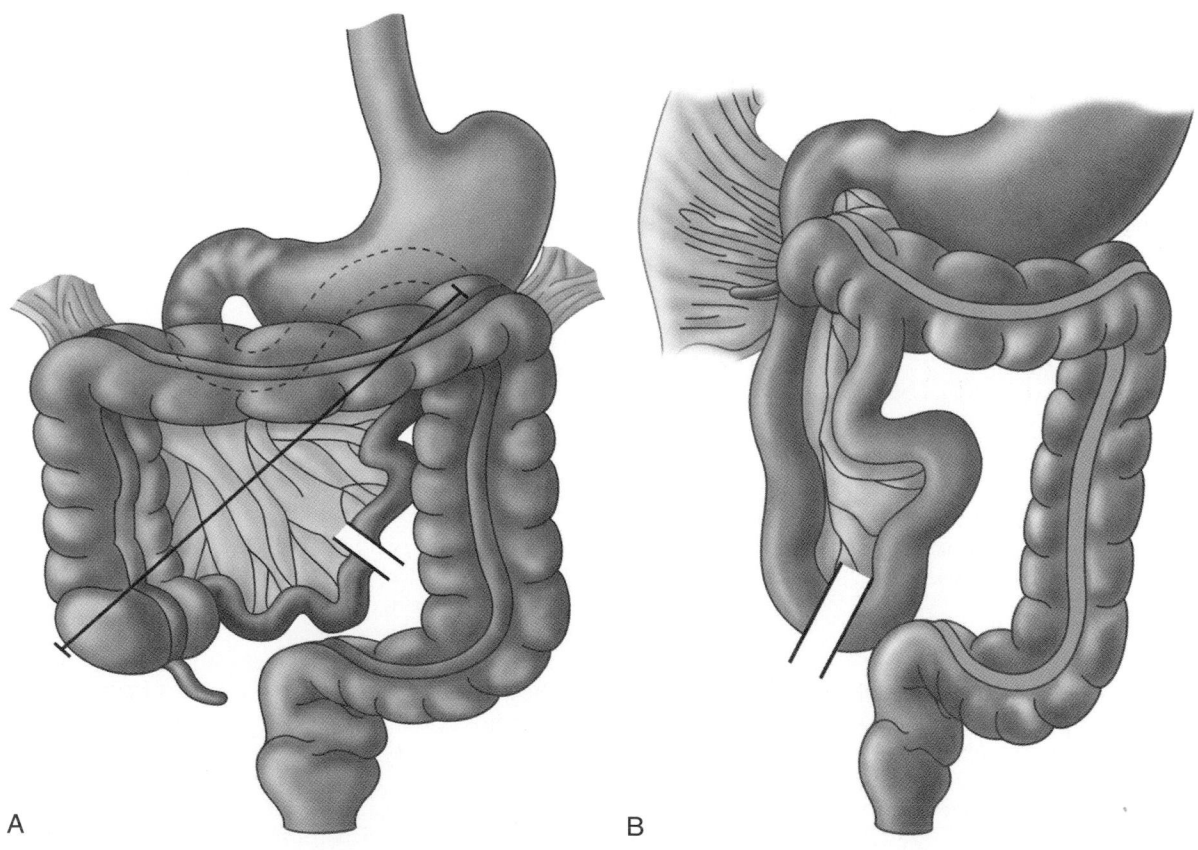

A                                                    B

**FIGURE 129-1**

**A,** Normal rotation of the midgut. Note the long axis of mesenteric attachment (*line*). **B,** Midgut malrotation. Note the narrow mesentery, which predisposes to volvulus, and the presence of Ladd bands extending across the duodenum from the abnormally elevated cecum. (From Donellan WJ [ed]: Abdominal Surgery of Infancy and Childhood. Luxembourg, *Harwood Academic Publishers*, 1996, pp 43/6, 43/8.)

**FIGURE 129-3**

**Types of intestinal atresia.** I, internal web; II, cordlike remnant connecting proximal and distal bowel; IIIa, interrupted bowel with V-shaped mesenteric defect; IIIb, "apple peel" atresia with surviving bowel spiraling around a marginal artery; IV, multiple atresias. (From Grosfeld JL, Ballantine TVN, Shoemaker R: Operative management of intestinal atresia based on pathologic findings. *J Pediatr Surg* 14:368, 1979.)

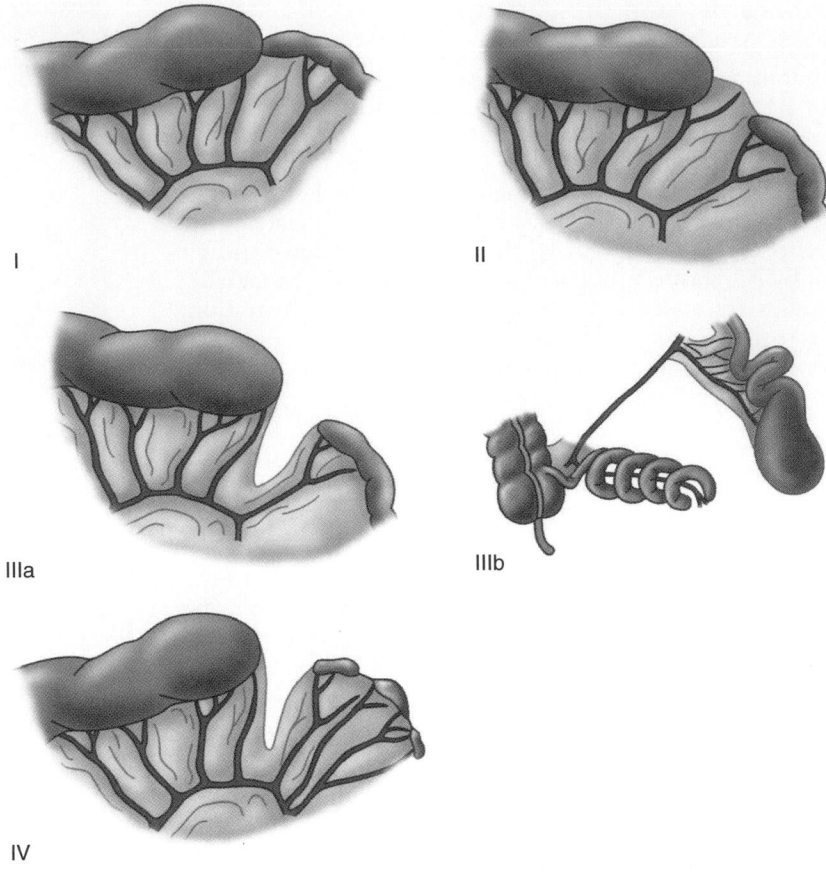

there may be varying degrees of obstruction caused by webs or stenosis, or there may be obliteration of the lumen in cordlike bowel remnants. The end result is obstruction with upstream dilation of the bowel and small, disused intestine distally. When obstruction is complete or high grade, bilious vomiting and abdominal distention are present in the newborn period. In lesser cases, as in *windsock* types of intestinal webs, the obstruction is partial, and symptoms are more subtle.

## Clinical Manifestations

Intestinal atresia presents with a history of polyhydramnios and with abdominal distention and bilious vomiting in the neonatal period. If intestinal perforation is present, peritonitis and sepsis are inevitable.

## Laboratory and Imaging Studies

Plain abdominal x-rays may localize the area of atresia and identify evidence of perforation, such as free air or calcifications typical of meconium peritonitis. Duodenal atresia appears as a double-bubble sign (gas in the stomach and enlarged proximal duodenum), with no gas distally. Atresias of the distal intestine are characterized by longer segments of dilated, air-filled bowel. Contrast studies are helpful if plain films are not sufficient. Atresia may also be a complication of **meconium ileus** associated with cystic fibrosis. Laboratory evaluation for **cystic fibrosis** (see Chapter 137) is indicated in cases of small bowel

atresia. Other laboratory studies are not specific for atresia, but a complete blood count, serum electrolytes, liver functions, and amylase should be measured to identify dehydration, pancreatitis, and other complications.

## Treatment

The treatment of intestinal atresia is surgical, but surgery must be preceded by adequate stabilization of the patient. Iintravenous (IV) fluids, nasogastric suction, and broad-spectrum antibiotics should be given.

## OTHER CONGENITAL DISORDERS

**Gastroschisis** is an abdominal wall defect not involving the umbilicus, through which intestinal contents have herniated. In contrast to omphalocele, the bowel is not covered by peritoneum or amniotic membrane. As a result, prolonged contact with the amniotic fluid typically causes a thick, exudative *peel* on the exposed bowel. Gastroschisis is not associated with extraintestinal anomalies, but segments of intestinal atresia are common. After surgical reduction of the defect, return of normal bowel function may be slow and requires prolonged parenteral nutrition for infants with long atretic segments (short bowel syndrome) and infants with a thick peel.

**Omphalocele** is an abdominal wall defect at the umbilicus caused by failure of the intestine to return to the abdomen during fetal life. The bowel remains within the umbilical cord and is covered by peritoneum and amniotic membranes. This defect is associated with other congenital anomalies, especially cardiac defects, **Beckwith-Wiedemann syndrome** (somatic overgrowth, hyperinsulinemic hypoglycemia, risk for Wilms tumor), and intestinal complications. Treatment is surgical closure, which sometimes must be performed in stages to fit the bowel into a congenitally small abdominal cavity.

**Anorectal malformations,** including imperforate anus and its variants, are embryologic defects recognized at birth by the absence of a normal anal opening. Evaluation of these infants should include observation for emergence of meconium from the urethra or from fistulas on the perineum. A urinary catheter should be placed if urinary distention is present. In low lesions, a fistulous opening that drains meconium is present on the perineum. Low lesions commonly are also associated with fistulization between the bowel and bladder, vagina, or urethra. Lateral plain x-rays show the level of the defect and show gas in the bladder caused by a fistula. These children are treated initially by colostomy to divert the fecal flow, with subsequent anogenital reconstruction. The internal sphincter muscle is functionally absent in high lesions, and continence after repair is difficult to achieve. All children with imperforate anus require magnetic resonance imaging (MRI) of the lumbosacral spinal cord because of high incidence of tethered spinal cord. Urologic dysfunction is common and should be evaluated appropriately.

**Hirschsprung disease** is a motility defect caused by failure of ganglion cell precursors to migrate into the distal bowel during fetal life. The aganglionic distal segment does not exhibit normal motility and is obstructed secondary to spasm. In 75% of cases, the involved segment is limited to the rectosigmoid; total colonic involvement is seen in 8%. Rarely, long segments of small bowel also are aganglionic. *Ultrashort* segments involve only a few centimeters of distal rectum. Hirschsprung disease typically presents in the newborn period with failure to pass meconium by 24 hours of age. About 95% of normal infants pass stool spontaneously by this age; 95% of infants with Hirschsprung disease do not. Symptoms of distal bowel obstruction occur with distention and bilious vomiting. If the diagnosis is not made quickly, **enterocolitis** can result, associated with a high rate of mortality. Diagnosis is based on examination and one or more diagnostic studies. Abdominal distention is present in most cases. Digital rectal examination reveals an empty rectum that clenches around the examiner's finger, giving the impression of an elongated sphincter. When the finger is withdrawn, a gush of retained stool is often expelled. A deep **rectal biopsy** specimen obtained surgically or by using a suction biopsy instrument is required for diagnosis. When no ganglion cells are shown in the submucosal plexus, accompanied by nerve trunk hyperplasia, the diagnosis is certain. **Barium enema** and **anorectal manometry** can demonstrate abnormalities, but false negative and false positive results occur. Therapy is surgical. When the bowel is markedly distended or inflamed, an initial colostomy usually is performed above the aganglionic segment, followed weeks later by one of several definitive repair procedures. With rectosigmoid involvement, transanal pull-through excises the aganglionic bowel and creates a primary colorectal anastomosis without laparotomy.

**Meckel diverticulum** is a remnant of the fetal omphalomesenteric duct and is an outpouching of the distal ileum present in 1% to 2% of the population. Although most are asymptomatic throughout life, some cause massive, painless GI bleeding due to acid secretion by ectopic gastric tissue. A Meckel diverticulum can also be a lead point for intussusception or may enable twisting (volvulus) of neighboring bowel around its vascular supply. Diverticulitis mimics appendicitis. Diagnosis may be made in most cases by technetium scan (Meckel scan), which labels the acid-producing mucosa. Because not all diverticula are seen, ultrasound and barium enteroclysis may be useful. When the level of suspicion is high, surgical or laparoscopic investigation is warranted. The treatment is surgical excision.

## INFLAMMATORY BOWEL DISEASE

### Epidemiology and Etiology

The peak incidence of inflammatory bowel disease (IBD) in children is in the second decade of life. IBD includes Crohn's disease (CD), which can involve the entire gut, and ulcerative colitis (UC), which affects only the colon. The incidence of IBD is increasing, especially in industrialized countries, for reasons that are unclear. IBD is uncommon in tropical and developing countries. It is more common in Jewish than in other ethnic populations. Genetic factors play a role in susceptibility, with significantly higher risk if there is a family history of IBD. Having a first-degree relative with IBD increases the risk about 30-fold. Susceptibility has been linked to some HLA subtypes, and linkage analysis has identified multiple other susceptibility loci on several chromosomes. Environmental factors also play a role, because there is often nonconcordance among monozygotic twins. The environmental agents responsible have not been identified. Dietary triggers are unproved. Smoking doubles the risk of CD and halves the risk for UC.

**Clinical manifestations** depend on the region of involvement. UC involves only the colon, whereas CD can involve the entire gut, from mouth to anus. **Colitis** from either condition results in diarrhea, blood, and mucus in the stool; urgency; and *tenesmus,* a sensation of incomplete emptying after defecation. When colitis is severe, the child often awakens from sleep to pass stool. **Toxic megacolon** is a life-threatening complication characterized by fever, abdominal distention and pain, massively dilated colon, anemia, and low serum albumin owing to fecal protein losses. Symptoms of colitis always are present in UC and usually suggest the diagnosis early in its course. Extraintestinal manifestations of UC occur in a few patients and may include primary sclerosing cholangitis, arthritis, uveitis, and pyoderma gangrenosum (Table 129-1).

Symptoms can be subtle in CD. **Small bowel involvement** is associated with loss of appetite, crampy postprandial pain, poor growth, delayed puberty, anemia, and lethargy. Some symptoms may be present for some time before the diagnosis is made. Severe CD may cause partial or complete small bowel obstruction. Perineal abnormalities, including skin tags and fistulas, distinguish CD from UC. Other extraintestinal manifestations of CD include arthritis, erythema nodosum, and uveitis or iritis.

**TABLE 129-1 Comparison of Crohn's Disease and Ulcerative Colitis**

| Feature | Crohn's Disease | Ulcerative Colitis |
|---|---|---|
| Malaise, fever, weight loss | Common | Common |
| Rectal bleeding | Sometimes | Usual |
| Abdominal mass | Common | Rare |
| Abdominal pain | Common | Common |
| Perianal disease | Common | Rare |
| Ileal involvement | Common | None (backwash ileitis) |
| Strictures | Common | Unusual |
| Fistula | Common | Very rare |
| Skip lesions | Common | Not present |
| Transmural involvement | Usual | Not present |
| Crypt abscesses | Variable | Usual |
| Intestinal granulomas | Common | Rarely present |
| Risk of cancer* | Increased | Greatly increased |
| Erythema nodosum | Common | Less common |
| Mouth ulceration | Common | Rare |
| Osteopenia at onset | Yes | No |
| Autoimmune hepatitis | Rare | Yes |
| Sclerosing cholangitis | Rare | Yes |

*Colonic cancer, cholangiocarcinoma.

**TABLE 129-2 Diagnostic Studies for Inflammatory Bowel Disease**

| Study | Interpretation |
|---|---|
| **BLOOD TESTS** | |
| CBC with WBC differential | Anemia, elevated platelets suggest IBD |
| ESR | Elevated in many, but not all, IBD patients |
| C-reactive protein | Elevated in many, but not all, IBD patients |
| ASCA | Found in most CD patients and few UC patients |
| Atypical p-ANCA | Found in most UC patients and few CD patients |
| Anti-OmpC | Found in some UC and CD patients, rare in non-IBD |
| **IMAGING STUDIES** | |
| Upper GI series with SBFT | Essential to rule out ileal and jejunal CD |
| CT scan | Used to detect abscess, small bowel involvement |
| Tagged WBC scan | Sometimes helpful in determining extent of disease |
| **ENDOSCOPY** | |
| Upper endoscopy | Evaluate for CD of esophagus, stomach, and duodenum; obtain tissue for histologic diagnosis |
| Colonoscopy | Show presence or absence of colitis and terminal ileal CD; obtain tissue for histology |
| Capsule endoscopy | Emerging role in diagnosis of small bowel CD, more sensitive than upper GI series with SBFT |

Anti-OmpC, antibody to outer membrane protein C; ASCA, anti–*Saccharomyces cerevisiae* antibody; atypical p-ANCA, atypical perinuclear staining by antineutrophil cytoplasmic antibody; CBC, complete blood count; CD, Crohn's disease; ESR, erythrocyte sedimentation rate; GI, gastrointestinal; IBD, inflammatory bowel disease; SBFT, small bowel follow-through; WBC, white blood cell.

## Laboratory and Imaging Studies

Blood tests should include complete blood count, erythrocyte sedimentation rate, and C-reactive protein and possibly serologic tests for IBD (Table 129-2). Anemia and elevated platelet counts are typical. Testing for abnormal serum antibodies can be helpful in diagnosing IBD and in discriminating between the colitis of CD and UC. **Atypical perinuclear staining by antineutrophil cytoplasmic antibody** is found in about 66% of UC patients and in only a few CD cases. **Anti-*Saccharomyces cerevisiae* antibody** is present in most CD patients and is uncommon in UC. Another IBD-specific antibody is anti-OmpC, directed against an *Escherichia coli* membrane protein. Because there is overlap between CD and UC, none of these tests can discriminate absolutely between the two conditions.

In patients with suspected IBD, an **upper GI series with small bowel follow-through** or **computed tomography (CT) scan** is needed to detect small bowel involvement. **Colonoscopy** is preferred over contrast enema because biopsy specimens can be obtained and visual features can be diagnostic. Findings in UC include diffuse carpeting of the distal or entire colon with tiny ulcers and loss of haustral folds. Within the involved segment, no skip areas are present. In CD, ulcerations tend to be much larger with a linear, branching, or aphthous appearance; skip areas are usually present. **Upper endoscopy** cannot evaluate the jejunum and ileum, but is more sensitive than contrast studies in identifying proximal CD involvement. The capsule endoscope, a swallowed device that can visualize the entire small bowel, is potentially useful to visualize subtle small bowel disease (Fig. 126-1) when radiologic findings are absent.

## Treatment

### Ulcerative Colitis

UC is treated with the aminosalicylate drugs, which deliver **5-aminosalicylic acid** (5-ASA, mesalamine) to the distal gut. Because it is rapidly absorbed, pure mesalamine must be specially packaged in coated capsules or pills or taken as a suppository to be effective in the colon.

Other aminosalicylates (sulfasalazine, olsalazine, and balsalazide) use 5-ASA covalently linked to a carrier molecule. Sulfasalazine is the least expensive, but side effects resulting from its sulfapyridine component are common. When aminosalicylates alone cannot control the disease, steroid therapy may be required to induce remission. Whenever possible, steroids should not be used for long-term therapy. An immunosuppressive drug, such as **6-mercaptopurine** or **azathioprine**, is useful to spare excessive steroid use in difficult cases. More potent immunosuppressives, such as cyclosporine or tacrolimus, are under investigation as rescue therapy when other treatments fail. Surgical colectomy with ileoanal anastomosis is curative and is an option for unresponsive severe disease or electively to end chronic symptoms and to reduce the risk of colon cancer, which is increased in patients with UC.

### Crohn's Disease

Inflammation in CD typically responds less well to aminosalicylates; oral or IV steroids are more important in inducing remission. To avoid the need for repetitive steroid therapy, immunosuppressive drugs, usually either azathioprine or 6-mercaptopurine, are started soon after diagnosis. CD that is difficult to control also may be treated with methotrexate or with agents that block the action of tumor necrosis factor-α. **Infliximab** is the most effective drug. Other drugs that inhibit white blood cell (WBC) migration or action, such as natalizumab, show promise. As with UC, surgery is sometimes necessary, usually because of obstructive symptoms, abscess, or severe, unremitting symptoms. Because surgery is not curative in CD, its use must be limited, and the length of bowel resection must be minimized.

## CELIAC DISEASE

### Etiology and Epidemiology

Celiac disease, or celiac sprue, is an immune-mediated injury to the mucosa of the small intestine triggered by the ingestion of **gluten** (a protein component) from wheat, rye, barley, and related grains. Rice does not contain *toxic* gluten and can be eaten freely, as can special pure preparations of oats not contaminated by other grains. In its severe form, celiac disease causes malabsorption and malnutrition. Nonetheless, many patients have few or no obvious or classic symptoms. Approximately 1 in 250 persons in the United States have celiac disease, only a few of which have been diagnosed due to severe manifestations. The disease is seen in association with diabetes and trisomy 21.

### Clinical Manifestations

Symptoms can begin at the age when gluten-containing foods are given. Diarrhea, abdominal bloating, failure to thrive, irritability, decreased appetite, and ascites caused by hypoproteinemia are classic. Children may be minimally symptomatic or may be severely malnourished. Constipation is found in a few patients, probably because of reduced intake. A careful inspection of the child's growth curve and determination of reduced subcutaneous fat and abdominal distention are crucial. Celiac disease should be considered in any child with chronic abdominal complaints.

### Laboratory and Imaging Studies

Serologic markers include IgA antiendomysial antibody and IgA tissue transglutaminase antibody. Because IgA deficiency is common in celiac disease, total serum IgA also must be measured to document the accuracy of these tests. In the absence of IgA deficiency, either test yields a sensitivity and specificity of 95%. An endoscopic **small bowel biopsy** is essential to confirm the diagnosis and should be performed while the patient is still taking gluten. The biopsy specimen shows varying degrees of villous atrophy (short or absent villi), mucosal inflammation, crypt hyperplasia, and increased numbers of intraepithelial lymphocytes. When there is any question about response to treatment, a repeat biopsy specimen may be obtained several months later. Other laboratory studies should be performed to rule out complications, including complete blood count, calcium, phosphate, total protein and albumin, and liver function tests. Mild elevations of the transaminases are common and should normalize with dietary therapy.

### Treatment

Treatment is complete elimination of gluten from the diet. The role of gluten in causing intestinal injury must be explained carefully. Consultation with a dietitian experienced in celiac disease is helpful, as is membership in a celiac disease support group. Lists of prepared foods that contain hidden gluten are particularly important for patients to use. Starchy foods that are safe include rice, soy, tapioca, buckwheat, potatoes, and (pure) oats. Many resources also are available via the Internet to help families cope with the large changes in diet and cooking that are required. Most patients respond clinically within a few weeks with weight gain, improved appetite, and improved sense of well-being. Histologic improvement lags behind clinical response, requiring several months to normalize.

## MILK AND SOY PROTEIN INTOLERANCE (ALLERGIC COLITIS)

### Etiology and Epidemiology

Dietary proteins are a common cause of intestinal inflammation with rectal bleeding in infants. The most commonly implicated agents are cow's milk and, less often, soy proteins. Other dietary antigens are possible in breastfed infants; breast milk also contains a sampling of protein fragments from the entire range of foods consumed by the mother. Symptoms can appear from 1 to 2 weeks to 12 months of age.

### Clinical Manifestations

Most infants with dietary protein intolerance appear healthy despite the presence of streaks of bloody mucus in their stools. This presentation often leads to an erroneous diagnosis of anal fissure. Careful examination of the anus is essential. There is no abdominal tenderness or distention and no vomiting. If these are present, other diagnoses, such as intussusception or volvulus, should be considered. Some children develop severe iron deficiency anemia; intestinal protein loss produces edema and a **protein-losing enteropathy**.

## Laboratory and Imaging Studies

No blood test is particularly helpful. Peripheral eosinophilia generally is not present on complete blood count, which nevertheless should be performed to rule out an associated iron deficiency anemia. Most children are diagnosed clinically and treated empirically. For children with persistent symptoms or other concerns, the diagnosis can be confirmed safely and easily by rectal mucosal biopsy; this shows eosinophilic inflammation of the mucosa. Visual findings at proctoscopy usually include mucosal friability and **lymphoid hyperplasia**, giving a lumpy, *mosquito-bitten* appearance to the rectal mucosa.

## Treatment

Infants who are bottle-fed should be switched to a **hydrolyzed protein formula** (e.g., Nutramigen, Pregestamil, or Alimentum). Breastfed infants may continue breastfeeding, but the mother should restrict dairy and soy products from her diet. Visible blood in stools typically resolves within a few days, although occult blood persists for several weeks. For infants with persistent bleeding, an amino acid–based formula is occasionally necessary. Nearly all of these infants lose their sensitivity to the offending protein by 1 year of age. The first intentional exposure to cow's milk should be performed in the physician's office because of a small risk of anaphylaxis. Treatment of iron deficiency also is indicated (see Chapter 150).

## INTUSSUSCEPTION

### Etiology and Epidemiology

Intussusception is the *telescoping* of a segment of proximal bowel into downstream bowel. Most cases occur in infants 1 to 2 years old. In infants younger than 2 years old, nearly all cases are idiopathic. In older children, the proportion of cases caused by a pathologic lead point increases. In young children, **ileocolonic** intussusception is common; the ileum invaginates into the colon, beginning at or near the ileocecal valve. When pathologic lead points are present, the intussusception may be ileoileal, jejunoileal, or jejunojejunal.

### Clinical Manifestations

An infant with intussusception has sudden onset of crampy abdominal pain; the infant's knees draw up, and the infant cries out and exhibits pallor with a colicky pattern occurring every 15 to 20 minutes. Feedings are refused. As the intussusception progresses, and obstruction becomes prolonged, bilious vomiting becomes prominent, and the dilated, fatigued intestine generates less pressure and less pain. As the intussuscepted bowel is drawn further into the downstream intestine by normal motility, the mesentery is pulled with it and becomes stretched and compressed. The venous outflow from the intussusceptum is obstructed, leading to edema, weeping of fluid, and congestion with bleeding. Third space fluid losses and "currant jelly" stools result. An unexpected feature of intussusception is **lethargy**. Between episodes of pain, the infant typically is glassy-eyed and groggy and appears to have been sedated. A sausage-shaped mass caused by the swollen, intussuscepted bowel may be palpable in the right upper quadrant or epigastrium.

## Laboratory and Imaging Studies

The diagnosis depends on the direct demonstration of bowel-within-bowel. A simple and direct way of showing this is by abdominal ultrasound. If the ultrasound is positive, or if good visualization has not been achieved, a pneumatic or contrast enema under fluoroscopy is indicated. This is the most direct and potentially useful way to show and **treat** intussusception. Air and barium can show the intussusception quickly and, when administered with controlled pressure, usually can reduce it completely. The success rate for pneumatic reduction may be higher than hydrostatic reduction with barium and approaches 90% if done when symptoms have been present for less than 24 hours. The pneumatic enema has the additional advantage over barium of not preventing subsequent radiologic studies, such as upper GI series or CT scan. Nonoperative reduction should not be attempted if the patient is unstable or has evidence of perforation or peritonitis.

## Treatment

Therapy must begin with placement of an IV catheter and a nasogastric tube. Before radiologic intervention is attempted, the child must have adequate **fluid resuscitation** to correct the often severe dehydration caused by vomiting and third space fluid losses. Ultrasound may be performed before the fluid resuscitation is complete. Surgical consultation should be obtained early as surgeons often prefer to be present during nonoperative reduction. If pneumatic or hydrostatic reduction is successful, the child should be admitted to the hospital for overnight observation of possible recurrence (risk is 5–10%). If reduction is not complete, emergency surgery is required. During surgery, gentle manual reduction is attempted, but resection of involved bowel because of severe edema, perforation, a pathologic lead point (polyp, Meckel diverticulum), or necrosis may be necessary.

## APPENDICITIS

### Etiology and Epidemiology

Appendicitis is the most common surgical emergency in childhood. The incidence peaks in the late teenage years, with only 5% of cases occurring in children younger than 5 years of age. Appendicitis begins with obstruction of the lumen, most commonly by fecal matter (fecalith), but appendiceal obstruction can occur secondary to hyperplasia of lymphoid tissue associated with viral infections or, rarely, the presence of neoplastic tissue (classically an appendiceal carcinoid tumor). Trapped bacteria proliferate and begin to invade the appendiceal wall, inducing inflammation and secretion. The obstructed appendix becomes engorged, its blood supply is compromised, and it finally ruptures. The entire process is rapid, with appendiceal rupture usually occurring within 48 hours of the onset of symptoms.

## Clinical Manifestations

Classic appendicitis begins with **visceral pain**, localized to the periumbilical region. Nausea and vomiting occur soon after, triggered by appendiceal distention. As the inflammation begins to irritate the parietal peritoneum adjacent to the appendix, **somatic pain** fibers are activated, and the pain localizes to the right lower quadrant which is tender to palpation. Voluntary guarding is present initially, progressing to rigidity with rebound tenderness with onset of peritonitis. These classic findings may not be present in young children. The nature and location of pain can vary if the appendix is retrocecal, covered by omentum, or is located elsewhere. If typical history and physical examination findings are present, the patient is taken to the operating room. When doubt exists, imaging is helpful to rule out complications (right lower quadrant abscess, liver disease) and other disorders, such as mesenteric adenitis and ovarian or fallopian tube disorders. If some doubt remains following a negative workup, the child should be admitted to the hospital for close observation and serial examinations.

## Laboratory and Imaging Studies

The history and examination are often enough to make the diagnosis, but laboratory and imaging studies are helpful when the diagnosis is uncertain. A WBC count greater than $10,000/mm^3$ is found in 89% of patients with appendicitis and 93% with perforated appendicitis. Unfortunately, this criterion is met by 62% of abdominal pain patients without appendicitis. Urinalysis is done to look for urinary tract infection, and a chest x-ray rules out pneumonia presenting as abdominal pain. Amylase, lipase, and liver enzymes are done to look for pancreatic or liver and gallbladder disease. The plain abdominal x-ray may reveal a calcified fecalith, which strongly suggests the diagnosis. When these studies are inconclusive, imaging is indicated with an abdominal ultrasound or CT scan, which may reveal the presence of an enlarged, thick-walled appendix with surrounding fluid. An appendiceal diameter of more than 6 mm is considered diagnostic.

## Treatment

Treatment of appendicitis is surgical. Simple appendectomy is curative if performed before perforation. With perforation, a course of postoperative IV broad-spectrum antibiotics is required to cover the mixed bowel flora.

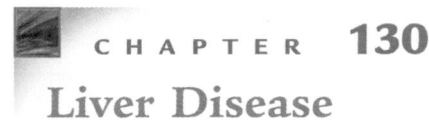

# CHAPTER 130
# Liver Disease

## CHOLESTASIS

### Etiology and Epidemiology

Cholestasis is defined as reduced bile flow and is characterized by elevation of the conjugated (direct) bilirubin fraction. This condition must be distinguished from ordinary neonatal jaundice, in which the direct bilirubin is never elevated (see Chapter 62). When direct bilirubin is elevated, many potentially serious disorders must be considered (Fig. 130-1). Emphasis must be placed on the rapid diagnosis of treatable disorders, especially biliary atresia and metabolic disorders such as galactosemia or tyrosinemia.

### Clinical Manifestations

Cholestasis is caused by many different disorders, the common characteristic of which is cholestatic jaundice. Clinical features of several of the most common causes are given.

The jaundice of **biliary atresia** usually is not evident immediately at birth, but develops in the first 1 to 2 weeks of life. In this disorder, bile ducts are usually present at birth, but are then destroyed by an inflammatory process. Aside from jaundice, these infants do not initially appear ill. The liver injury progresses rapidly to cirrhosis; symptoms of portal hypertension with splenomegaly, ascites, muscle wasting, and poor weight gain are evident by a few months of age. If surgical drainage is not performed successfully early in the course (ideally by 2 months), progression to liver failure is inevitable.

**Neonatal hepatitis** is characterized by an ill-appearing infant with an enlarged liver and jaundice. There is no specific laboratory test, but if liver biopsy is performed, the presence of hepatocyte giant cells is characteristic. Hepatobiliary scintigraphy typically shows slow hepatic uptake with eventual excretion of isotope into the intestine. These infants have a good prognosis overall, with spontaneous resolution occurring in most.

$\alpha_1$-**Antitrypsin deficiency** presents with clinical findings indistinguishable from neonatal hepatitis. Only about 20% of all infants with the genetic defect exhibit neonatal cholestasis. Of these affected infants, about 30% go on to have severe chronic liver disease resulting in cirrhosis and liver failure. $\alpha_1$-Antitrypsin deficiency is the leading metabolic disorder requiring liver transplantation.

**Alagille syndrome** is characterized by chronic cholestasis with the unique liver biopsy finding of paucity of bile ducts in the portal triads. Associated abnormalities include peripheral pulmonary stenosis or other cardiac anomalies; hypertelorism; unusual facies with deep-set eyes, prominent forehead, and a pointed chin; butterfly vertebrae; and a defect of the ocular limbus (*posterior embryotoxon*). Cholestasis is variable but is usually lifelong and associated with hypercholesterolemia and severe pruritus. Progression to end-stage liver disease is uncommon.

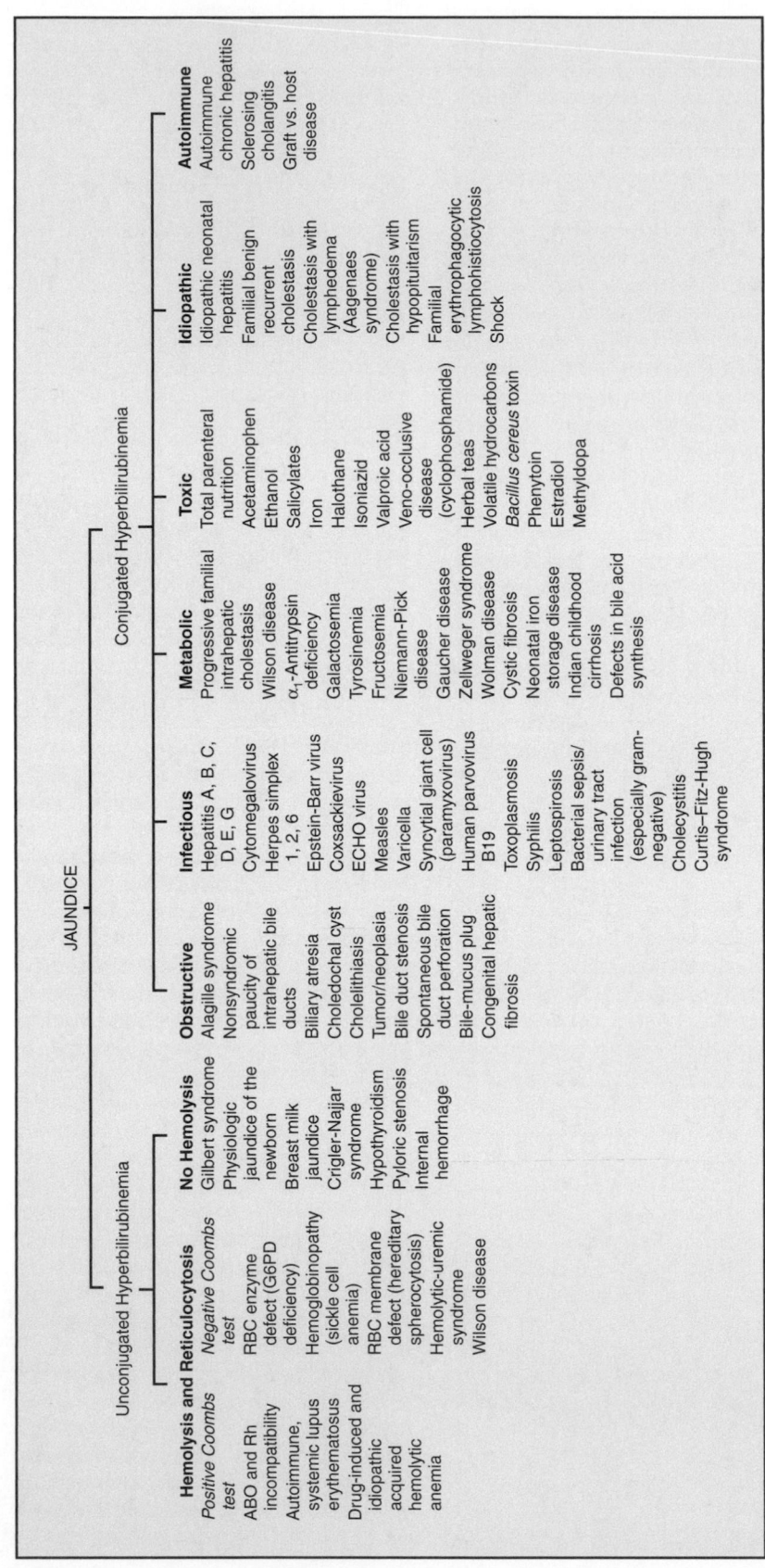

**FIGURE 130-1**

**Differential diagnosis of jaundice in childhood.** G6PD, glucose-6-phosphate dehydrogenase; RBC, red blood cell.

**TABLE 130-1 Laboratory and Imaging Evaluation of Neonatal Cholestasis**

| Evaluation | Rationale |
| --- | --- |
| **INITIAL TESTS** | |
| Total and direct bilirubin | Elevated direct fraction confirms cholestasis |
| AST, ALT | Hepatocellular injury |
| GGT | Biliary obstruction/injury |
| RBC galactose-1-phosphate uridyltransferase | Galactosemia |
| $\alpha_1$-Antitrypsin level | $\alpha_1$-Antitrypsin deficiency |
| Urinalysis and urine culture | Urinary tract infection can cause cholestasis in neonates |
| Blood culture | Sepsis can cause cholestasis |
| Serum amino acids | Aminoacidopathies |
| Urine organic acids | Zellweger syndrome, lysosomal disorders |
| Sweat chloride or CF mutation analysis | Cystic fibrosis |
| Urine culture for cytomegalovirus | Congenital cytomegalovirus infection |
| **INITIAL IMAGING STUDY** | |
| Abdominal ultrasound | Choledochal cyst, gallstones, mass lesion, Caroli disease |
| **SECONDARY IMAGING STUDY** | |
| Hepatobiliary scintigraphy | Rule out biliary atresia |

ALT, alanine aminotransferase; AST, aspartate aminotransferase; CF, cystic fibrosis; GGT, γ-glutamyltransferase; RBC, red blood cell.

## Laboratory and Imaging Studies

The laboratory approach to diagnosis of a neonate with cholestatic jaundice is presented in Table 130-1. Noninvasive studies are performed immediately. Imaging studies also are performed early to rule out biliary obstruction and other anatomic lesions that may be surgically treatable. When necessary to rule out biliary atresia or to obtain prognostic information, liver biopsy is a final option (Fig. 130-2).

## Treatment

Treatment of extrahepatic biliary atresia is the surgical **Kasai procedure.** The damaged bile duct remnant is removed and replaced with a roux-en-Y loop of jejunum. This operation must be performed before 2 to 3 months of age to have the best chance of success. Even so, the success rate is low; many children eventually require liver transplantation. Some metabolic causes of neonatal cholestasis are treatable by dietary manipulation (galactosemia) or medication (tyrosinemia); all affected patients require supportive care. This includes fat-soluble vitamin supplements (vitamins A, D, E, and K) and formula containing medium-chain triglycerides, which can be absorbed without bile salt–induced micelles. Choleretic agents, such as ursodeoxycholic acid and phenobarbital, may improve bile flow in some conditions.

## VIRAL HEPATITIS

Please see Chapter 113.

## FULMINANT LIVER FAILURE

### Etiology and Epidemiology

Fulminant liver failure is defined as severe liver disease with onset of hepatic encephalopathy within 8 weeks after initial symptoms, in the absence of chronic liver disease.

Etiology includes viral hepatitis, metabolic disorders, ischemia, neoplastic disease, and toxins (Table 130-2).

## Clinical Manifestations

Liver failure is a multisystem disorder with complex interactions among the liver, kidneys, vascular structures, gut, central nervous system (CNS), and immune function. Hepatic encephalopathy is characterized by varying degrees of impairment (Table 130-3). Respiratory compromise occurs as severity of the failure increases and requires early institution of ventilatory support. Hypoglycemia resulting from impaired glycogenolysis and gluconeogenesis must be prevented. Renal function is impaired, and frank renal failure, or **hepatorenal syndrome**, may occur. This syndrome is characterized by low urine output, azotemia, and low urine sodium content. Ascites develops secondary to hypoalbuminemia and disordered regulation of fluid and electrolyte homeostasis. Increased risk of infection occurs and may cause death. Portal hypertension causes an enlarged spleen with thrombocytopenia, aggravating the risk of hemorrhage from esophageal varices.

## Laboratory and Imaging Studies

Laboratory studies are used to follow the severity of the liver injury and to monitor the response to therapy. Coagulation tests and serum albumin are used to monitor hepatic synthetic function but are confounded by administration of blood products and clotting factors. Vitamin K should be administered to maximize the liver's ability to synthesize factors II, VII, IX, and X. In addition to monitoring prothrombin time and partial thromboplastin time, many centers measure factor V serially as a sensitive index of synthetic function. Renal function tests, electrolytes, serum ammonia, blood counts, and urinalysis also

**FIGURE 130-2**

Flow chart for evaluation of neonatal cholestasis.

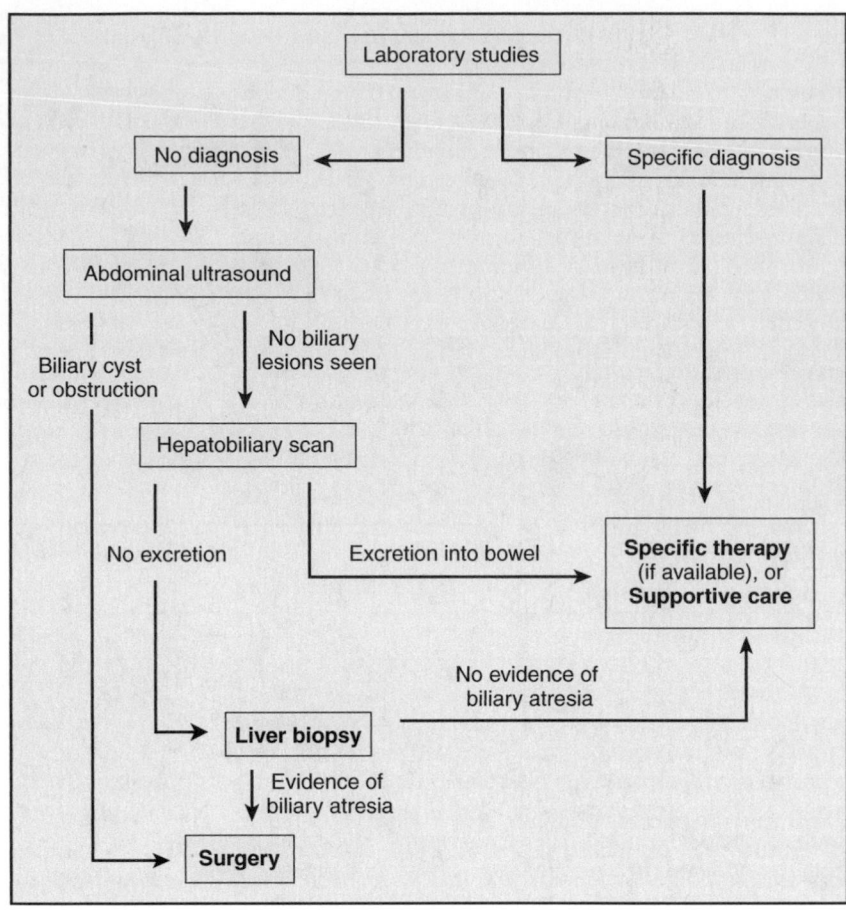

should be followed. In the setting of acute liver failure, liver biopsy may be indicated to ascertain the nature and degree of injury and estimate the likelihood of recovery. In the presence of coagulopathy, biopsy must be done using a transjugular or surgical approach.

## Treatment

Because of the life-threatening and complex nature of this condition, management must be carried out in an intensive care unit (ICU) at a liver transplant center. Treatment of acute liver failure is supportive; the definitive lifesaving therapy is liver transplantation. Supportive measures are listed in Table 130-4. Efforts are made to treat metabolic derangements, avoid hypoglycemia, support respiration, minimize hepatic encephalopathy, and support renal function.

## CHRONIC LIVER DISEASE

### Etiology and Epidemiology

Chronic liver disease in childhood is characterized by the development of cirrhosis and its complications and by progressive hepatic failure. Causative conditions may be congenital or acquired. Major congenital disorders leading to chronic disease include biliary atresia, tyrosinemia, untreated galactosemia, and $\alpha_1$-antitrypsin deficiency. In older children, hepatitis B virus (HBV), hepatitis C virus

(HCV), autoimmune hepatitis, Wilson disease, primary sclerosing cholangitis, cystic fibrosis, and biliary obstruction secondary to choledochal cyst are leading causes.

### Clinical Manifestations

Chronic liver disease is characterized by the consequences of portal hypertension, impaired hepatocellular function, and cholestasis. **Portal hypertension** caused by cirrhosis results in risk of gastrointestinal (GI) bleeding, ascites, and reduced hepatic blood flow. Blood entering the portal vein from the splenic and mesenteric veins is diverted to collateral circulation that bypasses the liver, enlarging these previously tiny vessels in the esophagus, stomach, and abdomen. **Esophageal varices** are particularly prone to bleed, but bleeding also can occur from hemorrhoidal veins, congested gastric mucosa, and gastric varices. **Ascites** develops as a result of weeping from pressurized visceral veins and from excessive renal water and salt retention. Ascitic fluid often becomes quite massive, interfering with patient comfort and respiration, and is easily infected (spontaneous bacterial peritonitis). The spleen enlarges secondary to impaired splenic vein outflow, causing excessive scavenging of platelets and white blood cells (WBCs); decreased cell counts increase the patient's susceptibility to bleeding and infection.

Impaired hepatocellular function is associated with coagulopathy unresponsive to vitamin K, low serum albumin,

## TABLE 130-2 Causes of Fulminant Liver Failure in Childhood

### METABOLIC

Neonatal hemochromatosis
Electron chain transport defects
Disorders of fatty acid oxidation
Galactosemia
Hereditary fructose intolerance
Bile acid synthesis disorders
Wilson disease

### CARDIOVASCULAR

Shock, hypotension
Congestive heart failure
Budd-Chiari syndrome

### INFECTIOUS

Hepatitis viruses (A, B, C, D)
Echovirus
Coxsackievirus
Adenovirus
Parvovirus
Cytomegalovirus
Sepsis
Herpes simplex

### NEOPLASTIC

Acute leukemia
Lymphoproliferative disease

### TOXIC

Acetaminophen
Valproic acid
Phenytoin
Isoniazid
Halothane
*Amanita* mushrooms

## TABLE 130-3 Stages of Hepatic Encephalopathy

### STAGE I

Alert and awake
Agitated and distractible
Infants and young children—irritable and fussy
Normal reflexes
Tremor, poor handwriting
Obeys age-appropriate commands

### STAGE II

Confused and lethargic
Combative or inappropriate euphoria
Hyperactive reflexes
Asterixis present
Purposeful movements, but may not obey commands

### STAGE III

Stuporous but arousable
Sleepy
Incoherent speech
Motor response to pain
Hyperreflexic
Hyperventilation
Asterixis present

### STAGE IV

Unconscious, not arousable
Unresponsive or responds nonpurposefully to pain
Reflexes hyperactive
Irregular respirations
Pupil response sluggish

### STAGE V

Unconscious
Hypoactive reflexes
Flaccid muscle tone
Apneic
Pupils fixed

---

elevated ammonia, and **hepatic encephalopathy**. The diversion of portal blood away from the liver via collateral circulation worsens this process. Malaise develops and contributes to poor nutrition, leading to muscle wasting and other consequences.

**Chronic cholestasis** causes debilitating pruritus and deepening jaundice. The reduced excretion of bile acids impairs absorption of fat and fat-soluble vitamins. Deficiency of vitamin K impairs production of clotting factors II, VII, IX, and X and increases the risk of bleeding. Vitamin E deficiency leads to hematologic and neurologic consequences unless corrected.

### Laboratory and Imaging Studies

Laboratory studies include specific tests for diagnosis of the underlying illness and testing to monitor the status of the patient. Children presenting for the first time with evidence of chronic liver disease should have a standard investigation (Table 130-5). Monitoring should include coagulation tests, electrolytes and renal function testing, complete blood count with platelet count, transaminases, alkaline phosphatase, and γ-glutamyltransferase at appropriate intervals. Frequency of testing should be tailored to the pace of the patient's illness. Ascites fluid can be tested for infection by culture and cell count and generally is found to have an albumin concentration lower than that of serum, with a serum-ascites albumen gradient (SAAG) greater than 1.1 g/dL.

### Treatment

Treatment of chronic liver disease is complex. Supportive care for each of the many problems encountered in these patients is outlined in Table 130-6. Ultimately, survival depends on the availability of a donor liver and the patient's candidacy for transplantation. When transplantation is not possible or is delayed, portal hypertension can be treated by a **portosystemic shunt**. The transjugular intrahepatic portosystemic shunt (TIPS) consists of an expandable stent placed between the hepatic vein and a

## TABLE 130-4 Treatment of Fulminant Liver Failure

| Problem | Management |
|---|---|
| Hepatic encephalopathy | Avoid sedatives |
| | Lactulose via nasogastric tube: start with 1-2 mL/kg/day; adjust dose to yield several loose stools per day |
| | Enemas if constipated |
| | Mechanical ventilation if stage III or IV |
| Coagulopathy | Fresh frozen plasma only if active bleeding, monitor coagulation studies frequently |
| | Platelet transfusions as required |
| Hypoglycemia | Intravenous glucose supplied with ≥10% dextrose solution, electrolytes as appropriate |
| Ascites | Restrict fluid intake to 50%–60% maintenance |
| | Restrict sodium intake to 0.5-1 mEq/kg/day |
| | Monitor central venous pressure to maintain adequate intravascular volume (avoid renal failure) |
| Renal failure | Maintain adequate intravascular volume, give albumin if low |
| | Diuretics |
| | Vasoconstrictors |
| | Dialysis or hemofiltration |
| | Exchange transfusion |
| | Liver transplantation |

branch of the portal vein within the hepatic parenchyma. This procedure is performed using catheters inserted via the jugular vein and is entirely nonsurgical. All portosystemic shunts carry increased risk of hepatic encephalopathy.

# SELECTED CHRONIC HEPATIC DISORDERS

## Wilson Disease

Wilson disease is characterized by abnormal storage of copper in the liver, leading to hepatocellular injury, CNS dysfunction, and hemolytic anemia. It is an autosomal recessive trait caused by mutations in the *ATP7B* gene, which codes for an ATP-driven copper pump. The **diagnosis** is made by identifying depressed serum levels of ceruloplasmin, elevated 24-hour urine copper excretion, the presence of Kayser-Fleischer rings in the iris, evidence of hemolysis, and elevated hepatic copper content. In any single patient, one or more of these measures may be normal. **Clinical presentation** also varies, but seldom occurs before age 3 years. Neurologic abnormalities may predominate, including tremor, decline in school performance, worsening handwriting, and psychiatric disturbances. Anemia may be the first noted symptom. Hepatic presentations include appearance of jaundice, spider hemangiomas, portal hypertension, and fulminant hepatic failure. **Treatment** consists of administration of copper chelating drugs (penicillamine or trientine), monitoring of urine

## TABLE 130-5 Laboratory and Imaging Investigation of Chronic Liver Disease

### METABOLIC TESTING

Serum $\alpha_1$-antitrypsin level
$\alpha_1$-Antitrypsin phenotype if low serum level
Serum ceruloplasmin
Sweat chloride, CF gene tests if CF suspected
Testing for other specific conditions as indicated by clinical/laboratory findings

### VIRAL HEPATITIS

HBsAg
Hepatitis B viral DNA, HBeAg if HBsAg positive
Hepatitis C antibody
Hepatitis C antibody confirmatory test if positive
Hepatitis C viral RNA, genotype if antibody confirmed

### AUTOIMMUNE HEPATITIS

Antinuclear antibody
Liver-kidney microsomal antibody
Anti–smooth muscle antibody
Antineutrophil cytoplasmic antibody
Total serum IgG (usually elevated)

### TESTS TO EVALUATE LIVER FUNCTION AND INJURY

Prothrombin time and partial thromboplastin time
Serum ammonia
CBC with platelet count
Serum albumin
AST, ALT, GGT, alkaline phosphatase
Total and direct bilirubin
Serum cholylglycine or bile acids
Serum cholesterol
Ultrasound examination of liver and bile ducts
Doppler ultrasound of hepatic vessels*
Magnetic resonance cholangiography*
Magnetic resonance angiography of hepatic vessels*
Percutaneous or endoscopic cholangiography*
Liver biopsy*

### ANATOMIC EVALUATION

Ultrasound of liver, pancreas, and biliary tree
Consider magnetic resonance cholangiography or ERCP if evidence of biliary process
Liver biopsy—as required for diagnosis or prognosis

### TESTS TO EVALUATE NUTRITIONAL STATUS

Height, weight, skinfold thickness
25-Hydroxyvitamin D level
Vitamin A level
Prothrombin time and partial thromboplastin time before and after vitamin K administration
Serum albumin and prealbumin

*Perform when indicated to obtain specific anatomic information.
ALT, alanine aminotransferase; AST, aspartate aminotransferase; CBC, complete blood count; CF, cystic fibrosis; ERCP, endoscopic retrograde cholangiopancreatography; GGT, γ-glutamyltransferase; HBeAg, hepatitis B early antigen; HBsAg, hepatitis B surface antigen.

**TABLE 130-6 Management of Chronic Liver Disease**

| Problem | Clinical Manifestations | Diagnostic Testing | Treatment |
|---|---|---|---|
| Gastrointestinal variceal bleeding* | Hematemesis, rectal bleeding, melena, anemia | CBC, coagulation tests, Doppler ultrasound, magnetic resonance angiography, endoscopy | Somatostatin (octreotide) infusion, variceal band ligation or sclerotherapy, propranolol to reduce portal pressure, acid-blocker therapy, TIPSS or surgical portosystemic shunt if transplant not possible |
| Ascites | Abdominal distention, shifting dullness and fluid wave, respiratory compromise, spontaneous bacterial peritonitis | Abdominal ultrasound, diagnostic paracentesis; measure ascites fluid albumin (and serum albumin), cell count, WBC differential, culture fluid in blood culture bottles | Restrict sodium intake to 0.5–1 mEq/kg/day, restrict fluids, monitor renal function, treat peritonitis and portal hypertension<br>Central portosystemic shunt may be required |
| Nutritional compromise | Muscle wasting, fat-soluble vitamin deficiencies, poor or absent weight gain, fatigue | Coagulation studies, serum albumin, 25-hydroxyvitamin D level, vitamin E level, vitamin A level | Fat-soluble vitamin supplements: vitamins A, D, E, and K; use water-soluble form of vitamins<br>Supplemental feedings— nasogastric or parenteral if necessary |
| Hepatic encephalopathy | Irritability, confusion, lethargy, somnolence, coma | Serum ammonia | Lactulose orally or via nasogastric tube, avoid narcotics and sedatives, liver transplantation |

*May also have peptic ulcerations.
CBC, complete blood count; TIPSS, transjugular intrahepatic portosystemic shunt; WBC, white blood cell.

copper excretion at intervals. Zinc salts inhibit intestinal copper absorption and are increasingly being used, especially after initial chelation therapy has reduced the excessive body copper stores. Adequate therapy must be continued for life to prevent liver and CNS deterioration.

## Autoimmune Hepatitis

Immune-mediated liver injury may be primary or occur in association with other autoimmune disorders, such as inflammatory bowel disease or systemic lupus erythematosus. **Diagnosis** is made on the basis of elevated serum total IgG and the presence of an autoantibody, most commonly antinuclear, anti–smooth muscle, or anti–liver-kidney microsomal antibody. Liver biopsy reveals a plasma cell–rich portal infiltrate with piecemeal necrosis. **Treatment** consists of corticosteroids initially, usually with the addition of an immunosuppressive drug after remission is achieved. Steroids are tapered gradually as tolerated to minimize glucocorticoid side effects. Many patients require lifelong immunosuppressive therapy, but some may be able to stop medications after several years under careful monitoring for recurrence.

## Primary Sclerosing Cholangitis

Primary sclerosing cholangitis typically occurs in association with ulcerative colitis. It may be accompanied by evidence of autoimmune hepatitis; this is termed **overlap syndrome.** Antineutrophil cytoplasmic antibody (p-ANCA) is present in most cases. **Diagnosis** is by liver biopsy and cholangiography, generally performed as endoscopic retrograde cholangiopancreatography (ERCP) or noninvasively by magnetic resonance cholangiopancreatography (MRCP). Treatment consists of ursodiol administration, which seems to slow progression and improves indices of hepatic injury; dilation of major biliary strictures during ERCP; and liver transplantation for end-stage liver disease.

## Steatohepatitis

**Nonalcoholic fatty liver disease** or **nonalcoholic fatty hepatitis** is characterized by the presence of macrovesicular fatty change in hepatocytes on biopsy. Varying degrees of inflammation and portal fibrosis may be present. This disorder occurs in obese children, sometimes in association with insulin-resistant (type 2) diabetes and hyperlipidemia. Children with marked obesity, with or without type 2 diabetes, who have elevated liver enzymes and no other identifiable liver disease, are likely to have this condition. Nonalcoholic fatty liver disease can progress to significant fibrosis. Treatment is with diet and exercise. Vitamin E may have some benefit. Efforts should be made to control blood glucose and hyperlipidemia and promote weight loss. In general, the rate of progression to end-stage liver disease is slow.

# CHAPTER 131

# Pancreatic Disease

## PANCREATIC INSUFFICIENCY

### Etiology and Epidemiology

The cause of inadequate pancreatic digestive function in 95% of cases is **cystic fibrosis** (see Chapter 137). The defect in *CFTR* chloride channel function results in thick secretions in the lungs, intestines, pancreas, and bile ducts. In the pancreas, there is destruction of pancreatic function, often before birth. Some mutations result in less severe defects in *CFTR* function and later onset of lung disease and pancreatic insufficiency. Less common causes of pancreatic insufficiency are Shwachman-Diamond syndrome and Pearson syndrome in developed countries and severe malnutrition in developing countries.

### Clinical Manifestations

Children with pancreatic exocrine insufficiency have **steatorrhea**—many bulky, foul-smelling stools each day, usually with visible oil or fat. They typically have voracious appetites because of massive malabsorption of calories from fat, complex carbohydrates, and proteins. Failure to thrive is uniformly present if diagnosis and treatment are not accomplished rapidly. It is important to distinguish children with malabsorption due to pancreatic disease from children with intestinal disorders that interfere with digestion or absorption. Appropriate testing should be performed to rule out conditions such as celiac disease and inflammatory bowel disease (IBD) if any doubt about the state of pancreatic sufficiency exists.

### Laboratory and Imaging Studies

Testing pancreatic function is difficult. Direct measurement of enzyme concentrations in aspirated pancreatic juice is not routine and is technically difficult. Stools can be tested for the presence of maldigested fat. The presence of fecal fat usually indicates poor fat digestion. Measuring fecal fat is relatively simple and, depending on method, can give either a qualitative assessment of fat absorption (fecal Sudan stain) or a semiquantitative measurement (72-hour fecal fat determination) of fat maldigestion. Another way to assess pancreatic function is to test for the presence of pancreatic enzymes in the stool. Of these, measuring fecal elastase-1 seems to be the most accurate method of assessment. Depressed fecal elastase-1 concentration correlates well with the presence of pancreatic insufficiency.

### Treatment

Replacement of missing pancreatic enzymes is the best available therapy. Pancreatic enzymes in powder form can be mixed with formula for infants, and administered as capsules containing enteric-coated microspheres for older children. For children unable to swallow capsules, the contents may be sprinkled on a spoonful of soft food. Excessive use of enzymes must be avoided because high doses (usually > 6000 U/kg/meal) can cause colonic fibrosis. In infants, typical dosing is 2000 to 4000 U of lipase in 120 mL of formula. In children younger than 4 years of age, 1000 U/kg/meal is given. For older children, 500 U/kg/meal is usual. This dose may be adjusted upward as required to control steatorrhea, but a dose of 2500 U/kg/meal should not be exceeded. Use of $H_2$ receptor antagonists or proton-pump inhibitors can increase the efficacy of pancreatic enzymes by enhancing their release from the microspheres and reducing inactivation by acid.

## ACUTE PANCREATITIS

### Etiology and Epidemiology

The exocrine pancreas produces numerous digestive enzymes, including trypsin, chymotrypsin, and carboxypeptidase. These are produced as inactive proenzymes to protect the pancreas from autodigestion. Trypsin is activated after leaving the pancreas by enterokinase, an intestinal brush border enzyme. After activation, trypsin cleaves other proteolytic proenzymes into their active states. Protease inhibitors found in pancreatic juice inhibit early activation of trypsin; the presence of self-digestion sites on the trypsin molecule allows for feedback inactivation. Pancreatitis occurs when digestive enzymes are activated inside the pancreas, causing injury. Triggers for acute pancreatitis differ between adults and children. In the adult patient, most episodes are related to alcohol abuse or gallstones. In children, most cases are idiopathic. Some cases are caused by medications, hypertriglyceridemia, biliary microlithiasis, trauma, or viral infection. Collagen vascular disorders and parasite infestations are responsible for the remainder.

### Clinical Manifestations

Acute pancreatitis presents with relatively rapid onset of pain, usually in the epigastric region. The pain may radiate to the back and is aggravated by eating. Nausea and vomiting occur in most cases. Pain is continuous and quite severe, usually requiring narcotics. Severe pancreatitis can lead to hemorrhage, visible as ecchymoses in the flanks (Grey Turner sign) or periumbilical region (Cullen sign). Rupture of a pancreatic duct can lead to development of a pancreatic **pseudocyst**, characterized by persistent severe pain, tenderness, and a palpable mass. Because of tissue necrosis and fluid collections, patients with severe pancreatitis are prone to infectious complications which may present with fever and signs of sepsis.

### Laboratory and Imaging Studies

Acute pancreatitis can be difficult to diagnose. Elevations in total serum amylase or lipase support the diagnosis. These pancreatic enzymes are released into the blood during pancreatic injury. As acute pancreatitis progresses, the amylase level tends to decline faster than lipase, making the latter a better choice for diagnostic testing late in the course of the disease.

Serial measurement of laboratory studies is important to monitor for severe complications. At diagnosis, baseline complete blood count, C-reactive protein, electrolytes, blood urea nitrogen (BUN), creatinine, glucose, calcium, and phosphorus should be obtained. These should be followed at least daily, along with amylase and lipase, until the patient has recovered.

Imaging studies are important to evaluate suspected pancreatitis. Ductal dilation secondary to obstruction by gallstones or other lesions must be ruled out. The liver, gallbladder, and common bile duct all should be visualized. In acute pancreatitis, edema is present in all but the mildest cases. Ultrasound is capable of detecting this edema and should be performed as part of the overall diagnostic approach. If overlying bowel gas obscures the pancreas, a computed tomography (CT) scan allows complete visualization of the gland. CT scans should be done with oral and intravenous contrast agents to facilitate interpretation. With persistent symptoms, ultrasound and CT also can detect pseudocysts.

### Treatment

There are no proven specific therapies for acute pancreatitis. If a predisposing etiology is found, such as a gallstone obstructing the ampulla of Vater, it should be specifically treated. Pain relief should be provided. Narcotics are necessary despite the theoretical disadvantage of increasing sphincter of Oddi pressure and trapping pancreatic secretions. Nutritional support should be provided. Once pain and emesis subside, enteral feeding is begun. Feedings administered downstream from the duodenum via a nasojejunal tube are generally well tolerated. If this is not possible, parenteral nutrition is an option. Broad-spectrum antibiotics should be administered if the patient is febrile, has extensive pancreatic necrosis, or has laboratory evidence of infection (sepsis, pancreatic abscess).

## CHRONIC PANCREATITIS

### Etiology and Epidemiology

Chronic pancreatitis is defined as recurrent or persistent attacks of pancreatitis, which have resulted in irreversible morphologic changes in pancreatic structure. Most patients have discrete attacks of acute symptoms occurring repeatedly, but chronic pain may be present. The causes of chronic pancreatitis include hereditary pancreatitis and milder phenotypes of cystic fibrosis associated with pancreatic sufficiency. Familial disease is caused by one of several known mutations in the trypsinogen gene. These mutations favor intrapancreatic activation of trypsin. Less commonly, mutations in the *SPINK1* gene, which codes for pancreatic trypsin inhibitor, have been found. Genetic testing is readily available for these mutations and for cystic fibrosis.

### Clinical Manifestations

Children with chronic pancreatitis initially present with recurring attacks of acute pancreatitis. Injury to the pancreatic ducts predisposes these children to continued attacks owing to scarring of small and large pancreatic ducts, stasis of pancreatic secretions, stone formation, and inflammation. Loss of pancreatic exocrine and endocrine tissue over time can lead to exocrine and endocrine deficiency. More than 90% of the pancreatic mass must be destroyed before steatorrhea becomes clinically apparent; this is a late complication that does not occur in all cases.

### Laboratory and Imaging Studies

Laboratory diagnosis of chronic pancreatitis is similar to acute pancreatitis. Monitoring also should include looking for consequences of chronic injury, including diabetes mellitus and compromise of the pancreatic and biliary ducts. Endoscopic retrograde cholangiopancreatography (ERCP) offers the possibility of therapeutic intervention to remove gallstones, dilate strictures, and place stents to enhance flow of pancreatic juice. Plain abdominal x-rays may show pancreatic calcifications.

### Treatment

Treatment is largely supportive. Potential but unproven therapies include the use of daily pancreatic enzyme supplements, octreotide (somatostatin) to abort early attacks, low-fat diets, and daily antioxidant therapy. Care must be taken that extreme diets do not result in nutritional deprivation. Interventional ERCP may be used to dilate large strictures and remove stones. Surgical pancreatic drainage to decompress dilated pancreatic ducts by creating a side-to-side pancreaticojejunostomy (Puestow procedure) has some value.

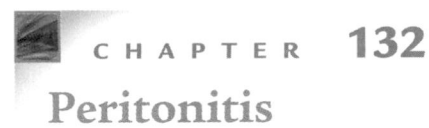

CHAPTER **132**

# Peritonitis

## ETIOLOGY AND EPIDEMIOLOGY

The peritoneum consists of a single layer of mesothelial cells that covers all intra-abdominal organs. The portion that covers the abdominal wall is derived from the underlying somatic structures and is innervated by somatic nerves. The portion covering the viscera is derived from visceral mesoderm and is innervated by nonmyelinated visceral afferents. Inflammation of the peritoneum, or peritonitis, usually is caused by infection, but may result from exogenous irritants introduced by penetrating injuries or surgical procedures, radiation, and endogenous irritants, such as meconium. Infectious peritonitis can be an acute complication of intestinal inflammation and perforation, as in appendicitis, or it can occur secondary to contamination of preexisting ascites associated with renal, cardiac, or hepatic disease. In this setting, when there is no other intra-abdominal source, it is referred to as **spontaneous bacterial peritonitis** and is usually due to pneumococcal infection.

## CLINICAL MANIFESTATIONS

Peritonitis is characterized on examination by marked abdominal tenderness. Rebound tenderness generally is quite pronounced. The patient tends to move very little owing to intense peritoneal irritation and pain. Fever is not always present, and absence of fever should not be regarded as contradictory to the diagnosis. Patients who are taking corticosteroids for an underlying condition, such as nephrotic syndrome, are likely to have little fever and reduced tenderness.

## LABORATORY AND IMAGING STUDIES

Blood tests should focus on identifying the nature of the inflammation and its underlying cause. An elevated white blood cell (WBC) count, erythrocyte sedimentation rate, and C-reactive protein suggest infection. In children older than 5 years, appendicitis is the leading cause. Total serum protein, albumin, and urinalysis should be ordered to rule out nephrotic syndrome. Liver function tests should be performed to rule out chronic liver disease causing ascites. When a large amount of ascites fluid is found on physical examination or imaging studies, **paracentesis** should be performed. Peritoneal fluid in spontaneous bacterial peritonitis has a high neutrophil count ($>250$ cells/mm$^3$). Other tests that should be run on the peritoneal fluid include amylase (to rule out pancreatic ascites), bacterial culture, albumin, and lactate dehydrogenase concentration. For culture, a large sample of fluid should be placed into aerobic and anaerobic blood culture bottles immediately on obtaining the sample.

Appendicitis may be identified by ultrasound or computed tomography (CT) scan (see Chapter 129). When other intra-abdominal emergencies are suspected, such as midgut volvulus, meconium ileus, peptic disease, or any other condition predisposing to intestinal perforation, specific testing should be performed.

## TREATMENT

Peritonitis caused by an intra-abdominal surgical process, such as appendicitis or a penetrating wound, must be managed surgically. Spontaneous bacterial peritonitis should be treated with a broad-spectrum antibiotic with good coverage of resistant pneumococcus and enteric bacteria. Cefotaxime is generally effective as initial therapy while awaiting culture and sensitivity results. Anaerobic coverage with metronidazole should be added whenever a perforated viscus is suspected.

---

 **SUGGESTED READING**

Kliegman RM, Behrman RE, Jenson HB, et al: Nelson Textbook of Pediatrics, 18th ed, Philadelphia, 2007, *Elsevier Health Sciences.*

Shneider BL, Mieli-Vergani G, Sherman P, et al: Walker's Pediatric Gastrointestinal Disease, ed 5, Hamilton, Ontario, 2008, *BC Decker..*

Suchy FJ, Sokol RJ, Balistreri WF: Liver Disease in Children, 3rd ed, Cambridge, 2007, *Cambridge University Press.*

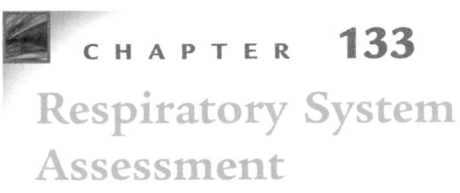

CHAPTER 133

# Respiratory System Assessment

## ANATOMY OF THE RESPIRATORY SYSTEM

Air enters the **nose** and passes over the large surface area of the **nasal turbinates.** The large surface area and convoluted patterns of airflow warm, humidify, and filter the inspired air. Secretions draining from the paranasal sinuses are carried to the **pharynx** by the mucociliary action of the ciliated respiratory epithelium. Lymphoid tissue (**adenoids**) can obstruct the orifices of the eustachian tubes, which extend from the middle ear to the posterior aspect of the nasopharynx.

The **epiglottis** helps to protect the larynx during swallowing by deflecting material toward the esophagus. The **arytenoid cartilages**, which assist in opening and closing the glottis, are less prominent in children than in adults. The opening formed by the vocal cords (the glottis) is V-shaped with the apex of the V being anterior. Below the vocal cords, the walls of the **subglottic space** converge toward the **cricoid** portion of the trachea. In children under 3 years of age, the cricoid ring (first tracheal ring and a complete ring) is the narrowest portion of the airway, and in older children and adults the glottis is the most narrow. Rings of cartilage extending approximately 320 degrees around the airway circumference support the **trachea** and mainstem **bronchi**. The posterior wall of the trachea is membranous. Beyond the lobar bronchi, the cartilaginous support for the airways becomes discontinuous.

The right lung has three lobes (upper, middle, lower) and comprises approximately 55% of the total lung volume. The left lung has two lobes (upper, lower). The inferior division of the left upper lobe, the lingula, is analogous to the right middle lobe.

The lung has a tremendous capacity for growth. A full-term infant has approximately 25 million alveoli; an adult nearly 300 million alveoli. Most growth of new alveoli occurs during the first 2 years of life and is complete by 8 years of age after which lung volume increases with linear growth, but new alveoli are not usually formed.

## PULMONARY PHYSIOLOGY

### Pulmonary Mechanics

The major function of the lungs is to **exchange oxygen** ($O_2$) and **carbon dioxide** ($CO_2$) between the atmosphere and the blood. The anatomy of the airways, mechanics of the respiratory muscles and rib cage, nature of the alveolar-capillary interface, pulmonary circulation, tissue metabolism, and neuromuscular control of ventilation all influence gas exchange.

Air enters the lungs when the pressure in the thorax is less than that of the surrounding atmosphere. During inspiration, negative intrathoracic pressure is generated by contraction and lowering of the **diaphragm**. The accessory muscles of inspiration (**external intercostal, scalene, and sternocleidomastoid muscles**) are not used during quiet breathing but are recruited during exercise or in disease states to raise and enlarge the rib cage. Exhalation is normally passive but, with active exhalation, the **abdominal** and **internal intercostal muscles** are recruited.

**Airway resistance** is influenced by the diameter and length of the conducting airways, the viscosity of gas, and the nature of the airflow. During quiet breathing, airflow in the smaller airways may be laminar (streamlined), and resistance is then inversely proportional to the fourth power of the radius of the airway. At higher flow rates, turbulent flow, especially in the larger airways, increases resistance. Relatively small changes in airway diameter can result in large changes in airway resistance. When mechanical forces acting on the lung are at equilibrium (at the end of a normal relaxed breath), the volume of gas in the lung is termed the **functional residual capacity (FRC)** (Fig. 133-1). This gas volume maintains exchange of $O_2$ during exhalation. **Lung compliance** (change in volume for a given change in pressure) is a measure of the ease with which the lung can be inflated. Processes that decrease **lung compliance** (surfactant deficiency, pulmonary fibrosis, pulmonary edema) may lead to decreases in FRC. Conversely, FRC may be increased in obstructive lung diseases (asthma and cystic fibrosis) secondary to gas trapping in the lungs.

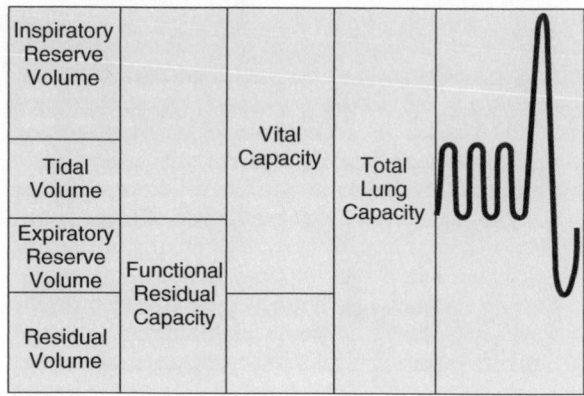

**FIGURE 133-1**

**Lung volumes and capacities.** Vital capacity and its subdivisions can be measured by spirometry, but calculation of residual volume requires measurement of functional residual capacity by body plethysmography, helium dilution, or nitrogen washout. (From Andreoli TE, Bennett JC, Carpenter CJ, et al [eds]: Cecil Essentials of Medicine, 4th ed. Philadelphia, *WB Saunders*, 1997, p 127.)

During normal tidal breathing, lung volumes are usually in the mid-range of inflation (see Fig. 133-1). **Residual volume (RV)** is the volume of gas left in the lungs at the end of a maximal exhalation, and **total lung capacity (TLC)** is the volume of gas in the lungs at the end of maximal inhalation. **Vital capacity (VC)** is the maximal amount of air that can be expelled from the lungs and is the difference between TLC and RV.

**Alveolar ventilation** is defined as the exchange of carbon dioxide between the alveoli and external environment. Normally, about 30% of each tidal breath fills the conducting (non-gas-exchanging) airways (**anatomic dead space**). Because the anatomic dead space is relatively constant, increasing the tidal volume may increase the efficiency of ventilation. Conversely, if tidal volume decreases, then the dead space/tidal volume ratio increases, and alveolar ventilation decreases.

Excessive airway secretions, bronchospasm, mucosal edema and inflammation, airway stenosis, foreign bodies, loss of airway wall integrity (as with bronchiectasis), and airway compression may all produce symptomatic **airway obstruction**. Asthma and bronchiolitis are common causes of airway obstruction. **Restrictive lung disease** is less common and is characterized by normal to low FRC and RV, low TLC and VC, decreased lung compliance, and relatively normal flow rates. Restrictive lung disease can result from neuromuscular weakness, an alveolar filling process (lobar pneumonia, pulmonary edema), pleural disease (pleural effusion, inflammation, or mass), thoracic narrowing/stiffness (scoliosis, severe pectus excavatum), and abdominal distention.

### Respiratory Gas Exchange

Gas exchange depends upon **alveolar ventilation**, **pulmonary capillary blood flow**, and the **diffusion** of gases across the alveolar-capillary membrane. Exchange of $CO_2$ is determined by alveolar ventilation, while the exchange of $O_2$ is influenced primarily by the regional matching of ventilation (V) with pulmonary blood flow (Q) (V/Q matching). V/Q matching is maintained, in part, by **hypoxic pulmonary vasoconstriction** (local constriction of the pulmonary vessels in areas that are hypoventilated). There are five causes of **hypoxemia** (Table 133-1). Disorders resulting in **V/Q mismatching** are the most common causes of hypoxemia.

### Lung Defense Mechanisms

The lungs are constantly exposed to particles and infectious agents. The **nose** is the primary filter for large particles. The **ciliated epithelium** of the paranasal sinuses and nasal turbinates propagate filtered particles toward the pharynx. Particles less than 10 μm in diameter may reach the trachea and bronchi and deposit on the mucosa. Particles less than 1 μm may reach the alveoli. Ciliated cells lining the airways from the larynx to the bronchioles continuously propel a thin layer of mucus toward the mouth. **Alveolar macrophages** and **polymorphonuclear cells** engulf particles and pathogens that have been opsonized by locally secreted IgA antibodies or transudated serum antibodies.

**Cough**, important in protecting the lungs, is a forceful expiration that can clear the airways of debris and secretions. Cough may be voluntary or generated by reflex irritation of the nose, sinus, pharynx, larynx, trachea, bronchi, and bronchioles. The loss of the ability to cough results in poor secretion clearance and predisposes to atelectasis and pneumonia.

## HISTORY

The complete respiratory history includes **onset, duration, and frequency** of respiratory symptoms (cough, noisy breathing, work of breathing/exercise tolerance, nasal congestion, sputum production), swallowing function (especially in infants), and exposure to others with respiratory illness. It is important to obtain information concerning the severity (hospitalizations, emergency department visits, missed school days) and pattern (acute, chronic, or intermittent) of symptoms. For infants, a feeding history should be obtained. **Family history** should include questions about asthma and atopy, immune deficiencies, and cystic fibrosis (CF). The **environmental history** includes exposure to smoke, pets, and pollutants. Travel history may also be relevant.

## PHYSICAL EXAMINATION

Clothing should be removed from the upper half of the child's body so that the thorax may be inspected. It is best to observe the respiratory pattern, rate, and work of breathing while the child is quiet, noting the shape and symmetry of the chest wall and the anteroposterior (AP) diameter.

Any factor that impairs respiratory mechanics is likely to increase the **respiratory rate**. However, nonrespiratory causes of tachypnea include fever, pain, and anxiety. Respiratory rates vary with age and activity (Table 133-2).

It is important to observe the respiratory **pattern** and **degree of effort** (work of breathing). **Hyperpnea** (increased depth of respiration) may be observed with fever, metabolic acidosis, pulmonary and cardiac disease,

**TABLE 133-1  Causes of Hypoxemia**

| Cause | Example(s) | $Pa_{O_2}$ | $Pa_{CO_2}$ | $Pa_{O_2}$ Improves with Supplemental Oxygen |
|---|---|---|---|---|
| Ventilation-perfusion mismatch | Asthma<br>Bronchopulmonary dysplasia<br>Pneumonia | ↓ | Normal, ↓, or ↑ | Yes |
| Hypoventilation | Apnea<br>Narcotic overdose<br>Neuromuscular disease | ↓ | ↑ | Yes |
| Extrapulmonary shunt | Cyanotic heart disease | ↓ | Normal or ↑ | No |
| Intrapulmonary shunt | Pulmonary arteriovenous malformation<br>Pulmonary edema | ↓ | Normal or ↑ | No |
| Low $F_{IO_2}$ | High altitude | ↓ | ↓ | Yes |
| Diffusion defect | Scleroderma<br>Hepatopulmonary syndrome<br>Pulmonary fibrosis | ↓ | Normal | Yes |

**TABLE 133-2  Breathing Patterns**

| Pattern | Features |
|---|---|
| Normal rate (breaths/min) | Preterm: 40–60; term: 30–40; 5 yr: 25; 10 yr: 20; 15 yr: 16; adult: 12 |
| Obstructive | |
|   Mild | Reduced rate, increased tidal volume, slightly prolonged expiratory phase |
|   Severe | Increased rate, increased use of accessory muscles, prolonged expiratory phase |
| Restrictive | Rapid rate, decreased tidal volume |
| Kussmaul respiration | Increased rate, increased tidal volume, regular deep respiration; consider metabolic acidosis or diabetic ketoacidosis |
| Cheyne-Stokes respiration | Cyclic pattern of waxing and waning of breathing interposed by central apneas/hypopneas; consider CNS injury, depressant drugs, heart failure, uremia (rare in children) |
| Biot respiration | Ataxic or periodic breathing with a respiratory effort followed by apnea; consider brainstem injury or posterior fossa mass |
| Gasping | Slow rate, variable tidal volume; consider hypoxia, shock, sepsis, or asphyxia |

or extreme anxiety. Hyperpnea without signs of respiratory distress suggests an extrapulmonary etiology (metabolic acidosis, fever, pain). When the work of breathing is increased, **intercostal, supraclavicular, or substernal retractions** are often observed. In children, increased inspiratory effort is also manifested by **nasal flaring**. **Grunting** (forced expiration against a partially closed glottis) suggests respiratory distress, but it may also be a manifestation of pain.

Causes of increased work of breathing during inspiration include upper airway obstruction (laryngomalacia), subglottic narrowing (croup, stenosis), and decreased pulmonary compliance (pneumonia, pulmonary edema). Increased expiratory work of breathing usually indicates intrathoracic airway obstruction (see Table 133-2).

**Stridor**, usually heard on inspiration, is a harsh sound emanating from the upper airway and caused by a partially obstructed extrathoracic airway. **Wheezing** is produced by partial obstruction of the lower airways and is usually heard more prominently during exhalation but may be present on inspiration. Wheezes can be harsh, monophonic, and low-pitched (usually from large, central airways) or high-pitched and musical (from small peripheral airways). Secretions in the intrathoracic airways may produce wheezing but more commonly result in irregular sounds called **rhonchi**. Fluid or secretions in small airways may produce sounds characteristic of crumpling cellophane (**fine crackles or rales**). Having the child take a deep breath and exhale forcefully will accentuate many abnormal lung sounds. Crackles may disappear after a few deep inspirations or a cough.

Normal breath sounds (**vesicular**) are characterized by long inspiratory and short expiratory phases. **Bronchial** breath sounds have short inspiratory and long expiratory phases and are normally heard over the trachea but suggest pulmonary consolidation or compression of the lung when heard elsewhere. Decreased breath sounds may be due to atelectasis, lobar consolidation (pneumonia), thoracic mass, or a pleural effusion. Observation of respiratory rate, work of breathing, tracheal and cardiac deviation, and chest wall motion, combined with percussion and auscultation help to identify intrathoracic disease (Table 133-3).

**TABLE 133-3  Physical Signs of Pulmonary Disease**

| Disease Process | Mediastinal Deviation | Chest Motion | Vocal Fremitus | Percussion | Breath Sounds | Adventitious Sounds | Voice Signs |
|---|---|---|---|---|---|---|---|
| Consolidation | No | Reduced over area | Increased | Dull | Bronchial or reduced | None or crackles | Egophony* Pectoriloquy† |
| Bronchospasm | No | Hyperexpansion with limited motion | Normal or decreased | Hyperresonant | Normal to decreased | Wheezes, crackles | Normal to decreased |
| Atelectasis | Shift toward affected side | Reduced over area | Decreased | Dull | Reduced | None or crackles | None |
| Pneumothorax | With tension pneumothorax: shift to the opposite side | Reduced over PMI | None | Resonant | None | None | None |
| Pleural effusion | Deviation to opposite side | Reduced over area | None or reduced | Dull | None | Egophony Friction rub | Muffled |
| Interstitial process | No | Reduced | Normal to increased | Normal | Normal | Inspiratory crackles | None |

*In egophony, e sounds like a (may be a sign of consolidation but also is associated with moderate-sized pleural effusions).
†In pectoriloquy, words/voice sounds clearer over the affected site (associated with consolidation and cavitary lesions).
PMI, point of maximum impulse.
Adapted from Andreoli TE, Bennett JC, Carpenter CJ, et al (eds): Cecil Essentials of Medicine, 4th ed. Philadelphia, WB Saunders, 1997, p 115.

**Digital clubbing** is seen in CF and in some patients with other chronic pulmonary diseases. However, it may also be present in nonpulmonary chronic diseases (cyanotic heart disease, endocarditis, celiac disease, inflammatory bowel disease, chronic active hepatitis) or, rarely, as a familial trait.

**Cough** results from stimulation of irritant receptors in the airway mucosa. Acute cough generally is associated with respiratory infections or irritant exposure (smoke) and subsides as the infection resolves or the exposure is eliminated. The characteristics of the cough and the circumstances under which the cough occurs help in determining the cause. Sudden onset after a choking episode suggests foreign body aspiration. Morning cough may be due to the accumulation of excessive secretions during the night from sinusitis, allergic rhinitis, or bronchial infections. Nighttime coughing is a hallmark of asthma and can also be caused by gastroesophageal reflux disease. Cough exacerbated by lying flat may be due to postnasal drip, sinusitis, or allergic rhinitis. Recurrent coughing with exercise is suggestive of exercise-induced asthma/bronchospasm. Paroxysmal cough suggests pertussis or foreign body aspiration. A repetitive, staccato cough occurs in chlamydial infections in infants. A harsh, brassy, *seal-like* cough suggests croup, tracheomalacia, or psychogenic cough. The latter, which is most common in teenagers, disappears during sleep. Younger children can develop a throat-clearing, habit cough, which also disappears during sleep.

**Chronic cough** is defined as a daily cough lasting longer than 3 weeks. Common causes of chronic cough are asthma, postnasal drip syndromes (allergic rhinitis, sinusitis), and postinfectious tussive syndromes. It can also be caused by gastroesophageal reflux disease, swallowing dysfunction (infants), anatomic abnormalities (tracheoesophageal fistula, tracheomalacia), and chronic infection. Persistent cough may also be caused by exposure to irritants (tobacco and wood stove smoke), foreign body aspiration, or may be psychogenic in origin.

During the first several years of life, children experience frequent viral respiratory infections, especially if they attend day care or preschool. Cough that resolves promptly and is clearly associated with a viral infection does not require further diagnostic workup. However, cough persisting longer than 3 weeks warrants further evaluation.

# DIAGNOSTIC MEASURES

## Imaging Techniques

**Chest radiographs** are useful in assessing respiratory disease in children. In addition to determining lung abnormalities, they provide information about the bony thorax (rib or vertebral abnormalities), the heart (cardiomegaly, pericardial effusion), and the great vessels (right aortic arch/vascular rings, rib notching). Chest radiographs should be obtained in both the posteroanterior (PA) and lateral projections. Estimation of lung hyperinflation based on a single PA view is unreliable, whereas flattened diaphragms and an increased AP diameter on a lateral projection indicates hyperinflation. Expiratory views and fluoroscopy may detect partial bronchial obstruction due to an aspirated foreign body resulting in regional hyperinflation because the lung or lobe does not deflate on exhalation. Routine chest radiographs should be obtained after a full inspiration. Crowding of the blood vessels with poor inspiration can be misinterpreted as increased markings or infiltrates. External skin folds, rotation, and motion may produce distorted or unclear images.

A **barium esophagogram** is valuable in diagnosing disorders of swallowing (dysphagia) and esophageal motility, vascular rings (esophageal compression), tracheoesophageal fistulas, and, to a lesser extent, gastroesophageal reflux. When evaluating for a tracheoesophageal fistula, contrast material must be instilled under pressure via a catheter with the distal tip situated in the esophagus (see Chapter 128).

A **computed tomography (CT) scan of the chest** is the imaging test of choice for evaluating pleural masses, bronchiectasis, and mediastinal lesions as well as delineating pleural from parenchymal lesions. CT scans with intravenous contrast material provide excellent information about the pulmonary and great vessel vasculature and pulmonary embolism. High-resolution CT scans are used to assess lung parenchyma (pulmonary fibrosis, interstitial fluid) and the airways (bronchiectasis). The speed of current CT scanners makes it possible to scan most children without sedating them. However, sedation may be required to decrease motion artifact. **Magnetic resonance imaging (MRI)**, useful in visualizing cardiac anatomy, is less useful for evaluation of pulmonary lesions.

**Ultrasonography** can be used to delineate some intrathoracic masses and is the imaging procedure of choice for assessing parapneumonic effusion/empyema. It is useful when assessing diaphragmatic motion.

## Measures of Respiratory Gas Exchange

Measurements of oxygenation ($Po_2$ and $O_2$ saturation) and ventilation ($Pco_2$) are important in the management of pulmonary diseases. A properly performed **arterial blood gas** analysis provides information about the effectiveness of both oxygenation and ventilation. However, arterial samples are more difficult to obtain, so capillary and venous blood samples are more commonly used. The $Pco_2$ from a capillary sample is similar to that from arterial blood. The $Pco_2$ in venous samples is approximately 6 mm Hg higher than arterial $Pco_2$. The ratio of the serum bicarbonate concentration to $Pco_2$ determines the pH. Capillary or venous samples should not be used to assess oxygenation.

There are both respiratory and metabolic causes of acidosis (see Chapter 37). In the presence of an alkalosis or acidosis, respiratory compensation (decreasing $Pco_2$ to maintain a normal pH) can occur within minutes, but renal compensation (increasing the serum bicarbonate level) may not be complete for several days.

**Pulse oximetry** measures the $O_2$ saturation of hemoglobin by measuring the blood absorption of two or more wavelengths of light. It is noninvasive, easy to use, and reliable. Because of the shape of the oxyhemoglobin dissociation curve, $O_2$ saturation does not decrease much until the $Po_2$ reaches approximately 60 mm Hg. Pulse oximetry may not accurately reflect true $O_2$ saturation when abnormal hemoglobin is present (carboxyhemoglobin, methemoglobin), when perfusion is poor, or if no light passes through to the photodetector (nail polish).

The measurement of $P_{CO_2}$ is accomplished most reliably by blood gas analysis. However, there are noninvasive monitors that record end-expiratory $P_{CO_2}$ (**end-tidal $CO_2$**), which is representative of alveolar $P_{CO_2}$. End-tidal $P_{CO_2}$ measurements are most commonly used in intubated and mechanically ventilated patients, but some devices can measure $P_{CO_2}$ at the nares. **Transcutaneous electrodes** can be used to monitor $P_{CO_2}$ and $P_{O_2}$ at the skin surface, but are not particularly accurate. Noninvasive techniques of $CO_2$ measurement are best suited for detecting trends rather than for providing absolute values.

## Pulmonary Function Testing

Measurement of lung volumes and airflow rates using spirometry are important in assessing pulmonary disease. The patient inhales to TLC and then forcibly exhales until no more air can be expelled. This test is often referred to as spirometry. During the forced expiratory maneuver the **VC**, the forced expired volume in the first second (**$FEV_1$**), and **forced expiratory flow (FEF) rates** are measured. The predicted values for lung functions are based on patient age, gender, and race, but rely mostly on height. Most children above 6 years of age can perform spirometry. It is possible to perform these tests in infants using sedation and sophisticated equipment.

Airway resistance, FRC, and RV cannot be measured with spirometry and require other techniques. **Body plethysmography** can be used to measure airway resistance and lung volumes. Helium dilution can measure TLC and RV by determining the magnitude of dilution of inhaled helium in the air within the lung.

Abnormal results on pulmonary function testing can be categorized as indicating **obstructive airway disease** (low flow rates and increased RV or FRC) or a **restrictive defect** (low VC and TLC, with relative preservation of flow rates and FRC). When the $FEV_1$ and flow rates are decreased to a greater extent than the VC, then airway obstruction is likely, but a proportional decrease in VC, $FEV_1$, and flow rates suggests a restrictive lung defect. The mean midexpiratory flow rate (**$FEF_{25-75\%}$**) is a more sensitive measure of small airways disease than the $FEV_1$, but is also more variable. The VC, $FEV_1$, and $FEF_{25-75\%}$ can be obtained with a simple spirometer. Pulmonary function testing can detect reversible airway obstruction characteristic of asthma with a significant improvement in $FEV_1$ (>12%) or in $FEF_{25-75\%}$ (>25%) following inhalation of a bronchodilator. Spirometry is also useful for longitudinal patient management. The **peak expiratory flow rate (PEFR)** can be obtained with a simple handheld device and may be useful for home monitoring of older children with asthma. However, it is highly dependent on patient effort and values must be interpreted with caution. **Inhalation challenge tests** using methacholine, histamine, or cold, dry air are used to assess airway hyperreactivity, but require sophisticated equipment and special expertise and should be performed only in a pulmonary function laboratory with experienced technicians.

## Endoscopic Evaluation of the Airways

Endoscopic evaluation of the upper airways (**nasopharyngoscopy**) is performed with a flexible fiberoptic nasopharyngocope to assess adenoid size, patency of the nasal passages, and abnormalities of the larynx. It is especially useful in evaluating stridor and assessing vocal motion/function. Endoscopic evaluation of the intrathoracic airways can be done with either a flexible or rigid bronchoscope. **Bronchoscopy** is useful in identifying airway abnormalities (stenosis, malacia, endobronchial lesions, excessive secretions) and in obtaining airway samples for culture (bronchoalveolar lavage), especially in immunocompromised patients. Rigid bronchoscopy is the method of choice for removing foreign bodies from the airways and performing other interventions, and flexible bronchoscopy is most useful as a diagnostic tool and for obtaining lower airway cultures. Bronchoscopy requires deep sedation, but flexible nasopharyngoscopy can be performed without anesthesia. There are few absolute contraindications to bronchoscopy. Relative contraindications include bleeding diatheses, thrombocytopenia ($<50,000/cm^3$), and clinical conditions too unstable to tolerate the procedure.

## Examination of Sputum

Sputum specimens may be useful in evaluating lower respiratory tract infections, but they are difficult to obtain in young children. In addition, an expectorated specimen may not provide a representative sample of lower airway secretions. Specimens containing large numbers of squamous epithelial cells are either not from the lower airways or are heavily contaminated with upper airway secretions and may yield misleading results. Sputum in patients with lower respiratory tract bacterial infections often contains polymorphonucleated leukocytes and one predominant organism on culture. If sputum cannot be obtained, then bronchoalveolar lavage specimens (obtained by bronchoscopy) may be used for microbiologic diagnosis in selected situations. In patients with CF who cannot produce sputum, specially processed throat cultures are often used as surrogates for lower airway cultures.

## Lung Biopsy

When less invasive methods fail to provide diagnoses in patients with pulmonary disease, a lung biopsy may be required. Although **transbronchial lung biopsy** through a bronchoscope is useful in adults, it is seldom done in children. Either a **thoracoscopic procedure** or a **thoracotomy** is preferred in children. Thoracotomy allows the surgeon to inspect and palpate the lung, which aids in choosing the best site for biopsy, but it is more invasive than thoracoscopy. In most cases, infants and children tolerate lung biopsy well.

# THERAPEUTIC MEASURES

## Oxygen Administration

Any child in respiratory distress should be treated with **supplemental $O_2$** to maintain normal $O_2$ saturation levels. A nasal cannula is the easiest way to provide supplemental $O_2$, but the oxygen concentration provided is variable and affected by the child's own respiratory pattern. Supplemental $O_2$ may also be delivered by a variety of facemask systems ranging from a simple facemask, which can provide 30 to 40% $O_2$, to a nonrebreather mask with reservoir that can provide nearly 100% $O_2$. For long-term administration of $O_2$, a **nasal cannula** is the most widely used device, as it enables patients to eat and speak unhindered by the $O_2$ delivery system.

The concentration of administered $O_2$ should be high enough to relieve hypoxemia. Inspired $O_2$ concentrations less than 40% are usually safe for long-term use. Patients requiring supplemental $O_2$ should be monitored with pulse oximetry, either intermittently or continuously, or with arterial blood gas measurements of $P_{O_2}$ to allow titration to the lowest possible $O_2$ concentration.

The *acceptable* $O_2$ saturation depends on the patient and clinical situation. Generally, supplemental $O_2$ should be administered to achieve a goal saturation level above 90%. Normal oxygen saturation is greater than 95%. It is unnecessary to achieve 100% saturation, especially if this requires potentially toxic levels of inspired $O_2$ for extended periods of time.

## Aerosol Therapy

Delivering therapeutic agents to the lower respiratory tract can be accomplished by inhalation of aerosol forms of the agents via dry powder inhalers (DPIs), metered dose inhalers (MDIs), or nebulizers. All of these devices are designed to generate relatively small particles that can bypass the filtering action of the upper airway and deposit in the lower airways. Many factors influence drug deposition including patient technique, the device used, age of the child (cooperation, inspiratory flow, and tidal volume), and breathing pattern. Plastic holding chambers (spacers) should be used with MDIs. Dry powder inhalers require a single rapid deep inhalation for optimal drug delivery, which is difficult for children under 6 years of age. MDIs and nebulizers can be used in children of all ages and are equally effective in delivering medications. The drugs most often delivered as aerosols are bronchodilators (albuterol, levalbuterol, ipratropium) and inhaled corticosteroids. Occasionally antibiotics (tobramycin) are delivered by aerosol.

## Chest Physiotherapy and Clearance Techniques

When disease processes impair clearance of pulmonary secretions, airway clearance techniques may help maintain airway patency. One method is **chest percussion**, which moves secretions toward the central airways, from which they can be expectorated. **Chest physiotherapy** can also be performed effectively with the **flutter valve, acapella device,** and **pneumatic vests**. Chest physiotherapy is most beneficial in children with chronic airway secretions, especially those with CF. Children who are too weak to generate an effective cough benefit from the use of a mechanical cough assist device, used in conjunction with chest physiotherapy. Chest physiotherapy is not generally beneficial for patients with asthma or pneumonia, and its effectiveness in patients with atelectasis has not been clearly established.

## Intubation

If the upper airway is obstructed or mechanical ventilation is needed, it may be necessary to provide the patient with an **artificial airway**. This is best done by placing an endotracheal tube via the mouth or nose into the trachea (**intubation**). Intubation alters the physiology of the respiratory tract in many ways, not all of which are beneficial. It interferes with the humidification, warming, and filtration of inspired air and prevents phonation. Intubation also stimulates secretion production. However, intubation with an endotracheal tube can be lifesaving.

**Endotracheal tubes** can damage the larynx and the airways if the tubes are of improper size and are not carefully maintained. The cricoid ring is the narrowest segment of a child's airway and is completely surrounded by cartilage, which makes it vulnerable to damage, leading to subglottic stenosis. If the pressure created by the tube against the airway mucosa exceeds capillary filling pressure (roughly 35 cm $H_2O$), mucosal ischemia develops, leading to necrosis. Therefore, a small air leak should be maintained around the endotracheal tube to minimize the risk of mucosal damage.

Artificial airways must be kept clear of secretions as mucous plugs in artificial airways can be fatal. Providing adequate humidification of inspired air and appropriate suctioning of the tube reduce the probability of occlusion by secretions. In addition to endotracheal tubes, the laryngeal mask can provide an artificial airway. This device consists of a tube with a soft mask at the distal end. The mask is placed over the larynx, creating a seal and allowing mechanical ventilation without the trachea being instrumented.

## Tracheostomy

Tracheostomy is the surgical placement of an artificial airway into the trachea below the larynx. If prolonged intubation is anticipated, elective tracheostomy may be used to prevent laryngeal trauma, obviate the danger of accidental extubation, increase patient comfort, and facilitate nursing care. No clear guidelines are available as to how long patients can be intubated without sustaining airway damage or when a tracheostomy is indicated.

Children with severe chronic upper airway obstruction or those requiring long-term mechanical ventilation may benefit from tracheostomies. Because the tracheostomy tube hampers the ability to phonate and communicate, the child must be monitored carefully at all times. As with endotracheal tubes, tracheostomy tubes must be kept clear. Occlusion of the tube with secretions or accidental dislodgment of the tube can be fatal. Many children with tracheostomy tubes can be cared for at home provided the caregivers are well trained and adequately equipped.

## Mechanical Ventilation

Patients who are unable to maintain adequate gas exchange may require mechanical ventilation. Most modes of mechanical ventilation involve inflation of the lungs with gas using positive-pressure ventilators. The inspiratory phase is active (air is pushed in) and exhalation is passive.

**Positive-pressure ventilation** often requires endotracheal intubation or tracheostomy, though it can be provided *noninvasively* via nasal or full facemasks. **Noninvasive ventilation** is particularly useful in patients with neuromuscular disease, but it can also be used to assist ventilation in patients in acute respiratory failure from a variety of causes.

No method of mechanical ventilation truly simulates natural breathing. All methods have their drawbacks and complications. Positive pressure is transmitted to the entire thorax and may impede venous return to the heart during inspiration. The airways and lung parenchyma may be damaged by inflation pressures and high concentrations of inspired $O_2$. In general, inflation pressures should be limited to those necessary to provide sufficient lung expansion for adequate ventilation and the prevention of atelectasis. Pressure-cycled and volume-cycled ventilators (conventional ventilation) are the most widely used modalities in pediatrics, but high-frequency jet ventilation and high-frequency oscillation ventilators may be used in patients with severe lung disease who are failing conventional mechanical ventilation.

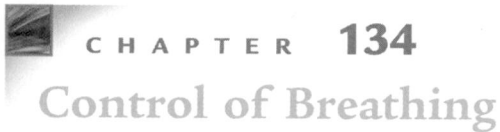

CHAPTER **134**

# Control of Breathing

## CONTROL OF VENTILATION

Ventilation is controlled primarily by **central chemoreceptors** located in the medulla that respond to intracellular pH and $P_{CO_2}$ levels (Fig. 134-1). To a lesser extent, ventilation is modulated by **peripheral receptors** located in the carotid and aortic bodies, which respond predominantly to $P_{O_2}$. The central receptors are quite sensitive.

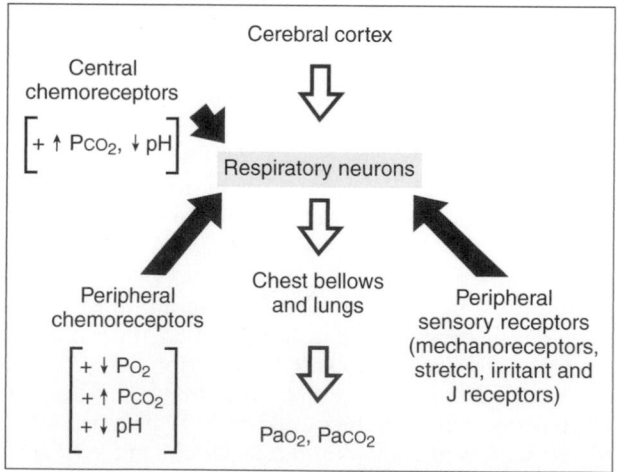

**FIGURE 134-1**

**Schematic representation of the respiratory control system.** The respiratory neurons in the brainstem receive information from the chemoreceptors, peripheral sensory receptors, and cerebral cortex. This information is integrated, and the resulting neural output is transmitted to the diaphragms and lungs. The "+" sign denotes stimulation of the receptor. (From Andreoli TE, Bennett JC, Carpenter CJ, et al [eds]: Cecil Essentials of Medicine, 4th ed. Philadelphia, *WB Saunders,* 1997, p 171.)

Small changes in $Pa_{CO_2}$ normally result in significant changes in **minute ventilation**. When the $P_{CO_2}$ is chronically elevated, the intracellular pH returns to normal levels because of compensatory increases in the bicarbonate level, and the ventilatory drive is not increased. The peripheral receptors do not stimulate ventilation until the $Pa_{O_2}$ decreases to approximately 60 mm Hg. These receptors become important in patients with chronic $Pa_{CO_2}$ elevation who may have a blunted ventilatory response to $CO_2$.

The output of the central respiratory center also is modulated by reflex mechanisms. Full lung inflation inhibits inspiratory effort (**Hering-Breuer reflex**) through vagal afferent fibers. Other reflexes from the airways and intercostal muscles may influence the depth and frequency of respiratory efforts (see Fig. 134-1).

## DISORDERS OF CONTROL OF BREATHING

### Acute Life-Threatening Events

#### Etiology

An acute life-threatening event (ALTE) is defined as any unexpected and frightening change in condition characterized by apnea, color change (usually blue or pale), sudden limpness, or choking or gagging. The incidence of such events is 0.05% to 1%. Specific causes can be identified in more than 50% of the cases. Gastroesophageal reflux and laryngospasm are the most common causes of ALTE, and they are associated with emesis, choking, or gagging. Central nervous system (CNS) causes (e.g., seizures, breath-holding spells, intracranial bleeding from accidental or nonaccidental trauma) account for approximately 15% of cases, and cardiovascular events and metabolic derangements account for smaller percentages.

#### Diagnostic Studies

The history obtained for infants with an ALTE should include questions concerning premature birth, prior apnea, level of consciousness at the time of the event, intercurrent illnesses, limpness or stiff/jerking (seizure), feeding history, any trauma, and the social situation of the family. The physical examination should focus on bruising and injury, the general and neurologic condition of the infant, nutritional status, respiratory pattern, and cardiac status. The laboratory evaluation should include serum electrolytes, serum glucose, blood urea nitrogen (BUN) and creatinine, hemoglobin, hematocrit, white blood cell (WBC) count, a chest radiograph, and blood gas analysis. Consider testing for respiratory syncytial virus (RSV)and pertussis in patients with evidence of respiratory infection. If gastroesophageal reflux is suspected, a barium swallow or pH probe study may be useful. Cardiorespiratory monitoring for 12 to 24 hours in the hospital can provide information on respiratory and cardiac patterns and feeding difficulties (choking, gagging, emesis); provide time to get more history and assess the home situation; and alleviate parental anxiety. Useful tests to determine CNS causes include a head computed tomography (CT) scan, magnetic resonance imaging (MRI) of the brain, and an electroencephalogram (for seizures).

## Treatment and Prevention

There are no standard recommendations for when home monitoring should be prescribed. Polysomnography is not useful in predicting which children with ALTE are likely to progress to sudden infant death syndrome (SIDS). The key to prevention of future events is to identify the underlying cause and treat it. Teaching the parents infant cardiopulmonary resuscitation (CPR) and attempting to alleviate anxiety surrounding the event are recommended.

## Sudden Infant Death Syndrome

### Etiology and Epidemiology

SIDS is defined as the **unexpected death** of an infant younger than 1 year of age in which the cause remains unexplained after an autopsy, death scene investigation, and review of clinical history. The risk of SIDS is higher in premature and low-birth-weight infants, infants of young impoverished mothers who smoke cigarettes, African-American and Native American infants, and in infants whose mothers have abused drugs. The risk of SIDS is increased three- to fivefold in siblings of infants who have died of SIDS and is highest during the winter. SIDS is rare before 4 weeks or after 6 months of age and is most common between 2 and 4 months of age. The incidence of SIDS has decreased dramatically since the 1980s.

A variety of mechanisms have been proposed to explain SIDS, although none have been proved. SIDS is associated with the prone position during sleep, especially on soft bedding. The widely advocated supine sleeping position (**back-to-sleep**) explains, in part, the decreased incidence of SIDS during the past two decades. Current theories for a predisposition to SIDS include cellular brainstem abnormalities and maturational delay related to neural or cardiorespiratory control. A portion of SIDS deaths may be due to prolongation of the Q-T interval, abnormal CNS control of respiration, and $CO_2$ rebreathing from sleeping face down (especially in soft bedding).

### Differential Diagnosis

See Table 134-1 for the differential diagnosis of SIDS.

### Prevention

There has been a significant decline in SIDS with the back-to-sleep program and avoiding soft bedding. Thus, all parents should be instructed to place their infants in the supine position unless there are medical contraindications. All soft bedding should be avoided, and parents who share beds with their infants should be counseled on the risks. Decreasing maternal cigarette smoking, both during and after pregnancy, is recommended.

## Apnea

### Etiology

Apnea is defined as the cessation of airflow, which can be due to either lack of respiratory effort (**central apnea**) or upper airway obstruction (**obstructive apnea**). Central

**TABLE 134-1 Differential Diagnosis of Sudden Infant Death Syndrome**

Fulminant infection*†
Infant botulism‡
Seizure disorder†
Brain tumor*
Hypoglycemia††
Medium-chain acyl-coenzyme A dehydrogenase deficiency‡
Carnitine deficiency*‡
Urea cycle defect‡
Child abuse*†
Accidental suffocation†
Hemosiderosis/pulmonary hemorrhage syndrome
Exposure to toxic environmental fungus
Drug intoxication‡
Cardiac arrhythmia
Gastroesophageal reflux*†
Midgut volvulus/shock*
Laryngospasm

*Obvious or suspected at autopsy.
†Relatively common.
‡Diagnostic test required.

apnea lasting less than 10 seconds is common in healthy infants and can be present in normal children during sleep, especially after a sigh breath. Central pauses lasting longer than 15 to 20 seconds are considered abnormal. Central apnea is more common in infants, and obstructive apnea, especially during sleep (**obstructive sleep apnea**) is more common in older children.

Premature infants can have **apnea of prematurity**, which consists of recurrent apneic episodes that are often of central origin, though they can be mixed central/obstructive. Apnea of prematurity should resolve by 44 weeks postconceptional age. Older infants and children with apnea warrant thorough investigation (Table 134-2).

**Obstructive sleep apnea syndrome (OSA),** which affects 2% to 3% of young children, is caused by complete or partial upper airway obstruction during sleep. It presents as episodes of respiratory pauses, gasping, and restless sleep that can result in hypoxia and hypercarbia. As a result of poor sleep quality, children may have difficulty awakening in the morning, daytime somnolence, behavioral changes, failure to thrive, and poor school performance. The nighttime hypoxia or hypercarbia can lead to morning headaches and, in severe cases, to pulmonary hypertension and cor pulmonale. Adenotonsillar hypertrophy is the most common cause of OSA in young children, but other risk factors for OSA include obesity, craniofacial malformations, glossoptosis, and neuromuscular diseases. Not all children who snore have OSA, and many young children with OSA do not have the classic findings of daytime somnolence and gasping respirations. Thus, when the diagnosis is in question, it should be confirmed with a polysomnogram.

Treatment of OSA starts with determining whether the child will benefit from an adenoidectomy, with or without

**TABLE 134-2  Categories of Apnea**

| Disease | Example | Mechanism | Signs | Treatment |
|---|---|---|---|---|
| Apnea of prematurity | Premature (<36 wk) | Central control, upper airway obstruction | Apnea, bradycardia | Theophylline, caffeine, nasal CPAP, intubation |
| Disorders of respiratory control | Congenital central hypoventilation syndrome (CCHS) | Abnormal central control | Apnea | Mechanical ventilation |
| Obesity hypoventilation | Morbid obesity, Prader-Willi syndrome | Airway obstruction, blunted central control | Somnolence, cor pulmonale | Theophylline, weight loss |
| Obstructive sleep apnea | Adenotonsillar hypertrophy, Pierre Robin syndrome, Down syndrome | Airway obstruction by enlarged tonsils or adenoids, large tongue, micrognathia, mid-face hypoplasia | Daytime sleepiness, snoring, restless sleep, enuresis, poor school performance, behavior problems, mouth breathing | Tonsillectomy, adenoidectomy, nasal trumpets, CPAP, uvuloveloplasty |
| Cyanotic breath-holding spells | Breath holder <3 yr old | Prolonged expiratory apnea; cerebral anoxia | Cyanosis, syncope, brief tonic-clonic movements | Reassurance that the condition is self-limiting; must exclude seizure disorder |
| Pallid breath-holding spells | Breath holder | Asystole; reflex anoxic seizures | Rapid onset, with or without crying; pallor; bradycardia; seizures | Must exclude seizure disorder |
| SIDS | Previously normal infant; increased incidence with prematurity, SIDS in sibling, maternal drug abuse, cigarette smoking, males; may have preceding minor URI | Central respiratory control; cardiac arrhythmia unknown; proposed: suffocation; central cardiac control problems(?) Overheating Chemoreceptor dysfunction Child abuse | 2- to 4-mo-old child found cyanotic, apneic, and pulseless in bed | No treatment Prevention with home apnea monitoring is unproved Supine sleep position (back to sleep) reduces risk |

(?), unproven contributing factor; CPAP, continuous positive airway pressure (by facial mask or nasal prongs); SIDS, sudden infant death syndrome; URI, upper respiratory infection.

Data from Southall D: Role of apnea in the sudden infant death syndrome. *Pediatrics* 81:73, 1988; Mark J, Brooks J: Sleep-associated airway problems in children. *Pediatr Clin North Am* 31:907, 1984; and Gordon N: Breath-holding spells. *Dev Med Child Neurol* 29:811, 1987.

a tonsillectomy. If surgical intervention is not indicated or fails to alleviate the problem, then the use of continuous positive airway pressure (CPAP) or bi-level positive airway pressure (BiPAP) via nasal interfaces can be used to distend the upper airway during sleep. This requires a tight-fitting nasal mask, which may not be well tolerated in children less than 2 years of age.

Congenital central alveolar hypoventilation (**CCHS**) is a rare disorder in which there is profound loss of respiratory control during sleep leading to central apnea, hypercarbia, and hypoxemia. Most patients with CCHS have a defect in the **PHOX2B** gene, which is necessary for autonomic nervous system development. Most infants with CCHS have respiratory difficulties within the first several weeks of life, although CCHS can also present later in childhood. CCHS is associated with an increased risk of Hirschsprung disease and neural crest tumors. Secondary causes of central hypoventilation include medications impairing central respiratory drive (narcotics), Arnold-Chiari malformation (meningomyelocele), dysautonomia, increased intracranial pressure, CNS tumors, and mitochondrial/metabolic disorders.

# CHAPTER 135

# Upper Airway Obstruction

## ETIOLOGY

Upper airway obstruction, which is defined as blockage of any part of the airway located above the thoracic inlet, can range from nasal obstruction due to the common cold to life-threatening obstruction of the larynx or upper trachea (subglottic space). In children, nasal obstruction is usually more of a nuisance than a danger because the mouth can serve as an airway, but it may be a serious problem for neonates, who breathe predominantly through their noses. The differential diagnosis of airway obstruction varies with patient age and can also be subdivided into **supraglottic** and **subglottic** causes (Tables 135-1, 135-2, and 135-3).

## CLINICAL MANIFESTATIONS

Upper airway obstruction is more pronounced during inspiration because the negative pressure generated tends to collapse the upper airway, which increases resistance to airflow and leads to inspiratory noise. The respiratory noise most commonly associated with upper airway obstruction is **stridor**, a harsh sound caused by the vibration of the airway structures. Occasionally stridor may also be present on exhalation. **Laryngomalacia** (floppy larynx) is the most common cause of inspiratory stridor in infants and may be aggravated by swallowing problems and gastroesophageal reflux. Hoarseness suggests **vocal cord** involvement. Stridor often decreases during sleep due to lower inspiratory flow rates and less negative pressure and airway wall vibration. Children with upper airway obstruction may have increased inspiratory work of breathing manifested by **suprasternal retractions**.

## DIAGNOSTIC STUDIES

**Radiographic evaluation** of a child with stridor may not be helpful. However, lateral views of the neck and nasopharynx can assess for adenoid hypertrophy. On anteroposterior (AP) views of the neck taken with the head in extension, the subglottic space should be symmetrical and the lateral walls of the airway should fall away steeply. Asymmetry suggests subglottic stenosis or a mass lesion, while tapering suggests subglottic edema. However, these findings may be subtle. Computed tomography (CT) scans of the upper airway can help delineate the site of the obstruction but may require sedation in younger children. Flexible nasopharyngoscopy, which can be done without sedation, is extremely useful in assessing airway patency, the presence of adenoid tissue, vocal cord and other airway lesions, and laryngomalacia. Bronchoscopy can be useful in assessing the subglottic space and intrathoracic large airways, but this procedure requires deep sedation.

| TABLE 135-1 Age-Related Differential Diagnosis of Upper Airway Obstruction |
| --- |
| **NEWBORN** |
| Congenital subglottic stenosis (uncommon) |
| Choanal atresia |
| Micrognathia (Pierre Robin syndrome, Treacher Collins syndrome, DiGeorge syndrome) |
| Macroglossia (Beckwith-Wiedemann syndrome, hypothyroidism, Pompe disease, trisomy 21, hemangioma) |
| Laryngeal web, clefts, atresia |
| Laryngospasm (intubation, aspiration, transient) |
| Vocal cord paralysis/paresis (weak cry; unilateral or bilateral, with or without increased intracranial pressure from Arnold Chiari malformation or other central nervous system pathology) |
| Pharyngeal collapse |
| Dislocated nasal cartilage |
| Nasal piriform aperture stenosis |
| Nasal encephalocele |
| **INFANCY** |
| Laryngomalacia (most common etiologic disorder) |
| Subglottic stenosis (congenital, acquired, e.g., after intubation) |
| Airway hemangioma |
| Tongue (macroglossia, tumor (dermoid, teratoma, ectopic thyroid) |
| Laryngeal dyskinesia |
| Laryngeal papillomatosis |
| Vascular rings/slings |
| Rhinitis |
| **TODDLERS** |
| Viral croup (most common etiology in children 6 mo to 4 yr of age) |
| Spasmodic/recurrent croup |
| Bacterial tracheitis (toxic, high fever) |
| Foreign body (airway or esophageal) |
| Laryngeal papillomatosis |
| Retropharyngeal abscess |
| Hypertrophied tonsils and adenoids |
| **OLDER CHILDREN** |
| Epiglottitis (infection, uncommon) |
| Inhalation injury (burns, toxic gas, hydrocarbons) |
| Foreign bodies |
| Angioedema (familial history, cutaneous angioedema) |
| Anaphylaxis (allergic history, wheezing, hypotension) |
| Trauma (tracheal or laryngeal fracture) |
| Peritonsillar abscess (adolescents) |
| Mononucleosis |
| Ludwig angina |

## DIFFERENTIAL DIAGNOSIS

### Adenoidal and Tonsillar Hypertrophy

#### Etiology

The most common cause of chronic upper airway obstruction in children is hypertrophy of the adenoids and tonsils. The adenoids are lymphoid tissue arising from the posterior

TABLE 135-2 Differential Diagnosis of Acute Upper Airway Obstruction

| Clinical/Historical Feature | Laryngotracheobronchitis (Croup) | Laryngitis | Spasmodic Croup | Epiglottitis | Membranous Croup (Bacterial Tracheitis) |
|---|---|---|---|---|---|
| Age | 6 mo–3 yr | 5 yr–teens | 3 mo–3 yr | 2–6 yr | Any age (3–10 yr) |
| Location | Subglottic | Subglottic | Subglottic | Supraglottic | Trachea |
| Etiologic agent(s) | Parainfluenza virus, influenza virus, RSV, rarely Mycoplasma, measles, adenovirus | As per croup | Noninfectious | Haemophilus influenzae type b inflammation | Respiratory virus with secondary bacterial infection (Staphylococcus aureus, Moraxella catarrhalis) |
| Prodrome/onset | Fever, URI | URI, sore throat at night | Sudden onset, short prodrome, prior episodes | Rapid onset; High fever | High fever with rapid deterioration |
| Stridor | Yes | None | Yes | Rarely | Yes |
| Retractions | Yes | None | Yes | Yes | Yes |
| Voice | Hoarse | Hoarse | Hoarse | Muffled | Normal or hoarse |
| Body positioning | Normal | Normal | Normal | Tripod sitting; leaning forward | Normal |
| Appearance | Normal to anxious | Normal | Anxious | Agitated; toxic | Anxious; toxic |
| Swallowing | Normal | Normal | Normal | Drooling | Normal |
| Barking cough | Yes | Rare | Yes | No | Sometimes |
| Toxicity | Rare | No | No | Severe | Severe |
| Fever | Body temperature usually <38.5°C | Body temperature usually <38.5°C | None | Body temperature usually >39°C | Body temperature usually >39°C |
| Radiographic appearance | Subglottic narrowing; steeple sign | Normal | Subglottic narrowing of the epiglottis | Thumb sign of thickened epiglottis | Ragged irregular tracheal border; steeple sign |
| WBC count | Normal | Normal | Normal | Leukocytosis with elevated band count | Leukocytosis with elevated % bands |
| Therapy | Racemic epinephrine aerosol, systemic steroids, aerosolized steroids, cold mist | None | Same as for viral croup | Endotracheal intubation; antibiotics | Antibiotics; intubation if needed |
| Prevention | None | None | None | H. influenzae type b conjugated vaccine | None |

| Clinical/Historical Feature | Retropharyngeal Abscess | Foreign Body | Angioedema | Peritonsillar Abscess | Laryngeal Papillomatosis |
|---|---|---|---|---|---|
| Age | <6 yr | 6 mo–5 yr | All ages | >10 yr | 3 mo–3 yr |
| Location | Posterior pharynx | Supra- or subglottic, variable | Variable | Oropharynx | Larynx, vocal cords, trachea |
| Etiology | *Streptoccus aureus* anaerobes | Small objects, vegetables, toys, coins | C1-esterase deficiency; anaphylaxis | Group A streptococci anaerobes | HPV |
| Prodrome/onset | Insidious or sudden | Sudden | Sudden | Biphasic with sudden worsening | Chronic |
| Stridor | None | Yes | Yes | No | Possible |
| Retractions | Yes | Yes—variable | Yes | No | No |
| Voice | Muffled | Complete obstruction—aphonic | Hoarse, may be normal | *Hot potato*, muffled | Hoarse |
| Body positioning | Arching of neck or normal | Normal | Normal; may have facial edema, anxiety | Normal | Normal |
| Appearance | Drooling | Variable, usually normal | Normal | Drooling, trismus | Normal |
| Cough | None | Variable; brassy if tracheal | Possible | None | Variable |
| Toxicity | Moderate-severe | None, but dyspneic | None, unless anaphylactic shock or severe anoxia is present | Dyspnea | None |
| Fever | Body temperature usually >38.5°C | None | None | Body temperature usually >38.5°C | None |
| Radiographic appearance | Thickened retropharyngeal space | Radiopaque object may be seen | Same as for viral croup | None needed | May be normal |
| WBC count | Leukocytosis with increased band count | Normal | Normal | Leukocytosis with increased % bands | Normal |
| Therapy | Antibiotics; surgical drainage of abscess | Endoscopic removal | Anaphylaxis: epinephrine, IV fluids, steroids; C1-esterase deficiency: danazol, C1 esterase infusion | Antibiotics; aspiration | Laser therapy, repeated excision, interferon |
| Prevention | None | Avoid small objects; supervision | Avoid allergens; FFP for congenital angioedema | Treat group A streptococcal infections promptly | Treat maternal genitourinary lesions; possible cesarean section? |

RSV, respiratory syncytial virus; URI, upper respiratory tract infection, coryza, sneezing; WBC, white blood cell. FFP, fresh frozen plasma; HPV, human papillomavirus; RSV, respiratory syncytial virus; URI, upper respiratory tract infection (with coryza, sneezing); WBC, white blood cell.
Modified from Arnold JE: Airway obstruction in children. In Kliegman RM, Nieder ML, Super DM (eds): Practical Strategies in Pediatric Diagnosis and Therapy. Philadelphia, *WB Saunders*, 1996, p 126. Modified from Arnold JE: Airway obstruction in children. In Kliegman RM, Nieder ML, Super DM (eds): Practical Strategies in Pediatric Diagnosis and Therapy. Philadelphia, *WB Saunders*, 1996, p 126.

**TABLE 135-3  Differentiating Supraglottic from Subglottic Causes of Airway Obstruction**

| Feature | Supraglottic Obstruction | Subglottic Obstruction |
| --- | --- | --- |
| Common clinical syndromes | Epiglottitis, peritonsillar and retropharyngeal abscess | Croup, angioedema, foreign body, tracheitis |
| Stridor | Quiet | Loud |
| Voice | Muffled | Hoarse |
| Dysphagia | Yes | No |
| Sitting-up or arching posture | Yes | No |
| Barking cough | No | Yes |
| Fever | High (temperature >39°C) | Low grade (temperature 38°-39°C) |
| Toxic | Yes | No, unless tracheitis is present |
| Trismus | Yes | No |
| Drooling | Yes | No |
| Facial edema | No | No, unless angioedema is present |

Adapted from Davis H, Gartner JC, Galvis AG, et al: Acute upper airway obstruction: Croup and epiglottitis. *Pediatr Clin North Am* 28:859–880, 1981.

and superior walls of the nasopharynx in the region of the choanae. Adenoid and tonsillar hyperplasia may be aggravated by recurrent infection, allergy, and inhaled irritants.

## Clinical Manifestations

The signs of adenoidal and tonsillar hypertrophy are mouth breathing, snoring, and, in some patients, obstructive sleep apnea (see Chapter 134). The eustachian tubes enter the nasopharynx at the choanae and can be obstructed by enlarged adenoids, predisposing to recurrent or persistent otitis media.

## Diagnostic Studies

Adenoidal hypertrophy is assessed by a lateral radiograph of the nasopharynx or by flexible nasopharyngoscopy.

## Treatment

If the adenoids or tonsils are large and thought to be significantly contributing to upper airway obstruction, then the most effective treatment is removal. Because the adenoids are not a discrete organ but rather consist of lymphoid tissue, regrowth after adenoidectomy is possible. Tonsils may enlarge to the point of producing airway obstruction, but often an adenoidectomy alone will suffice. However, if the tonsils are large and the obstruction is severe, then removing the tonsils in addition to the adenoids may be necessary.

## Choanal Stenosis (Atresia)

Choanal stenosis/atresia is a congenital problem that presents in the neonatal period. It may be bilateral or unilateral and is a relatively rare cause of respiratory distress in newborns. Neonates are generally obligate nose breathers, so obstruction of nasal passages can cause significant respiratory distress. Crying bypasses the obstruction because crying infants breathe though their mouths. Inability to easily pass a small catheter through the

nostrils should raise the suspicion of choanal atresia. The diagnosis is confirmed by CT scan and by inspecting the area directly with a flexible nasopharyngoscope. An oral airway may be useful in the short term, but the definitive treatment is surgery (see Chapter 61).

## Croup (Laryngotracheobronchitis)

See Chapter 107.

## Epiglottitis

See Chapter 107.

## Bacterial Tracheitis

See Chapter 107.

## Laryngomalacia (Floppy Larynx)

### Etiology

**Laryngomalacia** is due to exaggerated collapse of the glottic structures, especially the epiglottis and arytenoid cartilages, during inspiration, but its precise cause is not known. It may be due to decreased muscular tone of the larynx and surrounding structures or to immature cartilaginous structures. Inspiratory stridor beginning at or shortly after birth should raise the suspicion of laryngomalacia (see Table 135-1). This is a relatively common condition and is the most common cause of stridor in infants. It usually does not result in much respiratory distress, but occasionally it is severe enough to cause hypoventilation ($CO_2$ retention), hypoxemia, and difficulty with feeding.

### Clinical Manifestations

The primary sign of laryngomalacia is **inspiratory stridor** with little to no expiratory component. The stridor is typically loudest when the infant is feeding or active and decreases when the infant is relaxed, supine, or the neck is flexed. Any condition that increases upper airway inflammation will exacerbate laryngomalacia, including viral respiratory infections, dysphagia (swallowing dysfunction), and gastroesophageal reflux. Laryngomalacia normally peaks by 3 to 5 months of age and resolves between 6 and 12 months of age. However, occasionally it can persist in otherwise normal children up until 24 months of age and even longer in children with underlying conditions, especially neurologic diseases affecting control of upper airway muscles.

## Diagnostic Studies

In many infants with presumed laryngomalacia, the diagnosis can be tentatively established by history and physical examination. If the patient follows the typical course for laryngomalacia, then no further work-up is necessary. However, to firmly establish the diagnosis, which is important in more severe or atypical cases, the patient should undergo flexible nasopharyngoscopy/laryngoscopy to assess the patency and dynamic movement (collapse) of the larynx and surrounding structures. It can also identify vocal cord abnormalities and airway lesions.

## Treatment

In most cases, no therapy is required for laryngomalacia. The infant should be observed closely during times of respiratory infection for evidence of respiratory compromise, although most infants with laryngomalacia tolerate infections fairly well. Infants with severe laryngomalacia that results in hypoventilation, hypoxia, or growth failure may benefit from a surgical procedure (aryoepiglottoplasty) or, in extreme cases, a tracheostomy to bypass the upper airway.

## Subglottic Stenosis

### Etiology

**Subglottic stenosis** is the narrowing of the portion of the trachea immediately below the vocal cords. It may be congenital but more often is acquired. Endotracheal intubation, especially prolonged or repeated intubation required in some premature infants, can lead to inflammation and scarring of the subglottic space.

### Clinical Manifestations

Subglottic stenosis can present as stridor that is frequently biphasic (on both expiration and inspiration). However, the stridor is usually more prominent on inspiration. With increasing respiratory effort, the stridor becomes louder. Subglottic stenosis may also be associated with a barky cough similar to that noted with croup. Respiratory infections can cause subglottic edema, exacerbating the clinical manifestations of subglottic stenosis.

### Diagnostic Studies

Definitive diagnosis requires endoscopic evaluation, either by flexible or rigid bronchoscopy.

## Treatment

Mild subglottic stenosis can be managed conservatively and may improve sufficiently with airway growth alone. More severe cases require surgical intervention. Depending on the nature of the lesion, endoscopic laser treatment may be effective. Other surgical options include tracheoplasty and cricoid split procedures. A tracheostomy tube may be required to bypass the subglottic space until the airway is patent enough to allow adequate airflow.

## Mass Lesions

Upper airway mass lesions are relatively uncommon. The most common laryngeal tumor in childhood is the **hemangioma,** which usually presents before 6 months of age. Infants with stridor, especially if it is biphasic, should be examined carefully for cutaneous hemangiomas in a beardlike distribution about the face, which occurs in 50% of children with laryngeal hemangiomas. Subglottic lesions produce asymmetrical narrowing of the subglottic space on AP radiographs of the larynx, but definitive diagnosis requires endoscopy. The treatment of hemangiomas is controversial, but **laser therapy** and **corticosteroids** (both direct injection and systemic) have been used with moderate success. If the obstruction is severe, then a tracheostomy tube may be needed until the lesion spontaneously involutes or improves with therapy. As with cutaneous hemangiomas, spontaneous regression occurs but may take up to several years.

**Juvenile laryngeal papillomatosis** is a condition of benign tumors caused by human papillomavirus (HPV-6 and HPV-11) acquired at birth from maternal genital warts. Clinical manifestations usually start in infancy and include biphasic stridor and hoarse voice/cry. The lesions are most commonly located in the larynx, but can spread distally into the trachea, large bronchi, and even to the lung parenchyma. Treatment options, which are limited and rarely curative, include laser therapy and interferon. Tracheostomy may be required to ensure an adequate airway, but it should be avoided when possible because it predisposes to seeding of the distal airways with tumor.

## Vocal Cord Paralysis

### Etiology

Vocal cord paralysis is an important cause of laryngeal dysfunction. Paralysis may be unilateral or bilateral and is more often caused by damage to the recurrent laryngeal nerve than by a central lesion. The left recurrent laryngeal nerve passes around the aortic arch and is more susceptible to damage than the right laryngeal nerve. Peripheral nerve injury can be caused by trauma (neck traction during delivery of infants or thoracic surgical procedures), and mediastinal lesions. Central causes include Arnold-Chiari malformation (meningomyelocele), hydrocephalus, and intracranial hemorrhage.

### Clinical Manifestations

Vocal cord paralysis presents as biphasic stridor and alterations in voice and cry, including a weak cry (in infants), hoarseness, and aphonia. Unilateral paralysis may be relatively asymptomatic, although often the voice is affected. The airway protective role of the vocal cords during swallowing puts children with vocal cord paralysis at risk for aspiration, often manifested as coughing/choking with drinking and coarse airway sounds.

## Treatment and Prognosis

Patients with traumatic injury to the recurrent laryngeal nerve often have spontaneous improvement over time, usually within 3 to 6 months. If the paralyzed vocal cord has not recovered within 1 year of the injury, then it is likely permanently damaged. In some cases, Gelfoam injection of a paralyzed vocal cord can reposition the cord to improve phonation and airway protection. Patients with vocal cord paralysis resulting in severe airway obstruction and aspiration may require tracheostomy tube placement.

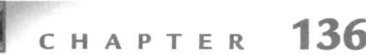

CHAPTER 136

# Lower Airway, Parenchymal, and Pulmonary Vascular Diseases

## ETIOLOGY

There are many causes of lower airway diseases ranging from acute and chronic infections, inflammatory processes (asthma, aspiration), lesions within the lumen (endobronchial), and those that extrinsically compress the airways (Table 136-1). Lower airway diseases often result in airway obstruction. The most common lower airway disease is **asthma**, which results in diffuse bronchial obstruction from airway inflammation, constriction of bronchial smooth muscle, and excessive secretions. Viral-induced wheezing episodes are common, especially in children under 3 years of age. These episodes often respond to asthma therapy, and two thirds of toddlers will outgrow their wheezing episodes by 3 years of age. The other third will go on to have asthma symptoms as older children. Wheezing that begins in the first weeks or months of life or that persists despite aggressive asthma therapy is likely not due to asthma, and further diagnostic evaluation may be warranted. Wheezing that is localized to one area of the chest suggests focal airway narrowing (foreign body aspiration or extrinsic compression by masses or lymph nodes).

## CLINICAL MANIFESTATIONS

In contrast to upper airway obstruction, obstruction below the thoracic inlet causes more wheezing on **expiration** than on inspiration. A **wheeze** is a continuous sound that is produced by vibration of airway walls and generally has a more musical quality than does stridor. Intrathoracic

| TABLE 136-1 Causes of Wheezing in Childhood |
|---|
| **ACUTE** |
| Reactive airway disease |
|   Asthma |
|   Exercise-induced asthma |
|   Hypersensitivity reactions |
| Bronchial edema |
|   Infection (e.g., bronchiolitis) |
|   Inhalation of irritant gases or particulates |
|   Increased pulmonary venous pressure |
| Bronchial hypersecretion |
|   Infection |
|   Inhalation of irritant gases or particulates |
|   Cholinergic drugs |
| Aspiration |
|   Foreign body |
|   Aspiration of gastric contents |
| **CHRONIC OR RECURRENT** |
| Reactive airway disease (see under Acute) |
| Hypersensitivity reactions, allergic bronchopulmonary aspergillosis (seen only in children with either asthma or cystic fibrosis) |
| Dynamic airway collapse |
|   Bronchomalacia/tracheomalacia |
|   Vocal cord adduction (paradoxical vocal cord motion) |
| Airway compression by mass or blood vessel |
|   Vascular ring/sling |
|   Anomalous innominate artery |
|   Pulmonary artery dilatation (absent pulmonary valve) |
|   Bronchial or pulmonary cysts |
|   Lymph nodes (tuberculosis, lymphoma) |
| Aspiration |
|   Foreign body |
|   Gastroesophageal reflux |
|   Swallowing dysfunction (dysphagia) |
|   Tracheoesophageal fistula |
| Bronchial hypersecretion or failure to clear secretions |
|   Bronchitis, bronchiectasis |
|   Cystic fibrosis |
|   Primary ciliary dyskinesia |
| Intrinsic airway lesions |
|   Endobronchial tumors (carcinoid) |
|   Endobronchial granulation tissue |
| Endobronchial tuberculosis |
|   Bronchial or tracheal stenosis |
|   Bronchiolitis obliterans |
| Congestive heart failure |

pressure is increased relative to atmospheric pressure during exhalation, which tends to collapse the intrathoracic airways and accentuates airway narrowing on expiration. This manifests as expiratory wheeze, prolonged expiratory phase, and increased expiratory work of breathing. In patients with chronic airway infection (e.g., cystic fibrosis [CF]), the bronchial tubes become permanently damaged and dilated **(bronchiectasis)**. Patients with bronchiectasis have episodes of cough, often productive of purulent sputum, and may have inspiratory crackles that are caused by the airways popping open during inspiration and air moving through bronchial secretions.

## DIAGNOSTIC STUDIES

When asthma is suspected, empiric trials of therapy (bronchodilators, short courses of oral corticosteroids, long-term use of inhaled corticosteroids) are useful in making a diagnosis. In children older than 6 years of age, pulmonary function tests (spirometry) can be used to assess airflow obstruction and response to bronchodilators. Evidence of airway obstruction and a bronchodilator response on pulmonary function tests, while not necessarily diagnostic, is suggestive of asthma. However, normal values do not rule out asthma. Radiographs are not particularly useful in diagnosing asthma. During an acute asthma exacerbation, the chest radiograph may show hyperinflation and patchy densities due to atelectasis, which are often mistaken for pneumonia. Thus, children with recurrent asthma exacerbations may be labeled as having recurrent pneumonia. Most children with asthma do not need **radiographic evaluation** with each episode of wheezing, but those with significant respiratory distress, fever, history consistent with foreign body aspiration, or focal auscultatory findings should have posteroanterior (PA) and lateral chest radiographs obtained. Generalized **hyperinflation**, indicated by flattening of the diaphragms and an increased anteroposterior (AP) diameter of the chest, suggests diffuse obstruction of the small airways. Localized hyperinflation, especially on expiratory views, suggests localized bronchial obstruction (foreign body or an anatomic anomaly). Dysphagia leading to aspiration and airway inflammation can present with persistent wheezing. This is best assessed with a **videofluoroscopic swallowing study.** Gastroesophageal reflux can also lead to wheezing by predisposing to aspiration or aggravating asthma. For a further discussion of asthma, see Chapter 78.

## DIFFERENTIAL DIAGNOSIS

### Tracheomalacia

#### Etiology

Tracheomalacia is a floppy trachea due to lack of structural integrity of the tracheal wall. The tracheal cartilaginous rings normally extend through an arc of approximately 320 degrees, maintaining rigidity of the trachea during changes in intrathoracic pressure. With tracheomalacia, the cartilaginous rings may not extend as far around the circumference, may be completely absent, or may be present but damaged, and often the membranous posterior trachea is wider than usual. These abnormalities can result in excessive collapse of the trachea during expiration. Tracheomalacia may be congenital (tracheoesophageal fistula or bony dysplasia syndromes) or acquired (long-term mechanical ventilation). Tracheomalacia must be differentiated from extrinsic tracheal compression by masses or vascular structures. In some patients, localized tracheomalacia may persist after the trachea has been relieved of compression by a mass lesion or abnormal blood vessels. Viral infections may exacerbate tracheomalacia, leading to coarse expiratory wheezing and barky cough. The expiratory noises of tracheomalacia are often mistakenly ascribed to asthma or bronchiolitis, and the barky cough is often misdiagnosed as croup.

#### Clinical Manifestations

With tracheomalacia, the tracheal collapse may only be apparent during forced exhalation or with cough. It is commonly aggravated by respiratory infections. The airway collapse may cause recurrent coarse expiratory wheeze and a prolonged expiratory phase. Infants with severe tracheomalacia may completely collapse their tracheas during agitation, resulting in cyanotic episodes that resemble breath-holding spells. The voice is normal, as is inspiratory effort. In older children, the hallmark sign is a brassy, barky cough due to the vibration of the tracheal walls. This cough can be loud, persistent, and it is often misdiagnosed as croup.

#### Treatment

Infants with mild-moderate tracheomalacia usually require no intervention. Tracheomalacia improves with airway growth as the lumen increases in diameter and the tracheal wall becomes more firm. In older children, tracheomalacia may manifest as a severe brassy cough, which is often aggravated by respiratory infections. The treatment of these older children is geared toward treating any precipitating cause for cough and providing supportive care. Children, especially infants, with severe tracheomalacia may require tracheostomy tubes to administer continuous positive airway pressure (CPAP), which serves to stent open the airway.

### Tracheoesophageal Fistula

See Chapter 128.

### Extrinsic Tracheal Compression

Compression of the trachea by vascular structures or masses can cause significant respiratory compromise. Tracheal compression by aberrant great vessels (aorta, innominate artery) may cause wheezing, stridor, cough, and dyspnea. The most common cause of tracheal compression is anterior compression from an **anomalous innominate artery** that arises more distally than normal from the aortic arch. This usually results in mild respiratory symptoms, and surgical correction is rarely necessary. Complete vascular rings, which compress the esophagus posteriorly and the trachea anteriorly, include the double aortic arch and a right aortic arch with a persistent ligamentum arteriosum (most common). Both lesions have right-sided aortic arches, which may be visible on chest radiograph. In addition to respiratory symptoms, complete vascular rings may cause dysphagia as a result of esophageal compression. The diagnosis of vascular anomalies can often be made by a barium swallow, which identifies the esophageal compression, but the diagnostic procedure of choice is a computed tomography (CT) angiogram of the chest and great vessels. Complete vascular rings almost always require surgical repair. Other causes of extrinsic tracheal compression include enlarged mediastinal lymph nodes (tuberculosis), mediastinal masses (teratoma, lymphoma, thymoma, germ cell tumors), and, rarely, cystic hygromas.

## Foreign Body Aspiration

### Epidemiology

Aspiration of foreign bodies into the trachea and bronchi is relatively common. The majority of children who aspirate foreign bodies are under 4 years of age. Most deaths secondary to foreign body aspiration occur in this age group. Because the right mainstem bronchus takes off at a less acute angle than the left mainstem bronchus, foreign bodies tend to lodge in right-sided airways. Some foreign bodies, especially nuts, can also lodge more proximally in the larynx or subglottic space totally occluding the airway. Many foreign bodies are not radiopaque, which makes them difficult to detect radiographically. The most common foreign bodies aspirated by young children are food (especially nuts) and small toys. Coins more often lodge in the esophagus than in the airways. Older children have been known to aspirate rubber balloons, which can be life-threatening.

### Clinical Manifestations

Many children who aspirate foreign bodies have clear histories of choking, witnessed aspiration, or physical or radiographic evidence of foreign body aspiration. However, a small percentage of patients have a negative history because the aspiration went unrecognized. Physical findings observed with acute foreign body aspiration include cough, localized wheezing, unilateral absence of breath sounds, stridor, and, rarely, bloody sputum.

Most foreign bodies are small and quickly expelled, but some may remain in the lung for long periods of time and may come to medical attention because of persistent cough, sputum production, or recurrent pneumonia. Foreign body aspiration should be in the differential diagnosis of patients with persistent wheezing unresponsive to bronchodilator therapy, persistent atelectasis, recurrent or persistent pneumonia, or chronic cough without another explanation. Foreign bodies may also lodge in the esophagus and compress the trachea, thus producing respiratory symptoms. Therefore, esophageal foreign bodies should be included in the differential diagnosis of infants or young children with persistent stridor or wheezing, particularly if dysphagia is present.

### Diagnostic Studies

Radiographic studies will reveal the presence of radiopaque objects and can also identify focal air trapping, especially on expiratory views. Thus, when foreign body aspiration is suspected, expiratory or lateral decubitus chest radiographs should be ordered. In addition, fluoroscopy may be helpful, especially in children who cannot perform expiratory views. If there is strong evidence of foreign body aspiration, the patient should undergo rigid bronchoscopy. Flexible bronchoscopy can be used to locate an aspirated foreign body and may be useful when the presentation is not straightforward, but foreign body removal is best performed via rigid bronchoscopy.

### Prevention

The best approach to preventing foreign body aspiration is to educate parents and caregivers. Before molar teeth have erupted, infants and children should not be given nuts, uncooked carrots, or other foods that may be easily broken into small pieces and aspirated. Additionally, tiny toys are at risk for being aspirated by young children. Sound parental judgment is required to determine at what age and stage of development small objects should be accessible to children.

## Bronchiolitis

See Chapter 109.

## Bronchopulmonary Dysplasia

See Chapter 61.

## Endobronchial Mass Lesions

Endobronchial mass lesions are relatively uncommon in children. The most common lesion is **granulation tissue**, which usually results from local inflammation. Tuberculosis can cause endobronchial granulomas. Primary tumors of the lung are extremely rare in children. The most common airway malignancy is the nonsecreting carcinoid tumor. Endobronchial lesions that partially obstruct an airway present with wheezing or obstructive emphysema and occasionally with hemoptysis. If the lesion completely occludes the airway, then atelectasis may result. Radiographs and CT scans of the chest aid in making the diagnosis. Bronchoscopy is often used to confirm the diagnosis.

## Emphysema

Emphysema is a condition due to disruption or destruction of alveolar septa. In pediatrics, the term emphysema often refers to hyperinflation or to leakage of air into the pulmonary interstitial spaces (interstitial emphysema, which may be seen in mechanically ventilated premature infants) or the subcutaneous tissue (subcutaneous emphysema). Although emphysema is common in adults, it is rare in children. However, generalized or localized **hyperinflation**, which can be caused by airway obstruction from a variety of causes, is common. Emphysema is commonly observed in the disease $\alpha_1$-**antitrypsin deficiency**, but it rarely appears before the second decade of life.

**Congenital lobar overdistention** (formally referred to as congenital lobar emphysema) consists of overinflation of one lobe of a lung. This overdistention may cause severe respiratory distress in the neonatal period due to compression of surrounding normal lung tissue, but it can also be asymptomatic and remain undiagnosed for years. Radiographically, it may be mistaken for a pneumothorax. Lobectomy may be required if respiratory distress is severe or progressive, but if the patient is asymptomatic, then surgical resection may not be indicated.

## Primary Ciliary Dyskinesia

### Etiology

Primary ciliary dyskinesia (PCD, immotile cilia syndrome) is an inherited disorder in which ultrastructural abnormalities in the cilia result in absent or disordered movement of the cilia. This disorder affects approximately 1:19,000 persons.

There are many reported abnormalities in ciliary structure, but the most common are due to defects in the dynein arms, ultrastructural features that provide energy via adenosine triphosphatase (ATPase), which is necessary for ciliary motility.

## Clinical Manifestations

The classic presentation is recurrent otitis media, chronic sinusitis, and bronchiectasis. Kartagener syndrome, the triad of **situs inversus**, **pansinusitis**, and **bronchiectasis**, accounts for approximately 50% of cases. Males are infertile as a result of immotile sperm. Because the cilia fail to beat normally, secretions accumulate in the airways, and endobronchial infection results. Chronic infection, if untreated, leads to bronchiectasis by early adulthood. Primary ciliary dyskinesia should be suspected in patients with early-onset chronic bronchitis or bronchiectasis associated with recurrent/persistent sinusitis and/or frequent otitis media.

## Diagnostic Studies

PCD is confirmed by electron microscopy of respiratory cilia. The cilia may be obtained from scrapings/biopsy of nasal or airway epithelium, although results may be difficult to interpret because chronic infection and inflammation may lead to ultrastructural abnormalities in nasal cilia. The measurement of nasal nitric oxide has been used as a screening tool for PCD. Low nasal nitric oxide values (<200 parts per billion) are consistent with PCD, while values greater than 400 parts per billion make the diagnosis less likely. However, the validity of nasal nitric oxide assays as a diagnostic test for PCD has not been fully substantiated.

## Treatment

Treatment is geared toward treating infections and improving clearance of respiratory secretions. Sinus surgical procedures are often done to manage chronic sinusitis, but their benefit is questionable. Most children require placement of pressure equalization (PE) tubes for management of recurrent otitis media. Chest physiotherapy and prompt treatment of bacterial infections are helpful, but the course of the disease tends to be slowly progressive.

## Pneumonia

See Chapter 110.

## Pulmonary Edema

### Etiology

Pulmonary edema is the seepage of fluid into the alveolar and interstitial spaces. At the alveolar-capillary interface, capillary hydrostatic forces and interstitial osmotic pressures tend to push fluid into the airspaces, while plasma osmotic pressures and tissue mechanical forces tend to move fluid away from the airspaces. Under normal circumstances, the sum of these forces favors absorption, so the alveolar and interstitial spaces remain dry. Fluid entering the alveoli is normally removed by pulmonary lymphatics. Pulmonary edema forms when transcapillary fluid flux exceeds lymphatic drainage. Reduced left ventricular function leads to pulmonary venous hypertension and increased capillary hydrostatic pressure, and fluid moves into the interstitial space and alveoli. Fluid initially enters the interstitial space around the terminal bronchioles, alveoli, and arterioles (**interstitial edema**), causing increased lung stiffness and premature closure of bronchioles on expiration. If the process continues, fluid then enters the alveoli, further reducing compliance and resulting in **intrapulmonary shunting** (alveolar units that are perfused but not ventilated). Decreased ventilation (hypercarbia) is a late finding.

Pulmonary edema is most commonly due to heart failure from left ventricular or biventricular dysfunction. Pulmonary hypertension and associated cor pulmonale (right ventricular dysfunction) do not usually cause pulmonary edema as the increased vascular resistance is proximal to the capillary bed. Pulmonary edema may occur with excessive swings in intrathoracic pressure, as seen after tracheal foreign body aspiration or severe obstruction from hypertrophied tonsils and adenoids (**postobstructive pulmonary edema**). Pulmonary edema may also be present in conditions with decreased serum oncotic pressure (hypoalbumenemia), after administration of large volumes of intravenous (IV) fluids, especially if there is capillary injury, with ascent to high altitude (**high altitude pulmonary edema**), and after CNS injury (**neurogenic pulmonary edema**).

### Clinical Manifestations

The clinical manifestations of pulmonary edema are **dyspnea**, tachypnea, and cough (often with frothy, pink-tinged sputum). As the edema worsens, there is increased work of breathing, hypoxemia, and diffuse inspiratory crackles can be heard on auscultation.

### Diagnostic Studies

Chest radiographs may reveal diffuse hazy infiltrates, classically in a perihilar pattern, but these findings may be obscured by underlying lung disease. Interstitial edema (**Kerley B lines**) may be seen, especially at the lung bases.

### Treatment and Prognosis

Treatment and prognosis depend on the cause of the pulmonary edema and response to therapy. Patients should be positioned in an upright posture and given supplemental $O_2$. Diuretic therapy and rapidly acting IV inotropic agents may be helpful in cardiogenic pulmonary edema. Continuous positive airway pressure (CPAP) or intubation with positive pressure ventilation using high positive end-expiratory pressures (PEEP) may be required.

## Acute Respiratory Distress Syndrome

See Chapter 39.

## Pulmonary Arterial Hypertension and Cor Pulmonale

### Etiology

Pulmonary arterial hypertension (PAH) may be primary or acquired. The most common cause is chronic hypoxia. Alveolar hypoxia results in local pulmonary vasoconstriction and PAH. Pulmonary hypertension is also seen with chronic lung disease, upper airway obstruction resulting in obstructive sleep apnea and hypoxemia, pulmonary thromboembolism, exposure to high altitude, and in autoimmune diseases (e.g., scleroderma). Acquired PAH can also be due to excessive pulmonary blood flow due to left-to-right cardiac shunting (see Chapter 143). With prolonged PAH, irreversible changes may occur in the intima and media of the pulmonary arterioles. **Idiopathic pulmonary arterial hypertension** (previously called primary pulmonary hypertension) is a disorder in which the changes in the pulmonary vasculature are not due to an identifiable underlying cause. It has been associated with mutations in the bone morphogenetic receptor 2 (*BMPR2*) gene and the use of anorectic weight loss drugs. There is an approximately 2:1 female predominance.

Pulmonary arterial hypertension strains the right side of the heart, which leads to hypertrophy and dilation of the right ventricle. This may result in **cor pulmonale,** a condition in which right-sided heart failure leads to hepatic congestion, fluid retention, and tricuspid insufficiency. In severe cor pulmonale, the ventricular septum may be displaced toward the left ventricle, hindering left ventricular function. The most common causes of cor pulmonale in children are chronic lung diseases, especially severe bronchopulmonary dysplasia and scleroderma, and severe untreated obstructive sleep apnea (with chronic hypoxia).

### Clinical Manifestations and Diagnostic Studies

Pulmonary arterial hypertension should be suspected whenever there is prolonged hypoxemia or hemodynamically significant left-to-right cardiac shunting. In addition to the other physical findings associated with pulmonary and cardiac diseases, an accentuated pulmonary component of the second heart sound may be heard in the left second intercostal space. Definitive diagnosis is made by cardiac catheterization, but echocardiography may confirm the presence of right ventricular hypertrophy, ventricular dysfunction, and tricuspid insufficiency and can be used to estimate the pulmonary artery pressures.

### Treatment and Prognosis

In acquired pulmonary arterial hypertension, it is important to treat the underlying condition. The relief of hypoxemia with supplemental $O_2$ therapy is essential. Heart failure may require treatment with diuretics and restrictions of salt and fluid intake. Vasodilator therapy (sildenafil) is helpful in some patients, and inhaled nitric oxide can be used short term. Continuous IV infusions of prostacyclin may be helpful both acutely and chronically. The use of endothelium antagonists may be beneficial.

Unfortunately, many patients with the idiopathic form of PAH have progressive courses, and lung or heart-lung transplantation may be the only treatment option.

## Pulmonary Hemorrhage

### Etiology

Pulmonary hemorrhage is a rare but potentially life-threatening condition in children. It can be due to bleeding from the airways (hemangiomas, bronchial vessel bleeds) or from diffuse capillary bleeding (alveolar hemorrhage). Alveolar hemorrhage is usually due to diffuse capillary disruption/inflammation caused by autoimmune disorders and after bone marrow transplantation. Airway bleeding can be due to airway hemangiomas, pulmonary arteriovenous malformations (as with hereditary hemorrhagic telangectasia), and bronchial artery collaterals, which develop in some patients with chronic lung infections, especially cystic fibrosis. **Idiopathic pulmonary hemosiderosis** is a rare disorder characterized by recurrent alveolar bleeding, iron deficiency anemia, and hemosiderin-laden macrophages in the lung. Red blood cells are phagocytosed by alveolar macrophages and the hemoglobin is converted to hemosiderin, which, with the use of special iron-staining techniques can be identified microscopically within the alveolar macrophages. Hemosiderin-laden macrophages may be identified in bronchoalveolar lavage or lung biopsy specimens. Although the term *hemosiderosis* is sometimes used interchangeably with pulmonary hemorrhage, it is a pathologic finding that results from bleeding anywhere in the lung, airway, pharynx, nasopharynx, or mouth leading to hemosiderin accumulation in the lung. **Pulmonary hemorrhage** is a preferable term for bleeding from an intrathoracic source.

### Clinical Manifestations

Most children with pulmonary hemorrhage present with **hemoptysis**. When evaluating a child with hemoptysis, it is important to rule out extrapulmonary sources of bleeding, including hematemesis and bleeding from the nasopharynx or mouth, as these are more common than true pulmonary hemorrhage. In addition to hemoptysis, the presenting signs and symptoms of pulmonary hemorrhage include cough, wheezing, shortness of breath, pallor, fatigue, cyanosis, and fever. Episodic pulmonary hemorrhage frequently manifests as recurrent respiratory symptoms associated with pulmonary infiltrates on chest radiographs. Symptomatic **airway hemorrhage** may result in significant hemoptysis with few radiographic changes, while **alveolar bleeding** often causes profound respiratory symptoms, hypoxemia, diffuse infiltrates on radiographs, and minimal hemoptysis. Some patients experience a localized bubbling sensation in the chest, which may be helpful in differentiating local from diffuse sources of pulmonary bleeding. Physical examination findings may include locally or diffusely decreased breath sounds, cyanosis, and crackles on auscultation.

The **differential diagnosis** of pulmonary hemorrhage includes alveolar and airway bleeding. The causes of alveolar (capillary) bleeding include idiopathic pulmonary hemosiderosis, diffuse alveolitis (capillaritis) secondary to autoimmune disease (Goodpasture syndrome, Wegener granulomatosis, systemic lupus erythematosus, polyarteritis nodosa), clotting disorders, veno-occlusive disease, diffuse alveolar injury (smoke inhalation), and cardiac conditions associated with elevated pulmonary venous and capillary pressures (mitral stenosis). Rarely, a previously well infant will present with life-threatening acute alveolar hemorrhage. Often no cause is found, and once the acute episode resolves, the infant returns to normal. Most of these infants never have a second bleeding episode. Hemoptysis can have cardiovascular, pulmonary, or immunologic causes (Table 136-2).

## Diagnostic Studies

It is important to perform a thorough upper airway examination to rule out epistaxis. Sometimes this requires nasopharyngoscopy. If extrapulmonary sources of bleeding have been excluded, then other diagnostic tests to consider are chest radiographs, CT angiogram of the chest, bronchoscopy, echocardiogram, and evaluation for rheumatologic/autoimmune diseases, especially Goodpasture disease, Wegener granulomatosis, Schönlein-Henoch purpura, and systemic lupus erythematosus.

## Treatment

The management of acute episodes of pulmonary bleeding includes the administration of supplemental $O_2$, blood transfusions, and, as is often the case with acute alveolar hemorrhages, mechanical ventilation with PEEP to tamponade the bleeding. Attempts should be made to identify the cause of the bleeding. Treatment is directed toward the underlying disorders and providing supportive care. In bronchial arterial bleeding, arteriography with vessel embolization has been shown to be successful.

## Pulmonary Embolism

### Etiology

Pulmonary embolism is rare in children. When it occurs, it is often associated with indwelling central venous catheters, oral contraceptives, or hypercoagulable states. In adolescents, trauma, obesity, abortion, and malignancy may lead to deep vein thromboses (DVT) and pulmonary embolism.

### Clinical Manifestations

Because the pulmonary vascular bed is distensible, small emboli, even if multiple, may be asymptomatic unless they are infected (septic emboli) and cause pulmonary infection. Large emboli may cause acute dyspnea, pleuritic chest pain, cough, and hemoptysis. **Hypoxia** is common, as are nonspecific ST-segment and T-wave changes on the electrocardiogram (ECG). The $P_2$ heart sound may be increased, and an $S_4$ sound may be present.

### Diagnostic Studies

Although the chest x-ray is usually normal, atelectasis or cardiomegaly may be seen. The measurement of D-dimers can be used as a screening test, but it must be interpreted in light of the probability of a pulmonary embolism. If the D-dimer is normal and the probability for embolism is low, then no further workup may be necessary. However, if the D-dimer is elevated, or if it is normal but the probability of embolism is moderate or high, then the diagnostic test of choice is a **CT angiogram of the chest.** Ventilation-perfusion scans may be helpful in the diagnosis by revealing defects in perfusion without matching ventilation defects, but they are difficult to perform in young children. Doppler or compression ultrasonography can be useful in assessing patients for lower extremity deep vein thromboses (DVTs). For definitive diagnosis of pulmonary embolism, the gold standard is still **pulmonary angiography,** though with the improvement in CT angiography, angiograms are now rarely necessary. Children with pulmonary embolism without an obvious

---

**TABLE 136-2  Differential Diagnosis of Hemoptysis–Pulmonary Hemorrhage**

### CARDIOVASCULAR DISORDERS

Heart failure
Eisenmenger syndrome
Mitral stenosis
Veno-occlusive disease
Arteriovenous malformation (Osler-Weber-Rendu syndrome)
Pulmonary embolism

### PULMONARY DISORDERS

Respiratory distress syndrome
Bronchogenic cyst
Sequestration
Pneumonia (bacterial, mycobacterial, fungal, or parasitic)
Cystic fibrosis
Tracheobronchitis
Bronchiectasis
Lung abscess
Tumor (adenoma, carcinoid, hemangioma, metastasis)
Foreign body retention
Contusion—trauma

### IMMUNE DISORDERS

Henoch-Schonlein purpura
Idiopathic pulmonary hemosiderosis
Goodpasture syndrome
Wegener granulomatosis
Systemic lupus erythematosus
Polyarteritis nodosa

### OTHER CONDITIONS/FACTORS

Hyperammonemia
Kernicterus
Intracranial hemorrhage (in preterm infant)
Toxins
Diffuse alveolar injury (smoke inhalation)
Post–bone marrow transplantation

cause should be evaluated for hypercoagulable states, the most common of which is factor V Leiden.

## Treatment

Once a pulmonary embolism is suspected, the patient should be anticoagulated, usually with low-molecular-weight heparin. All patients should receive supplemental $O_2$, and it is important to treat the predisposing factors. Thrombolytic therapy and surgical resection of emboli are rarely indicated. Occasionally an inferior vena caval filter needs to be placed to prevent recurrent emboli.

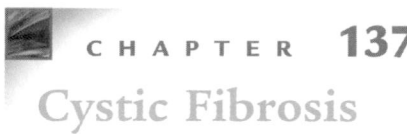

CHAPTER **137**

# Cystic Fibrosis

## ETIOLOGY AND EPIDEMIOLOGY

Cystic fibrosis (CF) is an autosomal recessive disorder that is the most common life-limiting genetic disease in whites. In the United States, the incidence of CF is approximately 1 in 3200 for whites, 1 in 15,000 African Americans, and 1 in 31,000 persons of Asian heritage. The gene for CF, which is located on the long arm of chromosome 7, encodes for a polypeptide, the **cystic fibrosis transmembrane regulator (CFTR)**. CFTR is a chloride channel located on the apical surface of epithelial cells. CFTR is important for the proper movement of salt and water across cell membranes and maintaining the appropriate composition of various secretions, especially in the airway, liver, and pancreas. The most common mutation is a deletion of three base pairs resulting in the absence of phenylalanine at the 508 position ($\Delta$F508). More than 1000 mutations of the *CFTR* gene have been identified.

The secretory and absorptive characteristics of epithelial cells are affected by abnormal CFTR, resulting in the clinical manifestations of CF. The lack of normal CFTR function alters chloride ion conductance in the sweat gland, resulting in excessively high sweat sodium and chloride levels. This is the basis of the sweat chloride test, which is still the standard diagnostic test for this disorder. It is positive (elevated sweat chloride > 60 mEq/L) in 99% of patients with CF. It is not completely understood how the abnormal chloride conductance accounts for all of the clinical manifestations of CF, but it is known that abnormal airway secretions make the airway more prone to colonization with bacteria. Defects in CFTR may also reduce the function of airway defenses and promote bacterial adhesion to the airway epithelium. This all leads to chronic airway infections and eventually to bronchial damage (bronchiectasis).

## CLINICAL MANIFESTATIONS

CF is a chronic progressive disease that can present with protein and fat malabsorption (failure to thrive, hypoalbuminemia, steatorrhea), liver disease (cholestatic jaundice),

or chronic respiratory infection (Table 137-1). Infants often present with failure to thrive, while pulmonary manifestations predominate in older children. The respiratory epithelium of patients with CF exhibits marked impermeability to chloride and an excessive reabsorption of sodium. These alterations in the bioelectrical properties of the epithelium lead to a relative dehydration of airway secretions, which results in airway obstruction and impaired mucociliary transport. This, in turn, leads to endobronchial colonization with bacteria, especially *Staphylococcus aureus* and

| TABLE 137-1  Complications of Cystic Fibrosis |
|---|
| **RESPIRATORY COMPLICATIONS** |
| Bronchiectasis, bronchitis, bronchiolitis, pneumonia |
| Atelectasis |
| Hemoptysis |
| Pneumothorax |
| Nasal polyps |
| Sinusitis |
| Airway reactivity |
| Cor pulmonale (associated with chronic hypoxemia) |
| Respiratory failure |
| Mucoid impaction of the bronchi |
| Allergic bronchopulmonary aspergillosis |
| **GASTROINTESTINAL COMPLICATIONS** |
| Meconium ileus (infants) |
| Meconium peritonitis (infants) |
| Volvulus (infants) |
| Intestinal atresia (infants) |
| Distal intestinal obstruction syndrome (non-neonatal obstruction) |
| Rectal prolapse |
| Intussusception |
| Fibrosing colonopathy (strictures) |
| Appendicitis |
| Pancreatitis |
| Hepatic cirrhosis (portal hypertension: esophageal varices, hypersplenism) |
| Neonatal obstructive jaundice |
| Hepatic steatosis |
| Gastroesophageal reflux |
| Cholelithiasis |
| Growth failure (malabsorption) |
| Fat soluble vitamin deficiency states (vitamins A, K, E, D) |
| Insulin deficiency, symptomatic hyperglycemia, diabetes |
| Malignancy (rare) |
| **OTHER COMPLICATIONS** |
| Infertility |
| Delayed puberty |
| Edema-hypoproteinemia (due to protein malabsorption) |
| Dehydration–heat exhaustion |
| Electrolyte disturbances (hyponatremia, hypokalemia, hypochloremia, and metabolic alkalosis) |
| Hypertrophic osteoarthropathy–arthritis |
| Digital clubbing |

*Pseudomonas aeruginosa. Pseudomonas aeruginosa* predominates in older patients with advanced disease. Chronic bronchial infection results in persistent or recurrent cough that is often productive of sputum, especially in older children. Chronic airway infection leads to airway obstruction and bronchiectasis and eventually to pulmonary insufficiency and premature death. The median age of survival (years) is currently in the mid-30s. **Digital clubbing** is common in patients with CF, even in those without significant lung disease. Chronic sinusitis and **nasal polyposis** are common. Any child with nasal polyps, especially if younger than 12 years of age, should be evaluated for CF.

Pulmonary infections with virulent strains of *Burkholderia cepacia* are difficult to treat and may be associated with accelerated clinical deterioration. **Allergic bronchopulmonary aspergillosis (ABPA)** is a hypersensitivity reaction to *Aspergillus* in the CF airways. It causes airway inflammation/obstruction and aggravates CF lung disease. The treatment for ABPA is parenteral corticosteroids (prednisone) and antifungal agents (itraconazole). Minor hemoptysis is usually due to airway infection, but major hemoptysis is caused by bleeding from bronchial artery collateral vessels in damaged/chronically infected portions of the lung. Pneumothoraces can occur in patients with advanced lung disease.

Ninety percent of patients with CF are born with **exocrine pancreatic insufficiency**. The inspissation of mucus and subsequent destruction of the pancreatic ducts result in the inability to excrete pancreatic enzymes into the intestine. This leads to malabsorption of proteins, sugars (to a lesser extent), and especially fat. Fat malabsorption manifests clinically as **steatorrhea** (large foul-smelling stools), deficiencies of fat-soluble vitamins (A, D, E, and K), and failure to thrive. Protein malabsorption can present early in infancy as hypoproteinemia and peripheral edema. Approximately 10% of patients with CF are born with intestinal obstruction caused by inspissated meconium (**meconium ileus**). In older patients, intestinal obstruction may result from thick inspissated mucus in the intestinal lumen (**distal intestinal obstruction syndrome**). In adolescent or adult patients, progressive pancreatic damage can lead to enough islet cell destruction to cause **insulin deficiency.** This initially presents as glucose intolerance, but true diabetes that requires insulin therapy (**CF-related diabetes**) may develop. The failure of the sweat ducts to conserve sodium and chloride may lead to hyponatremia and hypochloremic metabolic alkalosis, especially in infants. Inspissation of mucus in the reproductive tract leads to reproductive dysfunction in both males and females. In males, congenital absence of the vas deferens and azoospermia are nearly universal. In females, secondary amenorrhea is often present as a result of chronic illness and reduced body weight. Fertility is also diminished by abnormal secretions in the fallopian tubes and cervix, but women with CF can conceive.

The diagnosis of CF should be seriously considered in any infant presenting with failure to thrive, cholestatic jaundice, chronic respiratory symptoms, or electrolyte abnormalities (hyponatremia, hypochloremia, metabolic alkalosis). CF should be in the differential diagnosis of children with chronic respiratory or gastrointestinal symptoms, especially if there is digital clubbing. Any child with nasal polyps should be evaluated for CF.

## DIAGNOSTIC STUDIES

There are readily available commercial DNA tests that detect up to 100 CF mutations, but because there are more than 1000 identified mutations and some that have yet to be identified, DNA analysis will not detect all cases of CF. Many states now have newborn screening for CF, which is based either on elevated immunoreactive trypsinogen (IRT) levels or DNA tests. Newborn screening identifies the majority of infants with CF, but there are both false positive and false negative results. Therefore, the diagnostic test of choice is still the sweat test. Indications for performing a **sweat test** are listed in Table 137-2. The following criteria should be met to establish the diagnosis of CF:

The presence of one or more typical clinical features of CF (chronic pulmonary disease, characteristic gastrointestinal and nutritional abnormalities, salt loss syndromes, and obstructive azoospermia) OR

1. A positive result from a newborn screening test *and* at least one of the following: Positive results on at least two sweat chloride tests performed at a CF

---

**TABLE 137-2  Indications for Sweat Testing**

### RESPIRATORY

Chronic or recurrent cough
Chronic or recurrent pneumonia
Recurrent bronchiolitis
Recurrent or persistant atelectasis
Hemoptysis
*Pseudomonas aeruginosa* in the respiratory tract (if not explained by other factors, e.g. tracheostomy or prolonged intubation)

### GASTROINTESTINAL

Meconium ileus
Neonatal intestinal obstruction (meconium plug, atresia)
Steatorrhea, malabsorption
Hepatic cirrhosis in childhood (including any manifestations such as esophageal varices or portal hypertension)
Cholestatic jaundice in infancy
Pancreatitis
Rectal prolapse
Fat-soluble vitamin deficiency states (A, D, E, K)
Hypoproteinemia, hypoalbuminemia, peripheral edema unexplained by other causes
Prolonged, direct-reacting neonatal jaundice

### MISCELLANEOUS

Digital clubbing
Failure to thrive
Family history of cystic fibrosis (e.g., in sibling or cousin)
Salty taste of skin (typically noted by parent on kissing affected child—from salt crystals formed after evaporation of sweat)
Hyponatremic hypochloremic alkalosis in infants
Nasal polyps
Recurrent sinusitis
Aspermia
Absent vas deferens

### TABLE 137-3  Causes of False Positive and False Negative Results on Sweat Testing

**FALSE POSITIVE**

Adrenal insufficiency
Eczema
Ectodermal dysplasia
Nephrogenic diabetes insipidus
Hypothyroidism
Fucosidosis
Mucopolysaccharidosis
Dehydration
Malnutrition
Poor technique/inadequate sweat collection
Type I glycogen storage disease
Panhypopituitarism
Pseudohypoaldosteronism
Hypoparathyroidism
Prostaglandin $E_1$ administration

**FALSE NEGATIVE**

Edema
Poor technique/inadequate sweat collection
Atypical cystic fibrosis (unusual gene mutations—uncommon)

Foundation certified laboratory (positive if the value is > 60 mEq/L with adequate sweat collection, borderline if 40 to 60 mEq/L, and negative if < 40 mEq/L) or

2. Two mutations known to cause CF identified by DNA analysis or

3. A characteristic abnormality in ion transport across nasal epithelium demonstrated in vivo (nasal potential difference testing)

Although the sweat test is both specific and sensitive for CF, it is subject to technical problems, and there are false positive and false negative results (Table 137-3). Other supportive tests include the measurement of bioelectrical potential differences across nasal epithelium (not widely available) and measurement of fecal elastase levels. Low fecal elastase levels indicate exocrine pancreatic insufficiency. Detection of a known CF mutation by DNA analysis is useful but not foolproof. CF genotyping done by commercial laboratories identifies approximately 95% of patients with CF, but there are mutations that are not identified by standard testing.

Identification of carriers (heterozygotes) and prenatal diagnosis of children with the ΔF508 and other common mutations is currently offered at most medical centers. Present testing techniques can identify more than 90% of carriers. Prenatal detection of a known CF genotype may be accomplished by amniotic fluid or chorionic villus sampling.

## TREATMENT

The treatment of CF is multifactorial, but it is primarily directed toward the gastrointestinal and pulmonary complications. Presently there is no effective treatment for the underlying defect (abnormal salt and water transit across epithelial cells due to the abnormal CFTR chloride channel). However, medications that improve the function of defective CFTR and gene replacement therapy are both being actively investigated. The current management of pulmonary complications is directed toward facilitating clearance of secretions from the airways and minimizing the effects of chronic bronchial infection. Airway secretion clearance techniques (**chest physiotherapy**) help remove mucus from the airways, and aerosolized DNAse and 7% hypertonic saline, both delivered by nebulizer, decrease the viscosity of mucus. **Antibiotic therapy** is important in controlling chronic infection. Monitoring pulmonary bacterial flora via airway cultures and providing aggressive therapy with appropriate antibiotics (oral, aerosolized, and parenteral) help to slow the progression of lung disease. Patients often require 2- to 3-week courses of high-dose intravenous antibiotics and aggressive chest physiotherapy to treat pulmonary exacerbations. Antibiotics are selected based on organisms identified by sputum culture. If patients are unable to provide sputum, then a throat culture for CF pathogens can be used to direct therapy. Common infecting organisms are *Pseudomonas aeruginosa* and *Staphylococcus aureus*.

**Exocrine pancreatic insufficiency** is treated with enteric-coated pancreatic enzyme capsules, which contain lipase and proteases. Patients with CF are encouraged to follow high-calorie diets, often with the addition of nutritional supplements. Even with optimal pancreatic enzyme replacement, stool losses of fat and protein may be high. Fat should not be withheld from the diet, even when significant steatorrhea exists. Rather, pancreatic enzyme doses should be titrated to optimize fat absorption, although there is a limit to the doses that should be used. Lipase dosages exceeding 2500 U/kg/meal are contraindicated because they have been associated with **fibrosing colonopathy**. Fat-soluble vitamins (A, E, D, and K) are recommended, preferably in a water-miscible form.

Newborns with **meconium ileus** may require surgical intervention, but some can be managed with contrast (Gastrografin) enemas. Intestinal obstruction in CF patients beyond the neonatal period is often due to distal intestinal obstruction syndrome (DIOS), which may need to be treated with courses of oral laxatives (polyethelyne glycol) or, in more refractory cases, with balanced intestinal lavage solutions (GoLYTELY). Pancreatic enzyme dosage adjustment, adequate hydration, and dietary fiber may help prevent recurrent episodes. Patients with CF-related diabetes are treated with insulin, primarily to improve nutrition and prevent dehydration, as ketoacidosis is rare. Although transaminase elevation is common in patients with CF, only 1 to 3% of patients have progressive cirrhosis resulting in portal hypertension. Cholestasis is treated with the bile salt, ursodeoxycholic acid. Portal hypertension and esophageal varices due to cirrhosis of the liver are managed, when necessary, with portal vein shunting procedures or liver transplantation. Patients with symptomatic sinus disease and nasal polyps may require sinus surgical procedures.

The management of CF is complex and is best coordinated by personnel at accredited CF centers. As with other severe chronic diseases, management of patients with CF requires a multidisciplinary team. Physicians and other care providers, including nurses, respiratory therapists, nutritionists, and social workers must work with patients and their families to maintain an optimistic, comprehensive, and aggressive approach to treatment.

# Chest Wall and Pleura

## SCOLIOSIS

**Thoracic scoliosis** is curvature of the thoracic spine. When it is severe (curve > 60 degrees) it can be associated with chest wall deformity and limitation of chest wall movement. This, in turn, can lead to decreased lung volumes (restrictive lung disease), ventilation/perfusion mismatching, hypoventilation, and even respiratory failure (see Chapter 202). Surgical correction of scoliosis may prevent further loss of lung function, but it rarely improves pulmonary function above presurgical levels.

## PECTUS EXCAVATUM AND CARINATUM

### Pectus Excavatum

Sternal concavity (**pectus excavatum**) is a common chest wall deformity in children, and is usually not associated with significant pulmonary compromise. However, occasionally, if severe, it can result in restrictive lung disease and decreased right-sided heart output. Often it comes to attention because of concerns over the appearance of the chest (cosmetic reasons). Adolescents with pectus excavatum may complain of exercise intolerance, and formal exercise testing may be indicated. Routine spirometry is often normal but may show a decreased vital capacity consistent with restrictive lung disease. The main reason for surgical correction is to improve appearance (cosmetic reasons), although in some cases surgical repair is justified to improve cardiac output and exercise tolerance. Surgical correction is best done during young adolescence before the bones have achieved full skeletal maturity. Surgical repair may improve exercise tolerance, but it does not improve lung function.

### Pectus Carinatum

Pectus carinatum is an abnormality of chest wall shape in which the sternum bows out. It is not associated with abnormal pulmonary function. However, underlying pulmonary disease may contribute to the deformity, and it can be observed after open heart surgery performed via midsternal approaches. Surgical correction of this condition is rarely indicated, but occasionally it is done for cosmetic purposes.

## PNEUMOTHORAX

### Etiology

Pneumothorax, which is the accumulation of air in the pleural space, may result from external trauma or from leakage of air from the lungs or airways. **Spontaneous primary pneumothorax** (no underlying cause) occurs in teenagers and young adults, more commonly in tall, thin males and smokers. Factors predisposing to **secondary pneumothorax** (underlying cause identified) include barotrauma from mechanical ventilation, asthma, cystic fibrosis, trauma to the chest, and severe necrotizing pneumonia.

### Clinical Manifestations

The most common signs and symptoms of pneumothorax are chest and shoulder pain and dyspnea. If the pneumothorax is large and compresses functional lung (**tension peumothorax**), then severe respiratory distress and cyanosis may be present. Subcutaneous emphysema may result when the air leak communicates with the mediastinum. Physical findings associated with pneumothorax include decreased breath sounds on the affected side, a tympanitic percussion note, and evidence of mediastinal shift (deviation of the PMI and trachea away from the side of the pneumothorax) (see Table 133-3). If the pneumothorax is small, then there may be few or no clinical findings. However, the patient's clinical condition can deteriorate rapidly if the pneumothorax expands and especially if the air in the pleural space is under pressure (**tension pneumothorax**). This is a life-threatening condition that can result in death if the pleural space is not decompressed by evacuation of the pleural air.

### Diagnostic Studies

The presence of a pneumothorax can usually be confirmed by chest radiographs. Computed tomography (CT) scans of the chest are useful in quantifying the size of pneumothoraces and differentiating air within the lung parenchyma (cystic lung disease) from air in the pleural space. In infants, transillumination of the chest wall may be of some use in making a rapid diagnosis of pneumothorax.

### Treatment

The type of intervention depends on the size of the pneumothorax and the nature of the underlying disease. Small pneumothoraces (<20% of thorax occupied with pleural air) may not require intervention as they often resolve spontaneously. Inhaling high concentrations of supplemental $O_2$ may enhance reabsorption of pleural air by washing out nitrogen from the blood, thus establishing a higher nitrogen pressure gradient between pleural air and the blood. Larger pneumothoraces and any tension pneumothorax require immediate drainage of the air, preferably via chest tube. In an emergency situation, a simple needle aspiration may suffice, though placement of a chest tube is often required for resolution. In patients with recurrent or persistent pneumothoraces, sclerosing the pleural surfaces to obliterate the pleural space (pleurodesis) may be necessary. This can be done either chemically, by instilling talc or sclerosis agents (doxycycline) through the chest tube or by surgical abradement. Surgical approaches, open thoracotomy and video-assisted thoracoscopic surgery (VATS), enable visualization of the pleural space and resection of pleural blebs, when indicated.

## PNEUMOMEDIASTINUM

Pneumomediastinum results from the dissection of air from the pulmonary parenchyma into the mediastinum. It is usually a mild, self-limited process that does not require aggressive intervention. The most common causes in children are severe forceful coughing and acute asthma exacerbations. Common symptoms are chest pain and dyspnea. There are often no physical findings, although a crunching noise over the sternum can sometimes be noted on auscultation, and subcutaneous emphysema may be detected about the neck. The diagnosis is confirmed by chest radiograph, and treatment is directed toward the underlying lung disease.

## PLEURAL EFFUSION

### Etiology

Fluid accumulates in the pleural space when the local hydrostatic forces that are pushing fluid out of the vascular space exceed the oncotic forces that are drawing fluid back into the vascular space. Pleural effusions can be transudates (intact membrane but abnormal hydrostatic or oncotic forces) or exudates (decreased integrity of the membrane primarily due to inflammatory processes). There are relatively few causes of transudates, the primary ones being congestive heart failure and hypoproteinemia states, while the causes of exudates are legion. Almost any pulmonary inflammatory process can result in pleural fluid accumulation. Among the most common causes of exudates are infection (tuberculosis [TB], bacterial pneumonia), collagen vascular diseases (systemic lupus erythematosus), and malignancy. Chylous pleural effusions (elevated triglyceride levels) are seen with thoracic duct injury (thoracic surgery, chest trauma) and abnormalities of lymphatic drainage. Bacterial pneumonia can lead to an accumulation of pleural fluid (**parapneumonic effusion**). When this fluid is purulent or infected, then it is called an **empyema,** though often the terms parapneumonic effusion and empyema are used interchangeably. Parapneumonic effusion/empyema is the most common effusion in children. Most parapneumonic effusions are due to pneumonia caused by *Streptococcus pneumoniae,* group A streptococci, or *Staphylococcus aureus.*

### Clinical Manifestations

Small pleural effusions may be asymptomatic, but if they are large enough to compress lung tissue, then they can cause dyspnea, tachypnea, and occasionally chest pain. Effusions due to infection are usually associated with fever, malaise, poor appetite, pleuritic chest pain, and splinting. Physical findings include tachypnea, dullness to percussion, decreased breath sounds, mediastinal shift (with large effusions), and decreased tactile fremitus.

### Diagnostic Studies

The presence of pleural fluid can often be confirmed by chest radiograph. In addition to anteroposterior and lateral projections, a decubitus view should be done to assess for layering of fluid. Chest ultrasonography is useful for confirming the presence of the effusion and quantifying its size. CT scans of the chest can help differentiate pleural fluid from parenchymal lesions and pleural masses. Both ultrasonography and CT scans can determine whether parapneumonic effusions contain loculations (fibrous strands that compartmentalize the effusion).

The analysis of pleural fluid is useful in differentiating a transudate (low pleural fluid to serum lactate dehydrogenase and protein ratios) from an exudate. It is also useful in diagnosing chylous, tuberculous, and malignant effusions. However, the yield of pleural fluid cultures is low. Transudative pleural effusions have a low specific gravity ($<1.015$) and protein content ($<2.5$ g/dL), low lactate dehydrogenase activity ($<200$ IU/L), and a low WBC count with few polymorphonuclear cells. In contrast, exudates are characterized by high specific gravity and high protein ($>3$ g/dL) and lactate dehydrogenase ($>250$ IU/L) levels. They may also have a low pH ($<7.2$); low glucose level ($<40$ mg/dL); and a high white blood cell count with many lymphocytes or polymorphonuclear leukocytes.

### Treatment

Therapy is directed at the underlying condition causing the effusion and at relief of the mechanical consequences of the fluid collection. For small effusions, especially if they are transudates, no pleural drainage is required. Large effusions that are causing respiratory compromise should be drained. Transudates and most exudates other than parapneumonic effusions can be drained with a **chest tube**. With parapneumonic effusions/empyema, a chest tube alone is often not sufficient because the fluid may be thick and loculated. In such cases, pleural drainage is best achieved with either the administration of fibrinolytic agents via chest tubes or **video-assisted thoracoscopic surgery (VATS)**. Both fibrinolytic therapy via chest tubes and VATS can reduce morbidity and length of hospital stay, but many patients with small to moderate-sized parapneumonic effusions can be managed conservatively with intravenous antibiotics alone.

  **SUGGESTED  READING**

Balfour-Lynn IM, Abrahamson E, Cohen G, et al: BTS guidelines for the management of pleural infection in children, *Thorax* 60(suppl 1):1–21, 2005.

Chernick V, Boat TF, Wilmott RW, et al: Kendig's Disorders of the Respiratory Tract in Children, 7th ed, Philadelphia, 2006, *WB Saunders.*

Gibson RL: Cystic fibrosis. In Osborn L, DeWitt T, First L, Zenel J, editors: *Pediatrics.* Philadelphia, 2004, *Mosby Inc.,* pp 1198–1207.

Kliegman RM, Behrman RE, Jenson HB, et al, editors: Nelson Textbook of Pediatrics, 18th ed, Philadelphia, 2007, *WB Saunders.*

Levitzky MG: *Pulmonary Physiology,* 7th ed, New York, 2007, *McGraw-Hill.*

# THE CARDIOVASCULAR SYSTEM

**Daniel S. Schneider**

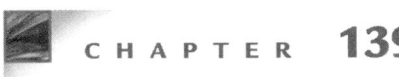

CHAPTER **139**

# Cardiovascular System Assessment

## HISTORY

The focus of the cardiovascular history depends on patient's age and is directed by the chief complaint. The **prenatal history** may reveal a maternal infection early in pregnancy (possibly teratogenic) or later in pregnancy (causing myocarditis or myocardial dysfunction in infants). A **maternal history** of medication, drug, or alcohol use or excessive smoking may contribute to cardiac and other systemic findings. While **growth** is a valuable sign of cardiovascular health, the birth weight is an indicator of the prenatal health of the fetus and the mother. Infants with **heart failure** grow poorly, with weight being more significantly affected than height and head circumference.

Heart failure may present with **fatigue** or **diaphoresis** with feeds or fussiness. Feeding may be difficult and prolonged because of tachypnea. **Tachypnea** without significant dyspnea may be present. Older children with heart failure may have easy fatigability, **shortness of breath** on exertion, and sometimes orthopnea. **Exercise intolerance** may be determined by asking how well children keep up while playing or exercising. Patients may have been misdiagnosed with recurrent pneumonia, bronchitis, wheezing, or asthma before heart failure is recognized.

A history of a **heart murmur** is important, but many well children have an innocent murmur at some time in their lives. Other cardiac symptoms include cyanosis, palpitations, chest pain, syncope, and near-syncope. A review of systems assesses for possible systemic diseases or congenital malformation syndromes that may cause cardiac abnormalities (Tables 139-1 and 139-2). Current and past medication use as well as history of drug use, is important. **Family history** should be reviewed for hereditary diseases, early atherosclerotic heart disease, congenital heart disease, sudden unexplained deaths, thrombophilia, rheumatic fever, hypertension, and hypercholesterolemia.

## PHYSICAL EXAMINATION

A complete cardiovascular examination starts in the supine position and includes evaluation in sitting and standing positions when possible. Much information regarding the cardiovascular status can be gained by **inspection**, which is supplemented by **palpation** and **auscultation.**

The examination starts with vital signs. The normal **heart rate** varies with age and activity. Newborn resting heart rates are approximately 120 beats/minute. It is slightly higher in infants 3 to 6 months of age and then gradually declines through adolescence when the average resting rate is near 80 beats/minute. The range of normal for any given age is relatively wide, approximately 30 beats/minute above or below the average. Tachycardia may be a manifestation of anemia, dehydration, shock, heart failure, or dysrhythmia. Bradycardia can be a normal finding in patient with high vagal tone (athletes), but may be a manifestation of atrioventricular block. The **respiratory rate** of infants is best assessed while observing the infant sitting quietly with the parent. Respiratory rate may be increased when there is a left-to-right shunt or pulmonary venous congestion.

Normal **blood pressure** also varies with age. A properly sized cuff, needed to obtain reliable information, should have a bladder width that is at least 90% of the arm circumference and a length that is 80% to 100% of the arm circumference. Initially, blood pressure in the right arm is measured. If elevated, measurements in the left arm and legs are indicated to evaluate for possible coarctation of the aorta. The **pulse pressure** is determined by subtracting the diastolic pressure from the systolic pressure. It is normally below 50 mm Hg or half the systolic pressure, whichever is less. A wide pulse pressure may be seen with aortopulmonary connections (patent ductus arteriosus [PDA], truncus arteriosus, arteriovenous malformations), aortic insufficiency, or relative intravascular volume depletion (anemia, vasodilation with fever or sepsis). A narrow pulse pressure is seen with pericardial tamponade, aortic stenosis, and heart failure.

**Inspection** includes general appearance, nutritional status, circulation, and respiratory effort. Many chromosomal abnormalities and syndromes associated with cardiac defects have dysmorphic features or failure to thrive (see Table 139-2). Skin color must be assessed for

### TABLE 139-1 Cardiac Manifestations of Systemic Diseases

| Systemic Disease | Cardiac Complications |
| --- | --- |
| Hunter-Hurler syndrome | Valvular insufficiency, heart failure, hypertension |
| Fabry disease | Mitral insufficiency, coronary artery disease with myocardial infarction |
| Pompe disease | Short PR interval, cardiomegaly, heart failure, arrhythmias |
| Friedreich ataxia | Cardiomyopathy, arrhythmias |
| Duchenne dystrophy | Cardiomyopathy, heart failure |
| Juvenile rheumatoid arthritis | Pericarditis |
| Systemic lupus erythematosus | Pericarditis, Libman-Sacks endocarditis, congenital AV block |
| Marfan syndrome | Aortic and mitral insufficiency, dissecting aortic aneurysm |
| Homocystinuria | Coronary thrombosis |
| Kawasaki disease | Coronary artery aneurysm, thrombosis, myocardial infarction, myocarditis |
| Lyme disease | Arrhythmias, myocarditis, heart failure |
| Graves disease (hyperthyroidism) | Tachycardia, arrhythmias, heart failure |
| Tuberous sclerosis | Cardiac rhabdomyoma |
| Neurofibromatosis | Pulmonic stenosis, coarctation of aorta |

AV, atrioventricular.

### TABLE 139-2 Congenital Malformation Syndromes Associated with Congenital Heart Disease

| Syndrome | Cardiac Features |
| --- | --- |
| Trisomy 21 (Down syndrome) | Endocardial cushion defect, VSD, ASD, PDA |
| Trisomy 18 | VSD, ASD, PDA, PS |
| Trisomy 13 | VSD, ASD, PDA, dextrocardia |
| XO (Turner syndrome) | Coarctation of aorta, aortic stenosis |
| CHARGE association (*c*oloboma, *h*eart, *a*tresia choanae, *r*etardation, *g*enital and *e*ar anomalies) | TOF, aortic arch and conotruncal anomalies* |
| 22q11 (DiGeorge) syndrome | Aortic arch anomalies, conotruncal anomalies* |
| VACTERL association[†] (*v*ertebral, *a*nal, *c*ardiac, *t*racheoesophageal, *r*adial, *r*enal, *l*imb anomalies) | VSD |
| Congenital rubella | PDA, peripheral pulmonic stenosis, mitral regurgitation (in infancy) |
| Marfan syndrome | Dilated and dissecting aorta, aortic valve regurgitation, mitral valve prolapse |
| Williams syndrome | Supravalvular aortic stenosis, peripheral pulmonary stenosis |
| Infant of diabetic mother | Hypertrophic cardiomyopathy, VSD, conotruncal anomalies |
| Holt-Oram syndrome | ASD, VSD |
| Asplenia syndrome | Complex cyanotic heart lesions, anomalous pulmonary venous return, dextrocardia, single ventricle, single AV valve |
| Polysplenia syndrome | Azygos continuation of inferior vena cava, pulmonary atresia, dextrocardia, single ventricle |
| Fetal alcohol syndrome | VSD, ASD |
| Ellis–van Creveld syndrome | Single atrium |
| Zellweger syndrome | PDA, VSD, ASD |
| Fetal hydantoin syndrome | TGA, VSD, TOF |

*Conotruncal—tetralogy of Fallot, pulmonary atresia, truncus arteriosus, transposition of great arteries.
[†]VACTERL association is also known as VATER association, in which the limb anomalies are not included.
ASD, atrial septal defect; AV, atrioventricular; PDA, patent ductus arteriosus; PS, pulmonic stenosis; TGA, transposition of great vessels; TOF, tetralogy of Fallot; VSD, ventricular septal defect.

**cyanosis** and pallor. Central cyanosis (tongue, lips) is associated with arterial desaturation; isolated peripheral cyanosis (hands, feet) is associated with normal arterial saturation and increased peripheral extraction of oxygen. Perioral cyanosis is a common finding, especially in pale infants or when infants and toddlers become cold. Chronic arterial desaturation results in **clubbing** of the fingernails and toenails. Inspection of the chest may reveal asymmetry or a prominent left precordium suggesting chronic cardiac enlargement.

After inspection, **palpation** of pulses in all four extremities, the precordial activity, and the abdomen is performed. Pulses are assessed for rate, regularity, intensity, symmetry, and timing between upper and lower extremities. A good pedal pulse with normal right arm blood pressure effectively rules out coarctation of the aorta. Precordial palpation may suggest significant cardiovascular disease in the absence of obvious auscultatory findings. The precordium should be assessed for apical impulse, **point of maximum impulse**, hyperactivity, and presence of a **thrill**. Abdominal palpation assesses liver and spleen size. The liver size provides an assessment of intravascular volume and is enlarged with systemic venous congestion. The spleen may be enlarged with infective endocarditis.

**Auscultation** is the most important part of the cardiovascular examination, but should supplement what already has been found by inspection and palpation. Systematic listening in a quiet room allows assessment of each portion of the cardiac cycle. In addition to heart rate and regularity, the heart sounds, clicks, and murmurs need to be timed and characterized.

## Heart Sounds

**$S_1$** is associated with closure of the mitral and tricuspid valves, is usually single, and is best heard at the lower left sternal border (LLSB) or apex (Fig. 139-1). Although it can normally be split, if a split **$S_1$** is heard, the possibility of an ejection click or, much less commonly, an **$S_4$** should be considered. **$S_2$** is associated with closure of the aortic and pulmonary valves. It should normally split with inspiration and be single with exhalation. Abnormalities of splitting and intensity of the pulmonary component are associated with significant anatomic and physiologic abnormalities (Table 139-3). **$S_3$** is heard in early diastole and is related to rapid ventricular filling. It is best heard at the LLSB or apex and may be a normal sound. A loud $S_3$ is abnormal and heard in conditions with dilated ventricles. **$S_4$** occurs late in diastole just before $S_1$, is best heard at the LLSB/apex, and is associated with decreased ventricular compliance. It is rare and is always abnormal.

## Clicks

A click implies a valvular abnormality or dilated great artery. It may be ejection or midsystolic in timing and may or may not be associated with a murmur. A midsystolic click is associated with mitral valve prolapse. **Ejection clicks** occur early in systole. Pulmonary ejection clicks are best heard at the left upper sternal border and vary in intensity with respiration. Aortic clicks are often louder at the apex, left midsternal border, or right upper sternal border and do not vary with respiration.

## Murmurs

Murmur evaluation should determine timing, duration, location, intensity, radiation, and frequency or pitch of the murmur. The timing is most important in determining a murmur's significance and can be used to develop a differential diagnosis and determine the need for further evaluation (see Fig. 139-1). Murmurs should be classified as **systolic**, **diastolic**, or **continuous**. Most murmurs are systolic and can be divided further into systolic ejection murmurs or holosystolic (also called pansystolic or regurgitant) murmurs. **Ejection murmurs** are crescendo-decrescendo with a short time between $S_1$ and the onset of the murmur (isovolumic contraction). Systolic ejection

**FIGURE 139-1**

Timing of heart murmurs. A-V, atrioventricular.

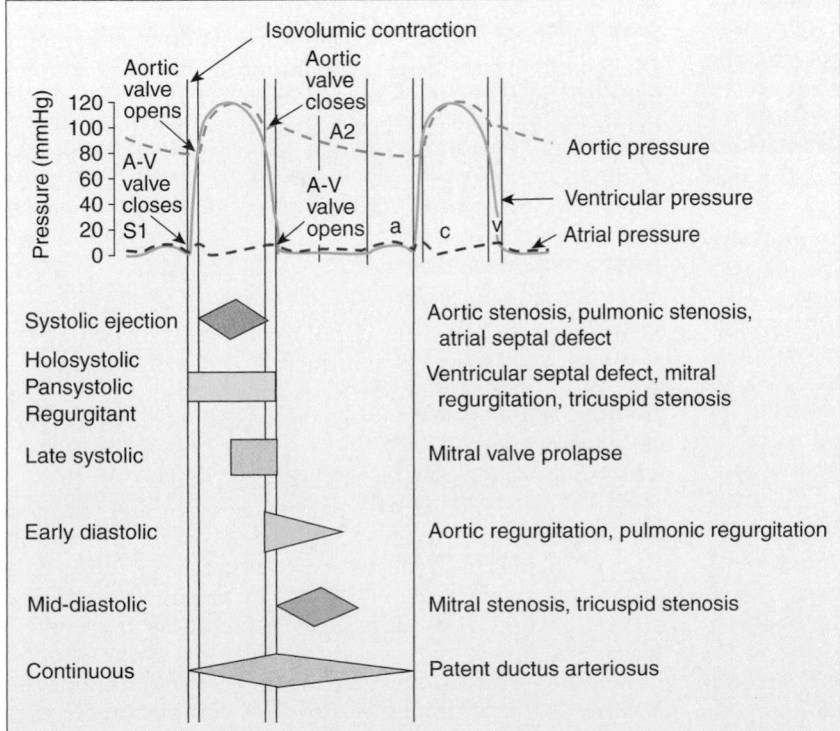

## TABLE 139-3  Abnormal Second Heart Sound

### SINGLE S₂

Pulmonary hypertension (severe)
One semilunar valve (aortic atresia, pulmonary atresia, truncus arteriosus)
Malposed great arteries (d-TGA, l-TGA)
Severe aortic stenosis

### WIDELY SPLIT S₂

Increased flow across valve (ASD, PAPVR)
Prolonged flow across valve (pulmonary stenosis)
Electrical delay (right bundle branch block)
Early aortic closure (severe mitral regurgitation)

### PARADOXICALLY SPLIT S₂

Severe aortic stenosis

### ABNORMAL INTENSITY OF P₂

Increased in pulmonary hypertension
Decreased in severe pulmonary stenosis, tetralogy of Fallot

ASD, atrial septal defect; d-TGA, dextro-transposition of the great arteries; l-TGA, levo-transposition of the great arteries; PAPVR, partial anomalous pulmonary venous return.

murmurs require the ejection of blood from the ventricle and may occur with aortic stenosis, pulmonary stenosis, atrial septal defects (ASDs), and coarctation of the aorta. **Holosystolic murmurs** have their onset with $S_1$. The murmur has a plateau quality and may be heard with ventricular septal defects (VSDs) and mitral or tricuspid regurgitation. A *late regurgitant* murmur may be heard after a midsystolic click in mitral valve prolapse.

Murmurs are often heard along the path of blood flow. Ejection murmurs usually are best heard at the base of the heart, whereas holosystolic murmurs are louder at the LLSB and apex. Pulmonary ejection murmurs radiate to the back and axilla. Aortic ejection murmurs radiate to the neck. The **intensity** or loudness of a heart murmur is assessed as grade I through VI (Table 139-4). The **frequency** or pitch of a murmur provides information regarding the pressure gradient. The higher the pressure gradient across a narrowed area (valve, vessel, or defect), the faster the flow and higher the frequency of the

## TABLE 139-4  Heart Murmur Intensity

| Grade | Description |
|---|---|
| Grade I | Very soft, heard in quiet room with cooperative patient |
| Grade II | Easily heard but not loud |
| Grade III | Loud but no thrill |
| Grade IV | Loud with palpable thrill |
| Grade V | Loud with thrill, audible with stethoscope at 45-degree angle |
| Grade VI | Loud with thrill, audible with stethoscope off chest 1 cm |

murmur. Low-frequency murmurs imply low pressure gradients and mild obstruction or less restriction to flow.

**Diastolic murmurs** are much less common than systolic murmurs, and should be considered abnormal. Early diastolic murmurs occur when there is regurgitation through the aortic or pulmonary valve. Mid-diastolic murmurs are caused by increased flow (ASD, VSD) or anatomic stenosis across the mitral or tricuspid valves.

**Continuous murmurs** are heard when there is flow through the entire cardiac cycle and are abnormal with one common exception, the **venous hum.** A PDA is the most common abnormal continuous murmur. Continuous murmurs can also be heard with coarctation of the aorta when collateral vessels are present.

Normal physiologic or **innocent murmurs** are common, occurring in at least 80% of normal infants and children. They have also been called benign, functional, vibratory, and flow murmurs. These normal murmurs are heard most often during the first 6 months of life, from 3 to 6 years of age, and in early adolescence. Characteristic findings of innocent murmurs include the quality of the sound, lack of significant radiation, and significant alteration in the intensity of the murmur with positional changes (Table 139-5). Most important, the cardiovascular history and examination are otherwise normal. The presence of symptoms, including failure to thrive or dysmorphic features should make one more cautious about diagnosing a *normal* murmur. Diastolic, holosystolic, late systolic, and continuous (except for the venous hum) murmurs and the presence of a thrill are not normal.

## LABORATORY AND IMAGING TESTS

### Pulse Oximetry

Recognizing cyanosis depends on experience and the patient's hemoglobin. Mild desaturation that is not clinically apparent may be the only early finding in complex congenital heart defects. Comparing pulse oximetry between the right arm and a lower extremity may allow diagnosis of a ductal dependent lesion in which desaturated blood flows right to left across a PDA to perfuse the lower body.

### Electrocardiography

The 12-lead electrocardiogram (ECG) provides information about the **rate, rhythm, depolarization**, and **repolarization** of the cardiac cells and the size and wall thickness of the chambers. It should be assessed for rate, rhythm, axis (P wave, QRS, and T wave), intervals (PR, QRS, QTc) (Fig. 139-2), and voltages (left atrial, right atrial, left ventricular, right ventricular) adjusted for the child's age.

The **P wave** represents atrial depolarization. A criterion for right atrial enlargement is an increase of the amplitude of the P wave, reflected best in lead II. The diagnosis of left atrial enlargement is made by prolongation of the second portion of the P wave, exhibited best in the chest leads.

The **PR interval,** measured from the beginning of the P wave to the beginning of the QRS complex, represents the time it takes for electricity to travel from the high

## TABLE 139-5 Normal or Innocent Heart Murmurs

| Murmur | Timing/Location/Quality | Usual Age at Diagnosis |
|---|---|---|
| Still's murmur/vibratory murmur | Systolic ejection murmur<br>LLSB or between LLSB and apex<br>Grades I–III/VI<br>Vibratory, musical quality<br>Intensity decreases in upright position | 3–6 yr |
| Venous hum | Continuous murmur<br>Infraclavicular region (right > left)<br>Grades I–III/VI<br>Louder with patient in upright position<br>Changes with compression of jugular vein or turning head | 3–6 yr |
| Carotid bruit | Systolic ejection murmur<br>Neck, over carotid artery<br>Grade Is–III/VI | Any age |
| Adolescent ejection murmur | Systolic ejection murmur<br>LUSB<br>Grades I–III/VI<br>Usually softer in upright position<br>Does not radiate to back | 8–14 yr |
| Peripheral pulmonary stenosis | Systolic ejection murmur<br>Axilla and back, LUSB/RUSB<br>Grades I–II/VI<br>Harsh, short, high-frequency | Newborn–6 mo |

LLSB, left lower scapular border; LUSB, left upper scapular border; RUSB, right upper scapular border.

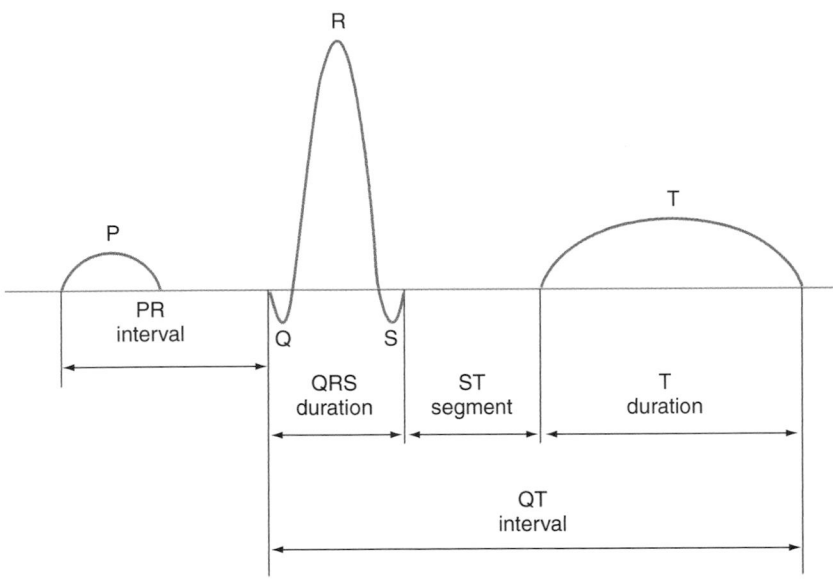

**FIGURE 139-2**

Nomenclature of electrocardiogram (ECG) waves and intervals.

right atrium to the ventricular myocardium. The PR interval increases with age. Conduction time is shortened when the conduction velocity is increased (glycogen storage disease) or when the atrioventricular node is bypassed (Wolff-Parkinson-White syndrome). A prolonged PR interval usually indicates slow conduction through the atrioventricular node. Diseases in the atrial myocardium, bundle of His, or Purkinje system may also contribute to prolonged PR intervals.

The **QRS complex** represents ventricular depolarization. A specific sequence of activation can be observed on the ECG. A greater ventricular volume or mass causes a greater magnitude of the complex. The proximity of the right ventricle to the chest surface accentuates that ventricle's contribution to the complex. Changes in the normal ECG occur with age. Normative data for each age group must be known to make a diagnosis from the ECG.

The **QT interval** is measured from the beginning of the QRS complex to the end of the T wave. The corrected QT interval (corrected for rate) should be less than 0.45 second ($QTc = QT/\sqrt{\text{preceding R to R interval}}$). The interval may be prolonged in children with hypocalcemia or severe hypokalemia. It is also prolonged in a group of children at risk for severe ventricular arrhythmias and sudden death (**prolonged QT syndrome**). Drugs such as quinidine and erythromycin may prolong the QT interval.

## Chest Radiography

A systematic approach to reading a chest radiograph includes assessment of extracardiac structures, the shape and size of the heart, and the size and position of the pulmonary artery and aorta (Fig. 139-3). Abnormalities of the thoracic skeleton, diaphragms, lungs, or upper abdomen may be associated with congenital heart defects. Assessment of the location and size of the heart and **cardiac silhouette** may suggest a cardiac defect. On a good inspiratory film, the cardiothoracic ratio should be less than 55% in infants under 1 year of age and less than 50% in older children and adolescents. An enlarged heart may be due to an increased volume load (left-right shunt) or due to myocardial dysfunction (dilated cardiomyopathy). A normal heart size virtually rules out heart failure; however, a large heart is not diagnostic of heart failure. The shape of the heart may suggest specific congenital heart defects. The most common examples are the *boot-shaped* heart seen with tetralogy of Fallot, the *egg-on-a-string* seen with dextroposed transposition of the great arteries, and the "snowman" seen with supracardiac total anomalous pulmonary venous return. The chest x-ray can aid in the assessment of **pulmonary blood flow**. Defects associated with left-to-right shunting have increased pulmonary blood flow (*shunt vascularity*) on x-ray. Right-to-left shunts have decreased pulmonary blood flow.

## Echocardiography

Echocardiography has become the most important noninvasive tool in the diagnosis and management of cardiac disease. Using ultrasound, two-dimensional echocardiography provides a full anatomic evaluation in most congenital heart defects (Fig. 139-4). Physiologic data on the direction of blood flow can be obtained with the use of pulsed, continuous wave, and color flow Doppler. Imaging from multiple views provides an assessment of spatial relationships. Three-dimensional (3D) and four-dimensional (4D) imaging now allows reconstruction of the heart and manipulation of the images to provide more detail, especially with regard to valve structure and function. Prenatal or fetal echocardiography can diagnose congenital heart disease by 18 weeks of gestation and allows for delivery of the infant at a tertiary care hospital, improving the timeliness of therapy. Many congenital heart defects now are surgically repaired based on the echocardiogram without need for cardiac catheterization.

Transesophageal echocardiography (TEE) provides better imaging when transthoracic imaging is inadequate. It is used intraoperatively to assess results and cardiac function after surgery. TEE and intracardiac echocardiography are used to guide interventional catheterization and radiofrequency ablation of dysrhythmias.

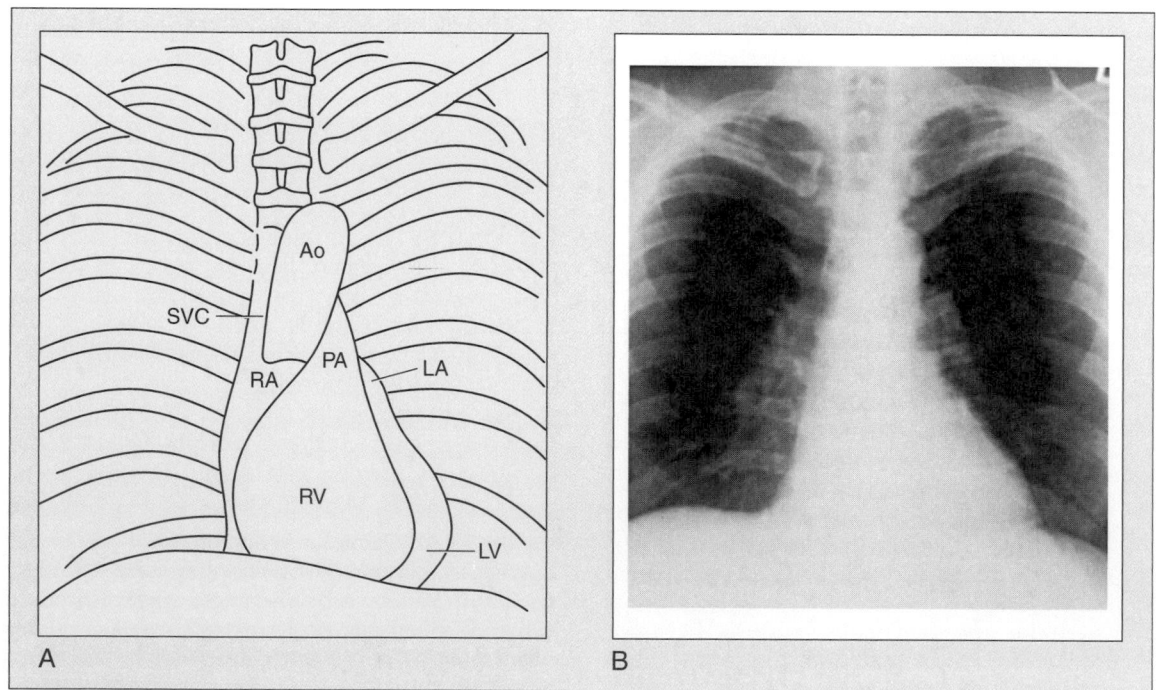

**FIGURE 139-3**

**A,** Parts of the heart whose outlines can be identified on a routine chest x-ray. **B,** Routine posteroanterior x-ray of the normal cardiac silhouette. Ao, aorta; LA, left atrium; LV, left ventricle; PA, pulmonary artery; RA, right atrium; RV, right ventricle; SVC, superior vena cava. (From Andreoli TE, Carpenter CCJ, Plum F, et al [eds]: Cecil Essentials of Medicine, 2nd ed. Philadelphia, *WB Saunders*, 1990.)

and pulmonary blood flow and systemic and pulmonary vascular resistance. Angiography is performed by injecting contrast material into selected sites to define anatomy and supplement noninvasive information. An increasing percentage of cardiac catheterizations are done to perform an intervention including balloon dilation of stenotic valves and vessels, ballooning and stenting of stenotic lesions, closure of collateral vessels by coil embolization, and device closure of PDAs, secundum ASDs, patent foramen ovales, and muscular VSDs. Catheterization with electrophysiologic studies allows for precise mapping of the electrical activity, can assess the risk of abnormal heart rhythms, and often are done in anticipation of radiofrequency ablation. Radiofrequency ablation alters the site of a dysrhythmia so that it no longer can cause the dysrhythmia.

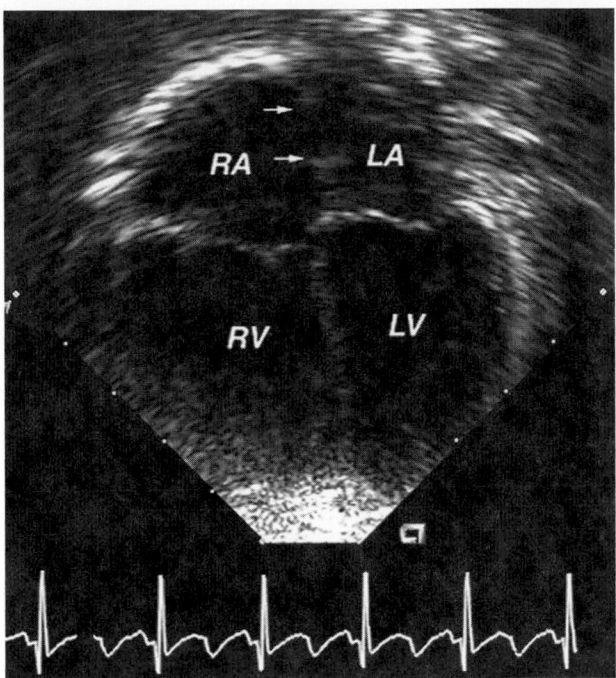

**FIGURE 139-4**

**Four-chamber echocardiogram of an atrial septal defect.** The defect margins are identified by the two arrows. LA, left atrium; LV, left ventricle; RA, right atrium; RV, right ventricle.

## Cardiac Catheterization

Cardiac catheterization is performed in patients who need additional anatomic information or precise hemodynamic information before operating or establishing a management plan. Pressures, oxygen saturations, and oxygen content are measured in each chamber and blood vessel entered (Fig. 139-5). This information is used to calculate systemic

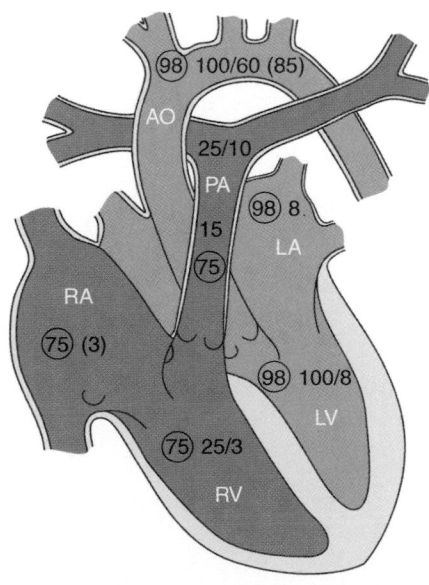

**FIGURE 139-5**

**The normal heart.** AO, aorta; LA, left atrium; LV, left ventricle; PA, pulmonary artery; RA, right atrium; RV, right ventricle. Circled values are oxygen saturations.

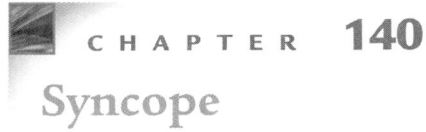

CHAPTER **140**

# Syncope

## ETIOLOGY

Syncope is the transient loss of consciousness and muscle tone that, by history, does not suggest other altered states of consciousness. Presyncope or near-syncope has many or all of the prodromal symptoms without loss of consciousness. Syncope is relatively common (Table 140-1). The frequency of episodes, amount of stress, and functional impairment caused by syncope vary. Most syncopal events are relatively benign, but can represent a serious cardiac condition that may lead to death.

## CLINICAL MANIFESTATIONS

**Typical syncopal events** usually occur in the upright position or are related to changing position. Syncope may be associated with anxiety, pain, blood drawing or the sight of blood, fasting, a hot environment, or crowded places. The patient often appears pale. A prodrome, consisting of *dizziness*, lightheadedness, nausea, diaphoresis, visual changes (blacking out), or possibly palpitations, warns the patient and often prevents injury. Unconsciousness lasts for less than 1 minute. A return to normal consciousness occurs relatively quickly. Most of these syncopal episodes are vasovagal or neurocardiogenic in origin. The physical examination is normal.

## DIAGNOSTIC STUDIES

Depending on the number, frequency, and amount of functional impairment, syncopal episodes may require no more than reassurance to the patient and family. If the episodes have a significant impact on daily activities, further evaluation may be indicated. An electrocardiogram (ECG) should be obtained with attention to the QTc and PR intervals (see Chapter 139). Although reassurance and increasing fluid and salt intake may be adequate to treat most cases of syncope, medical management is sometimes indicated.

**TABLE 140-1 Syncope and Dizziness: Etiology**

| Diagnosis | History | Signs/Symptoms | Description | Heart Rate/ Blood Pressure | Duration | Postsyncope | Recurrence |
|---|---|---|---|---|---|---|---|
| Neurocardiogenic (vasodepressor) | At rest | Pallor, nausea, visual changes | Brief ± convulsion | ↓/↓ | <1 min | Residual pallor, sweaty, hot; recurs if child stands | Common |
| Other vagal Vasovagal | Needle stick | Pallor, nausea | Brief ± convulsion | ↓/↓ | <1 min | Residual pallor; may recur if child stands | Situational |
| Micturition | Postvoiding | Pallor, nausea | Brief; convulsions rare | ↓/↓ | <1 min | | (+) |
| Cough (deglutition) | Paroxysmal cough | Cough | Abrupt onset | May not change | <5 min | Fatigue or baseline | (+) |
| Carotid sinus | Tight collar, turned head | Vague, visual changes | Sudden onset, pallor | Usually ↓/↓ | <5 min | Fatigue or baseline | (+) |
| Metabolic Hypoglycemia | Fasting, insulin use | Gradual hunger | Pallor, sweating; loss of consciousness rare | No change or mild tachycardia | Variable | Relieved only by eating | (+) |
| Neuropsychiatric Hyperventilation | Anxiety | SOB, fear, claustrophobia | Agitated, hyperpneic ± Pallor | Mild ↓/↓ | <5 min | Fatigue or baseline | (+) |
| Syncopal migraine | Headache | Aura, migraine, nausea | | No change | <10 min | Headache, often occipital | (+) |
| Seizure disorder | Anytime | ± Aura | Convulsion ± incontinence | No change or mild tachycardia | Any duration | Postictal lethargy + confusion | (+) |
| Hysterical | Always an "audience" present | Psychological distress | Gentle, graceful swoon | No change | Any duration | Normal baseline | (+) |
| Breath holding (hypoxic) | Agitation or injury | Crying | Cyanosis ± brief convulsion | ↓/↓ Frequent asystole | <10 min | Fatigue, residual pallor | (+) |

**TABLE 140-1 Syncope and Dizziness: Etiology—cont'd**

| Diagnosis | History | Signs/Symptoms | Description | Heart Rate/ Blood Pressure | Duration | Postsyncope | Recurrence |
|---|---|---|---|---|---|---|---|
| Cardiac syncope | | | | | | | |
| LVOT obstruction | Exercise | ± Chest pain, SOB | Abrupt during or after exertion, pallor | ↑/↓ | Any duration | Fatigue, residual pallor, and sweating | (+) |
| Pulmonary hypertension | Any time, especially exercise | SOB | Cyanosis and pallor | ↑/↓ | Any duration | Fatigue, residual cyanosis | (+) |
| Myocarditis | Post-viral infection exercise | SOB, chest pain, palpitations | Pallor | ↑/↓ | Any duration | Fatigue | (+) |
| Tumor or mass | Recumbent, paroxysmal | SOB ± chest pain | Pallor | ↑/↓ | Any duration | Baseline | (+) |
| Coronary artery disease | Exercise | SOB ± chest pain | Pallor | ↑/↓ | Any duration | Fatigue, chest pain | (+) |
| Dysrhythmia | Any time | Palpitations ± chest pain | Pallor | ↑ or ↑/↓ | Usually <10 min | Fatigue or baseline | (+) |

LVOT, left ventricular outflow tract; SOB, shortness of breath; ±, with or without; (+), yes but not consistent or predictable.
From Lewis DA: Syncope and dizziness. In Kliegman RM (ed): Practical Strategies in Pediatric Diagnosis and Therapy. Philadelphia, *WB Saunders*, 1996.

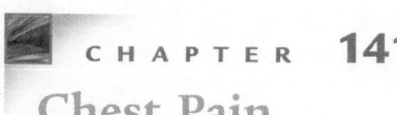

# CHAPTER 141
# Chest Pain

## ETIOLOGY

Chest pain in the pediatric patient often generates a significant amount of patient and parental concern. Although chest pain is rarely cardiac in origin in children, common knowledge about atherosclerotic heart disease

---

**TABLE 141-1  Differential Diagnosis of Pediatric Chest Pain**

### COMMON

Musculoskeletal
  Costochondritis
  Trauma or muscle overuse/strain
Pulmonary
  Asthma (often exercise-induced)
  Severe cough
  Pneumonia
Gastrointestinal
  Reflux esophagitis
Psychogenic
  Anxiety, hyperventilation
Miscellaneous
  Precordial catch syndrome (Texidor's twinge)
  Sickle cell vaso-occlusive crisis
  Idiopathic

### UNCOMMON/RARE

Cardiac
  Ischemia (coronary artery abnormalities, severe AS or PS, HOCM, cocaine)
  Infection/inflammation (myocarditis, pericarditis, Kawasaki disease)
  Dysrhythmia
  Mitral valve prolapse
Musculoskeletal
  Abnormalities of rib cage/thoracic spine
  Tietze syndrome
  Slipping rib
  Tumor
Pulmonary
  Pleurisy
  Pneumothorax, pneumomediastinum
  Pleural effusion
  Pulmonary embolism
Gastrointestinal
  Esophageal foreign body
  Esophageal spasm
Psychogenic
  Conversion symptoms
  Somatization disorders
  Depression

---

AS, aortic stenosis; HOCM, hypertrophic obstructive cardiomyopathy; PS, pulmonary stenosis.

---

raises concerns about a child experiencing chest pain. Most diagnosable chest pain in childhood is musculoskeletal in origin. A significant amount remains idiopathic; however. Knowledge of the complete differential diagnosis is necessary to make an accurate assessment (Table 141-1).

## CLINICAL MANIFESTATIONS

Assessment of a patient with chest pain includes a thorough history to determine activity at the onset; the location, radiation, quality, and duration of the pain; what makes the pain better and worse during the time that it is present; and any associated symptoms. A family history and assessment of how much anxiety the symptom is causing are important and often revealing. Although the history alone often determines the etiology, a careful general physical examination should focus on the chest wall, heart, lungs, and abdomen. A history of chest pain associated with exertion, syncope, or palpitations, or acute onset associated with fever suggests a cardiac etiology. Cardiac causes of chest pain are generally ischemic, inflammatory, or arrhythmic in origin.

## DIAGNOSTIC STUDIES

Tests rarely are indicated based on the history. A chest x-ray, electrocardiogram (ECG), 24-hour Holter monitoring, echocardiogram, and exercise stress testing may be obtained based on history and examination. Referral to a pediatric cardiologist is based on the history, physical examination findings, family history, and frequently the level of anxiety in the patient or family members regarding the pain.

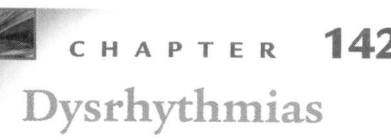

# CHAPTER 142
# Dysrhythmias

## ETIOLOGY AND DIFFERENTIAL DIAGNOSIS

Cardiac dysrhythmias or abnormal heart rhythms are uncommon in pediatrics, but may be caused by infection and inflammation, structural lesions, metabolic abnormalities, and intrinsic conduction abnormalities (Table 142-1). Many pediatric dysrhythmias are normal variants that do not require treatment or even further evaluation.

**Sinus rhythm** originates in the sinus node and has a normal axis P wave (upright in leads I and AVF) preceding each QRS complex. Because normal rates vary with age, sinus bradycardia and sinus tachycardia are defined based on age. **Sinus arrhythmia** is a common finding in children and represents a normal variation in the heart rate associated with breathing. The heart rate increases with inspiration and decreases with expiration, producing a recurring pattern on the electrocardiogram (ECG) tracing. Sinus arrhythmia does not require further evaluation or treatment.

## TABLE 142-1 Etiology of Dysrhythmias

### DRUGS

Intoxication (cocaine, tricyclic antidepressants, and others)
Antiarrhythmic agents (proarrhythmic agents [quinidine])
Sympathomimetic agents (caffeine, theophylline, ephedrine, and others)
Digoxin

### INFECTION AND POSTINFECTION

Endocarditis
Lyme disease
Diphtheria
Myocarditis
Guillain-Barré syndrome
Rheumatic fever

### METABOLIC-ENDOCRINE

Cardiomyopathy
Electrolyte disturbances ($\downarrow\uparrow K^+$, $\downarrow\uparrow Ca^{2+}$, $\downarrow Mg^{2+}$)
Uremia
Thyrotoxicosis
Pheochromocytoma
Porphyria
Mitochondrial myopathies

### STRUCTURAL LESIONS

Mitral valve prolapse
Ventricular tumor
Ventriculotomy
Pre-excitation and aberrant conduction system (Wolff-Parkinson-White syndrome)
Congenital heart defects
Arrhythmogenic right ventricle (dysplasia)

### OTHER CAUSES

Adrenergic-induced
Prolonged QT interval
Maternal SLE
Idiopathic
Central venous catheter

SLE, systemic lupus erythematosus.

## Atrial Dysrhythmias

A **wandering atrial pacemaker** is a change in the morphology of the P waves with variable PR interval and normal QRS complex. This is a benign finding, requiring no further evaluation or treatment.

**Premature atrial contractions** are relatively common prenatally and in infants. A premature P wave, usually with an abnormal axis consistent with its ectopic origin, is present. The premature atrial activity may be blocked (no QRS following it), conducted normally (normal QRS present), or conducted aberrantly (a widened, altered QRS complex). Premature atrial contractions are usually benign and, if present around the time of delivery, often disappear during the first few weeks of life.

**Atrial flutter** and **atrial fibrillation** are uncommon dysrhythmias in pediatrics and usually present after surgical repair of complex congenital heart disease. They may also be seen in patients with myocarditis or in association with drug toxicity.

**Supraventricular tachycardia** (SVT) is the most common symptomatic dysrhythmia in pediatric patients. The rhythm has a rapid, regular rate with a narrow QRS complex. SVT in infants is often 280 to 300 beats/minute with slower rates for older children and adolescents. The tachycardia has an abrupt onset and termination. In a child with a structurally normal heart, most episodes are relatively asymptomatic other than a pounding heart beat. If there is structural heart disease or the episode is prolonged (>12 hours), there may be alteration in the cardiac output and development of symptoms of heart failure. Although most patients with SVT have structurally normal hearts and normal baseline ECGs, some children have Wolff-Parkinson-White syndrome or pre-excitation as the cause of the dysrhythmia.

## Ventricular Dysrhythmias

**Premature ventricular contractions** (PVCs) are less common than premature atrial contractions in infancy but more common in older children and adolescents (Table 142-2). The premature beat is not preceded by a P wave and the QRS complex is wide and bizarre. If the heart is structurally normal, and the PVCs are singleton, uniform in focus, and disappear with increased heart rate, the PVCs are usually benign and require no treatment. Any deviation from the presentation (history of syncope or a family history of sudden death) requires further investigation and possibly treatment with antiarrhythmic medications.

**Ventricular tachycardia,** defined as three or more consecutive PVCs, is also relatively rare in pediatric patients. Although there are multiple causes of ventricular tachycardia, it usually is a sign of serious cardiac dysfunction or disease. Rapid rate ventricular tachycardia results in decreased cardiac output and cardiovascular instability. Treatment in symptomatic patients is synchronized cardioversion. Medical management with lidocaine or amiodarone may be appropriate in a conscious asymptomatic patient. Complete evaluation of the etiologic picture is necessary, including electrophysiologic study.

## Heart Block

**First-degree heart block** is the presence of a prolonged PR interval. It is asymptomatic and when present in otherwise normal children requires no evaluation or treatment. **Second-degree heart block** is when some, but not all, of the P waves are followed by a QRS complex. Mobitz type I (also known as Wenckebach) is characterized by a progressive prolongation of the PR interval until a QRS complex is dropped. It is often seen during sleep, usually does not progress to other forms of heart block, and does not require further evaluation or treatment in otherwise normal children. Mobitz type II is present when the PR interval does not change, but a QRS is intermittently dropped. This form may progress to complete heart block and may require pacemaker placement. **Third-degree heart**

| TABLE 142-2 Dysrhythmias in Children | | |
|---|---|---|
| **Type** | **ECG Characteristics** | **Treatment** |
| Supraventricular tachycardia | Rate usually >200 beats/min (range, 180–320 beats/min); abnormal atrial rate for age; ventricular rate may be slower because of AV block; P waves usually present and are related to QRS complex; normal QRS complexes unless aberrant conduction is present | Increase vagal tone (bag of ice water to face, Valsalva maneuver); adenosine; digoxin; sotalol; electrical cardioversion if acutely ill; catheter ablation |
| Atrial flutter | Atrial rate usually 300 beats/min, with varying degrees of block; sawtooth flutter waves | Digoxin, sotalol, cardioversion |
| Premature ventricular contraction | Premature, wide, unusually shaped QRS complex, with large inverted T wave | None if normal heart and if premature ventricular contractions disappear on exercise; lidocaine, procainamide |
| Ventricular tachycardia | ≥3 Premature ventricular beats; AV dissociation; fusion beats, blocked retrograde AV conduction; sustained if > 30 sec; rate 120–240 beats/min | Lidocaine, procainamide, propranolol, amiodarone, cardioversion |
| Ventricular fibrillation | No distinct QRS complex or T waves; irregular undulations with varied amplitude and contour, no conducted pulse | Nonsynchronized cardioversion |
| Complete heart block | Atria and ventricles have independent pacemakers; AV dissociation; escape-pacemaker is at atrioventricular junction if congenital | Awake rate < 55 beats/min in neonate or < 40 beats/min in adolescent or hemodynamic instability requires permanent pacemaker |
| First-degree heart block | Prolonged PR interval for age | Observe, obtain digoxin level if on therapy |
| Mobitz type I (Wenckebach) second-degree heart block | Progressive lengthening of PR interval until P wave is not followed by conducted QRS complex | Observe, correct underlying electrolyte or other abnormalities |
| Mobitz type II second-degree heart block | Sudden nonconduction of P wave with loss of QRS complex without progressive PR interval lengthening | Consider pacemaker |
| Sinus tachycardia | Rate < 240 beats/min | Treat fever, remove sympathomimetic drugs |

AV, atrioventricular; ECG, electrocardiogram.

**block**, whether congenital or acquired, is present when there is no relationship between atrial and ventricular activity. The ventricular rate is much slower than the atrial rate. **Congenital complete heart block** is associated with maternal collagen vascular disease (systemic lupus erythematosus) or congenital heart disease. The acquired form most often occurs after cardiac surgery, but may be secondary to infection, inflammation, or drugs.

## TREATMENT

Most atrial dysrhythmias require no intervention. Treatment of SVT depends on presentation and symptoms. Acute treatment of SVT in infants usually consists of **vagal maneuvers**, such as application of cold (ice bag) to the face. Intravenous (IV) **adenosine** usually converts the dysrhythmia because the atrioventricular node forms a part of the reentry circuit in most patients with SVT. In patients with cardiovascular compromise at the time

of presentation, **synchronized cardioversion** is indicated using 1 to 2 J/kg. In patients with palpitations, it is important to document heart rate and rhythm during their symptoms before considering therapeutic options. The frequency, length, and associated symptoms during the episodes, as well as what is required to convert the rhythm, determine the need for treatment. Some patients require only education regarding the dysrhythmia and follow-up. Ongoing pharmacologic management with either digoxin or a β-blocker is usually the first choice. However, digoxin is contraindicated in patients with Wolff-Parkinson-White syndrome. Additional antiarrhythmic medications rarely may be needed. In patients who are symptomatic or those not wanting to take daily medications, **radiofrequency ablation** may be performed.

A variety of antiarrhythmic agents are used to treat ventricular dysrhythmias that require intervention (Table 142-3). Management of third-degree heart block depends on the ventricular rate and presence of symptoms. Treatment, if needed, often requires placement of a pacemaker.

**TABLE 142-3  Classification of Drugs for Antiarrhythmia**

| Class | Action | Example(s) |
|---|---|---|
| I | Depression of phase of depolarization (velocity of upstroke of action potential); sodium channel blockade | |
| Ia | Prolongation of QRS complex and QT interval | Quinidine, procainamide, disopyramide |
| Ib | Significant effect on abnormal conduction | Lidocaine, mexiletine, phenytoin, tocainide |
| Ic | Prolongation of QRS complex and PR interval | Flecainide, propafenone, moricizine? |
| II | β blockade; slowing of sinus rate; prolongation of PR interval | Propranolol, atenolol, acebutolol |
| III | Prolongation of action potential; prolongation of PR, QT intervals, QRS complex; sodium and calcium channel blockade | Bretylium, amiodarone, sotalol |
| IV | Calcium channel blockade; reduction in sinus and AV node pacemaker activity and conduction; prolongation of PR interval | Verapamil and other calcium channel blocking agents |

AV, atrioventricular.

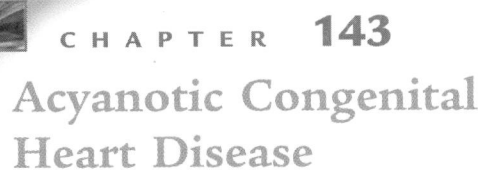

# CHAPTER 143

# Acyanotic Congenital Heart Disease

## ETIOLOGY AND EPIDEMIOLOGY

Congenital heart disease occurs in 8 per 1000 births. The spectrum of lesions ranges from asymptomatic to fatal. Although most cases of congenital heart disease are multifactorial, some lesions are associated with chromosomal disorders, single gene defects, teratogens, or maternal metabolic disease (see Table 139-2).

Congenital heart defects can be divided into three pathophysiologic groups (Table 143-1):

1. Left-to-right shunts
2. Right-to-left shunts
3. Obstructive stenotic lesions

Acyanotic congenital heart disease includes left-to-right shunts resulting in an increase in pulmonary blood flow (patent ductus arteriosus [PDA], ventricular septal defect [VSD], atrial septal defect [ASD]) and obstructive lesions (aortic stenosis, pulmonary stenosis, coarctation of the aorta), which usually have normal pulmonary blood flow.

## VENTRICULAR SEPTAL DEFECT

### Etiology and Epidemiology

The ventricular septum is a complex structure that can be divided into four components. The largest component is the **muscular septum**. The inlet or posterior septum comprises **endocardial cushion tissue**. The subarterial or **supracristal septum** comprises conotruncal tissue. The **membranous septum** is below the aortic valve and is relatively small. VSDs occur when any of these components fails to develop normally (Fig. 143-1). VSD, the most common congenital heart defect, accounts for 25% of all congenital heart disease. **Perimembranous VSDs** are the most common of all VSDs (67%).

Although the location of the VSD is important prognostically and in approach to repair, the amount of flow crossing a VSD depends on the size of the defect and the pulmonary vascular resistance. Large VSDs are not symptomatic at birth because the pulmonary vascular resistance is normally elevated at this time. As the pulmonary vascular resistance decreases over the first 6 to 8 weeks of life the amount of shunt increases, and symptoms may develop.

**TABLE 143-1  Classification of Congenital Cardiac Defects**

| Stenotic | Shunting | | Mixing |
|---|---|---|---|
| | Right → Left | Left → Right | |
| Aortic stenosis | Tetralogy | Patent ductus arteriosus | Truncus |
| Pulmonary stenosis | Transposition | Ventricular septal defect | TAPVR |
| Coarctation of the aorta | Tricuspid atresia | Atrial septal defect | HLH |

HLH, hypoplastic left heart syndrome; TAPVR, total anomalous pulmonary venous return.

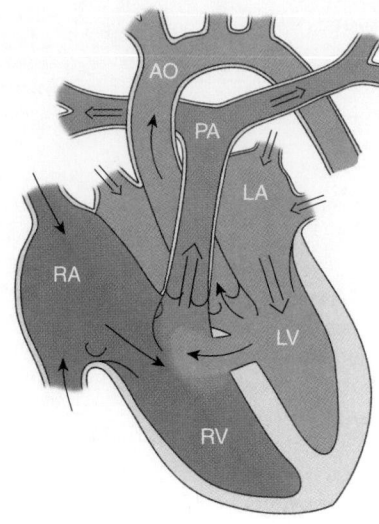

**FIGURE 143-1**

**Ventricular septal defect.** AO, aorta; LA, left atrium; LV, left ventricle; PA, pulmonary artery; RA, right atrium; RV, right ventricle.

## Clinical Manifestations

The size of the VSD affects the clinical presentation. Small VSDs with little shunt are often asymptomatic but have a loud murmur. Moderate to large VSDs result in pulmonary overcirculation and heart failure, presenting as fatigue, diaphoresis with feedings, and poor growth. The typical physical finding with a VSD is a **pansystolic murmur**, usually heard best at the lower left sternal border. There may be a thrill. Large shunts increase flow across the mitral valve causing a **mid-diastolic murmur** at the apex. The splitting of $S_2$ and intensity of $P_2$ depend on the pulmonary artery pressure.

## Imaging Studies

Electrocardiogram (ECG) and chest x-ray findings depend on the size of the VSD. Small VSDs usually have normal studies. Larger VSDs cause volume overload to the left side of the heart, resulting in ECG findings of left atrial and ventricular enlargement and hypertrophy. A chest x-ray may reveal cardiomegaly, enlargement of the left ventricle, an increase in the pulmonary artery silhouette, and increased pulmonary blood flow. Pulmonary hypertension due to either increased flow or increased pulmonary vascular resistance may lead to right ventricular enlargement and hypertrophy.

## Treatment

Approximately one third of all VSDs close spontaneously. Small VSDs usually close spontaneously and, if they do not close, surgical closure may not be required. Initial treatment for moderate to large VSDs includes **diuretics, digoxin,** and **afterload reduction.** Continued poor growth or pulmonary hypertension despite therapy requires closure of the defect. Most VSDs are closed surgically, but some VSDs, especially muscular defects, can be closed with **devices** placed at cardiac catheterization.

## ATRIAL SEPTAL DEFECT

### Etiology and Epidemiology

During the embryologic development of the heart, a septum grows toward the endocardial cushions to divide the atria. Failure of septal growth or excessive reabsorption of tissue leads to ASDs (Fig. 143-2). ASDs represent approximately 10% of all congenital heart defects. A secundum defect, with the hole in the region of the foramen ovale, is the most common ASD. A **primum ASD**, located near the endocardial cushions, may be part of a complete atrioventricular canal defect or may be present with an intact ventricular septum. The least common ASD is the **sinus venosus defect**, which may be associated with anomalous pulmonary venous return.

### Clinical Manifestations

Regardless of the site of the ASD, the pathophysiology and amount of shunting depend on the size of the defect and the relative compliance of the both ventricles. Even with large ASDs and significant shunts, infants and children are rarely symptomatic. A prominent **right ventricular impulse** at the left lower sternal border (LLSB) often can be palpated. A soft (grade I or II) **systolic ejection murmur** in the region of the right ventricular outflow tract and a **fixed split $S_2$** (due to overload of the right ventricle with prolonged ejection into the pulmonary circuit) are often audible. A larger shunt may result in a mid-diastolic murmur at the left lower sternal border as a result of the increased volume passing across the tricuspid valve.

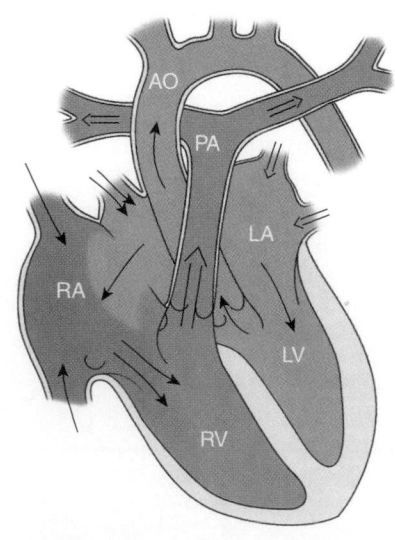

**FIGURE 143-2**

**Atrial septal defect.** AO, aorta; LA, left atrium; LV, left ventricle; PA, pulmonary artery; RA, right atrium; RV, right ventricle.

## Imaging Studies

ECG and chest x-ray findings reflect the **increased blood flow** through the right atrium, right ventricle, pulmonary arteries, and lungs. The ECG may show **right axis deviation** and **right ventricular enlargement**. A chest radiograph may show cardiomegaly, right atrial enlargement, and a prominent pulmonary artery.

## Treatment

Medical management is rarely indicated. If a significant shunt is still present at around 3 years of age, closure is usually recommended. Many secundum ASDs can be closed with an ASD **closure device** in the catheterization laboratory. Primum and sinus venosus defects require **surgical closure**.

## PATENT DUCTUS ARTERIOSUS

### Etiology and Epidemiology

The ductus arteriosus allows blood to flow from the pulmonary artery to the aorta during fetal life. Failure of the normal closure of this vessel results in a PDA (Fig. 143-3). With a falling pulmonary vascular resistance after birth, left-to-right shunting of blood and increased pulmonary blood flow occur. Excluding premature infants, PDAs represent approximately 5% to 10% of congenital heart disease.

### Clinical Manifestations

Symptoms depend on the amount of pulmonary blood flow. The magnitude of the shunt depends on the size of the PDA (diameter, length, and tortuosity) and the pulmonary vascular resistance. Small PDAs are asymptomatic; moderate to large shunts can produce the symptoms of heart failure as the pulmonary vascular resistance decreases.

The physical examination findings depend on the size of the shunt. A **widened pulse pressure** is often present as a result of the runoff of blood into the pulmonary circulation during diastole. A **continuous, machine-like murmur** can be heard at the left infraclavicular area. The murmur radiates along the pulmonary arteries and is often well heard over the left side of the back. Larger shunts with increased flow across the mitral valve may result in a mid-diastolic murmur at the apex and a **hyperdynamic precordium**. Splitting of $S_2$ and intensity of $P_2$ depend on the pulmonary artery pressure. A thrill may be palpable.

### Imaging Studies

ECG and chest x-ray findings are normal with small PDAs. Moderate to large shunts may result in a **full pulmonary artery silhouette** and **increased pulmonary vascularity**. ECG findings vary from normal to evidence of left ventricular hypertrophy. If pulmonary hypertension is present, there is also right ventricular hypertrophy.

### Treatment

Spontaneous closure of a PDA after a few weeks of age is uncommon in full-term infants. Moderate and large PDAs may be managed initially with **diuretics**, but eventually require closure. Elective closure of small, hemodynamically insignificant PDAs is controversial. Most PDAs can be closed in the catheterization laboratory by either **coil embolization** or a PDA **closure device**.

## ENDOCARDIAL CUSHION DEFECT

### Etiology and Epidemiology

Endocardial cushion defects, also referred to as **atrioventricular canal defects**, may be complete or partial (Fig. 143-4). Abnormal development of the endocardial

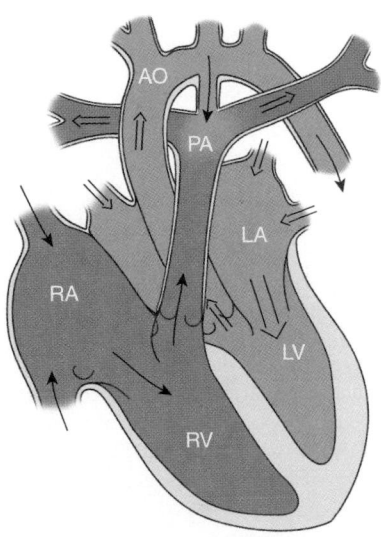

**FIGURE 143-3**

**Patent ductus arteriosus.** AO, aorta; LA, left atrium; LV, left ventricle; PA, pulmonary artery; RA, right atrium; RV, right ventricle.

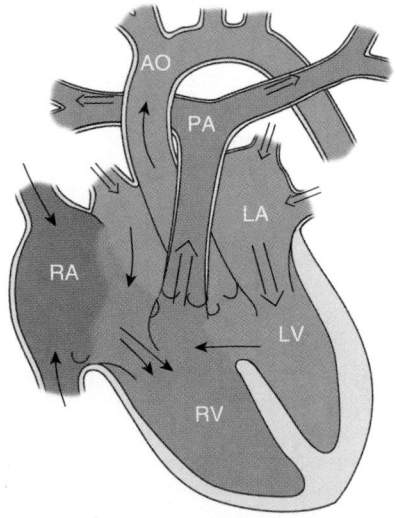

**FIGURE 143-4**

**Atrioventricular canal defects.** AO, aorta; LA, left atrium; LV, left ventricle; PA, pulmonary artery; RA, right atrium; RV, right ventricle.

cushion tissue results in failure of the septum to fuse with the endocardial cushion; this results in **abnormal atrioventricular valves** as well. The complete defect results in a primum ASD, a posterior or inlet VSD, and clefts in the anterior leaflet of the mitral and septal leaflet of the tricuspid valves. In addition to left-to-right shunting at both levels, there may be **atrioventricular valve insufficiency**.

## Clinical Manifestations

The symptoms of heart failure usually develop as the pulmonary vascular resistance decreases over the first 6 to 8 weeks of life. Symptoms may be earlier and more severe with significant atrioventricular valve insufficiency. Pulmonary hypertension resulting from increased pulmonary circulation often develops early. The presence of murmurs varies depending on the amount of shunting at both atrial and ventricular levels. If there is a large VSD component, $S_2$ will be single. Growth is usually poor. Some children with Down syndrome have complete endocardial cushion defects.

## Imaging Tests

The diagnosis usually is made with echocardiography. A chest radiograph reveals cardiomegaly with enlargement of all chambers and the presence of **increased vascularity**. An ECG reveals **left axis deviation** and **combined ventricular hypertrophy** and may show combined atrial enlargement.

## Treatment

Initial management includes diuretics (± digoxin) and afterload reduction for treatment of heart failure. **Surgical repair** of the defect ultimately is required.

# PULMONARY STENOSIS

## Etiology

Pulmonary stenosis accounts for approximately 10% of all congenital heart disease and can be **valvular, subvalvular**, or **supravalvular** in nature. Pulmonary stenosis results from the failure of the development, in early gestation, of the three leaflets of the valve, insufficient resorption of infundibular tissue, or insufficient canalization of the peripheral pulmonary arteries.

## Clinical Manifestations

Symptoms depend on the degree of obstruction present. Infants and children with mild pulmonary stenosis are asymptomatic. Moderate to severe stenosis results in **exertional dyspnea** and easy **fatigability**. Newborns with severe stenosis may be more symptomatic and even cyanotic because of right-to-left shunting at the atrial level.

Pulmonary stenosis causes a systolic ejection murmur at the second left intercostal space which radiates to the back. A thrill may be present. $S_2$ may be widely split with a quiet pulmonary component. With more severe pulmonary stenosis, an impulse at the lower left sternal border

results from **right ventricular hypertrophy**. Valvular stenosis may result in a **click** that varies with respiration. Worsening stenosis causes an increase in the duration of the murmur and a higher frequency of the sound. Murmurs of **peripheral pulmonary stenosis** vary with the location of the lesions. The systolic ejection murmur is heard distal to the obstruction along the course of blood flow in the pulmonary circulation including radiation to the back.

## Imaging Tests

ECG and chest x-ray findings are normal in mild stenosis. Moderate to severe stenosis results in **right axis deviation** and **right ventricular hypertrophy**. The heart size is usually normal on chest x-ray, although the main pulmonary artery segment may be prominent because of **poststenotic dilation of the main pulmonary artery**. Echocardiography provides assessment of the site of stenosis, degree of hypertrophy, and valve morphology and an estimate of the pressure gradient.

## Treatment

Valvular pulmonary stenosis usually does not progress, especially if it is mild. **Balloon valvuloplasty** is usually successful in reducing the gradient to acceptable levels for more significant or symptomatic stenosis. **Surgical repair** is required if balloon valvuloplasty is unsuccessful or when subvalvular (muscular) stenosis is present.

# AORTIC STENOSIS

## Etiology and Epidemiology

**Valvular, subvalvular**, or **supravalvular** aortic stenosis represents approximately 5% of all congenital heart disease. Lesions result from failure of development of the three leaflets or failure of resorption of tissue around the valve.

## Clinical Manifestations

Symptoms depend on the degree of stenosis. Mild to moderate obstructions cause no symptoms. More severe stenosis results in easy fatigability, exertional chest pain, and syncope. Infants with critical aortic stenosis may present with symptoms of heart failure.

A **systolic ejection murmur** is heard at the right second intercostal space along the sternum and radiating into the neck. The murmur increases in length and becomes higher in frequency as the degree of stenosis increases. With valvular stenosis, a **systolic ejection click** often is heard, and a thrill may be present at the right upper sternal border or in the suprasternal notch. The aortic component of $S_2$ may be decreased in intensity.

## Imaging Studies

ECG and chest x-ray findings are normal with mild degrees of stenosis. **Left ventricular hypertrophy** develops with moderate to severe stenosis and is detected on the ECG and chest x-ray. **Poststenotic dilation** of the ascending aorta or aortic knob may be seen on chest radiographs. Echocardiography shows the site of stenosis, valve morphology, and presence of left ventricular hypertrophy and allows an estimate of the pressure gradient.

## Treatment

The degree of aortic stenosis frequently progresses with growth and age. Aortic insufficiency often develops or progresses. Serial follow-up with echocardiography is indicated. **Balloon valvuloplasty** is usually the first interventional procedure for significant stenosis. It is not as successful as pulmonary balloon valvuloplasty and has a higher risk of significant valvular insufficiency. **Surgical management** is necessary when balloon valvuloplasty is unsuccessful, or significant valve insufficiency develops.

## COARCTATION OF THE AORTA

### Etiology and Epidemiology

Coarctation of the aorta occurs in approximately 10% of all congenital heart defects. It is almost always **juxtaductal** in position. During development of the aortic arch, the area near the insertion of the ductus arteriosus fails to develop correctly, resulting in a narrowing of the aortic lumen.

### Clinical Manifestations

Timing of presentation depends on the severity of obstruction and associated cardiac defects. Infants presenting with coarctation of the aorta frequently have hypoplastic aortic arches, abnormal aortic valves, and VSDs. They may be **dependent on a patent ductus arteriosus** to provide descending aortic flow. Symptoms develop when the aortic ampulla of the ductus closes. Less severe obstruction causes no symptoms because blood flow into the descending aorta is not dependent on the ductus.

Symptoms, including poor feeding, respiratory distress, and shock, may develop before 2 weeks of age. Classically the **femoral pulses** are weaker and delayed compared with the right radial pulse. The blood pressure in the lower extremities is lower than that in the upper extremities. If cardiac function is poor, however, these differences may not be as apparent until appropriate resuscitation is accomplished. In this situation, there may be no murmur, but an $S_3$ is often present.

Older children presenting with coarctation of the aorta are usually asymptomatic. There may be a history of **leg discomfort** with exercise, headache, or epistaxis. Decreased or absent lower extremity pulses, **hypertension** (upper extremity), or a murmur may be present. The murmur is typically best heard in the left interscapular area of the back. If significant collaterals have developed, continuous murmurs may be heard throughout the chest. An abnormal aortic valve is present approximately 50% of the time, causing a systolic ejection click and systolic ejection murmur of aortic stenosis.

### Imaging Studies

The ECG and chest x-ray show evidence of right ventricular hypertrophy in infantile coarctation with marked **cardiomegaly** and **pulmonary edema**. Echocardiography shows the site of coarctation and associated lesions. In older children, the ECG and chest x-ray usually show left ventricular hypertrophy and a mildly enlarged heart. **Rib notching** may also be seen in older children (>8 years of age) with large collaterals. Echocardiography shows the site and degree of coarctation, presence of left ventricular hypertrophy, and aortic valve morphology and function.

### Treatment

Management of an infant presenting with cardiac decompensation includes intravenous infusion of **prostaglandin $E_1$** (chemically opens the ductus arteriosus), inotropic agents, diuretics, and other supportive care. **Balloon angioplasty** has been done, especially in critically ill infants, but **surgical repair** of the coarctation is most commonly performed. Ballooning and stenting of older patients with coarctation has also been performed, but surgical repair remains the most common form of management.

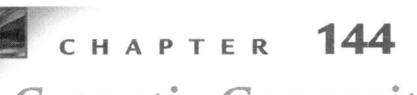

# CHAPTER 144
# Cyanotic Congenital Heart Disease

Cyanotic congenital heart disease occurs when some of the systemic venous return crosses from the right side of the heart to the left and returns to the body without going through the lungs (**right-to-left shunt**). **Cyanosis**, the visible sign of this shunt, occurs when approximately 5 g/100 mL of reduced hemoglobin is present in systemic blood. The patient's hemoglobin level determines the presentation of clinical cyanosis. A polycythemic patient appears cyanotic with a lower percentage of reduced hemoglobin. A patient with anemia requires a higher percentage of reduced hemoglobin for the recognition of cyanosis.

The most common cyanotic congenital heart defects are the five Ts:

Tetralogy of Fallot
Transposition of the great arteries
Tricuspid atresia
Truncus arteriosus
Total anomalous pulmonary venous return

Other congenital heart defects that allow complete mixing of systemic and pulmonary venous return can present with cyanosis depending on the amount of pulmonary blood flow that is present. Many cyanotic heart lesions present in the neonatal period (Table 144-1).

**TABLE 144-1 Categories of Presenting Symptoms and Signs in the Neonate**

| Symptom/Sign | Physiologic Category | Anatomic Cause | Lesion |
|---|---|---|---|
| Cyanosis with respiratory distress | Increased pulmonary blood flow | Transposition | *d*-Transposition with or without associated lesions |
| Cyanosis without respiratory distress | Decreased pulmonary blood flow | Right heart obstruction | Tricuspid atresia<br>Ebstein anomaly<br>Pulmonary atresia<br>Pulmonary stenosis<br>Tetralogy of Fallot |
| Hypoperfusion | Poor cardiac output | Left heart obstruction | Total anomalous pulmonary venous return with obstruction<br>Aortic stenosis<br>Hypoplastic left heart syndrome |
|  | Poor cardiac function | Normal anatomy | Cardiomyopathy<br>Myocarditis |
| Respiratory distress with desaturation (not visible cyanosis) | Bidirectional shunting | Complete mixing | Truncus arteriosus<br>AV canal<br>Complex single ventricle (including heterotaxias) without pulmonary stenosis |
| Respiratory distress with normal saturation | Left-to-right shunting | Simple intracardiac shunt | ASD<br>VSD<br>PDA<br>Aortopulmonary window<br>AVM |

ASD, atrial septal defect; AV, atrioventricular; AVM, arteriovenous malformation; PDA, patent ductus arteriosus; VSD, ventricular septal defect.

## TETRALOGY OF FALLOT

### Etiology and Epidemiology

Tetralogy of Fallot is the most common cyanotic congenital heart defect, representing about 10% of all congenital heart defects (Fig. 144-1). Anatomically, there are four structural defects: **ventricular septal defect (VSD), pulmonary stenosis, overriding aorta**, and **right ventricular hypertrophy.** Tetralogy of Fallot is due to abnormal septation of the truncus arteriosus into the aorta and pulmonary artery that occurs early in gestation (3–4 weeks). The VSD is large and the pulmonary stenosis is most commonly subvalvular or infundibular. It may also be valvular, supravalvular, or, frequently, a combination of levels of obstruction.

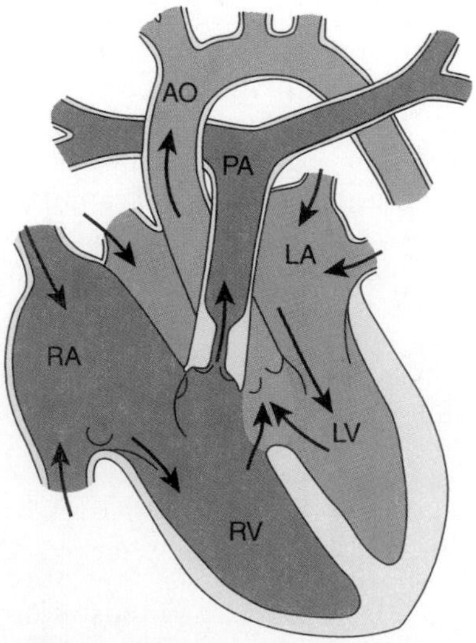

### Clinical Manifestations

The degree of cyanosis depends on the amount of pulmonary stenosis. Infants initially may be acyanotic. A **pulmonary stenosis murmur** is the usual initial abnormal finding. If the pulmonary stenosis is more severe, or as it becomes more severe over time, the amount of right-to-left shunting at the VSD increases and the patient becomes more cyanotic. With increasing severity of pulmonary stenosis, the murmur becomes shorter and softer. In addition to varying degrees of cyanosis and a murmur, a **single $S_2$** and **right ventricular impulse** at the left sternal border are typical findings.

When **hypoxic (Tet) spells** occur, they are usually progressive. During a spell, the child typically becomes restless and agitated and may cry inconsolably. An ambulatory toddler may squat. Hyperpnea occurs with gradually increasing cyanosis and loss of the murmur. In severe spells, prolonged unconsciousness and convulsions, hemiparesis, or death may occur. Independent of hypoxic spells, patients with tetralogy of Fallot are at increased risk for

**FIGURE 144-1**

**Tetralogy of Fallot.** AO, aorta; LA, left atrium; LV, left ventricle; PA, pulmonary artery; RA, right atrium; RV, right ventricle.

cerebral thromboembolism and cerebral abscesses resulting in part from their right-to-left intracardiac shunt.

## Imaging Studies

The electrocardiogram (ECG) usually has **right axis deviation** and **right ventricular hypertrophy**. The classic chest x-ray finding is a **boot-shaped heart** created by the small main pulmonary artery and upturned apex secondary to right ventricular hypertrophy. Echocardiography shows the anatomic features, including the levels of pulmonary stenosis, and provides quantification of the degree of stenosis. Coronary anomalies, most commonly a left anterior descending coronary artery crossing the anterior surface of the right ventricular outflow tract, are present in 5% of patients with tetralogy of Fallot.

## Treatment

The natural history of tetralogy of Fallot is progression of pulmonary stenosis and cyanosis. Treatment of hypoxic spells consists of oxygen administration (although this has minimal benefit) and placing the child in the knee-chest position (to increase venous return). Traditionally, giving morphine sulfate (to relax the pulmonary infundibulum and for sedation) is given. If necessary, the systemic vascular resistance can be increased acutely through the administration of an α-adrenergic agonist (phenylephrine). The occurrence of a cyanotic spell is an indication to proceed with surgical repair.

**Complete surgical repair** with VSD closure and removal or patching of the pulmonary stenosis can be performed in infancy. Occasionally, **palliative shunt surgery** between the subclavian artery and pulmonary artery is performed for complex forms of tetralogy of Fallot and more complete repair is done at a later time. **Subacute bacterial endocarditis prophylaxis** is indicated until 6 months after complete repair unless there is a residual VSD. Prophylaxis is then continued as long as there is a residual VSD.

## TRANSPOSITION OF THE GREAT ARTERIES

### Etiology and Epidemiology

Although dextroposed transposition of the great arteries represents only about 5% of congenital heart defects, it is the most common cyanotic lesion to present in the newborn period (Fig. 144-2). Transposition of the great arteries is ventriculoarterial discordance secondary to abnormalities of septation of the truncus arteriosus. In dextroposed transposition, the aorta arises from the right ventricle, anterior and to the right of the pulmonary artery, which arises from the left ventricle. This results in desaturated blood returning to the right side of the heart and being pumped back out to the body, while well-oxygenated blood returning from the lungs enters the left side of the heart and is pumped back to the lungs. Without mixing of the two circulations, death occurs quickly. Mixing can occur at the atrial (patent foramen ovale/atrial septal defect [ASD]), ventricular [VSD], or great vessel (patent ductus arteriosus [PDA]) level.

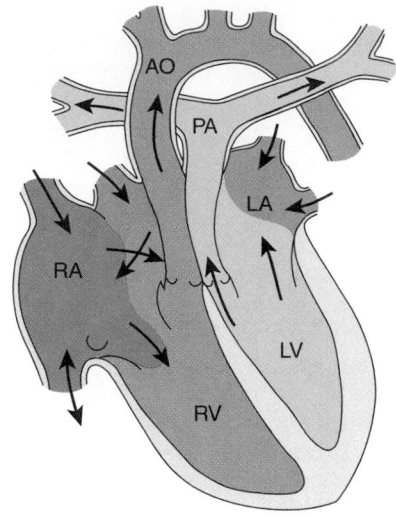

**FIGURE 144-2**

**Transposition of the great vessels.** AO, aorta; LA, left atrium; LV, left ventricle; PA, pulmonary artery; RA, right atrium; RV, right ventricle.

## Clinical Manifestations

A history of **cyanosis** is always present, although it depends on the amount of mixing. **Quiet tachypnea** and a **single S₂** are typically present. If the ventricular septum is intact, there may be no murmur.

Children with transposition and a large VSD have improved intracardiac mixing and less cyanosis. They may present with signs of heart failure. The heart is hyperdynamic, with palpable left and right ventricular impulses. A loud VSD murmur is heard. S₂ is single.

## Imaging Studies

ECG findings typically include **right axis deviation** and **right ventricular hypertrophy**. The chest x-ray reveals **increased pulmonary vascularity**, and the cardiac shadow is classically an **egg on a string** created by the narrow superior mediastinum. Echocardiography shows the transposition of the great arteries, the sites and amount of mixing, and any associated lesions.

## Treatment

Initial medical management includes **prostaglandin E₁** to maintain ductal patency. If significant hypoxia persists on prostaglandin therapy, a **balloon atrial septostomy** improves mixing between the two circulations. Complete surgical repair is most often an **arterial switch**. The arterial switch usually is performed within the first 2 weeks of life, when the left ventricle can still maintain systemic pressure.

## TRICUSPID ATRESIA

### Etiology and Epidemiology

Tricuspid atresia accounts for approximately 2% of all congenital heart defects (Fig. 144-3), occurring when normal development of the valve from endocardial cushions

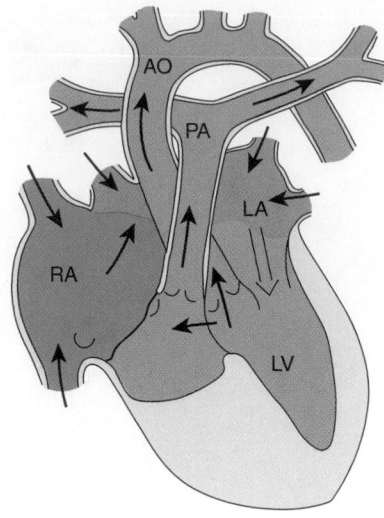

**FIGURE 144-3**

**Tricuspid atresia with ventricular septal defect.** AO, aorta; LA, left atrium; LV, left ventricle; PA, pulmonary artery; RA, right atrium, VSD, ventricular septal defect.

and septal tissue fails. The absence of the tricuspid valve results in a **hypoplastic right ventricle**. All systemic venous return must cross the atrial septum into the left atrium. A PDA or VSD is necessary for pulmonary blood flow and survival.

## Clinical Manifestations

Infants with tricuspid atresia are usually **severely cyanotic** and have a **single $S_2$**. If a VSD is present, there may be a murmur. A diastolic murmur across the mitral valve may be audible. Frequently there is no significant murmur.

## Imaging Studies

The ECG shows **left ventricular hypertrophy** and a **superior QRS axis** (between 0 and −90 degrees). The chest x-ray reveals a normal or mildly enlarged cardiac silhouette with **decreased pulmonary blood flow**. Echocardiography shows the anatomy, associated lesions, and source of pulmonary blood flow.

## Treatment

Management initially depends on the presence of a VSD and the amount of blood flow to the lungs. If there is no VSD, or it is small, prostaglandin $E_1$ maintains pulmonary blood flow until surgery. Surgery is staged with an initial subclavian artery-to-pulmonary shunt (**Blalock-Taussig procedure**) typically followed by a two-stage procedure: **bidirectional cavopulmonary shunt (bidirectional Glenn)** and **Fontan procedure**. These surgeries direct systemic venous return directly to the pulmonary arteries.

# TRUNCUS ARTERIOSUS

## Etiology and Epidemiology

Truncus arteriosus occurs in less than 1% of all cases of congenital heart disease (Fig. 144-4). It results from the failure of septation of the truncus, which normally occurs during the first 3 to 4 weeks of gestation. Anatomically, a single arterial trunk arises from the heart with a large VSD immediately below the truncal valve. The pulmonary arteries arise from the single arterial trunk either as a single vessel that divides or individually from the arterial trunk to the lungs.

## Clinical Manifestations

Varying degrees of cyanosis depend on the amount of pulmonary blood flow. If not diagnosed at birth, the infant may develop signs of heart failure as pulmonary vascular resistance decreases. The signs then include tachypnea and cough. Peripheral pulses are usually bounding as a result of the diastolic runoff into the pulmonary arteries. A single $S_2$ is due to the single valve. There may be a systolic ejection click, and there is often a **systolic murmur** at the left sternal border.

## Imaging Studies

ECG findings include **combined ventricular hypertrophy** and **cardiomegaly.** A chest x-ray usually reveals **increased pulmonary blood** and may show displaced pulmonary arteries.. Echocardiography defines the anatomy, including the VSD, truncal valve function, and origin of the pulmonary arteries.

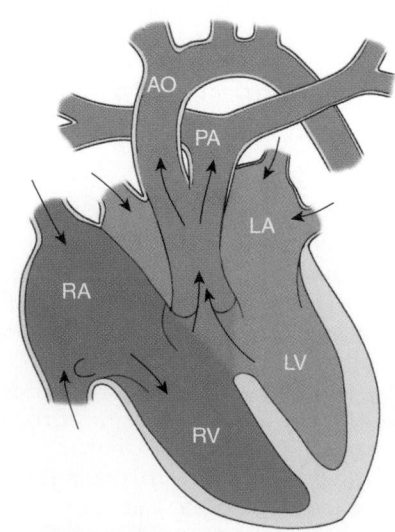

**FIGURE 144-4**

**Truncus arteriosus.** AO, aorta; LA, left atrium; LV, left ventricle; PA, pulmonary artery; RA, right atrium; RV, right ventricle.

### Treatment

Medical management is usually needed and includes **anticongestive medications**. **Surgical repair** includes VSD closure and placement of a conduit between the right ventricle and pulmonary arteries.

## TOTAL ANOMALOUS PULMONARY VENOUS RETURN

### Etiology and Epidemiology

Total anomalous pulmonary venous return accounts for about 1% of congenital heart disease (Fig. 144-5). Disruption of the development of normal pulmonary venous drainage during the third week of gestation results in one of four abnormalities. All of the pulmonary veins fail to connect to the left atrium and return abnormally via the right side of the heart. They may have **supracardiac**, **infracardiac, cardiac**, or **mixed drainage**. An atrial level communication is required for systemic cardiac output and survival.

### Clinical Manifestations

The most important determinant of presentation is the presence or absence of **obstruction** to the pulmonary venous drainage. Infants without obstruction have minimal cyanosis and may be asymptomatic. There is a hyperactive **right ventricular impulse** with a **widely split S₂** (owing to increased right ventricular volume) and a **systolic ejection murmur** at the left upper sternal border. There is usually a mid-diastolic murmur at the lower left sternal border (LLSB) from the increased flow across the tricuspid valve. Growth is relatively poor. Infants with **obstruction** present with cyanosis, marked tachypnea and dyspnea, and signs of right-sided heart failure including hepatomegaly. The obstruction results in little, if any, increase in right ventricular volume so there may be no murmur or changes in S₂.

### Imaging Studies

For infants without obstruction, the ECG is consistent with right ventricular volume overload. Cardiomegaly with increased pulmonary blood flow is seen on chest x-ray. Infants with obstructed veins have right axis deviation and right ventricular hypertrophy on ECG. On chest x-ray, the heart is normal or mildly enlarged with varying degrees of pulmonary edema that can appear similar to hyaline membrane disease or pneumonia. Echocardiography shows the volume-overloaded right side of the heart, right-to-left atrial level shunting, and common pulmonary vein site of drainage and degree of obstruction.

### Treatment

At **surgery**, the common pulmonary vein is opened into the left atrium, and there is ligation of any vein or channel that had been draining the common vein.

## HYPOPLASTIC LEFT HEART SYNDROME

### Etiology and Epidemiology

Hypoplastic left heart syndrome accounts for 1% of all congenital heart defects (Fig. 144-6) but is the most common cause of death from cardiac defects in the first month of life. Hypoplastic left heart syndrome occurs when there is failure of development of the mitral or aortic valve or the aortic arch. A small left ventricle that is

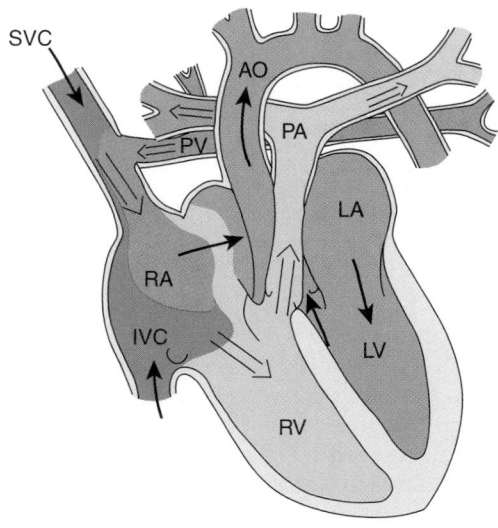

**FIGURE 144-5**

**Total anomalous pulmonary venous return.** AO, aorta; IVC, inferior vena cava; LA, left atrium; LV, left ventricle; PA, pulmonary artery; PV, pulmonary vein; RA, right atrium; RV, right ventricle; SVC, superior vena cava.

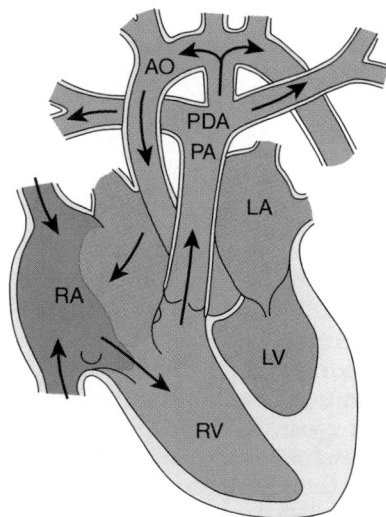

**FIGURE 144-6**

**Hypoplastic left side of the heart.** AO, aorta; LA, left atrium; LV, left ventricle; PA, pulmonary artery; PDA, patent ductus arteriosus; RA, right atrium; RV, right ventricle.

**TABLE 144-2 Extracardiac Complications of Cyanotic Congenital Heart Disease**

| Problem | Etiology | Therapy |
|---|---|---|
| Polycythemia | Persistent hypoxia | Phlebotomy |
| Relative anemia | Nutritional deficiency | Iron replacement |
| CNS abscess | Right-to-left shunting | Antibiotics, drainage |
| CNS thromboembolic stroke | Right-to-left shunting or polycythemia | Phlebotomy |
| Gingival disease | Polycythemia, gingivitis, bleeding | Dental hygiene |
| Gout | Polycythemia, diuretic agents | Allopurinol |
| Arthritis, clubbing | Hypoxic arthropathy | None |
| Pregnancy | Poor placental perfusion, poor ability to increase cardiac output | Bed rest |
| Infectious disease | Associated asplenia, DiGeorge syndrome | Antibiotics |
|  | Fatal RSV pneumonia with pulmonary hypertension | Ribavirin, RSV immune globulin |
| Growth | Failure to thrive, increased oxygen consumption, decreased nutrient intake | Treat heart failure; correct defect early |
| Psychosocial adjustment | Limited activity, peer pressure; chronic disease, multiple hospitalizations, cardiac surgical techniques | Counseling |

CNS, central nervous system; RSV, respiratory syncytial virus.

unable to support normal systemic circulation is a central finding of hypoplastic left heart syndrome, regardless of etiology. Associated degrees of hypoplasia of the ascending aorta and aortic arch are present. Left-to-right shunting occurs at the atrial level.

## Clinical Manifestations

After delivery, the infant is dependent on right-to-left shunting at the ductus arteriosus for systemic blood flow. As the ductus arteriosus constricts, the infant becomes critically ill with signs and symptoms of heart failure from excessive pulmonary blood flow and obstruction of pulmonary venous return. Pulses are diffusely weak or absent. $S_2$ is single and loud. There is usually no heart murmur. Cyanosis may be minimal, but **low cardiac output** gives a grayish color to the cool, mottled skin.

## Imaging Studies

ECG findings include **right ventricular hypertrophy** with **decreased left ventricular forces**. The chest x-ray reveals **cardiomegaly** (with right-sided enlargement) and pulmonary venous congestion or pulmonary edema. Echocardiography shows the small left side of the heart, the degree of stenosis of the aortic and mitral valves, the hypoplastic ascending aorta, and the adequacy of left-to-right atrial flow.

## Treatment

Medical management includes **prostaglandin $E_1$** to open the ductus arteriosus, correction of acidosis, and ventilatory and blood pressure support as needed. **Surgical repair** is staged with the first surgery (Norwood procedure) done in the newborn period. Subsequent procedures

create a systemic source for the pulmonary circulation (bidirectional Glenn and Fontan procedures), leaving the right ventricle to supply systemic circulation. There have been many modifications to all three stages of the repair. Prognosis for survival has improved significantly over the past two decades.

## COMPLICATIONS OF CONGENITAL HEART DISEASE

Extracardiac complications are summarized in Table 144-2.

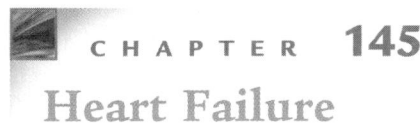

## CHAPTER 145

# Heart Failure

## ETIOLOGY AND EPIDEMIOLOGY

Myofibril contraction is translated into cardiac work or pump performance. The force generated by the muscle fiber depends on its contractile status and basal length, which is equivalent to the preload. As the preload (fiber length, left ventricular filling pressure or volume) increases, myocardial performance (stroke volume and wall tension) increases up to a point (the normal Starling curve). The relationship is the **ventricular function curve** (Fig. 145-1). Alterations in the contractile state of the muscle lower the relative position of the curve, but retain the relationship of fiber length to muscle work. Heart rate is another important determinant of cardiac work because the cardiac output equals stroke volume times the heart rate. Additional factors also affect cardiac performance (Table 145-1).

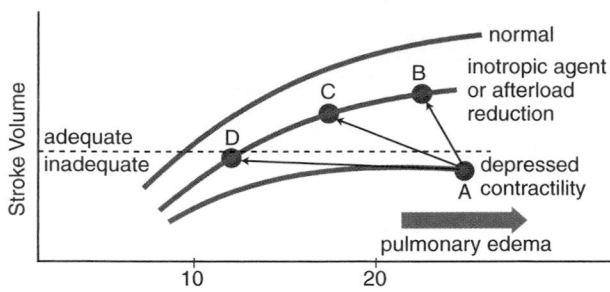

**FIGURE 145-1**

**Ventricular function curve illustrating the effect of inotropic agents or arterial vasodilators.** In contrast to diuretics, the effect of digitalis or arterial vasodilator therapy in a patient with heart failure is movement onto another ventricular function curve intermediate between the normal and the depressed curves. When the patient's ventricular function moves from A to B by the administration of one of these agents, the left ventricular end-diastolic pressure may also decrease because of improved cardiac function; further administration of diuretics or venodilators may shift the function further to the left along the same curve from B to C and eliminate the risk of pulmonary edema. A vasodilating agent that has arteriolar and venous dilating properties (e.g., nitroprusside) would shift this function directly from A to C. If this agent shifts the function from A to D because of excessive venodilation or administration of diuretics, the cardiac output may decrease too much, even though the left ventricular end-diastolic pressure would be normal (10 mm Hg) for a normal heart. Left ventricular end-diastolic pressures of 15 to 18 mm Hg are usually optimal in the failing heart to maximize cardiac output, but to avoid pulmonary edema. (From Andreoli TE, Carpenter CCJ, Griggs RC, Loscalzo J [eds]: Cecil Essentials of Medicine, 5th ed. Philadelphia, *WB Saunders*, 2001.)

| TABLE 145-1 Factors Affecting Cardiac Performance |
| --- |
| **PRELOAD (LEFT VENTRICULAR DIASTOLIC VOLUME)** |
| Total Blood Volume |
| Venous tone (sympathetic tone) |
| Body position |
| Intrathoracic and Intrapericardial Pressure |
| Atrial contraction |
| Pumping action of skeletal muscle |
| **AFTERLOAD (IMPEDANCE AGAINST WHICH THE LEFT VENTRICLE MUST EJECT BLOOD)** |
| Peripheral vascular resistance |
| Left ventricular volume (preload, wall tension) |
| Physical characteristics of the arterial tree (elasticity of vessels or presence of outflow obstruction) |
| **CONTRACTILITY (CARDIAC PERFORMANCE INDEPENDENT OF PRELOAD OR AFTERLOAD)** |
| Sympathetic nerve impulses* |
| Circulating catecholamines* |
| Digitalis, calcium, other inotropic agents* |
| Increased heart rate or postextrasystolic augmentation* |
| Anoxia, acidosis[†] |
| Pharmacologic depression[†] |
| Loss of myocardium[†] |
| Intrinsic depression[†] |
| **HEART RATE** |
| Autonomic nervous system |
| Temperature, metabolic rate |

*Increases contractility.
[†]Decreases contractility.
From Andreoli TE, Carpenter CCJ, Griggs RC, Loscalzo J: Cecil Essentials of Medicine, 5th ed. Philadelphia, *WB Saunders*, 2001.

Heart failure occurs when the heart is unable to pump blood at a rate commensurate with metabolic needs (oxygen delivery). It may be due to a change in **myocardial contractility** that results in low cardiac output or to **abnormal loading conditions** being placed on the myocardium. The abnormal loading conditions may be **afterload** (pressure overload, such as with aortic stenosis, pulmonary stenosis, or coarctation of the aorta) or **preload** (volume overload, such as in ventricular septal defect (VSD), patent ductus arteriosus (PDA), or valvular insufficiency). Volume overload is the most common cause of heart failure in children.

It is helpful to approach the differential diagnosis of heart failure based on age of presentation (Table 145-2). In the first weeks of life, heart failure is most commonly due to an excessive afterload being placed on the myocardium. Heart failure presenting around 2 months of age is usually due to increasing left-to-right shunts that become apparent as the pulmonary vascular resistance decreases. Acquired heart disease, such as myocarditis and cardiomyopathy, can present at any age.

## CLINICAL MANIFESTATIONS

Heart failure presents in infants as poor feeding, failure to thrive, tachypnea, and diaphoresis with feeding. Older children may present with shortness of breath, easy fatigability, and edema. The physical examination findings depend on whether pulmonary venous congestion, systemic venous congestion, or both are present. Tachycardia, a gallop rhythm, and thready pulses may be present with either cause. If left-sided failure is predominant, tachypnea, orthopnea, wheezing, and pulmonary edema are seen. Hepatomegaly, edema, and distended neck veins are signs of right-sided failure.

## IMAGING STUDIES

Noninvasive studies, such as chest radiography, are not specific, but the absence of cardiomegaly on a chest x-ray usually rules out the diagnosis of heart failure. An echocardiogram assesses the heart chamber sizes, measures myocardial function, and diagnoses congenital heart defects when present.

## TREATMENT

Initial treatment is directed at improving myocardial function and optimizing preload and afterload. Diuretics, inotropic support, and, often, **afterload reduction** are employed (Table 145-3). Long-term therapy usually consists of diuretics and afterload reduction frequently is added. Long-term therapy with **β-blockers** also may be beneficial, although this remains somewhat controversial in pediatric patients.

## TABLE 145-2 Etiology of Heart Failure by Age Group

### FETUS

Severe anemia (hemolysis, fetal-maternal transfusion, hypoplastic anemia)
Supraventricular tachycardia
Ventricular tachycardia
Complete heart block
Atrioventricular valve insufficiency
High-output cardiac failure (arteriovenous malformation, teratoma)

### PREMATURE NEONATE

Fluid overload
PDA
VSD
Cor pulmonale (BPD)

### FULL-TERM NEONATE

Asphyxial cardiomyopathy
Arteriovenous malformation (vein of Galen, hepatic)
Left-sided obstructive lesions (coarctation of aorta, hypoplastic left heart, critical aortic stenosis)
Transposition of great arteries
Large mixing cardiac defects (single ventricle, truncus arteriosus)
Viral myocarditis
Anemia
Supraventricular tachycardia
Complete heart block

### INFANT/TODDLER

Left-to-right cardiac shunts (VSD)
Hemangioma (arteriovenous malformation)
Anomalous left coronary artery
Metabolic cardiomyopathy
Acute hypertension (hemolytic uremic syndrome)
Supraventricular tachycardia
Kawasaki disease
Postoperative repair of congenital heart disease

### CHILD/ADOLESCENT

Rheumatic fever
Acute hypertension (glomerulonephritis)
Viral myocarditis
Thyrotoxicosis
Hemochromatosis/hemosiderosis
Cancer therapy (radiation, doxorubicin)
Sickle cell anemia
Endocarditis
Cor pulmonale (cystic fibrosis)
Arrhythmias
Chronic upper airway obstruction (cor pulmonale)
Unrepaired or palliated congenital heart disease
Cardiomyopathy

BPD, bronchopulmonary dysplasia; PDA, patent ductus arteriosus; VSD, ventricular septal defect.

## TABLE 145-3 Treatment of Heart Failure

| Therapy | Mechanism |
| --- | --- |
| **GENERAL CARE** | |
| Rest | Reduces cardiac output |
| Oxygen | Improves oxygenation in presence of pulmonary edema |
| Sodium, fluid restrictions | Decreases vascular congestion; decreases preload |
| **DIURETICS** | |
| Furosemide | Salt excretion by way of ascending loop of Henle; reduces preload; afterload reduced with control of hypertension; may also cause venodilation |
| Combination of distal tubule and loop diuretics | Greater sodium excretion |
| **INOTROPIC AGENTS** | |
| Digitalis | Inhibits membrane $Na^+,K^+$-ATPase and increases intracellular $Ca^{2+}$, improves cardiac contractility, increases myocardial oxygen consumption |
| Dopamine | Releases myocardial norepinephrine plus direct effect on β-receptor, may increase systemic blood pressure; at low infusion rates, dilates renal artery, facilitating diuresis |
| Dobutamine | $β_1$-Receptor agent; often combined with dopamine |
| Amrinone/milrinone | Nonsympathomimetic, noncardiac glycosides with inotropic effects; may cause vasodilation |
| **AFTERLOAD REDUCTION** | |
| Hydralazine | Arteriolar vasodilator |
| Nitroprusside | Arterial and venous relaxation; venodilation reduces preload |
| Captopril/enalapril | Inhibition of angiotensin-converting enzyme; reduces angiotensin II production |
| **OTHER MEASURES** | |
| Mechanical counterpulsation | Improves coronary flow, afterload |
| Transplantation | Removes diseased heart |
| Extracorporeal membrane oxygenation | Bypasses heart |
| Carvedilol | β-Blocking agent |

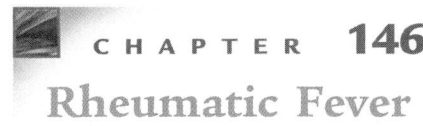

# CHAPTER 146
# Rheumatic Fever

## ETIOLOGY AND EPIDEMIOLOGY

Although uncommon in the United States, acute rheumatic fever remains an important preventable cause of cardiac disease. It is most common in children 6 to 15 years of age. It is due to an immunologic reaction that is a delayed sequela of group A beta-hemolytic streptococcal infections of the pharynx. A family history of rheumatic fever and lower socioeconomic status are additional factors.

## CLINICAL MANIFESTATIONS

Acute rheumatic fever is diagnosed using the clinical and laboratory findings of the **revised Jones criteria** (Table 146-1). The presence of either two **major criteria** or one major and two **minor criteria**, along with evidence of an antecedent **streptococcal infection**, confirm a diagnosis of acute rheumatic fever. The infection often precedes the presentation of rheumatic fever by 2 to 6 weeks. Streptococcal antibody tests, such as the antistreptolysin O titer, are the most reliable laboratory evidence of prior infection.

**Arthritis** is the most common major manifestation. It usually involves the large joints and is migratory. Arthralgia cannot be used as a minor manifestation if arthritis is used as a major manifestation. **Carditis** occurs in about 50% of patients. Tachycardia, a new murmur (mitral or aortic regurgitation), pericarditis, cardiomegaly, and signs of heart failure are evidence of carditis. **Erythema marginatum**, a serpiginous, nonpruritic, and evanescent rash, is uncommon, occurs on the trunk, and is brought out by warmth. **Subcutaneous nodules** are seen predominantly with chronic or recurrent disease. They are firm, painless, nonpruritic, mobile nodules found on the extensor surfaces of the large and small joints, the scalp, and the spine. **Chorea** (Sydenham chorea or St. Vitus dance) consists of neurologic and psychiatric signs. It also is uncommon and often presents long after the infection.

## TREATMENT AND PREVENTION

Management of acute rheumatic fever consists of **benzathine penicillin** to eradicate the beta-hemolytic streptococcus, anti-inflammatory therapy with **salicylates** after the diagnosis is established, and **bed rest**. Additional supportive therapy for heart failure or chorea may be necessary during the acute presentation. **Long-term penicillin prophylaxis**, preferably with intramuscular benzathine penicillin G, 1.2 million U every 28 days, is required. Oral regimens for prophylaxis generally are not as effective. The prognosis of acute rheumatic fever depends on the degree of permanent cardiac damage. Cardiac involvement may resolve completely, especially if it is the first episode and the prophylactic regimen is followed. The severity of cardiac involvement worsens with each recurrence of rheumatic fever.

**TABLE 146-1  Major Jones Criteria for Diagnosis of Acute Rheumatic Fever*†**

| Sign | Comments |
|---|---|
| Polyarthritis | Common; swelling, limited motion, tender, erythema |
| | Migratory; involves large joints but rarely small or unusual joints, such as vertebrae |
| Carditis | Common; pancarditis, valves, pericardium, myocardium |
| | Tachycardia greater than explained by fever; new murmur of mitral or aortic insufficiency; Carey-Coombs mid-diastolic murmur; heart failure |
| Chorea (Sydenham disease) | Uncommon; manifests long after infection has resolved; more common in females; antineuronal antibody positive |
| Erythema marginatum | Uncommon; pink macules on trunk and proximal extremities, evolving to serpiginous border with central clearing; evanescent, elicited by application of local heat; nonpruritic |
| Subcutaneous nodules | Uncommon; associated with repeated episodes and severe carditis; located over extensor surface of elbows, knees, knuckles, and ankles or scalp and spine; firm, nontender |

*Minor criteria include fever (temperatures of 101°–102°F [38.2°–38.9°C]), arthralgias, previous rheumatic fever, leukocytosis, elevated erythrocyte sedimentation rate/C-reactive protein, and prolonged PR interval.

†One major and two minor, or two major, criteria with evidence of recent group A streptococcal disease (e.g., scarlet fever, positive throat culture, or elevated antistreptolysin O or other antistreptococcal antibodies) strongly suggest the diagnosis of acute rheumatic fever.

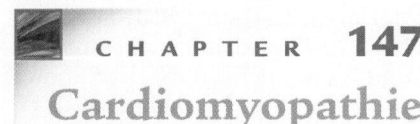

CHAPTER **147**

# Cardiomyopathies

## ETIOLOGY

A cardiomyopathy is an intrinsic disease of the heart muscle and is not associated with other forms of heart disease (Table 147-1). There are three types of cardiomyopathy based on anatomic and functional features:

1. Dilated
2. Hypertrophic
3. Restrictive

Dilated cardiomyopathies are the most common. They are often idiopathic, but may be due to infection (echovirus or Coxsackie B virus) or be postinfectious, familial, or secondary to systemic disease or to cardiotoxic drugs. Hypertrophic cardiomyopathies are usually familial with autosomal dominant inheritance, but may occur sporadically.

Restrictive cardiomyopathies are rare; they may be idiopathic or associated with systemic disease (Table 147-2).

## CLINICAL MANIFESTATIONS

Dilated cardiomyopathies result in enlargement of the left ventricle only or both ventricles. Myocardial contractility is variably decreased. Clinically, children with dilated cardiomyopathy present with signs and symptoms of inadequate cardiac output and **heart failure**. Tachypnea and tachycardia are present on examination. Peripheral pulses are often weak because of a **narrow pulse pressure**. Rales may be audible on auscultation. The heart sounds may be muffled and an $S_3$ is often present. Concurrent infectious illness may result in circulatory collapse and shock in children with dilated cardiomyopathies.

Hypertrophic cardiomyopathy is initially difficult to diagnose. Infants, but not older children, frequently present with signs of heart failure. Sudden death may be the initial presentation in older children. Dyspnea, fatigue, chest pain, syncope or near-syncope, and palpitations may be present. A murmur is heard in more than 50% of

---

### TABLE 147-1  Etiology of Myocardial Disease

#### FAMILIAL/HEREDITARY

Duchenne muscular dystrophy
Other muscular dystrophies (Becker, limb-girdle)
Myotonic dystrophy
Kearns-Sayre syndrome (progressive external ophthalmoplegia)
Friedreich ataxia
Hemochromatosis
Fabry disease
Pompe disease (glycogen storage)
Carnitine deficiency syndromes
Endocardial fibroelastosis
Mitochondrial myopathy syndromes
Familial restrictive cardiomyopathy
Familial hypertrophic cardiomyopathy
Familial dilated cardiomyopathy (dominant, recessive, X-linked)

#### INFECTIOUS (MYOCARDITIS)

Viral (e.g., coxsackievirus infection, mumps, Epstein-Barr virus infection, influenza, parainfluenza infection, measles, varicella, HIV infection)
Rickettsial (e.g., psittacosis, Coxiella infection, Rocky Mountain spotted fever)
Bacterial (e.g., diphtheria, Mycoplasma infection, meningococcal disease, leptospirosis, Lyme disease)
Parasitic (e.g., Chagas disease, toxoplasmosis)

#### METABOLIC/NUTRITIONAL/ENDOCRINE

Beriberi (thiamine deficiency)
Keshan disease (selenium deficiency)
Hypothyroidism
Hyperthyroidism
Carcinoid

Pheochromocytoma
Mitochondrial myopathies and oxidative respiratory chain defects
Type II, X-linked 3-methylglutaconic aciduria

#### CONNECTIVE TISSUE/GRANULOMATOUS DISEASE

SLE
Scleroderma
Churg-Strauss syndrome
Rheumatoid arthritis
Rheumatic fever
Sarcoidosis
Amyloidosis
Dermatomyositis

#### DRUGS/TOXINS

Doxorubicin (Adriamycin)
Ipecac
Iron overload (hemosiderosis)
Irradiation
Cocaine
Amphetamines

#### CORONARY ARTERIES

Anomalous left coronary artery
Kawasaki disease

#### OTHER DISORDERS/CONDITIONS

Sickle cell anemia
Hypereosinophilic syndrome
Endomyocardial fibrosis
Asymmetrical septal hypertrophy
Right ventricular dysplasia
Idiopathic

SLE, systemic lupus erythematosus.

**TABLE 147-2  Anatomic and Functional Features of Cardiomyopathies**

| Feature | Dilated | Hypertrophic | Restrictive |
|---|---|---|---|
| Etiology | Infectious | Sporadic | Infiltrative (amyloidosis, sarcoidosis) |
| | Metabolic | Inherited (autosomal dominant) | Noninfiltrative (idiopathic, familial) |
| | Toxic | | Storage disease (hemachromatosis, Fabry disease) |
| | Idiopathic | | Endomyocardial disease |
| Hemodynamics | Decreased systolic function | Diastolic dysfunction (impaired ventricular filling) | Diastolic dysfunction (impaired ventricular filling) |
| Treatment | Positive inotropes | β-Blockers | Diuretics |
| | Diuretics | Calcium channel blockers | Anticoagulants |
| | Afterload reduction | | Cardiac transplantation |
| | β-Blockers | | |
| | Antiarrhythmics | | |
| | Anticoagulants | | |
| | Cardiac transplantation | | |

children referred after identification of an affected family member. Restrictive cardiomyopathies are relatively rare in pediatrics. Presenting symptoms usually include dyspnea exacerbated by a respiratory illness, syncope, hepatomegaly, and an $S_4$ heart sound on examination.

## IMAGING STUDIES

Cardiomegaly usually is seen on chest radiographs for all three types of cardiomyopathies. The electrocardiogram (ECG) in dilated cardiomyopathy may have nonspecific ST-T wave changes and left ventricular hypertrophy. ECG evidence of right ventricular hypertrophy is present in 25% of children with cardiomyopathy. The ECG with hypertrophic cardiomyopathy is universally abnormal, but changes are nonspecific. Primary hypertrophic cardiomyopathy is associated with a prolonged QT interval. Children with restrictive cardiomyopathies may show atrial enlargement on the ECG. Echocardiography features vary by type of cardiomyopathy. Dilated cardiomyopathies result in left atrial and ventricular dilation, a decreased shortening fraction, and globally depressed contractility. Asymmetrical septal hypertrophy and left ventricular outflow tract obstruction are seen in hypertrophic cardiomyopathies. Massive atrial dilation is seen in restrictive cardiomyopathies. Endomyocardial biopsy specimens, obtained while the patient is hemodynamically stable, identify histologic type and allow tests for mitochondrial or infiltrative diseases.

## TREATMENT

Supportive therapy, including **diuretics, inotropic medications**, and **afterload reduction**, is provided for all three types of cardiomyopathy and depends on the degree of symptoms and severity of cardiovascular compromise. If a specific etiology can be identified, treatment is directed at the etiology. Symptomatic therapy with close monitoring and follow-up is crucial. Because of the high mortality rate associated with all forms of cardiomyopathy, **cardiac transplantation** must be considered.

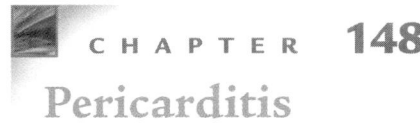

## CHAPTER 148
# Pericarditis

## ETIOLOGY AND EPIDEMIOLOGY

Pericarditis is inflammation of the parietal and visceral surfaces of the pericardium. It is most often viral in origin with many viruses identified as causative agents. A bacterial etiology is rare, but usually bacteria cause a much more serious and symptomatic pericarditis. *Staphylococcus aureus* and *Streptococcus pneumoniae* are the most likely bacterial causes. Pericarditis is associated with collagen vascular diseases, such as rheumatoid arthritis, and is seen with uremia (Table 148-1). **Postpericardiotomy syndrome** is a relatively common form of pericarditis that follows heart surgery.

## CLINICAL MANIFESTATIONS

The symptoms of pericarditis (Table 148-2) depend on the amount of fluid in the pericardial space and how fast it accumulates. A small effusion usually is well tolerated. A large effusion may be remarkably well tolerated if it accumulates slowly. The faster the fluid accumulates, the sooner the patient is hemodynamically compromised and develops symptoms.

## IMAGING AND LABORATORY STUDIES

Echocardiography is the most specific and useful diagnostic test for detection of pericardial effusions. A chest x-ray may reveal cardiomegaly. A large effusion creates a rounded, globular cardiac silhouette. The electrocardiogram (ECG) may show tachycardia, elevated ST segments, reduced QRS voltage or electrical alternans (variable QRS amplitude). The causative organism may be identified through viral titers, antistreptolysin O (ASO) titers, or diagnostic testing of the pericardial fluid.

## TABLE 148-1 Etiology of Pericarditis and Pericardial Effusion

### IDIOPATHIC (PRESUMED VIRAL) INFECTIOUS AGENTS

*Bacterial*
Group A streptococci
*Staphylococcus aureus*
Pneumococcus, meningococcus*
*Haemophilus influenzae**
*Salmonella*
*Mycoplasma pneumoniae*
*Borrelia burgdorferi*
*Mycobacterium tuberculosis*
*Rickettsia*
Tularemia
*Viral*[†]
Coxsackievirus (group A, B)
Echovirus
Mumps
Influenza
Epstein-Barr
Cytomegalovirus
Herpes simplex
Herpes zoster
Hepatitis B
*Fungal*
*Histoplasma capsulatum*
*Coccidioides immitis*
*Blastomyces dermatitidis*
*Cryptococcus neoformans*
*Candida*
*Aspergillus*
*Parasitic*
*Toxoplasma gondii*
*Entamoeba histolytica*
Schistosomes

### COLLAGEN VASCULAR–INFLAMMATORY AND GRANULOMATOUS DISEASES

Rheumatic fever
Systemic lupus erythematosus (idiopathic and drug-induced)
Rheumatoid arthritis
Kawasaki disease
Scleroderma
Mixed connective tissue disease
Reiter syndrome
Inflammatory bowel disease
Wegener granulomatosis

Dermatomyositis
Behçet syndrome
Sarcoidosis
Vasculitis
Familial Mediterranean fever
Serum sickness
Stevens-Johnson syndrome

### TRAUMATIC

Cardiac contusion (blunt trauma)
Penetrating trauma
Postpericardiotomy syndrome
Radiation

### CONTIGUOUS SPREAD

Pleural disease
Pneumonia
Aortic aneurysm (dissecting)

### METABOLIC

Hypothyroidism
Uremia
Gaucher disease
Fabry disease
Chylopericardium

### NEOPLASTIC

Primary
Contiguous (lymphoma)
Metastatic
Infiltrative (leukemia)

### OTHER ETIOLOGIC DISORDERS/FACTORS

Drug reaction
Pancreatitis
After myocardial infarction
Thalassemia
Central venous catheter perforation
Heart failure
Hemorrhage (coagulopathy)
Biliary-pericardial fistula

*Infectious or immune complex.
[†]Common (viral pericarditis or myopericarditis is probably the most common cause of acute pericarditis in a previously normal host).
From Sigman G: Chest pain. In Kliegman RM, Nieder ML, Super DM (eds): Practical Strategies in Pediatric Diagnosis and Therapy. Philadelphia, *WB Saunders*, 1996.

## TREATMENT

**Pericardiocentesis** is indicated for treatment of hemodynamically significant effusions and to determine the etiology of the pericarditis. Additional treatment is directed at the specific etiology. There is no specific treatment for viral pericarditis other than **anti-inflammatory medications**.

**TABLE 148-2  Manifestations of Pericarditis**

### SYMPTOMS

Chest pain (worsened if lying down or with inspiration)
Dyspnea
Malaise
Patient assumes sitting position

### SIGNS

*Nonconstrictive*
Fever
Tachycardia
Friction rub (accentuated by inspiration, body position)
Enlarged heart by percussion and x-ray examination
Distant heart sounds
*Tamponade*
*As above, plus:*
Distended neck veins

Hepatomegaly
Pulsus paradoxus (>10 mm Hg with inspiration)
Narrow pulse pressure
Weak pulse, poor peripheral perfusion
*Constrictive*
Distended neck veins
Kussmaul sign (inspiratory increase in jugular venous pressure)
Distant heart sounds
Pericardial knock
Hepatomegaly
Ascites
Edema
Tachycardia

# SUGGESTED READING

Doniger SJ, Sharieff GQ: Pediatric dysrhythmias, *Pediatr Clin North Am* 53:85–105, vi, 2006.
Kliegman RM, Behrman RE, Jenson HB, et al, editors: Nelson Textbook of Pediatrics, 18th ed, Philadelphia, 2007, *WB Saunders.*
Margossian R: Contemporary management of pediatric heart failure. *Exp Rev Cardiovasc Ther* 6(2):187–197, 2008.
Park MK: Pediatric Cardiology for Practitioners, 5th ed, Philadelphia, 2008, *Mosby.*
Walsh EP: Interventional electrophysiology in patients with congenital heart disease, *Circulation* 115:3224–3234, 2007.

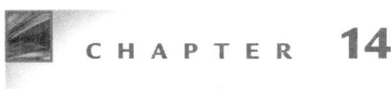

C H A P T E R  149

# Hematology Assessment

## HISTORY

A detailed, careful history of the onset, severity, progression, associated symptoms, presence of systemic complaints, and exacerbating factors is crucial to the diagnosis of a blood disorder. In many blood disorders, a **detailed pedigree** is essential because a pattern of inheritance can point to the diagnosis.

## PHYSICAL EXAMINATION AND COMMON MANIFESTATIONS

The physical examination of patients with blood disorders first focuses on hemodynamic stability. Acute episodes of anemia may be life-threatening, presenting with impairment of perfusion and cognitive status. The two most common findings of anemia include **pallor** and **jaundice**. The presence of **petechiae**, **purpura**, or deeper sites of **bleeding**, including generalized hemorrhage, indicates abnormalities of platelets, coagulation factors, or a consumptive coagulopathy. **Growth parameters** point to whether anemia is an acute or chronic process. Severe types of anemia, thrombocytopenia, and pancytopenia are associated with congenital anomalies and a pattern of growth delay. The presence or absence of other organ system involvement or systemic illness (especially **hepatosplenomegaly** and **lymphadenopathy**), point to a generalized illness as the cause for hematologic abnormalities (Table 149-1).

## INITIAL DIAGNOSTIC EVALUATION

The basis for the diagnosis of blood disorders is laboratory testing. Diagnosis of pediatric blood disorders requires a detailed knowledge of normal hematologic values during infancy and childhood which varies according to age and, after puberty, according to sex (Table 149-2). From the history, physical examination, and screening laboratory studies, the astute clinician can use specific diagnostic testing to confirm the diagnosis.

## DEVELOPMENTAL HEMATOLOGY

Hematopoiesis begins by 3 weeks of gestation with **erythropoiesis** in the yolk sac. By 2 months' gestation, the primary site of hematopoiesis has migrated to the liver. By 5 to 6 months' gestation, the process of hematopoiesis shifts from the liver to the bone marrow. An extremely premature infant may have significant **extramedullary hematopoiesis** due to limited bone marrow hematopoiesis. During infancy, virtually all marrow cavities are actively hematopoietic and the proportion of hematopoietic to stromal elements is quite high. As the child grows, hematopoiesis moves to the central bones of the body (vertebrae, sternum, ribs, and pelvis), and the marrow is gradually replaced with fat. This replacement is partially reversible. Hemolysis or marrow damage may lead to marrow repopulation of cavities where hematopoiesis previously had ceased or may cause a delay in the shift of hematopoiesis. Children with thalassemia and other chronic hemolytic diseases may have large head circumferences and prominent skull bones as a result of increased erythropoiesis within the medullary cavities of the skull. Hepatosplenomegaly in patients with chronic hemolysis may signify extramedullary hematopoiesis. When a patient with cytopenia is being evaluated, a **bone marrow examination** provides valuable information about processes that lead to underproduction of circulating cells. Additionally, bone marrow infiltration by neoplastic elements or storage cells often occurs in concert with infiltration in the spleen, liver, and lymph nodes.

The hematopoietic cells consist of the following:

1. Small compartment of **pluripotential progenitor stem cells** that morphologically resemble small lymphocytes and are capable of forming all myeloid elements
2. Large compartment of committed, **proliferating cells of myeloid, erythroid, and megakaryocytic lineage**
3. Large compartment of **postmitotic maturing cells** (Fig. 149-1)

Hematopoiesis is controlled by numerous cytokines. The bone marrow is the major storage organ for mature neutrophils and contains about seven times the intravascular pool of neutrophils. It contains 2.5 to 5 times as many cells of

| TABLE 149-1 Presentation of Hematologic Disorders | | |
|---|---|---|
| **Condition** | **Symptoms and Signs** | **Common Examples** |
| Anemia | Pallor, fatigue, heart failure, jaundice | Iron deficiency, hemolytic anemia |
| Polycythemia | Irritability, cyanosis, seizures, jaundice, stroke, headache | Cyanotic heart disease, infant of diabetic mother, cystic fibrosis |
| Neutropenia | Fever, pharyngitis, oral ulceration, cellulitis, lymphadenopathy, bacteremia, gingivitis | Congenital or drug-induced agranulocytosis, leukemia |
| Thrombocytopenia | Petechiae, ecchymosis, gastrointestinal hemorrhage, epistaxis | ITP, leukemia |
| Coagulopathy | Bruising, hemarthrosis, mucosal bleeding | von Willebrand disease, hemophilia, DIC |
| Thrombosis | Pulmonary embolism, deep vein thrombosis | Lupus anticoagulant; protein C, protein S, or antithrombin III deficiency; factor V Leiden, prothrombin 20210 |

DIC, disseminated intravascular coagulation; ITP, idiopathic thrombocytopenic purpura.

myeloid lineage as cells of erythroid lineage. Smaller numbers of megakaryocytes, plasma cells, histiocytes, lymphocytes, and stromal cells are also stored in the marrow.

**Erythropoiesis** (red blood cell [RBC] production) is controlled by erythropoietin, a glycoprotein that stimulates primitive pluripotential stem cells to differentiate along the erythroid line and is made by the juxtaglomerular apparatus of the kidney in response to local tissue hypoxia. The normally high hemoglobin level of the fetus is a result of fetal erythropoietin production in the liver in response to low $Po_2$ in utero. Control of erythropoiesis by erythropoietin begins at the time of hepatic hematopoiesis in early gestation. Erythropoietin leads to production of the **erythroid colony-forming unit**. The earliest recognizable erythroid cell in vivo is the erythroblast, which forms eight or more daughter cells. The immature RBC nucleus becomes gradually pyknotic as the cell matures and eventually is extruded before being released from the marrow as a **reticulocyte**. The reticulocyte maintains residual mitochondrial and protein synthetic capacity. These highly specialized RBC precursors are engaged primarily in the production of **globin chains**, **glycolytic enzymes**, and **heme**. Iron is taken up via transferrin receptors and incorporated into the heme ring, which combines with globin chains synthesized within the immature RBC. When the messenger RNA and mitochondria are gone from the RBC, heme or protein synthesis is no longer possible; however, the RBC continues to function for its normal life span of about 120 days in older children and adults.

During embryonic and fetal life, the globin genes are sequentially activated and inactivated. Embryonic hemoglobins are produced during yolk sac erythropoiesis, then replaced by **fetal hemoglobin** (hemoglobin F, $\alpha_2\gamma_2$) during the hepatic phase. During the third trimester, gamma chain production gradually diminishes, and gamma chains are replaced by beta chains, resulting in **hemoglobin A** ($\alpha_2\beta_2$). Some fetal factors (e.g., infant of a diabetic mother) delay onset of beta chain production, but premature birth does not. Just after birth, with the expansion of the lungs and rapid increases in oxygen saturation, erythropoietin production stops and, thus, erythropoiesis ceases. Fetal RBCs have a shorter survival time (60 days).

Fetal RBCs have less deformable membranes as well as enzymatic differences from the red blood cells of older children. Senescent RBCs are destroyed in the liver and spleen due to changes in their membrane sialic acid content and the metabolic depletion that occurs as they age. During the first few months of postnatal life, rapid growth, shortened RBC survival, and cessation of erythropoiesis cause a gradual decline in hemoglobin levels, with a nadir at 8 to 10 weeks of life. This so-called **physiologic nadir** is accentuated in premature infants. Erythropoietin is produced in response to the decline in hemoglobin and decreased oxygen delivery. Erythropoiesis subsequently resumes with an increase in the reticulocyte count. The hemoglobin level gradually increases, accompanied by synthesis of increasing amounts of hemoglobin A. By 6 months of age in healthy infants, only trace gamma chain synthesis occurs.

Production of **neutrophil precursors** is controlled predominantly by two different colony-stimulating factors (see Fig. 149-1). The most immature neutrophil precursors are controlled by **granulocyte-monocyte colony-stimulating factor** (GM-CSF), produced by monocytes and lymphocytes. GM-CSF increases the entry of primitive precursor cells into the myeloid line of differentiation. **Granulocyte colony-stimulating factor** (G-CSF) augments the production of more mature granulocyte precursors. GM-CSF and G-CSF, working in concert, can augment production of neutrophils, shorten the usual baseline 10- to 14-day production time from stem cell to mature neutrophil, and stimulate functional activity. The rapid increase in neutrophil count that occurs with infection is caused by release of stored neutrophils from the bone marrow. This activity also is under the control of GM-CSF. During maturation, a mitotic pool of neutrophil precursors exists—myeloblasts, promyelocytes, and myelocytes possessing primary granules. The postmitotic pool consists of metamyelocytes, bands, and mature polymorphonuclear leukocytes containing secondary or specific granules that define the cell type. Only bands and mature neutrophils are fully functional with regard to phagocytosis, chemotaxis, and bacterial killing. Neutrophils migrate from the bone marrow, circulate for 6 to 7 hours, and enter the tissues, where they become end-stage cells that do not

## TABLE 149-2 Hematologic Values During Infancy and Childhood

| Age | Hemoglobin (g/dL) Mean | Range | Hematocrit (%) Mean | Range | Reticulocytes (%) Mean | Leukocytes (per mm³) Mean | Range | Differential Counts Neutrophils (%) Mean | Range | Lymphocytes (%) Mean | Eosinophils (%) Mean | Monocytes (%) Mean | Nucleated Red Cells/ 100 WBCS |
|---|---|---|---|---|---|---|---|---|---|---|---|---|---|
| Cord blood | 16.8 | 13.7–20.1 | 55 | 45–65 | 5 | 18,000 | 9000–30,000 | 61 | 40–80 | 31 | 2 | 6 | 7 |
| 2 wk | 16.5 | 13–20 | 50 | 42–66 | 1 | 12,000 | 5000–21,000 | 40 | | 48 | 3 | 9 | 3–10 |
| 3 mo | 12.0 | 9.5–14.5 | 36 | 31–41 | 1 | 12,000 | 6000–18,000 | 30 | | 63 | 2 | 5 | 0 |
| 6 mo–6 yr | 12.0 | 10.5–14 | 37 | 33–42 | 1 | 10,000 | 6000–15,000 | 45 | | 48 | 2 | 5 | 0 |
| 7–12 yr | 13.0 | 11–16 | 38 | 34–40 | 1 | 8000 | 4500–13,500 | 55 | | 38 | 2 | 5 | 0 |
| Adult | | | | | | | | | | | | | |
| Female | 14.0 | 12–16 | 42 | 37–47 | 1.6 | 7500 | 5000–10,000 | 55 | 35–70 | 35 | 3 | 7 | 0 |
| Male | 16.0 | 14–18 | 47 | 42–52 | | | | | | | | | |

WBCs, white blood cells.
From Behrman RE (ed): Nelson Textbook of Pediatrics, 14th ed. Philadelphia, *WB Saunders*, 1992.

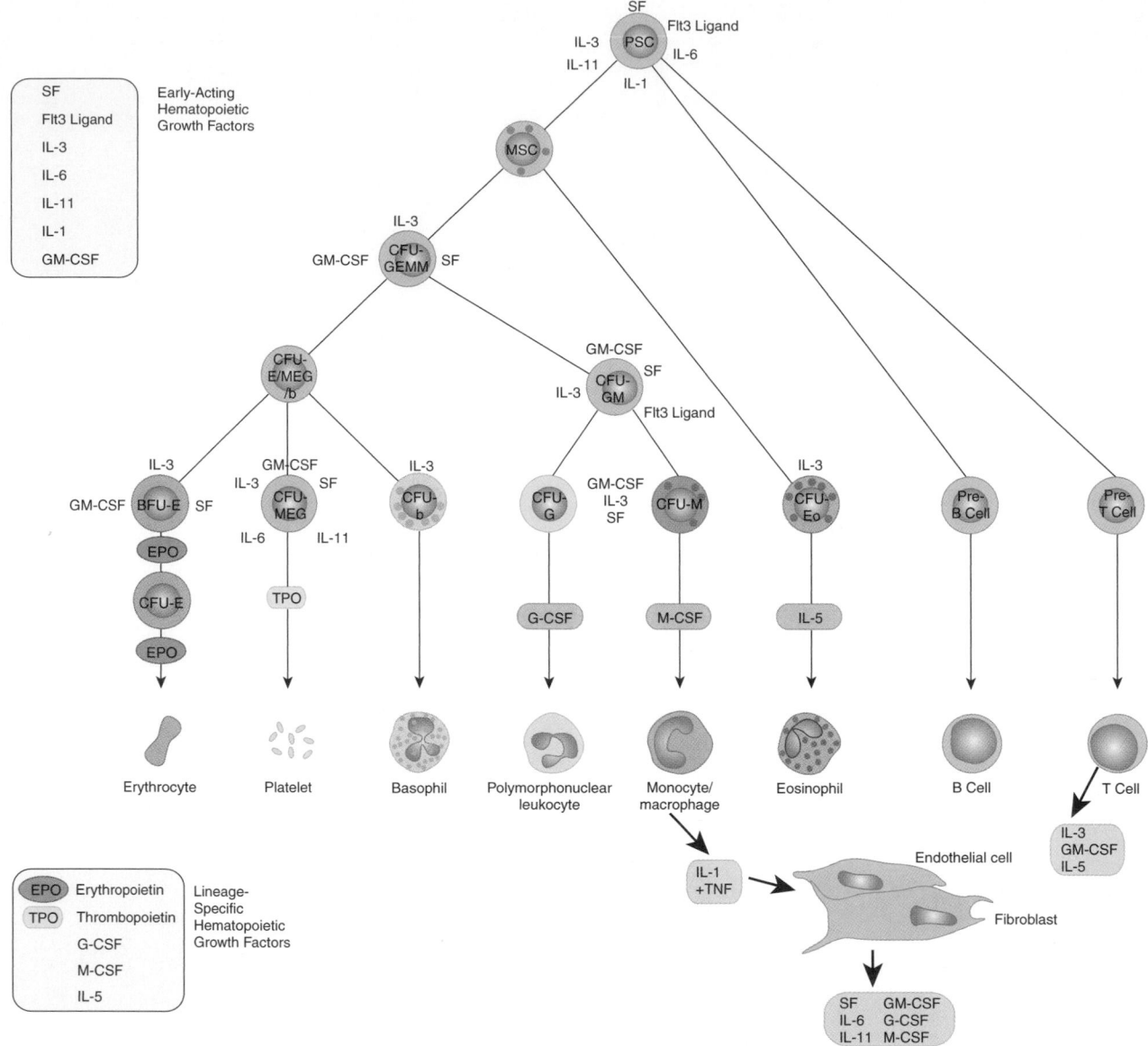

**FIGURE 149-1**

**Major cytokine sources and actions to promote hematopoiesis.** Cells of the bone marrow microenvironment, such as macrophages, endothelial cells, and reticular fibroblasts, produce macrophage colony-stimulating factor (M-CSF), granulocyte-macrophage colony-stimulating factor (GM-CSF), and granulocyte colony-stimulating factor (G-CSF) after stimulation. These cytokines and others as listed in the text have overlapping interactions during hematopoietic differentiation, as indicated; for all lineages, optimal development requires a combination of early and late acting factors. BFU, burst-forming unit; CFU, colony-forming unit; EPO, erythropoietin; IL, interleukin; MSC, myeloid stem cells; PSC, pluripotent stem cells; TNF, tumor necrosis factor; TPO, thrombopoietin. (From Sieff CA, Nathan DG, Clark SC: The anatomy and physiology of hematopoiesis. In Orkin SH, Nathan DG [eds]: Hematology of Infancy and Childhood, 5th ed. Philadelphia, *WB Saunders*, 1998, p 168.)

recirculate. Eosinophil production is under the control of a related glycoprotein hormone, interleukin 3. Eosinophils, which play a role in host defense against parasites, also are capable of living in tissues for prolonged periods.

**Megakaryocytes** are giant, multinucleated cells that derive from the primitive stem cell and are polyploid (16–32 times the normal DNA content) because of nuclear but not cytoplasmic cell division. Platelets form by invagination of the megakaryocytic cell membrane and bud off from the periphery. **Thrombopoietin** is the primary regulator of platelet production. Platelets adhere to damaged

endothelium and subendothelial surfaces via specific receptors for the adhesive proteins, von Willebrand factor (vWF), and fibrinogen. Platelets also have specific granules that readily release their contents after stimulation and trigger the process of platelet aggregation. Platelets circulate for 7 to 10 days and have no nucleus.

**Lymphocytes** are particularly abundant in the bone marrow of young children, although they are a significant component of normal bone marrow at all ages. These are primarily B lymphocytes arising in the spleen and lymph nodes, but T lymphocytes also are present.

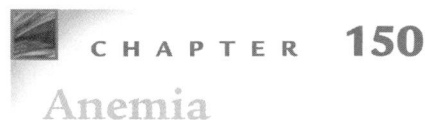

CHAPTER 150

# Anemia

## ETIOLOGY

Anemia may be defined either quantitatively or physiologically. The diagnosis of anemia is determined by comparison of the patient's **hemoglobin level** with age-specific and sex-specific normal values (see Table 149-2). The production of androgens at the onset of puberty in boys causes males to maintain a normal hemoglobin value about 1.5 to 2 g/dL higher than girls. The easiest quantitative definition of anemia is any hemoglobin or

hematocrit value that is 2 standard deviations (SDs) (95% confidence limits) below the mean for age and gender. Nevertheless, in certain pathologic states, anemia may be present with a normal hemoglobin level, such as in cyanotic cardiac or pulmonary disease or when a hemoglobin with an abnormally high affinity for oxygen is present. In these circumstances, the physiologic definition is more appropriate. Anemia is often not a disease per se, but rather a manifestation of some other primary process and may accentuate other organ dysfunction.

Anemias are classified based on the size and hemoglobin content of the cells (Fig. 150-1). **Hypochromic, microcytic anemia** is caused by an inadequate production of hemoglobin. The most common causes of this type of anemia are iron deficiency and thalassemia. Most **normocytic anemias** are associated with a systemic

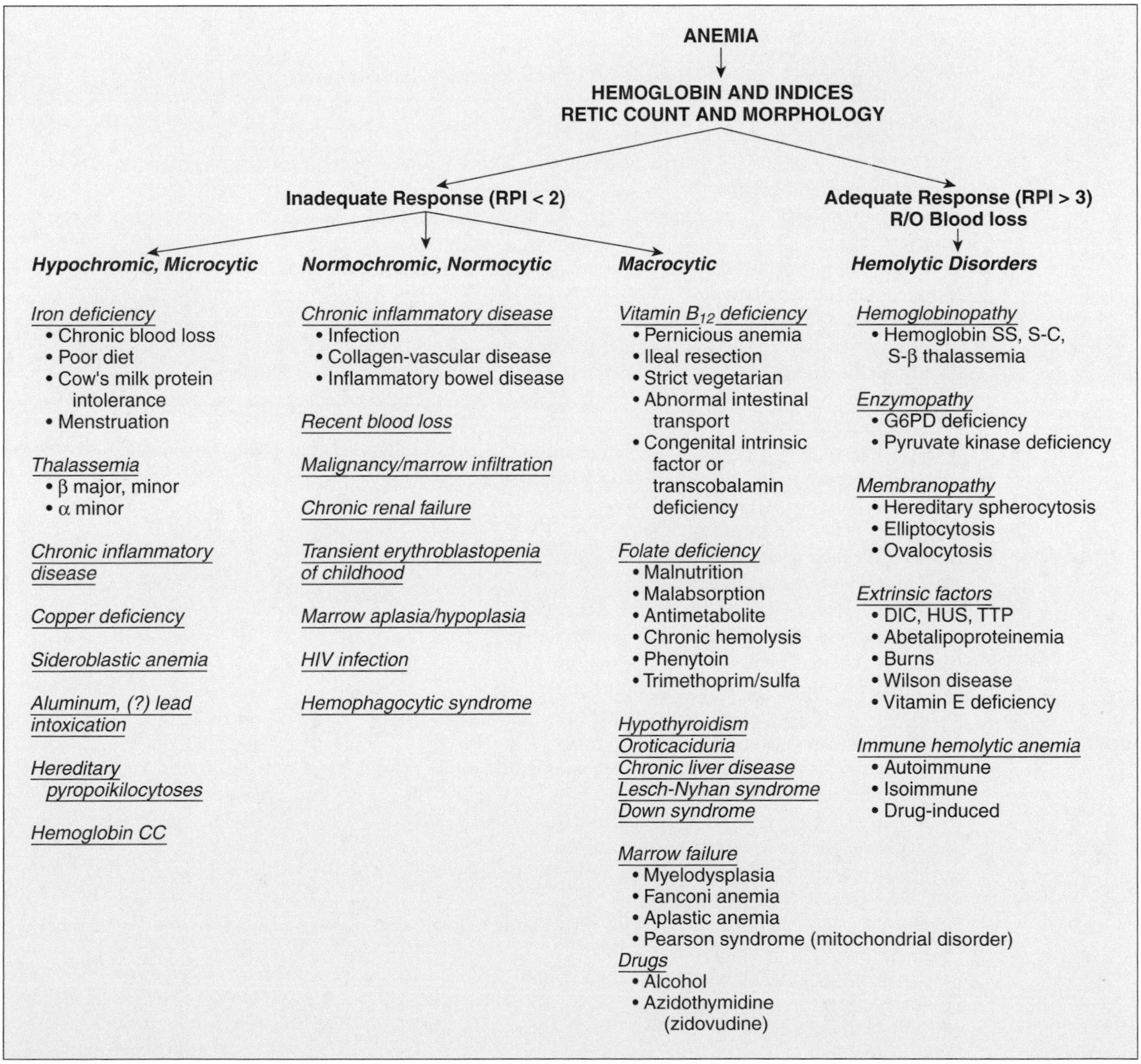

---

**ANEMIA**

↓

**HEMOGLOBIN AND INDICES**
**RETIC COUNT AND MORPHOLOGY**

**Inadequate Response (RPI < 2)** | **Adequate Response (RPI > 3)** / **R/O Blood loss**

| **Hypochromic, Microcytic** | **Normochromic, Normocytic** | **Macrocytic** | **Hemolytic Disorders** |
|---|---|---|---|
| *Iron deficiency* <br> • Chronic blood loss <br> • Poor diet <br> • Cow's milk protein intolerance <br> • Menstruation | *Chronic inflammatory disease* <br> • Infection <br> • Collagen-vascular disease <br> • Inflammatory bowel disease | *Vitamin B₁₂ deficiency* <br> • Pernicious anemia <br> • Ileal resection <br> • Strict vegetarian <br> • Abnormal intestinal transport <br> • Congenital intrinsic factor or transcobalamin deficiency | *Hemoglobinopathy* <br> • Hemoglobin SS, S-C, S-β thalassemia |
| *Thalassemia* <br> • β major, minor <br> • α minor | *Recent blood loss* <br><br> *Malignancy/marrow infiltration* | | *Enzymopathy* <br> • G6PD deficiency <br> • Pyruvate kinase deficiency |
| *Chronic inflammatory disease* | *Chronic renal failure* | *Folate deficiency* <br> • Malnutrition <br> • Malabsorption <br> • Antimetabolite <br> • Chronic hemolysis <br> • Phenytoin <br> • Trimethoprim/sulfa | *Membranopathy* <br> • Hereditary spherocytosis <br> • Elliptocytosis <br> • Ovalocytosis |
| *Copper deficiency* | *Transient erythroblastopenia of childhood* | | *Extrinsic factors* <br> • DIC, HUS, TTP <br> • Abetalipoproteinemia <br> • Burns <br> • Wilson disease <br> • Vitamin E deficiency |
| *Sideroblastic anemia* | *Marrow aplasia/hypoplasia* | | |
| *Aluminum, (?) lead intoxication* | *HIV infection* | *Hypothyroidism* <br> *Oroticaciduria* <br> *Chronic liver disease* <br> *Lesch-Nyhan syndrome* <br> *Down syndrome* | *Immune hemolytic anemia* <br> • Autoimmune <br> • Isoimmune <br> • Drug-induced |
| *Hereditary pyropoikilocytoses* | *Hemophagocytic syndrome* | | |
| *Hemoglobin CC* | | *Marrow failure* <br> • Myelodysplasia <br> • Fanconi anemia <br> • Aplastic anemia <br> • Pearson syndrome (mitochondrial disorder) <br> *Drugs* <br> • Alcohol <br> • Azidothymidine (zidovudine) | |

**FIGURE 150-1**

**Use of the complete blood count, reticulocyte count, and blood smear in the diagnosis of anemia.** DIC, disseminated intravascular coagulation; G6PD, glucose-6-phosphate dehydrogenase; HUS, hemolytic uremic syndrome; R/O, rule out; RPI, reticulocyte production index; TTP, thrombotic thrombocytopenic purpura.

illness that impairs adequate marrow synthesis of red blood cells (RBCs). Vitamin $B_{12}$ and folic acid deficiencies lead to **macrocytic anemia**. Anemias may also occur from increased destruction. **Hemolytic diseases** are mediated either by intrinsic disorders of the RBC or by disorders extrinsic to the RBC itself. The most common RBC membrane disorders are **hereditary spherocytosis** and **hereditary elliptocytosis**. In both of these disorders, abnormalities of proteins within the cytoskeleton lead to abnormal RBC shape and function. Numerous RBC enzyme deficiencies may lead to hemolysis, but only two are common: **glucose-6-phosphate dehydrogenase (G6PD) deficiency** and **pyruvate kinase deficiency**. Immune-mediated hemolysis may be extravascular when RBCs coated with antibodies or complement are phagocytosed by the reticuloendothelial system. The hemolysis may be intravascular when antibody binding leads to complement fixation and lysis of RBCs.

## CLINICAL MANIFESTATIONS

Acute onset of anemia can result in a poorly compensated state and may be manifested as an elevated heart rate, a flow murmur, poor exercise tolerance, headache, excessive sleeping (especially in infants) or fatigue, irritability, poor feeding, and syncope. In contrast, chronic anemia often is exceptionally well tolerated in children because of their cardiovascular reserve. Usually, children with chronic anemia will have tachycardia and a flow murmur on examination. The urgency of diagnostic and therapeutic intervention, especially the use of packed RBC transfusion, should be dictated by the extent of cardiovascular or functional impairment more than the absolute level of hemoglobin.

The causes of anemia often can be suspected from a careful history adjusted for the patient's age (Tables 150-1 and 150-2). Anemia at any age demands a search for

### TABLE 150-1 Historical Clues in Evaluation of Anemia

| Variable | Comments |
|---|---|
| Age | Iron deficiency rare in the absence of blood loss before 6 mo or in term infants or before doubling of birth weight in preterm infants |
| | Neonatal anemia with reticulocytosis suggests hemolysis or blood loss; with reticulocytopenia, suggests bone marrow failure |
| | Sickle cell anemia and β-thalassemia appear as fetal hemoglobin disappears (4–8 mo of age) |
| Family history and genetic considerations | X-linked: G6PD deficiency |
| | Autosomal dominant: spherocytosis |
| | Autosomal recessive: sickle cell anemia, Fanconi anemia |
| | Family member with history of cholecystectomy (for bilirubin stones) or splenectomy at an early age |
| | Ethnicity (thalassemia in persons of Mediterranean origin; G6PD deficiency in blacks, Greeks, and people of Middle Eastern origin) |
| | Race (β-thalassemia in persons of Mediterranean, African, or Asian descent; α-thalassemia in those of African and Asian descent; SC and SS in African descent) |
| Nutrition | Cow's milk diet: iron deficiency |
| | Strict vegetarian: vitamin $B_{12}$ deficiency |
| | Goat's milk diet: folate deficiency |
| | Pica: plumbism, iron deficiency |
| | Cholestasis, malabsorption: vitamin E deficiency |
| Drugs | G6PD: oxidants (e.g., nitrofurantoin, antimalarials) |
| | Immune-mediated hemolysis (e.g., penicillin) |
| | Bone marrow suppression (e.g., chemotherapy) |
| | Phenytoin, increasing folate requirements |
| Diarrhea | Malabsorption of vitamin $B_{12}$ or E or iron |
| | Inflammatory bowel disease and anemia of inflammation (chronic disease) with or without blood loss |
| | Milk protein intolerance–induced blood loss |
| | Intestinal resection: vitamin $B_{12}$ deficiency |
| Infection | *Giardia lamblia* infection: iron malabsorption |
| | Intestinal bacterial overgrowth (blind loop): vitamin $B_{12}$ deficiency |
| | Fish tapeworm: vitamin $B_{12}$ deficiency |
| | Epstein-Barr virus, cytomegalovirus infection: bone marrow suppression, hemophagocytic syndromes |
| | *Mycoplasma* infection: hemolysis |
| | Parvovirus infection: bone marrow suppression |
| | HIV infection |
| | Chronic infection |
| | Endocarditis |
| | Malaria: hemolysis |
| | Hepatitis: aplastic anemia |

G6PD, glucose-6-phosphate dehydrogenase.

## TABLE 150-2  Physical Findings in the Evaluation of Anemia

| System/Structure | Observation | Significance |
|---|---|---|
| Skin | Hyperpigmentation | Fanconi anemia, dyskeratosis congenita |
| | Café au lait spots | Fanconi anemia |
| | Vitiligo | Vitamin $B_{12}$ deficiency |
| | Partial oculocutaneous albinism | Chédiak-Higashi syndrome |
| | Jaundice | Hemolysis |
| | Petechiae, purpura | Bone marrow infiltration, autoimmune hemolysis with autoimmune thrombocytopenia, hemolytic uremic syndrome, hemophagocytic syndromes |
| | Erythematous rash | Parvovirus or Epstein-Barr virus infection |
| | Butterfly rash | SLE antibodies |
| | Bruising | Bleeding disorder, nonaccidental trauma, scurvy |
| Head | Frontal bossing | Thalassemia major, severe iron deficiency, chronic subdural hematoma |
| | Microcephaly | Fanconi anemia |
| Eyes | Microphthalmia | Fanconi anemia |
| | Retinopathy | Hemoglobin SS, SC disease (see Table 150-7) |
| | Optic atrophy | Osteopetrosis |
| | Blocked lacrimal gland | Dyskeratosis congenita |
| | Kayser-Fleischer ring | Wilson disease |
| | Blue sclera | Iron deficiency |
| Ears | Deafness | Osteopetrosis |
| Mouth | Glossitis | Vitamin $B_{12}$ deficiency, iron deficiency |
| | Angular stomatitis | Iron deficiency |
| | Cleft lip | Diamond-Blackfan syndrome |
| | Pigmentation | Peutz-Jeghers syndrome (intestinal blood loss) |
| | Telangiectasia | Osler-Weber-Rendu syndrome (blood loss) |
| | Leukoplakia | Dyskeratosis congenita |
| Chest | Shield chest or widespread nipples | Diamond-Blackfan syndrome |
| | Murmur | Endocarditis: prosthetic valve hemolysis; severe anemia |
| Abdomen | Hepatomegaly | Hemolysis, infiltrative tumor, chronic disease, hemangioma, cholecystitis, extramedullary hematopoiesis |
| | Splenomegaly | Hemolysis, sickle cell disease, (early) thalassemia, malaria, leukemia/lymphoma, Epstein-Barr virus, portal hypertension |
| | Nephromegaly | Fanconi anemia |
| | Absent kidney | Fanconi anemia |
| Extremities | Absent thumbs | Fanconi anemia |
| | Triphalangeal thumb | Diamond-Blackfan syndrome |
| | Spoon nails | Iron deficiency |
| | Beau line (nails) | Heavy metal intoxication, severe illness |
| | Mees line (nails) | Heavy metals, severe illness, sickle cell anemia |
| | Dystrophic nails | Dyskeratosis congenita |
| Rectal | Hemorrhoids | Portal hypertension |
| | Heme-positive stool | Gastrointestinal bleeding |
| Nerves | Irritable, apathy | Iron deficiency |
| | Peripheral neuropathy | Deficiency of vitamins $B_1$, $B_{12}$, and E; lead poisoning |
| | Dementia | Deficiency of vitamins $B_{12}$ and E |
| | Ataxia, posterior column signs | Vitamin $B_{12}$ deficiency |
| | Stroke | Sickle cell anemia, paroxysmal nocturnal hemoglobinuria |
| General | Small stature | Fanconi anemia, HIV infection, malnutrition |

SLE, systemic lupus erythematosus.

**blood loss**. A history of jaundice, pallor, previously affected siblings, drug ingestion by the mother, or excessive blood loss at the time of birth provides important clues to the diagnosis in newborns. A careful **dietary history** is crucial. The key findings in patients with hemolytic anemias are **jaundice**, **pallor**, and **splenomegaly**. Because of increased bilirubin production, **gallstones** (bilirubinate), a result of chronic hemolysis, are a common complication. Systemic complaints suggest acute or chronic illnesses as probable causes of anemia. In later childhood and adolescence, the presence of constitutional symptoms, unusual diets, drug ingestion, or blood loss, especially from menstrual bleeding, often points to a diagnosis. **Congenital hemolytic disorders** (enzyme deficiencies and membrane problems) often present in the first 6 months of life and frequently are associated with neonatal jaundice, although these disorders often go undiagnosed. A careful **drug history** is essential for detecting problems that may be drug-induced. Pure dietary iron deficiency is rare except in infancy, when cow's milk protein intolerance causes gastrointestinal blood loss and further complicates an already inadequate iron intake.

The physical examination also suggests the presence of anemia and may point to the potential causes (see Table 150-2). The first step is to assess the **physiologic stability** of the patient. Acute blood loss and acute hemolysis may manifest with tachycardia, blood pressure changes, and, most ominously, an altered state of consciousness. The presence of **jaundice** suggests hemolysis. **Petechiae** and **purpura** indicate a bleeding tendency. **Hepatosplenomegaly** and **adenopathy** suggest infiltrative disorders. **Growth failure** or poor weight gain suggests an anemia of chronic disease. An essential element of the physical examination in a patient with anemia is the investigation of the stool for the presence of **occult blood**.

## LABORATORY STUDIES

The initial laboratory evaluation of anemia involves a hemoglobin or hematocrit test to indicate the severity of the anemia. When the diagnosis of anemia has been substantiated, the workup should include a **complete blood count** with differential, platelet count, indices, and reticulocyte count. Examination of the peripheral blood smear assesses the **morphology** of RBCs (Fig. 150-2), white blood cells (WBCs), and platelets. All cell lines should be scrutinized to determine whether anemia is the result of a process limited to the erythroid line or a process that

### FIGURE 150-2

**Morphologic abnormalities of the red blood cell. A,** Normal. **B,** Hypochromic microcytes (iron deficiency). **C,** Schistocytes (hemolytic uremic syndrome **D,** Blister cells (glucose-6-phosphate dehydrogenase deficiency). **E,** Sickle cells (hemoglobin SS disease). **F,** Spherocytes (autoimmune hemolytic anemia. *(Courtesy of B. Trost and J.P. Scott.)*

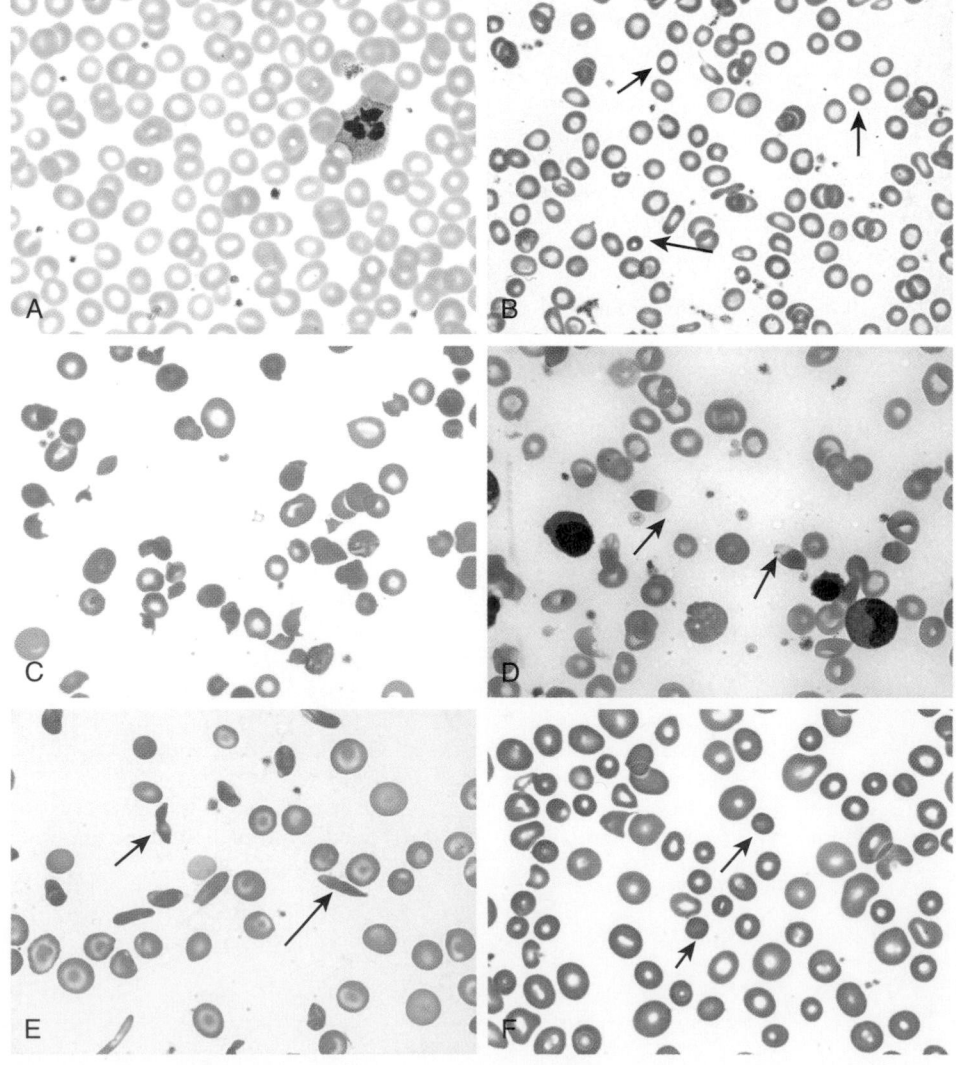

affects other marrow elements. Using data obtained from the **indices** and **reticulocyte count**, the workup can be organized on the basis of whether RBC production is adequate or inadequate and whether the cells are microcytic, normocytic, or macrocytic (see Fig. 150-1).

The **reticulocyte production index** (RPI), which corrects the reticulocyte count for the degree of anemia, indicates whether the bone marrow is responding appropriately. Reticulocytes routinely are counted per 1000 RBCs. A reduction in the denominator, which occurs in anemia, falsely increases the reticulocyte count. The formula for calculating the RPI is as follows:

$$RPI = \text{reticulocyte count} \times \text{hemoglobin}_{observed}/\text{hemoglobin}_{normal} \times 0.5$$

An RPI greater than 3 suggests increased production and implies either hemolysis or blood loss, whereas an index below 2 suggests decreased or ineffective production for the degree of anemia. Reticulocytopenia signifies that the anemia is so acute in onset that the marrow has not had adequate time to respond, that reticulocytes are being destroyed in the marrow (antibody-mediated), or that intrinsic bone marrow disease is present. Some machines that perform complete blood counts report an absolute reticulocyte number that corrects the artifact caused by the degree of anemia.

When conducting a workup for hemolysis, the best indicators of the severity of hemolysis are the hemoglobin level and the elevation of the **reticulocyte count**. Biochemical evidence of hemolysis includes an increase in levels of bilirubin and lactate dehydrogenase and a decrease in haptoglobin.

## DIFFERENTIAL DIAGNOSIS

Hypochromic, Microcytic Anemia

### Iron Deficiency Anemia

**Etiology.** Infants fed cow's milk when younger than 1 year of age, toddlers fed large volumes of cow's milk, and menstruating teenage girls who are not receiving supplemental iron are at high risk for iron deficiency. **Dietary** iron deficiency anemia is most common in bottle-fed toddlers who are receiving large volumes of cow's milk and ingest few dietary substances high in iron

(see Chapters 28 and 31). Iron deficiency anemia also may be found in children with chronic inflammatory diseases, even without **chronic blood loss**.

**Epidemiology.** The prevalence of iron deficiency, the most common cause of anemia in the world, is about 9% in toddlers, 9% to 11% in adolescent girls, and less than 1% in teenage boys. Iron deficiency anemia occurs in about one third of children who are iron deficient (Table 150-3). Some underprivileged minority populations in the United States may be at increased risk for iron deficiency because of poor dietary intake (see Chapter 31). Breastfed infants are less likely to have iron deficiency than bottle-fed infants because, although there is less iron in breast milk, this iron is more efficiently absorbed.

**Clinical Manifestations.** In addition to manifestations of anemia, central nervous system (CNS) abnormalities (**apathy, irritability, poor concentration**) have been linked to iron deficiency, presumably resulting from alterations of iron-containing enzymes (monoamine oxidase) and cytochromes. Poor muscle endurance, gastrointestinal dysfunction, and impaired WBC and T cell function have been associated with iron deficiency. Iron deficiency in infancy may be associated with later **cognitive deficits** and poor school performance.

**Treatment.** In an otherwise healthy child, a **therapeutic trial of iron** is the best diagnostic study for iron deficiency as long as the child is re-examined and a response is documented. The response to oral iron includes rapid subjective improvement, especially in neurologic function (within 24–48 hours) and reticulocytosis (48–72 hours); increase in hemoglobin levels (4–30 days); and repletion of iron stores (in 1–3 months). A usual therapeutic dose of 4 to 6 mg/day of elemental iron induces an increase in hemoglobin of 0.25 to 0.4 g/dL/day (a 1%/day increase in hematocrit). If the hemoglobin level fails to increase within 2 weeks after institution of iron treatment, careful re-evaluation for ongoing blood loss, development of infection, poor compliance, or other causes of microcytic anemia is required (Table 150-4; see Fig. 150-1).

**Prevention.** Bottle-fed infants should receive an iron-containing formula until 12 months of age, and breastfed infants older than 6 months of age should receive an iron supplement. The introduction of iron-enriched solid foods at 6 months of age, followed by a transition to a

### TABLE 150-3 Stages in Development of Iron Deficiency Anemia

| Hemoglobin (g/dL) | Peripheral Smear | Serum Iron (μg/dL) | Bone Marrow Iron | Serum Ferritin (ng/mL) |
|---|---|---|---|---|
| 13+ (normal) | nc/nc | 50/150 | $Fe^{2+}$ | *Male*: 40–340<br>*Female*: 40–150 |
| 10–12 | nc/nc | ↓ | $Fe^{2+}$ absent, erythroid hyperplasia | <12 |
| 8–10 | hypo/nc | ↓ | $Fe^{2+}$ absent, erythroid hyperplasia | <12 |
| <8 | hypo/micro* | ↓ | $Fe^{2+}$ absent, erythroid hyperplasia | <12 |

*Microcytosis, determined by a mean corpuscular volume (in fL) <2 SD below the mean, must be adjusted for age (e.g., −2 SD at 3–6 mo = 74; at 0.5–2 yr = 70; at 2–6 yr = 75; at 6–12 yr = 77; and at 12–18 yr = 78).
hypo/micro, hypochromic, microcytic; hypo/nc, hypochromic, normocytic; nc/nc, normochromic, normocytic.
From Andreoli TE, Bennett JC, Carpenter CC, et al: Cecil Essentials of Medicine, 4th ed. Philadelphia *WB Saunders*, 1997.

**TABLE 150-4 Differentiating Features of Microcytic Anemias\***

| Test | Iron Deficiency Anemia | Thalassemia Minor[†] | Anemia of Inflammation[‡] |
|---|---|---|---|
| Serum iron | Low | Normal | Low |
| Serum iron-binding capacity | High | Normal | Low or normal |
| Serum ferritin | Low | Normal or high | Normal or high |
| Marrow iron stores | Low or absent | Normal or high | Normal or high |
| Marrow sideroblasts | Decreased or absent | Normal or increased | Normal or increased |
| Free erythrocyte protoporphyrin | High | Normal or slightly increased | High |
| Hemoglobin $A_2$ or F | Normal | High β-thalassemia; normal α-thalassemia | Normal |
| Red blood cell distribution width[§] | High | Normal | Normal/↑ |

\*See Table 150-3 for definition of microcytosis.
[†]α-Thalassemia minor can be diagnosed by the presence of Bart hemoglobin on newborn screening.
[‡]Usually normochromic; 25% of cases are microcytic.
[§]Red blood cell distribution width quantitates the degree of anisocytosis (different sizes) of red blood cells.

limited amount of cow's milk and increased solid foods at 1 year, can help prevent iron deficiency anemia. Teenage girls who are menstruating should have a diet enriched with iron-containing foods. A vitamin with iron may also be used.

## Thalassemia Minor

**Etiology and Epidemiology. α-Thalassemia** and **β-thalassemia minor** are common causes of microcytosis, either with or without a mild hypochromic, microcytic anemia. They are prevalent in certain ethnic groups (Mediterranean, Southeast Asian, African Americans). Individuals of Asian descent are at risk of having three or four α genes deleted, resulting in hemoglobin H disease ($\gamma_4$) or hydrops fetalis with only Bart ($\alpha_4$) hemoglobin. (Table 150-5 and Fig. 150-3)

**Laboratory Testing.** The thalassemia minor syndromes are characterized by a mild hypochromic, microcytic anemia with a low RPI (see Table 150-5). The RBC count is usually elevated. As a result, if the mean corpuscular volume (MCV) divided by the RBC count is less than 12.5 (Mentzer index), the diagnosis is suggestive of thalassemia trait. The blood smear reveals only microcytosis with α-thalassemia trait. Outside the neonatal period, when Bart hemoglobin is detectable, hemoglobin electrophoresis usually is normal in α-thalassemia minor (see Fig. 150-3). Blood smears of patients with β-thalassemia minor show microcytic RBCs. Target cells and basophilic stippled RBCs, caused by precipitation of alpha chain tetramers, also may be present. The diagnosis is based on an elevation of hemoglobin $A_2$ and F levels in **β-thalassemia**.

**TABLE 150-5 Thalassemic Syndromes**

| Disorder | Genotypic Abnormality | Clinical Phenotype |
|---|---|---|
| **β-THALASSEMIA** | | |
| Thalassemia major (Cooley's anemia) | Homozygous $\beta^0$-thalassemia | Severe hemolysis, ineffective erythropoiesis, transfusion dependency, iron overload |
| Thalassemia intermedia | Compound heterozygous $\beta^0$- and $\beta^+$-thalassemia | Moderate hemolysis, severe anemia, but not transfusion-dependent; main life-threatening complication is iron overload |
| Thalassemia minor | Heterozygous $\beta^0$- and $\beta^+$-thalassemia | Microcytosis, mild anemia |
| **α-THALASSEMIA** | | |
| Silent carrier | α–/αα | Normal complete blood count |
| α-Thalassemia trait | αα/– – (α-thalassemia 1) *or* α –/α – (α-thalassemia 2) | Mild microcytic anemia |
| Hemoglobin H | α –/– – | Microcytic anemia and mild hemolysis; not transfusion-dependent |
| Hydrops fetalis | – –/– – | Severe anemia, intrauterine anasarca from congestive heart failure; death in utero or at birth |

From Andreoli T, Carpenter C, Griggs R, et al: Andreoli and Carpenter's Cecil Essentials of Medicine, 7th ed. Philadelphia, *Saunders*, 2007.

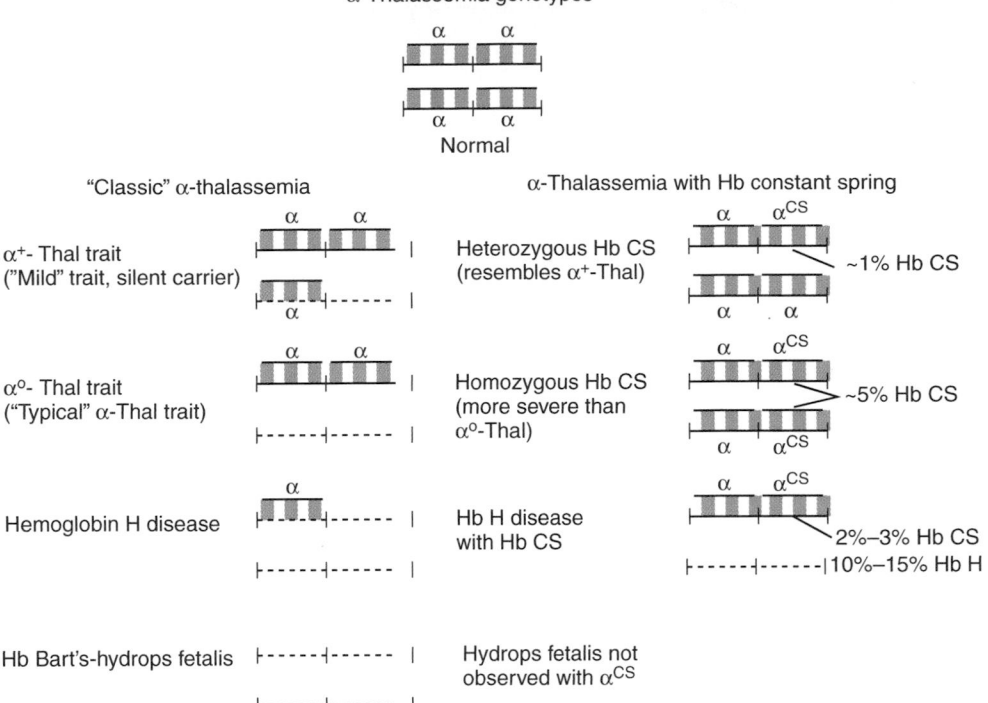

α-Thalassemia genotypes

Normal

"Classic" α-thalassemia

α-Thalassemia with Hb constant spring

α+- Thal trait
("Mild" trait, silent carrier)

Heterozygous Hb CS
(resembles α+-Thal)

~1% Hb CS

α°- Thal trait
("Typical" α-Thal trait)

Homozygous Hb CS
(more severe than
α°-Thal)

~5% Hb CS

Hemoglobin H disease

Hb H disease
with Hb CS

2%–3% Hb CS
10%–15% Hb H

Hb Bart's-hydrops fetalis

Hydrops fetalis not
observed with α^CS

**FIGURE 150-3**

**Genetic origins of the classic α-thalassemia syndromes due to gene deletions in the α-globin gene cluster.** Hb Constant Spring (Hb CS) is an α-globin chain variant synthesized in such small amounts (1%–2% of normal) that it has the phenotypic impact of a severe nondeletion α-thalassemia allele; however, the α^CS allele is always linked to a functioning α-globin gene, so it has never been associated with hydrops fetalis. (From Hoffman: Hematology: Basic Principles and Practice, 5th ed. Philadelphia, *Churchill Livingstone*, 2008.)

**Treatment.** No treatment is required for children with **thalassemia minor**. However, children with hemoglobin H disease ($\gamma_4$) or hydrops fetalis with only Bart ($\alpha_4$) hemoglobin are likely to require chronic transfusion therapy.

## Lead Poisoning

Lead poisoning may be associated with a hypochromic, microcytic anemia. Most patients have concomitant iron deficiency. The history of living in an older home (built before 1980) with chipped paint or lead dust should raise suspicion of lead poisoning, especially in a child with **pica. Basophilic stippling** on the blood smear is common. Lead intoxication rarely causes hemolytic anemia. Detection by routine screening, removal from exposure, chelation therapy, and correction of iron deficiency are crucial to the potential development of affected children.

## Normocytic Anemia

**Etiology and Treatment.** Anemia is a common component of chronic inflammatory disease. Hepcidin, a protein made in the liver, plays a key role in iron homeostasis. Inflammation causes an increase in the production of hepcidin which interrupts the process of iron release by macrophages and also interrupts the absorption of iron from the intestines leading to anemia. The **anemia of inflammation** may be normocytic or, less often, microcytic. At times, this situation poses a clinical challenge, when children with inflammatory disorders that may be associated with blood loss (inflammatory bowel disease) exhibit a microcytic anemia. In these circumstances, the only specific diagnostic test that can differentiate the two entities clearly is a bone marrow aspiration with

staining of the sample for iron (see Table 150-4). Low **ferritin** levels indicate concurrent iron deficiency. A trial of iron therapy is not indicated without a specific diagnosis in children who appear to be systemically ill.

Bone marrow **infiltration by malignant cells** commonly leads to a normochromic, normocytic anemia. The mechanism by which neoplastic cells interfere with RBC and other marrow cell synthesis is multifactorial. The reticulocyte count is often low. Immature myeloid elements may be released into the peripheral blood due to the presence of the offending tumor cells. An examination of the peripheral blood may reveal lymphoblasts; when solid tumors metastasize to the marrow, these cells are seldom seen in the peripheral blood. Teardrop cells may be seen in the peripheral blood. A bone marrow examination is frequently necessary in the face of normochromic, normocytic anemia.

**Congenital pure RBC aplasia** (Diamond-Blackfan syndrome), a lifelong disorder, usually presents in the first few months of life or at birth with severe anemia and mild macrocytosis or a normocytic anemia. It is due to a deficiency of bone marrow red blood cell precursors (see Table 150-6). More than a third of patients have short stature. Many patients (50–66%) respond to corticosteroid treatment, but must receive therapy indefinitely. Patients who do not respond to corticosteroid treatment are transfusion-dependent and are at risk of the multiple complications of long-term transfusion therapy, especially iron overload. These patients have a higher rate of developing leukemia or other hematologic malignancies than the general population.

In contrast to the congenital hypoplastic anemias, **transient erythroblastopenia of childhood**, a normocytic anemia caused by suppression of RBC synthesis, usually appears after 6 months of age in an otherwise normal infant. Viral

**TABLE 150-6 Differentiation of Red Blood Cell Aplasias and Aplastic Anemias**

| Disorder | Age at Onset | Characteristics | Treatment |
|---|---|---|---|
| **CONGENITAL** | | | |
| Diamond-Blackfan syndrome (congenital hypoplastic anemia) | Newborn–1 mo; 90% of patients are <1 yr of age | Pure red blood cell aplasia, autosomal recessive trait, elevated fetal hemoglobin, fetal i antigen present, macrocytic, short stature, webbed neck, cleft lip, triphalangeal thumb; late-onset leukemia | Prednisone, transfusion |
| **ACQUIRED** | | | |
| Transient erythroblastopenia | 6 mo–5 yr of age; 85% of patients are >1 yr of age | Pure red blood cell defect; no anomalies, fetal hemoglobin, or i antigen; spontaneous recovery, normal MCV | Expectant transfusion for symptomatic anemia |
| Idiopathic aplastic anemia (status post hepatitis, drugs, unknown) | All ages | All cell lines involved; exposure to felbamate, chloramphenicol, radiation | Hematopoietic stem cell transplantation, antithymocyte globulin, cyclosporine, androgens |
| **FAMILIAL** | | | |
| Fanconi anemia | Before 10 yr of age; mean is 8 yr | All cell lines; microcephaly, absent thumbs, café au lait spots, cutaneous hyperpigmentation, short stature; chromosomal breaks, high MCV and hemoglobin F; horseshoe or absent kidney; leukemic transformation; autosomal recessive trait | Androgens, corticosteroids, hematopoietic stem cell transplantation |
| Paroxysmal nocturnal hemoglobinuria | After 5 yr | Initial hemolysis followed by aplastic anemia; increased complement-mediated hemolysis; thrombosis; iron deficiency; CD59 low | Iron, hematopoietic stem cell transplantation, androgens, steroids, eculizumab |
| Dyskeratosis congenita | Mean is 10 yr for skin; mean is 17 yr for anemia | Pancytopenia; hyperpigmentation, dystrophic nails, leukoplakia; X-linked recessive; lacrimal duct stenosis; high MCV and fetal hemoglobin | Androgens, splenectomy, bone marrow transplantation |
| Familial hemophagocytic lymphohistiocytosis | Before 2 yr | Pancytopenia; fever, hepatosplenomegaly, hypertriglyceridemia, CSF pleocytosis | Transfusion; often lethal; VP-16, bone marrow transplantation, IVIG, cyclosporine |
| **INFECTIOUS** | | | |
| Parvovirus | Any age | Any chronic hemolytic anemia, typically sickle cell; new-onset reticulocytopenia | Transfusion |
| Epstein-Barr virus (EBV) | Any age; usually < 5 yr of age | X-linked immunodeficiency syndrome, pancytopenia | Transfusion, bone marrow transplantation |
| Virus-associated hemophagocytic syndrome (CMV, HHV-6, EBV) | Any age | Pancytopenia; hemophagocytosis in marrow, fever, hepatosplenomegaly | Transfusion, antiviral therapy, IVIG |

CMV, cytomegalovirus; CSF, cerebrospinal fluid; HHV-6, human herpesvirus 6; IVIG, intravenous immune globulin; MCV, mean corpuscular volume; VP-16, etoposide.

infections are thought to be the trigger, although the mechanism leading to RBC aplasia is poorly understood. The onset is gradual, but anemia may become severe. Recovery usually is spontaneous. Differentiation from Diamond-Blackfan syndrome, in which erythroid precursors also are absent or diminished in the bone marrow, may be challenging. Transfusion of packed RBCs may be necessary if the anemia becomes symptomatic before recovery.

**Aplastic crises** may complicate any chronic hemolytic anemia. These periods of severe reticulocytopenia, during which the usual high rate of RBC destruction leads to an acute exacerbation of the anemia, may precipitate a cardiovascular decompensation. Human parvovirus B19 (the cause of fifth disease) infects erythroid precursors and shuts down erythropoiesis. Transient erythroid aplasia is without consequence in individuals with normal RBC survival. Recovery from parvovirus infection in hemolytic disease is spontaneous, but patients may need transfusion if the anemia is severe.

## Macrocytic Anemia

See Figure 150-1.

### Marrow Failure/Pancytopenia

**Etiology.** Pancytopenia is a quantitative decrease in formed elements of the blood—erythrocytes, leukocytes, and platelets. Patients more often exhibit symptoms of infection or bleeding than anemia because of the relatively short life span of WBCs and platelets compared with the life span of RBCs. Causes of pancytopenia include failure of production (implying intrinsic bone marrow disease), sequestration (hypersplenism), and increased peripheral destruction.

**Differential Diagnosis.** Features that suggest **bone marrow failure** and mandate an examination of bone marrow include a low reticulocyte count, teardrop forms of RBCs (implying marrow replacement, not just failure), presence of abnormal forms of leukocytes or myeloid elements less mature than band forms, small platelets, and an elevated mean corpuscular volume in the face of a low reticulocyte count. Pancytopenia resulting from bone marrow failure is usually a gradual process, starting with one or two cell lines, but later involving all three cell lines. Features suggesting **increased destruction** include reticulocytosis, jaundice, immature erythroid or myeloid elements on the blood smear, large platelets, and increased serum bilirubin and lactic dehydrogenase.

### Aplastic Anemia

**Etiology and Epidemiology.** In a child with aplastic anemia, pancytopenia evolves as the hematopoietic elements of the bone marrow disappear and the marrow is replaced by fat. In developed countries, aplastic anemia is most often idiopathic. The disorder may be induced by drugs such as chloramphenicol and felbamate or by toxins such as benzene. Aplastic anemia also may follow infections, particularly hepatitis and infectious mononucleosis (Table 150-6). Immunosuppression of hematopoiesis is postulated to be an important mechanism in patients with postinfectious and idiopathic aplastic anemia.

**Laboratory Studies.** A **bone marrow biopsy** is crucial to determine cellularity or the extent of depletion of the hematopoietic elements.

**Treatment.** Survival rate is about 20% in severe aplastic anemia with supportive care alone, although the duration of survival may be years when vigorous blood product and antibiotic support is provided. For children with severe aplastic anemia—defined by an RPI less than 1%, absolute neutrophil count less than 500/mm³, platelet count less than $20,000/mm^3$, and bone marrow cellularity on biopsy specimen less than 25% of normal—the treatment of choice is **hematopoietic stem cell transplantation (HSCT)** from a sibling with identical HLA and compatible mixed lymphocytes. When HSCT occurs before the recipient is sensitized to blood products, survival rate is greater than 80%. The treatment of aplastic anemia without an HLA-matched donor for HSCT is evolving, with two major options: potent immunosuppressive therapy or unrelated or partially matched HSCT. Results of trials using immunosuppressive therapy with antithymocyte globulin, cyclosporine, and corticosteroids in combination with hematopoietic growth factors have been encouraging. Such therapy is often toxic, and relapses often occur when therapy is stopped.

### Fanconi Anemia

**Etiology and Epidemiology.** Fanconi anemia is a constitutional form of aplastic anemia that usually presents in the latter half of the first decade of life and may evolve over years. A group of genetic defects in proteins involved in **DNA repair** have been identified in Fanconi anemia which is inherited in an autosomal recessive manner. The diagnosis is based on demonstration of increased chromosomal breakage after exposure to agents that damage DNA. The repair mechanism for DNA damage is abnormal in all cells in Fanconi anemia, which may contribute to the increased risk of malignancies. Terminal acute leukemia develops in 10% of cases. Other malignancies include solid tumors of the head and neck, gastrointestinal tumors, and gynecologic tumors.

**Clinical Manifestations.** Patients with Fanconi anemia have numerous characteristic clinical findings (see Table 150-6).

**Treatment.** Hematopoietic stem cell transplantation can cure the pancytopenia caused by bone marrow aplasia. Many patients with Fanconi anemia and about 20% of children with aplastic anemia seem to respond for a time to **androgenic therapy**, which induces masculinization and may cause liver injury and liver tumors. Androgenic therapy increases RBC synthesis and may diminish transfusion requirements. The effect on granulocytes, and especially the platelet count, is less impressive.

**Marrow Replacement.** Marrow replacement may occur as a result of **leukemia**, **solid tumors** (especially neuroblastoma), **storage diseases**, **osteopetrosis** in infants, and **myelofibrosis**, which is rare in childhood. The mechanisms by which malignant cells impair marrow synthesis of normal hematopoietic elements are complex and incompletely understood. Bone marrow aspirate and biopsy are needed for precise diagnosis of the etiology of marrow synthetic failure.

**Pancytopenia Resulting from Destruction of Cells.** Pancytopenia resulting from destruction of cells may be caused by **intramedullary destruction** of hematopoietic elements (myeloproliferative disorders, deficiencies of folic acid and vitamin $B_{12}$) or by the **peripheral destruction** of mature cells. The usual site of peripheral destruction of blood cells is the spleen, although the liver and other parts of the reticuloendothelial system may participate. **Hypersplenism** may be the result of anatomic causes (portal hypertension or splenic hypertrophy from thalassemia); infections (including malaria); or storage diseases (Gaucher disease; lymphomas; or histiocytosis). Splenectomy is indicated only when the pancytopenia is of clinical significance (e.g., increased susceptibility to bleeding or infection or produces high transfusion requirements).

## Hemolytic Anemias

### Major Hemoglobinopathies

**Etiology.** Because alpha chains are needed for fetal erythropoiesis and production of hemoglobin F ($\alpha_2\gamma_2$), **alpha chain hemoglobinopathies** are present in utero. Four alpha genes are present on the two number 16 chromosomes (see Fig. 150-3 and Table 150-5). Single gene deletions produce no disorder (silent carrier state), but can be detected by measuring the rates of $\alpha$ and $\beta$ synthesis or by using molecular biologic techniques. Deletion of two genes produces **α-thalassemia minor** with mild or no anemia and microcytosis. In individuals of African origin, the gene deletions occur on different chromosomes (*trans*), and the disorder is benign. In the Asian population, deletions may occur on the same chromosome (*cis*), and infants may inherit two number 16 chromosomes lacking three or even four genes. Deletion of all four genes leads to hydrops fetalis, severe intrauterine anemia, and death, unless intrauterine transfusions are administered. Deletion of three genes produces moderate hemolytic anemia with $\gamma_4$ tetramers (**Bart hemoglobin**) in the fetus and $\beta_4$ tetramers (hemoglobin H) in older children and adults (see Table 150-5).

**Beta chain hemoglobinopathies** are more prevalent than alpha chain disorders possibly because these abnormalities are not symptomatic in utero. The major beta hemoglobinopathies include those that alter hemoglobin function, including **hemoglobins S, C, E, and D**, and those that alter beta chain production, the β-thalassemias. Because each RBC has two copies of chromosome 11 and they express both β-globin genes, most disorders of beta chains are not clinically severe, unless both beta chains are abnormal. By convention, when describing β-thalassemia genes, $\beta^0$ indicates a thalassemic gene resulting in absent beta chain synthesis, whereas $\beta^+$ indicates a thalassemic gene that permits reduced but not absent synthesis of normal β chains. Disorders of the beta chain usually manifest themselves clinically between 4 and 12 months of age, unless they have been detected prenatally or by cord blood screening.

### β-Thalassemia Major (Cooley Anemia)

**Etiology and Epidemiology.** β-Thalassemia major is caused by mutations that impair **beta chain synthesis**. Because of unbalanced synthesis of alpha and beta chains, alpha chains precipitate within the cells, resulting in RBC destruction either in the bone marrow or in the spleen. β-Thalassemia major is seen most commonly in individuals of Mediterranean or Asian descent. The clinical severity of the illness varies on the basis of the molecular defect.

**Clinical Manifestations.** Signs and symptoms of β-thalassemia major result from the combination of chronic hemolytic disease, decreased or absent production of normal hemoglobin A, and ineffective erythropoiesis. The anemia is severe and leads to growth failure and high-output heart failure. **Ineffective erythropoiesis** causes increased expenditure of energy and expansion of the bone marrow cavities of all bones, leading to osteopenia, pathologic fractures, extramedullary erythropoiesis, and an increase in the rate of iron absorption.

**Treatment.** Treatment of β-thalassemia major is based on a **hypertransfusion program** that corrects the anemia and suppresses the patient's own ineffective erythropoiesis, limiting the stimulus for increased iron absorption. This suppression permits the bones to heal, decreases metabolic expenditures, increases growth, and limits dietary iron absorption. Splenectomy may reduce the transfusion volume, but adds to the risk of serious infection. Chelation therapy with deferoxamine or deferasirox should start when laboratory evidence of iron overload (**hemochromatosis**) is present and before there are clinical signs of iron overload (nonimmune diabetes mellitus, cirrhosis, heart failure, bronzing of the skin, and multiple endocrine abnormalities). Hematopoietic stem cell transplantation in childhood, before organ dysfunction induced by iron overload, has had a high success rate in β-thalassemia major and is the treatment of choice.

### Sickle Cell Disease

**Etiology and Epidemiology.** The common sickle cell syndromes are **hemoglobin SS disease**, **hemoglobin S-C disease**, **hemoglobin S-β thalassemia**, and rare variants (Table 150-7). The specific hemoglobin phenotype must be identified because the clinical complications differ in frequency, type, and severity. As a result of a single **amino acid substitution** (valine for glutamic acid at the β6 position), sickle hemoglobin crystallizes and forms a gel in the deoxygenated state. When reoxygenated, the sickle hemoglobin is normally soluble. The so-called reversible sickle cell is capable of entering the microcirculation. As the oxygen is extracted and saturation declines, sickling may occur, occluding the microvasculature. The surrounding tissue undergoes infarction, inducing pain and dysfunction. This sickling phenomenon is exacerbated by hypoxia, acidosis, fever, hypothermia, and dehydration.

**Clinical Manifestations and Treatment.** A child with sickle cell anemia is vulnerable to **life-threatening infection** by 4 months of age. By that time, **splenic dysfunction** is caused by sickling of the RBCs within the spleen, resulting in an inability to filter microorganisms from the bloodstream in most patients. Splenic dysfunction is followed, eventually, by **splenic infarction**, usually by 2 to 4 years of age. The loss of normal splenic function makes the patient susceptible to overwhelming infection by encapsulated organisms, especially *Streptococcus pneumoniae* and other pathogens (see Table 150-8). The hallmark of infection is fever. A febrile patient with a sickle cell syndrome (temperature > 38.5°C) must be evaluated immediately (see Chapter 96). Current precautions to

### TABLE 150-7 Comparison of Sickle Cell Syndromes

| Genotype | Clinical Condition | Percent Hemoglobin | | | | | Other Finding(s) |
|---|---|---|---|---|---|---|---|
| | | Hb A | Hb S | Hb A$_2$ | Hb F | Hb C | |
| SA | Sickle cell trait | 55–60 | 40–45 | 2–3 | — | — | Usually asymptomatic |
| SS | Sickle cell anemia | 0 | 85–95 | 2–3 | 5–15 | — | Clinically severe anemia; Hb F heterogeneous in distribution |
| S-β$^0$ thalassemia | Sickle cell–β$^0$ thalassemia | 0 | 70–80 | 3–5 | 10–20 | — | Moderately severe anemia; splenomegaly in 50%; smear: hypochromic, microcytic anemia |
| S-β$^+$ thalassemia | Sickle cell–β$^+$ thalassemia | 10–20 | 60–75 | 3–5 | 10–20 | | Hb F distributed heterogeneously; mild microcytic anemia |
| SC | Hb SC disease | 0 | 45–50 | — | — | 45–50 | Moderately severe anemia; splenomegaly; target cells |
| S-HPFH | Sickle-hereditary persistence of Hb F | 0 | 70–80 | 1–2 | 20–30 | — | Asymptomatic; Hb F is uniformly distributed |

From Andreoli TE, Bennett JC, Carpenter CC, et al: Cecil Essentials of Medicine, 4th ed. Philadelphia, *WB Saunders*, 1997.

### TABLE 150-8 Clinical Manifestations of Sickle Cell Anemia*

| Manifestation | Comments |
|---|---|
| Anemia | Chronic, onset 3–4 mo of age; may require folate therapy for chronic hemolysis; hematocrit usually 18–26% |
| Aplastic crisis | Parvovirus infection, reticulocytopenia; acute and reversible; may need transfusion |
| Sequestration crisis | Massive splenomegaly (may involve liver), shock; treat with transfusion |
| Hemolytic crisis | May be associated with G6PD deficiency |
| Dactylitis | Hand-foot swelling in early infancy |
| Painful crisis | Microvascular painful vaso-occlusive infarcts of muscle, bone, bone marrow, lung, intestines |
| Cerebrovascular accidents | Large and small vessel occlusion → thrombosis/bleeding (stroke); requires chronic transfusion |
| Acute chest syndrome | Infection, atelectasis, infarction, fat emboli, severe hypoxemia, infiltrate, dyspnea, absent breath sounds |
| Chronic lung disease | Pulmonary fibrosis, restrictive lung disease, cor pulmonale, pulmonary hypertension |
| Priapism | Causes eventual impotence; treated with transfusion, oxygen, or corpora cavernosa-to-spongiosa shunt |
| Ocular | Retinopathy |
| Gallbladder disease | Bilirubin stones; cholecystitis |
| Renal | Hematuria, papillary necrosis, renal concentrating defect; nephropathy |
| Cardiomyopathy | Heart failure |
| Skeletal | Osteonecrosis (avascular) of femoral or humeral head |
| Leg ulceration | Seen in older patients |
| Infections | Functional asplenia, defects in properdin system; pneumococcal bacteremia, meningitis, and arthritis; deafness from meningitis; *Salmonella* and *Staphylococcus aureus* osteomyelitis; severe *Mycoplasma* pneumonia |
| Growth failure, delayed puberty | May respond to nutritional supplements |
| Psychological problems | Narcotic addiction (rare), dependence unusual; chronic illness, chronic pain |

*Clinical manifestations with sickle cell trait are unusual but include renal papillary necrosis (hematuria), sudden death on exertion, intraocular hyphema extension, and sickling in unpressurized airplanes.
G6PD, glucose-6-phosphate dehydrogenase.

prevent infections include prophylactic daily oral penicillin begun at diagnosis and vaccinations against pneumococcus, *Haemophilus influenzae* type b, hepatitis B virus, and influenza virus.

The anemia of SS disease is usually a chronic, moderately severe, hemolytic anemia that is not routinely transfusion dependent. The severity depends in part on the patient's phenotype. Manifestations of chronic anemia include jaundice, pallor, variable splenomegaly in infancy, a cardiac flow murmur, and delayed growth and sexual maturation. Decisions about transfusion should be made on the basis of the patient's clinical condition, the hemoglobin level, and the reticulocyte count.

Sickle cell disease is complicated by sudden, occasionally severe and life-threatening events caused by the acute intravascular sickling of the RBCs, with resultant pain or organ dysfunction (so-called **crisis**). In two different clinical situations, an acute, potentially life-threatening decline in the hemoglobin level may be superimposed on the chronic compensated anemia. **Splenic sequestration crisis** is a life-threatening, hyperacute decline in the hemoglobin level (blood volume) secondary to splenic pooling of the patient's RBCs and sickling within the spleen. The spleen is moderately to markedly enlarged and the reticulocyte count is elevated. In an **aplastic crisis**, parvovirus B19 infects RBC precursors in the bone marrow and induces transient RBC aplasia with reticulocytopenia and a rapid worsening of anemia. Simple transfusion therapy is indicated for sequestration and aplastic crises when the anemia is symptomatic.

**Vaso-occlusive painful events** may occur in any organ of the body and are manifested by pain or significant dysfunction (Table 150-8). The **acute chest syndrome** is a vaso-occlusive crisis within the lungs with evidence of a new infiltrate on chest radiograph. It is often associated with infection and infarction. The patient may first complain of chest pain but within a few hours develops cough, increasing respiratory and heart rates, hypoxia, and progressive respiratory distress. Physical examination reveals areas of decreased breath sounds and dullness on chest percussion. Treatment involves early recognition and prevention of arterial hypoxemia. Oxygen, fluids, judicious use of analgesic medications, antibiotics, bronchodilators, and RBC transfusion (rarely exchange transfusion) are indicated in therapy for acute chest syndrome. *Incentive spirometry* may help reduce the incidence of acute chest crisis in patients presenting with pain in the chest or abdomen.

**Pain crisis** is the most common type of vaso-occlusive event. The pain usually localizes to the long bones of the arms or legs, but may occur in smaller bones of the hands or feet in infancy (dactylitis) or in the abdomen. Painful crises usually last 2 to 7 days. Vaso-occlusive crises within the femur may lead to avascular necrosis of the femoral head and chronic hip disease. Treatment of pain crises includes administration of fluids, analgesia (usually narcotics and nonsteroidal anti-inflammatory drugs) and oxygen if the patient is hypoxic. Although pain is often impossible to quantitate, the risk for drug dependency is highly overrated and appropriate use of analgesics is necessary.

**Priapism** occurs most typically in boys between 6 and 20 years old. The child experiences a sudden, painful onset of a tumescent penis that will not relax. Therapeutic steps for priapism include the administration of oxygen, fluids, transfusion to achieve a hemoglobin S less than 30% (often by partial exchange transfusion), and analgesia when appropriate. Fluid management requires recognition that renal medullary infarction results in loss of the ability to concentrate urine.

Overt **stroke** occurs in approximately 8% to 10% of patients with SS disease. These events may present as the sudden onset of an altered state of consciousness, seizures, or focal paralysis. **Silent stroke**, which is defined as evidence of cerebral infarction on imaging studies but a normal neurologic examination, is more common and occurs in approximately 20% of patients with SS disease. A significant change in school performance or behavior has been associated with silent stroke. Children with Hg SS disease over 3 years of age should be screened for increased risk of stroke using transcranial doppler (TCD).

**Laboratory Diagnosis.** The diagnosis of hemoglobinopathies is made by identifying the precise amount and type of hemoglobin using **hemoglobin electrophoresis**, **isoelectric focusing**, or **high-performance liquid chromatography**. Every member of an at-risk population should have a precise hemoglobin phenotype performed at birth (preferably) or during early infancy. Most states perform newborn screening for sickle cell disease.

**Treatment.** Direct therapy of sickle cell anemia is evolving. The mainstay of care are supportive measures. The use of chronic RBC transfusions to treat patients who have had a stroke has been very successful. Chronic RBC transfusions have also been used successfully for short time periods to prevent recurrent vaso-occlusive painful events, including acute chest syndrome and priapism. **Hydroxyurea**, which increases hemoglobin F, decreases the number and severity of vaso-occlusive events. **Hematopoietic stem cell transplantation**, utilizing a haploidentical sibling match, has cured many children with sickle cell disease. HSCT using alternative donors for children, without a suitable sibling match, is being studied.

## Enzymopathies

**Etiology.** **Glucose-6-phosphate dehydrogenase (G6PD) deficiency** is an abnormality in the **hexose monophosphate shunt pathway** of glycolysis that results in the depletion of reduced nicotinamide adenine dinucleotide phosphate (NADPH) and the inability to regenerate reduced glutathione. Reduced glutathione protects sulfhydryl groups in the RBC membrane from oxidation. When a patient with G6PD is exposed to significant oxidant stress, hemoglobin is oxidized, forming precipitates of sulfhemoglobin (**Heinz bodies**), which are visible on specially stained preparations. The gene for G6PD deficiency is on the X chromosome.

The severity of hemolysis depends on the enzyme variant. In many G6PD variants, the enzymes become unstable with aging of the RBC and cannot be replaced because the cell is anucleated. Older cells are most susceptible to oxidant-induced hemolysis. In other variants, the enzyme is kinetically abnormal.

**Epidemiology.** The most common variants of G6PD deficiency have been found in areas where malaria is endemic. G6PD deficiency protects against parasitism of the erythrocyte. The most common variant with normal activity is termed **type B** and is defined by its electrophoretic mobility. The approximate gene frequencies in African Americans are 70% type B, 20% type A, and 10% type A−. Only the **A− variant**, termed the *African variant*, is unstable. Ten percent of black males are affected. A group of variants found in Sardinians, Sicilians, Greeks, Sephardic and Oriental Jews, and Arabs is termed the **Mediterranean variant** and is associated with chronic hemolysis and potentially life-threatening hemolytic disease. Because the gene for G6PD deficiency is carried on the X chromosome, clinical hemolysis is most common in males. Heterozygous females who have randomly inactivated a higher percentage of the normal gene may become symptomatic, as may homozygous females with the A− variant (0.5% to 1% of females of African descent).

**Clinical Manifestations.** G6PD deficiency has two common presentations. Individuals with the A− variant have normal hemoglobin values when well, but develop an **acute episode of hemolysis** triggered by serious (bacterial) infection or ingestion of an oxidant drug. The RBC morphology during episodes of acute hemolysis is striking. RBCs appear to have "bites" (cookie cells) taken out of them. These are areas of absent hemoglobin that are produced by phagocytosis of Heinz bodies by splenic macrophages; as a result, the RBCs appear blistered. Clinically evident jaundice, dark urine resulting from bilirubin pigments, hemoglobinuria when hemolysis is intravascular, and decreased haptoglobin levels are common during hemolytic episodes. Early on, the hemolysis usually exceeds the ability of the bone marrow to compensate, so the reticulocyte count may be low for 3 to 4 days.

**Laboratory Studies.** The diagnosis of G6PD deficiency is based on decreased NADPH formation. G6PD levels during an acute, severe hemolytic episode may be normal, however, because the most deficient cells have been destroyed and reticulocytes are enriched with G6PD. Repeating the test at a later time when the patient is in a steady-state condition, testing the mothers of boys with suspected G6PD deficiency, or performing electrophoresis to identify the precise variant present aids in diagnosis.

**Treatment and Prevention.** The treatment of G6PD deficiency is supportive. Transfusions are indicated when significant cardiovascular compromise is present. Maintaining hydration and urine alkalization protects the kidneys against damage from precipitated free hemoglobin. Hemolysis is prevented by avoidance of known oxidants, particularly long-acting sulfonamides, nitrofurantoin, primaquine, dimercaprol and moth balls (naphthalene). Fava beans (favism) have triggered hemolysis, particularly in patients with the Mediterranean variant. Infection also is a major precipitant of hemolysis in G6PD-deficient young children.

**Pyruvate kinase deficiency** is much less common than G6PD deficiency and represents a clinical spectrum of disorders caused by the functional deficiency of pyruvate kinase. Some individuals have a true deficiency state, and others have abnormal enzyme kinetics. The metabolic consequence of pyruvate kinase deficiency is adenosine triphosphate (ATP) depletion, impairing RBC survival. Pyruvate kinase deficiency is usually an autosomal disorder, and most children who are affected (and are not products of consanguinity) are double heterozygotes for two abnormal enzymes. Hemolysis is not aggravated by oxidant stress because patients with this condition tend to have a profound reticulocytosis. Aplastic crises are potentially life-threatening. The spleen is the site for RBC removal in pyruvate kinase deficiency. Most patients have amelioration of the anemia and a reduction of transfusion requirements after splenectomy.

## Membrane Disorders

**Etiology.** The biochemical basis of **hereditary spherocytosis** and **hereditary elliptocytosis** are similar. Both conditions appear to have a defect in the protein lattice (spectrin, ankyrin, protein 4.2, band 3) that underlies the RBC lipid bilayer and provides stability of the membrane shape. In hereditary spherocytosis, pieces of membrane bud off as microvesicles because of abnormal vertical interaction of the cytoskeletal proteins and uncoupling of the lipid bilayer from the cytoskeleton. When the RBC loses membrane, cell shape changes from a biconcave disc to a spherocyte, which has the lowest ratio of surface area to volume. The RBC is less deformable when passing through narrow passages in the spleen. Hereditary elliptocytosis is a disorder of spectrin dimer interactions that occurs primarily in individuals of African descent. The transmission of the two variants is usually autosomal dominant, but spontaneous mutations causing hereditary spherocytosis are common. **Hereditary pyropoikilocytosis** (unusual instability of the erythrocytes when they are exposed to heat at 45°C) is the result of a structural abnormality of spectrin.

**Clinical Manifestations.** Hereditary spherocytosis varies greatly in clinical severity, ranging from an asymptomatic, well-compensated, mild hemolytic anemia that may be discovered incidentally to a severe hemolytic anemia with growth failure, splenomegaly, and chronic transfusion requirements in infancy necessitating early splenectomy. The most common variant of hereditary elliptocytosis is a clinically insignificant, morphologic abnormality without shortened RBC survival. The less common variant is associated with spherocytes, ovalocytes, and elliptocytes with a moderate, usually compensated, hemolysis. Far more significant hemolysis occurs in hereditary pyropoikilocytosis. The peripheral blood smear in hereditary pyropoikilocytosis often includes elliptocytes, spherocytes, fragmented RBCs, and striking microcytosis. Such patients may have bizarre blood smears in the newborn period with small, fragmented RBCs.

**Laboratory Diagnosis.** The clinical diagnosis of hereditary spherocytosis should be suspected in patients with even a few spherocytes found on the blood smear because the spleen preferentially removes spherocytes. An incubated **osmotic fragility test** confirms the presence of spherocytes and increases the likelihood of the diagnosis. The osmotic fragility test result is abnormal in any hemolytic disease in which spherocytes are present, however, especially antibody-mediated hemolysis.

**Treatment. Splenectomy** corrects the anemia and normalizes the RBC survival in patients with hereditary spherocytosis, but the morphologic abnormalities persist. Splenectomy should be considered for any child with symptoms referable to anemia or growth failure, but should be deferred until age 5 years, if possible, to minimize the risk of overwhelming postsplenectomy sepsis and to maximize the antibody response to the polyvalent pneumococcal vaccine. In several reports, partial splenectomy seems to improve the hemolytic anemia and maintain splenic function in host defense.

## Hemolytic Anemia Caused by Disorders Extrinsic to the Red Blood Cell

**Etiology and Clinical Manifestations. Isoimmune hemolysis** is caused by active maternal immunization against fetal antigens that the mother's erythrocytes do not express (see Chapter 62). Examples are antibodies to the A, B, and Rh D antigens; other Rh antigens; and the Kell, Duffy, and other blood groups. Anti-A and anti-B hemolysis is caused by the placental transfer of naturally occurring maternal antibodies from mothers who lack A or B antigen (usually blood type O). Positive results of the direct antiglobulin (**Coombs**) test on the infant's RBCs (Fig. 150-4), the indirect antiglobulin test on the mother's serum and the presence of spherocytes and immature erythroid precursors (erythroblastosis) on the infant's blood smear confirm this diagnosis. Isoimmune hemolytic disease varies in clinical severity. There may be no clinical manifestations or the infant may exhibit jaundice, severe anemia, and hydrops fetalis.

**Autoimmune hemolytic anemia** is usually an acute, self-limited process that develops after an infection (*Mycoplasma,* Epstein-Barr, or other viral infections). Autoimmune hemolytic anemia may also be the presenting symptom of a chronic autoimmune disease (systemic lupus erythematosus, lymphoproliferative disorders, or immunodeficiency). Drugs may induce a Coombs-positive hemolytic anemia by forming a hapten on the RBC membrane (penicillin) or by forming immune complexes (quinidine) that attach to the RBC membrane. Antibodies then activate complement-induced intravascular hemolysis. The third type of drug-induced immune hemolysis occurs during treatment with α-methyldopa and a few other drugs. In this type, prolonged drug exposure alters the RBC membrane, inducing neoantigen formation. Antibodies are produced that bind to the neoantigen; this produces a positive antiglobulin test result far more commonly than it actually induces hemolysis. In each of these conditions, the erythrocyte is an *innocent bystander.*

A second form of acquired hemolytic disease that is not antibody mediated is caused by mechanical damage to the RBC membrane during circulation. In **thrombotic microangiopathy**, the RBCs are trapped by fibrin strands in the circulation and physically broken by shear stress as they pass through these strands. Hemolytic uremic syndrome, disseminated intravascular coagulation (DIC), thrombotic thrombocytopenic purpura, malignant hypertension, toxemia, and hyperacute renal graft rejection all produce thrombotic microangiopathy. The platelets are usually large, indicating that they are young, but have a decreased survival even if the numbers are normal. Consumption of clotting factors is more prominent in DIC than in the other forms of thrombotic microangiopathy. The smear shows RBC fragments (schistocytes), microspherocytes, teardrop forms, and polychromasia. Other examples of mechanical injury to RBCs include damage by exposure to nonendothelialized surfaces (as in artificial heart valves) or as a result of high flow and shear rates in giant hemangiomas (**Kasabach-Merritt syndrome**).

**Alterations in the plasma lipids**, especially cholesterol, may lead to damage to the RBC membrane and shorten RBC survival. Lipids in the plasma are in equilibrium with lipids in the RBC membrane. High cholesterol levels increase the membrane cholesterol and the total membrane surface without affecting the volume of the cell. This condition produces **spur cells** that may be seen in abetalipoproteinemia and liver diseases. Hemolysis

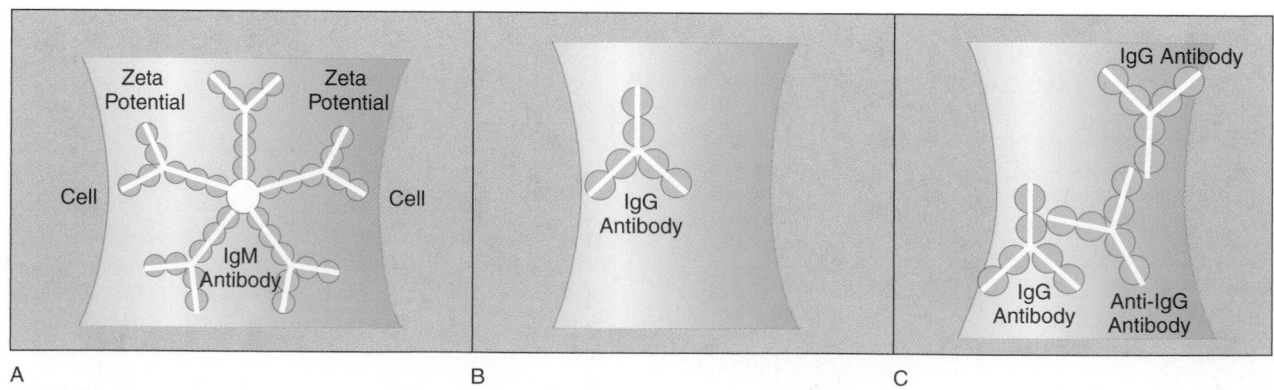

A                                    B                                    C

**FIGURE 150-4**

**Coombs or direct antiglobulin test (DAT).** In the DAT, so-called Coombs serum that recognizes human immunoglobulin (Ig) or complement (C) is used to detect the presence of antibody or C on the surface of the red blood cells (RBCs) by agglutination. **A,** An IgM antibody can bind two RBCs simultaneously because of its multiple antigen-binding sites. The great size of the IgM allows it to bridge the surface repulsive forces (zeta potential) between RBCs and cause agglutination. **B,** An IgG antibody is too small to bridge the zeta potential and cause agglutination. **C,** On the addition of Coombs serum, the zeta potential is bridged successfully, and RBCs agglutinate. (Modified from Ware RE, Rosse WF: Autoimmune hemolytic anemia. In Orkin SH, Nathan DG, Look AT, Ginsburg D [eds]: Hematology of Infancy and Childhood, 6th ed. Philadelphia, *WB Saunders,* 2003, p 530.)

occurs in the spleen, where poor RBC deformability results in erythrocyte destruction. **Circulating toxins** (e.g., snake venoms and heavy metals) that bind sulfhydryl groups may damage the RBC membrane and induce hemolysis. Irregularly spiculated RBCs (burr cells) are seen in renal failure. **Vitamin E deficiency** can also cause an acquired hemolytic anemia as a result of abnormal sensitivity of membrane lipids to oxidant stress. Vitamin E deficiency may occur in premature infants who are not being supplemented with vitamin E or who have insufficient nutrition, in infants with severe malabsorption syndromes (including cystic fibrosis), and in infants with transfusional iron overload, which can lead to severe oxidant exposure.

**Laboratory Diagnosis.** The peripheral blood smear in autoimmune hemolytic anemia usually reveals spherocytes and occasionally nucleated RBCs. The reticulocyte count varies because some patients have relatively low reticulocyte counts as a result of autoantibodies which cross-reacts with RBC precursors.

**Treatment and Prognosis.** Transfusion for the treatment of autoimmune hemolysis is challenging because crossmatching is difficult, as the autoantibodies react with virtually all RBCs. In addition to **transfusion**, which may be lifesaving, management of autoimmune hemolytic anemia depends on antibody type. Management may involve administration of **corticosteroids** and, at times, **intravenous immunoglobulin**. Corticosteroids reduce the clearance of sensitized RBCs in the spleen. In drug-induced hemolysis, withdrawal of the drug usually leads to resolution of the hemolytic process. More than 80% of children with autoimmune hemolytic anemia recover spontaneously.

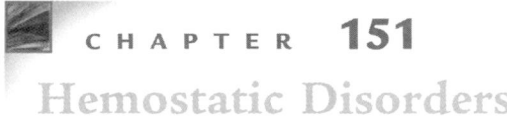

CHAPTER **151**

# Hemostatic Disorders

## NORMAL HEMOSTASIS

Hemostasis is the dynamic process of **coagulation** as it occurs in areas of vascular injury. This process involves the carefully modulated interaction of platelets, vascular wall, and procoagulant and anticoagulant proteins. After an injury to the vascular endothelium, subendothelial collagen induces a conformational change in von Willebrand factor (**vWF**), an adhesive protein to which platelets bind via their glycoprotein Ib receptor. After adhesion, platelets undergo activation and release numerous intracellular contents, including adenosine diphosphate (ADP). These **activated platelets** subsequently induce aggregation of additional platelets. Simultaneously, tissue factor, collagen, and other matrix proteins in the tissue activate the coagulation cascade, leading to the formation of the enzyme **thrombin** (Fig. 151-1). Thrombin has multiple effects on the coagulation mechanism, such as further aggregation of platelets, a positive feedback activation of factors 5 and 8, the conversion of fibrinogen to fibrin, and the activation of factor 11. A **platelet plug** forms,

and bleeding ceases, usually within 3 to 7 minutes. The generation of thrombin leads to formation of a permanent clot by the activation of factor 13, which cross-links fibrin forming a stable thrombus. As a final element to this process, contractile elements within the platelet mediate **clot retraction**. Thrombin also contributes to the eventual limitation of clot size by binding to the protein thrombomodulin on intact endothelial cells, converting protein C into activated protein C. Thrombin contributes to the eventual lysis of the thrombus by activating plasminogen to plasmin. All of the hemostatic processes are closely interwoven and occur on biologic surfaces that mediate coagulation by bringing the critical *players*: platelets, endothelial cells, and subendothelium into close proximity with pro- and anticoagulant proteins.

Although it is convenient to think of coagulation as having **intrinsic and extrinsic pathways**, the reality is that these pathways are closely interactive and do not react independently (Fig. 151-2). For ease of use all coagulation factors are denoted using Arabic rather than Roman numerals to prevent misreading factor VII (7) as factor VIII (8). In vivo, factor 7 autocatalyzes to form small amounts of factor 7a. When tissue is injured, **tissue factor** is released and causes a burst of factor 7a generation. In vivo, tissue factor, in combination with calcium and factor 7a, activates factor 9 and factor 10. The major physiologic pathway is the activation of factor 9 by factor 7a, with eventual generation of thrombin. Thrombin then feeds back on factor 11, generating factor 11a and accelerating thrombin formation. This process explains why deficiency of factor 8 or factor 9 leads to severe bleeding disorders, whereas deficiency of factor 11 is usually mild, and deficiency of factor 12 is asymptomatic.

As the procoagulant proteins are activated, a series of inhibitory factors serve to tightly regulate the activation of coagulation. **Antithrombin III** inactivates thrombin and factors 10a, 9a, and 11a. The **protein C and protein S** system inactivates the activated factors 5 and 8, which are cofactors localized in the "tenase" and "prothrombinase" complexes. The **tissue factor pathway inhibitor**, an anticoagulant protein, limits the activation of the coagulation cascade by factor 7a and factor 10a. **Fibrinolysis** is initiated by the action of tissue plasminogen activator on plasminogen, producing plasmin, the active enzyme that degrades fibrin into split products. Fibrinolysis eventually dissolves the clot and allows normal flow to resume. Deficiencies of anticoagulant proteins may lead to thrombosis.

## DEVELOPMENTAL HEMOSTASIS

In the fetus, fibrinogen, factor 5, factor 8, and platelets approach normal levels during the second trimester. Levels of other clotting factors and anticoagulant proteins increase gradually throughout gestation. The premature infant is simultaneously at increased risk of bleeding or clotting complications that are exacerbated by many of the medical interventions needed for care and monitoring, especially indwelling arterial or venous catheters. Most children attain normal levels of procoagulant and anticoagulant proteins by 1 year of age, although levels of protein C lag and normalize in adolescence.

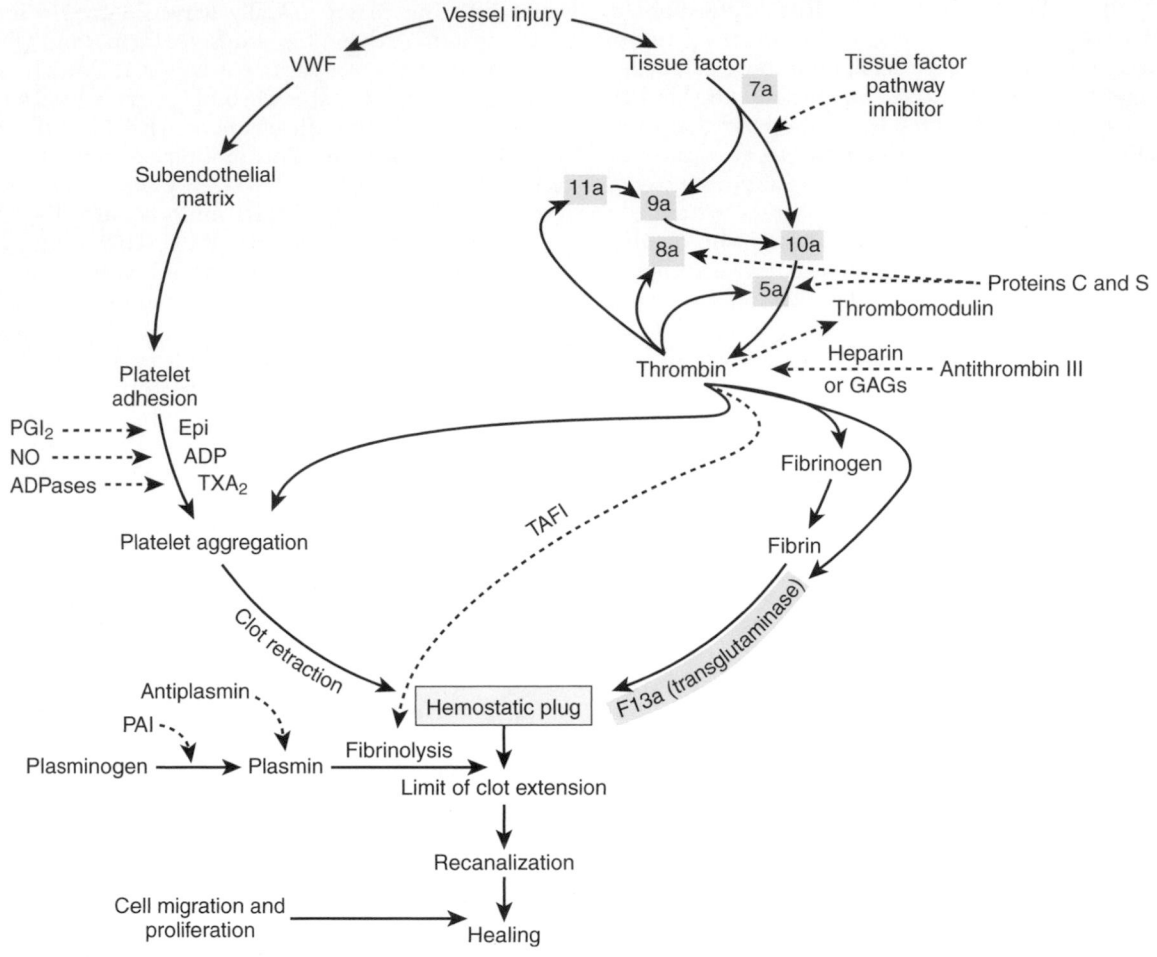

**FIGURE 151-1**

**Diagram of the multiple interactions of the hemostatic mechanism.** Solid lines indicate reactions that favor coagulation, and dashed lines indicate reactions that inhibit clotting. Epi, epinephrine; GAGs, glycosaminoglycans; NO, nitric oxide; PAI, plasminogen activator inhibitor; $PGI_2$, prostaglandin $I_2$ (prostacyclin); TAFI, thrombin-activated fibrinolytic inhibitor; $TXA_2$, thromboxane $A_2$; VWF, von Willebrand factor. (Modified from, Scott JP, Montgomery RR: Hemorrhagic and thrombotic diseases. In Kliegman RM, Behrman RE, Jenson HB, Stanton BF [eds]: Nelson Textbook of Pediatrics, 18th ed. Philadelphia, *WB Saunders*, 2007, p 2062.)

## HEMOSTATIC DISORDERS

### Etiology and Epidemiology

A detailed **family history** is crucial for bleeding and thrombotic disorders. **Hemophilia** is X-linked, and almost all affected children are boys. **von Willebrand disease** usually is inherited in an autosomal dominant fashion. In the investigation of thrombotic disorders, a personal or family history of blood clots in the legs or lungs, early-onset stroke, or heart attack suggests a hereditary predisposition to thrombosis. The causes of bleeding may be hematologic in origin or due to vascular, nonhematologic causes (Fig. 151-3). Thrombotic disorders can be congenital or acquired (Table 151-1) and frequently present after an initial event (central catheter, trauma, malignancy, infection, pregnancy, treatment with estrogens) provides a nidus for clot formation or a procoagulant stimulus.

### Clinical Manifestations

Patients with hemostatic disorders may have complaints of either bleeding or clotting. Age at onset of bleeding indicates whether the problem is congenital or acquired. The **sites of bleeding** (mucocutaneous or deep) and **degree of trauma** (spontaneous or significant) required to induce injury suggest the type and severity of the disorder. Certain medications (aspirin and valproic acid) are known to exacerbate preexisting bleeding disorders by interfering with platelet function.

The **physical examination** should characterize the presence of skin or mucous membrane bleeding and deeper sites of hemorrhage into the muscles and joints or internal bleeding sites. The term **petechia** refers to a non-blanching lesion less than 2 mm in size. **Purpura** is a group of adjoining petechiae, **ecchymoses** (bruises) are

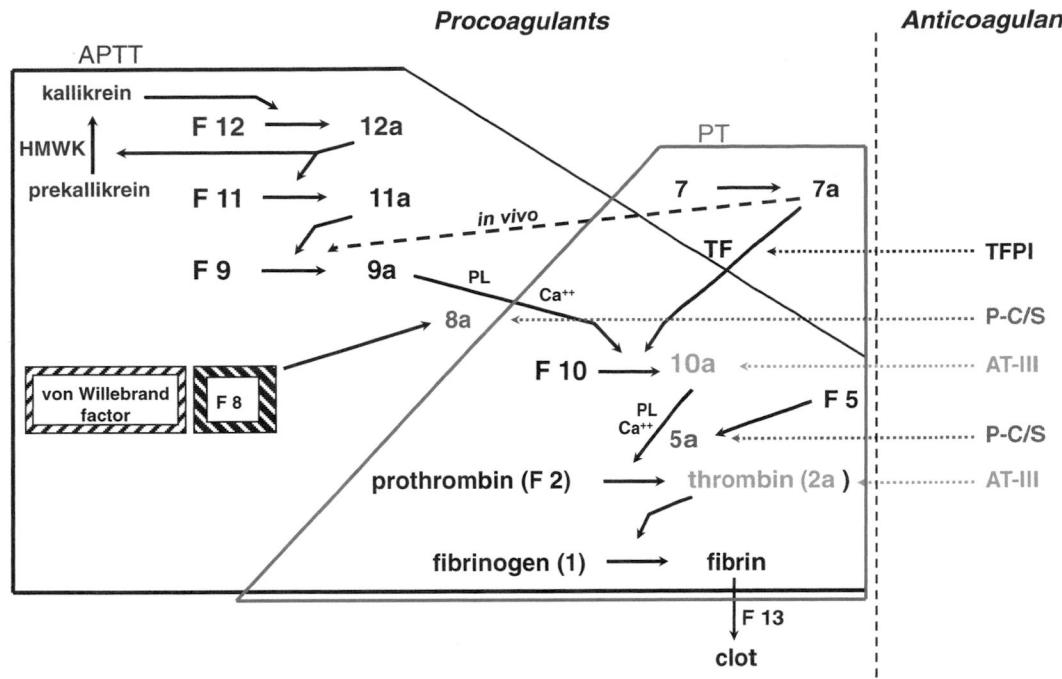

**FIGURE 151-2**

**Simplified pathways of blood coagulation.** The area inside the solid black line is the intrinsic pathway measured by the activated partial thromboplastin time (APTT). The area inside the green line is the extrinsic pathway, measured by the prothrombin time (PT). The area encompassed by both lines is the common pathway. AT-III, antithrombin III; F, factor; HMWK, high-molecular-weight kininogen; P-C/S, protein C/S; PL, phospholipid; TFPI, tissue factor pathway inhibitor. (Modified from Scott JP, Montgomery RR: Hemorrhagic and thrombotic diseases. In Kliegman RM, Behrman RE, Jenson HB, Stanton, BF [eds]: Nelson Textbook of Pediatrics, 18th ed. Philadelphia, *WB Saunders*, 2007, p 2061.)

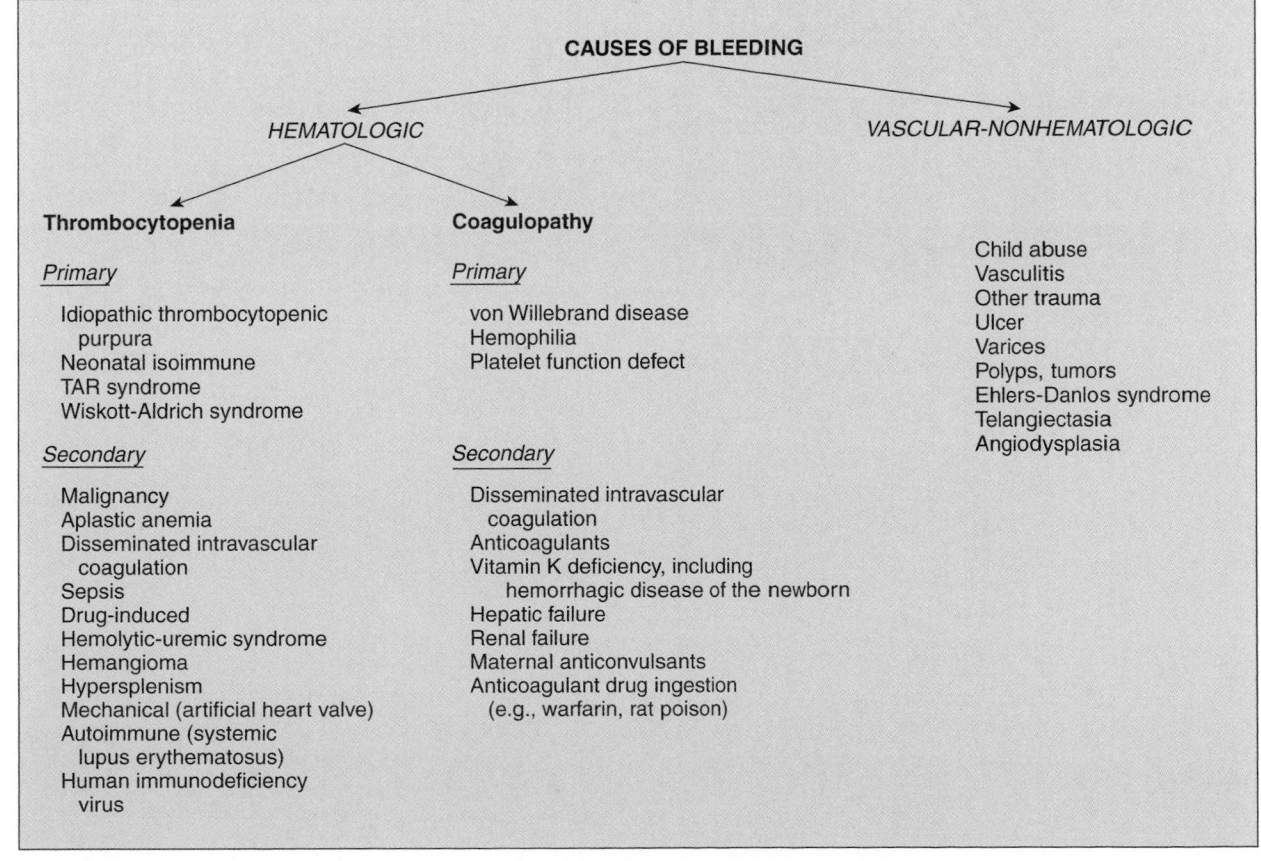

**FIGURE 151-3**

**Common causes of bleeding.** TAR, thrombocytopenia with absence of radius (syndrome).

**TABLE 151-1 Common Hypercoagulable States**

### CONGENITAL DISORDERS

Factor V Leiden (activated protein C resistance)
Prothrombin 20210
Protein C deficiency
Protein S deficiency
Antithrombin III deficiency
Plasminogen deficiency
Dysfibrinogenemia
Homocystinuria

### ACQUIRED DISORDERS

Indwelling catheters
Lupus anticoagulant/antiphospholipid syndrome
Nephrotic syndrome
Malignancy
Pregnancy
Birth control pills
Autoimmune disease
Immobilization/surgery
Trauma
Infection
Inflammatory bowel disease

From Scott JP: Bleeding and thrombosis. In Kliegman RM (ed): Practical Strategies in Pediatric Diagnosis and Therapy. Philadelphia, *WB Saunders*, 1996.

isolated lesions larger than petechiae, and **hematomas** are raised, palpable ecchymoses.

Because systemic disorders may induce either hemorrhagic or thrombotic disorders, the physical examination should search for manifestations of an underlying disease, lymphadenopathy, hepatosplenomegaly, vasculitic rash, or chronic hepatic or renal disease. **Deep venous thrombi** may cause warm, swollen (distended), tender, purplish discolored extremities or organs or *no findings*. **Arterial clots** cause acute, painful, pale, and poorly perfused extremities. Arterial thrombi of the internal organs present with signs and symptoms of infarction.

## Laboratory Testing

Screening laboratory studies for bleeding patients include a **platelet count**, **prothrombin time**, **partial thromboplastin time**, **fibrinogen**, and **bleeding time** or other screening test of platelet function. Many laboratories have adopted the platelet function analyzer (PFA) to replace the bleeding time as a screening test for platelet function abnormalities and von Willebrand disease. The PFA has variable sensitivity and specificity for common bleeding disorders. No single laboratory test can screen for all bleeding disorders. The findings on screening tests for bleeding vary with the specific disorder (Table 151-2).

## Differential Diagnosis

### Disorders of Platelets

Platelet counts less than 150,000/mm$^3$ constitute **thrombocytopenia**. Mucocutaneous bleeding is the hallmark of platelet disorders, including thrombocytopenia. The risk of bleeding correlates imperfectly with the platelet count. Children with platelet counts greater than 80,000/mm$^3$ are able to withstand all but the most extreme hemostatic challenges, such as surgery or major trauma. Children with platelet counts less than 20,000/mm$^3$ are at risk for spontaneous bleeding. These generalizations are modified by factors such as the age of the platelets (young, large

**TABLE 151-2 Screening Tests for Bleeding Disorders**

| Test | Mechanism Tested | Normal Values | Disorder |
|---|---|---|---|
| Prothrombin time | Extrinsic and common pathway | <12 sec beyond neonate; 12–18 sec in term neonate | Defect in vitamin K–dependent factors; hemorrhagic disease of newborn, malabsorption, liver disease, DIC, oral anticoagulants, ingestion of rat poison |
| Activated partial thromboplastin time | Intrinsic and common pathway | 25–40 sec beyond neonate; 70 sec in term neonate | Hemophilia; von Willebrand disease, heparin; DIC; deficient factors 12 and 11; lupus anticoagulant |
| Thrombin time | Fibrinogen to fibrin conversion | 10–15 sec beyond neonate; 12–17 sec in term neonate | Fibrin split products, DIC, hypofibrinogenemia, heparin, uremia |
| Bleeding time | Hemostasis, capillary and platelet function | 3–7 min beyond neonate | Platelet dysfunction, thrombocytopenia, von Willebrand disease, aspirin |
| Platelet count | Platelet number | 150,000–450,000/mL | Thrombocytopenia differential diagnosis (Fig. 151-4) |
| PFA | Closure time | | |
| Blood smear | Platelet number and size; RBC morphology | — | Large platelets suggest peripheral destruction; fragmented, bizarre RBC morphology suggests microangiopathic process (e.g., hemolytic uremic syndrome, hemangioma, DIC) |

DIC, disseminated intravascular coagulation; PFA, platelet function analyzer-100; RBC, red blood cell.

platelets usually function better than old ones) and the presence of inhibitors of platelet function, such as antibodies, drugs (especially aspirin), fibrin degradation products, and toxins formed in the presence of hepatic or renal disease. The size of platelets is routinely measured as the mean platelet volume (MPV). The etiology of thrombocytopenia (Fig. 151-4) may be organized into three mechanisms:

1. Decreased platelet production
2. Increased destruction
3. Sequestration

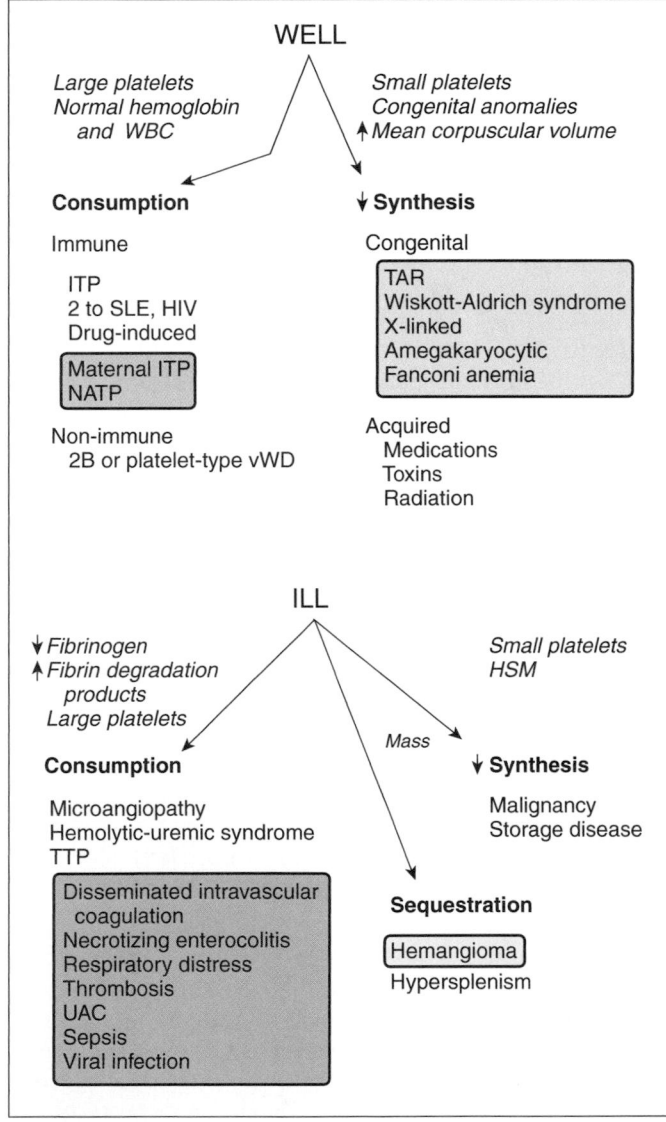

**FIGURE 151-4**

**Differential diagnosis of childhood thrombocytopenic syndromes.** The syndromes initially are separated by their clinical appearances. Clues leading to the diagnosis are presented in italics. The mechanisms and common disorders leading to these findings are shown in the lower part of the figure. Disorders that commonly affect neonates are listed in the shaded boxes. HSM, hepatosplenomegaly; ITP, idiopathic immune thrombocytopenic purpura; NATP, neonatal alloimmune thrombocytopenic purpura; SLE, systemic lupus erythematosus; TAR, thrombocytopenia with absence of radius (syndrome); TTP, thrombotic thrombocytopenic purpura; UAC, umbilical artery catheter; WBC, white blood cell. (From Scott JP: Bleeding and thrombosis. In Kliegman RM, Greenbaum LA, Lye PS [eds]: Practical Strategies in Pediatric Diagnosis and Therapy. Philadelphia, *WB Saunders*, 2004, p 920.)

## Sequestration Thrombocytopenia Resulting from Decreased Platelet Production

Primary disorders of megakaryopoiesis (platelet production) are rare in childhood, other than as part of an aplastic syndrome. **Thrombocytopenia with absent radii syndrome** is characterized by severe thrombocytopenia in association with orthopedic abnormalities, especially of the upper extremity. The thrombocytopenia usually improves over time. **Amegakaryocytic thrombocytopenia** presents at birth or shortly thereafter with findings of severe thrombocytopenia, but no other congenital anomalies. The marrow is devoid of megakaryocytes and usually progresses to aplasia of all hematopoietic cell lines.

Acquired thrombocytopenia as a result of decreased production is rarely an isolated finding. It is seen more often in the context of **pancytopenia resulting from bone marrow failure** caused by infiltrative or aplastic processes. Certain chemotherapeutic agents may affect megakaryocytes selectively more than other marrow elements. **Cyanotic congenital heart disease with polycythemia** often is associated with thrombocytopenia, but this is rarely severe or associated with significant clinical bleeding. Congenital (TORCH [toxoplasmosis, other agents, rubella, cytomegalovirus, herpes simplex]) and acquired **viral infections** (human immunodeficiency virus [HIV], Epstein-Barr virus, and measles) and some **drugs** (anticonvulsants, antibiotics, cytotoxic agents, heparin, and quinidine) may induce thrombocytopenia. Postnatal infections and drug reactions usually cause transient thrombocytopenia, whereas congenital infections may produce prolonged suppression of bone marrow function.

## Thrombocytopenia Resulting from Peripheral Destruction

**Etiology.** In a child who appears well, **immune-mediated mechanisms** are the most common cause of thrombocytopenia resulting from rapid peripheral destruction of antibody-coated platelets by reticuloendothelial cells. **Neonatal alloimmune thrombocytopenic purpura** (NATP) occurs as a result of sensitization of the mother to antigens present on fetal platelets. Antibodies cross the placenta and attack the fetal platelet (see Chapter 59). Many platelet alloantigens have been identified and sequenced, permitting prenatal diagnosis of the condition in an at-risk fetus. Mothers with idiopathic thrombocytopenic purpura (**maternal ITP**) or with a history of ITP may have passive transfer of antiplatelet antibodies that bind to fetal platelets, with resultant neonatal thrombocytopenia (see Chapter 59). The maternal platelet count is sometimes a useful indicator of the probability that the infant will be affected. If the mother has had a splenectomy, her platelet count may be normal and is a poor predictor of the likelihood of severe neonatal thrombocytopenia because maternal antibody triggers destruction of the fetal platelets in the fetal spleen.

**Clinical Manifestations.** The infant with NATP is at risk for **intracranial hemorrhage** in utero and during the immediate delivery process. In ITP, the greatest risk seems to be present during passage through the birth canal, during which molding of the head may induce intracranial hemorrhage. Fetal scalp sampling or percutaneous umbilical blood sampling may be performed to measure the fetal platelet count.

**Treatment.** Administration of intravenous (IV) immunoglobulin before delivery increases fetal platelet counts and may alleviate thrombocytopenia in the infant in cases of NATP and ITP. Delivery by cesarean section is recommended to prevent central nervous system (CNS) bleeding (see Chapter 59). Neonates with severe thrombocytopenia (platelet counts < 20,000/mm$^3$) may be treated with IV immunoglobulin or corticosteroids or both until the period of thrombocytopenia remits. If necessary, infants with NATP may receive washed maternal platelets.

## Idiopathic Thrombocytopenic Purpura

**Etiology.** Autoimmune thrombocytopenic purpura of childhood (childhood ITP) is a common disorder in children that usually follows an acute viral infection. Childhood ITP is caused by an antibody (IgG or IgM) that binds to the platelet membrane. The condition results in Fc receptor–mediated splenic destruction of antibody-coated platelets. Rarely, ITP may be the presenting symptom of an autoimmune disease, such as systemic lupus erythematosus.

**Clinical Manifestations.** Young children typically exhibit ITP 1 to 4 weeks after viral illness, with abrupt onset of petechiae, purpura, and epistaxis. The thrombocytopenia usually is severe. Significant adenopathy or hepatosplenomegaly is unusual, and the red blood cell (RBC) and white blood cell (WBC) counts are normal.

**Diagnosis.** The diagnosis of ITP usually is based on clinical presentation and the platelet count and does not often require a bone marrow examination. If atypical findings are noted, however, marrow examination is indicated to rule out an infiltrative disorder (leukemia) or an aplastic process (aplastic anemia). In ITP, an examination of the bone marrow reveals increased megakaryocytes and normal erythroid and myeloid elements.

**Treatment and Prognosis.** Therapy is seldom indicated for platelet counts greater than 30,000/mm$^3$. Therapy does not affect the long-term outcome of ITP but is intended to increase the platelet count acutely. For moderate and severe clinical bleeding with severe thrombocytopenia (platelet count < 10,000/mm$^3$), therapeutic options include **prednisone**, 2 to 4 mg/kg/24 hours for 2 weeks; IV immunoglobulin, 1 g/kg/24 hours for 1 to 2 days; or **IV anti-D** (WinRho SD), 50 to 75 µg/kg/dose for Rh-positive individuals. All of these approaches seem to decrease the rate of clearance of sensitized platelets, rather than decreasing production of antibody. The optimal choice for therapy (if any) is controversial. Splenectomy is indicated in acute ITP only for life-threatening bleeding. Approximately 80% of children have a spontaneous resolution of ITP within 6 months after diagnosis. Serious bleeding, especially intracranial bleeding, occurs in less than 1% of patients with ITP. There is no evidence that treatment prevents intracranial bleeding.

ITP that persists for 6 to 12 months is classified as **chronic ITP**. Repeated treatments with IV immunoglobulin, IV anti-D, or high-dose pulse steroids are effective in delaying the need for splenectomy. Secondary causes of chronic ITP, especially systemic lupus erythematosus and HIV infection, should be ruled out. Splenectomy induces a remission in 70% to 80% of childhood chronic ITP cases. The risks of splenectomy (surgery, sepsis from encapsulated bacteria, pulmonary hypertension) must be weighed against the risk of severe bleeding.

## Other Disorders

**Wiskott-Aldrich syndrome** is an X-linked disorder characterized by hypogammaglobinemia, eczema, and thrombocytopenia caused by a molecular defect in a cytoskeletal protein common to lymphocytes and platelets (see Chapter 74). Small platelets are seen on a peripheral blood smear. Nevertheless, thrombocytopenia often is improved by splenectomy. Hematopoietic stem cell transplantation cures the immunodeficiency and thrombocytopenia. Familial X-linked thrombocytopenia can be seen as a variant of Wiskott-Aldrich syndrome or a mutation in the *GATA1* gene. Autosomal macrothrombocytopenia is due to deletions in chromosomes 22q11 or mutations in 22q12.

**Thrombotic microangiopathy** causes thrombocytopenia, anemia secondary to intravascular RBC destruction, and, in some cases, depletion of clotting factors. Children with thrombotic microangiopathy usually are quite ill. In a child with **DIC**, the deposition of fibrin strands within the vasculature and activation of thrombin and plasmin result in a wide-ranging hemostatic disorder with activation and clearance of platelets. **Hemolytic uremic syndrome** occurs as a result of exposure to a toxin that induces endothelial injury, fibrin deposition, and platelet activation and clearance (see Chapter 164). In **thrombotic thrombocytopenic purpura**, platelet consumption, precipitated by a congenital or acquired deficiency of a metalloproteinase that cleaves von Willebrand factor, seems to be the primary process, with a modest deposition of fibrin and RBC destruction.

## Disorders of Platelet Function

**Etiology.** Primary disorders of platelet function may involve receptors on platelet membranes for adhesive proteins. Deficiency of glycoprotein Ib complex (vWF receptor) causes **Bernard-Soulier syndrome**. A deficiency of glycoprotein IIb-IIIa (the fibrinogen receptor) causes **Glanzmann thrombasthenia**. Mild abnormalities of platelet aggregation and release, detectable by platelet aggregometry, are far more common. Secondary disorders caused by toxins and drugs (uremia, valproic acid, aspirin, nonsteroidal anti-inflammatory drugs, and infections) may cause a broad spectrum of platelet dysfunction.

**Clinical Manifestations.** Disorders of platelet function present with mucocutaneous bleeding and a prolonged bleeding time or long PFA closure time and may be primary or secondary. The bleeding time is an insensitive screen for mild and moderate platelet function disorders, but is usually prolonged in severe platelet function disorders, such as Bernard-Soulier syndrome or Glanzmann thrombasthenia.

## Disorders of Clotting Factors

**Etiology.** Hereditary deficiencies of most procoagulant proteins lead to bleeding. The genes for factor 8 and factor 9 are on the X chromosome, whereas virtually all the other clotting factors are coded on autosomal chromosomes. **Factor 8 and factor 9 deficiencies** are the most common severe inherited bleeding disorders. **von Willebrand disease** is the most common congenital bleeding disorder. Of the procoagulant proteins, low levels of the so-called contact factors (prekallikrein, high-molecular-weight kininogen, and Hageman factor [factor 12]) cause a prolonged activated partial thromboplastin time (aPTT) but are not associated with a predisposition to bleeding.

## Hemophilia

**Etiology. Hemophilia A** (factor 8 deficiency) occurs in 1 in 5000 males. **Hemophilia B** (factor 9 deficiency) occurs in approximately 1 in 25,000. Clinically the two disorders are indistinguishable other than by their therapy (Table 151-3). The lack of factor 8 or factor 9 delays the generation of thrombin, which is crucial to forming a normal, functional fibrin clot and solidifying the platelet plug that has formed in areas of vascular injury. The severity of the disorder is determined by the degree of clotting factor deficiency.

**Clinical Manifestations.** Patients with less than 1% (severe hemophilia) factor 8 or factor 9 may have **spontaneous bleeding** or bleeding with minor trauma. Patients with 1% to 5% (moderate hemophilia) factor 8 or factor 9 usually require moderate trauma to induce bleeding episodes. In mild hemophilia (>5% factor 8 or factor 9), significant trauma is necessary to induce bleeding; spontaneous bleeding does not occur. Mild hemophilia may go undiagnosed for many years, whereas severe hemophilia manifests in infancy when the child reaches the toddler stage.

In severe hemophilia, spontaneous bleeding occurs, usually in the muscles or joints (**hemarthroses**).

**Laboratory Studies.** The diagnosis of hemophilia is based on a **prolonged activated partial thromboplastin time** (aPTT). In the aPTT, a surface-active agent activates the intrinsic system of coagulation, of which factors 8 and 9 are crucial components. In factor 8 or factor 9 deficiency, the aPTT is quite prolonged, but should correct to normal when the patient's plasma is mixed 1:1 with normal plasma. When an abnormal aPTT is obtained, **specific factor assays** are needed to make a precise diagnosis (see Table 151-2) to determine the appropriate factor replacement therapy. Prenatal diagnosis and carrier diagnosis are possible using molecular techniques.

**Treatment.** Early, appropriate **replacement therapy** is the hallmark of excellent hemophilia care. Acute bleeding episodes are best treated in the home when the patient has attained the appropriate age, and the parents have learned home treatment. Bleeding associated with surgery, trauma, or dental extraction often can be anticipated, and excessive bleeding can be prevented with appropriate replacement therapy. For life-threatening bleeding, levels of 80% to 100% of normal factor 8 or factor 9 are necessary. For mild to moderate bleeding episodes (hemarthroses), a 40% level for factor 8 or a 30 to 40% level for factor 9 is appropriate. The dose can be calculated using the knowledge that 1 U/kg body weight of factor 8 increases the plasma level 2%, whereas 1.5 U/kg of recombinant factor 9 increases the plasma level 1%:

$$\text{Dose for factor 8} = \text{desired level (\%)} \times \text{weight (kg)} \times 0.5$$

or

$$\text{Dose for recombinant factor 9} = \text{desired level (\%)} \times \text{weight (kg)} \times 1.5$$

**TABLE 151-3 Comparison of Hemophilia A, Hemophilia B, and von Willebrand Disease**

| Feature | Hemophilia A | Hemophilia B | von Willebrand Disease |
|---|---|---|---|
| Inheritance | X-linked | X-linked | Autosomal dominant |
| Factor deficiency | Factor 8 | Factor 9 | von Willebrand factor, factor 8 |
| Bleeding site(s) | Muscle, joint, surgical | Muscle, joint, surgical | Mucous membranes, skin, surgical, menstrual |
| Prothrombin time | Normal | Normal | Normal |
| Activated partial thromboplastin time | Prolonged | Prolonged | Prolonged or normal |
| Bleeding time/PFA-100 | Normal | Normal | Prolonged or normal |
| Factor 8 coagulant activity | Low | Normal | Low or normal |
| von Willebrand factor antigen | Normal | Normal | Low |
| von Willebrand factor activity | Normal | Normal | Low |
| Factor 9 | Normal | Low | Normal |
| Ristocetin-induced platelet agglutination | Normal | Normal | Normal, low, or increased at low-dose ristocetin |
| Platelet aggregation | Normal | Normal | Normal |
| Treatment | DDAVP* or recombinant factor 8 | Recombinant factor 9 | DDAVP* or vWF concentrate |

*Desmopressin (DDAVP) for mild to moderate hemophilia A or type 1 von Willebrand disease.
PFA, platelet function analyzer-100.

**Desmopressin acetate** is a synthetic vasopressin analog with minimal vasopressor effect. Desmopressin triples or quadruples the initial factor 8 level of a patient with mild or moderate (not severe) hemophilia A, but has no effect on factor 9 levels. When adequate hemostatic levels can be attained, desmopressin is the treatment of choice for individuals with mild and moderate hemophilia A. Aminocaproic acid is an inhibitor of fibrinolysis that may be useful for oral bleeding.

Patients treated with older factor 8 or 9 concentrates derived from large pools of plasma donors were at high risk for **hepatitis B**, **C**, and **D** and **HIV**. Recombinant factor 8 and factor 9 concentrates are safe from virally transmitted illnesses. Older patients who were exposed to factor concentrates, cryoprecipitate, or both before modern viral testing have a high prevalence of HIV infection. Acquired immunodeficiency syndrome (AIDS) is the most common cause of death in older hemophilia patients. Many older patients also have chronic hepatitis C.

**Inhibitors** are IgG antibodies directed against transfused factor 8 or factor 9 in congenitally deficient patients. Inhibitors arise in 15% of severe factor 8 hemophiliacs and less commonly in factor 9 hemophiliacs. They may be high or low titer and show an anamnestic response to treatment. The treatment of bleeding patients with an inhibitor is difficult. For low titer inhibitors, options include continuous factor 8 infusions. For high titer inhibitors, it is usually necessary to administer a product that bypasses the inhibitor, preferably recombinant factor 7a. Activated prothrombin complex concentrates, used in the past to treat inhibitor patients, paradoxically increased the risks of thrombosis, resulting in fatal complications, such as myocardial infarction. For long-term treatment of inhibitor patients, induction of immune tolerance by repeated infusion of the deficient factor with or without immunosuppression may be beneficial.

Prevention of long-term crippling orthopedic abnormalities is a major goal of hemophilic care. Early institution of factor replacement and continuous prophylaxis beginning in early childhood should prevent the chronic joint disease associated with hemophilia.

## von Willebrand disease

**Etiology.** Von Willebrand disease is a common disorder (found in 1% of the population) caused by a deficiency of **vWF**. vWF is an adhesive protein that serves two functions: vWF acts as a bridge between subendothelial collagen and platelets and it binds and protects circulating factor 8 from rapid clearance from circulation. Von Willebrand disease usually is inherited as an autosomal dominant trait and rarely as an autosomal recessive trait. vWF may be either quantitatively deficient (partial = type 1 or absolute = type 3) or qualitatively abnormal (type 2 = dysproteinemia). Approximately 80% of patients with von Willebrand disease have classic (type 1) disease (i.e., a mild to moderate deficiency of vWF). Several other subtypes are clinically important, each requiring different therapy.

**Clinical Manifestations.** Mucocutaneous bleeding, epistaxis, gingival bleeding, cutaneous bruising, and menorrhagia occur in patients with von Willebrand

disease. In severe disease, factor 8 deficiency may be profound, and the patient may also have manifestations similar to hemophilia A (hemarthrosis). Findings in classic von Willebrand disease differ from findings in hemophilia A and B (see Table 151-3).

**Laboratory Testing.** vWF testing involves measurement of the amount of protein, usually measured immunologically as the **vWF antigen** (vWF:Ag). vWF activity (vWF:Act) is measured functionally in the **ristocetin cofactor assay** (vWFR:Co), which uses the antibiotic ristocetin to induce vWF to bind to platelets.

**Treatment.** The treatment of von Willebrand disease depends on the severity of bleeding. **Desmopressin** is the treatment of choice for most bleeding episodes in patients with type 1 disease and some patients with type 2 disease. When high levels of vWF are needed but cannot be achieved satisfactorily with desmopressin, treatment with a virally attenuated, **vWF-containing concentrate** (Humate P) may be appropriate. The dosage can be calculated as for factor 8 in hemophilia. Cryoprecipitate should not be used because it is not virally attenuated. Hepatitis B vaccine should be given before the patient is exposed to plasma-derived products. As in all bleeding disorders, aspirin should be avoided.

## Vitamin K Deficiency

For discussion of vitamin K deficiency, see Chapters 27 and 31.

## Disseminated Intravascular Coagulation

**Etiology.** Disseminated intravascular coagulation (DIC) is a disorder in which widespread activation of the coagulation mechanism is usually associated with shock. Bleeding and clotting manifestations may be present. Normal hemostasis is a balance between hemorrhage and thrombosis. In DIC, this balance is altered by the severe illness, so the patient has activation of coagulation mediated by thrombin and fibrinolysis mediated by plasmin. Coagulation factors—especially platelets, fibrinogen, and factors 2, 5, and 8—are consumed, as are the anticoagulant proteins, especially antithrombin, protein C, and plasminogen. Endothelial injury, tissue release of thromboplastic procoagulant factors, or, rarely, exogenous factors (snake venoms) directly activate the coagulation mechanism (Table 151-4).

**Clinical Manifestations.** The diagnosis of DIC usually is suspected clinically and is confirmed by laboratory findings of a **decline in platelets and fibrinogen** associated with elevated prothrombin time, partial thromboplastin time, and elevated levels of D-dimer, formed when fibrinogen is clotted and then degraded by plasmin (Table 151-5). In some patients, DIC may evolve more slowly and there may be a degree of compensation. In a severely ill patient, the sudden occurrence of bleeding from a venipuncture or incision site, gastrointestinal or pulmonary hemorrhage, petechiae, or ecchymosis or evidence of peripheral gangrene or thrombosis suggests the diagnosis of DIC.

## TABLE 151-4  Causes of Disseminated Intravascular Coagulation

### INFECTIOUS

Meningococcemia (purpura fulminans)
Other gram-negative bacteria (*Haemophilus, Salmonella, Escherichia coli*)
Rickettsiae (Rocky Mountain spotted fever)
Virus (cytomegalovirus, herpes, hemorrhagic fevers)
Malaria
Fungus

### TISSUE INJURY

Central nervous system trauma (massive head injury)
Multiple fractures with fat emboli
Crush injury
Profound shock or asphyxia
Hypothermia or hyperthermia
Massive burns

### MALIGNANCY

Acute promyelocytic leukemia
Acute monoblastic or myelocytic leukemia
Widespread malignancies (neuroblastoma)

### VENOM OR TOXIN

Snake bites
Insect bites

### MICROANGIOPATHIC DISORDERS

"Severe" thrombotic thrombocytopenic purpura
Hemolytic uremic syndrome
Giant hemangioma (Kasabach-Merritt syndrome)

### GASTROINTESTINAL DISORDERS

Fulminant hepatitis
Severe inflammatory bowel disease
Reye syndrome

### HEREDITARY THROMBOTIC DISORDERS

Antithrombin III deficiency
Homozygous protein C deficiency

### NEONATAL PERIOD

Maternal toxemia
Group B streptococcal infections
Abruptio placentae
Severe respiratory distress syndrome
Necrotizing enterocolitis
Congenital viral disease (e.g., cytomegalovirus infection or herpes)
Erythroblastosis fetalis

### MISCELLANEOUS CONDITIONS/DISORDERS

Severe acute graft rejection
Acute hemolytic transfusion reaction
Severe collagen vascular disease
Kawasaki disease
Heparin-induced thrombosis
Infusion of "activated" prothrombin complex concentrates
Hyperpyrexia/encephalopathy, hemorrhagic shock syndrome

From Scott JP: Bleeding and thrombosis. In Kliegman RM (ed): Practical Strategies in Pediatric Diagnosis and Therapy. Philadelphia, *WB Saunders,* 1996.

## TABLE 151-5  Differential Diagnosis of Coagulopathies That Can Be Confused with Disseminated Intravascular Coagulation

|  | Prothrombin Time | Partial Thromboplastin Time | Fibrinogen | Platelets | D-dimer | Clinical Key(s) |
|---|---|---|---|---|---|---|
| DIC | ↑ | ↑ | ↓ | ↓ | ↑ | Shock |
| Liver failure | ↑ | ↑ | ↓ | Normal or ↓ | ↑ | Jaundice |
| Vitamin K deficiency | ↑ | ↑ | Normal | Normal | Normal | Malabsorption, liver disease |
| Sepsis without shock | ↑ | ↑ | Normal | Normal | ↑ or normal | Fever |

DIC, disseminated intravascular coagulation.
From Scott JP: Bleeding and thrombosis. In Kliegman RM (ed): Practical Strategies in Pediatric Diagnosis and Therapy. Philadelphia, *WB Saunders,* 1996.

**Treatment.** The treatment of DIC is challenging. General guidelines include the following: treat the disorder inducing the DIC first; **support** the patient by correcting hypoxia, acidosis, and poor perfusion; and replace depleted blood-clotting factors, platelets, and anticoagulant proteins by transfusion. **Heparin** may be used to treat significant arterial or venous thrombotic disease unless sites of life-threatening bleeding coexist. **Drotrecogin alfa** (recombinant activated protein C) reduces mortality rate in adults with DIC and sepsis, but these results have not been confirmed in children.

Thrombosis

**Etiology.** A hereditary predisposition to **thrombosis** (see Table 151-1) may be caused by a deficiency of an anticoagulant protein (**protein C or S, antithrombin,** or **plasminogen**) (Fig. 151-5), by an abnormality of a procoagulant protein making it resistant to proteolysis by its respective inhibitor (**factor 5 Leiden**), by a mutation resulting in an increased level of a procoagulant protein (prothrombin 20210), or by damage to endothelial cells (**homocysteinemia**). Neonates with deficiency syndromes may be particularly vulnerable to thrombosis. Neonates with homozygous protein C deficiency present with purpura fulminans or thrombosis of the major arteries and veins or both. Many individuals with an inherited predisposition to thrombosis exhibit symptoms in adolescence or early adulthood. Protein C deficiency presenting in adulthood usually is inherited as an autosomal dominant trait, whereas the homozygous form usually is autosomal recessive. Protein S and antithrombin III deficiencies are inherited as autosomal dominant traits. Factor 5 Leiden is the most common hereditary cause of a predisposition to thrombosis, appearing in 3% to 5% of whites. **Acquired antiphospholipid antibodies** (anticardiolipin and lupus anticoagulant) also predispose to thrombosis.

**Clinical Manifestations.** Neonates and adolescents are the most likely pediatric patients to present with thromboembolic disease. Indwelling catheters, vasculitis, sepsis, immobilization, nephrotic syndrome, coagulopathy, trauma, infection, surgery, inflammatory bowel disease, oral contraceptive agents, pregnancy, and abortion all predispose to thrombosis. The manifestations of pulmonary emboli vary from no findings to chest pain, diminished breath sounds, increased $S_2$, cyanosis, tachypnea, and hypoxemia.

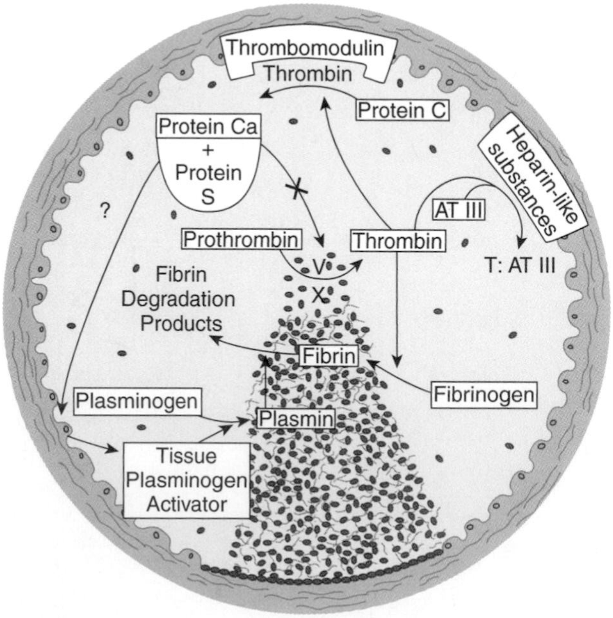

**Diagnostic and Imaging Studies.** Venous thrombosis can be detected noninvasively by ultrasound Doppler flow compression studies. The gold standard for diagnosis is the venogram. An abnormal (*high probability*) ventilation-perfusion scan or detection of an intravascular thrombus on helical computed tomography (CT) is diagnostic of pulmonary emboli. There are no appropriate screening studies for thrombotic disorders. Diagnosis of a congenital or acquired predisposition to thrombosis requires a battery of specific assays.

**Treatment.** Therapy of thrombotic disorders depends on the underlying condition and usually involves standard or low-molecular-weight **heparin** and then longer term anticoagulation with **warfarin**. Major vessel thrombosis or life-threatening thrombosis may necessitate treatment with **fibrinolytic agents** (recombinant tissue plasminogen activator). In newborns, inherited deficiency syndromes may present as emergencies and necessitate **replacement** with plasma, antithrombin III concentrates, or protein C concentrates.

CHAPTER **152**

Blood Component Therapy

**Transfusion** of red blood cells (RBCs), granulocytes, platelets, and coagulation factors can be lifesaving or life maintaining (Table 152-1). **Whole blood** is indicated only when acute hypovolemia and reduced oxygen-carrying capacity are present. Otherwise, **packed RBCs** are indicated to treat anemia by increasing oxygen-carrying capacity. Blood cell transfusions should not be used to treat asymptomatic nutritional deficiencies that can be corrected by administering the appropriate deficient nutrient (iron or folic acid). Blood component therapy requires proper anticoagulation of the blood, screening for a variety of infectious agents, and blood group compatibility testing before administration. Typical **transfusion reactions** are listed in Table 152-2. Filtering of blood products to remove white blood cells (WBCs) may prevent febrile reactions. Long-term complications of transfusions include iron overload, alloimmunization to RBCs and WBCs or platelets and plasma proteins (1:100), graft-versus-host disease, and **infectious diseases**, such as **hepatitis B and C** (<1:250,000), **human immunodeficiency virus (HIV,** <1:1 million), malaria, syphilis, babesiosis, brucellosis, and Chagas disease. Transfusion therapy may result in circulatory overload, especially in the presence of chronic cardiopulmonary deficiency. Recombinant factor 7a has been used off label to treat uncontrolled bleeding after surgery, trauma, and massive transfusion.

**FIGURE 151-5**

**Formation of the hemostatic plug at the site of vascular injury.** Three major physiologic anticoagulant mechanisms—antithrombin III (AT III), protein C, and the fibrinolytic system—are activated to limit clot formation to the site of damage and to prevent generalized thrombosis. T, thrombin. (From Schafer A: The hypercoaguable state. *Ann Intern Med* 102:814–828, 1985.)

### TABLE 152-1 Commonly Used Transfusion Products

| Component | Content | Indication | Dose | Expected Outcome |
|---|---|---|---|---|
| Packed RBCs | 250–300 mL/unit | ↓ Oxygen-carrying RBCs | 10–15 mL/kg | 4 mL/kg → 1 g/dL ↑ |
| Platelet concentrate | $5–7 \times 10^{10}$ platelets/unit | Severe thrombocytopenia ± bleeding | 1 unit/10 kg | ↑ Platelet count by 50,000/μL |
| Fresh frozen plasma | 1 unit/mL of each clotting factor | Multiple clotting factor deficiency | 10–15 mL/kg | Improvement in prothrombin and partial thromboplastin times |
| Cryoprecipitate | Fibrinogen, factor 8, vWF, factor 13 | Hypofibrinogenemia, factor 13 deficiency | 1 bag/5 kg | ↑ Fibrinogen by 50–100 mg/dL |
| Recombinant factor concentrates | Units as labeled | Hemophilic bleeding or prophylaxis | F8: 20–50 units/kg* F9: 40–120 units/kg* | F8: ↑ 2%/unit/kg F9: ↑ 0.7 unit/kg |
| Recombinant factor VIIa (NovoSeven) | Micrograms (μg) | Hemophilic bleeding in patient with inhibitor; uncontrolled postoperative hemorrhage | 90 μg/kg/ dose | Cessation of bleeding |

*Should be clinically significant.
Hgb, hemoglobin; RBCs, red blood cells; vWF, von Willebrand factor.

### TABLE 152-2 Evaluation of Transfusion Reactions

| Type of Reaction | Clinical Signs | Management of Problems |
|---|---|---|
| Major hemolytic (incidence of 1:100,000) (incompatibility) | Acute shock, back pain, flushing, early fever, intravascular hemolysis, hemoglobinemia, hemoglobinuria; may be delayed 5–10 days and less severe if anamnestic response is present | 1. Stop transfusion; return blood to bank with fresh sample of patient's blood 2. Hydrate intravenously; support blood pressure, maintain high urine flow, alkalinize urine 3. Check for hemoglobinemia, hemoglobinuria, hyperkalemia 4. Jaundice, anemia if delayed |
| Delayed hemolytic transfusion reaction | Onset 7–14 days after transfusion: pain, fever, jaundice, hemoglobinuria; fall in hemoglobin; reticulocytopenia | Corticosteroids; erythropoietin?; avoid transfusion if possible |
| Febrile (incidence of 1:100) | Fever at end of transfusion, urticaria (usually because of sensitization to WBC HLA antigens), chills | Pretreat with hydrocortisone, antipyretics, diphenhydramine (Benadryl), or all three; use leukocyte-poor RBCs, washed RBCs, filtered or frozen RBCs |
| Allergic | Fever, urticaria, anaphylactoid reaction (often because of sensitivity to donor plasma proteins) | Benadryl, hydrocortisone; use washed RBCs or frozen RBCs |

HLA, human leukocyte antigen; RBCs, red blood cells; WBC, white blood cell.
Adapted from Andreoli TE, Bennett JC, Carpenter CC, Plum F, et al: Cecil Essentials of Medicine, 4th ed. Philadelphia, *WB Saunders*, 1997.

## SUGGESTED READING

Blanchette V, Bolton-Maggs P: Childhood immune thrombocytopenic purpura: Diagnosis and management, *Pediatr Clin North Am* 55(2):393–420, 2008.

Gluckman E, Wagner JE: Hematopoietic stem cell transplantation in childhood inherited bone marrow failure syndrome, *BMT* 41:127–132, 2008.

Key NS, Negrier C, Klein HG, et al: Transfusion medicine 1, 2, 3, *Lancet* 370 (9585):415–426, 2007 427–438, 439–448.

Kliegman RM, Behrman RE, Jenson HB, et al: Nelson Textbook of Pediatrics, 18th ed, Philadelphia, 2007, *WB Saunders*, pp 1997–2053, 2060–2094.

Krishnamurti L, Bunn FH, Williams AM, et al: Hematopoietic cell transplantation for hemoglobinopathies, *Curr Probl Pediatr Adolesc Health Care* 38:6–18, 2008.

Levi M, Peters M, Buller HR: Efficacy and safety of recombinant factor VIIa for treatment of severe bleeding: A systematic review, *Crit Care Med* 33(4): 883–890, 2005.

Monagle P, Chalmers E, Chan A, et al: Antithrombotic therapy in neonates and children: Evidence-based clinical practice guidelines, *Chest* 133(6 Suppl): 887S–968S, 2008.

Robertson J, Lillicrap D, James PD: Von Willebrand disease, *Pediatr Clin North Am* 55(2):377–392, 2008.

Young NS, Scheinberg P, Calado RT: Aplastic anemia, *Curr Opin Hematol* 15:162–168, 2008.

## CHAPTER 153

# Oncology Assessment

Childhood cancer is rare; only about 1% of new cancer cases in the United States occur among children younger than 19 years of age. Hematopoietic tumors (leukemia, lymphoma) are the most common childhood cancers, followed by brain/central nervous system (CNS) tumors and sarcomas of soft tissue and bone (Fig. 153-1). There is wide variability in the age-specific incidence of childhood cancers. Embryonal tumors, such as neuroblastoma and retinoblastoma, peak during the first 2 years of life; acute lymphoblastic leukemia peaks during early childhood (age 2–5 years); osteosarcoma peaks during adolescence; and Hodgkin disease peaks during late adolescence (Fig. 153-2). The overall incidence of cancer among white children is higher than that among other ethnic groups.

Childhood cancers differ significantly from adult cancers. Solid organ carcinomas are the most common type of adult cancer, whereas carcinomas are relatively rare in individuals under 20 years of age. Acute leukemias, lymphomas, and brain tumors are the most common pediatric and young adult cancers. Leukemias, including acute lymphoblastic leukemia (ALL) and acute myeloblastic leukemia (AML), and various embryonal tumors such as Wilms tumor, neuroblastoma, retinoblastoma, and hepatoblastoma are more common in infancy and early childhood, whereas Hodgkin disease, bone cancers, and gonadal malignancies are more common in adolescents.

## HISTORY

Many signs and symptoms of childhood cancer are non-specific. Although most children with fever, fatigue, weight loss, or limp do not have cancer, each of these symptoms may be a manifestation of an underlying malignancy. Uncommonly, a child with cancer will have no symptoms at all. An abdominal mass may be palpated on routine examination, or a complete blood count may be unexpectedly abnormal. Some children have a genetic susceptibility to cancer and should be screened appropriately (Table 153-1).

It is important to explore quality, duration, location, severity, and precipitating events of the chief complaint. A prominent lymph node that does not resolve (with or without antibiotics) may warrant a biopsy. A limp that does not improve within weeks should prompt a complete blood count and a radiograph or a bone scan. Persistent headaches or morning vomiting should prompt a computed tomography (CT) or magnetic resonance imaging (MRI) scan of the head. Fever, night sweats, or weight loss should raise the concern for lymphoma. In addition, it is important to obtain the birth history, past medical and surgical history, growth history, developmental history, family history, and social history.

## PHYSICAL EXAMINATION

Growth parameters and vital signs are important to obtain in all patients. Pulse oximetry should be obtained if respiratory symptoms are present. The overall appearance of the patient should be noted, particularly general appearance, pain, cachexia, pallor, and respiratory distress. Palpable masses should be measured. Lymphadenopathy and organomegaly should be quantified, if present. A thorough examination of the skin may reveal rashes, bruises, and petechiae. Careful neurologic and ophthalmologic examinations are crucial if headache or vomiting is present, as the vast majority of patients with CNS tumors have abnormal neurologic examinations.

## COMMON MANIFESTATIONS

The most common manifestations of childhood cancer are fatigue, anorexia, malaise, pain, fever, abnormal lump or mass, pallor, bruising, petechiae, bleeding, headache, vomiting, visual changes, weight loss, and night sweats (Table 153-2).

Patients with leukemia or a tumor that has infiltrated the bone marrow typically have one or more of the following signs/symptoms: fever, pallor, bruising, petechiae, and bleeding. Lymphadenopathy and organomegaly are also common in leukemia, particularly with T-cell ALL or non-Hodgkin lymphoma (NHL). Patients with solid tumors

585

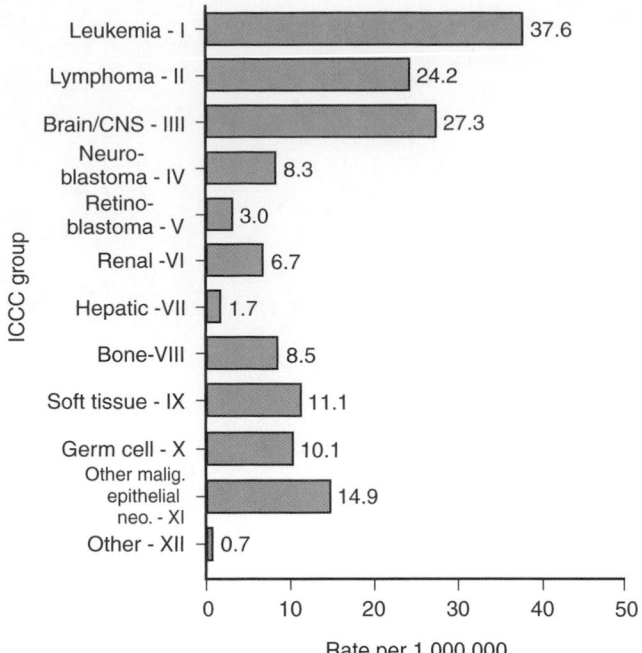

## DIFFERENTIAL DIAGNOSIS

Distinguishing a malignant process from another disease can be difficult. Ultimately, a tissue diagnosis (from bone marrow or solid tumor biopsy) with pathologic confirmation is required to confirm a diagnosis of cancer. Infection commonly masquerades as a potential malignancy. In particular, Epstein-Barr virus (EBV), cytomegalovirus (CMV), and mycobacterial infections can mimic leukemia or lymphoma by causing fever, lymphadenopathy, organomegaly, weight loss, and abnormal blood counts. Trauma may produce swelling that can mimic solid tumors. Idiopathic thrombocytic purpura (ITP) and iron deficiency can produce thrombocytopenia and anemia, respectively. Immune deficiencies or irregularities (autoimmune hemolytic anemia or neutropenia) can also produce cytopenias. Juvenile idiopathic arthritis and other collagen vascular disease can cause musculoskeletal pain and anemia, mimicking leukemia. Benign tumors are relatively common in children, including mature germ cell tumors/ hamartomas, hemangiomas or other vascular tumors, mesoblastic nephromas, and bone cysts.

**FIGURE 153-1**

Cancer SEER incidence rates, 1975–2006, by ICCC group, in children under 20 years of age, both sexes, all races. (From Steliarova-Foucher E, Stiller C, Lacour B, et al: International Classification of Childhood Cancer, 3rd ed. Bethesda, MD, *National Cancer Institute*, 2005; Cancer 103(7):1457–1467, 2005. Accessed at http://seer.cancer.gov/csr/ 1975_2006/browse_csr.php?section=29&page=sect_29_zfig.01.html.) SEER, Surveillance Epidemiology and End Results.

## INITIAL DIAGNOSTIC EVALUATION

### Screening Tests

A complete blood count (CBC) with differential and review of the peripheral blood smear is the best screening test for many pediatric malignancies. Leukopenia, (with or without neutropenia), anemia, or thrombocytopenia may be present in leukemia or any cancer that invades the bone marrow (e.g., neuroblastoma, rhabdomyosarcoma, or Ewing sarcoma). Leukemia may also produce leukocytosis, usually with blasts present on the peripheral blood smear. An isolated cytopenia (neutropenia, anemia, or thrombocytopenia) widens the differential diagnosis, but still could be the only abnormal laboratory finding. Of note, a patient with leukemia may also have a normal CBC.

usually have a palpable or measurable mass. Other signs and symptoms may include pain, limp, cough, dyspnea, headache, vomiting, cranial nerve palsies, and papilledema. In general, malignant masses are firm, fixed, and nontender, whereas masses that are infectious or inflammatory in nature are relatively softer, mobile, and tender to palpation.

**FIGURE 153-2**

Incidence of the most common types of cancer in children by age. The cumulative incidence is shown as a dashed line. (From Kliegman RM, Behrman RE, Jenson HB, et al (eds): Nelson Textbook of Pediatrics, 18th ed. Philadelphia, *WB Saunders*, 2007.)

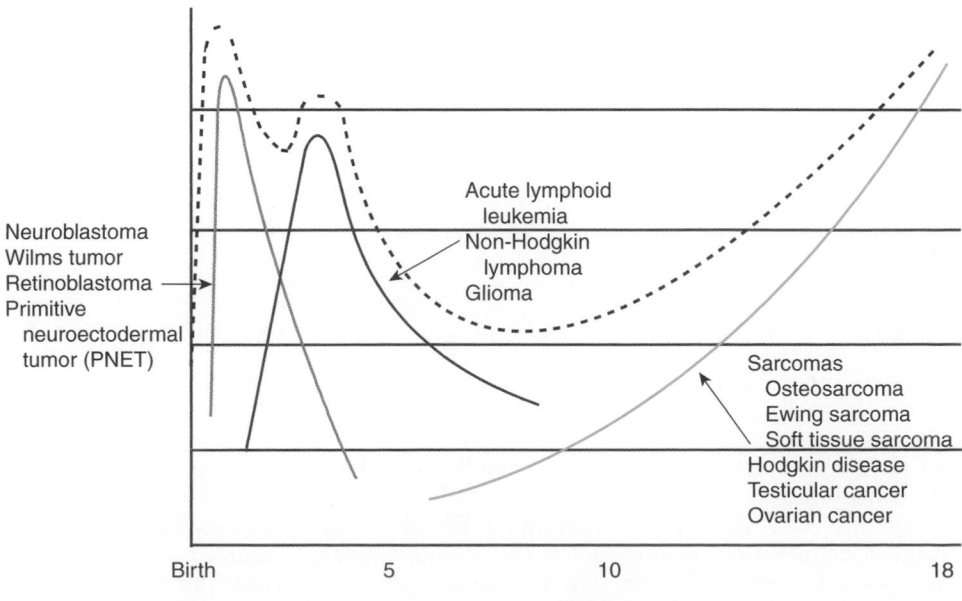

**TABLE 153-1  Known Risk Factors for Selected Childhood Cancers**

| Cancer Type | Risk Factor | Comments |
|---|---|---|
| Acute lymphoid leukemia | Ionizing radiation | Although primarily of historical significance, prenatal diagnostic x-ray exposure increases risk. |
| | | Therapeutic irradiation for cancer treatment also increases risk. |
| | Race | Rate in white children is twice that in black children in the USA. |
| | Genetic conditions | Down syndrome is associated with an estimated 10- to 20-fold increased risk. |
| | | Neurofibromatosis type 1, Bloom syndrome, ataxia-telangiectasia, and Langerhans cell histiocytosis, among others, are associated with an elevated risk. |
| Acute myeloid leukemias | Chemotherapeutic agents | Alkylating agents and epipodophyllotoxins increase risk. |
| | Genetic factors | Down syndrome and neurofibromatosis type 1 are strongly associated. Familial monosomy 7 and several other genetic syndromes are also associated with increased risk. |
| Brain cancers | Therapeutic ionizing radiation to the head | Patients treated with radiation therapy for leukemia or brain tumors. |
| | Genetic factors | Neurofibromatosis type 1 is strongly associated with optic gliomas, and, to a lesser extent, with other central nervous system tumors. Tuberous sclerosis and several other genetic syndromes are associated with increased risk. |
| Hodgkin disease | Family history | Monozygotic twins and siblings are at increased risk. |
| | Infections | Epstein-Barr virus is associated with increased risk. |
| Non-Hodgkin lymphoma | Immunodeficiency | Acquired and congenital immunodeficiency disorders and immunosuppressive therapy increase risk. |
| | Infections | Epstein-Barr virus is associated with increased risk. |
| Osteosarcoma | Ionizing radiation | Cancer radiation therapy and high radium exposure increase risk. |
| | Chemotherapy | Alkylating agents increase risk. |
| | Genetic factors | Increased risk is apparent with Li-Fraumeni syndrome and hereditary retinoblastoma. |
| Ewing sarcoma | Race | Incidence is about 9 times higher in white children than in black children in the USA. |
| Neuroblastoma | Genetic factors | Chromosome 6p22 variants are associated with increased risk. |
| Retinoblastoma | Genetic factors | No other established risk factors have been recognized. |
| Wilms tumor | Congenital anomalies | Aniridia, Beckwith-Wiedemann syndrome, and other congenital and genetic conditions are associated with increased risk. |
| | Race | Reported rates in Asian children are about half those in white and black children. |
| Renal medullary carcinoma | Sickle cell trait | Etiology is unknown. |
| Rhabdomyosarcoma | Congenital anomalies and genetic conditions | Li-Fraumeni syndrome and neurofibromatosis type 1 are believed to be associated with increased risk. Some concordance with major birth defects has been recognized. |
| Hepatoblastoma | Genetic factors | Beckwith-Wiedemann syndrome, hemihypertrophy, Gardner syndrome, and family history of adenomatous polyposis are associated with increased risk. |
| Hepatocellular carcinoma | Infections | Hepatitis B virus infection increases risk. |
| Leiomyosarcoma | Immunosuppression and Epstein-Barr virus infection | Epstein-Barr virus is associated with leiomyosarcoma for all forms of congenital and acquired immunosuppression but not leiomyosarcoma among immunocompetent persons. |
| Malignant germ cell tumors | Cryptorchidism | Cryptorchidism is a risk factor for testicular germ cell tumors. |

Modified from Kadan-Lottick NS: Epidemiology of childhood and adolescent cancer. In Kliegman RM, Behrman RE, Jenson HB, et al (eds): Nelson Textbook of Pediatrics, 18th ed. Philadelphia, *Saunders*, 2007.

### TABLE 153-2 Common Manifestations of Childhood Malignancies

| Sign/Symptom | Significance | Example |
|---|---|---|
| **HEMATOLOGIC** | | |
| Pallor, anemia | Bone marrow infiltration | Leukemia, neuroblastoma |
| Petechiae, thrombocytopenia | Bone marrow infiltration | Leukemia, neuroblastoma |
| Fever, pharyngitis, neutropenia | Bone marrow infiltration | Leukemia, neuroblastoma |
| **SYSTEMIC** | | |
| Bone pain, limp, arthralgia | Primary bone tumor, metastasis to bone | Osteosarcoma, Ewing sarcoma, leukemia, neuroblastoma |
| Fever of unknown origin, weight loss, night sweats | Lymphoreticular malignancy | Hodgkin disease, non-Hodgkin lymphoma |
| Painless lymphadenopathy | Lymphoreticular malignancy, metastatic solid tumor | Leukemia, Hodgkin disease, non-Hodgkin lymphoma, Burkitt lymphoma, thyroid carcinoma |
| Cutaneous lesion | Primary or metastatic disease | Neuroblastoma, leukemia, Langerhans cell histiocytosis, melanoma |
| Abdominal mass | Adrenal-renal tumor | Neuroblastoma, Wilms tumor, lymphoma |
| Hypertension | Sympathetic nervous system tumor | Neuroblastoma, pheochromocytoma, Wilms tumor |
| Diarrhea | Vasoactive intestinal polypeptide | Neuroblastoma, ganglioneuroma |
| Soft tissue mass | Local or metastatic tumor | Ewing sarcoma, osteosarcoma, neuroblastoma, thyroid carcinoma, rhabdomyosarcoma, eosinophilic granuloma |
| Diabetes insipidus, galactorrhea, poor growth | Neuroendocrine involvement of hypothalamus or pituitary gland | Adenoma, craniopharyngioma, prolactinoma, Langerhans cell histiocytosis |
| Emesis, visual disturbances, ataxia, headache, papilledema, cranial nerve palsies | Increased intrathecal pressure | Primary brain tumor; metastasis |
| **OPHTHALMOLOGIC** | | |
| Leukocoria | White pupil | Retinoblastoma |
| Periorbital ecchymosis | Metastasis | Neuroblastoma |
| Miosis, ptosis, heterochromia | Horner syndrome: compression of cervical sympathetic nerves | Neuroblastoma |
| Opsomyoclonus, ataxia | Neurotransmitters (?) Autoimmunity (?) | Neuroblastoma |
| Exophthalmos, proptosis | Orbital tumor | Rhabdomyosarcoma, lymphoma |
| **THORACIC** | | |
| Anterior mediastinal mass | Cough, stridor, pneumonia, tracheal-bronchial compression | Germ cell tumor, T-cell lymphoma, Hodgkin disease |
| Posterior mediastinal mass | Vertebral or nerve root compression; dysphagia | Neuroblastoma, neuroenteric cyst |

Lactate dehydrogenase (LDH) and uric acid are often elevated in fast-growing tumors (leukemia or lymphoma) and occasionally in sarcomas or neuroblastoma. In many cases, it is appropriate to assess electrolytes and renal and hepatic function in the screening process. Elevated blood pressure, if confirmed by repeat measurements, should prompt a urine analysis, as should the palpation of an abdominal mass.

## Diagnostic Imaging

A chest x-ray (CXR) (posteroanterior and lateral) is the best screening radiographic study for a patient with suspicious cervical lymphadenopathy, fever, and weight loss. Mediastinal masses and pleural effusions can often be detected on CXR. Abdominal signs or symptoms warrant an ultrasound or CT. Persistent headache, vomiting, or abnormal neurologic findings should lead to a head CT

**TABLE 153-3 Minimum Workup Required for Common Pediatric Malignancies to Assess Primary Tumor and Potential Metastases***

| Malignancy | BMA/bx | CXR | CT Scan | MRI | Bone Scan | CSF Analysis | Marker(s) | Other |
|---|---|---|---|---|---|---|---|---|
| Leukemia | Yes | Yes | | | | Yes | | |
| Non-Hodgkin lymphoma | Yes | Yes | Yes | | Yes | Yes | | |
| Hodgkin lymphoma | Yes | Yes | Yes | | Yes | | | PET or gallium scan |
| CNS tumors | | | | Yes | | Yes | | |
| Neuroblastoma | Yes | | Yes | | Yes | | VMA, HVA | mIBG scan |
| Wilms tumor | | Yes | Yes | | | | | |
| Rhabdomyosarcoma | Yes | Yes | Yes | | Yes | Yes, for parameningeal tumors only | | |
| Osteosarcoma | | Yes | Yes (chest) | Yes (primary) | Yes | | | |
| Ewing sarcoma | Yes | Yes | Yes (chest) | Yes (primary) | Yes | | | |
| Germ cell tumors | | Yes | Yes | | | | AFP, β-hCG | Consider brain MRI |
| Liver tumors | | Yes | Yes | | | | AFP | |
| Retinoblastoma | ± | | Yes, if MRI not available | Yes (brain) | ± | Yes | | Rb gene analysis |

*Individual cases may require additional studies.

AFP, alpha-fetoprotein; BMA/bx, bone marrow aspirate/biopsy; CSF, cerebrospinal fluid; CNS, central nervous system; CT, computed tomography; CXR, chest x-ray study; HVA, homovanillic acid; β-hCG, beta-human chorionic gonadotropin; mIBG, meta-iodobenzylguanidine; MRI, magnetic resonance imaging; PET, positron emission tomography; Rb, retinoblastoma; VMA, vanillylmandelic acid.

or MRI. For suspected bone tumors, plain radiographs are indicated and will usually reveal the lesion(s), if present. Radiographs may be normal when a bony pelvic lesion is suspected; a CT or MRI should be obtained. Other imaging studies to delineate a mass and to search for suspected metastases are often indicated, but these decisions are usually best left to the pediatric oncology team. Table 153-3 shows the general use of diagnostic imaging following confirmation of a diagnosis of cancer, assessing for the primary tumor and for metastases. Positron emission tomography (PET) has proved useful for staging and assessing response for some pediatric cancers, especially lymphomas. The use of total body MRI for detection of metastases in pediatric malignancies is currently under investigation.

# CHAPTER 154

# Principles of Cancer Treatment

The overall goal of pediatric oncology is to cure all patients with minimal toxicity. Overall outcomes have been shown to be superior for patients treated in clinical trials compared to those not treated in clinical trials. Treatment for children with cancer is often multimodal and may involve surgery, radiation therapy, and chemotherapy. Surgery and radiation are generally local treatment modalities (an exception is total body irradiation as part of a bone marrow or stem cell transplant), whereas chemotherapy has both local and systemic effects.

Primary prevention strategies for most pediatric malignancies are unknown. Two exceptions are the use of hepatitis B vaccine to lower the rates of hepatocellular carcinoma and the use of human papillomavirus vaccine to reduce the risk of cervical, vulvar, and vaginal cancers. Childhood malignancies are not associated with tobacco or alcohol use, dietary factors, or sun exposure. Treatment with certain chemotherapy agents and radiation therapy increases the rate of second malignancies. Secondary prevention may be accomplished by screening the at-risk child (e.g., a child with Beckwith-Wiedemann syndrome or twin of a leukemia patient) but these opportunities are rare.

## ONCOLOGIC EMERGENCIES

Adverse effects of tumors and treatments may result in oncologic emergencies in children and adolescents (Table 154-1). Mediastinal masses from lymphoma can cause life-threatening airway obstruction. Tumors with a large tumor burden (e.g., Burkitt lymphoma, germ cell tumors) may affect renal function adversely from tubular deposition of uric acid crystals. Allopurinol or rasburicase can be administered before chemotherapy to minimize this effect.

## TABLE 154-1 Oncologic Emergencies

| Condition | Manifestations | Etiology | Malignancy | Treatment |
|---|---|---|---|---|
| **METABOLIC** | | | | |
| Hyperuricemia | Uric acid nephropathy; gout | Tumor lysis syndrome | Lymphoma, leukemia | Allopurinol, alkalinize urine; hydration and diuresis, rasburicase |
| Hyperkalemia | Arrhythmias, cardiac arrest | Tumor lysis syndrome | Lymphoma, leukemia | Kayexalate; sodium bicarbonate, glucose, and insulin; check for pseudohyperkalemia from leukemic cell lysis in test tube |
| Hyperphosphatemia | Hypocalcemic tetany; metastatic calcification, photophobia, pruritus | Tumor lysis syndrome | Lymphoma, leukemia | Hydration, forced diuresis; stop alkalinization; oral aluminum hydroxide to bind phosphate |
| Hyponatremia | Seizure, lethargy, asymptomatic | SIADH; fluid, sodium losses with vomiting | Leukemia, CNS tumor | Restrict free water for SIADH; replace sodium if depleted |
| Hypercalcemia | Anorexia, nausea, polyuria, pancreatitis, gastric ulcers; prolonged PR/ shortened QT interval | Bone resorption; ectopic parathormone, vitamin D, or prostaglandins | Metastasis to bone, rhabdomyosarcoma | Hydration and furosemide diuresis; corticosteroids; mithramycin; calcitonin, diphosphonates |
| **HEMATOLOGIC** | | | | |
| Anemia | Pallor, weakness, heart failure | Bone marrow suppression or infiltration; blood loss | Any with chemotherapy | Packed red blood cell transfusion |
| Thrombocytopenia | Petechiae, hemorrhage | Bone marrow suppression or infiltration | Any with chemotherapy | Platelet transfusion |
| Disseminated intravascular coagulation | Shock, hemorrhage | Sepsis, hypotension, tumor factors | Promyelocytic leukemia, others | Fresh frozen plasma; platelets, treat infection |
| Neutropenia | Infection | Bone marrow suppression or infiltration | Any with chemotherapy | If patient is febrile, administer broad-spectrum antibiotics, with G-CSF if appropriate |
| Hyperleukocytosis (>50,000/mm$^3$) | Hemorrhage, thrombosis; pulmonary infiltrates, hypoxia; tumor lysis syndrome | Leukostasis; vascular occlusion | Leukemia | Leukapheresis; chemotherapy |
| Graft-versus-host disease | Dermatitis, diarrhea, hepatitis | Immunosuppression and nonirradiated blood products; bone marrow transplantation | Any with immunosuppression | Corticosteroids; cyclosporine; antithymocyte globulin |
| **SPACE-OCCUPYING LESIONS** | | | | |
| Spinal cord compression | Back pain ± radicular *Cord above T10*: symmetrical | Metastasis to vertebra and extramedullary space | Neuroblastoma; medulloblastoma | MRI or myelography for diagnosis; corticosteroids; |

**TABLE 154-1 Oncologic Emergencies—cont'd**

| Condition | Manifestations | Etiology | Malignancy | Treatment |
|---|---|---|---|---|
| | weakness, increased deep tendon reflex; sensory level present; toes up *Conus medullaris (T10-L2)*: symmetrical weakness, increased knee reflexes, decreased ankle reflexes; saddle sensory loss; toes up or down *Cauda equina (below L2)*: asymmetrical weakness, loss of deep tendon reflex and sensory deficit; toes down | | | radiotherapy; laminectomy; chemotherapy |
| Increased intracranial pressure | Confusion, coma, emesis, headache, hypertension, bradycardia, seizures, papilledema, hydrocephalus; cranial nerve III and VI palsies | Primary or metastatic brain tumor | Neuroblastoma, astrocytoma; glioma | CT or MRI for diagnosis; corticosteroids; phenytoin; ventriculostomy tube; radiotherapy; chemotherapy |
| Superior vena cava syndrome | Distended neck veins, plethora, edema of head and neck, cyanosis, proptosis; Horner syndrome | Superior mediastinal mass | Lymphoma | Chemotherapy; radiotherapy |
| Tracheal compression | Respiratory distress | Mediastinal mass compressing trachea | Lymphoma | Irradiation, corticosteroids |

CNS, central nervous system; CT, computed tomography; G-CSF, granulocyte colony-stimulating factor; MRI, magnetic resonance imaging; SIADH, syndrome of inappropriate antidiuretic hormone [secretion].

A common metabolic emergency is **tumor lysis syndrome**, often seen in treatment of leukemia and lymphoma. Large amounts of phosphate, potassium, and uric acid are released into the circulation from lysed cells. Overwhelming infection and spinal cord compression with neurologic compromise are other oncologic emergencies.

## SURGERY

Appropriate imaging (usually with computed tomography [CT] or magnetic resonance imaging [MRI]) for solid tumors presenting as a palpable mass or mass-related symptoms (pain, respiratory distress, intestinal obstruction) should be obtained and followed by resection (when possible) or a biopsy (if complete resection is not feasible). An exception to this is a suspected lymphoma, for which a biopsy may be needed. However, almost all pediatric lymphomas are chemosensitive and do not require surgical resection.

Many pediatric solid tumors (non-Hodgkin lymphoma, neuroblastoma, Ewing sarcoma, and rhabdomyosarcoma) may have very similar appearances on light microscopic examination. This group of tumors is referred to as **small, round blue cell tumors**. To diagnose the particular tumor type adequately, surface marker analysis, immunohistochemistry, and electron microscopy may be required. Cytogenetic evaluations should be carried out, because many types of leukemia and certain solid tumors show either specific chromosomal translocations or other recurring cytogenetic abnormalities that can lead to the correct diagnosis. It is crucial to determine the amount of tissue required and the appropriate distribution of the tissue for testing so that all necessary studies are performed. A general oncologic surgery principle is to resect not just the tumor, but in most cases a surrounding margin of normal tissue to ensure the entire tumor has been resected.

## CHEMOTHERAPY

Because most pediatric solid tumors have a high risk for micrometastatic disease at the time of diagnosis, chemotherapy is used in almost all cases (Table 154-2). Exceptions

## TABLE 154-2 Cancer Chemotherapy

| Drug* | Action | Metabolism | Excretion | Indication | Toxicity |
|---|---|---|---|---|---|
| **ANTIMETABOLITES** | | | | | |
| Methotrexate | Folic acid antagonist; inhibits dihydrofolate reductase | Hepatic | Renal, 50%–90% excreted unchanged; biliary | ALL, lymphoma, medulloblastoma, osteosarcoma | Myelosuppression (nadir 7–10 days), mucositis, stomatitis, dermatitis, hepatitis, renal and CNS effects with high-dose administration; prevent with leucovorin, monitor levels |
| 6-Mercaptopurine | Purine analog | Hepatic; allopurinol inhibits metabolism | Renal | ALL | Myelosuppression; hepatic necrosis; mucositis; allopurinol increases toxicity |
| Cytosine arabinoside (Ara-C) | Pyrimidine analog; inhibits DNA polymerase | Hepatic | Renal | ALL, lymphoma, sarcoma | Myelosuppression, conjunctivitis, mucositis, CNS dysfunction |
| **ALKYLATING AGENTS** | | | | | |
| Cyclophosphamide (Cytoxan) | Alkylates guanine; inhibits DNA synthesis | Hepatic | Renal | ALL, lymphoma, sarcoma | Myelosuppression; hemorrhagic cystitis; pulmonary fibrosis, inappropriate ADH secretion, bladder cancer, anaphylaxis |
| Ifosfamide | Similar to cyclophosphamide | Hepatic | Renal | Lymphoma, Wilms tumor, sarcoma, germ cell and testicular tumors | Similar to cyclophosphamide; CNS dysfunction, cardiac toxicity |
| **ANTIBIOTICS** | | | | | |
| Doxorubicin (Adriamycin) and daunorubicin (Cerubidine) | Binds to DNA, intercalation | Hepatic | Biliary, renal | ALL, AML, osteosarcoma, Ewing sarcoma, lymphoma, neuroblastoma | Cardiomyopathy, red urine, tissue necrosis on extravasation, myelosuppression, conjunctivitis, radiation dermatitis, arrhythmia |
| Dactinomycin | Binds to DNA, inhibits transcription | — | Renal, stool, 30% excreted as unchanged drug | Wilms tumor, rhabdomyosarcoma, Ewing sarcoma | Tissue necrosis on extravasation, myelosuppression, radiosensitizer, stomatitis |
| Bleomycin | Binds to DNA, cuts DNA | Hepatic | Renal | Hodgkin disease, lymphoma, germ cell tumors | Pneumonitis, stomatitis, Raynaud phenomenon, pulmonary fibrosis, dermatitis |
| **VINCA ALKALOIDS** | | | | | |
| Vincristine (Oncovin) | Inhibits microtubule | Hepatic | Biliary | ALL, lymphoma, Wilms tumor, Hodgkin disease, Ewing sarcoma, neuroblastoma, rhabdomyosarcoma, brain tumors | Local cellulitis, peripheral neuropathy, constipation, ileus, jaw pain, inappropriate ADH secretion, seizures, ptosis, minimal myelosuppression |
| Vinblastine (Velban) | Inhibits microtubule formation | Hepatic | Biliary | Hodgkin disease, Langerhans cell histiocytosis | Local cellulitis, leukopenia |

## TABLE 154-2  Cancer Chemotherapy—cont'd

| Drug* | Action | Metabolism | Excretion | Indication | Toxicity |
|-------|--------|-----------|-----------|------------|----------|
| **ENZYMES** | | | | | |
| Asparaginase | Depletion of asparagine | — | Reticuloendothelial system | ALL | Allergic reaction; pancreatitis, hyperglycemia, platelet dysfunction and coagulopathy, encephalopathy |
| **HORMONES** | | | | | |
| Prednisone | Direct lymphocyte cytotoxicity | Hepatic | Renal | ALL; Hodgkin disease, lymphoma | Cushing syndrome, cataracts, diabetes, hypertension, myopathy, osteoporosis, infection, peptic ulceration, psychosis |
| **MISCELLANEOUS** | | | | | |
| BCNU (carmustine, nitrosourea) | Carbamylation of DNA; inhibits DNA synthesis | Hepatic; phenobarbital increases metabolism, decreases activity | Renal | CNS tumors, lymphoma, Hodgkin disease | Delayed myelosuppression (4–6 wk); pulmonary fibrosis, carcinogenic, stomatitis |
| Cisplatin | Inhibits DNA synthesis | — | Renal | Gonadal tumors; osteosarcoma, neuroblastoma, CNS tumors, germ cell tumors | Nephrotoxic; myelosuppression, ototoxicity, tetany, neurotoxicity, hemolytic uremic syndrome; aminoglycosides may increase nephrotoxicity, anaphylaxis |
| Carboplatin | Inhibits DNA synthesis | — | Renal | Same as for cisplatin | Myelosuppression |
| Etoposide (VP-16) | Topoisomerase inhibitor | — | Renal | ALL, lymphoma, germ cell tumor | Myelosuppression, secondary leukemia |
| Tretinoin (vitamin A analog) and isotretinoin | Enhances normal differentiation | Liver | Liver | M3 AML; neuroblastoma | Dry mouth, hair loss, pseudotumor cerebri, premature epiphyseal closure |

*Many drugs produce nausea and vomiting during administration, and many cause alopecia with repeated doses.
ADH, antidiuretic hormone; ALL, acute lymphoblastic leukemia; AML, acute myeloid leukemia; BCNU, bis-chloronitrosourea; CNS, central nervous system.

include low-stage neuroblastoma (particularly in infants) and low-grade central nervous system (CNS) tumors. For patients with localized solid tumors, chemotherapy administered after removal of the primary tumor is referred to as **adjuvant therapy.** Chemotherapy administered while the primary tumor is still present is referred to as **neoadjuvant chemotherapy**. Neoadjuvant chemotherapy has a number of potential benefits, including an early attack on presumed micrometastatic disease, shrinkage of the primary tumor to facilitate local control, and additional time to plan for definitive surgery. In patients with osteosarcoma and Ewing sarcoma who undergo surgical removal of the primary tumor following neoadjuvant chemotherapy, a higher degree of necrosis following chemotherapy correlates with better prognosis.

Resistance to a particular chemotherapeutic agent can develop in a number of ways: decreased influx or increased efflux of the chemotherapeutic agent from the malignant cell; mutation in the target tissue so that it cannot be inhibited by the drug; amplification of a drug target to overcome inhibition; and blockade of normal cellular processes, which leads to programmed cell death or apoptosis. Because mutation is an ongoing process in malignant tumors, it follows that certain subpopulations of tumor cells within a tumor may be more or less sensitive to any particular chemotherapy drug. Given this fact, combinations of chemotherapy drugs are used, as opposed to sequential single agents, to treat the various forms of childhood cancer.

The blood-brain barrier prevents the penetration of chemotherapeutic drugs into the CNS; instillation of the chemotherapeutic agent directly into the cerebrospinal fluid (by lumbar puncture) may be necessary. Radiation therapy also circumvents the blood-brain barrier.

## RADIATION THERAPY

Radiation therapy is the process of delivering ionizing radiation to malignant cells in order to kill them directly or, more commonly, prevent them from dividing by interfering with DNA replication. Conventional radiation therapy uses photons, but atomic particles such as electrons, protons, and neutrons can also be used. Not all tumors are radiosensitive, and radiation therapy is not necessary in all tumors that are radiosensitive.

## OTHER THERAPIES

Certain cancers have been treated with cytokines, biologic response modifiers, or monoclonal antibodies in addition to standard treatments. **Targeted therapies** specifically target the tumor cells, sparing normal host cells. Imatinib mesylate is a protein kinase inhibitor that targets the effects of the t(9;22) translocation of chronic myeloid leukemia and acute lymphoblastic leukemia.

Supportive care also plays an important role in pediatric oncology, including the use of appropriate antimicrobial agents, blood products, nutritional support, intensive care, and complementary and alternative therapies.

## ADVERSE EFFECTS

Because chemotherapy agents are cellular toxins, numerous adverse effects are associated with their use. Bone marrow suppression, immunosuppression, nausea, vomiting, and alopecia are general adverse effects of commonly used chemotherapy drugs. Each chemotherapy drug also has specific toxicities. Doxorubicin can cause cardiac damage; cisplatin can cause renal damage and ototoxicity; bleomycin can cause pulmonary fibrosis; cyclophosphamide and ifosfamide can cause hemorrhagic cystitis; and vincristine can cause peripheral neuropathy. Radiation therapy produces many adverse effects such as mucositis, growth retardation, organ dysfunction, and the later development of secondary cancers. Significant therapy-related **late effects** may develop in pediatric cancer patients (Table 154-3).

| TABLE 154-3 Long-Term Sequelae of Cancer Therapy | |
|---|---|
| **Problem** | **Etiologic Agent(s)** |
| Infertility | Alkylating agents; irradiation |
| Second cancers | Genetic predisposition; irradiation; alkylating agents, VP-16, topoisomerase II inhibitors |
| Sepsis | Splenectomy |
| Hepatotoxicity | Methotrexate, 6-mercaptopurine; radiation |
| Hepatic veno-occlusive disease | High-dose, intensive chemotherapy (busulfan, cyclophosphamide) ± bone marrow transplant |
| Scoliosis | Radiation |
| Pulmonary (pneumonia, fibrosis) | Radiation; bleomycin, busulfan |
| Cardiomyopathy, pericarditis | Doxorubicin (Adriamycin), daunomycin; radiation |
| Leukoencephalopathy | Cranial irradiation ± methotrexate |
| Cognition/intelligence | Cranial irradiation ± methotrexate |
| Pituitary dysfunction (isolated growth hormone deficiency, panhypopituitary) | Cranial irradiation |
| Psychosocial | Stress, anxiety, death of peers; conditioned responses to chemotherapy |
| Thyroid dysfunction | Radiation |
| Osteonecrosis | Corticosteroids |

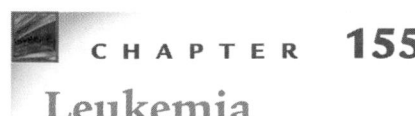

# CHAPTER 155

# Leukemia

## ETIOLOGY

The etiology of childhood leukemia is unknown and is probably multifactorial. Genetics and environmental factors play important roles. There are many recurrent non-random chromosomal translocations in leukemia cells. A translocation may lead to the formation of a new gene, whose expression may lead to a novel protein with transforming capabilities. In chronic myeloid leukemia (CML), a translocation between chromosomes 9 and 22 results in a fusion gene incorporating parts of two genes, *BCR* and *ABL*. The protein formed by this novel gene plays an important role in the development of CML. In addition, certain constitutional genotypes can predispose a child to the development of acute leukemia. Patients with Down syndrome, Fanconi anemia, Bloom syndrome, ataxia-telangiectasia, Wiskott-Aldrich syndrome, and neurofibromatosis type 1 all have an increased risk of acute leukemia. Siblings of children with leukemia are also at increased risk of developing leukemia (approximately two- to fourfold above the childhood population). This risk increases for twin siblings (up to 25% for monozygotic twins). In certain patients with leukemia, the unique antigen receptor gene rearrangement or the specific chromosomal translocation characterizing the patient's leukemic clone can be demonstrated in cord blood cells and neonatal blood spots used for screening for metabolic diseases, suggesting a possible in utero etiology. There are reports of familial leukemia. Environmental factors that may increase the risk of leukemia include ionizing radiation and exposure to certain chemotherapy agents, particularly the topoisomerase II inhibitors.

## EPIDEMIOLOGY

Each year, 2500 to 3500 new cases of childhood leukemia occur in the United States. The disease affects about 40 per 1 million children under the age of 15 years. **Acute lymphoblastic leukemia (ALL)** accounts for approximately 75% of cases. The various subtypes of **acute myelogenous leukemia (AML)** account for 15% to 20%, and types of **chronic myelogenous leukemia (CML)** account for less than 5% of cases. Other chronic leukemias, including juvenile myelomonocytic leukemia, chronic myelomonocytic leukemia, and chronic lymphocytic leukemia, are rare in childhood.

ALL and AML are classified according to the World Health Organization (WHO) system (Table 155-1), although many clinicians and pathologists still use the FAB (French-American-British) system for AML. ALL is classified according to cell lineage as either B-lineage or T-lineage. The incidence of ALL peaks at 2 to 5 years of age and is higher in boys than in girls. T-cell ALL, in particular, is associated with a male predominance as well as an older age of peak incidence. In the United States, ALL is more common in white than in African-American children.

| TABLE 155-1 Classification of Acute Lymphoblastic and Acute Myeloid Leukemias |
| --- |
| **ACUTE LYMPHOBLASTIC LEUKEMIA (ALL)** |
| ALL—L1/L2 morphology |
|   Precursor B-cell ALL |
|   Precursor T-cell ALL |
| ALL, B cell—L3 morphology (i.e., Burkitt's leukemia) |
| **ACUTE MYELOID LEUKEMIA (AML)** |
| AMLs with recurrent cytogenetic translocations |
|   AML with t(8;21)(q22;q22), AML1(CBF-alpha)/ETO |
|   Acute promyelocytic leukemia—AML with t(15;17)(q22; q11-12) and variants, PML/RAR-alpha) (i.e., M3*) |
|   AML with abnormal bone marrow eosinophils—inv(16) (p13q22) or t(16;16)(p13;q11), CBFb/MYH11 |
|   AML with 11q23/MLL abnormalities |
| AML with multilineage dysplasia |
|   With prior myelodysplasic syndrome |
|   Without prior myelodysplastic syndrome |
| AML and myelodysplastic syndromes, therapy-related |
|   Alkylating agent–related |
|   Epipodophyllotoxin-related (some may be lymphoid) |
|   Other types |
| AML not otherwise categorized |
|   AML minimally differentiated (M1) |
|   AML without maturation (M0) |
|   AML with maturation (M2) |
|   Acute myelomonocytic leukemia (M4) |
|   Acute monocytic leukemia (M5) |
|   Acute erythroid leukemia (M6) |
|   Acute megakaryocytic leukemia (M7) |
|   Acute basophilic leukemia |
|   Acute panmyelosis with myelofibrosis |

*The designations M0 to M7 are those of the French-American-British (FAB) classification system for AML, which predated the World Health Organization system and is still used by many clinicians and pathologists. (Modified from World Health Organization Classification.)
MLL, mixed lineage leukemia.

The incidence of AML is relatively high in the neonatal period, then drops and stabilizes until adolescence when there is a slight increase, which continues into adulthood, especially beyond 55 years of age. Males and females are equally affected by AML. Hispanic and African-American children have slightly higher incidence rates than white children.

## CLINICAL MANIFESTATIONS

Signs and symptoms of acute leukemias are related to the infiltration of leukemic cells into normal tissues, resulting in either bone marrow failure (anemia, neutropenia, thrombocytopenia) or specific tissue infiltration (lymph nodes, liver, spleen, brain, bone, skin, gingiva, testes). Common presenting symptoms are fever, pallor, petechiae or ecchymoses, lethargy, malaise, anorexia, and bone or joint pain. **Physical examination** frequently reveals lymphadenopathy and hepatosplenomegaly. Symptomatic central nervous system (CNS) involvement is rare at the time of presentation. The testes are a common extramedullary site for ALL; a painless enlargement of one or both testes may be seen. Patients with **T-cell ALL** are frequently older males (8–10 years), and often have high white blood cell (WBC) counts, anterior mediastinal masses, bulky disease with cervical lymphadenopathy, hepatosplenomegaly, and CNS involvement. In patients with AML, extramedullary soft tissue tumors may be found in various sites. The presence of myeloperoxidase in these tumors may impart a greenish hue; such tumors are known as chloromas.

## LABORATORY AND IMAGING STUDIES

The diagnosis of acute leukemia is confirmed by findings of immature blast cells on either the peripheral blood smear, bone marrow aspirate, or both. With rare exception (a physiologically unstable patient), a bone marrow aspirate should be done urgently to confirm the diagnosis. Most patients have abnormal blood counts; anemia and thrombocytopenia are common. The WBC count may be low, normal, or high; 15% to 20% of patients have WBC count greater than 50,000/mm$^3$. The likely diagnosis of the particular type of leukemia (lymphoid or myeloid) can often be determined by evaluating blast morphology on a peripheral smear or a bone marrow aspirate. Definitive diagnosis requires the evaluation of cell surface markers (**immunophenotype**) by flow cytometry and evaluation of cytochemical staining patterns. **Cytogenetic analysis** should be undertaken in all cases of acute leukemia. Certain types of both lymphoid and myeloid leukemias have specific chromosomal abnormalities. In ALL, the t(12;21) translocation is most common (approximately 20% of all cases) and is associated with a favorable prognosis. The t(9;22) translocation occurs in less than 5% of cases and is associated with a poor prognosis. The t(4;11) translocation (and other translocations involving the *MLL* gene on chromosome 11) often occurs in infants and patients with secondary AML and is generally associated with a poor prognosis. Fluorescence in situ hybridization (FISH) or polymerase chain reaction (PCR) techniques are now employed in most cases of leukemia because many chromosomal abnormalities may not be apparent on routine karyotypes. A **lumbar puncture** should always be performed at the time of diagnosis to evaluate the possibility of CNS involvement. A chest x-ray should be obtained in all patients to exclude an anterior mediastinal mass, which is commonly seen in T-cell ALL. Electrolytes, calcium, phosphorus, uric acid, and renal and hepatic function should be monitored in all patients.

## DIFFERENTIAL DIAGNOSIS

The differential diagnosis of acute leukemia includes nonmalignant and malignant diseases. Infection is probably the most common mimicker of acute leukemia, particularly Epstein-Barr virus infection. Other infections (cytomegalovirus, pertussis, mycobacteria) also can produce signs and symptoms common to leukemia. Noninfectious diagnostic considerations include aplastic anemia, juvenile rheumatoid arthritis, immune thrombocytopenic purpura, and congenital or acquired conditions that lead to neutropenia or anemia. Several malignant diagnoses also can mimic leukemia, including neuroblastoma, rhabdomyosarcoma, and Ewing sarcoma. These all may appear to be small, round, blue cell tumors. Newborns with trisomy 21 may have a condition known as **transient myeloproliferative disorder**, which produces elevated WBC counts with peripheral blasts, anemia, and thrombocytopenia. It usually resolves with supportive care only, but these children have a significantly increased risk (30%) of developing true acute leukemia (ALL or AML) within the next few months and years of life.

Proliferation and accumulation of histiocytes produces the **histiocytoses.** Langerhans cell histiocytosis manifests with varying degrees of bone, skin, lung, liver, and bone marrow (pancytopenia) involvement; familial erythrophagocytic lymphohistiocytosis and infection-associated (e.g., Epstein-Barr virus, cytomegalovirus, herpes simplex viruses, malaria) hemophagocytic syndromes manifest with fever, weight loss, irritability, hepatosplenomegaly, rash, hypertriglyceridemia, cytopenias, and aseptic meningitis. These histiocytic diseases should be included in the differential diagnosis of leukemia.

## TREATMENT

Patients with ALL generally receive three- or four-agent **induction chemotherapy** based on their initial risk group assignment. Low- and standard-risk patients receive vincristine, prednisone, and L-asparaginase for 4 weeks; high-risk patients also receive an anthracycline (daunorubicin or doxorubicin). During induction, intrathecal instillation of some combination of methotrexate, cytarabine, and hydrocortisone is given to treat existing CNS leukemia or prevent its development. Following induction of successful remission, which is achieved in nearly all patients with ALL, the remission is **consolidated** along with **CNS-directed therapy**. For patients with CNS disease detected at diagnosis and those with T-cell ALL, cranial radiation therapy is usually provided. For high-risk patients, the use of intensive systemic chemotherapy in addition to the CNS-directed therapy during consolidation results in significant improvement in overall outcome. Systemic chemotherapy during this phase often includes cyclophosphamide, cytarabine, and 6–mercaptopurine. A delayed intensification improves outcomes in most groups.

After delayed intensification, all patients receive **continuation therapy** for a total duration of therapy of 2 to 3 years. Continuation therapy generally consists of a monthly dose of vincristine and short courses (5–7 days) of oral corticosteroid therapy, plus daily oral 6-mercaptopurine, and weekly methotrexate (orally or intramuscularly). In most protocols, intrathecal chemotherapy is given approximately every 3 months during continuation therapy.

The **treatment of AML** is quite different from that of ALL because nonmyelosuppressive drugs (vincristine, prednisone, and asparaginase) are not effective. Several cycles of extremely intensive myelosuppressive chemotherapy are necessary to cure childhood AML; there is little evidence that low-dose continuation therapy is helpful in AML (with the exception of acute promyelocytic leukemia).

Induction therapy for AML usually consists of cytarabine, daunomycin, and etoposide (or 6-thioguanine). Induction is most effective for long-term outcome when two courses of drugs are given consecutively (1 to 2 weeks apart) regardless of blood counts, as opposed to waiting for counts to recover after the first course. If a patient has an HLA-matched sibling donor, most experts recommend a stem cell transplantation in the first remission, except in patients with Down syndrome and those with relatively favorable cytogenetics such as inv(16), t(15;17), and t(8;21). Gemtuzumab ozogamicin, a drug composed of recombinant humanized anti-CD33 antibody and the cytotoxic antibiotic calicheamicin, and haplo-identical natural killer cell transplantation are being studied as an adjuvant therapy for newly diagnosed childhood AML.

## COMPLICATIONS

Major short-term complications associated with the treatment of leukemia result from bone marrow suppression caused by chemotherapy. Patients may have bleeding and significant anemia that necessitates transfusion of platelets or blood. Neutropenia with fewer than 500 neutrophils/mm$^3$, and especially fewer than 100 neutrophils/mm$^3$, greatly predispose the patient to significant bacterial infection. Cell-mediated immunosuppression increases the risk of *Pneumocystis jiroveci* (*carinii*) pneumonia. Prophylaxis with oral trimethoprim-sulfamethoxazole or aerosolized pentamidine can prevent this. Patients who have not previously had varicella or the varicella vaccine are at risk for severe infection. On exposure, a nonimmune patient should receive varicella-zoster immune globulin. Patients with AML have prolonged periods of neutropenia, which increases the risk of bacterial and fungal infections. Prophylaxis with penicillin and fluconazole is frequently instituted. Long-term sequelae of therapy are less common than in previous treatment eras, but are prevalent in long-term survivors treated in the 1980s and earlier. These sequelae include neurocognitive impairment, short stature, obesity, cardiac dysfunction, infertility, second malignant neoplasms, and psychosocial problems (see Table 154-3).

## PROGNOSIS

Patients with ALL are classified into four prognostic risk groups (low, standard, high, and very high) based on age, initial WBC count, genetic characteristics, and response to induction therapy. Classification systems are complex and evolving (Table 155-2). In general, low-risk patients are 1 to 9 years old with an initial WBC count less than 50,000/mm$^3$ and favorable cytogenetic findings such as t(12;21). High-risk patients are younger than 1 year of age or 10 years of age and older, have an initial WBC count greater than 50,000/mm$^3$, have CNS or testicular disease at diagnosis, or have unfavorable cytogenetics such as t(4;11). Very high risk patients have a hypodiploid DNA index, a t(9;22) translocation, or fail to achieve remission after 4 weeks of therapy. All other patients are considered to have standard-risk ALL. Immunophenotype, minimal residual disease, and early response to therapy are other factors that influence risk stratification. Infants with ALL generally have a highly undifferentiated immunophenotype, often have a translocation involving the mixed lineage leukemia gene (e.g., t(4;11)), and have a poor prognosis. It was suggested previously that African-American, Native American, and Hispanic children have poorer outcomes compared with white and Asian children; these results have not been confirmed in all studies.

The overall **cure rate** for childhood **ALL** with current therapy approximates 80%. Relapse of ALL occurs most commonly in the bone marrow, but also may occur in the CNS, testes, or other extramedullary sites. If relapse occurs while the patient is still receiving treatment, the prognosis is worse than if relapse occurs after discontinuation of therapy. Longer first remissions are associated with higher cure rates with salvage therapy compared with shorter first remissions. Stem cell transplant from a matched sibling donor, matched unrelated donor, or cord blood currently is recommended for patients who have a relapse while receiving initial chemotherapy. The current overall **cure rate** for childhood **AML** is approximately 50%. It is higher for patients who receive a matched sibling stem cell transplant in first remission than for patients treated with chemotherapy alone. The prognosis for relapsed AML is poor.

**TABLE 155-2  General Prognostic Factors in Acute Lymphoblastic Leukemia**

| Factor | Favorable (Lower Risk) | Unfavorable (Higher Risk) |
|---|---|---|
| Age | 1–9.99 years | <1 or ≥10 years |
| Initial WBC count | <50,000/mm$^3$ | >50,000/mm$^3$ |
| CNS disease at diagnosis | Absent | Present |
| DNA index | >1.16 | ≤1.16 |
| Cytogenetics | t(12;21) | t(4;11), t(9;22) |
| Response to therapy | Rapid | Slow |

CNS, central nervous system; WBC, white blood cell.

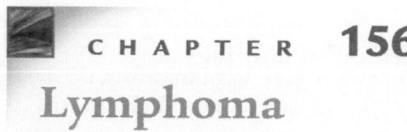

# CHAPTER 156

# Lymphoma

## ETIOLOGY

Lymphomas, or malignancies of lymphoid tissues, are the third most common malignancy in childhood, behind leukemias and central nervous system (CNS) tumors. There are two major types of lymphoma: **Hodgkin disease** and **non-Hodgkin lymphoma (NHL)**. The etiologies are unknown, but evidence in many cases suggests that Epstein-Barr virus plays a causal role in both conditions.

Almost all cases of NHL in childhood are diffuse, are highly malignant, and show little differentiation. NHL has three histologic subtypes: small noncleaved cell (Burkitt lymphoma), lymphoblastic, and large cell. For simplicity, these may be regarded as B cell, T cell, and large cell (which may be of either B-cell or T-cell origin) (Table 156-1).

Chromosomal translocation may move an oncogene from its normal site to a new, unregulated site, leading to increased expression. In Burkitt lymphoma, translocation occurs between chromosome 8 (c-*myc* oncogene) and the immunoglobulin gene locus on chromosome 2, 14, or 22, such that the c-*myc* oncogene comes to reside next to an immunoglobulin gene. The c-*myc* gene turns on the immunoglobulin gene, leading to a malignant B-cell lymphoma.

## EPIDEMIOLOGY

The incidence of Hodgkin disease has a bimodal distribution with peaks in the adolescent/young adult years and again after age 50; it is rarely seen in children younger than 5 years of age. In children, boys are affected more commonly than girls; in adolescents, the gender ratio is approximately equal. The incidence of NHL increases with age. It is more common in whites than in African Americans and in males than in females. NHL has been described in association with congenital or acquired immunodeficiency states and after organ or stem cell transplantation. Burkitt lymphoma commonly is divided into two forms: a sporadic form commonly seen in North America and an endemic form commonly seen in Africa, which has a strong association with Epstein-Barr virus.

## CLINICAL MANIFESTATIONS

The most common clinical presentation of Hodgkin disease is painless, firm lymphadenopathy often confined to one or two lymph node areas, usually the supraclavicular and cervical nodes. Mediastinal lymphadenopathy producing cough or shortness of breath is another frequent initial presentation. The presence of one of three **B symptoms** has prognostic value: fever (>38°C for 3 consecutive days), drenching night sweats, and unintentional weight loss of 10% or more within 6 months of diagnosis.

The **sporadic (North American) form** of Burkitt lymphoma more commonly has an abdominal presentation (typically with pain), whereas the **endemic (African) form** frequently presents with tumors of the jaw. The anterior mediastinum and cervical nodes are the usual primary sites for T-cell lymphomas. These lymphomas may cause airway or superior vena cava obstruction, pleural effusion, or both.

The **diagnosis** of lymphoma is established by tissue biopsy or examination of pleural or peritoneal fluid. Systemic symptoms, such as fever and weight loss, may be present and are particularly prominent in patients with anaplastic large cell lymphoma, which can be insidious in onset. If the bone marrow contains 25% or greater blasts, the disease is classified as acute leukemia (either B-cell ALL or T-cell ALL). This distinction makes little prognostic or therapeutic difference as both require aggressive, systemic therapy in addition to CNS-directed therapy.

## LABORATORY/IMAGING STUDIES

Patients suspected to have lymphoma should have a complete blood count (CBC), erythrocyte sedimentation rate, and measurement of serum electrolytes, calcium, phosphorus, lactate dehydrogenase, and uric acid. A chest x-ray assesses for a mediastinal mass (Fig. 156-1). The diagnosis ultimately requires a pathologic confirmation from tissue or fluid sampling. For staging purposes, a bone marrow aspirate, bone scan, and positron emission tomography (PET) or gallium scan also are indicated. The pathologic hallmark of Hodgkin disease is the identification of **Reed-Sternberg cells**. Histopathologic subtypes in childhood Hodgkin disease are similar to those in adults; 10% to 15% have lymphocyte predominant, 50% to 60% have nodular sclerosis, 30% have mixed cellularity, and less than 5% have lymphocyte depletion. All subtypes are responsive to treatment. Staging of Hodgkin disease is according to

| TABLE 156-1 Subtypes of Non-Hodgkin Lymphoma in Children | | | |
|---|---|---|---|
| **Histologic Category** | **Immunophenotype** | **Usual Primary Site** | **Most Common Translocation(s)** |
| Small noncleaved (Burkitt lymphoma) | Mature B-cell (surface immunoglobulin present) | Abdomen (sporadic form)<br>Head and neck (endemic form) | t(8;14)(q24;q32)<br>t(2;8)(p11;q24)<br>t(8;22)(q24;q11) |
| Lymphoblastic | T-cell (rarely pre-B-cell) | Neck and/or anterior mediastinum | Many |
| Large cell | T-cell, B-cell, or indeterminate | Lymph nodes, skin, soft tissue, bone | t(2;5)(p23;q35) |

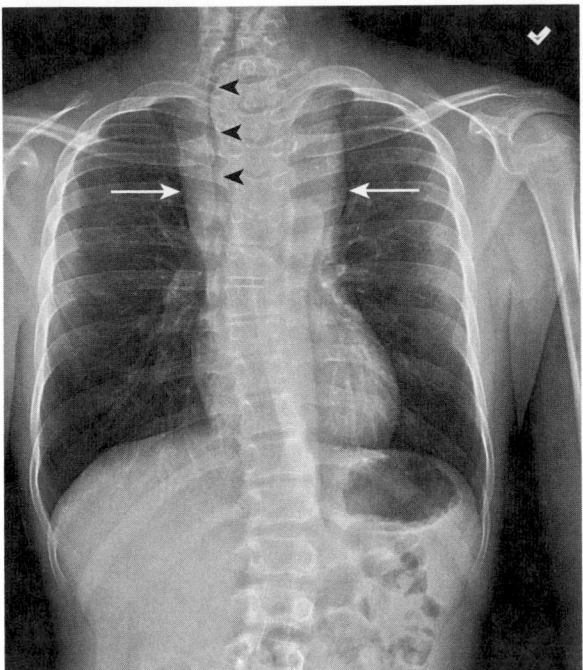

**FIGURE 156-1**

Chest x-ray of a 15-year-old boy demonstrating a large superior anterior mediastinal mass (*large arrows*) compressing the trachea and deviating it rightward (*arrowheads*). Biopsy revealed non-Hodgkin lymphoma.

the Ann Arbor system. Staging laparotomy is rarely used in children today because computed tomography (CT) scans often identify abdominal (lymph nodes, liver, spleen) involvement.

## DIFFERENTIAL DIAGNOSIS

The differential diagnosis for lymphomas in children includes leukemia, rhabdomyosarcoma, nasopharyngeal carcinoma, germ cell tumors, and thymomas. Nonmalignant diagnoses include infectious mononucleosis (Epstein-Barr virus infection), branchial cleft and thyroglossal duct cysts, cat scratch disease (*Bartonella henselae*), bacterial or viral lymphadenitis, mycobacterial infection, toxoplasmosis, and even tinea capitis, all of which can produce significant lymphadenopathy that can mimic lymphoma. Patients with acute abdominal pain from Burkitt lymphoma may be misdiagnosed as having appendicitis.

## TREATMENT

The generally accepted treatment for childhood Hodgkin disease is a combination of chemotherapy and low-dose, involved-field radiation therapy. Chemotherapy usually consists of some combination of cyclophosphamide, vincristine, procarbazine, doxorubicin, bleomycin, vinblastine, prednisone, and etoposide. In general, four to six courses of combination chemotherapy are given. The successful treatment of select low-risk patients with chemotherapy without radiation therapy is well documented and being investigated for select intermediate-risk patients.

Distant, noncontiguous metastases are common in childhood NHL. Systemic chemotherapy is mandatory and should be administered to all children with NHL, even those with clinically localized disease at diagnosis.

T-cell lymphoblastic lymphoma and T-cell anaplastic large cell lymphoma generally are treated with aggressive multidrug regimens similar to the regimens used in ALL. The main drugs used in the treatment of mature B-cell NHL are cyclophosphamide, moderate- to high-dose methotrexate, cytarabine, doxorubicin, ifosfamide, and etoposide. Surgery and radiation therapy rarely are used because the disease is rarely localized and is highly sensitive to chemotherapy.

## COMPLICATIONS

The short-term complications from the treatment of lymphoma are similar to other pediatric malignancies and commonly include immunosuppression, related sequelae from myelosuppression, nausea, vomiting, and alopecia. **Late adverse effects** include second malignant neoplasms (AML or myelodysplasia, thyroid malignancies, and breast cancer in women), hypothyroidism, impaired soft tissue and bone growth, cardiac dysfunction, and pulmonary fibrosis.

## PROGNOSIS

Children and adolescents with **Hodgkin disease** are classified as low, intermediate, or high risk according to stage and nodal bulk. The prognosis is excellent. There is an approximately 90% 5-year overall survival rate; approaching 100% for low-risk patients and 70% to 90% for high-risk patients. For **NHL**, prognosis also is related to stage. The overall 3-year survival rates for B-cell, T-cell, and large cell NHL are 70% to 90%.

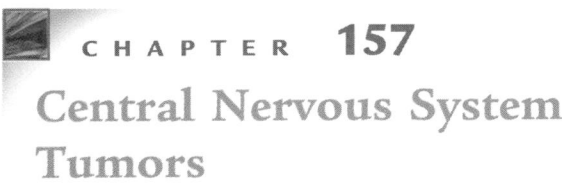

# CHAPTER 157

# Central Nervous System Tumors

## ETIOLOGY

Most central nervous system (CNS) tumors in children and adolescents are **primary tumors** that originate in the CNS and include low-grade astrocytomas or embryonic neoplasms (medulloblastoma, ependymoma, germ cell tumor). In contrast, CNS tumors in adults are high-grade astrocytomas or **secondary tumors** that are metastatic from other carcinomas. CNS tumors also may arise in patients previously treated with radiation therapy. CNS tumors are likely multifactorial in etiology. The classification of CNS tumors is complex and evolving, with the World Health Organization classification the most complete and accurate system.

## EPIDEMIOLOGY

CNS tumors are the most common solid tumors in children and are second to leukemia in overall incidence during childhood. About 1700 new cases occur each year in the United States; the rate is approximately 33 cases per 1 million children under 15 years of age. The incidence peaks before age 10 years, then decreases until a second peak after age 70. For medulloblastoma and ependymoma, males are more affected than females; for other tumor types, no gender differences exist. In the first 2 to 3 years of life, whites are affected more than multiracial children; otherwise, incidence rates are essentially equal for whites and multiracial children.

Children with certain inherited syndromes, including neurofibromatosis (types 1 and 2), Li-Fraumeni syndrome, tuberous sclerosis, Turcot syndrome, and von Hippel–Lindau syndrome have an increased risk for developing a CNS tumor. Most CNS tumors arise in children with no known underlying disorder or risk factor.

## CLINICAL MANIFESTATIONS

Brain tumors can cause symptoms by impingement on normal tissue (usually cranial nerves) or by an increase in intracranial pressure caused either by obstruction of cerebrospinal fluid (CSF) flow or by a direct mass effect. Tumors that obstruct the flow of CSF become symptomatic quickly. Symptoms of **increased intracranial pressure** are lethargy, headache, and vomiting (particularly in the morning on awakening). Irritability, anorexia, poor school performance, and loss of developmental milestones all may be signs of slow-growing CNS tumors. In young children with open cranial sutures, an increase in head circumference may occur. Optic pathway tumors may lead to loss of visual acuity or visual field defects. Inability to abduct the eye as the result of sixth cranial nerve palsy is a common sign of increased intracranial pressure. Cranial nerve deficits other than sixth nerve palsy suggest involvement of the brainstem. Seizures occur in 20% to 50% of patients with supratentorial tumors; focal weakness or sensory changes also may be seen. Pituitary involvement produces neuroendocrine effects (galactorrhea with prolactinoma, excessive growth with growth hormone secretory tumors, precocious puberty). Cerebellar tumors are associated with ataxia and diminished coordination. A history and physical examination are fundamental for evaluation, which should include a careful neurologic assessment, including visual fields and a funduscopic examination.

## LABORATORY/IMAGING STUDIES

If an intracranial lesion is suspected, **magnetic resonance imaging (MRI)** is currently the examination of choice (Fig. 157-1); a computed tomography (CT) scan may be more easily obtained, especially in an emergency. Examination of CSF by cytocentrifuge histologic testing is essential to determine the presence of metastatic disease in primitive neuroectodermal tumors, germ cell tumors, and pineal region tumors. A lumbar puncture should not be performed before a CT scan or MRI has been obtained to evaluate for evidence of increased intracranial

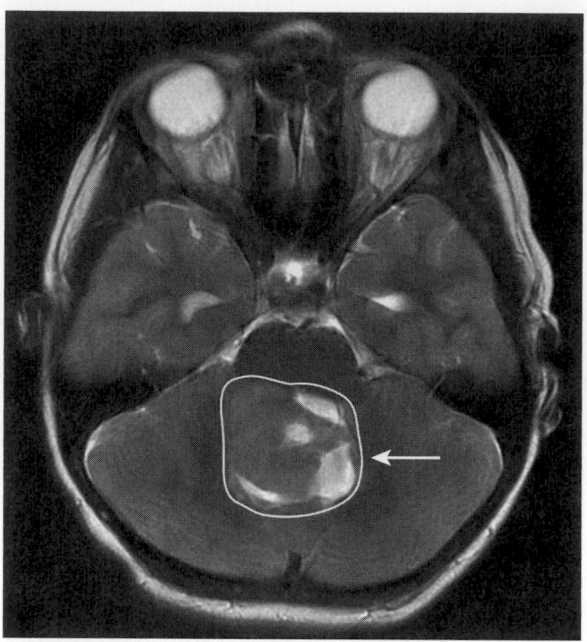

**FIGURE 157-1**

Magnetic resonance imaging scan of a 9-year-old boy showing a heterogeneously enhancing fourth ventricular mass (*arrow*). It was resected and pathology revealed medulloblastoma.

pressure. If a tumor is suspected to have metastatic potential (medulloblastoma), MRI of the entire spine should be obtained before surgery to assess for neuraxial dissemination. A postoperative MRI study of the brain (and spine, if not done preoperatively) should be obtained within 24 to 48 hours of surgery to assess the extent of resection. During follow-up, magnetic resonance spectroscopy can help distinguish recurrent tumor from radiation necrosis.

## DIFFERENTIAL DIAGNOSIS

The differential diagnosis of a CNS mass lesion includes malignant tumor, benign tumor, arteriovenous malformation, aneurysm, brain abscess, cysticercosis, granulomatous disease (tuberculosis, sarcoid), intracranial hemorrhage, pseudotumor cerebri, vasculitis, and, rarely, metastatic tumor.

## TREATMENT

The therapy for children with CNS tumors is individualized and depends on the tumor type, location, size, and associated symptoms. High-dose **dexamethasone** often is administered immediately to reduce tumor-associated edema. Surgical objectives are complete excision, if possible, and maximal debulking if a complete excision is not possible. In children, radiation therapy often is combined with chemotherapy; in young children, radiation therapy may be delayed or avoided altogether. Primitive neuroectodermal tumors (including medulloblastoma) and germ cell tumors are sensitive to chemotherapy; gliomas are less sensitive to chemotherapy. Chemotherapy plays an especially important role, particularly in infants in whom the effects of high-dose CNS radiation may have devastating effects on growth and neurocognitive development.

## COMPLICATIONS

Short-term adverse effects of therapy include nausea, vomiting, anorexia, fatigue, immunosuppression, and cushingoid features. Long-term adverse effects include neurocognitive deficits, endocrinologic sequelae, decreased bone growth, ototoxicity, renal insufficiency, cataracts, infertility, and second malignant neoplasms (including myelodysplasia). The neurocognitive deficits can be significant, particularly in infants and young children, and are the primary reason for the continued search for the lowest efficacious radiation therapy dose and the most conformal delivery methods for the radiation therapy boosts. **Cerebellar mutism syndrome** occurs in 25% of patients after resection of a posterior fossa tumor and is characterized by an acute decrease in speech (often mutism), behavioral changes (e.g., irritability, apathy, or both), diffuse cerebellar dysfunction, and other neurologic abnormalities. It may begin within hours to days of surgery and is usually self-resolving within weeks to months; cerebellar ataxia and dysmetria often persist. **Somnolence syndrome**, which is characterized by excessive fatigue and sleepiness, may occur in the months after completion of radiation therapy and is self-limited. **Posterior fossa syndrome** manifests as headache and aseptic meningitis days to weeks after surgery in this area.

## PROGNOSIS

Improvements in neurodiagnosis, neurosurgical techniques, chemotherapy regimens, and radiation therapy techniques have improved overall outcome. The 5-year overall survival rate associated with all childhood CNS tumors is approximately 50% to 60%, resulting in large measure from the high curability of cerebellar astrocytomas and the increasing cure rate for patients with medulloblastoma (Table 157-1). Intrinsic brainstem gliomas and glioblastoma multiforme have extremely poor prognoses.

### TABLE 157-1 Location, Incidence, and Prognosis of CNS Tumors in Children

| Location | Incidence (%) | 5-Year Survival (%) |
|---|---|---|
| **Infratentorial (posterior fossa)** | 55–60 | |
| Astrocytoma (cerebellum) | 20 | 90 |
| Medulloblastoma | 20 | 50–80 |
| Glioma (brainstem) | 15 | High grade: 0–5; low grade: 30 |
| Ependymoma | 5 | 50–60 |
| **Supratentorial (cerebral hemispheres)** | 40–55 | |
| Astrocytoma | 15 | 50–75 |
| Glioblastoma multiforme | 10 | 0–5 |
| Ependymoma | 2.5 | 50–75 |
| Choroid plexus papilloma | 1.5 | 95 |
| **Midline** | | |
| Craniopharyngioma | 6 | 70–90 |
| Pineal (germinoma) | 1 | 65–75 |
| Optic nerve glioma | 3 | 90 |

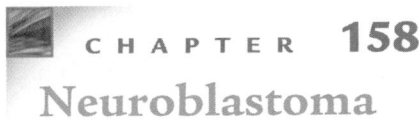

## CHAPTER 158
# Neuroblastoma

## ETIOLOGY

Neuroblastoma is derived from **neural crest cells** that form the adrenal medulla and the sympathetic nervous system. The cause is unknown. Because most cases occur in young children, it is likely that neuroblastoma results from prenatal and perinatal events. Genetic mutations at chromosome 6p22 increase the risk of neuroblastoma and are also associated with high-risk disease.

## EPIDEMIOLOGY

Neuroblastoma is the most common extracranial solid tumor of childhood and the most common malignancy in infancy. The median age at diagnosis is 20 months. In the United States, there are approximately 650 new cases of neuroblastoma each year. The incidence is estimated to be 1 in 7000 live births. The tumor usually occurs sporadically, but in 1% to 2% of cases, there is a family history of neuroblastoma.

## CLINICAL MANIFESTATIONS

Neuroblastoma is remarkable for its broad spectrum of clinical prognosis ranging from spontaneous regression to rapid progression and metastasis resulting in death. Children with localized disease are often asymptomatic at diagnosis, whereas children with metastases often appear ill and have systemic complaints, such as fever, weight loss, and pain. The most common presentation is abdominal pain or mass. The mass is often palpated in the flank and is hard, smooth, and nontender. In the abdomen, 45% of tumors arise in the adrenal gland and 25% arise in the retroperitoneal sympathetic ganglia. Other sites of origin are the paravertebral ganglia of the chest and neck. Paraspinal tumors may invade through the neural foramina and cause spinal cord compression. Horner syndrome sometimes is seen with neck or apical masses. Several **paraneoplastic syndromes,** including secretory diarrhea, profuse sweating, and **opsomyoclonus** (*dancing eyes and dancing feet*), are associated with neuroblastoma.

Neuroblastoma may metastasize to multiple organs including the liver, bone, bone marrow, and lymph nodes. Periorbital ecchymoses is a sign of orbital bone involvement. A unique category of neuroblastoma, **stage 4S**, is defined in infants (<1 year old) with a small primary tumor and metastasis limited to skin, liver, or bone marrow. It is associated with a favorable outcome.

## LABORATORY/IMAGING STUDIES

A complete blood count (CBC) and plain films may help identify patients with neuroblastoma. Calcification within abdominal neuroblastoma tumors is often observed on plain films of the abdomen. About 90% of neuroblastomas produce **catecholamines (VMA, HVA)** that can be detected in the urine. Definitive diagnosis of neuroblastoma requires tissue for light microscopic, electron microscopic, and immunohistologic examination. Cytogenetic analysis and molecular studies to detect *MYCN* (also known as *N-myc*) amplification and mutations at chromosome 6p22 provide important prognostic information. A computed tomography (CT) scan of the chest, abdomen, and pelvis; a bone scan; bilateral bone marrow aspiration and biopsies; and urinary catecholamines complete the evaluation. Neuroblastoma cells concentrate metaiodobenzylguanidine (mIBG), a neurotransmitter precursor; thus mIBG scintography is a sensitive method for detecting metastatic disease.

## DIFFERENTIAL DIAGNOSIS

The abdominal presentation of neuroblastoma must be differentiated from Wilms tumor, which also presents as an abdominal flank mass. Ultrasound or CT examination differentiates the tumors. Periorbital ecchymoses from orbital metastases sometimes are mistaken for child abuse. Because children with bone marrow involvement may have anemia, thrombocytopenia, or neutropenia, leukemia is often considered in the differential.

## TREATMENT

Treatment of neuroblastoma is based on surgical staging and biologic features (Table 158-1). Complete surgical excision is the initial treatment of choice for localized neuroblastoma. Children with favorable biology who undergo a gross total resection require no further therapy. In patients with advanced disease, combination chemotherapy usually is given after confirmation of the diagnosis. The most commonly used agents are vincristine, cyclophosphamide, doxorubicin, cisplatin, and etoposide. Delayed resection of the primary tumor is undertaken after numerous courses of chemotherapy. Radiation therapy often is administered to the primary tumor bed and areas of metastatic disease. **High-dose chemotherapy with autologous stem cell rescue** has improved the outcome for patients with high-risk neuroblastoma. Survival has also improved with the addition of *cis*-**retinoic acid** (isotretinoin) after maximal reduction of tumor burden with chemotherapy, surgery and radiation therapy. Isotretinoin induces tumor differentiation in vitro and down-regulates *MYCN* mRNA expression.

## COMPLICATIONS

Spinal cord compression from neuroblastoma may cause an irreversible neurologic deficit and is an oncologic emergency. Children with the opsomyoclonus syndrome may suffer from developmental delay or mental retardation. The aggressive chemotherapy and radiation therapy currently used to treat high-risk neuroblastoma may result in complications such as ototoxicity, nephrotoxicity, growth problems, and second malignancies.

## PROGNOSIS

The prognosis for survival is affected by age at diagnosis, stage, primary site, presence or absence of metastasis, cytogenetics, DNA ploidy, *MYCN* status, chromosome 6p22 status, and histopathology. Currently, children with neuroblastoma can be divided into three groups: low, average, and high risk. Unfavorable biologic factors include lack of cell differentiation, amplification (>10 copies/cell) of the *MYCN*

**TABLE 158-1  Proposed Children's Oncology Group Neuroblastoma Risk Stratification Schema, by Stage**

| Stage | Age | MYCN | Ploidy | Histology | Other | Risk Group |
|---|---|---|---|---|---|---|
| 1 | | | | | | Low |
| 2A/2B | | Not amplified | | | >50% resection | Low |
| | | Not amplified | | | <50% resection | Intermediate |
| | | Not amplified | | | Biopsy only | Intermediate |
| | | Amplified | | | | High |
| 3 | <547 days | Not amplified | | | | Intermediate |
| | ≥547 days | Not amplified | | Favorable | | Intermediate |
| | | Amplified | | | | High |
| | ≥547 days | Not amplified | | Unfavorable | | High |
| 4 | <365 days | Amplified | | | | High |
| | <365 days | Not amplified | | | | Intermediate |
| | 365–547 days | Amplified | | | | High |
| | 365–547 days | | DI = 1 | | | High |
| | 365–547 days | | | Unfavorable | | High |
| | 365–547 days | Not amplified | DI > 1 | Favorable | | Intermediate |
| | ≥547 days | | | | | High |
| 4S | <365 days | Not amplified | DI > 1 | Favorable | Asymptomatic | Low |
| | <365 days | Not amplified | DI = 1 | | | Intermediate |
| | <365 days | Missing | Missing | Missing | | Intermediate |
| | <365 days | Not amplified | | | Symptomatic | Intermediate |
| | <365 days | Not amplified | | Unfavorable | | Intermediate |
| | <365 days | Amplified | | | | High |

DI, DNA index.

From Maris JM, Hogarty MD, Bagatell R, et al: Neuroblastoma. *Lancet* 369:2106–2120, 2007.

oncogene, lack of hyperdiploidy, and mutations of chromosome 1p, 11q, or 6p22. Patients with favorable biology tend to be younger and often have localized disease. Patients under 1 year of age generally have a better prognosis than older patients. Older patients with stage 4 disease most commonly have unfavorable biology and more than 50% will relapse due to drug-resistant residual disease. Although neuroblastoma represents only 8% of cases of childhood cancer, it is responsible for 15% of cancer deaths in children.

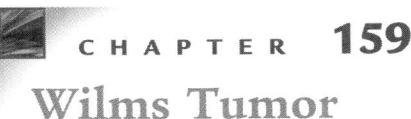

# CHAPTER 159
# Wilms Tumor

## ETIOLOGY

Wilms tumor is thought to arise from primitive, metanephric blastema, the precursor of normal kidney. Nephrogenic rests are foci of embryonal cells that may be rarely (<1%) found in normal infant kidneys and are commonly (25–40%) found in Wilms tumor-bearing kidneys. They may be perilobar, intralobar or both, and they are widely considered to be precursors to Wilms tumors. Although the cause of Wilms tumor is unknown, children with certain congenital anomalies or genetic conditions are at increased risk of developing the disease.

Multiple Wilms tumor or *WT* genes have been identified. The *WT1* gene at chromosomal band 11p13 is important in a minority of tumors, and other genes at 11p15, 16q, and 1p are also involved. The identification of several genes involved in the etiology or progression of Wilms tumor and the loss of heterozygosity (LOH) in normal tissues of some patients demonstrate that the genetic predisposition to Wilms tumor is heterogeneous.

## EPIDEMIOLOGY

Wilms tumor is the most common malignant **renal tumor** of childhood, with approximately 500 new cases per year in the United States. The mean age at diagnosis is 3 to 3.5 years of age, and no gender predilection is apparent. A hereditary form of Wilms tumor may be associated with bilateral presentation and younger age at onset. Many congenital anomalies are associated with Wilms tumor including sporadic aniridia, hemihypertrophy, and genitourinary abnormalities (hypospadias, cryptorchidism, horseshoe or fused kidneys, ureteral duplication, and polycystic kidneys). Patients with the WAGR syndrome (Wilms tumor, aniridia, genitourinary malformation, mental retardation) have Wilms tumor as a manifestation of the syndrome itself, resulting from a germline deletion at chromosome 11p. Patients with Beckwith-Wiedemann syndrome and some other overgrowth syndromes are at increased risk for developing Wilms tumor and should be screened with periodic renal imaging.

## CLINICAL MANIFESTATIONS

Most children with Wilms tumor are brought to medical attention because they have an **abdominal mass** that is discovered by their parents. Although many children do not have complaints at the time that the mass is first noted, associated symptoms may include abdominal pain, fever, hypertension, and hematuria.

## LABORATORY/IMAGING STUDIES

An abdominal ultrasound or computed tomography (CT) scan can usually distinguish an intrarenal mass from a mass in the adrenal gland or other surrounding structures. Evaluation of the inferior vena cava is crucial because tumor may extend from the kidney into the vena cava. A complete blood count (CBC), urinalysis, liver and renal function studies, and a chest radiograph (to identify pulmonary metastases) should be obtained. In most cases, a CT scan of the chest, abdomen, and pelvis is obtained. The diagnosis is confirmed by histologic examination of the tumor. Although most cases of Wilms tumor are classified as *favorable histology*, the presence of anaplasia is predictive of a worse prognosis and is considered *unfavorable*. The National Wilms Tumor Study Group has developed a staging system for Wilms tumor.

## DIFFERENTIAL DIAGNOSIS

The differential diagnosis of Wilms tumor includes hydronephrosis and polycystic disease of the kidney; benign renal tumors, such as mesoblastic nephroma and hamartoma; and other malignant tumors, such as renal cell carcinoma, neuroblastoma, lymphoma, and retroperitoneal rhabdomyosarcoma.

## TREATMENT

The timing of nephrectomy for unilateral, resectable Wilms tumor remains controversial. The North American approach is for immediate nephrectomy followed by adjuvant chemotherapy, whereas the European approach is to make a diagnosis by imaging and sometimes biopsy, give neoadjuvant chemotherapy followed by surgery and then adjuvant chemotherapy (plus radiation therapy, as indicated). The overall survival is comparable regardless of the approach. The Children's Oncology Group protocols for Wilms tumor with favorable histologic findings generally include vincristine and actinomycin, with or without doxorubicin. Radiation therapy is reserved for a minority of patients depending on stage, presence of metastases, response to therapy, and LOH status. Minimizing radiation effects to the liver is crucial because actinomycin potentiates radiation hepatotoxicity.

**Bilateral Wilms tumor** is present in about 5% of children on initial presentation, whereas recurrent disease affects the opposite kidney in 4% to 5% of patients. Treatment for patients with bilateral Wilms tumor should be individualized to retain as much normal kidney as possible.

## COMPLICATIONS

Survivors of Wilms tumor are at risk for several late effects including cardiomyopathy, scoliosis, hypertension and prehypertension, renal and bladder insufficiency, pulmonary dysfunction, hepatic dysfunction, infertility, and second malignancies. Patients with bilateral Wilms tumor are sometimes left with renal insufficiency or failure. Female survivors may have complicated pregnancies and deliveries.

## PROGNOSIS

In general, the prognosis for patients with Wilms tumor is very good. Prognostic factors include stage and histologic features. Anaplastic variants of Wilms tumor have a significantly worse outcome than classic Wilms tumor. In addition, LOH at chromosomes 1p or 16q confers an increased risk of relapse and death compared to tumors without LOH at either site. The 4-year relapse-free survival of patients with tumors of favorable histologic picture is directly related to stage. Cure rates for patients with localized Wilms tumor at diagnosis are greater than 85%, whereas patients with pulmonary metastases have event-free survival rates of approximately 70% to 80%.

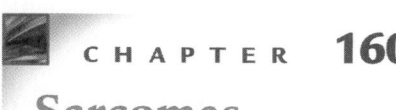

## CHAPTER 160

# Sarcomas

Sarcomas are divided into soft tissue sarcomas and bone cancers. Soft tissue sarcomas arise primarily from the connective tissues of the body, such as muscle tissue, fibrous tissue, and adipose tissue. **Rhabdomyosarcoma**, the most common soft tissue sarcoma in children, is derived from mesenchymal cells that are committed to skeletal muscle lineage. Less common soft tissue sarcomas include fibrosarcoma, synovial sarcoma, and extraosseous **Ewing sarcoma**. The most common malignant bone cancers in children are **osteosarcoma** and Ewing sarcoma. Osteosarcomas derive from primitive bone-forming mesenchymal stem cells. Ewing sarcomas are thought to be of neural crest cell origin.

## ETIOLOGY

The cause is unknown for most children diagnosed with sarcoma, although a few observations have been made regarding risks. Individuals with **Li-Fraumeni syndrome** (associated with a germline *p53* mutation) and **neurofibromatosis** (associated with *NF1* mutations) have an increased risk of soft tissue sarcomas. There is a 500-fold increased risk for osteosarcoma for individuals with hereditary retinoblastoma. Deletions on the long arm of chromosome 13, which can occur in patients with retinoblastoma, have been found in some patients with osteosarcoma. Li-Fraumeni syndrome and Rothmund-Thomson syndrome are associated with osteosarcoma. Prior treatment for childhood cancer with **radiation therapy** or chemotherapy, specifically alkylating agents, or both increases the risk for osteosarcoma as a second malignancy.

## EPIDEMIOLOGY

In the United States, 850 to 900 children and adolescents under 20 years of age are diagnosed with soft tissue sarcomas each year; approximately 350 are rhabdomyosarcoma. The incidence of rhabdomyosarcoma peaks in children 2 to 6 years old and in adolescents. Two thirds of all cases of rhabdomyosarcoma are diagnosed before 11 years of age. The early peak is associated with tumors in the genitourinary region, head, and neck; the later peak is associated with tumors in the extremities, trunk, and male genitourinary tract. Boys are affected 1.5 times more often than girls.

Of the 650 to 700 U.S. children and adolescents under 20 years of age diagnosed with bone tumors each year, approximately 400 are osteosarcoma and 200 are Ewing sarcoma. Osteosarcoma most commonly affects adolescents; the peak incidence occurs during the period of maximum growth velocity. The incidence of Ewing sarcoma peaks between ages 10 and 20 years, but may occur at any age. Ewing sarcoma affects primarily whites; it rarely occurs in African-American children or Asian children.

## CLINICAL MANIFESTATIONS

The clinical presentation of **rhabdomyosarcoma** varies depending on the site of origin, subsequent mass effect, and presence of metastatic disease. Periorbital swelling, proptosis, and limitation of extraocular motion may be seen with an orbital tumor. Nasal mass, chronic otitis media, ear discharge, dysphagia, neck mass, and cranial nerve involvement may be noted with tumors in other head and neck sites. Urethral or vaginal masses, paratesticular swelling, hematuria, and urinary frequency or retention may be noted with tumors in the genitourinary tract. Trunk or extremity lesions tend to present as rapidly growing masses that may or may not be painful. If there is metastatic disease to bone or bone marrow, limb pain and evidence of marrow failure may be present.

**Osteosarcoma** often is located at the epiphysis or metaphysis of anatomic sites that are associated with maximum growth velocity (distal femur, proximal tibia, proximal humerus), but any bone may be involved. It presents with pain and may be associated with a palpable mass. Because the pain and swelling often are initially thought to be related to trauma, radiographs of the affected region frequently are obtained, which usually reveal a lytic lesion, often associated with calcification in the soft tissue surrounding the lesion. Approximately 75% to 80% of patients with osteosarcoma have apparently localized disease at diagnosis, but the majority of patients are believed to have micrometastatic disease as well.

Although **Ewing sarcoma** can occur in almost any bone in the body, the femur and pelvis are the most common sites. In addition to local pain and swelling, clinical manifestations include systemic symptoms, such as fever and weight loss.

## LABORATORY/IMAGING STUDIES

Tissue biopsy is needed for definitive diagnosis of sarcomas. Selection of the biopsy site is important for each patient and has implications for future surgical resection and radiation therapy. Under light microscopy, rhabdomyosarcoma and Ewing sarcoma appear as **small, round, blue cell tumors**. Osteosarcomas are distinguishable by the presence of **osteoid substance**.

Immunohistochemical staining for muscle-specific proteins, such as actin and myosin, and other muscle-related proteins, such as desmin and vimentin, helps confirm the diagnosis of rhabdomyosarcoma. Two major histologic variants exist for rhabdomyosarcoma: **embryonal** and **alveolar**. Embryonal histologic variant is most common in younger children with head, neck and genitourinary primary tumors. Alveolar histologic variant occurs in older patients and is seen most commonly in trunk and extremity tumors. Alveolar rhabdomyosarcoma often is characterized by specific translocations: t(2;13) or t(1;13). Metastatic evaluation for patients with rhabdomyosarcoma should include a computed tomography (CT) scan of the chest, abdomen, and pelvis; a bone scan; and bone marrow aspiration and biopsy. In patients with a parameningeal primary site (the middle ear, nasopharynx, infratemporal fossa), a lumbar puncture is required.

Definitive diagnosis of osteosarcoma usually is established by carefully placed needle biopsy. The presence of osteoid and immunohistochemical analysis confirms the diagnosis of osteosarcoma. The extent of the primary tumor must be delineated carefully with magnetic resonance imaging (MRI) before starting chemotherapy. Osteosarcoma tends to metastasize to lung, most commonly, and also to bone; a metastatic evaluation consists of a chest CT scan and a bone scan.

The diagnosis of Ewing sarcoma is established with immunohistochemical analysis and cytogenetic and molecular diagnostic studies of the biopsy material. Ewing sarcoma is characterized by a specific chromosomal translocation, **t(11;22)**, which is seen in 95% of tumors. A variant translocation, t(21;22), is seen in approximately 5% of tumors. MRI of the primary lesion should be performed to delineate extent of the lesion and any associated soft tissue mass. Metastatic evaluation involves a bone scan, chest CT scan, and bone marrow aspiration and biopsy.

## DIFFERENTIAL DIAGNOSIS

Patients with Ewing sarcoma often are misdiagnosed as having **osteomyelitis**; children with osteogenic sarcoma often are thought initially to have pain and swelling related to trauma. The differential diagnosis for rhabdomyosarcoma depends on the location of the tumor. Tumors of the trunk and extremities often present as a painless mass and may be initially thought to be benign tumors. Periorbital rhabdomyosarcoma may be misdiagnosed as orbital cellulitis, and other head and neck rhabdomyosarcoma may be confused with chronic infection of ears or sinuses. The differential diagnosis for intraabdominal rhabdomyosarcoma includes other abdominal malignancies, such as Wilms tumor or neuroblastoma.

## TREATMENT

Treatment of rhabdomyosarcoma is currently based on a staging system that incorporates both the primary site and histologic picture. The staging system also involves a local tumor group assessment based on the extent of disease and surgical result. In the intergroup rhabdomyosarcoma studies, the most common chemotherapy agents used are cyclophosphamide, vincristine, and actinomycin. Doxorubicin, etoposide, ifosfamide, and topotecan are also active against rhabdomyosarcoma. Radiation is administered to patients who have residual disease after initial surgery or who have had a biopsy only of the primary tumor.

The current treatment of osteosarcoma involves neoadjuvant chemotherapy followed by limb salvage surgery or amputation and further postoperative chemotherapy. Agents effective against osteosarcoma are doxorubicin, cisplatin, high-dose methotrexate, ifosfamide, and etoposide. Pegylated interferon alfa-2b is being evaluated as an immunotherapy for osteosarcoma in the setting of minimal residual disease.

The treatment for Ewing sarcoma is similar to that for osteosarcoma; preoperative chemotherapy is given, followed by local control measures and then further chemotherapy. In contrast to osteosarcoma, Ewing sarcoma is **radiation sensitive**. Chemotherapy includes vincristine, cyclophosphamide, ifosfamide, etoposide, and doxorubicin.

## COMPLICATIONS

In addition to the risk of late effects from the chemotherapy, children with sarcomas have potential complications related to local control of the tumor. If the local disease is controlled with surgery, the long-term sequelae may include loss of limb or limitation of function. If local control is accomplished with radiation therapy, the late effects depend on the dose of radiation given, the extent of the site radiated, and the development of the child at the time of radiation therapy. Irradiating tissues interferes with growth and development so that radiation given to a young child can have significant adverse consequences.

## PROGNOSIS

For all children with sarcoma, presence or absence of **metastatic disease** at presentation is the most important prognostic factor. The outlook for patients who have distant metastasis from Ewing sarcoma, rhabdomyosarcoma, or osteosarcoma at diagnosis remains poor.

Patients with localized rhabdomyosarcomas in favorable sites have an excellent prognosis when treated with surgery followed by vincristine and actinomycin. In patients with osteosarcoma and Ewing sarcoma, another important prognostic factor is the **degree of tumor necrosis** after preoperative chemotherapy. In general, patients whose tumor specimens show a high degree (>90%) of necrosis following preoperative chemotherapy have an event-free survival rate greater than 80%. Patients who still have large amounts of viable tumor after presurgical chemotherapy have a much worse prognosis. The cure rate for patients with localized osteosarcoma and Ewing sarcoma is approximately 60% to 70%. Patients who have lung metastasis at diagnosis have a cure rate of approximately 30% to 35%. Patients with metastases to other bones have a poor prognosis.

## SUGGESTED READING

Dickerman JD: The late effects of childhood cancer therapy, *Pediatrics* 119:554–568, 2007.

Loeb DM, Thornton K, Shokek O: Pediatric soft tissue sarcomas, *Surg Clin North Am* 88:615–627, 2008.

Maris JM, Hogarty MD, Bagatell R, et al: Neuroblastoma, *Lancet* 369:2106–2120, 2007.

Packer RJ, MacDonald T, Vezina G: Central nervous system tumors, *Pediatr Clin North Am* 55:121–145, 2008.

Pui CH, Robison LL, Look AT: Acute lymphoblastic leukaemia, *Lancet* 371:1030–1043, 2008.

Rubnitz JE, Gibson B, Smith FO: Acute myeloid leukemia, *Pediatr Clin North Am* 55:21–51, 2008.

# NEPHROLOGY AND UROLOGY

**John D. Mahan**

---

CHAPTER **161**

## Nephrology and Urology Assessment

The kidneys provide a variety of functions to preserve homeostasis: they maintain fluid and electrolyte balance, excrete metabolic waste products though glomerular filtration and tubular secretion, generate energy (gluconeogenesis), and produce important endocrine hormones (renin, vitamin D metabolites, erythropoietin). Renal disorders, by disturbing homeostasis, can affect growth and development and result in a variety of clinical manifestations (Table 161-1). Renal disorders in children may be intrinsic renal diseases or derive from systemic conditions (Table 161-2).

### HISTORY

Fetal urine production contributes to amniotic fluid volume, lung maturation, and somatic development. Congenital renal disorders may be associated with reduced (oligohydramnios) or increased amniotic fluid volume (polyhydramnios). Pulmonary hypoplasia and fetal maldevelopment of the face and extremities occur with insufficient amniotic fluid (Potter's syndrome) (see Chapters 58 and 60).

A careful history can reveal risk factors for renal disease. Perinatal hypoxia-ischemia increases the risk of renal insufficiency from acute tubular necrosis or renal vein thrombosis. A detailed family history may identify hereditary conditions. A history of poor growth or poor feeding may identify children who have underlying renal disease without overt renal symptoms. Questions about fluid intake and output define body fluid status or altered renal function. A history of edema may indicate protein loss, poor protein production, or fluid overload. Fluid or metabolic imbalance may result in weight gain loss, respiratory distress, fatigue, irritability, fever, pallor, and a history of seizures. Urine color may provide clues to underlying glomerular disease, ingestions, or urinary tract infection (UTI). The voiding history (dysuria, frequency, nocturia, hesitancy or difficulty with stream, urinary

incontinence, gross hematuria or passage of calculi) may uncover symptoms of renal and urinary tract disease.

### PHYSICAL EXAMINATION

A number of renal diseases in children may be initially asymptomatic and detected during routine visits. Abnormal growth or hypertension may suggest occult renal disease. Dehydration or overhydration may be due to renal dysfunction (see Chapter 33). Abnormal skin findings may indicate systemic diseases with renal involvement. Abnormal facial features may suggest syndromes associated with renal disorders (fetal alcohol syndrome, Down syndrome). Preauricular tags and deformities of the external ear are sometimes present in children with congenital renal defects. Ophthalmologic examination may detect abnormalities associated with renal disease (keratoconus, aniridia, iridocyclitis, cataracts). Cardiac examination may reveal volume overload (cardiomegaly), murmurs (cardiac disease, anemia), or a pericardial friction rub (uremia). Rales may indicate extravascular volume overload or hypoalbuminemia. Abdominal examination may reveal ascites, masses or hepatomegaly (systemic lupus erythematosus, polycystic kidney disease, glomerular disorders). Bladder distention suggests polyuria from a urine-concentrating defect or urinary tract obstruction.

### RENAL PHYSIOLOGY

Normal renal function depends on intact **glomerular filtration** and **tubular function** (proximal tubule, loop of Henle, and distal tubule) which results in **urine formation** (Fig. 161-1). The net glomerular pressure favors movement of fluid out of the capillaries into Bowman's space. Intraglomerular pressure is regulated by afferent and efferent arteriolar tone, particularly the latter. **Renin** is generated by cells in the juxtaglomerular apparatus, located at the base of each glomerulus in proximity to the afferent/efferent arterioles and distal tubule of that nephron, in response to glomerular flow and perfusion.

The **proximal tubule** conducts isosmotic reabsorption (see Fig. 161-1) to reabsorb two thirds of the filtered volume, sodium, and chloride. Glucose, amino acids, potassium, and phosphate are almost completely reabsorbed. Approximately 75% of filtered bicarbonate is reabsorbed

**TABLE 161-1 Common Manifestations of Renal Disease by Age**

| Finding | Significance |
|---|---|
| **NEONATE** | |
| Flank mass | Multicystic dysplasia, urinary tract obstruction (hydronephrosis), polycystic disease, tumor |
| Hematuria | Acute tubular /cortical necrosis, urinary tract malformation, trauma, renal vein thrombosis |
| Anuria and oliguria | Renal agenesis, obstruction, acute tubular necrosis, vascular thrombosis |
| **CHILD/ADOLESCENT** | |
| Cola red–colored urine | Hemoglobinuria (hemolysis); myoglobinuria (rhabdomyolysis); pigmenturia (porphyria, urate, beets, drugs); hematuria (infection, glomerulonephritis, Schönlein-Henoch purpura, hypercalciuria, stones) |
| Gross hematuria | Infection, glomerulonephritis, trauma, benign hematuria, nephrolithiasis, tumor |
| Edema | Nephrotic syndrome, glomerulonephritis, acute/chronic renal failure, cardiac/liver disease |
| Hypertension | Acute glomerulonephritis, acute/chronic renal failure, obstruction, cysts, dysplasia, coarctation of the aorta, renal artery stenosis |
| Polyuria | Diabetes mellitus, central and nephrogenic diabetes insipidus, obstruction, dysplasia, hypokalemia, hypercalcemia, psychogenic polydipsia, sickle disease/trait, polyuric renal failure, diuretic abuse |
| Oliguria | Dehydration, acute tubular necrosis, acute glomerulonephritis, interstitial nephritis, hemolytic uremic syndrome |
| Urgency | Urinary tract infection, vaginitis, hypercalciuria, foreign body |

in the proximal tubule. When filtered bicarbonate exceeds the proximal tubular threshold, bicarbonate is spilled into the urine. The proximal tubule also secretes compounds, such as organic acids, penicillins, and other drugs. The most potent vitamin D analog—1,25(OH)$_2$-cholecalcifererol (**calcitriol**)—is produced by proximal tubular cells in response to parathyroid hormone and intracellular calcium/phosphorus concentrations.

The **loop of Henle** is the site of reabsorption of 25% of sodium chloride filtered in the glomerulus (see Fig. 161-1).

**TABLE 161-2 Primary and Systemic Causes of Renal Disease in Children**

| Primary | Secondary (Systemic) |
|---|---|
| Minimal change nephrotic syndrome | Postinfectious glomerulonephritis |
| Focal segmental glomerulosclerosis | IgA nephropathy |
| Membranoproliferative glomerulonephritis | Schönlein-Henoch purpura–related nephritis |
| Membranous nephropathy | Lupus nephritis |
| Congenital nephrotic syndrome | Wegener granulomatosis and other vasculitides |
| Alport syndrome | Tubular toxins |
| Intrinsic tubular disorders | Antibiotics |
| Structural renal disorders | Chemotherapeutic agents |
| Congenital urinary tract abnormalities | Hemoglobin/myoglobin |
| Polycystic kidney disease | Tubular disorders |
| Renal/urinary tract tumor | Cystinosis, oxalosis |
| | Galactosemia, hereditary fructose intolerance |
| | Stones |
| | Sickle disease/trait |
| | Trauma |
| | Extrarenal malignancy (leukemia, lymphoma) |

Active chloride transport drives the countercurrent multiplier and composes the medullary interstitial hypertonic gradient required for urinary concentration.

The **distal tubule** is composed of the **distal convoluted tubule** and **collecting ducts**. The distal convoluted tubule is water impermeable and contributes to urine dilution by active sodium chloride absorption. Some of this sodium-potassium exchange (sodium-hydrogen exchange) is regulated by aldosterone. The collecting duct is the primary site of **antidiuretic hormone** (**vasopressin**) response, which leads to urine concentration. Active hydrogen ion secretion, which is responsible for the final acidification of the urine, occurs in the collecting duct.

Renal **ammonia** production and intraluminal generation of ammonium ($NH_4^+$) facilitate hydrogen ion excretion in the urine. Urinary ammonia/ammonium is not measured easily, but levels can be inferred by the calculation of the **urinary anion gap**. The *gap* between measured anions and cations largely consists of ammonium. Problems with renal acid excretion or ammonia production decrease the urinary anion gap. A urinary gap of approximately 1 mEq/kg body weight is a reasonable expectation in urine produced by normal kidneys.

The maximum **urinary concentrating capacity** in a preterm newborn ($\sim$ 400 mOsm/L) is less than in a full-term newborn (600–800 mOsm/L), which is less than in older children and adults ($\sim$ 1200 mOsm/L). Neonates can dilute urine to the same degree as adults (75–90 mOsm/L), but because the glomerular filtration rate (GFR) is lower, the capacity to excrete a water load is less in infants. GFR reaches adult levels by 1 to 2 years of age. Tubular reabsorption of sodium, potassium, bicarbonate, and phosphate and excretion of hydrogen are all reduced in infants relative to adults. These functions mature independently and at different ages, so a neonate rapidly develops the ability to reabsorb sodium efficiently, but it takes 2 years for bicarbonate reabsorption to mature. **Erythropoietin** is secreted by interstitial cells in

**FIGURE 161-1**

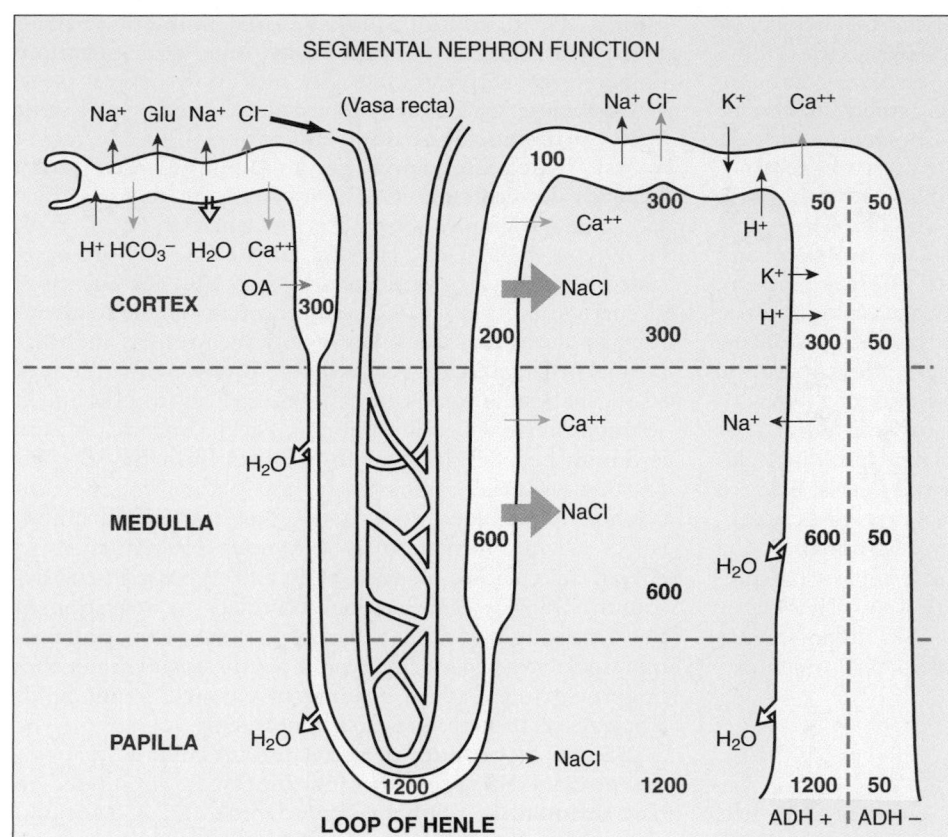

SEGMENTAL NEPHRON FUNCTION

Major transport functions of each nephron segment, including representative osmolalities in vasa recta, interstitium, and tubule at different levels within the kidney. ADH, antidiuretic hormone; Glu, glucose; OA, organic acid. (From Andreoli TE, Carpenter CCJ, Plum F, et al [eds]: Cecil Essentials of Medicine. Philadelphia, *WB Saunders,* 1986.)

the renal medulla in response to low oxygen delivery and helps regulate bone marrow red blood cell production.

## COMMON MANIFESTATIONS

Renal disorders can be classified as **primary** (originating in kidney or urinary tract) or **secondary** (due to systemic illnesses) (see Table 161-2). Renal diseases may present with obvious signs, such as hematuria or edema, or with more subtle signs and symptoms detected on screening examinations (abdominal or flank mass, hypertension, proteinuria). Fever, irritability, and vomiting may be the presenting symptoms in neonates and infants with **urinary tract infections** (UTIs), whereas frequency and dysuria suggest UTI in older children. Chronic renal disease often is associated with poor growth and feeding difficulties, but may be first detected on screening examinations (hypertension, hematuria). An abnormal urine stream may indicate posterior urethral valves or other bladder disorders and obstructive lesions.

## DIAGNOSTIC STUDIES

### Laboratory Studies

**Glomerular filtration rate** (GFR) is measured most accurately by infusion of a substance that is freely filtered by the glomerulus but is not metabolized, reabsorbed, or secreted in or by the tubules. The GFR is calculated as follows:

$$GFR = [U]V/[P]$$

where $[U]$ is urine concentration, $[P]$ is serum concentration of a substance (mg/dL) used to measure clearance, and $V$ is urine flow rate (mL/min)

By convention, GFR is corrected to body surface area of 1.73 m$^2$ to allow comparison between different sized individuals. In a full-term newborn, an uncorrected GFR of 4 to 5 mL/min corrects to approximately 40 mL/min/1.73 m$^2$. GFR increases rapidly during the first 2 years of life when it achieves adult values (100 to 120 mL/min/1.73 m$^2$). After that, GFR and body size increase proportionally, and GFR remains stable.

**Plasma creatinine** (Cr) reflects muscle mass, increases with age and is used to approximate GFR. Creatinine is also secreted by proximal tubules, resulting in less accurate measurement of GFR with immature kidneys or with decreased renal function. **Blood urea nitrogen (BUN)** also estimates renal function, but is greatly affected by hydration, nutrition, catabolism, and tissue breakdown. The correlation between creatinine and GFR can be used to estimate GFR. The most commonly used formula (Schwartz formula) is:

$$GFR \ (mL/min/1.73 \ m^2) = k \times L \ (cm)/P_{Cr} \ (mg/dL)$$

The value for $k$, derived from the creatinine-length-GFR correlation, is 0.33 in preterm infants, 0.45 in full-term infants, 0.55 in children and adolescent girls, and 0.7 in adolescent boys. This formula is most useful when body habitus and muscle mass are reasonably normal and when renal function is relatively stable. **Creatinine clearance** ($[U_{Cr}]V/[P_{Cr}]$) estimates GFR, but overestimates GFR when renal function is decreased.

**Urinalysis** is a useful screen for renal abnormalities. In addition to urine color and turbidity, **macroscopic**

**urinalysis** uses a **urine dipstick** for pH and the presence of protein, glucose, ketones, blood, and leukocytes. Dilute urine may result in a false negative result for protein; false positive results may occur with extremely alkaline or concentrated urine or if there is a delay in reading the test. Dipsticks are exquisitely sensitive to the presence of hemoglobin (or myoglobin); there are few, if any, false negative test results, but many false positive results. **Glucose** is detected via a glucose oxidase-peroxidase reaction, and leukocytes are detected via a **leukocyte esterase** reaction. The **nitrate test** may detect bacteriuria if the bacteria reduce nitrate to nitrite and have long contact time with the urine. False negative results occur with frequent voiding, low urine bacterial count, urinary tract obstruction, and infection with bacteria unable to generate nitrite. Gross hematuria or prolonged contact (uncircumcised boys) may result in a false positive nitrite test. **Microscopic urinalysis** is used to confirm pyuria and hematuria and detect casts and crystals.

Proteinuria can be further defined by determination of a **spot urine protein/creatinine** ($U_{Pr/Cr}$) in a single urine specimen. This unit-less value correlates very well with 24-hour urine protein excretion: spot $U_{Pr/Cr}$ – 0.2 approximates 24-hour urine protein/m²/day (normal < 0.20; nephrotic range > 2.0 in children).

## Imaging Studies

**Ultrasound** reliably assesses kidney presence and size, determines degree of dilation, and differentiates cortex and medulla. The bladder also can be visualized. **Pulsed Doppler studies** assess arterial and venous blood flow and can be used to calculate resistive index within the kidneys.

A **voiding cystourethrogram** (VCUG) involves repeated filling of the bladder to detect vesicoureteral reflux and to evaluate the urethra. **Computed tomography (CT)** and **magnetic resonance imaging (MRI)** have mostly replaced the **intravenous (IV) pyelogram** to evaluate kidney structure and function. Radionuclide studies can define renal size and scars and renal function/excretion.

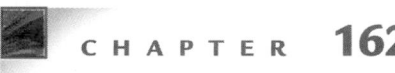

CHAPTER **162**

# Nephrotic Syndrome and Proteinuria

## ETIOLOGY AND EPIDEMIOLOGY

A small amount of protein is found in the urine of healthy children (<4 mg/m²/hour or $U_{Pr/Cr}$ < 0.2). **Nephrotic proteinuria** in children is defined as protein greater than 40 mg/m²/hour or $U_{Pr/Cr}$ greater than 2.0. Proteinuria between these two levels is mildly to moderately elevated, but not nephrotic.

Proteinuria may be **transient** or **persistent, asymptomatic or symptomatic,** and **orthostatic** (present in the upright position but not in the recumbent position) or **fixed** (present in all positions). Proteinuria may be **glomerular** (disruptions of the normal glomerular barrier to protein filtration) or **tubular** (increased filtration, impaired reabsorption or secretion of proteins).

**Nephrotic syndrome** (NS) is characterized by persistent heavy **proteinuria** (mainly albuminuria) (>2 g/m²/24 hours); **hypoproteinemia** (serum albumin <3.0 g/dL); **hypercholesterolemia** (>250 mg/dL); and **edema**. Age, race, and geography affect the incidence of NS. Certain HLA types (HLA-DR7, HLA-B8, and HLA-B12) are associated with an increased incidence of NS. The increased glomerular permeability to serum proteins is due to alterations in glomerular basement membrane proteins and their normal negative charge that restricts filtration of serum proteins. The resultant massive proteinuria leads to a decline in serum proteins, especially albumin. Plasma oncotic pressure is diminished, resulting in fluid shifts from the vascular to the interstitial compartment and plasma volume contraction. Renal blood flow and GFR are not usually diminished. Edema formation is enhanced by reduction in effective circulating blood volume and increase in tubular sodium chloride reabsorption secondary to activation of the renin-angiotensin-aldosterone system. Hypoproteinemia stimulates hepatic lipoprotein synthesis and diminishes lipoprotein metabolism, leading to elevated serum lipids (cholesterol, triglycerides) and lipoproteins.

NS may be **primary or secondary**. A child with apparent primary NS, prior to renal biopsy, is considered to have **idiopathic nephrotic syndrome** (INS). **Minimal change nephrotic syndrome** (MCNS) is the most common histologic form of primary nephrotic syndrome in children. More than 80% of children under 7 years of age with nephrotic syndrome have MCNS. Children 7 to 16 years old with NS have a 50% chance of having MCNS, and males are affected more frequently than females (2:1).

**Focal segmental glomerulosclerosis (FSGS)** accounts for approximately 10% to 20% of children with primary NS. It may present like MCNS or with less impressive proteinuria. FSGS may develop from MCNS or present as a separate entity. A circulating factor that increases glomerular permeability is found in some patients with FSGS. Over one third of children with FSGS progress to renal failure.

**Membranoproliferative glomerulonephritis** (MPGN) is characterized by hypocomplementemia with signs of glomerular renal disease. MPGN is present in 5% to 15% of children with primary NS, is typically persistent, and has a high likelihood of progression to renal failure over time.

Less than 5% of children with primary NS have **membranous nephropathy** histologic examination on biopsy. It is seen most commonly in adolescents and children with systemic infections, such as hepatitis B, syphilis, malaria, and toxoplasmosis, or who are receiving drug therapy (gold salts, penicillamine).

**Congenital nephrotic syndrome** presents during the first 2 months of life. There are two common types. The Finnish type is an autosomal recessive disorder most common in persons of Scandinavian descent and is due to a mutation in the nephrin protein component in the glomerular filtration slit. The second type is a heterogeneous group of abnormalities including diffuse mesangial sclerosis and conditions associated with drugs or infections. Prenatal onset is supported by elevated levels of maternal alpha-fetoprotein.

**Secondary NS** may be seen with systemic lupus erythematosus, Schönlein-Henoch purpura, infections (hepatitis B, hepatitis C, malaria), Wegener and other vasculitides, allergic reactions, diabetes, amyloidosis, malignancies, congestive heart failure, constrictive pericarditis, and renal vein thrombosis.

## CLINICAL MANIFESTATIONS

The sudden onset of dependent pitting edema or ascites is the most common presentation for children with NS. Anorexia, malaise, and abdominal pain are often present, especially with significant ascites. Blood pressure may be elevated in up to 25% of children on presentation; acute tubular necrosis and significant hypotension may occur with sudden decline in serum albumin and significant volume depletion. Diarrhea (due to intestinal edema) and respiratory distress (due to pulmonary edema or pleural effusion) may be present. Typical MCNS is characterized by the *absence* of hematuria as well as renal insufficiency, hypertension, and hypocomplementemia.

## DIAGNOSTIC STUDIES

Proteinuria of 1+ or higher on two to three random urine specimens suggests persistent proteinuria that should be further quantified. A $U_{Pr/Cr}$ above 0.2 on a first morning specimen excludes orthostatic proteinuria. $U_{Pr/Cr}$ greater than 2.0 is indicative of nephrotic range proteinuria.

In addition to demonstration of proteinuria, hypercholesterolemia, and hypoalbuminemia, routine testing typically includes a serum C3 complement level. A low level of C3 implies the presence of a lesion other than MCNS and a renal biopsy is indicated before a trial of steroid therapy. Microscopic hematuria may be present in up to 25% of cases of MCNS but does not predict response to steroids. Additional laboratory tests, including electrolytes, blood urea nitrogen (BUN), creatinine, total protein, and serum albumin level, are performed based on history and physical examination features. Renal ultrasound is often useful. Biopsy is performed when indicated.

## DIFFERENTIAL DIAGNOSIS

**Transient proteinuria** can be seen after vigorous exercise, fever, significant dehydration, seizures, and adrenergic agonist therapy. This type of proteinuria usually is mild ($U_{Pr/Cr} < 1$), is glomerular in origin, and always resolves within a few days. It does not indicate renal disease.

**Postural (orthostatic) proteinuria** is a benign condition defined by normal protein excretion while recumbent, but significant proteinuria when upright. It is glomerular in nature, more common in adolescents and tall, thin individuals and not associated with progressive renal disease. Many children with orthostatic proteinuria continue this process into adulthood.

**Tubular proteinuria** is characterized by preponderance of low-molecular-weight proteins in the urine and is typically suspected in conditions associated with acute tubular necrosis (ATN), pyelonephritis, structural renal disorders, polycystic kidney disease, and tubular toxins such as antibiotics or chemotherapeutic agents. The combination of tubular proteinuria, with evidence of tubular electrolyte wasting and glycosuria, is termed **Fanconi syndrome**.

**Glomerular proteinuria** is characterized by a combination of large- and small–molecular-weight proteins in the urine, variable levels of proteinuria, and often evidence of glomerular disease (hematuria, red blood cell [RBC] casts, hypertension, and renal insufficiency). Causes of glomerular proteinuria include glomerular capillary disruption (hemolytic uremic syndrome [HUS], cresentic glomerulonephritis); glomerular capillary immune complex deposition (poststreptococcal glomerulonephritis [PSGN] and lupus nephritis); and altered glomerular capillary permeability (MCNS, congenital NS).

## TREATMENT

Because more than 80% of children under 13 years of age with primary NS have steroid-responsive forms (chiefly MCNS), steroid therapy may be initiated without a renal biopsy if a child has typical features of NS. Typical therapy for MCNS is prednisone, 2 mg/kg/day (60 mg/m$^2$/24 hours, maximum 60 mg/day), divided into two to four doses per day. Over 90% of children who respond to steroids do so within 4 weeks. Responders should receive steroids for 12 weeks. A renal biopsy is indicated for nonresponders, as steroid resistance decreases the chance that MCNS is the underlying disease. Frequent relapses or steroid resistance in MCNS may necessitate additional immunosuppressive therapy.

No clearly effective therapy for FSGS has been identified. Approximately 35% respond to steroid therapy; others may respond to immunosuppressive therapy. MPGN and membranous GN may improve with chronic steroid or immunosuppressive therapy but do not reliably remit with standard NS steroid therapy. Aggressive medical therapy of familial congenital NS, with early nephrectomy, dialysis, and transplantation, is the only effective approach to this syndrome.

Edema due to nephrotic syndrome is treated by restricting salt intake. Severe edema may require the use of loop diuretics. When these therapies do not alleviate severe edema, cautious parenteral administration of 25% albumin (0.5–1.0 g/kg intravenously over 1–2 hours) with an intravenous (IV) loop diuretic usually results in diuresis. The administered albumin is excreted rapidly, and thus, salt restriction and diuretics must be continued. Significant pleural effusions may require drainage. Acute hypertension (HTN) is treated with β-blockers or calcium channel blockers. Persistent HTN usually responds to angiotensin-converting enzyme inhibitors.

## COMPLICATIONS

Infection is a major complication in children with NS. An increased incidence of serious infections, particularly **bacteremia** and **peritonitis** (particularly *Streptococcus pneumoniae*, *Escherichia coli*, or *Klebsiella*), is due to urinary loss of immunoglobulins and complement. Side effects of steroids are most common in steroid-dependent and frequently relapsing patients. Hypovolemia may result from diarrhea or diuretic use. The loss of coagulation factors, antithrombin, and plasminogen may lead to a hypercoagulable state with a risk of **thromboembolism** (TE). Warfarin, lovenox, low-dose aspirin, or dipyridamole may minimize the risk of clots in NS patients with a history of TE or high risk for TE. Hyperlipidemia promotes increased atherosclerotic vascular disease.

## PROGNOSIS

Most children with NS eventually go into remission. Nearly 80% of children with MCNS experience NS relapse, defined as heavy proteinuria that persists for 3 or more consecutive days. Transient (up to 3 days) proteinuria may occur with intercurrent infection in children with MCNS and is not considered a relapse. Steroid therapy is rapidly effective for true relapse. Steroid-responsive patients have little risk of chronic renal failure. Patients with FSGS may initially respond to steroids, but later not respond. Many children with FSGS progress to end-stage kidney failure (see Chapter 165). Recurrence of FSGS occurs in 30% of children who undergo renal transplantation.

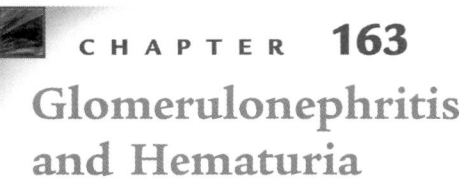

CHAPTER **163**

# Glomerulonephritis and Hematuria

## ETIOLOGY AND EPIDEMIOLOGY

A child with **gross hematuria** requires prompt evaluation. After a careful history and physical examination, a urinalysis is required. *Red urine, dipstick blood, but no red blood cells (RBCs) on (prompt) microscopy* suggest:

1. Ingested foods, medications, or chemicals
2. The presence of free hemoglobin or myoglobin

In infants, urate crystals can precipitate in diapers to give an orange-red color. **Hemoglobinuria** may result from acute intravascular hemolysis, disseminated intravascular coagulation, or other causes of hemolysis. **Myoglobinuria** results from rhabdomyolysis secondary to crush injury, burns, myositis, or asphyxia. *Red urine, dipstick blood, RBCs but no RBC casts on microscopy* suggest urinary tract bleeding from a site below the renal tubules. Examining urinary RBC morphology assists in localizing hematuria. Altered RBC morphology is typically seen in glomerular hematuria, but absence of casts or dysmorphic RBCs does not exclude a glomerular etiology. *Red urine, dipstick blood and dysmorphic RBCs with RBC casts on microscopy* suggest a glomerular disease.

Glomerular injury may result from **immunologic injury** (poststreptococcal acute glomerulonephritis, PSGN), **inherited disease** (Alport syndrome), or **toxins** (hemolytic uremic syndrome). Children with glomerular hematuria and any other cardinal features of glomerular injury (proteinuria, hypertension, edema, oliguria, renal insufficiency) are considered to have **glomerulonephritis** (GN). This contrasts clinically with children with nonglomerular

hematuria, minimal proteinuria, and signs of impaired water handling (polyuria or oliguria) who may have **tubulointerstitial nephritis** (TIN). These children typically do not have hypertension and only develop renal insufficiency with severe TIN.

Immune-mediated inflammation is the mechanism for proliferative GN, of which PSGN is the most common form. **PSGN** usually occurs during or after streptococcal pharyngitis or impetigo. Immunologic reaction to bacterial proteins trapped in the glomerular capillary wall, followed by in situ activation of complement, leads to cell proliferation and glomerular injury. Only certain nephritogenic strains of *group A streptococcus* cause this reaction. Age, gender, socioeconomic status, and genetic predisposition affect likelihood of PSGN. It occurs most frequently in children 2 to 12 years of age and more often in boys. Crowded conditions, poor hygiene, malnutrition, and delayed treatment may result in epidemic outbreaks.

## CLINICAL MANIFESTATIONS

**PSGN** may present with hematuria (gross in 65%), edema (75%), and hypertension (50%). Acute renal insufficiency may occur. Manifestations develop 5 to 21 days (average 10 days) after nephritogenic streptococcal infections. Many children still have active infection at time of clinical renal manifestations. As glomerular filtration rate (GFR) is reduced, distal sodium reabsorption is enhanced, elevating plasma volume and suppressing plasma renin. Oliguria, renal insufficiency, and consequent hypertension may lead to complications such as heart failure, seizures, and encephalopathy. **Acute postinfectious GN** is occasionally seen with other bacterial and viral pathogens.

**Urinary tract infection** (UTI) is the most common identifiable cause of hematuria in children. Hematuria without casts is seen in **sickle cell trait** or **disease**, after strenuous **exercise**, and after renal **trauma**. Coagulopathies can lead to hematuria. **Hypercalciuria** can cause isolated hematuria in children; 25% to 30% of children with isolated hematuria have elevated urinary calcium excretion. **Urolithiasis** may be associated with asymptomatic hematuria or with urinary tract symptoms, such as pain. Most common kidney stones in children are secondary to metabolic predisposition (familial hypercalciuria), urine stasis, or infection. **Structural abnormalities** of the urinary tract, such as cysts or obstruction, and malignant tumors must also be considered.

Hematuria may be due to renal parenchymal disorders. The most common from of chronic GN in children is **IgA nephropathy** (IgA GN), which often presents with microscopic hematuria or recurrent gross hematuria shortly after onset of upper respiratory infection. The course of IgA GN is usually benign, and occurs more frequently in boys and in school age children and young adults. IgA GN may progress to end-stage renal disease (ESRD) in up to 30% of children, particularly in patients with proteinuria or renal insufficiency at presentation. There are now promising results with chronic steroid therapy and anti-inflammatory strategies (fish oil, vitamin E) in IgA GN. Schönlein-Henoch purpura nephritis, lupus nephritis, and vasculitis-associated GN often have hematuria at presentation.

Asymptomatic microscopic hematuria may be due to undiagnosed structural disorders, mild forms of GN, or **benign familial hematuria.** The latter is a relatively common, nonprogressive, usually autosomal dominant disorder, characterized by thinning of the glomerular basement membrane (GBM). Other family members have benign hematuria. **Alport syndrome** may present with asymptomatic microscopic hematuria early in life. Several patterns of inheritance and several mutated genes are associated with significant GBM disruption over time. The most common form includes progressive high-tone bilateral **neurosensory deafness** and progressive renal failure during adolescence and young adulthood, particularly in males. Children with nonfamilial benign hematuria or the non-Alport form of idiopathic familial hematuria (thin GBM) have an excellent renal prognosis, but long-term follow-up is required to exclude progressive forms of familial hematuria.

A special form of GN is **rapidly progressive glomerulonephritis (RPGN)** which may present with rapidly progressing renal insufficiency, edema, gross hematuria, and hypertension (HTN). Renal biopsy shows glomerular epithelial cell proliferation with **crescents.** RPGN is more common in late childhood and adolescence. It may be idiopathic or associated with various conditions (MPGN, PSGN, IgA GN, antineutrophilic cytoplasmic antibody–associated vasculitis, and Schönlein-Henoch purpura). Therapy depends on the underlying disease and usually involves high-dose corticosteroids.

## DIAGNOSTIC STUDIES

Hematuria can be gross or microscopic. A positive urine dipstick requires microscopy to identify RBCs. Microscopic hematuria is defined as more than 3 to 5 RBCs per high-power field in freshly voided and centrifuged urine; the evaluation is summarized in Table 163-1.

Most pediatric nephrologists do not biopsy children with isolated microscopic hematuria, but concerns about a positive family history of renal disease or parental anxiety may justify biopsy in some children. In a child with hematuria and significant proteinuria, the diagnosis of GN should be considered until proved otherwise and, unless PSGN is likely, a diagnostic renal biopsy is warranted.

---

**TABLE 163-1 Evaluation of a Child with Hematuria**

1. Complete history and physical examination (particularly blood pressure, optic discs, skin, abdomen, genitalia)
2. Confirmation of true hematuria by urine microscopic examination
3. Urine culture
4. Urine calcium, protein, creatinine
5. Complete blood count including platelets, serum electrolytes, BUN/serum creatinine (calculate creatinine clearance), calcium, total protein and albumin
5. Streptozyme, C3, C4, ANA
6. Renal ultrasonography
7. Renal biopsy in selected cases

ANA, antinuclear antibody; BUN, blood urea nitrogen; C3, complement component 3; C4, complement component 4.

---

## THERAPY

Specific therapy for PSGN involves dietary sodium restriction, diuretics, and antihypertensive agents as needed. Therapies for children with other forms of GN are still evolving. In some cases, corticosteroid, immunosuppressive, and/or anti-inflammatory agents may be useful, often for extended treatment courses. Treatment with angiotensin-converting enzyme inhibitors or angiotensin receptor blockers may minimize proteinuria and glomerular hyperperfusion.

## PROGNOSIS AND PREVENTION

PSGN is a relatively benign disease in children. In typical cases, proteinuria and edema decline quickly (in 5–10 days). Microscopic hematuria may persist for months or even years; over 95% of children recover completely. Treating the streptococcal infection does not prevent PSGN; however, if the patient still has active streptococcal infection, antibiotic treatment is warranted. Few children with PSGN or other forms of postinfectious GN progress to ESRD.

Children with IgA GN and other forms of chronic GN have a real risk of progression to ESRD. In IgA GN, presence of persistent, heavy proteinuria, hypertension, reduced GFR, and severe glomerular lesions on biopsy have been associated with poor outcomes. Recurrence of IgA deposits in transplanted kidneys is often observed, but does not significantly alter graft survival. The prognosis for renal recovery in other forms of chronic GN and in RPGN is variable and related to the disorder and disease severity at diagnosis.

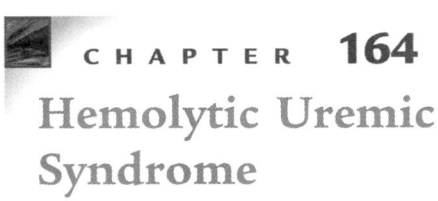

## CHAPTER 164

# Hemolytic Uremic Syndrome

---

## ETIOLOGY AND EPIDEMIOLOGY

HUS is characterized by the triad of **microangiopathic hemolytic anemia, thrombocytopenia,** and **renal injury** and is an important cause of acute renal failure (ARF) in children. The most common type, D+HUS, is associated with a prodromal diarrheal illness and may be sporadic, epidemic, or endemic. The disease typically occurs in children between 6 months and 4 years of age. Verotoxins (VTs) have been implicated in most D+HUS, especially the Shiga-like toxin from *Escherichia coli* O157:H7. VT binds to a specific globoceramide receptor on endothelial cells, producing endothelial cell injury, endothelial surface coagulation, and, in severe cases, widespread microvascular glomerular and interstitial vessel thrombosis. Contamination of meat, fruit, vegetables, and water with VT-producing *E. coli* is responsible for many outbreaks. VT causes hemorrhagic enterocolitis of variable severity and results in HUS in 5% to 25% of affected children. VT may be produced by other *E. coli* strains as well as other bacteria, such as *Shigella.*

HUS presenting without a prodrome of diarrhea (D-HUS) may occur at any age. More cases of D-HUS related to specific strains of *Streptococcus pneumoniae* infections are being recognized. Other cases of D-HUS have a genetic component (often autosomal recessive) and relapsing nature. Rare familial forms of HUS have been associated with abnormalities of complement factor H, plasminogen-activator inhibitor-1, and other molecules involved in the regulation of intravascular clotting and anticoagulation.

## CLINICAL MANIFESTATIONS

Classic D+HUS typically begins as gastroenteritis, often bloody, followed in 7 to 10 days by weakness, lethargy, irritability, and oliguria/anuria. Physical examination reveals irritability, pallor, edema, petechiae, and occasionally hepatosplenomegaly. Dehydration is often present; however, some children have volume overload. Hypertension may be due to volume overload or renin. The diagnosis is supported by the presence of microangiopathic hemolytic anemia, thrombocytopenia, and renal involvement (hematuria, renal insufficiency). Seizures may indicate central nervous system (CNS) involvement and occur in 20% of cases.

Children without evidence of a diarrheal prodrome may have a similar microangiopathic syndrome, identified as **thrombotic thrombocytopenic purpura** (TTP). Children with TTP typically have predominant CNS symptoms but may also have significant renal disease, and recurrent episodes are common. Increasingly, abnormalities of von Willebrand factor processing have been identified in affected children.

## DIAGNOSTIC STUDIES

Peripheral blood smear reveals schistocytes, helmet and burr cells, and fragmented erythrocytes, (**intravascular hemolysis**). Evidence for disseminated intravascular coagulation is rarely present. The reticulocyte count is elevated and plasma haptoglobin is low. Coombs test is negative. Leukocytosis is common. Urinalysis typically reveals hematuria, proteinuria, and casts. Stool can be cultured to identify VT-producing *E. coli* strains. Tests for demonstration of VT in stool are now also available. Diarrhea and the presence of toxin-producing *E. coli* may have resolved by the time HUS is diagnosed.

## TREATMENT AND PROGNOSIS

Therapy for HUS is supportive and includes volume repletion, control of hypertension, and early dialysis when indicated. Red blood cell transfusions are provided as needed but platelet transfusions are beneficial only during active hemorrhage. Antibiotics for the prodromal diarrhea may increase the risk of developing HUS. Antidiarrheal agents prolong exposure to VT-producing bacteria and should be avoided. Most children (>95%) survive the acute phase; more than 50% recover normal renal function. D+HUS has the best prognosis. D-HUS, familial cases, and sporadic HUS have poorer outcomes.

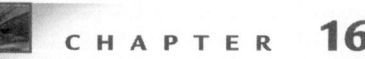

CHAPTER **165**

# Acute and Chronic Renal Failure

## ACUTE RENAL FAILURE

### Etiology and Pathophysiology

Acute renal failure (ARF) is defined as an abrupt and significant decrease in glomerular filtration rate (GFR) and tubular function. This may lead to decreased excretion of waste products (creatinine, urea, phosphate) and water, resulting in azotemia and altered body fluid homeostasis. Urine output may be low, normal, or high. Early recognition and management are crucial.

ARF may be **oliguric** (<1 mL/kg/hour in neonates and infants, <0.5 mL/kg/hour in children) or **nonoliguric**. Nonoliguric ARF can be easily missed. Despite normal urine output, electrolyte disturbances and uremia may become significant. Urine osmolality is typically similar to serum osmolality in such patients.

The major causes of ARF may be divided into **prerenal** (renal underperfusion); **intrinsic renal** (vascular, immunologic, ischemic, or toxic kidney injury); and **postrenal** (urinary tract obstruction or stasis) (Table 165-1).

---

**TABLE 165-1 Causes of Acute Renal Failure**

**PRERENAL**

Dehydration
Septic shock
Heart failure
Hemorrhage
Burns
Peritonitis, ascites, cirrhosis

**POSTRENAL (OBSTRUCTION)**

Urethral obstruction (stricture, posterior urethral valves, diverticulum)
Ureteral obstruction (calculi/crystals, clot)
Ureterocele
Extrinsic tumor compressing bladder outlet
Neurogenic bladder
Tumor lysis syndrome

**INTRINSIC**

Acute tubular necrosis
Nephrotoxins (drugs)
Acute cortical necrosis
Glomerulonephritis/interstitial nephritis
Vascular (renal vein thrombosis, arterial emboli—umbilical artery catheter)
Disseminated intravascular coagulation
Vasculitis (Schönlein-Henoch purpura, lupus, Wegener granulomatosis)
Hemoglobinuria/myoglobinuria

This classification is useful to apply to the differential diagnosis of oliguric states. If a child has an acute elevation in serum creatinine and no recent oliguria, the likelihood of a prerenal cause for ARF is low. Patients may migrate from one category to another; renal underperfusion (prerenal) or obstruction (postrenal) for an extended period may result in intrinsic renal damage and ARF.

**Acute tubular necrosis** (ATN) is the most common cause of ARF in children and is usually the consequence of renal underperfusion. Hypoxia-ischemia resulting from poor perfusion leads to early renal vasoconstriction and eventual tubular injury. Toxic injury secondary to drugs, exogenous toxins (ethylene glycol, methanol), or endogenous toxins (myoglobin, hemoglobin) also result in ATN. Severe vascular compromise with or without secondary arterial or venous thrombosis may result in **acute cortical necrosis**.

## Clinical Manifestations

The history, physical examination, and laboratory data usually allow proper classification of the child with ARF (Table 165-2). A precipitating illness associated with vomiting and diarrhea or inadequate oral intake resulting in oliguria are consistent with prerenal causes. Postrenal causes may be occult and are not associated with hypoperfusion or dehydration. With obstructive causes, flank masses or a distended bladder may be present on examination.

Intrinsic renal failure can be associated with signs of volume overload (hypertension, cardiac enlargement, a gallop rhythm). Urine output characteristically is decreased, and signs of systemic involvement may be evident. Urinalysis usually reveals red blood cells (RBCs) and granular casts, with mild to moderate proteinuria.

## Diagnostic Studies

In oliguric states, differentiation between prerenal azotemia and intrinsic renal disease is aided by determining the **fractional excretion of sodium** ($FE_{Na}$). The $FE_{Na}$ is the percentage of sodium filtered by the glomeruli that is reabsorbed by the tubules and is calculated by the following equation:

$$[U/P \text{ Na} \div U/P \text{ creatinine}] \times 100$$

where $U$ and $P$ are the urine and plasma concentrations. Values under 1% are consistent with prerenal azotemia (as the kidney maximizes water and salt reabsorption). Values greater than 2% are consistent with intrinsic renal dysfunction. A ratio of serum **blood urea nitrogen (BUN)** and **creatinine** greater than 20:1 is typical of prerenal states. **Urinalysis** may identify hematuria, proteinuria, or casts, which further support intrinsic or postrenal causes of ARF.

**Hyperkalemia** can be seen in patients with ARF as a result of decreased potassium excretion. **Acidosis** is due to impaired secretion of hydrogen ions and catabolic waste products. **Hypocalcemia** in ARF is often exacerbated by **hyperphosphatemia** and, if untreated, can lead to tetany or seizures.

Ultrasound imaging may reveal increased echogenicity with ATN and loss of corticomedullary differentiation with more severe involvement. Radiologic studies (ultrasound, voiding cystourethrogram [VCUG], computed tomography [CT], nuclear imaging) are often helpful in determining the cause of obstruction in postrenal cases.

**Renal biopsy**, usually performed percutaneously, may be indicated if the presentation of ARF is atypical to assess the severity of systemic disease involvement, to guide therapy, or establish a prognosis. Light microscopy should be augmented by immunofluorescence and electron microscopy.

## Treatment

Careful assessment of intake and output should be augmented with serial measurements of body weight. Initial fluid and electrolyte therapy provides water to equal insensible losses; water and electrolytes are then added to replace ongoing losses. If hypovolemia is present, intravascular volume should be expanded by intravenous (IV) administration of physiologic saline. If hypervolemia is present, 1 to 2 mg/kg of furosemide may be attempted. Severe fluid overload in the presence of marked oliguria or anuria is one indication for **dialysis**. Serum electrolyte levels should be determined frequently during the acute phase of ARF.

**TABLE 165-2 Laboratory and Clinical Differential Diagnosis of Renal Insufficiency**

| Laboratory/Clinical Feature | Prerenal | | Renal | | Postrenal |
|---|---|---|---|---|---|
| | Child | Neonate | Child | Neonate | |
| Urine Na⁺ (mEq/L) | <20 | <20–30 | >40 | >40 | Variable, may be >40 |
| $FE_{Na}$* (%) | <1 | <2–5 | >2 | >2–5 | Variable, may be >2 |
| Urine osmolality (mOsm/L) | >500 | >300–500 | ~300 | ~300 | Variable, may be <300 |
| BUN/serum Cr ratio | >20 | ≥10 | ~10 | ≥10 | Variable, may be >20 |
| Urinalysis | Normal | Normal | RBCs/WBCs, protein, casts | | Variable |
| History | Diarrhea, vomiting Diuretics | | Hypotension, anoxia Nephrotoxins | | Poor urine stream/output |
| Physical examination | Dehydration, hemorrhage | | Hypertension, edema | | Flank mass, distended bladder |

*$FE_{Na}$ (%) = [(urine sodium/plasma sodium) ÷ (urine creatinine/plasma creatinine)] × 100.

BUN, blood urea nitrogen; Cr, creatinine; $FE_{Na}$, fractional excretion of sodium; RBCs, red blood cells; WBCs, white blood cells.

Foods, fluids, and medications that contain potassium should be restricted until renal function is re-established or dialysis initiated. The major risk of hyperkalemia is arrhythmias (see Chapter 142). Intravenous calcium will block the acute cardiac toxicity of hyperkalemia while measures to shift potassium onto cells (bicarbonate, beta-agonists, glucose/insulin) and hasten removal (diuretics, sodium-potassium exchange resins, dialysis) are initiated. Although sodium bicarbonate counteracts acidosis, it engenders a risk of fluid overload, hypernatremia, and hypertension.

Treatment of hypocalcemia and hyperphosphatemia primarily involves efforts to lower the serum phosphorus by dietary phosphorus restriction and administration of phosphate binders (calcium acetate and calcium carbonate). Symptomatic hypocalcemia can be treated with IV calcium; it must be given cautiously to avoid precipitation with circulating phosphorus.

In children with ARF, **dialysis** has three major indications:

1. Hypervolemia unresponsive to fluid restriction or diuretics
2. Major electrolyte abnormalities unresponsive to medical therapy (hyperkalemia, acidosis)
3. Signs of uremia

Renal replacement therapies in children include peritoneal dialysis, hemodialysis, and continuous renal replacement therapy (continuous venovenous hemofiltration). Careful monitoring of blood levels of drugs excreted by the kidney and appropriate adjustment of either the total dose or dosing intervals are necessary to prevent complications or further renal injury.

## Prognosis

Recovery from ARF depends on the etiology, availability of specific treatments, and other aspects of the patient's clinical course. Sepsis and infections are major complications of ARF.

# CHRONIC KIDNEY DISEASE

## Etiology and Epidemiology

Congenital and obstructive abnormalities are the most common causes of chronic kidney disease (CKD) that present between birth and 10 years of age. After age 10, acquired diseases, such as FSGS and chronic GN, are more common causes of CKD. The risk of progression to ESRD is related to the cause of CKD and modifiable factors, such as UTI and hypertension. During puberty, renal function may deteriorate if the damaged kidneys are not able to grow and adapt to the increased demands of larger body size. CKD is staged to facilitate appropriate evaluation and monitoring (Table 165-3).

## Clinical Manifestations

The factors associated with **growth failure** in children with CKD include poor nutrition, renal osteodystrophy (ROD), acidosis, anemia, hormonal abnormalities, medication

**TABLE 165-3 Classification of the Stages of Chronic Kidney Disease**

| Stage | GFR (mL/min/ 1.73 m$^2$)* | Description |
|-------|---------------------------|-------------|
| 1 | ≥90 | Minimal kidney damage |
| 2 | 60–89 | Kidney damage with mild reduction of GFR |
| 3 | 30–59 | Moderate reduction of GFR |
| 4 | 15–29 | Severe reduction of GFR |
| 5 | <15 (or dialysis) | Kidney failure |

*GFR ranges apply for children 2 years of age and older.
GFR, glomerular filtration rate.
From National Kidney Foundation Kidney Disease Outcomes Quality Initiative.

toxicity (steroids), and the growth hormone/IGF-1 resistance seen in uremia. **Anemia** results primarily from a failure of the kidney to produce adequate **erythropoietin** and an impaired response to erythropoietin due to uremia. **Renal osteodystrophy** is common and is related to phosphate retention from low GFR and diminished 1,25-dihydroxyvitamin D production in the kidney. Secondary hyperparathyroidism and poor bone mineralization may ensue and lead to fractures and bone deformities. Delayed puberty may be due to altered gonadotropin secretion and feedback patterns. Hypertension is relatively common in CKD and may be asymptomatic or associated with headaches, left ventricular hypertrophy (LVH), and heart failure. Learning and school performance may also be impaired in CKD.

## Treatment

The management of children with CKD requires a multidisciplinary team of pediatric practitioners to address their growth and development. Adequate nutrition should be provided even if this requires dietary supplements and tube feedings. With very low GFR, maintenance dialysis may be needed for growing children to allow adequate fluid and recommended daily allowance of protein and calories. In infants with CKD, a low-solute formula with a phosphate binder may be indicated.

When acidosis develops, sodium bicarbonate or sodium citrate is indicated. Unless a child is oliguric, fluid restriction is not necessary. Sodium intake depends on the particular sodium handling aspects of the renal disease. Many children with congenital renal disorders waste sodium in their urine and require supplemental salt. Conversely, children with GN tend to retain sodium and may become hypertensive or edematous if given excess salt. High-potassium foods should be avoided in advanced CKD.

The initial therapy for ROD is to restrict phosphate in the diet. Oral phosphate binders are used if this is not sufficient. Supplemental calcium may be needed. Parathyroid hormone levels should be kept in the normal range and this may require supplemental vitamin D analog (calcitriol, paricalcital) therapy.

Recombinant-produced erythropoietin is used to maintain near normal hemoglobin levels in children with CKD. Effective erythropoiesis requires iron and typically depletes iron stores. Parenteral iron is often needed for children on erythropoietin. Growth failure is more common with advanced stages of CKD. Recombinant-produced growth hormone is useful in children with CKD who are not growing well despite proper management.

The optimal treatment of ESRD is **renal transplantation**. Identifying potential live donors should occur as the child reaches CKD stage 3 to 4. For children with slowly progressing CKD, preemptive renal transplantation can be used to avoid the stress of dialysis. Deceased and living donors can be used for renal transplantation. Live donor transplantation has several advantages and is often the first choice for children, when available. Living donors can be scheduled at the convenience of the donor and the recipient. Additionally, there is slightly better renal function and graft survival with live donor kidneys compared with cadaveric kidneys.

**Maintenance dialysis** is effective for a child awaiting renal transplantation or for whom renal transplantation is not possible. **Peritoneal dialysis** (PD) is effective in even small infants, and about 40% of children who require chronic dialysis use this modality in the United States. **Hemodialysis** is used more often for older and larger children, when intravascular access is less of a concern, and for children whose parents cannot provide home PD.

### Prognosis

Infants and children with ESRD have a good prognosis, given the effectiveness of dialysis and transplantation. Kidney transplants have an excellent success rate. More than 90% of transplants in children (living or deceased donor) function 1 year after transplant; more than 50% still function 20 years later. Lifelong immunosuppressive medications are necessary. The major complications relate to side effects of medications: infections, cardiac complications (left ventricular hypertrophy [LVH], atherosclerosis, arrhythmias), and increase in malignancies. Children after renal transplant who have not had prior Epstein-Barr virus (EBV) infection are more susceptible to develop an EBV-mediated post-transplant lymphoproliferative disorder (PTLD) that resembles malignant lymphoma. With early detection, PTLD and other malignancies can usually be treated successfully.

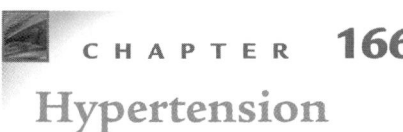

C H A P T E R  **166**

# Hypertension

## ETIOLOGY

Systolic and diastolic blood pressures normally increase gradually between 1 and 18 years of age. In children, hypertension (HTN) is defined as a blood pressure (BP) higher than the 95th percentile for age, gender, and height. Although not proven for children, it is assumed that the risk for sequelae of HTN increases as BP increases. HTN in children is either **primary** (*essential*) or **secondary**. **Essential HTN** is now the most common cause of HTN in children. **Renal disease** is the most common cause of secondary HTN in children. HTN in children has many causes (Table 166-1). Obese children are more likely to develop essential HTN than nonobese children.

**TABLE 166-1  Causes of Hypertension**

**CONGENITAL RENAL CAUSES**

Congenital anomalies
Dysplastic kidney
Polycystic kidney
Obstructive uropathy

**ACQUIRED RENAL CAUSES**

Wilms tumor
Glomerulonephritis
Hemolytic uremic syndrome
Reflux nephropathy
Drugs, toxins, systemic lupus erythematosus

**ENDOCRINE CAUSES**

Catecholamine-secreting tumors
Adrenogenital syndrome (11-hydroxylase deficiency)
Cushing syndrome
Hyperaldosteronism
Hyperthyroidism
Diabetic nephropathy
Liddle syndrome (pseudohyperaldosteronism)

**NEUROLOGIC CAUSES**

Stress, anxiety
Dysautonomia (Riley-Day syndrome)
Increased intracranial pressure
Guillain-Barré syndrome
Quadriplegia
Poliomyelitis
Encephalitis
Neurofibromatosis

**VASCULAR CAUSES**

Coarctation of the aorta
Renal artery embolism (from umbilical artery catheter)
Renal vein thrombosis
Renal artery stenosis
Arteritis (Takayasu arteritis, periarteritis nodosa)

**OTHER CAUSES**

Skeletal traction
Sympathomimetic drugs

## CLINICAL MANIFESTATIONS

Most children with HTN have no symptoms; the only way to diagnose HTN is to measure the BP. BP measurement should be done for all children over 3 years of age at every medical encounter. Cuff size selection is crucial (see Chapter 139). Neonatal history (low birth weight or use of umbilical artery catheter); family history of hypertension, stroke, or heart attacks; and dietary history (excessive salt or caffeine, drugs) are important. Signs and symptoms associated with HTN are heart failure, stroke, encephalopathy (seizures, headache, coma), polyuria, oliguria, edema, papilledema, and retinopathy (blurred vision). Additional findings that may suggest specific causes include abdominal bruits, diminished leg pressure (coarctation of aorta), café-au-lait spots (neurofibromatosis associated renal artery fibromuscular dysplasia), flank masses (hydronephrosis, Wilms tumor), ataxia/opsoclonus (neuroblastoma), tachycardia with flushing and diaphoresis (pheochromocytoma), and truncal obesity, acne, striae, and buffalo hump (Cushing syndrome). Signs of chronic kidney disease may be present (see Chapter 165).

## DIAGNOSTIC STUDIES

The evaluation of children with HTN, after several BP measurements have verified its presence, includes the following:

Assessment for target organ damage (echocardiogram for left ventricular hypertrophy)

Baseline etiologic assessment (urinalysis [UA], electrolytes, calcium, blood urea nitrogen [BUN]/creatinine, and renal ultrasound)

Focused studies based on specific findings (urinary catecholamines and metanephrines, thyroid studies, Doppler imaging)

Assessment of other cardiovascular risk factors (lipids, uric acid)

## TREATMENT

When a diagnosis of HTN has been established but no correctable cause is identified, therapy should be provided. For mild asymptomatic HTN without target organ damage, systemic diseases, or other risk factors therapeutic lifestyle changes (diet, exercise) should be initiated. Medical treatment should be started for moderate to severe or symptomatic HTN. Calcium channel blockers, angiotensin-converting enzyme inhibitors, β-blockers, or combined α/β-blockers may be used for mild to moderate HTN. Single-agent therapy usually suffices for these children. Combined therapy (diuretic and calcium channel blocker or angiotensin-converting enzyme inhibitor) might be needed for severe HTN. Hypertensive emergencies (encephalopathy and acute congestive heart failure) and hypertensive *urgencies* (extreme elevations of BP without neurologic or cardiac symptoms) require prompt hospitalization and, usually, parenteral antihypertensive treatment with nifedipine, labetalol, esmolol, or sodium nitroprusside. Renovascular HTN may require angioplasty.

## PROGNOSIS

Prognosis depends on the underlying etiology. Essential HTN, when present in adolescents, is usually not associated with morbidity at presentation. Left untreated, however, even asymptomatic essential HTN may contribute to the cardiovascular, central nervous system, and renal morbidity in adults.

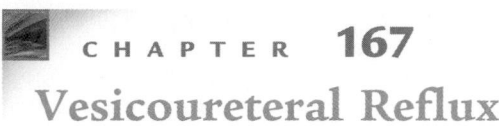

CHAPTER **167**

# Vesicoureteral Reflux

## ETIOLOGY AND EPIDEMIOLOGY

Vesicoureteral reflux (VUR) is the retrograde flow of urine from the bladder to the ureter or up to the kidney. Most VUR results from congenital incompetence of the ureterovesical (UV) junction that matures through early childhood. In a significant minority of children, structural UV abnormalities exist that never resolve. VUR may be familial; 30% to 40% of siblings of a child with VUR also have VUR. VUR may also be secondary to distal bladder obstruction or other urinary tract anomalies.

VUR exposes the kidney to increased hydrodynamic pressure during voiding and increases the likelihood of renal infection due to incomplete emptying of the ureter and bladder (see Chapter 114). **Reflux nephropathy** refers to development and progression of renal scarring. This is a particular risk if VUR is associated with infection or obstruction. Even though a single urinary tract infection (UTI) may result in renal scarring, the incidence is higher in children with recurrent UTIs. Renal scars noted in newborns, screened because of familial VUR, along with genetic studies, suggest that renal dysplasia is associated with congenital VUR. Because of the increasing use of maternal-fetal ultrasonography, a number of newborns are now identified with VUR before UTI has occurred, creating opportunities for early intervention and UTI prevention strategies. **Duplication of the ureters,** with or without an associated ureterocele, may obstruct the upper collecting system. Often the ureter draining the lower pole of a duplicated renal unit has VUR. **Neurogenic bladder,** with or without myelomeningocele, is accompanied by VUR in up to 50% of affected children. VUR may also be due to increased intravesicular pressure when the bladder outlet is obstructed from inflammation of the bladder (cystitis) or by acquired bladder obstruction.

## CLINICAL MANIFESTATIONS

VUR is most often identified during radiologic evaluation following a UTI (see Chapter 114). The younger the patient with a UTI, the more likely VUR is present. No clinical signs are reliable in differentiating children with UTI with and without VUR.

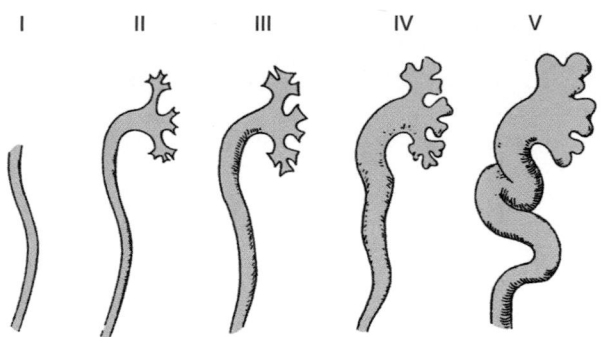

**FIGURE 167-1**

**International classification of vesicoureteral reflux.** Grade I: into a nondilated ureter; grade II: into the pelvis and calyces without dilatation; grade III: mild to moderate dilatation of the ureter, renal pelvis, and calyces with minimal blunting of the fornices; grade IV: moderate ureteral tortuosity and dilatation of the pelvis and calyces; grade V: gross dilatation of the ureter, pelvis, and calyces; loss of papillary impressions; and ureteral tortuosity. (From Wein A, Kavoussi L, Novick A, et al: Campbell-Walsh Urology, 9th ed. Philadelphia, *WB Saunders*, 2007.)

## DIAGNOSTIC STUDIES

A **voiding cystourethrogram** (VCUG) or **radionuclide cystogram** (NCG) should be performed in all infants and children up to 6 years of age with a documented first UTI, regardless of gender. An imaging study should be performed after initiation of UTI treatment, but there is no need to wait days or weeks before performing the test. The VCUG provides additional anatomic detail, but the NCG may detect a higher percentage of children with mild VUR and involves less radiation exposure. An international grading system has been used to describe reflux (Fig. 167-1). The incidence of renal scarring in patients with low-grade VUR is low (15%) and increases with grade IV or V reflux (65%). Grade I or II VUR is likely to resolve without surgical intervention, but VUR resolves in less than 50% grade IV or V. **Nuclear renal scanning** best identifies renal scars.

## TREATMENT

The presence of VUR is generally an indication for long-term prophylactic antibiotic therapy (trimethoprim-sulfamethoxazole or nitrofurantoin). Pivotal studies are under way to define the best evidence for appropriate observation versus prophylactic antibiotics versus corrective procedures in affected children. **Complications** of reflux nephropathy are hypertension and chronic kidney disease (CKD). CKD is typically heralded by mild proteinuria and involves development of focal and segmental glomerulosclerosis and interstitial scarring. Indications for surgical repair of VUR are controversial and have been made more complex by the development of dextranomer/hyaluronic acid copolymer (Deflux procedure), which appears to be a very successful minimally invasive correction of mild to moderate VUR.

## CHAPTER 168

# Congenital and Developmental Abnormalities of the Urinary Tract

## ETIOLOGY AND EPIDEMIOLOGY

Anomalies of the urinary tract occur in up to 4% of infants. **Bilateral renal agenesis** occurs in 1 in 4000 births. Renal agenesis is a component of **Potter syndrome** (flat facies, clubfoot, and pulmonary hypoplasia). Any intrauterine urinary tract disorder that results in little fetal urine and, therefore, little amniotic fluid can lead to Potter syndrome. **Unilateral renal agenesis** occurs in 1 in 3000 births and is more common in infants of diabetic mothers and African Americans. It is accompanied by normal or minimally reduced renal function. This condition can also be found with vesicoureteral reflux (VUR) and other anomalies of the genital tract, ear, skeletal system, and cardiovascular system. Unilateral renal agenesis can be a component of the Turner syndrome, Poland syndrome, or VACTERL association (vertebral abnormalities, anal atresia, cardiac abnormalities, tracheoesophageal fistula or esophageal atresia, renal agenesis and dysplasia, and limb defects).

**Renal hypoplasia/dysplasia** refers to kidneys that are congenitally small, malformed, or both. Over time, many affected children progress to chronic kidney disease (CKD) because of reduced nephron number. The kidneys are often unable to reabsorb sodium and water fully, requiring salt and water supplementation to optimize growth.

**Multicystic renal dysplasia** (MCD) is due to abnormal nephron development that occurs in 1 in 4000 births. There is minimal or no functioning renal tissue in the affected kidney; bilateral disease is lethal. There is an association with VUR in the contralateral kidney. MCD often spontaneously involutes over the first few years of life and is rarely associated with hypertension (HTN) or recurrent urinary tract infection (UTI).

**Polycystic kidney diseases** (PKDs) are a group of genetic diseases affecting the kidneys and other tissues. PKD may be primary (autosomal recessive or autosomal dominant) or associated with other syndromes. Autosomal recessive PKD occurs in 1 in 10,000 to 1 in 40,000 children and is due to genetic defects in fibrocystin. Autosomal dominant PKD, due to defects in polycystin 1 or 2, occurs in 1 in 1000 individuals, making it the most common inherited kidney disease. Although there is some overlap clinically, the two conditions differ morphologically. Both may appear in infancy or in older children. Renal cysts also are observed in other inherited disorders, such as von Hippel–Lindau syndrome, tuberous sclerosis, and Bardet-Biedl syndrome.

**TABLE 168-1 Site and Etiology of Urinary Tract Obstruction**

| Site | Etiologic Condition/Disorder |
|---|---|
| Infundibula/ pelvis | Congenital, calculi, infection, trauma/ hemorrhage, tumor |
| Ureteropelvic junction | Congenital stenosis,* calculi, trauma/ hemorrhage |
| Ureter | Obstructive megaureter,* ectopic ureter, ureterocele, calculi,* inflammatory bowel disease |
| | Retroperitoneal tumor (lymphoma), retroperitoneal fibrosis, chronic granulomatous disease |
| Bladder | Neurogenic dysfunction,* tumor (rhabdomyosarcoma), diverticula, ectopic ureter |
| Urethra | Posterior valves,* diverticula, strictures, atresia, ectopic ureter, foreign body |
| | Phimosis,* priapism |

*Relatively common.

**Urinary tract obstruction** can occur at any anatomic level of the genitourinary system (Table 168-1). Early in gestation, severe obstruction results in renal dysplasia. Ureteral obstruction later in fetal life or after birth results in dilation of the ureter and collecting system, often with subsequent renal parenchymal alterations. An obstructed urinary tract is susceptible to infections, which may worsen renal injury. **Posterior urethral valves** are the most common cause of **bladder outlet obstruction** in males, present in 1 in 50,000 boys. Parents may note a poor urine stream in affected children. The valves are sail-shaped membranes that arise from the verumontanum and attach to the urethral wall. The prostatic urethra becomes dilated, VUR may be present, and hypertrophied detrusor muscle develops. Renal dilation varies in severity. Some degree of renal dysplasia is often present. Severe obstruction may be associated with oligohydramnios, resulting in lethal pulmonary hypoplasia. Intrauterine rupture of the renal pelvis produces **urinary ascites**, which is the most common cause of ascites in the newborn period.

## CLINICAL MANIFESTATIONS

**Bilateral renal agenesis** results in insufficient lung development, due to oligohydramnios, and characteristic facial features (Potter syndrome). Respiratory distress is severe, pneumothoraces can occur, and severe pulmonary hypoplasia is fatal. Unilateral renal agenesis may be asymptomatic because the nonaffected kidney undergoes compensatory growth and provides normal renal function.

**Autosomal recessive PKD** is characterized by marked bilateral renal enlargement. Interstitial fibrosis and tubular atrophy progress over time. Kidney failure usually occurs in early childhood. **Hepatic fibrosis** is present and may lead to portal hypertension. Bile duct ectasia and biliary dysgenesis occur. Most affected infants have clinical manifestations such as flank masses, hepatomegaly, pneumothorax, proteinuria, or hematuria.

**Autosomal dominant PKD** typically presents in middle adulthood, but may present in infancy or childhood. Infants may have a clinical picture similar to autosomal recessive PKD, but older children show a pattern similar to that of adults, with large isolated cysts developing over time. The defect may occur anywhere along the nephron unit. Hepatic cysts are often present, and pancreatic, splenic, and ovarian cysts can also develop. **Cerebral aneurysms** may be present, and the risk of hemorrhage depends on size, blood pressure, and family history of intracranial hemorrhage.

Urinary tract obstruction may be silent, but usually is discovered during prenatal ultrasound or with UTI or flank mass in early childhood. In a newborn, the most common type of abdominal mass is renal (most commonly **ureteropelvic junction obstruction**).

## DIAGNOSTIC IMAGING

**Renal ultrasound** (RUS) and **radionuclide renography** (usually with a diuretic administered) are the standard tests for diagnosis of urinary tract obstruction. RUS allows identification of renal agenesis, hypoplasia, dysplasia, cysts, and urinary tract dilation. Obstruction may be suggested but a dilated urinary tract may also result from ureteral hypoplasia or neurogenic bladder. A voiding cystourethrogram (VCUG) is also a part of the evaluation. Many boys with posterior urethral valves are identified by prenatal ultrasound. Postnatally the diagnosis and extent of renal damage are established by RUS and VCUG.

## TREATMENT

Infants and children with bilateral dysplasia often require additional sodium and water due to renal wasting. With MCD, surgical removal of the kidney is rarely indicated unless severe HTN develops or recurrent UTI occurs.

Treatment of HTN due to renal disease can prolong maintenance of renal function. General therapy of CKD (see Chapter 165) can improve growth and development in such children.

Urinary tract obstruction always requires drainage or surgical correction. Treatment of posterior urethral valve (PUV) consists of either primary valve ablation or diversion (usually via vesicostomy) if ablation is not possible. Ectopic ureters are frequently obstructed; when this happens, surgical intervention is required.

Children with neurogenic bladder are prone to UTI and renal impairment from poor urine emptying. Clean intermittent catheterization or a urinary diversion is used to help minimize these complications.

# Other Urinary Tract and Genital Disorders

## URINARY TRACT STONES

### Etiology

Urinary tract calculi are called **nephrolithiasis** or **urolithiasis**. Primary bladder stones can be seen in children with recurrent urinary tract infections (UTIs), neurogenic bladder or bladder surgery (sutures serve as a nidus), and intestinal bladder augmentation. Renal stones can result from obstructive abnormalities or an underlying metabolic predisposition. In industrialized societies, most stones in children arise in the urinary tract (>90%) and become symptomatic with passage or if lodged (most commonly at the ureteropelvic junction or the ureterovesical junction). Metabolic causes include idiopathic familial hypercalciuria (IHC), hyperoxaluria, uric acid disorders, distal renal tubular acidosis, cystinuria, hypercalcemic hypercalciuria, and primary hyperparathyroidism. Some children with urinary tract abnormalities and stones have a concomitant metabolic predisposition.

### Clinical Manifestations

Acute obstruction of urine flow is the cause of renal colic, a severe sharp intermittent pain in the flank or lower abdomen often radiating to the groin. Vomiting, signs of distress, and inability to relieve pain with position changes are characteristic. In younger children, classic symptoms may not be apparent and fussiness and vomiting may be the only symptoms. Hematuria may be gross or microscopic and typically clears rapidly with passage of gravel or stone material.

### Diagnostic Studies

Ultrasound may identify kidney stones in the kidney, but can easily miss urinary tract stones. Computed tomography (CT), particularly a helical CT, can identify stones throughout the urinary tract, but stones can be obscured by the administration of oral or intravenous contrast material. If there is suspicion of stone disease, the CT scan should be performed before administering any contrast agents. Etiologic diagnosis is facilitated when stone material can be obtained and sent for analysis. Spot or 24-hour urine studies for mineral and electrolyte determinations, obtained on a typical diet for the child, are important to characterize any underlying metabolic predisposition and are valuable even when a stone is available for analysis.

### Treatment

Acute treatment of urinary calculi consists of hydration and analgesia. Chronic treatment for all types of metabolic stones involves vigorous fluid intake, usually twice maintenance rates. Infection-related stones require treatment of infection and often removal of the stone as well as correction of any predisposing anatomic abnormality. Specific metabolic conditions require specific treatments; for IHC, normal calcium intake with low sodium and low oxalate intake is prescribed. For some children with IHC, potassium citrate or thiazides are required to minimize stone recurrence. Lithotripsy or surgery by a pediatric urologist may be required for children with large, infected, or obstructing stones.

## VOIDING DYSFUNCTION

### Etiology

Voiding difficulties are frequent in pre–school age children due to delay in maturation of the bladder and micturition pathways. Normal micturition and continence rely on structural urinary tract integrity, neurologic maturation, and coordination between somatic and autonomic nervous system units, including the central nervous system, spinal cord pathways, nerves innervating the bladder/urinary sphincter, and the autonomic system. Daytime continence is usually achieved before night-time continence with most children dry, day and night, by 4 to 5 years of age. Nocturnal enuresis is the involuntary loss of urine during sleep. Children with primary enuresis have never had a prolonged (usually > 3 month) span of night-time continence. Up to 10% of 5-year-old children have primary enuresis with 15% spontaneous resolution per year. Boys are affected more than girls with increased incidence in families (40% at 6 years of age if one affected parent, 70% if two affected parents). Secondary enuresis involves loss of night-time control after an extended period of dryness and generally requires evaluation to uncover the cause.

### Clinical Manifestations

Dysfunctional voiding (DV) may manifest as incontinence, frequency, urgency, hesitancy, dysuria, lower abdominal pain, or recurrent UTI. The DV history should focus on types of symptoms, onset and pattern of incontinence, sensation with accidents, symptoms reflecting efforts to inhibit emptying (*curtsey* sign and leg movements), and signs of incontinence with stress (coughing, sneezing, giggling, exercise). Symptoms may vary over time and be associated with obvious neurologic problems (spinal cord injury, encephalitis), constipation, and/or behavioral problems. DV may vary depending on recent UTI or changes in family or school life/stressors. Physical examination may reveal obvious or occult signs of neurologic impairment, café au lait spots, or a sacral dimple. The majority of children with DV are anatomically, neurologically, and psychologically normal.

### Diagnostic Studies

Evaluation for DV may be performed at any age but isolated urinary incontinence in an otherwise normal child is not usually evaluated until 5 years of age. A urinalysis and urine culture should be done to exclude occult infection or signs of renal disease. Children with daytime incontinence should undergo renal/bladder ultrasound to exclude structural abnormalities. Urodynamic evaluation is typically reserved for children with a suspicion of a neurogenic bladder or those with a known neurologic etiology.

## Treatment

For children with recurrent UTI, prophylactic antibiotics may be useful. Timed voiding and anticholinergic medications are used to treat bladder hyperactivity and sensory defects. More complicated treatment regimens may include biofeedback, α-blockers, and intermittent catheterization. For children with simple primary enuresis, the bed wetting alarm provides safe and effective resolution of the problem for greater than 70% of affected children; medical therapy with anticholinergics, imipramine, or DDAVP may also be employed in selected children.

## ANOMALIES OF THE PENIS

### Etiology

**Hypospadias** occurs in approximately 1 in 500 newborn infants. In this condition, the urethral meatus is located ventrally and proximal to its normal position, secondary to failure of the urethral folds to fuse completely over the urethral groove. The ventral foreskin is also lacking, and the dorsal portion gives the appearance of a hood. Severe hypospadias with undescended testes is a form of ambiguous genitalia. Etiologies include congenital adrenal hyperplasia with masculinization of females or androgen insensitivity. Urinary tract anomalies are uncommon in association with hypospadias. Hypospadias may occur alone, but in severe cases can be associated with a **chordee** (a fixed ventral curvature of the penile shaft). Rarely when the urethra opens onto the perineum, the chordee is extreme, and the scrotum is bifid and sometimes extends to the dorsal base of the penis.

In 90% of uncircumcised males, the foreskin should be retractable by adolescence. Before this age, the prepuce may normally be tight and not need treatment. After this age, the inability to retract the prepuce is termed **phimosis**. The condition may be congenital or the result of inflammation. **Paraphimosis** occurs when the prepuce has been retracted behind the coronal sulcus, cannot resume its normal position, and causes swelling of the glans or pain.

### Clinical Manifestations and Treatment

The meatal opening in **hypospadias** may be located anteriorly (on the glans, coronal, or distal third of the shaft); on the middle third of the shaft; or posteriorly (near the scrotum). Testes are undescended in 10% of boys with hypospadias. Inguinal hernias are common. Males with hypospadias should not be circumcised, particularly if the meatus is proximal to the glans, because the foreskin may be necessary for later repair. Most pediatric urologists repair hypospadias before the patient is 18 months old.

**Phimosis** is rarely symptomatic, and parents should be reassured that loosening of the prepuce usually occurs during puberty. Treatment, if needed, is the application of topical steroids. If the narrowing is severe, gentle stretching may be useful. Circumcision is reserved for the most severe cases. **Paraphimosis** with venous stasis and edema leads to severe pain. When paraphimosis is discovered early, reduction of the foreskin may be possible with lubrication. In some cases, emergent circumcision is needed.

## DISORDERS AND ABNORMALITIES OF THE SCROTUM AND ITS CONTENTS

### Etiology

**Undescended testes** (cryptorchidism) are found in about 1% of boys after 1 year of age. It is more common in full-term newborns (3.4%) than in older children. In neonates, cryptorchidism is more common with shorter gestation (20% in 2000- to 2500-g infants and 100% in < 900-g infants). Cryptorchidism is bilateral in 30% of cases. Spontaneous testicular descent does not tend to occur after 1 year of age, but failure to find one or both testes in the scrotum does not indicate undescended testicles. **Retractile testes**, absent testes, and ectopic testes may resemble cryptorchidism in presentation.

### Clinical Manifestations

A history of maternal drug use (steroids) and family history are important in evaluation of a child for apparent cryptorchidism. Whether the testis was ever noted in the scrotum should be asked. The true undescended testis is found along the normal embryologic path of descent, usually in the presence of a patent processus vaginalis. An undescended testis is often associated with an inguinal hernia; it is also subject to **torsion**. There is a high incidence of infertility in adulthood. When bilateral and untreated, infertility is uniform. There is an increased malignancy risk (five times the normal rate) with undescended testis, usually presenting between the ages of 20 and 30. The risk is greater in untreated males or those with surgical correction during or after puberty.

Retractile testes are normal testes that retract into the inguinal canal from an exaggerated cremasteric reflex. The diagnosis of retractile testes is likely if testes are palpable in the newborn period but not at later examination. Frequently parents describe seeing their son's testes in his scrotum when he is in the bath and seeing one or both *disappear* when he gets cold.

### Complications

Torsion of the testis is an emergency requiring prompt diagnosis and treatment to save the affected testis. Torsion accounts for about 40% of cases of acute scrotal pain and swelling and is the major cause of the acute scrotum in boys younger than 6 years of age. It is thought to arise from abnormal fixation of the testis to the scrotum. On examination, the testicle is swollen and tender, and the cremasteric reflex is absent. The absence of blood flow on nuclear scan or Doppler ultrasound is consistent with torsion.

The differential diagnosis of testicular pain includes trauma, an incarcerated hernia, and torsion of the testicular epididymal appendix. Torsion of the appendix testis is associated with point tenderness over the lesion and minimal swelling. In adolescents, the differential diagnosis of testicular torsion also must include **epididymitis**, the most common cause of acute scrotal pain and swelling in older adolescents. Diagnosis is aided by an antecedent history of sexual activity or UTI. Testicular torsion must be considered as the principal diagnosis when severe acute testicular pain is present.

## Treatment

The undescended testis is usually histologically normal at birth. Atrophy and dysplasia are found after the first year of life. Some boys have congenital dysplasia in the contralateral descended testis. Surgical correction at an early age results in greater chance of adult fertility. Administration of human chorionic gonadotropin causes testosterone release from functioning testes and may result in descent of retractile testes.

**Orchidopexy** is usually done in the second year of life. Most extra-abdominal testes can be brought into the scrotum with correction of the associated hernia. If the testis is not palpable, ultrasound or magnetic resonance imaging (MRI) may determine its location. The closer the testis is to the internal inguinal ring, the better the chance of successful orchidopexy.

Surgical correction of testicular torsion is called *detorsion and fixation of the testis*. If performed within 6 hours of torsion, there is a greater than 90% chance of testicular salvage. The contralateral testis usually is fixed to the scrotum to prevent possible torsion. If torsion of the appendix is found, the necrotic tissue is removed.

## ACKNOWLEDGMENT

We gratefully acknowledge the useful contributions of Rama Jayanthi, MD, Pediatric Urology, Nationwide Children's Hospital, Columbus, Ohio.

## SUGGESTED READING

Avner E, Harmon W, Niaudet P: Pediatric Nephrology, 5th ed, Philadelphia, 2004, *Lippincott Williams & Wilkins.*

Feld LG, Corey H: Hypertension in childhood, *Pediatr Rev* 28:283–298, 2007.

Geary DF, Schaefer F: Comprehensive Pediatric Nephrology, Philadelphia, 2008, *Mosby.*

Gillespie RS, Stapleton FB: Nephrolithiasis in children, *Pediatr Rev* 25:131–139, 2004.

Gordillo R, Spitzer A: The nephrotic syndrome, *Pediatr Rev* 30:94–105, 2009.

Kher KK, Schnaper HW, Makker SP: Clinical Pediatric Nephrology, 2nd ed, Boca Raton, FL, 2007, *Taylor and Francis.*

Massengill SF: Hematuria, *Pediatr Rev* 29:342–348, 2008.

Schwaderer AL, Schwartz GJ: Back to basics: Acidosis and alkalosis, *Pediatr Rev* 25:350–357, 2004.

Schwartz GJ, Munoz A, Schneider MF, Mak RH, Kaskel F, Warady BA, Furth SL: New equation to estimate GFR in children with CKD, *J Am Soc Nephrology* 20:629–637, 2009.

Whyte DA, Fine RN: Acute renal failure in children, *Pediatr Rev* 29:299–307, 2008.

Whyte DA, Fine RN: Chronic kidney disease in children, *Pediatr Rev* 29:335–341, 2008.

## CHAPTER 170

# Endocrinology Assessment

The endocrine system regulates vital body functions by means of hormonal messengers. **Hormones** are defined as circulating messengers, with action at a distance from the organ (**gland**) of origin of the hormone. Hormones can be regulated by nerve cells; endocrine agents can serve as neural messengers. There is also a relationship between the endocrine system and the immune system; autoantibodies may cause an organ to produce an excess or deficiency of a hormone. Manifestations of an endocrine disorder are related to the response of the peripheral tissue to a hormone excess or deficiency.

Hormone action also may be **paracrine** (acting on adjacent neighboring cells to the cell of origin of the hormone) or **autocrine** (acting on the cell of origin of the hormone itself); agents acting in these ways are called *factors* rather than hormones (Fig. 170-1). Hormones generally are regulated in a feedback loop so that the production of a hormone is linked to its effect or its circulating concentration. Endocrine disorders generally manifest from one of four ways:

1. By **excess hormone**: In Cushing syndrome, there is an excess of glucocorticoid present; if the excess is secondary to autonomous glucocorticoid secretion by the adrenal gland, the trophic hormone adrenocorticotropic hormone (ACTH) is suppressed.
2. By **deficient hormone**: In glucocorticoid deficiency, the level of cortisol is inadequate; if the deficiency is at the adrenal gland, the trophic hormone is elevated (ACTH). In type 1 diabetes mellitus (DM1), the insulin secretion is low to absent.
3. By an abnormal **response of end organ** to hormone: In pseudohypoparathyroidism, there is resistance to parathyroid hormone (PTH).
4. By **gland enlargement** that may have effects as a result of size rather than function: With a large nonfunctioning pituitary adenoma, abnormal visual fields and other neurologic signs and symptoms result even though no hormone is produced by the tumor.

**Peptide hormones** act through specific cell membrane receptors; when the hormone is attached to the receptor, the complex triggers various intracellular second messengers that cause the biologic effects. Peptide hormone receptor number and avidity may be regulated by hormones. **Steroid hormones** exert their effects by attachment to intranuclear receptors, and the hormone-receptor complex translocates to the nucleus, where it binds with DNA, and leads to further gene activation.

The interpretation of serum hormone levels must be related to their controlling factors. For example, a given value of PTH may be normal in a eucalcemic patient, but inadequate in a hypocalcemic patient with partial hypoparathyroidism or excessive in a hypercalcemic patient with hyperparathyroidism.

## HYPOTHALAMIC-PITUITARY AXIS

The **hypothalamus** controls many endocrine systems either directly or through the pituitary gland. Higher central nervous system (CNS) centers control the hypothalamus. Hypothalamic releasing or inhibiting factors travel through capillaries of the pituitary portal system to control the anterior pituitary gland, regulating the hormones specific for the factor (Fig. 170-2). The pituitary hormones enter the peripheral circulation and exert their effects on target glands, which produce other hormones that feed back to suppress their controlling hypothalamic and pituitary hormones. (Insulin-like growth factor-1 [IGF-1], growth hormone (GH), cortisol, sex steroids, and thyroxine [$T_4$] all feed back on the hypothalamic-pituitary system.) Prolactin is the only pituitary hormone that is suppressed by a hypothalamic factor, prolactin inhibitory factor (dopamine). Hypothalamic deficiency leads to a decrease in most pituitary hormone secretions, but may lead to an increase in prolactin secretion. The hypothalamus is also the location of vasopressin-secreting axons that either terminate in the posterior pituitary gland and exert their effect via vasopressin secretion from this area or terminate in the mediobasal hypothalamus, from which they can exert effects on water balance, even in the absence of the posterior pituitary gland.

In childhood, **increased pituitary secretion** of various hormones as a result of an adenoma is rare, although

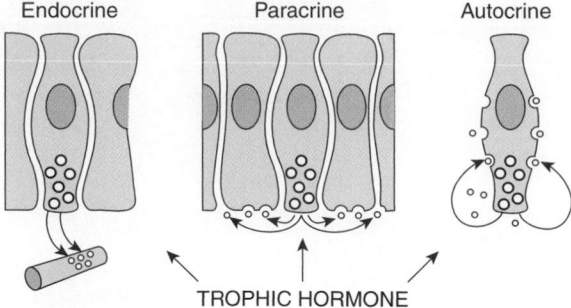

**FIGURE 170-1**

**Schematic representation of mechanisms of action of hormones and growth factors.** Although traditional hormones are formed in endocrine glands and transported to distant sites of action through the bloodstream (endocrine mechanism), peptide growth factors may be produced locally by the target cells themselves (autocrine modality of action) or by neighboring cells (paracrine action). (From Wilson JD, Foster DW [eds]: Williams Textbook of Endocrinology, 8th ed. Philadelphia, *WB Saunders*, 1992, p 1007.)

cases of pituitary gigantism (growth hormone [GH] excess from a pituitary adenoma) do occur. Destructive lesions of the pituitary gland or hypothalamus are more common in childhood. A **craniopharyngioma**, a tumor of the Rathke pouch, may descend into the sella turcica, causing erosion of the bone and destruction of pituitary and hypothalamic tissue. Acquired hypopituitarism also may result from pituitary infections; from infiltration, such as with Langerhans cell histiocytosis (histiocytosis X),

lymphoma, and sarcoidosis; after radiation therapy or trauma to the CNS; and as a consequence of autoimmunity against the pituitary gland.

**Congenital hypopituitarism** usually is caused by absence of hypothalamic releasing factors rather than anatomic absence of the pituitary gland itself. Without hypothalamic stimulation, the pituitary gland does not release its hormones but it can be primed for secretion by exogenous hypothalamic releasing factors. However, exogenous administration is of limited clinical value because the end products of the glands themselves can be given to treat hypopituitarism. Congenital defects associated with hypopituitarism range from **holoprosencephaly** (cyclopia, cebocephaly, orbital hypotelorism), to cleft palate (6% of cases of cleft palate are associated with GH deficiency). **Septo-optic dysplasia** (optic nerve hypoplasia, absent septum pellucidum, or variations of both, and hypopituitarism) may result in significant visual impairment with pendular nystagmus (to-and-fro nystagmus caused by an inability to focus on a target). The magnetic resonance imaging (MRI) findings of congenital hypopituitarism include an ectopic posterior pituitary gland *hot spot* and the appearance of a *pituitary stalk transection* and small pituitary gland.

The assessment of pituitary function may be determined by measuring some of the specific pituitary hormone in the basal state; other assessments require the measurement after stimulation. Indirect assessment of pituitary function can be obtained by measuring serum concentrations of the target gland hormones (Table 170-1). Several tests of pituitary function are listed in Table 170-2.

**FIGURE 170-2**

**Hormonal influences of the hypothalamus and pituitary gland.** *Solid line* represents stimulatory influence; *dotted line* represents inhibitory influence. ACTH, adrenocorticotropic hormone; CRH, corticotropin-releasing hormone or CRF; FSH, follicle-stimulating hormone; GH, growth hormone; GHRH, GH-releasing hormone or GRF; GnRH, gonadotropin-releasing hormone or luteinizing hormone releasing factor, LRF or LHRH; LH, luteinizing hormone; SRIF, somatotropin release–inhibiting factor, somatostatin or SS; TRH, thyrotropin-releasing hormone or TRF; TSH, thyroid-stimulating hormone; $T_3$, triiodothyronine; $T_4$, thyroxine.

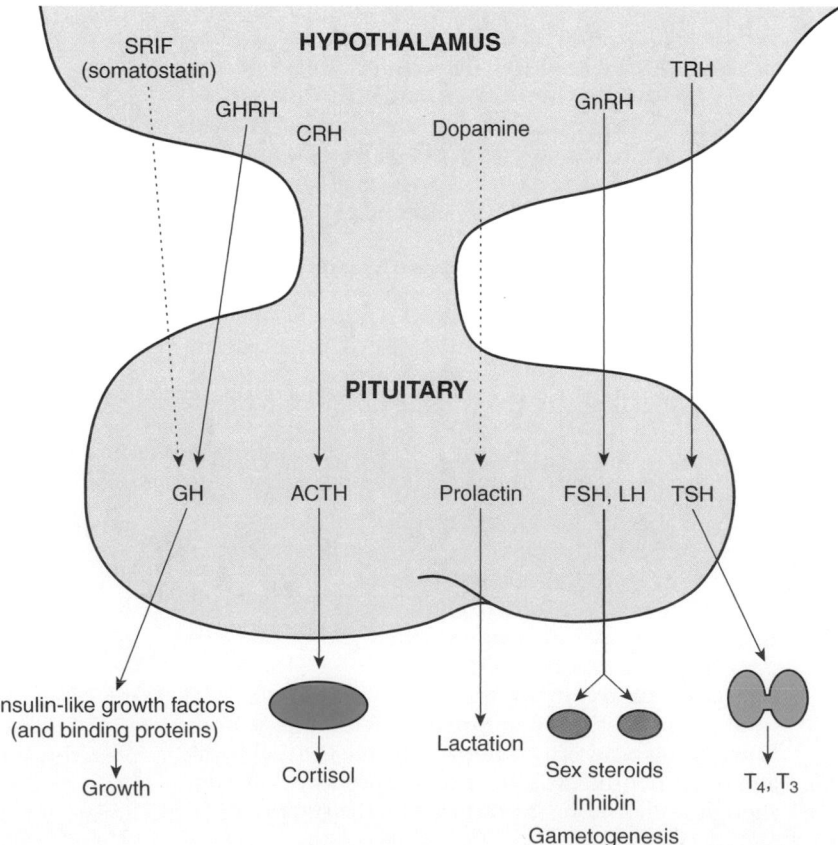

## TABLE 170-1 Diagnostic Evaluation of Hypopituitarism

| Manifestation | Cause | Tests* |
|---|---|---|
| Growth failure, hypothyroidism, or both | GH deficiency, TRH/TSH deficiency, or both | Provocative GH tests, free $T_4$, bone age, IGF-1, IGF-BP3 |
| Hypoglycemia | GH deficiency, ACTH insufficiency, or both | Provocative GH tests, test of ACTH secretion, IGF-1, IGF-BP3 |
| Micropenis, pubertal delay or arrest | Hypogonadotropic hypogonadism or GH deficiency | Sex steroids ($E_2$, testosterone), basal LH and FSH (analyzed by ultrasensitive assays) or after GnRH administration, provocative GH tests, IGF-1, IGF-BP3 |
| Polyuria, polydipsia | ADH deficiency | Urine analysis (specific gravity), serum electrolytes, urine and serum osmolality, water deprivation test |

*Each patient with hypopituitarism should have CNS MRI as part of evaluation to determine the etiology of the condition.
ADH, antidiuretic hormone; CNS, central nervous system; $E_2$, estradiol; FSH, follicle-stimulating hormone; GH, growth hormone; GnRH, gonadotropin-releasing hormone; IGF-1, insulin-like growth factor; IGF-BP3, insulin-like growth factor–binding protein 3; LH, luteinizing hormone; MRI, magnetic resonance imaging; $T_4$, thyroxine; TRH, thyrotropin-releasing hormone; TSH, thyroid-stimulating hormone.

## TABLE 170-2 Anterior Pituitary Hormone Function Testing

| Random Hormone Measurements | Provocative Stimulation Test | Target Hormone Measurement |
|---|---|---|
| GH (useless as a random determination except in newborns, and in GH resistance or in pituitary gigantism) | Arginine (a weak stimulus)<br>L-Dopa (useful clinically)<br>Insulin-induced hypoglycemia (a dangerous but accurate test)<br>Clonidine (useful clinically)<br>GRH<br>12- to 24-hr integrated GH levels (of questionable utility) | IGF-1, IGF-BP3 (affected by malnutrition as well as GH excess) |
| ACTH (early AM sample useful only if in high-normal range) | Cortisol after insulin-induced hypoglycemia (a dangerous test)<br>11-Desoxycortisol after metyrapone<br>CRH<br>ACTH stimulation test (may differentiate ACTH deficiency from primary adrenal insufficiency) | AM cortisol<br><br>24-hr urinary free cortisol |
| TSH* | TRH | $FT_4$ |
| LH, FSH* | GnRH (difficult to interpret in prepubertal subjects) | Testosterone<br>Estradiol |
| Prolactin (elevated in hypothalamic disease and decreased in pituitary disease) | TRH | None |

*New supersensitive assays allow determination of abnormally low values found in hypopituitarism.
ACTH, adrenocorticotropic hormone; CRH, corticotropin-releasing hormone; L-dopa, L-dihydroxyphenylalanine; FSH, follicle-stimulating hormone; $FT_4$, free thyroxine; GH, growth hormone; GnRH, gonadotropin-releasing hormone; GRH, growth hormone–releasing hormone; IGF-1, insulin-like growth factor-1; IGF-BP3, insulin-like growth factor-binding protein 3; LH, luteinizing hormone; TRH, thyrotropin-releasing hormone; TSH, thyroid-stimulating hormone.

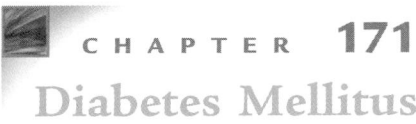

# CHAPTER 171
# Diabetes Mellitus

Diabetes mellitus (DM) is characterized by hyperglycemia and glycosuria and is an end point of a few disease processes (Table 171-1). The most common type occurring in childhood is type 1 DM, which is caused by autoimmune destruction of the insulin-producing beta cells (islets) of the pancreas leading to permanent insulin deficiency. Type 2 diabetes mellitus (DM2) is less common in children and often results from insulin resistance and relative insulin deficiency, usually in the context of exogenous obesity. The incidence of DM1 and DM2 in the United States is increasing. Less common subtypes of DM2 result from genetic defects of the insulin receptor or inherited abnormalities in sensing of ambient glucose concentration by pancreatic beta cells (see Table 171-1).

**TABLE 171-1  Classification of Diabetes Mellitus in Children and Adolescents**

| Type | Comment |
|---|---|
| **TYPE 1 (INSULIN-DEPENDENT)** ||
| Transient neonatal | Manifests immediately after birth; lasts 1–3 months |
| Permanent neonatal | Other pancreatic defects possible |
| Classic type 1 | Glycosuria, ketonuria, hyperglycemia, islet cell antibody to glutamic acid decarboxylase positive; genetic component |
| **TYPE 2 (NON–INSULIN-DEPENDENT)** ||
| Secondary | Cystic fibrosis, hemochromatosis, drugs (ʟ-asparaginase, tacrolimus) |
| Adult type (classic) | Associated with obesity, insulin resistance; genetic component |
| Maturity-onset diabetes of youth | Autosomal dominant, onset before age of 25 years; not associated with obesity or autoimmunity |
| | Single-gene mutations include hepatocyte nuclear factors 1β, 1α, 4α; glucokinase; insulin promoter factor 1 |
| Mitochondrial diabetes | Associated with deafness and other neurologic defects, maternal transmission—mtDNA point mutations |
| **OTHER** ||
| Gestational diabetes | Abnormal glucose tolerance only during pregnancy, which reverts to normal post partum; increased risk for later onset of diabetes |

mtDNA, mitochondrial DNA.

## DEFINITION

A **diagnosis** of diabetes mellitus is made when a fasting serum glucose concentration is at or above 126 mg/dL or a 2-hour postprandial serum glucose concentration is at or above 200 mg/dL on two separate occasions. A patient is considered **glucose intolerant** if fasting serum glucose concentrations is 100 to 125 mg/dL and 2-hour plasma glucose following an oral glucose tolerance test (OGTT) is 140 to 199 mg/dL. Sporadic hyperglycemia can occur in children, usually in the setting of an intercurrent illness. When the hyperglycemic episode is clearly related to an illness or other physiologic stress, the probability of incipient diabetes is small (< 5%). Sporadic hyperglycemia occurring without a clear precipitating physiologic stress is of more concern because diabetes develops in at least 30%.

## INSULIN-DEPENDENT (TYPE 1) DIABETES MELLITUS

### Etiology

DM1 results from the autoimmune destruction of insulin-producing beta cells (islets) of the pancreas. In addition to the presence of diabetes susceptibility genes, an unknown environmental insult presumably triggers the autoimmune process. A variety of studies have produced conflicting data regarding a host of environmental factors. These include cow's milk feeding before age 2 years, viral infectious agents (coxsackie B virus, cytomegalovirus, mumps, and rubella), and possibly vitamin D deficiency. DM1 is thought to be primarily a T cell–mediated disease; however, that knowledge is evolving.

Antibodies to islet cell antigens may be seen months to years before the onset of beta cell dysfunction (Fig. 171-1). These include islet cell antibodies, insulin autoantibodies, antibodies to tyrosine phosphatase IA-2, antibodies to glutamic acid decarboxylase, and others. The risk for diabetes increases with the number of antibodies detected in the serum. In individuals with only one detectable antibody, the risk is only 10% to 15%; in individuals with three or more antibodies, the risk is 55% to 90%. When 80% to 90% of the beta cell mass has been destroyed, the remaining beta cell mass is insufficient to maintain euglycemia, and clinical manifestations of diabetes result (see Fig. 171-1).

Diabetes in childhood also can result from rare inherited defects in **mitochondrial genes**. Other rare subtypes of DM2 are syndromes of severe insulin resistance caused by mutations in the insulin receptor gene and diabetes resulting from the secretion of abnormal forms of insulin or insulin action (e.g., lipoatrophic DM). Diseases of exocrine pancreas (e.g., cystic fibrosis related diabetes); endocrinopathies (e.g., Cushing syndrome); and drug therapies (e.g., glucocorticoids, chemotherapeutics) are other rare causes of diabetes or glucose intolerance.

### Epidemiology

In the United States, the annual incidence is approximately 20 in 100,000. The annual incidence in children ranges from a high of 40 in 100,000 among Scandinavian populations to less than 1 in 100,000 in China. The annual incidence of DM1 is increasing steadily but with significant geographic differences. The prevalence of DM1 in the United States is highest in whites and is lower in African Americans and Hispanic Americans.

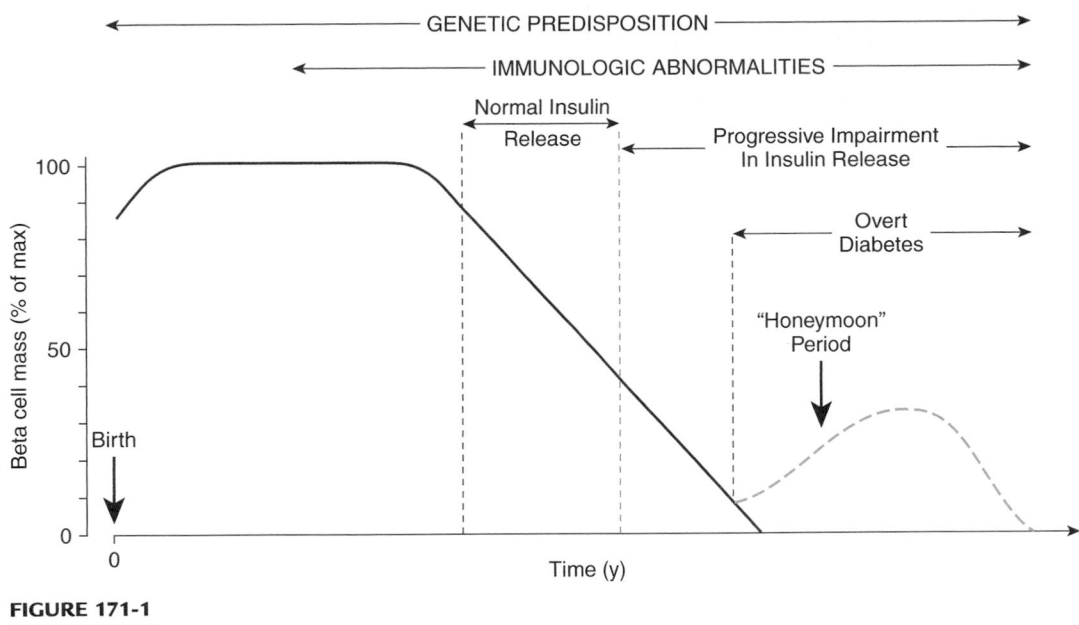

**FIGURE 171-1**

Schematic representation of the autoimmune evolution of diabetes in genetically predisposed individuals.

Genetic determinants play a role in the susceptibility to DM1, although the mode of inheritance is complex and clearly multigenic. Siblings or offspring of patients with diabetes have a risk of 3% to 6% for development of diabetes; an identical twin has a 30% to 50% risk. The HLA region on chromosome 6 provides the strongest determinant of susceptibility, accounting for approximately 40% of familial inheritance of DM1. Specific class II DR and DQ HLA alleles (HLA DR3 and HLA DR4) increase the risk of developing DM1, whereas other specific HLA alleles exert a protective effect. More than 90% of children with DM1 possess HLA DR3 alleles, HLA DR4 alleles, or both. The insulin gene region VNTR on chromosome 11 is also linked to DM1 susceptibility. There is evidence for association, beyond HLA, of more than 100 other loci with DM1. Genetic factors do not fully account for susceptibility to DM1; environmental factors also play a role.

## Clinical Manifestations

Hyperglycemia results when insulin secretory capacity becomes inadequate to enhance peripheral glucose uptake and to suppress hepatic and renal glucose production. Insulin deficiency usually first causes postprandial hyperglycemia, then fasting hyperglycemia. Ketogenesis is a sign of more complete insulin deficiency. Lack of suppression of gluconeogenesis and glycogenolysis further exacerbates hyperglycemia while fatty acid oxidation generates the ketone bodies: β-hydroxybutyrate, acetoacetate, and acetone. Protein stores in muscle and fat stores in adipose tissue are metabolized to provide substrates for gluconeogenesis and fatty acid oxidation.

Glycosuria occurs when the serum glucose concentration exceeds the renal threshold for glucose reabsorption (approximately 180 mg/dL). Glycosuria causes an osmotic diuresis (including obligate loss of sodium, potassium, and other electrolytes), leading to dehydration. Polydipsia occurs as the patient attempts to compensate for the excess fluid losses. Weight loss results from the persistent catabolic state and the loss of calories through glycosuria and ketonuria. The classic presentation of DM1 includes polyuria, polydipsia, polyphagia, and weight loss.

## Diabetic Ketoacidosis

If the clinical features of new-onset DM1 are not detected, diabetic ketoacidosis (DKA) will occur. DKA also can occur in patients with known DM1 if insulin injections are omitted or during an intercurrent illness when greater insulin requirements are unmet in the presence of elevated concentrations of the counter-regulatory and stress hormones (glucagon, growth hormone [GH], cortisol, and catecholamines). DKA can be considered to be present if (1) the arterial pH is below 7.25, (2) the serum bicarbonate level is below 15 mEq/L, and (3) ketones are elevated in serum or urine.

### Pathophysiology

In the absence of adequate insulin secretion, persistent partial hepatic oxidation of fatty acids to ketone bodies occurs. Two of these three ketone bodies are organic acids and lead to metabolic acidosis with an elevated anion gap. Lactic acid may contribute to the acidosis when severe dehydration results in decreased tissue perfusion. Hyperglycemia causes an osmotic diuresis that is initially compensated for by increased fluid intake. As the hyperglycemia and diuresis worsen, most patients are unable to maintain the large fluid intake, and dehydration occurs. Vomiting, as a result of increasing acidosis, and increased insensible water losses caused by tachypnea can worsen the dehydration. Electrolyte abnormalities occur through a loss of electrolytes in the urine and transmembrane alterations resulting from acidosis. As hydrogen ions accumulate as a result of ketoacidosis, intracellular potassium is exchanged for hydrogen ions. Serum concentrations of potassium increase initially with acidosis, then decrease as serum potassium is cleared by the kidney. Depending on the duration of ketoacidosis, serum potassium concentrations at diagnosis may be increased, normal, or decreased, but intracellular potassium concentrations are depleted. A decreased serum potassium concentration is an ominous sign of total body potassium depletion. Phosphate depletion also can occur as a result of the increased renal phosphate excretion required for elimination of excess hydrogen ions. Sodium depletion also is common in DKA, resulting from renal losses of sodium caused by osmotic diuresis and from gastrointestinal losses from vomiting (Fig. 171-2).

## Presentation

Patients with DKA present initially with polyuria, polydipsia, and nausea and vomiting. Abdominal pain occurs frequently and can mimic an acute abdomen. The abdomen may be tender from vomiting, or distended secondary to a paralytic ileus. The presence of polyuria, despite a state of clinical dehydration, indicates osmotic diuresis and differentiates patients with DKA from patients with gastroenteritis or other gastrointestinal disorders. Respiratory compensation for acidosis results in tachypnea with deep (**Küssmaul**) respirations. The *fruity* odor of acetone frequently can be detected on the patient's breath. An altered mental status can occur, ranging from disorientation to coma.

**Laboratory studies** reveal hyperglycemia (serum glucose concentrations ranging from 200 mg/dL to > 1000 mg/dL). Arterial pH is below 7.25, and the serum bicarbonate concentration is less than 15 mEq/L. Serum sodium concentrations may be elevated, normal, or low, depending on the balance of sodium and free water losses. The measured serum sodium concentration is artificially depressed, however, because of hyperglycemia (see Chapter 35). Hyperlipidemia also contributes to the decrease in measured serum sodium. The level of blood urea nitrogen (BUN) can be elevated with prerenal azotemia secondary to dehydration. The white blood cell count is usually elevated and can be left-shifted without implying the presence of infection. Fever is unusual and should prompt a search for infectious sources that may have triggered the episode of DKA.

## Treatment

Therapy for patients with DKA involves careful replacement of fluid deficits, correction of acidosis and hyperglycemia via insulin administration, correction of electrolyte imbalances, and monitoring for complications of treatment. The optimal approach to management of DKA must strike a balance between adequate correction of fluid losses and avoidance of rapid shifts in osmolality and fluid balance. The most serious complication of DKA and its treatment is **cerebral edema** and cerebral herniation.

**Dehydration.** A patient with severe DKA is assumed to be approximately 10% dehydrated. If a recent weight measurement is available, the precise extent of dehydration can be calculated. An initial intravenous (IV) fluid bolus of a glucose-free isotonic solution (normal saline, lactated Ringer's solution) at 10 to 20 mL/kg should be given to restore intravascular volume and renal perfusion. The remaining fluid deficit after the initial bolus should be added to maintenance fluid requirements, and the total should be replaced slowly over 36 to 48 hours. Ongoing losses resulting from osmotic diuresis usually do not need to be replaced unless urine output is large or signs of poor perfusion are present. Osmotic diuresis is usually minimal when the serum glucose concentration decreases to less than 300 mg/dL. To avoid rapid shifts in serum osmolality, 0.9% sodium chloride can be used as the replacement

**FIGURE 171-2**

Pathophysiology of diabetic ketoacidosis.

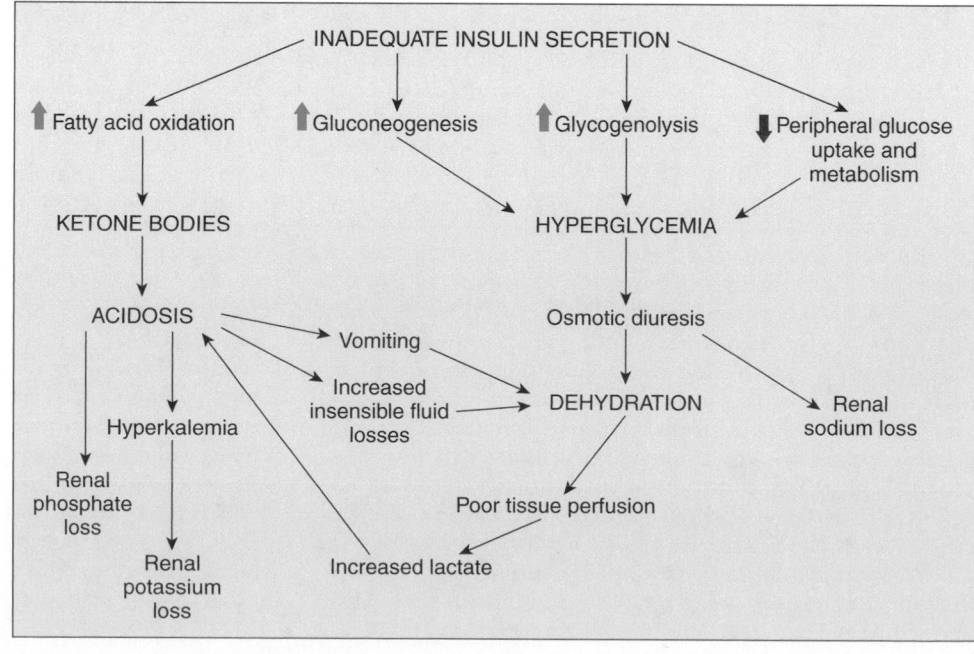

fluid for the initial 4 to 6 hours, followed by 0.45% sodium chloride.

**Hyperglycemia.** Fast-acting soluble insulin should be administered as a continuous IV infusion (0.1 U/kg/hour). Serum glucose concentrations should decrease at a rate no faster than 100 mg/dL/hour. When serum glucose concentrations decrease to less than 250 to 300 mg/dL, glucose should be added to the IV fluids. If serum glucose concentrations decrease to less than 200 mg/dL before correction of acidosis, the glucose concentration of the IV fluids should be increased, but the insulin infusion should not be decreased by more than half, and it should never be discontinued before resolution of acidosis.

**Acidosis.** Insulin therapy decreases the production of free fatty acids (FFAs) and protein catabolism, and enhances glucose usage in target tissues. These processes correct acidosis. Bicarbonate therapy should be avoided unless severe acidosis (pH < 7.0) results in hemodynamic instability, or when symptomatic hyperkalemia is present. Potential adverse effects of bicarbonate administration include paradoxical increases in central nervous system (CNS) acidosis caused by increased diffusion of carbon dioxide across the blood-brain barrier, potential tissue hypoxia caused by shifts in the oxyhemoglobin dissociation curve, abrupt osmotic changes, and increased risk of development of cerebral edema.

As acidosis is corrected, urine ketone concentrations may appear to rise. β-Hydroxybutyrate, which is not detected in urine ketone assays, is converted with treatment to what the assay most detects, acetoacetate. Hence, minute to minute urine ketone concentrations are not a required index of the adequacy of therapy.

**Electrolyte Imbalances.** Regardless of the serum potassium concentration at presentation, total body potassium depletion is likely. Potassium concentrations can decrease rapidly as insulin, and then glucose, therapy improves acidosis and potassium is exchanged for intracellular hydrogen ions. When adequate urine output is shown, potassium should be added to the IV fluids. Potassium replacement should be given as 50% potassium chloride and 50% potassium phosphate at a concentration of 20 to 40 mEq/L. This combination provides phosphate for replacement of deficits, but avoids excess phosphate administration, which may precipitate hypocalcemia. If the serum potassium level is greater than 6 mEq/L, potassium should not be added to IV fluids until the potassium level decreases.

**Monitoring.** A flow sheet should be used to record and monitor fluid balance and laboratory measurements. Initial laboratory measurements should include serum glucose, sodium, potassium, chloride, bicarbonate, BUN, creatinine, calcium, phosphate, and magnesium concentrations; arterial or venous pH; and a urinalysis. Serum glucose measurement should be repeated every hour during therapy; electrolyte concentrations should be repeated every 2 to 3 hours. Calcium, phosphate, and magnesium concentrations should be measured initially and every 4 to 6 hours during therapy. Neurologic and mental status should be assessed at frequent intervals. Any complaints of headache or deterioration of mental status should prompt rapid evaluation for possible **cerebral edema**. Indicative symptoms include a decreased sensorium, sudden severe headache, vomiting, change in vital signs (bradycardia, hypertension, apnea), a dilated pupil, ophthalmoplegia, or seizure.

## Complications

Clinically apparent **cerebral edema** occurs in 1% to 5% of cases of DKA. Cerebral edema is the most serious complication of DKA, with a mortality rate of 20% to 80%. The pathogenesis of cerebral edema likely involves osmolar shift resulting in fluid accumulation in the intracellular compartment and cell swelling. Subclinical cerebral edema is common in patients with DKA, but the factors that exacerbate this process leading to symptomatic brain swelling and possible cerebral herniation are not clearly defined. Cerebral edema typically occurs 6 to 12 hours after therapy for DKA is begun, often following a period of apparent clinical improvement. Factors that correlate with increased risk for cerebral edema include higher initial BUN concentration, lower initial $Pco_2$, failure of the serum sodium concentration to increase as glucose concentration decreases during treatment, and treatment with bicarbonate.

Signs of advanced cerebral edema include obtundation, papilledema, pupillary dilation or inequality, hypertension, bradycardia, and apnea. **Treatment** involves the rapid use of IV mannitol, endotracheal intubation, and hyperventilation, and may require the use of a subdural bolt. Other complications of DKA are intracranial thrombosis or infarction, acute tubular necrosis with acute renal failure caused by severe dehydration, pancreatitis, arrhythmias caused by electrolyte abnormalities, pulmonary edema, and bowel ischemia. Peripheral edema occurs commonly 24 to 48 hours after therapy is initiated and may be related to residual elevations in antidiuretic hormone and aldosterone.

## Transition to Outpatient Management

When the acidosis has been corrected and the patient tolerates oral feedings, the IV insulin infusion can be discontinued and a regimen of subcutaneous (SC) insulin injections can be initiated. The first SC insulin dose should be given 30 to 45 minutes before discontinuation of the IV insulin infusion. Further adjustment of the insulin dose should be made over the following 2 to 3 days. A patient already diagnosed with DM1 may be restarted on the prior doses if they were adequate. For a patient with new-onset DM1, typical starting total daily doses are approximately 0.7 U/kg/24 hours for prepubertal patients and approximately 1 U/kg/24 hours for adolescents, using any number of the available insulin combinations. The best and most common choice for making the transition to SC insulin is to begin by giving injections of fast-acting insulin (lispro or aspart or glulisine insulin) with each meal and long- or basal-acting insulin (glargine or detemir) at bedtime. This regimen of multiple daily injections (MDIs) provides the most flexibility but requires the patient to administer many injections per day and to count carbohydrates in food. An alternative to MDIs is a fixed mixed split dosing regimen, with two daily injections. Two thirds of the total daily dose is given in the morning, at breakfast, and one third given in the evening, with dinner (Fig. 171-3). The ratio of insulins in the morning dose should be two-thirds intermediate-acting insulin (NPH), and one-third fast-acting insulin. In the evening, one half of the evening insulin dose should be given as intermediate-acting insulin (NPH), and one half should be given as fast-acting insulin.

Externally worn pumps that provide a continuous SC infusion of fast-acting insulin are available, although not usually at the very onset of DM1. They may be used by all age groups who are highly motivated to achieve tight control.

Serum glucose concentrations should be assessed before each meal, at bedtime, and at 2 to 3 AM to provide information for adjustment of the regimen. Patients and their families should begin learning the principles of diabetes care as soon as possible. Demonstration of ability

to administer insulin injections and test glucose concentrations using a glucometer is necessary before discharge, as is knowledge of hypoglycemia management. Meal planning is crucial to control of glucose in DM1, and nutrition services must be part of the care delivered to the families from the outset.

## Honeymoon Period

In patients with new onset of DM1 who do not have DKA, the beta cell mass has not been completely destroyed. The remaining functional beta cells seem to recover function with insulin treatment. When this occurs, exogenous insulin requirements decrease. This is a period of stable blood glucose control, often with nearly normal glucose concentrations. This phase of the disease, known as the honeymoon period, usually starts in the first weeks of therapy and often continues for 3 to 6 months, but can last 2 years.

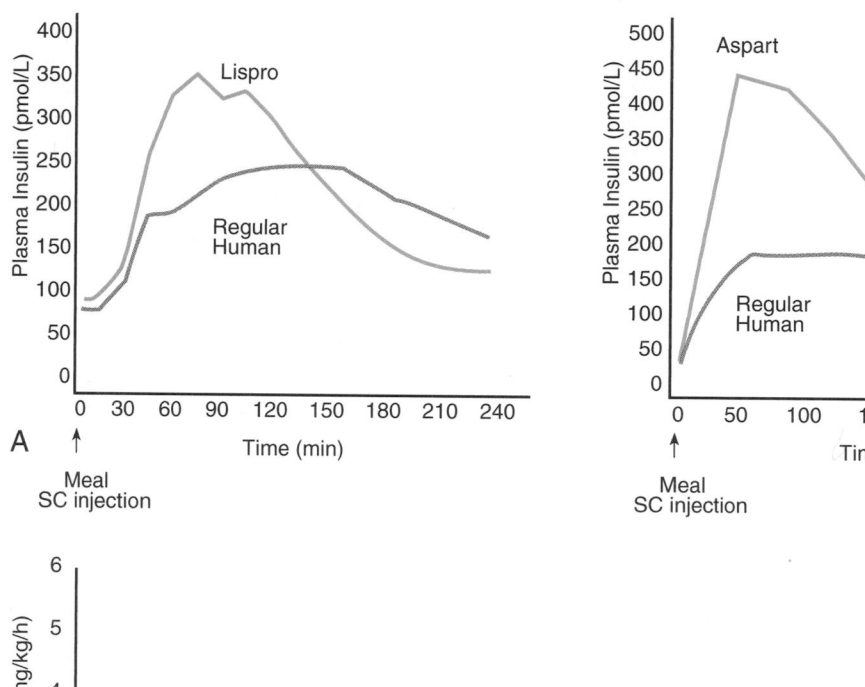
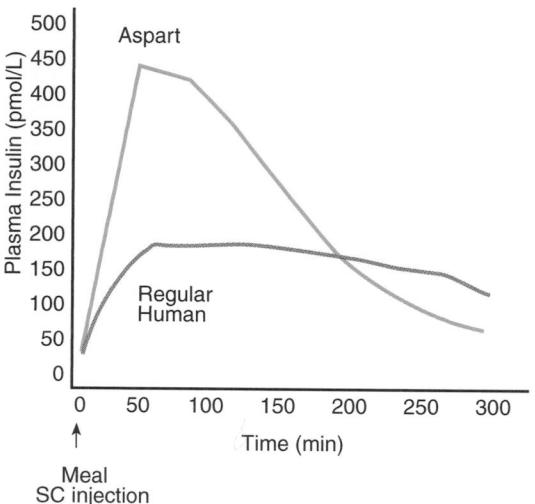
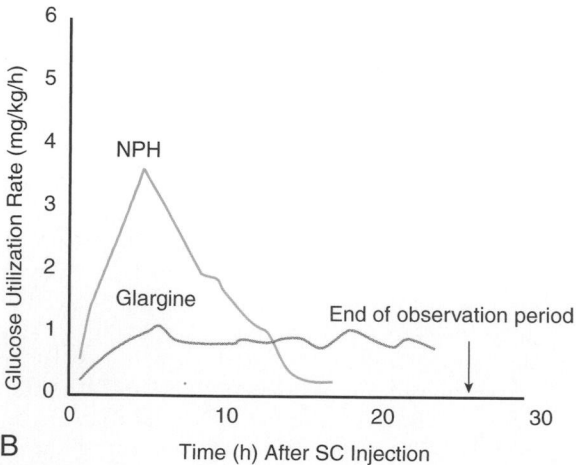

**FIGURE 171-3**

Representative profiles of insulin effect using combined injection regimens: intermediate-acting insulin (NPH or lente) and regular (short-acting) insulin. **A,** Short-acting lispro, regular, or aspart insulins. **B,** Long-acting NPH or glargine profiles. SC, subcutaneous. (Adapted from Mudaliar SR, Lindberg FA, Joyce M, et al: Insulin aspart [B28 asp-insulin]: A fast-acting analog of human insulin: Absorption kinetics and action profile compared with regular human insulin in healthy nondiabetic subjects. *Diabetes Care* 22:1501–1506, 1999; and Lepore M, Kurzals R, Pampanelli S, et al: Pharmacokinetics and dynamics of S.C. injection of the long-acting glargine [HOE 901] in T1DM. *Diabetes* 48[Suppl 1]:A97, 1999.)

## Outpatient Type 1 Diabetes Mellitus Management

Management of DM1 in children requires a comprehensive approach, with attention to medical, nutritional, and psychosocial issues. Therapeutic strategies should be flexible, with the individual needs of each patient and the family taken into account. Optimal care involves a team of diabetes professionals, including a physician, a diabetes nurse educator, a dietitian, and a social worker or psychologist.

### Goals

The Diabetes Control and Complications Trial established that intensive insulin therapy, with the goal of maintaining blood glucose concentrations as close to normal as possible, can delay the onset and slow the progression of complications of diabetes (retinopathy, nephropathy, neuropathy). Attaining this goal using intensive insulin therapy can increase the risk of hypoglycemia. The adverse effects of hypoglycemia in young children may be significant because the immature CNS may be more susceptible to glycopenia. Although the risk for diabetic complications increases with duration of diabetes, there is controversy as to whether the rate of increase of risk may be slower in the prepubertal years than in adolescence and adulthood. It is safe to establish goals to achieve tight control of blood glucose concentrations in childhood.

The goals of therapy differ, depending on the age of the patient. For children younger than 5 years old, an appropriate goal is maintenance of blood glucose concentrations between 80 and 180 mg/dL. For school age children, 80 to 150 mg/dL is a reasonable target range. For adolescents, the goal is 70 to 150 mg/dL. Goals of therapy also should take into account other individual characteristics, such as a past history of severe hypoglycemia and the abilities of the patient and family.

### Insulin Regimens

Many types of insulin differ in duration of action and time to peak effect (Table 171-2). These insulins can be used in various combinations, depending on the needs and goals of the individual patient. The most commonly used regimen is that of multiple injections of fast-acting insulin given with meals in combination with long-acting basal insulin given at bedtime. This regimen provides flexibility but requires administration of many injections per day and will require assistance for young children. After the total daily dose of insulin is determined, 50% is given usually at bed time as long-acting insulin, while the remainder is given as fast-acting insulin, divided according to the need for corrections of high glucose levels and for meals. To correct for hyperglycemia, one determines the insulin sensitivity using the 1800 rule, by dividing 1800 by the total daily dose of insulin to determine how many mg/dL of glucose will decrease with 1 unit of insulin. The insulin:carbohydrate ratio is used to calculate insulin for the carbohydrate content of food; 450 divided by the total daily dose determines the number of grams of carbohydrate that requires 1 unit of insulin.

| TABLE 171-2  Insulin Preparations | | | |
|---|---|---|---|
| Type of Insulin | Onset | Peak Action | Duration |
| **VERY SHORT-ACTING** | | | |
| Lispro, aspart | 10–20 min | 30–90 min | 3 hr |
| **SHORT-ACTING** | | | |
| Regular | 30 min–hr | 2–4 hr | 6–10 hr |
| **INTERMEDIATE-ACTING** | | | |
| NPH | 1–4 hr | 4–12 hr | 16–24 hr |
| Lente | 1–4 hr | 4–12 hr | 12–24 hr |
| **LONG-ACTING** | | | |
| Protamine zinc | 4–6 hr | 8–20 hr | 24–30 hr |
| Ultralente | 4–6 hr | 8–20 hr | 24–36 hr |
| Glargine | 1–2 hr | No peak | 24–30 hr |

When it is not possible for the patient to receive an insulin injection at midday (e.g., during school hours) one can use intermediate-acting insulin (NPH) in the morning along with the fast-acting insulin (see Fig. 171-3). Patients using this regimen must adhere to a meal schedule with consistent breakfast, lunch, and dinner and snacks as needed, and must receive a second evening injection of NPH; this can be difficult to coordinate with variations in daily activities. Pumps that provide a continuous SC infusion of short-acting insulin also are available and are being used by children and adolescents who are highly motivated to achieve tight control.

Lispro and aspart and glulisine insulins are synthetic human insulin analogs in which amino acid alterations result in fast absorption and onset of action (see Table 171-2). Because of the short duration of action, these are used in combination with long-acting insulin. Glargine and detemir are insulin analogs in which the amino acid alterations result in increased solubility at acidic pH and decreased solubility at physiologic pH. Glargine and detemir have been shown to have a duration of greater than 24 hours and act as a basal insulin.

Newly diagnosed patients in the honeymoon period may require 0.4 to 0.6 U/kg/24 hours. Prepubertal patients with diabetes longer than 1 to 2 years typically require 0.5 to 1 U/kg/24 hours. During middle adolescence, when elevated growth hormone (GH) concentrations produce relative insulin resistance, insulin requirements increase by 40% to 50%, and doses of 1 to 2 U/kg/24 hours are typical.

### Nutrition

Balancing the daily meal plan with the dosages of insulin is crucial for maintaining serum glucose concentrations within the target range and avoiding hypoglycemia or hyperglycemia. The content and schedule of meals vary according to the type of insulin regimen used; it is recommended that carbohydrates contribute 50% to 65% of the total calories; protein, 12% to 20%; and fat, less than 30%. Saturated fat should contribute less than 10% of the total caloric intake, and cholesterol intake should be less than 300 mg/24 hours. High fiber content is recommended.

Patients using MDIs or the insulin pump can maintain a more flexible meal schedule with regard to the timing of meals and the carbohydrate content. These patients give an injection of insulin before or immediately after each meal, with the total dose calculated according to the carbohydrate content of the meal. Further adjustments in the dose can be made based on the measured serum glucose concentration and plans for exercise during the day. Children using a twice a day combination of intermediate-acting and fast-acting insulins need to maintain a relatively consistent meal schedule so that carbohydrate absorption and insulin action peaks correspond. A typical meal schedule for a patient using this type of regimen involves three meals and three snacks daily. The total carbohydrate content of the meals and snacks should be kept constant.

## Blood Glucose Testing

Blood glucose should be routinely monitored (with rapid glucose meters) before each meal and at bedtime. Hypoglycemia during the night or excessive variability in the morning glucose concentrations should prompt additional testing at 2 or 3 AM to ensure that there is no consistent hypoglycemia or hyperglycemia. During periods of intercurrent illness or when blood glucose concentrations are higher than 300 mg/dL, urine ketones also should be tested.

## Long-Term Glycemic Control

Measurements of glycohemoglobin or hemoglobin $A_{1c}$ reflect the average blood glucose concentration over the preceding 3 months and provide a means for assessing long-term glycemic control. Glycohemoglobin should be measured four times a year, and the results should be used for counseling of patients. Table 171-3 summarizes the correlation between hemoglobin $A_{1c}$ or glycohemoglobin and daily blood glucose measurements. Measurements of glycohemoglobin or hemoglobin $A_{1c}$ are inaccurate in patients with hemoglobinopathies. Glycosylated albumin or fructosamine can be used in these cases.

### TABLE 171-3 Biochemical Indices of Glycemic Control

| Poor Control | Average Control | Intensive Control |
|---|---|---|
| HgbA$_{1c}$ > 10% | HgbA$_{1c}$ > 8–10% | HgbA$_{1c}$ 6–8% |
| Average blood glucose > 240 mg/dL | Average blood glucose 180–240 mg/dL | Average blood glucose 120–180 mg/dL |

HgbA$_{1c}$, hemoglobin A$_{1c}$.

## Complications

Patients with DM1 for more than 3 to 5 years should receive an annual ophthalmologic examination for retinopathy. Urine should be collected annually for assessment of microalbuminuria; if present, microalbuminuria suggests early renal dysfunction and indicates a high risk of progression to nephropathy. *Treatment* with angiotensin-converting enzyme inhibitors may halt the progression of microalbuminuria. In children with DM1, annual cholesterol measurements and periodic assessment of blood pressure are recommended. Early detection of hypertension and hypercholesterolemia with appropriate intervention can help to limit future risk of coronary disease.

## Other Disorders

Chronic lymphocytic thyroiditis is particularly common and can result in hypothyroidism. Because symptoms can be subtle, thyroid function tests should be performed annually. Other disorders that occur with increased frequency in children with DM1 include celiac disease, IgA deficiency, Addison disease, and peptic ulcer disease.

## Special Problems: Hypoglycemia

Hypoglycemia occurs commonly in patients with DM1. For patients in adequate or better control, it is expected to occur on average once or twice a week. Severe episodes of hypoglycemia, resulting in seizures or coma or requiring assistance from another person, occur in 10% to 25% of these patients per year.

Hypoglycemia in patients with DM1 results from a relative excess of insulin in relation to the serum glucose concentration. This excess can be caused by alterations in the dose, timing, or absorption of insulin; alterations of carbohydrate intake; or changes in insulin sensitivity resulting from exercise. Defective counter-regulatory responses also contribute to hypoglycemia. Abnormal glucagon responses to falling serum glucose concentrations develop within the first few years of the disease, and abnormalities in epinephrine release occur after a longer duration.

**Lack of awareness** of hypoglycemia occurs in approximately 25% of patients with diabetes. Recent episodes of hypoglycemia may play a role in the pathophysiology of hypoglycemia unawareness; after an episode of hypoglycemia, autonomic responses to subsequent episodes are reduced. A return of symptoms of hypoglycemia can be exhibited in these patients after 2 to 3 weeks of strict avoidance of hypoglycemic episodes.

Symptoms of hypoglycemia include symptoms resulting from neuroglycopenia (headache, visual changes, confusion, irritability, or seizures) and symptoms resulting from the catecholamine response (tremors, tachycardia, diaphoresis, or anxiety) (see Chapter 172). Mild episodes can be treated with administration of rapidly absorbed oral glucose (glucose gel or tablets, fruit juices, and non-diet or non–artificially sweetened sodas). More severe episodes that result in seizures or loss of consciousness at home should be treated with glucagon injections. IV glucose should be given in hospital settings.

## Prognosis

Long-term complications of DM1 include retinopathy, nephropathy, neuropathy, and macrovascular disease. Evidence of organ damage caused by hyperglycemia is rare in patients with duration of diabetes of less than 5 to 10 years, and clinically apparent disease rarely occurs before 10 to 15 years' duration. The eventual morbidity and fatality attributable to these disorders are substantial. Diabetic retinopathy is the leading cause of blindness in the United States. Nephropathy eventually occurs in 30% to 40% and accounts for approximately 30% of all new adult cases of end-stage renal disease. Neuropathy occurs in 30% to 40% of postpubertal patients with DM1 and leads to sensory, motor, or autonomic deficits. Macrovascular disease results in an increased risk of myocardial infarction and stroke among individuals with diabetes.

Intensive control of diabetes, employing frequent blood glucose testing and multiple daily injections of insulin or an insulin pump can reduce substantially the development or progression of diabetic complications. Intensive management resulted in a 76% reduction of risk for retinopathy, a 39% reduction in microalbuminuria, and a 60% reduction in clinical neuropathy. For pubertal and adult patients, these benefits of intensive therapy likely outweigh the increase in risk for hypoglycemia. For younger patients, in whom the risks for hypoglycemia are greater, and the benefits of tight glucose control may be lower, a less intensive regimen may be appropriate.

## NON–INSULIN-DEPENDENT (TYPE 2) DIABETES MELLITUS

### Pathophysiology

DM2 can occur as the result of various pathophysiologic processes; however, the most common form results from peripheral insulin resistance and compensatory hyperinsulinemia followed thereafter with failure of the pancreas to maintain adequate insulin secretion (see Table 171-1). The precise defects underlying the insulin-resistant state and the eventual pancreatic beta cell failure are complex and, while still poorly understood, are beginning to be understood at the genetic level. Other subtypes of DM2 also can occur in children. **Maturity-onset diabetes of youth (MODY)** comprises a group of dominantly inherited forms of relatively mild diabetes. Insulin resistance does not occur in these patients; instead the primary abnormality is an insufficient insulin secretory response to glycemic stimulation.

### Epidemiology

The prevalence of DM2 in children is increasing in parallel with childhood obesity and is highest in children of ethnic groups with a high prevalence of DM2 in adults, including Native Americans, Hispanic Americans, and African Americans. Obesity, the metabolic syndrome, ethnicity, and a family history of DM2 are thus risk factors. Among some clinically assumed to have DM2, autoantibodies to the pancreas are present, compounding the difficulty in differentiating DM1 from DM2 at the outset.

### Clinical Manifestations and Differential Diagnosis

Fasting and postprandial glucose levels for diagnosis of DM2 are the same as those for DM1. The diagnosis of DM2 may be suspected on the basis of polyuria and polydipsia and in a background of the metabolic syndrome. Differentiating DM2 from DM1 in children on clinical grounds only can be challenging. The possibility of DM2 should be considered in patients who are obese, have a strong family history of DM2, have other characteristics of the metabolic syndrome and acanthosis nigricans on physical examination, or have absence of antibodies to beta cell antigens at the time of diagnosis of diabetes. **Acanthosis nigricans,** a dermatologic manifestation of hyperinsulinism, presents as hyperkeratotic pigmentation in the nape of the neck and in flexural areas. Although ketoacidosis occurs far more commonly in DM1, it also can occur in patients with DM2 under conditions of physiologic stress and cannot be used as an absolute differentiating factor. DM2 can be confirmed by evaluation of insulin or C-peptide responses to stimulation with oral carbohydrate and in the absence of islet cell autoreactivity.

### Therapy

DM2 is the result of a combination of insulin resistance and relative insulin deficiency, and a secretory beta cell defect. Asymptomatic patients with mildly elevated glucose values (slightly > 126 mg/dL for fasting or slightly > 200 mg/dL for random glucose) may be managed initially with lifestyle modifications, including nutrition therapy (dietary adjustments) and increased exercise. Exercise has been shown to decrease insulin resistance. In most children with new-onset, uncomplicated DM2, oral hypoglycemic agents are usually the first line of therapy. These medications include insulin secretagogues and insulin sensitizers. The most common treatment is either metformin or one of the thiazolidinediones. A rare side effect of metformin is lactic acidosis, which occurs mainly in patients with compromised renal function. The most common side effect is gastrointestinal upset. If ketonuria or ketoacidosis occurs, insulin treatment is necessary at first to achieve adequate glycemic control, but may be discontinued within weeks with continuation of oral medications. Oral drugs may be used as combinations.

Because DM2 may have a long preclinical course, early diagnosis is possible, including prevention in subjects at risk who have the **metabolic syndrome**. Emerging data indicate that treatment with insulin sensitizers may delay or prevent development of the full-blown disease. Significant lifestyle modifications, such as improved eating habits and increased exercise, have a role in preventing or decreasing the morbidity of DM2. Finally, it is critical to monitor and manage the other components of the metabolic syndrome, such as advanced pubertal development, hypertension, hyperlipidemia, and polycystic ovary syndrome in females.

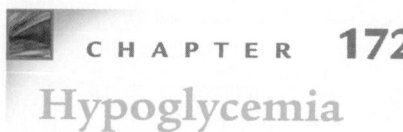

# CHAPTER 172

# Hypoglycemia

Hypoglycemia in infancy and childhood can result from a large variety of hormonal and metabolic defects (Table 172-1). Hypoglycemia occurs most frequently in the early neonatal period, often as a result of inadequate energy stores to meet the disproportionately large metabolic needs of premature or small for gestational age newborns. Hypoglycemia during the first few days of life in an otherwise normal newborn is less frequent and warrants concern (see Chapter 6). After the initial 2 to 3 days of life, hypoglycemia is far less common and is more frequently the result of endocrine or metabolic disorders.

## DEFINITION

The **diagnosis** of hypoglycemia should be made on the basis of a low serum glucose concentration, symptoms compatible with hypoglycemia, and resolution of the symptoms after administration of glucose.

Serum glucose concentrations less than 45 mg/dL are considered to be abnormal and necessitate treatment. Serum glucose concentrations greater than 55 mg/dL occasionally can occur in normal individuals, especially with prolonged fasting, but should be considered suspect, particularly if there are concurrent symptoms of hypoglycemia (Table 172-2).

## CLINICAL MANIFESTATIONS

The symptoms and signs of hypoglycemia result from direct depression of the central nervous system (CNS) owing to lack of energy substrate and the counter-regulatory adrenergic response to low glucose via catecholamine

---

**TABLE 172-1  Classification of Hypoglycemia in Infants and Children**

| ABNORMALITIES IN THE HORMONAL SIGNAL INDICATING HYPOGLYCEMIA | FATTY ACID OXIDATION |
|---|---|
| *Counterregulatory Hormone Deficiency* | Long-, medium-, or short-chain fatty acid acyl-CoA dehydrogenase deficiency |
| Panhypopituitarism | Carnitine deficiency (primary or secondary) |
| Isolated growth hormone deficiency | Carnitine palmitoyltransferase deficiency |
| ACTH deficiency | *Other* |
| Addison disease | Enzymatic defects |
| Glucagon deficiency |   Galactosemia |
| Epinephrine deficiency |   Hereditary fructose intolerance |
| *Hyperinsulinism* |   Propionicacidemia |
| Infant of a diabetic mother |   Methylmalonic acidemia |
| Infant with erythroblastosis fetalis |   Tyrosinosis |
| Persistent hyperinsulinemic hypoglycemias of infancy |   Glutaric aciduria |
| Beta cell adenoma (insulinoma) | Global hepatic dysfunction |
| Beckwith-Wiedemann syndrome | Reye syndrome |
| Anti-insulin receptor antibodies | Hepatitis |
| | Heart failure |
| **INADEQUATE SUBSTRATE** | Sepsis, shock |
| Prematurity/small for gestational age infant | Carcinoma/sarcoma (IGF-2 secretion) |
| Ketotic hypoglycemia | Malnutrition/starvation |
| Maple syrup urine disease | Hyperviscosity syndrome |
| **DISORDERS OF METABOLIC RESPONSE PATHWAYS** | **DRUGS/INTOXICATIONS** |
| *Glycogenolysis* | Oral hypoglycemic agents |
| Glucose-6-phosphatase deficiency | Insulin |
| Amylo-1,6-glucosidase deficiency | Alcohol |
| Liver phosphorylase deficiency | Salicylates |
| Glycogen synthase deficiency | Propranolol |
| *Gluconeogenesis* | Valproic acid |
| Fructose-1,6-diphosphatase deficiency | Pentamidine |
| Pyruvate carboxylase deficiency | Ackee fruit (unripe) |
| Phosphenolpyruvate carboxykinase deficiency | Quinine |
| | Trimethoprim-sulfamethoxazole (with renal failure) |

ACTH, adrenocorticotropic hormone; acyl-CoA, acyl coenzyme A; IGF-2, insulin-like growth factor-2.

**TABLE 172-2 Symptoms and Signs of Hypoglycemia**

| Features Associated with Epinephrine Release* | Features Associated with Cerebral Glycopenia |
|---|---|
| Perspiration | Headache |
| Palpitation (tachycardia) | Mental confusion |
| Pallor | Somnolence |
| Paresthesia | Dysarthria |
| Trembling | Personality changes |
| Anxiety | Inability to concentrate |
| Weakness | Staring |
| Nausea | Hunger |
| Vomiting | Convulsions |
| | Ataxia |
| | Coma |
| | Diplopia |
| | Stroke |

*These features and perceptions of the features may be blunted if the patient is receiving β-blocking agents.

secretion designed to correct hypoglycemia (see Table 172-2). Compared with older children, infants do not usually show adrenergic symptoms. The neuroglycopenic symptoms and signs of hypoglycemia in infants are relatively nonspecific and include jitteriness, feeding difficulties, pallor, hypotonia, hypothermia, episodes of apnea and bradycardia, depressed levels of consciousness, and seizures. In older children, symptoms and signs include confusion, irritability, headaches, visual changes, tremors, pallor, sweating, tachycardia, weakness, seizures, and coma.

Failure to recognize and treat severe prolonged hypoglycemia can result in serious long-term morbidity, including mental retardation and nonhypoglycemic seizures. Younger infants and patients with more severe or prolonged hypoglycemia are at greatest risk for adverse outcomes.

## PATHOPHYSIOLOGY

### Hormonal Signal

Normal regulation of serum glucose concentrations requires appropriate interaction of a number of hormonal signals and metabolic pathways. An overview of these pathways is presented in Figure 172-1. In a normal individual, a decrease in serum glucose concentrations leads to suppression of insulin secretion and increased secretion of the counter-regulatory hormones (growth hormone [GH], cortisol, glucagon, and epinephrine) (see Fig. 172-1). This hormonal signal promotes the release of amino acids (particularly alanine) from muscle to fuel gluconeogenesis and the release of triglyceride from adipose tissue stores to provide free fatty acids (FFAs) for hepatic ketogenesis. FFAs and ketones serve as alternate fuels for muscle; the brain cannot transport FFAs across the blood-brain barrier. This hormonal signal also stimulates the breakdown of hepatic glycogen and promotes gluconeogenesis. Failure of any of the components of this hormonal signal can lead to hypoglycemia.

### Hyperinsulinemia

A lack of suppression of insulin secretion in response to low serum glucose concentrations can occur in infants, but is uncommon beyond the neonatal period. This situation arises most frequently in infants of diabetic mothers who were exposed to high concentrations of maternally derived glucose in utero, resulting in fetal islet cell hyperplasia. The hyperinsulinemic state is transient, usually lasting hours to days.

Hyperinsulinism that persists beyond a few days of age can result from distinct genetic disorders affecting glucose-regulated insulin release. These were previously referred to as nesidioblastosis, or **persistent hyperinsulinemic hypoglycemia of the newborn**. In these infants, hyperplasia of the pancreatic islet cells develops in the absence of excess stimulation by maternal diabetes. Some patients with persistent hyperinsulinemic hypoglycemia of the newborn have genetic abnormalities of the islet cell sulfonylurea receptor or other genetic defects that alter the function of the adenosine triphosphate (ATP)-sensitive potassium channel that regulates insulin secretion. Hyperinsulinism also can occur in **Beckwith-Wiedemann syndrome**, a condition characterized by neonatal somatic gigantism: macrosomia, macroglossia, omphalocele, visceromegaly, and earlobe creases.

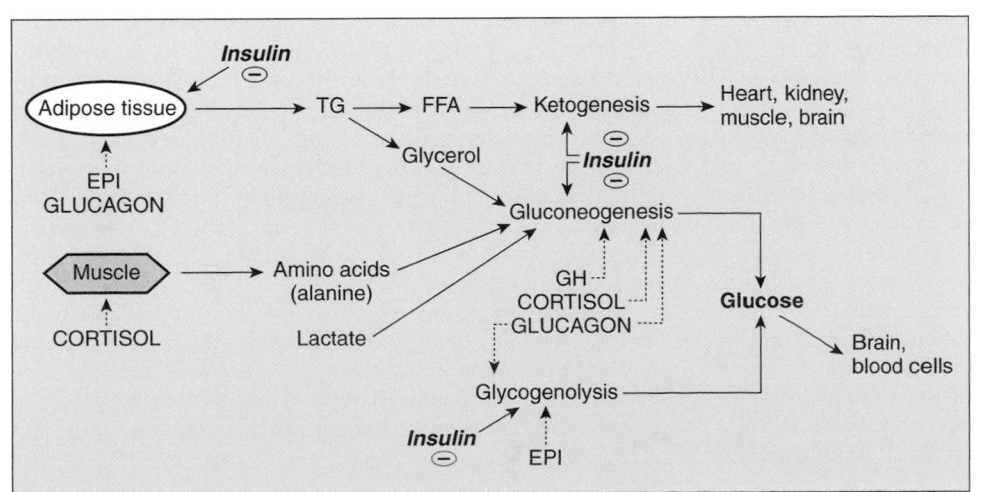

**FIGURE 172-1**

**Regulation of serum glucose.**
— represents inhibitions. EPI, epinephrine; FFA, free fatty acid; GH, growth hormone; TG, triglyceride.

Regardless of the cause, neonates with hyperinsulinism are characteristically large for gestational age (see Chapter 60). Hypoglycemia is severe and frequently occurs within 1 to 3 hours of a feeding. Glucose requirements are increased, often two to three times the normal basal glucose requirement of 6 to 8 mg/kg/min. The *diagnosis* of hyperinsulinism is confirmed by the detection of serum insulin concentrations greater than 5 µU/mL during an episode of hypoglycemia. The absence of serum and urine ketones at the time of hypoglycemia is an important diagnostic feature, distinguishing hyperinsulinism from defects in counter-regulatory hormone secretion.

*Treatment* initially involves the infusion of intravenous (IV) glucose at high rates and of diazoxide to suppress insulin secretion. If diazoxide therapy is unsuccessful because the receptor on which it acts is dysfunctional, long-acting somatostatin analogs can be tried. Often, medical therapy for persistent hyperinsulinemic hypoglycemia of the newborn is unsuccessful, and subtotal (90%) pancreatectomy is required to prevent long-term neurologic sequelae of hypoglycemia.

In children, hyperinsulinemia is rare and usually results from an **islet cell adenoma**. Children with this condition characteristically have a voracious appetite, obesity, and accelerated linear growth. As in infants, *diagnosis* requires demonstration of insulin concentrations greater than 5 µU/mL during an episode of hypoglycemia. Computed tomography (CT), magnetic resonance imaging (MRI), or radioisotope imaging of the pancreas should be attempted, but visualization of an adenoma is usually difficult. Surgical removal of the adenoma is curative.

## Factitious Hyperinsulinemia

In rare cases, insulin or a hypoglycemic medication is administered by a parent or caregiver to a child as a form of child abuse, which is a condition referred to as **Munchausen syndrome by proxy**. This *diagnosis* should be suspected if extremely high insulin concentrations are detected (>100 µU/mL). C-peptide concentrations are low or undetectable, which confirms that the insulin is from an exogenous source.

## Defects in Counter-regulatory Hormones

Abnormalities in the secretion of counter-regulatory hormones that produce hypoglycemia usually involve GH, cortisol, or both. Deficiencies in glucagon and epinephrine secretion are rare. GH and cortisol deficiency occur as a result of hypopituitarism. Hypopituitarism results from congenital hypoplasia or aplasia of the pituitary or, more commonly, from deficiency of hypothalamic releasing factors (see Chapter 173). Clues to this diagnosis in infants include the presence of hypoglycemia in association with midline facial or neurologic defects (e.g., cleft lip and palate or absence of the corpus callosum), pendular nystagmus (indicating visual impairment from possible abnormalities in the development of the optic nerves, which can occur in septo-optic dysplasia), and the presence of microphallus and cryptorchidism in boys (indicating abnormalities in gonadotropin secretion). Jaundice and hepatomegaly also can occur, simulating neonatal hepatitis. Despite the presence of GH deficiency, these infants are usually of normal size at birth. Older children with hypopituitarism usually have short stature and a subnormal growth velocity.

Deficient cortisol secretion also can occur in primary adrenal insufficiency resulting from a variety of causes. In infants, it often results from congenital adrenal hyperplasia (CAH), most frequently as a result of 21-hydroxylase deficiency (see Chapters 177 and 178). In older children, primary adrenal insufficiency is seen most frequently in **Addison disease**, but it also can occur in adrenoleukodystrophy and other disorders (see Chapter 178). Addison disease should be suspected if there is hyperpigmentation of the skin, a history of salt craving, and confirmation of hyponatremia, and hyperkalemia.

Confirmation of GH or cortisol deficiency as the cause of hypoglycemia requires the detection of low serum GH and cortisol concentrations during an episode of hypoglycemia or after other stimulatory testing. In contrast to hyperinsulinism, serum and urine ketones are positive at the time of hypoglycemia, and FFAs are elevated. Treatment involves supplementation of the deficient hormones, GH or cortisol, in physiologic doses.

## ENERGY STORES

Sufficient energy stores in the form of glycogen, adipose tissue, and muscle are necessary to respond appropriately to hypoglycemia. Deficiencies in these stores are a common cause of hypoglycemia in neonates who are small for gestational age or premature (see Chapter 60). Beyond the early neonatal period, energy stores are usually sufficient to meet the metabolic requirements except in malnourished children. Release of substrate from energy stores, for gluconeogenesis and fatty acid oxidation, is thought to be abnormal in one common form of childhood hypoglycemia, ketotic hypoglycemia.

## IDIOPATHIC KETOTIC HYPOGLYCEMIA

Idiopathic ketotic hypoglycemia is usually seen in children between 18 months and 5 years of age. It is a common cause of new-onset hypoglycemia in this age group. Patients have symptoms of hypoglycemia after a period of prolonged fasting, often in the setting of an intercurrent illness with decreased feeding. Children with this disorder are often thin and small and may have a history of being small for gestational age. Defective mobilization of alanine from muscle to fuel gluconeogenesis is thought to be the cause, although the condition may derive mostly from having lower fuel reserves. Because there are no specific diagnostic tests for this disorder, ketotic hypoglycemia is a *diagnosis of exclusion*.

*Treatment* involves avoidance of fasting and frequent feedings of a high-protein, high-carbohydrate diet. Patients may require hospitalization for IV glucose infusion if they cannot maintain adequate oral intake during a period of illness. The disorder usually resolves spontaneously by 7 to 8 years of age.

# METABOLIC RESPONSE PATHWAYS

Maintenance of normal serum glucose concentrations in the fasting state requires glucose production via glycogenolysis and gluconeogenesis and the production of alternative energy sources (FFAs and ketones) via lipolysis and fatty acid oxidation.

## Glycogenolysis

Glycogen storage diseases occur in a variety of subtypes that differ in severity (see Chapter 52). Among the subtypes that result in hypoglycemia, the most severe form is glucose-6-phosphatase deficiency which is characterized by severe hypoglycemia, massive hepatomegaly, growth retardation, and lactic acidosis. In contrast, deficiencies in the glycogen phosphorylase enzymes may cause isolated hepatomegaly with or without hypoglycemia.

The *diagnosis* of glycogen storage disease is suggested by a finding of hepatomegaly without splenomegaly. Ketosis occurs with hypoglycemic episodes. Confirmation of the diagnosis requires specific biochemical studies of leukocytes or liver biopsy specimens. *Treatment* involves frequent high-carbohydrate feedings during the day and continuous feedings at night via nasogastric tube. Feedings of uncooked cornstarch during bedtime are sufficient to maintain serum glucose concentrations in some patients. Treatment can prevent night-time hypoglycemia.

## Gluconeogenesis

Defects in gluconeogenesis are uncommon and include fructose-1,6-diphosphatase deficiency and phosphoenolpyruvate carboxykinase deficiency. Affected patients exhibit fasting hypoglycemia, hepatomegaly caused by fatty infiltration, lactic acidosis, and hyperuricemia. Ketosis occurs and FFA and alanine concentrations are high. *Treatment* involves frequent high-carbohydrate, low-protein feedings (see Chapter 52).

## Fatty Acid Oxidation

Fatty acid oxidation disorders of ketogenesis include the fatty acid acyl-coenzyme A (CoA) dehydrogenase deficiencies; long-chain, medium-chain, and short-chain acyl-CoA dehydrogenase deficiencies; and hereditary carnitine deficiency (see Chapter 55). Of these disorders, medium-chain acyl-CoA dehydrogenase deficiency is the most common; it occurs in 1 in 9000 to 1 in 15,000 live births. Patients often are well in infancy and have the first episode of hypoglycemia at 2 years of age or older. Episodes of hypoglycemia usually occur with prolonged fasting or during episodes of intercurrent illness.

Mild hepatomegaly may be present along with mild hyperammonemia, hyperuricemia, and mild elevations in hepatic transaminases. Ketone concentrations are low or undetected. The *diagnosis* is confirmed by the finding of elevated concentrations of dicarboxylic acids in the urine. *Treatment* involves avoidance of fasting.

# OTHER METABOLIC DISORDERS

Many metabolic disorders can lead to hypoglycemia, including galactosemia, hereditary fructose intolerance, and disorders of organic acid metabolism (see Table 172-1). Hypoglycemia in these disorders is usually a reflection of global hepatic dysfunction secondary to the buildup of hepatotoxic intermediates. Many of these disorders present with low concentrations of ketone bodies because ketogenesis also is affected. The finding of non–glucose-reducing substances in the urine suggests a diagnosis of galactosemia or hereditary fructose intolerance. Occurrence of symptoms after ingestion of fructose or sucrose **suggests hereditary fructose intolerance**. *Treatment* requires dietary restriction of the specific offending substances.

# MEDICATIONS AND INTOXICATION

Hypoglycemia can occur as an adverse effect of numerous medications, including insulin, oral hypoglycemic agents, and propranolol, and as a result of salicylate intoxication. Valproate toxicity can cause a disorder similar to that seen in the fatty acid oxidation defects. Ethanol ingestion also can cause hypoglycemia, especially in younger children, because the metabolism of ethanol results in the depletion of cofactors necessary for gluconeogenesis.

# DIAGNOSIS

While the list of causes of hypoglycemia is long and complex, establishing the *etiology* in a particular patient is important. Frequently, it is difficult to make an accurate diagnosis until one can obtain a *critical sample* of blood and urine at the time of the hypoglycemic episode. In a child with unexplained hypoglycemia, a serum sample should be obtained before treatment for the measurement of glucose and insulin, GH, cortisol, FFAs, and $\beta$-hydroxybutyrate and aceto-acetate. Measurement of serum lactate levels also should be considered. A urine specimen should be obtained for measuring ketones and reducing substances. Hypoglycemia without ketonuria suggests hyperinsulinism or a defect in fatty acid oxidation. The results of this initial testing can establish whether endocrine causes are responsible and, if not, provide initial information regarding which types of metabolic disorders are most likely. Whenever possible, additional samples of blood and urine should be frozen for further analysis if necessary.

# EMERGENCY MANAGEMENT

Acute care of a patient with hypoglycemia consists of rapid administration of IV glucose (2 mL/kg of 10% dextrose in water). After the initial bolus, an infusion of IV glucose should provide approximately 1.5 times the normal hepatic glucose production rate (8–12 mg/kg/min in infants, 6–8 mg/kg/min in children). This infusion allows for suppression of the catabolic state and prevents further decompensation in patients with certain metabolic disorders. Higher infusion rates may be needed for hyperinsulinemic states. If adrenal insufficiency is suspected, stress doses of glucocorticoids should be administered.

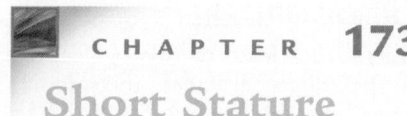

CHAPTER **173**

# Short Stature

## GROWTH

Normal growth is the final common pathway of many factors, including endocrine, environmental, nutritional, and genetic influences (see Chapter 5). A normal linear growth pattern is good evidence of overall health and can be considered a *bioassay* for the well-being of the whole child. The effects of certain hormones on growth and ultimate height are listed in Table 173-1. Just as various factors influence stature, stature itself influences psychological, social, and potentially economic well-being. Parental concern about the psychosocial consequences of abnormal stature often causes a family to seek medical attention. There is an increased bias toward *heightism*, particularly among males. Physicians must be sensitized to the overall context of a particular youngster's attention to stature.

### Growth Hormone Physiology

Growth hormone (GH) secretion is pulsatile, stimulated by hypothalamic GH-releasing factor (GRF) and inhibited by GH release inhibitory factor (somatostatin, SRIF), which interact with their individual receptors on the somatotrope in a noncompetitive manner. GH is also stimulated by ghrelin, produced in the stomach. GH circulates bound to a GH-binding protein (GHBP) which is the proteolytic product of the extracellular domain of the membrane-bound GH receptor; GHBP abundance reflects the abundance of GH receptors. GH has direct effects on tissue and also causes production and secretion of insulin-like growth factor-1 (IGF-1) in many tissues. IGF-1 is most closely associated with postnatal growth. GH stimulates IGF production in liver along with production of the acid-labile subunit (ALS) and the IGF-binding protein (IGF-BP3); this forms the complex that delivers IGF-1 to tissue. Serum concentrations of IGF-1 follow serum concentrations of GH. IGF-BP3 is measurable in clinical assays and is itself GH dependent, but less influenced by nutrition and age than is IGF-1; measuring IGF-1 and IGF-BP3 is useful in evaluating GH adequacy, particularly in infancy and early childhood. IGF-1 production is influenced by disease states such as malnutrition, chronic renal and liver disease, hypothyroidism, or obesity.

IGF-1 acts primarily as a paracrine and autocrine agent, so the IGF-1 measured in the peripheral circulation is far removed from the site of action and is an imperfect reflection of IGF-1 physiology. IGF-1 resembles insulin in structure, and the IGF-1 receptor resembles the insulin receptor, so cross-reaction of one agent, if present in excess, can cause physiologic effects usually attributed to the other agent. When IGF-1 attaches to its membrane-bound receptor, second messengers are stimulated to change the physiology of the cell and produce growth effects.

### Measurement of Growth

The correct measurement of an infant's length requires one adult to hold the infant's head still and another adult to extend the feet with the soles perpendicular to the lower legs. A caliper-like device, such as an infantometer, or the movable plates on an infant scale are used so that the exact distance between the two calipers or plates can be determined. Marking the position of the head and feet of an infant lying on a sheet of paper on the examining table leads to inaccuracies and may miss true disorders of growth or create false concerns about a disorder of growth in a normal child. Accurate measurements of height, or length, and weight should be plotted on the Centers for Disease Control and Prevention growth charts for the timely diagnosis of growth disorders (http://www.cdc.gov/growthcharts/).

After 2 years of age, the height of a child should be measured in the standing position. Children measured in the standing position should be barefoot against a hard surface. A Harpenden stadiometer or equivalent device is optimal for the measurement of stature, but the flexible bars that extend upward on some health scales are unreliable and may be misleading. A decrease of roughly 1.25 cm in height measurement may occur when the child is measured in the standing position rather than in the lying position; many children who appear to be *not growing* are referred to a subspecialist, but all the only change is the position of the child at the time of measurement.

Measurement of the **arm span** is essential when the diagnoses of Marfan or Klinefelter syndrome, short-limbed dwarfism, or other dysmorphic conditions are considered. Arm span is measured as the distance between

**TABLE 173-1 Hormonal Effects on Growth**

| Hormone | Bone Age | Growth Rate | Adult Height* |
|---|---|---|---|
| Androgen excess | Advanced | Increased | Diminished |
| Androgen deficiency | Normal or delayed | Normal or decreased | Increased slightly or normal |
| Thyroxine excess | Advanced | Increased | Normal or diminished |
| Thyroxine deficiency | Retarded | Decreased | Diminished |
| Growth hormone excess | Normal or advanced | Increased | Excessive |
| Growth hormone deficiency | Retarded | Decreased | Diminished |
| Cortisol excess | Retarded | Decreased | Diminished |
| Cortisol deficiency | Normal | Normal | Normal |

*Effect in most patients with treatment.
Adapted from Underwood LE, Van Wyk JJ: Normal and aberrant growth. In Wilson JD, Foster DW (eds): Textbook of Endocrinology, 8th ed. Philadelphia, *WB Saunders*, 1992.

the tips of the fingers when the patient holds both arms outstretched horizontally while standing against a solid surface. The **upper-to-lower segment ratio** is the ratio of the upper segment (determined by subtraction of the measurement from the symphysis pubis to the floor [known as the lower segment] from the total height) to the lower segment. This ratio changes with age. A normal term infant has an upper-to-lower ratio of 1.7:1, a 1-year-old has a ratio of 1.4:1, and a 10-year-old has a ratio of 1:1. Conditions of hypogonadism, not commonly discerned or suspected until after the normal age for onset of puberty, lead to greatly decreased upper-to-lower ratio in an adult, whereas long-lasting and untreated hypothyroidism leads to a high upper-to-lower ratio in the child.

### Endocrine Evaluation of Growth Hormone Secretion

GH, or somatotropin, is a 191–amino acid protein secreted by the pituitary gland under the control of GRF and SRIF (see Fig. 170-2). GH secretion is enhanced by α-adrenergic stimulation, hypoglycemia, starvation, exercise, early stages of sleep, and stress. GH secretion is inhibited by β-adrenergic stimulation and hyperglycemia. Because concentrations of GH are low throughout the day except for brief secretory peaks in the middle of the night or early morning, the daytime ascertainment of GH deficiency or sufficiency on the basis of a single determination of a random GH concentration is impossible. Adequacy of GH secretion may be determined by a stimulation test to measure peak GH secretion. A normal response is a vigorous secretory peak after stimulation; the lack of such a peak is consistent with GH deficiency. However, there is a high false positive rate (on any day, about 10% or more of normal children may not reach the normal GH peak after even two stimulatory tests). Indirect measurements of GH secretion, such as serum concentrations of IGF-1 and IGF-BP3, are replacing GH stimulatory tests.

The factors responsible for postnatal growth are not the same as the factors that mediate fetal growth. **Thyroid hormone** is essential for normal postnatal growth, although a thyroid hormone–deficient fetus achieves a normal birth length; similarly, a GH-deficient fetus has a normal birth length, although in IGF-1 deficiency resulting from GH resistance (**Laron dwarfism**), fetuses are shorter than control subjects. Adequate thyroid hormone is necessary to allow the secretion of GH. Hypothyroid patients may appear falsely to be GH deficient; with thyroid hormone repletion, GH secretion normalizes. Gonadal steroids are important in the pubertal growth spurt. The effects of other hormones on growth are noted in Table 173-1.

## ABNORMALITIES OF GROWTH

### Short Stature of Nonendocrine Causes

**Short stature** is defined as subnormal height relative to other children of the same gender and age, taking family heights into consideration. It can be caused by numerous conditions (Table 173-2). The Centers for Disease Control and Prevention growth charts use the 3rd percentile of the growth curve as the demarcation of the lower limit. **Growth failure** denotes a slow growth rate regardless of stature. Ultimately a slow growth rate leads to short

stature, but a disease process is detected sooner if the decreased growth rate is noted before the stature becomes short. Height velocity may be derived and plotted on special height velocity charts. Plotted on a growth chart, growth failure appears as a curve that crosses percentiles downward and is associated with a height velocity below the 5th percentile of height velocity for age (Fig. 173-1). A corrected mid-parental, or genetic target, height helps determine if the child is growing well for the family (see Chapter 6). To determine a range of normal height for the family under consideration, the corrected mid-parental height is bracketed by 2 standard deviations (SDs), which for the United States is approximately 10 cm (4 inches). The presence of a height 3.5 SDs below the mean, a height velocity below the 5th percentile for age, or a height below the target height corrected for mid-parental height requires a diagnostic evaluation.

Nutrition is the most important factor affecting growth on a worldwide basis (see Chapter 28). Failure to thrive may develop in the infant as a result of **maternal deprivation** (nutritional deficiency or aberrant psychosocial interaction) or as a result of organic illness (anorexia, nutrient losses through a form of malabsorption, or hypermetabolism caused by hyperthyroidism) (see Chapter 21). Psychological difficulties also can affect growth, as in **psychosocial** or **deprivation dwarfism**, in which the child develops functional temporary GH deficiency and poor growth as a result of psychological abuse; when placed in a different, healthier psychosocial environment, GH physiology normalizes, and growth occurs.

The common condition known as **constitutional delay** in growth or puberty or both is a variation of normal growth, caused by a reduced tempo, or cadence, of physiologic development and not a disease (see Fig. 173-1). Usually a family member had delayed growth or puberty but achieved a normal final height. The bone age is delayed, but the growth rate remains mostly within the lower limits of normal. Constitutional delay usually leads to a delay in secondary sexual development. **Genetic or familial short stature** (Table 173-3) refers to the stature of a child of short parents, who is expected to reach a lower than average height and yet normal for these parents. If the parents were malnourished as children, grew up in a zone of war, or suffered famine, the heights of the parents are less predictive. Although there are differences in height associated with ethnicity, the most significant difference in stature between ethnic groups is the result of nutrition. Growth curves exist for Asian children and for children with some chromosomal disorders.

Phenotypic features suggesting an underlying chromosomal disorder can occur in a host of syndromes. These syndromes can be suspected by attending to arm spans and upper-to-lower segment ratios. Genetic syndromes often combine obesity and decreased height, whereas otherwise normal obese children are usually taller than average and have advanced skeletal development and physical maturation (see Table 173-2). The **Prader-Willi syndrome** includes fetal and infantile hypotonia, small hands and feet (acromicria), postnatal acquired obesity with an insatiable appetite, developmental delay, hypogonadism, almond-shaped eyes, and abnormalities of the SNRP portion of the 15th chromosome at 15q11-q13. Most cases have deletion of the paternal sequence, but about 20% to 25%

## TABLE 173-2  Causes of Short Stature

### VARIATIONS OF NORMAL

Constitutional (delayed bone age)
Genetic (short familial height)

### ENDOCRINE DISORDERS

GH deficiency
  *Congenital*
  Isolated GH deficiency
  With other pituitary hormone deficiencies
  With midline defects
  Pituitary agenesis
  With gene deficiency
  *Acquired*
  Hypothalamic/pituitary tumors
  Histiocytosis X (Langerhans cell histiocytosis)
  CNS infections and granulomas
  Head trauma (birth and later)
  Hypothalamic/pituitary irradiation
  CNS vascular accidents
  Hydrocephalus
  Autoimmune
  Psychosocial dwarfism (functional GH deficiency)
  Amphetamine treatment for hyperactivity*
Laron dwarfism (increased GH and decreased IGF-1)
Pygmies (normal GH and IGF-2 but decreased IGF-1)
Hypothyroidism
Glucocorticoid excess
  Endogenous
  Exogenous
Diabetes mellitus under poor control
Diabetes insipidus (untreated)
Hypophosphatemic vitamin D–resistant rickets
Virilizing congenital adrenal hyperplasia (tall child, short adult)
  $P-450_{c21}$, $P-450_{c11}$ deficiencies

### SKELETAL DYSPLASIAS

Osteogenesis imperfecta
Osteochondroplasias

### LYSOSOMAL STORAGE DISEASES

Mucopolysaccharidoses
Mucolipidoses

### SYNDROMES OF SHORT STATURE

Turner syndrome (syndrome of gonadal dysgenesis)
Noonan syndrome (pseudo–Turner syndrome)
Autosomal trisomy 13, 18, 21
Prader-Willi syndrome
Laurence-Moon-Bardet-Biedl syndrome
Autosomal abnormalities
Dysmorphic syndromes (e.g., Russell-Silver or Cornelia de Lange syndrome)
Pseudohypoparathyroidism

### CHRONIC DISEASE

Cardiac disorders
  Left-to-right shunt
  Congestive heart failure
Pulmonary disorders
  Cystic fibrosis
  Asthma
Gastrointestinal disorders
  Malabsorption (e.g., celiac disease)
  Disorders of swallowing
  Inflammatory bowel disease
Hepatic disorders
Hematologic disorders
  Sickle cell anemia
  Thalassemia
Renal disorders
  Renal tubular acidosis
  Chronic uremia
Immunologic disorders
  Connective tissue disease
  Juvenile rheumatoid arthritis
  Chronic infection
  AIDS
Hereditary fructose intolerance
Malnutrition
Kwashiorkor, marasmus
Iron deficiency
Zinc deficiency
Anorexia caused by chemotherapy for neoplasms

*Only if caloric intake is severely diminished.
AIDS, acquired immunodeficiency syndrome; CNS, central nervous system; GH, growth hormone; IGF, insulin-like growth factor.
Modified from Styne DM: Growth disorder. In Fitzgerald PA (ed): Handbook of Clinical Endocrinology. Norwalk, CT, *Appleton & Lange*, 1986.

have uniparental disomy, in which both chromosomes 15 derive from the mother; when both chromosomes 15 come from the father, Angelman syndrome develops. **Laurence-Moon-Bardet-Biedl syndrome** is characterized by retinitis pigmentosa, hypogonadism and developmental delay with an autosomal dominant inheritance pattern. Laurence-Moon syndrome is associated with spastic paraplegia, however, and Bardet-Biedl syndrome is associated with obesity and polydactyly. **Pseudohypoparathyroidism** leads to short stature and developmental delay with short fourth and fifth digits (Albright hereditary osteodystrophy phenotype),

resistance to parathyroid hormone (PTH) and resultant hypocalcemia and elevated levels of serum phosphorus.

## Short Stature Caused by Growth Hormone Deficiency

### Etiology and Epidemiology

**Classic congenital** or **idiopathic GH deficiency** occurs in about 1 in 4000 to 1 in 10,000 children. Idiopathic GH deficiency, of unidentified specific etiology, is the

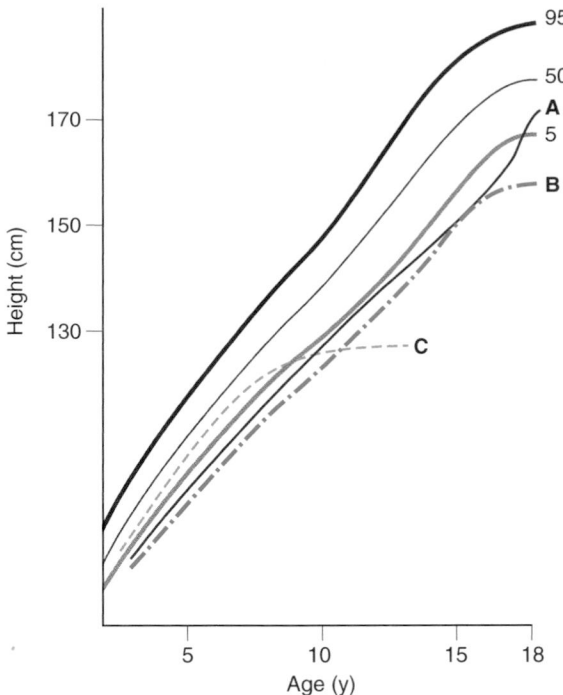

**FIGURE 173-1**

**Patterns of linear growth.** Normal growth percentiles (5th, 50th, and 95th) are shown along with typical growth curves for **A**, constitutional delay of growth and adolescence (short stature with normal growth rate for bone age, delayed pubertal growth spurt, and eventual achievement of normal adult stature); **B**, familial short stature (short stature in childhood and as an adult); and **C**, acquired pathologic growth failure (e.g., acquired untreated primary hypothyroidism) (see Chapter 5).

most common cause of both congenital GH deficiency and acquired GH deficiency. Less often, GH deficiency is caused by anatomic defects of the pituitary gland, such as pituitary aplasia or other midline defects with variable degrees of deficiency of other pituitary functions. Hereditary forms of GH deficiency that affect pituitary differentiation are the result of heterogeneous defects of the gene for GH, GRF, or GH receptor. *Classic GH deficiency* refers to very reduced to absent secretion of GH; numerous short children may have intermediate forms of decreased GH secretion. Acquired GH deficiency causing late-onset growth failure suggests the possibility of a **tumor** of the hypothalamus or pituitary (Table 173-4). Other rare causes of direct injury to the pituitary gland include infection, inflammation, and autoimmunity.

## Clinical Manifestations

Infants with congenital GH deficiency achieve a normal or near-normal birth length and weight at term, but the growth rate slows after birth, most noticeably after age 2 to 3 years, as these children become progressively shorter for age. They also tend to have an elevated weight-to-height ratio and appear chubby and short. Careful measurements in the first year of life may suggest the diagnosis, but most patients elude diagnosis until several years of age. A patient with classic GH deficiency has the appearance of a cherub (a chubby, immature appearance), with a high-pitched voice resulting from an immature larynx. Unless severe hypoglycemia occurs or dysraphism (midline defects) of the head includes a central nervous system (CNS) defect that affects mentation, the patient has normal intellectual growth and age-appropriate speech. Male neonates with isolated GH deficiency with or without gonadotropin deficiency may have a microphallus (a stretched penile length of <2 cm [normal is 3–5 cm]) and fasting hypoglycemia. Patients who lack adrenocorticotropic hormone (ACTH, cortisol) in addition to GH may have more profound hypoglycemia since cortisol also stimulates gluconeogenesis.

GH resistance or GH insensitivity is caused by abnormal number or function of GH receptors or by a postreceptor defect. Patients with the autosomal recessive **Laron syndrome**, involving mutations of the GH receptor, have a prominent forehead, hypoplastic nasal bridge, delayed dentition, sparse hair, blue sclerae, delayed bone maturation and osteoporosis, progressive adiposity, hypercholesterolemia, and low blood glucose. They have elevated serum GH concentrations, although serum IGF-1 and IGF-BP3 concentrations are low. The characteristic decrease in the number of GH receptors is reflected in the decreased serum concentration of GH-binding protein. The patients do not respond to the administration of GH with an increase in growth or an increase in serum concentrations of IGF-1 or IGF-BP3. Subjects with Laron syndrome have been treated experimentally with recombinant human IGF-1 with varying degrees of success. Malnutrition or severe liver disease may cause acquired GH resistance because serum GH is elevated, and IGF-1 is decreased.

## Diagnosis

If family or other medical history does not provide a likely diagnosis, screening tests should include a metabolic panel to evaluate kidney and liver function, a complete blood count (CBC) to rule out anemia, a celiac panel with antibodies to tissue transglutaminase to rule out celiac disease, and carotene and folate levels to reflect nutrition and rule out malabsorption. A urinalysis aids in evaluation of renal function. Urinary pH and serum bicarbonate can assess for renal tubular acidosis. In a girl without another explanation for short stature, a karyotype may rule out **Turner syndrome**. A bone age will establish skeletal maturation.

If chronic disease or familial short stature are ruled out and routine laboratory testing is normal (see Table 173-4), two GH stimulatory tests are commonly performed (see Table 170-2). GH testing should be offered to a patient who is short (<5th percentile and usually >3.5 SDs below the mean), growing poorly (<5th percentile growth rate for age), or whose height projection, based on current height and skeletal maturation as assessed by bone age, is below the target height when corrected for family height.

Classic GH-deficient patients do not show an increase in serum GH levels after stimulation by various secretagogues. Some patients release GH in response to secretagogue testing, but cannot release GH spontaneously during the day or night. Measuring serum IGF-1 and

**TABLE 173-3 Differential Diagnosis and Therapy of Short Stature**

| Diagnostic Feature | Hypopituitarism GH Deficiency* | Constitutional Delay | Familial Short Stature | Deprivational Dwarfism | Turner Syndrome | Hypothyroidism | Chronic Disease |
|---|---|---|---|---|---|---|---|
| Family history positive | Rare | Frequent | Always | No | No | Variable | Variable |
| Gender | Both | Males more often affected than females | Both | Both | Female | Both | Both |
| Facies | Immature or with midline defect (e.g., cleft palate or optic hypoplasias) | Immature | Normal | Normal | Turner facies or normal | Coarse (cretin if congenital) | Normal |
| Sexual development | Delayed | Delayed | Normal | May be delayed | Female prepubertal | Usually delayed, may be precocious if hypothyroidism is severe | Delayed |
| Bone age | Delayed | Delayed | Normal | Usually delayed; growth arrest lines present | Delayed | Delayed | Delayed |
| Dentition | Delayed | Normal; delay usual | Normal | Variable | Normal | Delayed | Normal or delayed |
| Hypoglycemia | Variable | No | No | No | No | No | No |
| Karyotype | Normal | Normal | Normal | Normal | 45,X or partial deletion of X chromosome or mosaic | Normal | Normal |
| Free $T_4$ | Low (with TRH deficiency) or normal | Normal | Normal | Normal or low | Normal: hypothyroidism may be acquired | Low | Normal |
| Stimulated GH | Low | Normal for bone age | Normal | Possibly low, or high if patient malnourished | Usually normal | Low | Usually normal |
| Insulin-like growth factor-1 | Low | Normal or low for chronologic age | Normal | Low | Normal | Low | Low or normal (depending on nutritional status) |
| Therapy | Replace deficiencies | Reassurance; sex steroids to initiate secondary sexual development in selected patients | None | Change or improve environment | Sex hormone replacement, GH; oxandrolone may be useful | $T_4$ | Treat malnutrition, organ failure (e.g., dialysis, transplant, cardiotonic drugs, insulin) |

*Possibly with GnRH, CRH, or TRH deficiency.

ACTH, adrenocorticotropic hormone; CRH, corticotropin-releasing hormone; GH, growth hormone; GnRH, gonadotropin-releasing hormone; $T_4$, thyroxine; TRH, thyrotropin-releasing hormone.

**TABLE 173-4 Growth Failure: Screening Tests**

| Test | Rationale |
|---|---|
| CBC | *Anemia:* nutritional, chronic disease, malignancy |
| | *Leukopenia:* bone marrow failure syndromes |
| | *Thrombocytopenia:* malignancy, infection |
| ESR, CRP | Inflammation of infection, inflammatory diseases, malignancy |
| Metabolic panel (electrolytes, liver enzymes, BUN) | Signs of acute or chronic hepatic, renal, adrenal dysfunction; hydration and acid-base status |
| Carotene, folate, and prothrombin time; celiac antibody panel | Assess malabsorption; detect celiac disease |
| Urinalysis with pH | Signs of renal dysfunction, hydration, water and salt homeostasis; renal tubular acidosis |
| Karyotype | Determines Turner (XO) or other syndromes |
| Cranial imaging (MRI) | Assesses hypothalamic-pituitary tumors (craniopharyngioma, glioma, germinoma) or congenital midline defects |
| Bone age | Compare with height age, and evaluate height potential |
| IGF-1, IGF-BP3 | Reflects growth hormone status or nutrition |
| Free thyroxine | Detects panhypopituitarism or isolated hypothyroidism |
| Prolactin | Elevated in hypothalamic dysfunction or destruction, suppressed in pituitary disease |

BUN, blood urea nitrogen; CBC, complete blood count; CRP, C-reactive protein; ESR, erythrocyte sedimentation rate; IGF-1, insulin-like growth factor-1; IGF-BP3, insulin-like growth factor–binding protein 3; MRI, magnetic resonance imaging.

IGF-BP3 is suggested but not consistently helpful in establishing a diagnosis of GH deficiency. Tests for GH secretion are insensitive, not very specific, and fairly variable. However, they do allow distinction of GH deficiency from GH insensitivity. In equivocal cases, an operational definition of GH deficiency might be that patients who require GH grow significantly faster when administered a normal dose of GH than before treatment.

## Treatment

GH deficiency is treated with biosynthetic recombinant DNA–derived GH. Dosage is titrated to the growth rate. Treatment with GH carries the risk of an increased incidence of slipped capital femoral epiphysis, especially in rapidly growing adolescents, and of pseudotumor cerebri.

Administration of GH to patients with normal GH responsiveness to secretagogues is controversial, but as noted earlier, diagnostic tests are imperfect; if the patient is growing extremely slowly without alternative explanation, GH therapy is sometimes used. GH is effective in increasing the growth rate and final height in Turner syndrome and in chronic renal failure; GH also is used for treatment of short stature and muscle weakness of Prader-Willi syndrome. Other indications include children born small for gestational age who have not exhibited catch-up growth by 2 years of age and the long-term treatment of idiopathic short stature with height 2.25 SDs or less below the mean. This condition also is called non–GH-deficient short stature.

Psychological support of children with severe short stature is important because of possible ridicule. Although there is controversy, marital status, satisfaction with life, and vocational achievement may be decreased in children of short stature who are not given supportive measures.

## CHAPTER 174

# Disorders of Puberty

The staging of pubertal changes and the sequence of events are discussed in Chapter 67. The onset of puberty is marked by pubarche and gonadarche. **Pubarche** results from adrenal maturation or adrenarche. With the appearance of pubic hair, other features include oiliness of hair and skin, acne, axillary hair, and body odor. Adrenarche does not include breast development in females or testicular enlargement in males. **Gonadarche** is characterized by increasing secretion of gonadal sex steroids as a result of the maturation of the hypothalamic-pituitary-gonadal axis. These sex steroids differ by gender, consisting of testosterone from the testes and estradiol and progesterone from the ovaries. In males, physical signs are pubic hair, axillary hair, facial hair, increased muscularity, deeper voice, increased penile size, and increased testicular volume. In females, the physical signs are breast development, development of the female body habitus, increased size of the uterus, and menarche with regular menstrual cycles. The third component is the growth spurt of puberty.

Hypothalamic gonadotropin-releasing hormone (GnRH), produced by cells in the arcuate nucleus, is secreted from the median eminence of the hypothalamus into the pituitary portal system and reaches the membrane receptors on the pituitary gonadotropes to cause the production and release of luteinizing hormone (LH) and follicle-stimulating hormone (FSH) into the circulation. In females, FSH stimulates the ovarian production of estrogen and, later in puberty, causes the formation and support of corpus luteum. In males, LH stimulates the production of testosterone from the Leydig cells; later in puberty, FSH stimulates the development and support of the seminiferous tubules. The gonads also produce the protein inhibin. Both sex steroids and inhibin suppress the secretion of gonadotropins. The interplay of the products of the gonads and GnRH modulates the serum concentrations of gonadotropins. GnRH is released in episodic pulses that vary during development and during the menstrual period. These pulses ensure that gonadotropins are released in a pulsatile manner. With the onset of puberty, the amplitude of the pulses of gonadotropins increases, first at night and then throughout the day. Sex steroids are secreted in response, first during the night and then throughout the day. The hypothalamic-pituitary-gonadal axis is active in the fetus and newborn, but is suppressed in the childhood years until activity increases again at the onset of puberty.

Adrenarche occurs several years earlier than gonadarche and is heralded by increasing circulating dehydroepiandrosterone (DHEA) or androstenedione. Serum DHEA increases years before the appearance of its effects, such as the development of pubic or axillary hair.

## DELAYED PUBERTY

Puberty is delayed when there is no sign of pubertal development by age 13 years in girls and 14 years in boys living in the United States (Tables 174-1 and 174-2).

### Constitutional Delay in Growth and Adolescence

Patients with constitutional delay have delayed onset of pubertal development and significant bone age delay (2 standard deviations [SDs] below the mean, which is equal to a 1.5- to 2-year delay as a teenager). The height of the patient should remain close to the genetic potential, based on the parental heights, when reinterpreted for that bone age (see Chapter 173). The bone age should be consistent with the somatic maturity of the patient. Usually, height gain is below, although fairly parallel to, the normal percentiles on the growth curve. The prepubertal nadir, or deceleration before their pubertal growth spurt, is prolonged or protracted. A family history of delayed puberty in a parent or sibling is reassuring. Spontaneous puberty usually begins in these patients by the time the bone age reaches 12 years in boys and 11 years in girls. Other causes of delayed puberty must be eliminated before a diagnosis of constitutional delay in puberty is made. Observation and reassurance are appropriate. Spontaneous progression into puberty occurs when the bone age reaches 12 to 13 years, and an adult height normal for the genetic potential is attained. In some cases, boys may be treated with low-dose testosterone for a few months if the bone age is at least 11 to 12 years. Treatment is not required for longer than 4 to 8 months since endogenous hormone production usually ensues. No similar form of therapy for constitutional delay is available for girls. Young women with delayed puberty may need to be evaluated for primary amenorrhea.

### TABLE 174-1 Classification of Delayed Puberty and Sexual Infantilism

**Constitutional delay in growth and puberty**

**Hypogonadotropic hypogonadism**

CNS disorders
  Tumors (craniopharyngioma, germinoma, glioma, prolactinoma)
  Congenital malformations
  Radiation therapy
  Other causes
Isolated gonadotropin deficiency
  Kallmann syndrome (anosmia-hyposmia)
  Other disorders
Idiopathic and genetic forms of multiple pituitary hormone deficiencies
Miscellaneous disorders
  Prader-Willi syndrome
  Laurence-Moon-Bardet-Biedl syndrome
  Functional gonadotropin deficiency
    Chronic systemic disease and malnutrition
    Hypothyroidism
    Cushing disease
    Diabetes mellitus
    Hyperprolactinemia
    Anorexia nervosa
    Psychogenic amenorrhea
    Impaired puberty and delayed menarche in female athletes and ballet dancers (exercise amenorrhea)

**Hypergonadotropic hypogonadism**

Klinefelter syndrome (syndrome of seminiferous tubular dysgenesis) and its variants
Other forms of primary testicular failure
Anorchia and cryptorchidism
Syndrome of gonadal dysgenesis and its variants (Turner syndrome)
Other forms of primary ovarian failure
XX and XY gonadal dysgenesis
  Familial and sporadic XX gonadal dysgenesis and its variants
  Familial and sporadic XY gonadal dysgenesis and its variants
Noonan syndrome
Galactosemia

CNS, central nervous system.
Modified from Grumbach MM, Styne DM: Puberty. In Wilson JD, Foster DW (eds): Williams Textbook of Endocrinology, 9th ed. Philadelphia, *WB Saunders*, 1998.

### Hypogonadotropic Hypogonadism

As a cause of delayed or absent puberty, hypogonadotropic hypogonadism may be difficult to distinguish from constitutional delay (see Tables 174-1 and 174-2). Hypogonadotropic hypogonadism precludes spontaneous entry into gonadarche; adrenarche usually occurs to some degree. Throughout childhood and in early puberty, patients with hypogonadotropic hypogonadism have normal proportions and growth. When these patients reach adulthood, *eunuchoid* proportions may ensue because their long bones grow for longer than normal, producing an upper-to-lower ratio below the lower limit of normal of 0.9

**TABLE 174-2  Differential Diagnostic Features of Delayed Puberty and Sexual Infantilism**

| Causative Condition/Disorder | Stature | Plasma Gonadotropins | GnRH Test: LH Response | Plasma Gonadal Steroids | Plasma DHEAS | Karyotype | Olfaction |
|---|---|---|---|---|---|---|---|
| Constitutional delay in growth and adolescence | Short for chronologic age, usually appropriate for bone age | Prepubertal, later pubertal | Prepubertal, later pubertal | Prepubertal, later normal | Low for chronologic age, appropriate for bone age | Normal | Normal |
| **HYPOGONADOTROPIC HYPOGONADISM** | | | | | | | |
| Isolated gonadotropin deficiency | Normal, absent pubertal growth spurt | Low | Prepubertal or no response | Low | Appropriate for chronologic age | Normal | Normal |
| Kallmann syndrome | Normal, absent pubertal growth spurt | Low | Prepubertal or no response | Low | Appropriate for chronologic age | Normal | Anosmia or hyposmia |
| Idiopathic multiple pituitary hormone deficiencies | Short stature and poor growth since early childhood | Low | Prepubertal or no response | Low | Usually low | Normal | Normal |
| Hypothalamic-pituitary tumors | Decrease in growth velocity of late onset | Low | Prepubertal or no response | Low | Normal or low for chronologic age | Normal | Normal |
| **PRIMARY GONADAL FAILURE** | | | | | | | |
| Syndrome of gonadal dysgenesis and variants | Short stature since early childhood | High | Hyperresponse for age | Low | Normal for chronologic age | XO or variant | Normal |
| Klinefelter syndrome and variants | Normal to tall | High | Hyperresponse at puberty | Low or normal | Normal for chronologic age | XXY or variant | Normal |
| Familial XX or XY gonadal dysgenesis | Normal | High | Hyperresponse for age | Low | Normal for chronologic age | XX or XY | Normal |

DHEAS, dehydroepiandrosterone sulfate; GnRH, gonadotropin-releasing hormone; LH, luteinizing hormone.
From Grumbach MM, Styne DM: Puberty. In Wilson JD, Foster DW (eds): Williams Textbook of Endocrinology, 9th ed. Philadelphia, WB Saunders, 1997.

and an arm span greater than their height. If a patient has concurrent growth hormone (GH) deficiency, however, stature is exceptionally short, and the condition may have been diagnosed in infancy with a microphallus.

## Isolated Gonadotropin Deficiency

Disorders that can cause hypogonadism include congenital hypopituitarism, such as midline defects, tumors, infiltrative disease (hemochromatosis), and many syndromes, including Laurence-Moon-Bardet-Biedl, Prader-Willi, and Kallmann syndromes. If there is an inability to release gonadotropins but no other pituitary abnormality, the patient has isolated gonadotropin deficiency (almost universally a result of absent GnRH). Patients grow normally until the time of the pubertal growth spurt, when they fail to experience the accelerated growth characteristic of the normal growth spurt.

**Kallmann syndrome** combines isolated gonadotropin deficiency with disorders of olfaction. There is genetic heterogeneity; some patients have a decreased sense of smell, others have abnormal reproduction, and some have both. Most cases are sporadic but a number of patients may have mutations in the *KAL1* gene at Xp 22.3 (X chromosome) or *KAL2* gene. The mutation causes the GnRH neurons to remain ineffectually located in the primitive nasal area, rather than migrating to the correct location at the medial basal hypothalamus. Olfactory bulbs and olfactory sulci are often absent on magnetic resonance imaging (MRI). Other symptoms include disorders of the hand, with one hand copying the movements of the other hand, shortened fourth metacarpal bone, and an absent kidney.

## Abnormalities of the Central Nervous System

Central nervous system (CNS) tumors, including pituitary adenoma, germinoma, glioma, prolactinoma, or craniopharyngioma, are important causes of gonadotropin deficiency. Craniopharyngiomas have a peak incidence in the teenage years and may cause any type of anterior or posterior hormone deficiency. Craniopharyngiomas usually calcify, eroding the sella turcica when they expand. They may impinge on the optic chiasm, leading to bitemporal hemianopsia and optic atrophy. Germinomas are noncalcifying hypothalamic or pineal tumors that frequently produce human chorionic gonadotropin (hCG), which may cause sexual precocity in prepubertal boys (hCG cross-reacts with the LH receptor because of the similarity of structure between LH and hCG). Other tumors that may affect pubertal development include astrocytomas and gliomas.

## Idiopathic Hypopituitarism

Congenital absence of various combinations of pituitary hormones may produce idiopathic hypopituitarism. Although this disorder may occur in family constellations, after X-linked or autosomal recessive patterns, sporadic types of congenital idiopathic hypopituitarism are more common. Congenital hypopituitarism may manifest in a male with GH deficiency and associated gonadotropin deficiency with a microphallus or with hypoglycemia with seizures, especially if adrenocorticotropic hormone (ACTH) and GH deficiency occurs as well.

## Syndromes of Hypogonadotropic Hypogonadism

Weight loss resulting from voluntary dieting, malnutrition, or chronic disease leads to decreased gonadotropin function when weight decreases to less than 80% of ideal weight. **Anorexia nervosa** is characterized by striking weight loss and psychiatric disorders (see Chapter 70). Primary or secondary amenorrhea frequently is found in affected girls, and pubertal development is absent or minimal, depending on the level of weight loss and the age at onset. Regaining weight to the ideal level may not immediately reverse the condition. Increased physical activity, even without weight loss, can lead to decreased menstrual frequency and gonadotropin deficiency in **athletic amenorrhea**; when physical activity is interrupted, menstrual function may return. Chronic or systemic illness (e.g., cystic fibrosis, diabetes mellitus, inflammatory bowel disease, or hematologic diseases) can lead to pubertal delay or to amenorrhea from hypothalamic dysfunction. **Hypothyroidism** inhibits the onset of puberty and delays menstrual periods. Conversely, severe primary hypothyroidism may lead to precocious puberty.

## Hypergonadotropic Hypogonadism

Hypergonadotropic hypogonadism is characterized by elevated gonadotropin and low sex steroid levels resulting from primary gonadal failure. This permanent condition is almost always diagnosed following the lack of entry into gonadarche and is not suspected throughout childhood. Gonadotropins do not increase to greater than normal until shortly before or around the normal time of puberty.

## Ovarian Failure

Turner syndrome or the syndrome of gonadal dysgenesis is a common cause of ovarian failure and short stature. The karyotype is classically 45,XO, but other abnormalities of the X chromosome or mosaicism are possible. The incidence of Turner syndrome is 1 in 2000 to 1 in 3000 births. The features of a girl with Turner syndrome need not be evident on physical examination or by history. The diagnosis must be considered in any girl who is short without a contributory history. Patients with other types of gonadal dysgenesis and galactosemia as well as patients treated with radiation therapy or chemotherapy for malignancy may develop ovarian failure.

## Testicular Failure

Klinefelter syndrome (seminiferous tubular dysgenesis) is the most common cause of testicular failure. The karyotype is 47,XXY, but variants with more X chromosomes are possible. The incidence is approximately 1 in 500 to 1 in 1000 in males. Testosterone levels may be close to normal, at least until mid-puberty, because Leydig cell function may be spared; however, seminiferous tubular function characteristically is lost, causing infertility. Commonly, LH levels may be normal to elevated, whereas FSH levels are usually more unequivocally elevated. The age of onset of puberty is usually normal, but secondary sexual changes may not progress because of inadequate Leydig cell function.

## Primary Amenorrhea

When it is determined that no secondary sexual development is present after the upper age limits of normal pubertal development, serum gonadotropin levels should be obtained to determine whether the patient has a hypogonadotropic or hypergonadotropic hypogonadism (see Table 174-2). Based only on gonadotropin measurements, the differentiation between constitutional delay in growth and hypogonadotropic hypogonadism is difficult; the gonadotropin levels are low in both conditions. Sometimes observation for months or years is necessary before the diagnosis is confirmed.

**Differential Diagnosis.** Lack of menstruation in the presence of normal pubertal development might be the result of physiologic variation. The entities leading to **hypogonadism** include congenital hypopituitarism; tumors such as a pituitary adenoma, germinoma, glioma, prolactinoma, and craniopharyngioma; infiltrative disease; and Laurence-Moon-Biedl, Prader-Willi, and Kallmann syndromes. In females, stress, competitive athletics, or inadequate nutrition from chronic or systemic illness or from an eating disorder can lead to extreme pubertal delay, or amenorrhea on the basis of hypothalamic dysfunction. When primary amenorrhea occurs, an anatomic defect may be responsible; the Mayer-Rokitansky-Kuster-Hauser syndrome of congenital absence of the uterus occurs in 1 in 4000 to 1 in 5000 female births. Anatomic obstruction by imperforate hymen or vaginal septum also presents with normal secondary sexual development without menstruation. The complete syndrome of **androgen insensitivity** includes normal feminization, absence of pubic or axillary hair, and primary amenorrhea. In this syndrome, all müllerian structures, including ovaries, uterus, fallopian tubes, and upper third of the vagina, are lacking; the karyotype is 46,XY, and subjects have intra-abdominal testes. Undiagnosed Turner syndrome is another relatively common cause of amenorrhea, resulting from abnormal ovarian function. Secondary sexual development also is absent or minimal.

**Treatment.** If a permanent condition is apparent, replacement with sex steroids is indicated. Females are given low-dose ethinyl estradiol (5–10 µg) or conjugated estrogens (starting at 0.3 mg daily, increasing to 0.625 or 0.9 by 6–12 months later) in low daily doses until breakthrough bleeding occurs, at which time cycling is started with a dose on the first 25 days of the month; on days 20 to 25 of the month, a progestational agent, such as medroxyprogesterone acetate (5 mg), is added to mimic the normal increases in gonadal hormones and to induce a normal menstrual period. In males, testosterone enanthate or cypionate (50 mg monthly with a progressive increase to 100–200 mg) is given intramuscularly once every 4 weeks. Transdermal administration also is possible. This starting regimen is appropriate for patients with hypogonadotropic or hypergonadotropic hypogonadism, and doses are increased gradually to adult levels. Oral agents are not used for fear of hepatotoxicity. Patients with apparent constitutional delay in puberty who have, by definition, passed the upper limits of normal onset of puberty may be given a 3-month course of low-dose, sex-appropriate gonadal steroids to see if spontaneous puberty occurs. This course of therapy might be repeated once without undue advancement of bone age. All patients with any form of delayed puberty are at risk for decreased bone density; adequate calcium intake is essential. Patients with hypogonadotropic hypogonadism may be able to achieve fertility by the administration of gonadotropin therapy or pulsatile hypothalamic-releasing hormone therapy administered by a programmable pump on an appropriate schedule. Subjects with hypergonadotropic hypogonadism, whether Turner syndrome or Klinefelter syndrome, have, by definition, a primary gonadal problem and are unlikely to achieve spontaneous fertility.

In subjects with Turner syndrome, the goals of therapy include promoting growth with exogenous human GH supplementation and induction of the secondary sexual characteristics and of menses with low-dose cyclic estrogen replacement therapy, with progestagen added at the end of each cycle. Patients with Turner syndrome have had successful pregnancies after in vitro fertilization with a donor ovum and endocrine support.

## SEXUAL PRECOCITY

### Classification

Sexual precocity (precocious puberty) is classically defined as secondary sexual development occurring before the age of 9 years in boys or 8 years in girls (Tables 174-3 and 174-4). The lower limit of normal puberty may be 7 years in white girls and 6 years in African-American girls. At present, the mean age at which girls exhibit Tanner II breast development (thelarche) is approximately 10 years for white girls and 9 years for African-American girls (normal range 8–13 years). The mean age at which girls exhibit Tanner II pubic hair development is 9 years for white girls and 10.5 years for African-American girls. Menarche usually occurs at 12.2 and 12.9 years (range 10–15 years). Pubertal progression results from two components: **gonadarche** (maturation of the gonad and secretion of sex steroid, estrogen in females, testosterone in males) and **adrenarche** (maturation of the adrenal and secretion of adrenal sex steroid, DHEA and androstenedione). The normal developmental sequence in girls is **thelarche** (due to gonadarche) followed closely by **pubarche** (due to adrenarche) and finally **menarche,** 2 to 3 years later. In boys, the first normal event is enlargement of testes followed by appearance of pubic hair (long diameter of the testis greater than 2.5 cm, volume greater than 4 mL).

**Central precocious puberty**, resulting in gonadarche, emanates from premature activation of the hypothalamic-pituitary-gonadal axis (GnRH-dependent). **Peripheral precocious puberty**, gonadarche or adrenarche, does not involve the hypothalamic-pituitary-gonadal axis (GnRH-independent).

### TABLE 174-3 Classification of Sexual Precocity

**TRUE PRECOCIOUS PUBERTY OR COMPLETE ISOSEXUAL PRECOCITY**

Idiopathic true precocious puberty
  CNS tumors
    Hamartomas (ectopic GnRH pulse generator)
  Other tumors
Other CNS disorders
True precocious puberty after late treatment of congenital virilizing adrenal hyperplasia

**INCOMPLETE ISOSEXUAL PRECOCITY (GNRH-INDEPENDENT SEXUAL PRECOCITY)**

*Males*
Chorionic gonadotropin-secreting tumors (hCG-dependent sexual precocity)
CNS tumors (e.g., germinoma, chorioepithelioma, teratoma)
Tumors in locations outside the CNS (hepatoblastoma)
LH-secreting pituitary adenoma
Increased androgen secretion by adrenal or testis
Congenital adrenal hyperplasia (21-hydroxylase deficiency, 11-hydroxylase deficiency)
Virilizing adrenal neoplasm
Leydig cell adenoma
Familial testotoxicosis (familial premature gonadotropin-independent Leydig cell and germ cell maturation)

*Females*
Estrogen-secreting ovarian or adrenal neoplasms
Ovarian cysts
*Males and females*
McCune-Albright syndrome
Primary hypothyroidism
Peutz-Jeghers syndrome
Iatrogenic sexual precocity

**VARIATIONS OF PUBERTAL DEVELOPMENT**

Premature thelarche
Premature menarche
Premature adrenarche
Adolescent gynecomastia

**CONTRASEXUAL PRECOCITY**

*Males* (feminization)
Adrenal neoplasm
Increased extraglandular conversion of circulating steroids to estrogen
*Females* (virilization)
(Congenital adrenal hyperplasia, P-450$_{c21}$ deficiency, P-450$_{c11}$ deficiency, 3β-Hydroxysteroid dehydrogenase deficiency)
Virilizing adrenal neoplasms
Virilizing ovarian neoplasms (e.g., arrhenoblastomas)

CNS, central nervous system; GnRH, gonadotropin-releasing hormone; hCG, human chorionic gonadotropin; LH, luteinizing hormone.
From Grumbach MM, Styne DM: Puberty. In Wilson JD, Foster DW (eds): Williams Textbook of Endocrinology, 9th ed. Philadelphia, *WB Saunders*, 1998.

### TABLE 174-4 Differential Diagnosis of Sexual Precocity

| Causative Disorder | Serum Gonadotropin Concentration* | LH Response to GnRH | Serum Sex Steroid Concentrations | Gonadal Size | Miscellaneous |
|---|---|---|---|---|---|
| True precocious puberty | Pubertal values | Pubertal | Pubertal values of testosterone or estradiol | Normal pubertal testicular enlargement or ovarian and uterine enlargement (by sonography) | MRI scan of brain to rule out CNS tumor or other abnormality; bone scan for McCune-Albright syndrome |
| Incomplete sexual precocity (pituitary gonadotropin-independent) *Males* | | | | | |
| Chorionic gonadotropin-secreting tumor in males | High hCG (low LH) | Prepubertal (suppressed) | Pubertal values of testosterone | Slight to moderate uniform enlargement of testes | Hepatomegaly suggests hepatoblastoma; MRI scan of brain if chorionic gonadotropin-secreting CNS tumor suspected |
| Leydig cell tumor in males | Suppressed | Suppressed | Very high testosterone | Irregular asymmetrical enlargement of testes | |

## TABLE 174-4 Differential Diagnosis of Sexual Precocity—cont'd

| Causative Disorder | Serum Gonadotropin Concentration* | LH Response to GnRH | Serum Sex Steroid Concentrations | Gonadal Size | Miscellaneous |
|---|---|---|---|---|---|
| Familial testotoxicosis | Suppressed | Suppressed | Pubertal values of testosterone | Testes symmetrical and >2.5 cm but smaller than expected for pubertal development; spermatogenesis may occur | Familial; probably sex-linked, autosomal dominant trait |
| Premature adrenarche | Prepubertal | Prepubertal | Prepubertal testosterone; DHEAS values appropriate for pubic hair stage 2 | Testes prepubertal | Onset usually after 6 yr of age; more frequent in brain-injured children |
| *Females* | | | | | |
| Granulosa cell tumor (presentation may be similar to that with follicular cysts) | Suppressed | Suppressed | Very high estradiol | Ovarian enlargement on physical examination, MRI, CT, or sonography | Tumor often palpable on abdominal examination |
| Follicular cyst | Suppressed | Suppressed | Prepubertal to very high estradiol values | Ovarian enlargement on physical examination, MRI, CT, or sonography | Single or repetitive episodes; exclude McCune-Albright syndrome (e.g., perform skeletal survey and inspect skin) |
| Feminizing adrenal tumor | Suppressed | Suppressed | High estradiol and DHEAS values | Ovaries prepubertal | Unilateral adrenal mass |
| Premature thelarche | Prepubertal | Prepubertal | Prepubertal or early pubertal estradiol | Ovaries prepubertal | Onset usually before 3 yr of age |
| Premature adrenarche | Prepubertal | Prepubertal | Prepubertal estradiol; DHEAS values appropriate for pubic hair Tanner stage 2 | Ovaries prepubertal | Onset usually after 6 yr of age; more frequent in brain-injured children |

*In supersensitive assays.

CNS, central nervous system; CT, computed tomography; DHEAS, dehydroepiandrosterone sulfate; GnRH, gonadotropin-releasing hormone; hCG, human chorionic gonadotropin; LH, luteinizing hormone; MRI, magnetic resonance imaging.

Modified from Grumbach MM, Styne DM: Puberty. In Wilson JD, Foster DW (eds): Williams Textbook of Endocrinology, 9th ed. Philadelphia, *WB Saunders*, 1997.

## Central Precocious Puberty (Constitutional or Familial Precocious Puberty)

In **central precocious puberty**, every endocrine and physical aspect of pubertal development is normal but too early; this includes tall stature, advanced bone age, increased sex steroid and pulsatile gonadotropin secretion, and increased response of LH to GnRH. The clinical course of central precocious puberty may wax and wane. Benign precocious puberty is the presumptive diagnosis in individuals who begin puberty early on a **constitutional** or **familial** basis. If no cause can be determined, the diagnosis is idiopathic precocious puberty; this condition occurs much more often in girls than in boys. Obese girls have earlier adrenarche, and sometimes menarche as well, than normal weight girls, and the high incidence of overweight and obesity in developed countries is contributing to a shift to earlier entry into puberty. Compared with girls, boys with precocious puberty have a higher incidence of CNS disorders, such as tumors and hamartomas, precipitating the precocious puberty. Almost any condition that affects the CNS, including hydrocephalus, meningitis, encephalitis, suprasellar cysts, head trauma, epilepsy, mental retardation and irradiation, can precipitate central precocious puberty.

A CNS tumor or disease must be considered in all children with precocious puberty before the condition is diagnosed as idiopathic. **Hamartomas** are nonmalignant tumors of the tuber cinereum with a characteristic appearance on computed tomography (CT) or MRI; biopsy is rarely required. The mass of GnRH neurons secrete GnRH and cause precocious puberty. While hamartomas are not true neoplasms they may require neurosurgical attention, such as ventriculoperitoneal shunting, if they lead to increased intracranial pressure. The resulting precocious puberty is responsive to medical therapy with GnRH agonists, and surgery is rarely indicated.

Other masses that cause precocious puberty are not benign. **Optic** or **hypothalamic gliomas** (with or without neurofibromatosis), astrocytomas, and ependymomas may cause precocious puberty by disrupting the negative restraint of the areas of the CNS that normally inhibit pubertal development throughout childhood. These tumors may require radiotherapy, which contributes to a significant risk for hypopituitarism. Growth is greater than that found in age-matched control subjects, but less than in GH-replete patients with precocious puberty. The GH deficiency is not as obvious as in GH-deficient patients without precocious puberty. With GnRH analog treatment, precocious puberty is controlled and the growth rate decreases to that of a GH-deficient child. GH is additional therapy.

## Gonadotropin-Releasing Hormone–Independent Precocious Puberty

The most common cause of GnRH-independent precocious puberty, **McCune-Albright syndrome**, is more frequent in girls than boys and includes precocious gonadarche, a bone disorder with polyostotic fibrous dysplasia, and hyperpigmented cutaneous macules (café au lait spots). The precocious gonadarche results from ovarian hyperfunction and sometimes cyst formation, leading to episodic estrogen secretion. This disorder results from a postconception somatic mutation in the G protein intracellular signaling system (specifically $G_{s\alpha}$, which leads to unregulated constitutive activation of adenylate cyclase, and of cAMP in the absence of trophic hormone stimulation), in the affected cells in ovary, bone, and skin; other endocrine organs may also autonomously hyperfunction for the same reason. Hyperthyroidism, hyperadrenalism, or acromegaly may occur. **Adrenal carcinomas** usually secrete adrenal androgens, such as DHEA; **adrenal adenomas** may virilize a child as a result of the production of androgen or may feminize a child as a result of the production of estrogen.

Boys may have precocious gonadarche on the basis of a rare entity called **familial GnRH-independent sexual precocity with premature Leydig cell maturation.** This condition, with germ cell maturation caused by an X-limited dominant defect, produces constitutive activation of the LH receptor which leads to continuous production and secretion of testosterone without requiring the presence of LH or hCG. Outside of the pituitary, gonadotropins can originate from a tumor. hCG-secreting tumors stimulate LH receptors and increase testosterone secretion. These tumors may be found in various places, including the pineal gland (dysgerminomas, which are radiosensitive) or the liver (hepatoblastoma, which may lead to death within a few months after diagnosis).

Ovarian cysts may occur once or may be recurrent. High serum estrogen values may mimic ovarian tumors. Congenital adrenal hyperplasia is a cause of virilization in girls and is discussed in the following sections.

## Evaluation of Sexual Precocity

The first step in evaluating sexual precocity is to determine which characteristics of normal puberty are apparent (Chapter 67) and whether estrogen effects, androgen effects or both are present (see Table 174-4). In girls, androgen effect manifests as adult odor, pubic and axillary hair, and facial skin oiliness and acne, whereas estrogen effect manifests as breast development, uterine increase, and eventually menarche. In boys, androgen effect manifests as adult odor, pubic and axillary hair, and facial skin oiliness and acne; it is also important to note whether the testes are enlarged more than 2.5 cm in length, which implies gonadarche. If the testes are not enlarged, but virilization is progressing, the source of the androgens may be the adrenal glands or exogenous sources. If the testes are slightly enlarged but not consistent with the stage of pubertal development, ectopic production of hCG or familial Leydig and germ cell maturation may be the cause. Most of the enlargement of testes during puberty is the result of seminiferous tubule maturation. If only Leydig cells are enlarged, as in these conditions, the testes make considerable testosterone, but show only minimal enlargement.

**Laboratory evaluation** includes determination of sex steroid (testosterone, estradiol, or DHEA-S or androstenedione) and baseline gonadotropin concentrations. The inherent nature of gonadotropin secretion is characterized by low secretory rates throughout childhood and pulsatile secretion in adolescents and adults. If baseline gonadotropin values are elevated into the normal pubertal range, central precocious puberty is likely. If baseline gonadotropins are low, however, no immediate conclusion may be drawn as to GnRH-dependent versus GnRH-independent precocious puberty. This distinction often requires assessment of gonadotropin responsiveness to GnRH stimulation. A prepubertal GnRH response is FSH predominant, whereas a pubertal response is more LH predominant. Thyroid hormone determination also is useful because severe primary hypothyroidism can cause incomplete precocious puberty. If there is a suggestion of a CNS anomaly or a tumor (CNS, hepatic, adrenal, ovarian, or testicular), MRI of the appropriate location is indicated. The diagnosis of central precocious puberty mandates that MRI of the CNS be performed.

## Treatment

Long-acting, superactive analogs of GnRH are the treatment of choice for central precocious puberty because they suppress gonadotropin secretion by down-regulating GnRH

**TABLE 174-5 Pharmacologic Therapy of Sexual Precocity**

| Disorder | Treatment | Action and Rationale |
|---|---|---|
| GnRH-dependent true or central precocious puberty | GnRH agonists | Desensitization of gonadotropes; blocks action of endogenous GnRH |
| GnRH-independent incomplete sexual precocity | | |
| *Girls* | | |
| Autonomous ovarian cysts | Medroxyprogesterone acetate | Inhibition of ovarian steroidogenesis; regression of cyst (inhibition of FSH release) |
| McCune-Albright syndrome | Medroxyprogesterone acetate* | Inhibition of ovarian steroidogenesis; regression of cyst (inhibition of FSH release) |
| | Testolactone* or fadrozole | Inhibition of P-450 aromatase; blocks estrogen synthesis |
| *Boys* | | |
| Familial testotoxicosis | Ketoconazole* | Inhibition of P-450$_{c17}$ (mainly 17,20-lyase activity) |
| | Spironolactone* or flutamide *and* testolactone or fadrozole | Antiandrogen Inhibition of aromatase; blocks estrogen synthesis |
| | Medroxyprogesterone acetate* | Inhibition of testicular steroidogenesis |

*If true precocious puberty develops, a GnRH agonist can be added.
FSH, follicle-stimulating hormone; GnRH, gonadotropin-releasing hormone.
Modified from Grumbach MM, Kaplan SL: Recent advances in the diagnosis and management of sexual precocity. *Acta Paediatr Jpn* 30(Suppl):155, 1988.

receptors in the pituitary gonadotropes (Table 174-5). After a brief (2–3 days) increase in gonadotropin secretion and, rarely, some withdrawal bleeding in girls, gonadotropin values decrease, and the gonadal secretion reverts to the prepubertal state. The early sexual development and increased height of a patient with precocious puberty mandate psychological support or even counseling for children and families. Boys with GnRH-independent premature Leydig cell and germ cell maturation do not respond to GnRH analogs, but require treatment with an inhibitor of testosterone synthesis (e.g., ketoconazole), an antiandrogen (e.g., spironolactone), or an aromatase inhibitor (e.g., testolactone or letrozole). Patients with precocious puberty from a hormone-secreting tumor require surgical removal, if possible. The precocious puberty of the McCune-Albright syndrome is GnRH independent and unresponsive to therapy with GnRH analog. Therapy is provided with testolactone and antiandrogens or antiestrogen, such as tamoxifen. After successful therapy for the latter conditions, central precocious puberty may develop secondarily; GnRH agonist administration is effective therapy.

## VARIATIONS IN PUBERTAL DEVELOPMENT

### Isolated Premature Thelarche (Premature Breast Development)

Benign **premature thelarche** is the isolated appearance of unilateral or bilateral breast tissue in girls, usually at ages 6 months to 3 years. There are no other signs of puberty and no evidence of excessive estrogen effect (vaginal bleeding, thickening of the vaginal secretions, increased height velocity, or bone age acceleration). Ingestion or dermal application of estrogen-containing compounds must be excluded. Laboratory investigations are not usually necessary, but a pelvic ultrasound study rarely may be indicated to exclude ovarian disease. Girls with

this condition should be re-evaluated at intervals of 6 to 12 months to ensure that apparent premature thelarche is not the beginning of progression into precocious puberty. The prognosis is excellent; if no progression occurs, no treatment other than reassurance is necessary. There is no indication for a breast biopsy in a patient with established premature thelarche.

### Gynecomastia

In males, breast tissue is termed *gynecomastia,* and it may occur to some degree in 45% to 75% of normal pubertal boys (see Chapter 67). Androgens normally are converted to estrogen by aromatization; in early puberty, only modest amounts of androgens are produced, and the estrogen effect can overwhelm the androgen effects at this stage. Later in pubertal development, the androgen production is so great that there is little effect from the estrogen produced by aromatization. Gynecomastia also can suggest the possibility of Klinefelter syndrome as puberty progresses. Prepubertal gynecomastia suggests an unusual source of estrogen either from exogenous sources (oral or dermal estrogen administration is possible from contamination of food or ointments) or from endogenous sources (from abnormal function of adrenal gland or ovary or from increased peripheral aromatization).

### Isolated Premature Adrenarche (Pubarche)

The isolated appearance of pubic hair before age 6 to 7 years in girls or before age 9 years in boys is termed **premature pubarche**, usually results from adrenarche, and is relatively common. If the pubic hair is associated with any other feature of virilization (clitoral or penile enlargement or advanced bone age) or other signs (acne, rapid growth, or voice change), a detailed investigation for a pathologic cause of virilization is indicated to rule out a life-threatening cause, such as an adrenocortical carcinoma. Measurements of serum testosterone, 17-hydroxyprogesterone (17-OHP), and DHEA in basal and ACTH-stimulated states are indicated in heavily virilized patients to investigate the possibility of **congenital adrenal hyperplasia (CAH)**. Ultrasound studies may reveal a hyperplastic adrenal gland or a virilizing adrenal or ovarian tumor. Most patients with isolated pubic hair do not have progressive virilization and simply have premature adrenarche (*pubarche*) resulting from premature activation of DHEA secretion from the adrenal gland. The skeletal maturation, as assessed by bone age, may be slightly advanced and the height slightly increased, but testosterone concentrations are normal. DHEA levels usually are high for prepubertal age, but are consistent with Tanner (sexuality maturity rating) stages II and III.

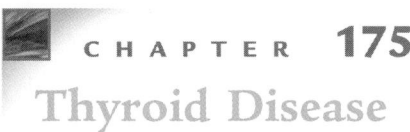

# CHAPTER 175
# Thyroid Disease

## THYROID PHYSIOLOGY AND DEVELOPMENT

Thyrotropin-releasing hormone (TRH), a tripeptide synthesized in the hypothalamus, stimulates the release of pituitary thyroid-stimulating hormone (TSH). Pituitary TSH is a glycoprotein that stimulates the synthesis and release of thyroid hormones by the thyroid gland. Thyroid function develops in three stages:

1. Embryogenesis begins on the floor of the primitive oral cavity. The gland descends to its definitive position in the anterior lower neck by the end of the first trimester. Thyroid glands that do not reach the normal location are ectopic but may retain function; however, the glands most often become insufficient by early to mid childhood to support full thyroid secretion (a lingual or sublingual site or even tissue found in a thyroglossal duct cyst may be the only functioning thyroid gland).
2. The hypothalamic-pituitary-thyroid axis becomes functional in the second trimester.
3. Peripheral metabolism of thyroid hormones matures in the third trimester.

Thyroxine ($T_4$), triiodothyronine ($T_3$), and TSH do not cross the placenta in significant amounts. Concentrations in fetal serum reflect primarily fetal secretion and metabolism. Maternal thyroid antibodies, iodides (including radioactive iodides), and medications given to mothers to treat hyperthyroidism (e.g., propylthiouracil, methimazole) cross the placenta and affect fetal thyroid function. An infant born prematurely or with intrauterine growth restriction may have an interruption of the normal maturational process and appear to have hypothyroidism by standard tests.

The thyroid gland (1) concentrates iodine and (2) binds it (organifies it) to tyrosine molecules to produce either monoiodotyrosine or diiodotyrosine, with subsequent (3) coupling of two tyrosines, $T_4$ or $T_3$. The major fraction of circulating $T_3$ (approximately two thirds) is derived from peripheral deiodination of $T_4$ to $T_3$, but some is produced by the thyroid gland itself. In Graves disease, a larger fraction originates in the thyroid gland. The conversion of $T_4$ to $T_3$ requires the removal of one iodine from the outer ring of tyrosine; removing an iodine from the inner ring results in reverse $T_3$, which has little biologic effect. Preferential conversion of $T_4$ to reverse $T_3$ rather than $T_3$ occurs in utero and in all forms of severe illness, including respiratory distress syndrome, fevers, anorexia, cachexia, and starvation. Conversion from $T_4$ to $T_3$ increases immediately after birth and throughout life. $T_4$ and $T_3$ are noncovalently bound to a specific serum carrier protein, **$T_4$-binding globulin**, and, to a lesser extent, albumin. Only small (<0.02%) fractions of $T_4$ and $T_3$ are not bound; free $T_4$ (as it is converted to free $T_3$) and free $T_3$ are biologically active. Free $T_3$ exerts metabolic effects and negative feedback on TSH release (Fig. 175-1).

Serum TSH increases just after birth, but soon decreases to lower values considered normal for later life. $T_4$ secretion increases after birth, partially as a result of the peak in TSH and partially because of maturation of thyroid metabolism. Serum thyroid hormone concentrations decrease, but only slowly reach values routinely found in adults. It is important to refer to age-adjusted normative data to interpret thyroid function tests properly, whether relative to making diagnoses of hyperthyroidism or hypothyroidism or when adjusting therapy. Free $T_4$ is the test of choice because it eliminates the effects of variation in protein binding, which can be substantial.

Table 175-1 summarizes laboratory test results in various types of thyroid abnormalities. In usual circumstances, plasma concentrations of TSH above the normal range indicate primary hypothyroidism, and concentrations below the normal range most often indicate the presence of hyperthyroidism. Although a thyroid scan rarely is indicated in the evaluation of pediatric thyroid disease, thyroid agenesis, ectopic thyroid tissue and the diagnoses of hyperfunctioning "hot" nodules or of non-functioning "cold" nodules may be detected by this test. A thyroid scan performed with the short-lived isotope radioactive iodine ($^{123}$I) indicates the size, shape, and location of the thyroid gland and iodine concentrating ability. A solitary nodule is a source of concern for the possibility of cancer, especially if it is solid and nonfunctional. Ultrasound may determine whether it is cystic or solid. If the nodule is solid, a $^{123}$I scan indicates its functional status. Excisional biopsies usually are performed on solitary nodules. Scans are rarely indicated in the diagnosis of Hashimoto thyroiditis or thyrotoxicosis.

## THYROID DISORDERS
### Hypothyroidism

Hypothyroidism is diagnosed by a decreased serum free $T_4$ and may be the result of diseases of the thyroid gland (primary hypothyroidism), abnormalities of the pituitary gland (secondary) or abnormalities of the hypothalamus (tertiary). Hypothyroidism is congenital or acquired and may be associated with a goiter (Table 175-2).

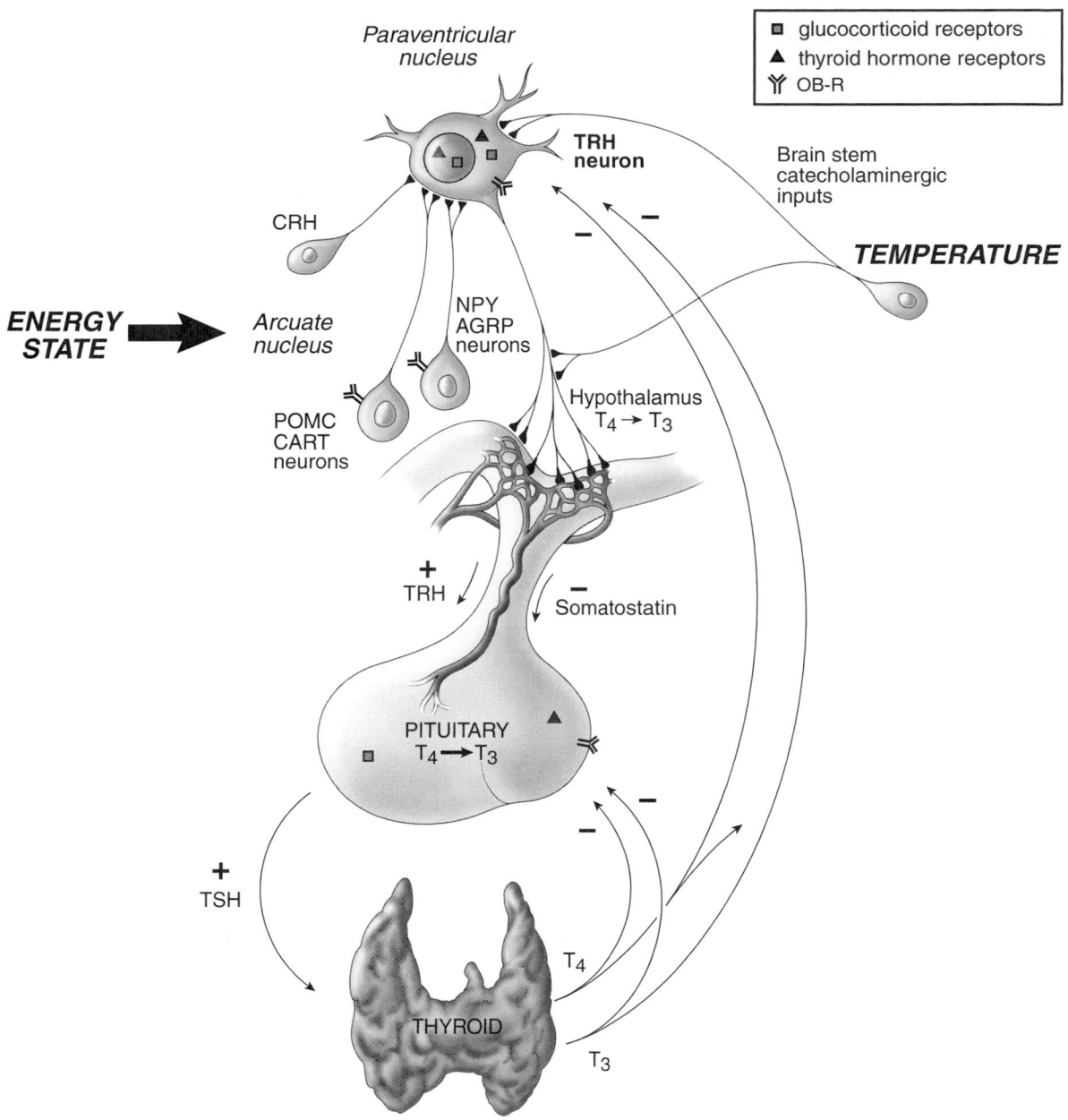

**FIGURE 175-1**

**Interrelationships of the hypothalamic-pituitary-thyroid axis.** Thyroid-stimulating hormone (TSH) from the pituitary gland stimulates the secretion of thyroxine ($T_4$) and triiodothyronine ($T_3$) from the thyroid gland. These act at the pituitary gland level to control secretion of TSH by a negative feedback mechanism. In addition, $T_4$ is metabolized to the potent $T_3$ within the pituitary gland by a monoiodinase. Secretion of TSH is stimulated by thyrotropin-releasing hormone (TRH) from the hypothalamus and inhibited by somatostatin. Thyroid hormone acts at the hypothalamus to stimulate secretion of somatostatin (somatostatin acts as a negative signal to the pituitary secretion of TSH). CRH, corticotropin-releasing hormone; OB-R, leptin receptor. (From Melmed S, Polonsky K, Kronenberg H, Larsen R [eds]: Williams Textbook of Endocrinology, 10th ed. Philadelphia, *Elsevier*, 2003, p 101.)

## Congenital Hypothyroidism

Congenital hypothyroidism occurs in approximately 1 in 4000 live births and is caused by dysgenesis, disorders of embryogenesis (agenesis, aplasia, ectopia), far more often than by dyshormonogenesis disorders (e.g., enzyme defects). Thyroid tissue usually is not palpable in these sporadic nongoitrous conditions. Dyshormonogenesis, disorders of intrathyroid metabolism or goitrous congenital hypothyroidism, occurs in about 1 in 30,000 live births. The goiter reflects an inborn error of metabolism in the pathway of iodide incorporation or thyroid hormone biosynthesis or reflects the transplacental passage of antithyroid drugs given to the mother. The free $T_4$ concentration is low, and the TSH level is elevated. Routine neonatal screening programs to measure cord blood or heel-stick TSH values occur in every state in the United States. An immediate confirmatory serum sample should be obtained from any infant having a positive result on a **screening test.** A low $T_4$ and high TSH confirm the finding.

**TABLE 175-1 Laboratory Test Results in Various Types of Thyroid Function Abnormalities in Children***

| Abnormality | Serum Total T₄ | Free T₄ | Serum TSH | Serum TBG |
|---|---|---|---|---|
| Primary hypothyroidism | ↓ | ↓ | ↑ | N |
| Hypothalamic (TRH) tertiary hypothyroidism | ↓ | ↓ | ↓ | N |
| Pituitary (TSH) secondary hypothyroidism | ↓ | ↓ | ↓ | N |
| TBG deficiency | ↓ | N | N | ↓ |
| TBG excess | ↑ | N | N | ↑ |

*TSH may be slightly elevated.

N, normal; ↓, decreased; ↑, increased; T₄, thyroxine; TBG, thyroxine-binding globulin; TRH, thyrotropin-releasing hormone; TSH, thyroid-stimulating hormone.

**TABLE 175-2 Causes of Hypothyroidism in Infancy and Childhood**

| Age Group | Manifestation | Cause |
|---|---|---|
| Newborn | No goiter | Thyroid gland dysgenesis or ectopic location |
| | | Exposure to iodides |
| | | TSH deficiency |
| | | TRH deficiency |
| | Goiter | Inborn defect in hormone synthesis* or effect |
| | | Maternal goitrogen ingestion, including propylthiouracil, methimazole, iodides |
| | | Severe iodide deficiency (endemic) |
| Child | No goiter | Thyroid gland dysgenesis |
| | | Cystinosis |
| | | Hypothalamic-pituitary insufficiency |
| | | Surgical after thyrotoxicosis or other thyroid surgery |
| | Goiter | Hashimoto thyroiditis: chronic lymphocytic thyroiditis |
| | | Inborn defect in hormone synthesis or effect |
| | | Goitrogenic drugs |
| | | Infiltrative (sarcoid, lymphoma) |

*Impaired iodide transport, defective thyroglobulin iodination, defective iodotyrosine dehalogenase, or defective thyroglobulin or its coupling to iodotyrosines.

TRH, thyrotropin-releasing hormone; TSH, thyroid-stimulating hormone.

Isolated secondary or tertiary hypothyroidism is rare, occurring in 1 in 100,000 live births; the free T₄ is normal to low. When tertiary or secondary hypothyroidism is detected, assessment of other pituitary hormones and investigation of pituitary-hypothalamic anatomy via magnetic resonance imaging (MRI) are indicated. Although not a hypothyroid condition, **congenital T₄-binding globulin deficiency** occurs in about 1 in 10,000 live births and is associated with a low serum total T₄ concentration, a normal TSH and serum free T₄, and a euthyroid status. This entity does not require treatment with thyroid hormone because it is merely a binding protein abnormality. It is commonly X-linked dominant.

**Clinical manifestations** of congenital hypothyroidism in the immediate newborn period usually are subtle but become more evident weeks or months after birth. By then, it is too late to ensure that there is not a detriment to the infant's cognitive development. Newborn screening is crucial to make an early diagnosis and initiate thyroid replacement therapy by younger than 1 month of age. Findings at various stages after birth include gestation greater than 42 weeks, birth weight greater than 4 kg, hypothermia, acrocyanosis, respiratory distress, large posterior fontanelle, abdominal distention, lethargy and poor feeding, jaundice more than 3 days after birth, edema, umbilical hernia, mottled skin, constipation, large tongue, dry skin, and hoarse cry. Thyroid hormones are crucial for maturation and differentiation of tissues such as bone (the bone age is often delayed at birth because of intrauterine hypothyroidism) and brain (most thyroid-dependent brain maturation occurs 2 to 3 years after birth) (Table 175-3).

When **treatment** is initiated within 1 month or less after birth, the prognosis for normal intellectual development is excellent; screening programs usually offer therapy within 1 to 2 weeks of birth. If therapy is instituted after 6 months, when the signs of severe hypothyroidism are present, the likelihood of normal intellectual function is markedly decreased. Growth improves after thyroid replacement, even in late diagnosed cases. The dose of T₄ changes with age; 10 to 15 μg/kg of T₄ is used for a newborn, but about 3 μg/kg is used later in childhood. In neonatal hypothyroidism, the goal is to bring the serum free T₄ rapidly into the upper half of the range of normal. Suppression of TSH is not seen in all cases and

## TABLE 175-3 Symptoms and Signs of Hypothyroidism

### ECTODERMAL

Poor growth
Dull facies: thick lips, large tongue, depressed nasal bridge, periorbital edema
Dry scaly skin
Sparse brittle hair
Diminished sweating
Carotenemia
Vitiligo

### CIRCULATORY

Sinus bradycardia/heart block
Cold extremities
Cold intolerance
Pallor
ECG changes: low-voltage QRS complex

### NEUROMUSCULAR

Muscle weakness
Hypotonia: constipation, potbelly
Umbilical hernia
Myxedema coma (carbon dioxide narcosis, hypothermia)
Pseudohypertrophy of muscles
Myalgia
Physical and mental lethargy
Developmental delay
Delayed relaxation of reflexes
Paresthesias (nerve entrapment: carpal tunnel syndrome)
Cerebellar ataxia

### SKELETAL

Delayed bone age
Epiphyseal dysgenesis, increased upper-to-lower segment ratio

### METABOLIC

Myxedema
Serous effusions (pleural, pericardial, ascites)
Hoarse voice (cry)
Weight gain
Menstrual irregularity
Arthralgia
Elevated CK
Macrocytosis (anemia)
Hypercholesterolemia
Hyperprolactinemia
Precocious puberty in severe cases

CK, creatine kinase; ECG, electrocardiographic.

is not necessary in all cases because such suppression may lead to excessive doses of $T_4$.

## Acquired Hypothyroidism

The **etiology** of acquired hypothyroidism is presented in Table 175-2. The **clinical manifestations** may be subtle. Hypothyroidism should be suspected in any child who has a decline in growth velocity, especially if not associated with weight loss (see Table 175-3). The most common cause of acquired hypothyroidism in older children in the United States is lymphocytic autoimmune thyroiditis (**Hashimoto thyroiditis**). In many areas of the world, iodine deficiency is the etiology of endemic goiter (**endemic cretinism**). The failure of the thyroid gland may be heralded by an increase of TSH before $T_4$ levels decrease. In contrast to untreated congenital hypothyroidism, acquired hypothyroidism is not a cause of permanent developmental delay.

**Hashimoto Thyroiditis.** Also known as autoimmune or *lymphocytic thyroiditis,* Hashimoto thyroiditis is a common cause of goiter and acquired thyroid disease in older children and adolescents. A family history of thyroid disease is present in 25% to 35% of patients. The *etiology* is an autoimmune process targeted against the thyroid gland with lymphocytic infiltration and lymphoid follicle and germinal center formation preceding fibrosis and atrophy.

**Clinical manifestations** include a firm, nontender euthyroid, hypothyroid, or, rarely, hyperthyroid (hashitoxicosis) diffuse goiter with a pebble-like feeling; an insidious onset after 6 years of age (the incidence peaks in adolescence, with a female predominance); and sometimes a pea-sized delphian lymph node above the thyroid isthmus. Associated autoimmune diseases include diabetes mellitus type 1 (DM1), adrenal insufficiency (Schmidt syndrome), and hypoparathyroidism. **Autoimmune polyglandular syndrome type I** consists of hypoparathyroidism, Addison disease, mucocutaneous candidiasis, and often hypothyroidism. **Autoimmune polyglandular syndrome type II** consists of Addison disease, DM1, and frequently autoimmune hypothyroidism. Trisomy 21 and Turner syndrome predispose to the development of autoimmune thyroiditis.

The **diagnosis** may be confirmed by serum antithyroid peroxidase (previously antimicrosomal) and antithyroglobulin antibodies. Neither biopsy nor thyroid scan is indicated in Hashimoto thyroiditis, although the thyroid scan with reduced uptake may differentiate hashitoxicosis from Graves disease.

**Treatment** with thyroid hormone sufficient to normalize TSH and free $T_4$ is indicated for hypothyroidism in Hashimoto thyroiditis. Patients without manifestation of hypothyroidism require periodic thyroid function testing (serum TSH and free $T_4$) every 6 to 12 months to detect the later development of hypothyroidism. Goiter with a normal TSH usually is not an indication for treatment.

## Hyperthyroidism

### Graves Disease

Most children with hyperthyroidism have Graves disease, the autonomous functioning of the thyroid caused by autoantibodies stimulating the thyroid stimulating immunoglobulins (TSIs). The resulting excessive synthesis, release, and peripheral metabolism of thyroid hormones produce the clinical features. Hashimoto thyroiditis and thyrotoxicosis are on a continuum of autoimmune diseases; there is overlap in their immunologic findings. Antimicrosomal and antithyroglobulin antibodies may be present in thyrotoxicosis, although the values are usually lower than in Hashimoto thyroiditis. Exceptionally high titers of antibodies may indicate the thyrotoxic phase of Hashimoto thyroiditis with the subsequent evolution toward permanent hypothyroidism. In Graves disease, serum $T_4$ or $T_3$ or both levels are elevated, whereas TSH is suppressed. Rare causes of hyperthyroidism include McCune-Albright syndrome, thyroid neoplasm, TSH hypersecretion, subacute thyroiditis, and iodine or thyroid hormone ingestion.

**Clinical Manifestations.** Graves disease presents as hyperthyroidism (Table 175-4) and is about five times more common in girls than in boys, with a peak incidence in adolescence. Personality changes, mood instability, and poor school performance are common initial problems. Tremor, anxiety, inability to concentrate, and weight loss may be insidious and confused with a psychological disorder until thyroid function tests reveal the elevated serum free $T_4$ level. Serum $T_4$ may be near-normal, whereas serum $T_3$ is selectively elevated ($T_3$ toxicosis, a rare entity). A firm, homogeneous goiter is usually present. Many patients complain of neck fullness and, in older subjects, a change in the size of their shirt collars. Thyroid gland enlargement is best visualized with the neck only slightly extended and with the examiner lateral to the patient; palpation of the thyroid gland is best performed with the examiner's hands around the neck from the back. The patient swallows so that the examiner can feel and examine the size, consistency, nodularity, and motion of the gland. The examiner should watch the patient swallow to note any discernible enlargement or asymmetry of the thyroid lobes. The thickness is estimated, and the dimensions of each lobe are measured vertically and laterally. Auscultation may reveal a bruit over the gland, which needs to be differentiated from a carotid bruit.

**Treatment.** Three treatment choices are available: pharmacologic, surgical, and radioactive iodine.

**Drugs.** Medical therapy to block thyroid hormone synthesis consists of propylthiouracil (5–7 mg/kg/24 hours orally in divided doses every 8 hours) or methimazole (0.5–0.7 mg/kg/24 hours orally in divided doses every 8–12 hours). Both medications are equally effective; methimazole may be easier to manage and titrate. Propranolol is started if symptoms are severe (2–3 mg/kg/24 hours orally) to control cardiac manifestations and is tapered as the propylthiouracil or methimazole takes effect. Propylthiouracil usually is continued for 1 to 2 years because the remission rate is approximately 25% per year. In patients complying with the treatment regimen, the 2-year course of treatment can be repeated. Propylthiouracil should suppress thyroid function to normal, without the need to add thyroid hormone replacement to normalize serum free $T_4$. Complications of propylthiouracil are lupus-like syndrome, rash, granulocytopenia, and jaundice. The granulocytopenia is an idiosyncratic complication of rapid onset, which is observed only in the early months after institution of antithyroid medication and which must be attended to promptly by monitoring the complete blood count (CBC). If a suppressed white blood cell count is observed, antithyroid therapy must be discontinued; this is potentially lethal (more rarely, thrombocytopenia or aplastic anemia) and is a rare complication that affects 3 in 10,000 users a year. After resolution, the other of the two antithyroid medications can be started because there is usually less than a 50% chance of a similar reaction from the other medication. These side effects are sometimes severe and usually reversible after discontinuation of antithyroid therapy; failure to monitor and then discontinue propylthiouracil when complications arise may be fatal. Iodine administration, which may suppress thyroid function but becomes ineffective in a few weeks, is sometimes used as a preparation for surgery but never for long-term therapy.

**Surgery.** Surgical treatment consists of partial or complete thyroidectomy. Risks associated with thyroidectomy include the use of anesthesia and the possibility that the thyroid removal will be excessive, causing hypothyroidism, or that it will be inadequate, resulting in persistent hyperthyroidism. In addition, keloid formation, recurrent laryngeal nerve palsy, and hypoparathyroidism (transient

### TABLE 175-4 Clinical Manifestations of Hyperthyroidism

| Associated Change | Sign/Symptom |
|---|---|
| Increased catecholamine effects | Nervousness |
| | Palpitations |
| | Tachycardia |
| | Atrial arrhythmias |
| | Systolic hypertension |
| | Tremor |
| | Brisk reflexes |
| Hypermetabolism | Increased sweating |
| | Shiny, smooth skin |
| | Heat intolerance |
| | Fatigue |
| | Weight loss—increased appetite |
| | Increased bowel movement (hyperdefecation) |
| | Hyperkinesis |
| Myopathy | Weakness |
| | Periodic paralysis |
| | Cardiac failure—dyspnea |
| Miscellaneous | Proptosis, stare, exophthalmos, lid lag, ophthalmopathy |
| | Hair loss |
| | Inability to concentrate |
| | Personality change (emotional lability) |
| | Goiter |
| | Thyroid bruit |
| | Onycholysis |
| | Painful gland* |
| | Acute thyroid storm (hyperpyrexia, tachycardia, coma, high-output heart failure, shock) |

*Unusual except in subacute thyroiditis with hyperthyroid phase.

postoperative or permanent) may occur. Thyroid storm caused by the release of large amounts of preformed hormone is a serious but rare complication. Even with optimal immediate postoperative results, patients may become hypothyroid within 10 years.

**Radioiodine. Radioiodine ($^{131}$I)** is slower in exerting therapeutic effects, may require repeated dosing, and is likely to cause permanent hypothyroidism. Ultimately, hypothyroidism is the desired outcome because it is easier and safer to treat than continued hyperthyroidism. Although studies reveal no long-term consequences, concern remains about possible sequelae in children. This method of treatment is entering the mainstream for adolescents and adults. Radioiodine given to a pregnant teenager renders the fetus hypothyroid and is contraindicated.

## Thyroid Storm

Thyroid storm (see Table 175-4) is a rare medical emergency consisting of tachycardia and hyperthermia. *Treatment* includes reducing the hyperthermia with a cooling blanket and administering propranolol to control the tachycardia, hypertension, and autonomic hyperfunction symptoms. Iodine may be given to block thyroid hormone release. Hydrocortisone may be indicated for relative adrenal insufficiency, and therapy for heart failure includes diuretics and digoxin.

## Congenital Hyperthyroidism

This disorder results from transplacental passage of maternal TSIs and may be masked for several days until the short-lived effects of transplacental maternal antithyroid medication wear off (assuming the mother was receiving such medication), at which time the effects of TSIs are observed. Irritability, tachycardia (often with signs of cardiac failure simulating *cardiomyopathy*), polycythemia, craniosynostosis, bone age advancement, poor feeding and, later, failure to thrive are the clinical hallmarks. This condition may be anticipated if the mother is known to be thyrotoxic in pregnancy. Cure of hyperthyroidism before pregnancy (surgery or radioiodine treatment) limits or curtails $T_4$ production but not the underlying immune disturbance producing TSIs; thus, the infant still may be affected, at least transiently.

**Treatment** for a severely affected neonate includes oral propranolol, 2 to 3 mg/kg/24 hours in divided doses, and propylthiouracil, approximately 5 mg/kg/24 hours orally in three divided doses. Because the half-life of the immunoglobulin is several weeks, spontaneous resolution of neonatal thyrotoxicosis resulting from transplacental passage of TSIs usually occurs by 2 to 3 months of age. Observation without treatment is indicated in patients who are minimally affected.

## TUMORS OF THE THYROID

Carcinoma of the thyroid is rare in children, but papillary and follicular carcinomas represent 90% of children's thyroid cancers. A history of therapeutic head or neck irradiation or radiation exposure from nuclear accidents predisposes a child to thyroid cancer. Carcinoma usually presents as a firm to hard, painless, nonfunctional solitary nodule and may spread to adjacent lymph nodes. Rapid growth, hoarseness (recurrent laryngeal nerve involvement), and lung metastasis may be present. If the nodule is solid on ultrasound, is *cold* on radioiodine scanning, and feels hard, the likelihood of a carcinoma is high. Excisional biopsy usually is performed, but fine needle aspiration biopsy also may be diagnostic.

**Treatment** includes total thyroidectomy, selective regional node dissection, and radioablation with $^{131}$I for residual or recurrent disease. The **prognosis** is usually good if the disease is diagnosed early.

**Medullary carcinoma of the thyroid** may be asymptomatic except for a mass. *Diagnosis* is based on the presence of elevated calcitonin levels, either in the basal state or after pentagastrin stimulation, and histologic examination. This tumor most often occurs with multiple endocrine neoplasia 2a or 2b, pheochromocytoma, or alone, possibly in a familial pattern. The presence of mutations of the *RET* proto-oncogene is predictive of the development of medullary carcinoma of the thyroid in some families. Screening the other members of the family is indicated after a proband is recognized. Prophylactic thyroidectomy is indicated for the family members with the same allele.

# CHAPTER 176

# Disorders of Parathyroid Bone and Mineral Endocrinology

## PARATHYROID HORMONE AND VITAMIN D

Calcium and phosphate are regulated mainly by diet and three hormones: parathyroid hormone (PTH), vitamin D, and calcitonin. PTH is secreted in response to a decrease in serum ionized calcium level. PTH attaches to its membrane receptor. It then acts via adenylate cyclase to mobilize calcium from bone into the serum and to enhance fractional reabsorption of calcium by the kidney while inducing phosphate excretion, all of which increase the serum calcium concentration and decrease serum phosphate. Lack of PTH effect is heralded by low serum calcium in the presence of elevated phosphate for age. PTH stimulates vitamin D secretion by increasing renal 1α-hydroxylase activity and acts indirectly to elevate serum calcium concentration by stimulating the production of 1,25-dihydroxyvitamin D from 25-hydroxyvitamin D. Calcitonin increases the deposition of calcium into bone; in normal states, the effect is subtle, but calcitonin may be used to suppress extremely elevated serum calcium values.

1,25-Dihydroxyvitamin D enhances calcium absorption from the gastrointestinal tract, resulting in increased serum calcium levels and increased bone mineralization. Vitamin D, derived from exposure of the skin to ultraviolet (UV) rays (usually via the sun) or from oral ingestion, must be modified sequentially first to 25-hydroxyvitamin D in the liver and then $1\alpha$-hydroxylated to the metabolically active form (1,25-dihydroxyvitamin D) in the kidney. The serum concentration of 25-hydroxyvitamin D is a better reflection of vitamin D sufficiency than the measurement of 1,25-hydroxyvitamin D (see Chapter 31).

## HYPOCALCEMIA

The **clinical manifestations** of hypocalcemia (ionized calcium < 4.5 mg/dL; total calcium < 8.5 mg/dL if serum protein is normal) result from increased neuromuscular irritability and include muscle cramps, carpopedal spasm (tetany), weakness, paresthesia, laryngospasm, and seizure-like activity. Tetany can be detected by the *Chvostek sign* (facial spasms produced by lightly tapping over the facial nerve just in front of the ear) or by the *Trousseau sign* (carpal spasms exhibited when arterial blood flow to the hand is occluded for 3 to 5 minutes with a blood pressure cuff inflated to 15 mm Hg above systolic blood pressure). Total serum calcium concentration is usually measured, although a determination of serum ionized calcium, the biologically active form, is preferable. Albumin is the major reservoir of protein-bound calcium. Disorders that alter plasma pH or serum albumin concentration must be considered when circulating calcium concentrations are being evaluated. The fraction of ionized calcium is inversely related to plasma pH; **alkalosis** can precipitate hypocalcemia by lowering ionized calcium without changing total serum calcium. Alkalosis may result from hyperpnea caused by anxiety or from hyperventilation related to physical exertion. Hypoproteinemia may lead to a false suggestion of hypocalcemia because the serum total calcium level is low even though the ionized $Ca^{2+}$ remains normal. It is best to measure serum ionized calcium if hypocalcemia or hypercalcemia is suspected.

**Primary hypoparathyroidism** causes hypocalcemia, but does not cause rickets. The etiology of primary hypoparathyroidism includes the following:

1. Congenital malformation (e.g., DiGeorge syndrome or other complex syndromes) resulting from developmental abnormalities of the third and fourth branchial arches (see Chapters 143 and 144)
2. Surgical procedures, such as thyroidectomy or parathyroidectomy, in which parathyroid tissue is removed either deliberately or as a complication of surgery for another goal
3. Autoimmunity (autoimmune polyglandular syndrome type 1), which may destroy the parathyroid gland

**Pseudohypoparathyroidism** may occur in one of four forms, all with hypocalcemia and hyperphosphatemia, as follows:

1. *Type Ia*—an abnormality of the $G_{s\alpha}$ protein linking the PTH receptor to adenylate cyclase; biologically active PTH is secreted in great quantities but does not stimulate its receptor
2. *Type Ib*—normal phenotype, normal $G_{s\alpha}$ with abnormalities in the production of adenylate cyclase
3. *Type Ic*—abnormal phenotype, normal production of adenylate cyclase, but a distal defect eliminates the effects of PTH
4. *Type II*—normal phenotype, normal production of adenylate cyclase, with a postreceptor defect, close to type Ib

Pseudohypoparathyroidism is an autosomal dominant condition that may present at birth or later. Other *clinical manifestations* of pseudohypoparathyroidism associated with **Albright hereditary osteodystrophy** include short stature, stocky body habitus, round facies, short fourth and fifth metacarpals, calcification of the basal ganglia, subcutaneous calcification, and, often, developmental delay. Albright hereditary osteodystrophy may be inherited separately so that a patient may have a normal appearance with hypocalcemia or may have the Albright hereditary osteodystrophy phenotype with normal serum calcium, phosphate, PTH, and response to PTH.

During the first 3 days after birth, serum calcium concentrations normally decline in response to withdrawal of the maternal calcium supply via the placenta. Sluggish PTH response in a neonate may result in a transient hypocalcemia. Hypocalcemia caused by attenuated PTH release is found in infants of mothers with hyperparathyroidism and hypercalcemia; the latter suppresses fetal PTH release, causing **transient hypoparathyroidism** in the neonatal period.

Normal serum magnesium concentrations are required for normal parathyroid gland function and action. **Hypomagnesemia** may cause a secondary hypoparathyroidism, which responds poorly to therapies other than magnesium replacement.

**Neonatal tetany** is most often noted in premature or asphyxiated infants and infants of diabetic mothers. Excessive phosphate retention, as occurs in renal failure, also produces hypocalcemia.

The **etiology** of hypocalcemia usually can be discerned by combining features of the clinical presentation with determinations of serum ionized calcium, phosphate, alkaline phosphatase, PTH (preferably at a time when the calcium is low), magnesium, and albumin. If the PTH concentration is not elevated appropriately relevant to low serum calcium, hypoparathyroidism (transient, primary, or caused by hypomagnesemia) is present. Vitamin D stores can be estimated by measuring serum 25-hydroxyvitamin D. Renal function is assessed by a serum creatinine measurement or determination of creatinine clearance (Table 176-1).

**Treatment** of severe tetany or seizures resulting from hypocalcemia consists of intravenous calcium gluconate (1–2 mL/kg of a 10% solution) given slowly over 10 minutes, while cardiac status is monitored by electrocardiogram (ECG) for bradycardia, which can be fatal. Long-term treatment of hypoparathyroidism involves administering vitamin D, preferably as 1,25-dihydroxyvitamin D, and calcium. Therapy is adjusted to keep the serum calcium in the lower half of the normal range to avoid episodes of hypercalcemia that might produce nephrocalcinosis and to avoid pancreatitis.

**TABLE 176-1 Important Physiologic Changes in Bone and Mineral Diseases**

| Condition | Calcium | Phosphate | Parathyroid Hormone | 25(OH)D |
|---|---|---|---|---|
| Primary hypoparathyroidism | ↓ | ↑ | ↓ | Nl |
| Pseudohypoparathyroidism | ↓ | ↑ | ↑ | Nl |
| Vitamin D deficiency | Nl(↓) | ↓ | ↑ | ↓ |
| Familial hypophosphatemic rickets | Nl | ↓ | Nl (sl↑) | Nl |
| Hyperparathyroidism | ↑ | ↓ | ↑ | Nl |
| Immobilization | ↑ | ↑ | ↓ | Nl |

↑, high; ↓, low; Nl, normal; 25(OH)D, 25-hydroxyvitamin D; sl, slight.

## RICKETS

Rickets is defined as decreased or defective bone mineralization in growing children; **osteomalacia** is the same condition in adults. The proportion of osteoid (the organic portion of bone) is excessive. As a result, the bone becomes soft and the metaphyses of the long bones widen. Very low birth weight infants have an increased incidence of rickets of prematurity. In older infants, poor linear growth, bowing of the legs on weight bearing (which can be painful), thickening at the wrists and knees, and prominence of the costochondral junctions (rachitic rosary) of the rib cage occur. At this stage, x-ray findings are diagnostic.

In **nutritional vitamin D deficiency**, calcium is not absorbed adequately from the intestine (see Chapter 31). Poor vitamin D intake (food fads or poor maternal diet affecting breast milk vitamin D) or avoidance of sunlight in infants exclusively breastfed may contribute to the development of rickets. Vitamin D–deficiency rickets occurs predominantly in the United States in African-American or Asian infants who are breastfed and have inadequate exposure to sun. Fat malabsorption resulting from hepatobiliary disease (biliary atresia, neonatal hepatitis) or other causes (cystic fibrosis) also may produce vitamin D deficiency because vitamin D is a fat-soluble vitamin. Defects in vitamin D metabolism by the kidney (renal failure, autosomal recessive deficiency of 1α-hydroxylation, **vitamin D–dependent rickets**) or liver (defect in 25-hydroxylation) also can cause rickets.

In **familial hypophosphatemic rickets**, the major defect in mineral metabolism is failure of the kidney to reabsorb filtered phosphate adequately so that serum phosphate decreases, and urinary phosphate is high. The *diagnosis* of this X-linked disease usually is made within the first few years of life. Disease typically is more severe in males.

The **etiology** of rickets usually can be determined by assessment of the mineral and vitamin D status (25-hydroxyvitamin D < 8 ng/mL suggests nutritional vitamin D deficiency) (see Table 176-1). Further testing of mineral balance or measurement of other vitamin D metabolites may be required.

Several chemical forms of vitamin D can be used for **treatment** of the different rachitic conditions, but their potencies vary widely. Required dosages depend on the condition being treated (see Chapter 31). Rickets usually is treated with 1,25-hydroxyvitamin D and supplemental calcium. In hypophosphatemic rickets, phosphate supplementation (not calcium) must accompany vitamin D therapy, which is given to suppress secondary hyperparathyroidism. Adequate therapy restores normal skeletal growth and produces resolution of the radiographic signs of rickets. Nutritional rickets is treated with vitamin D in one large dose or multiple smaller replacement doses. Surgery may be required to straighten legs in untreated patients with long-standing disease.

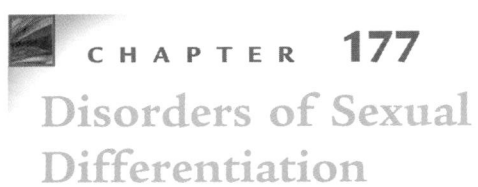

## CHAPTER 177

# Disorders of Sexual Differentiation

## NORMAL SEXUAL DEVELOPMENT

The successive sequence of chromosomal sex, gonadal sex, and phenotypic sex leads to gender identity of the individual. Genes usually determine the morphology of internal organs and of gonads (gonadal sex); this directs the appearance of the external genitalia which form the secondary sex characteristics (phenotypic sex); self-perception of the individual (gender identity) and the perception of the individual by others (gender role) follow last. In most children, these features blend and conform, but in some patients, one or more features may not follow this sequence, leading to an intersex condition (see Chapter 23).

**Ambiguous genitalia** in a newborn must be attended to with as little delay as possible and with informed sensitivity to the psychosocial context as required. The laboratory evaluations required might take days or weeks to complete, delaying a sex assignment and naming of the infant, such that choice often precedes diagnosis. Beyond infancy and childhood, and to offset any gender uncertainty in the patient and confusion in the parents, health care providers must help families come to an appropriate closure and gender choice.

**Diagnosis and treatment** of disorders of sex differentiation are best understood in terms of the embryology and hormonal control of normal sex differentiation. The internal and external genitalia are formed between 9 and 13 weeks of gestation. Fetal gonad and external genitalia are bipotential and have the capacity to support development of a normal male or female phenotype (Fig. 177-1).

**FIGURE 177-1**

**Differentiation of male and female external genitalia as proceeding from a common embryonic anlage.** Testosterone acts at 9 to 13 weeks of gestation to virilize the bipotential anlage. In the absence of testosterone action, the female phenotype develops. (From Grumbach MM, Conte FA: Disorders of sexual differentiation. In Wilson JD, Foster DW [eds]: Textbook of Endocrinology, 8th ed. Philadelphia, *WB Saunders*, 1990, p 873. Adapted from Spaulding MH: *Contrib Embryol Instit* 13:69–88, 1921.)

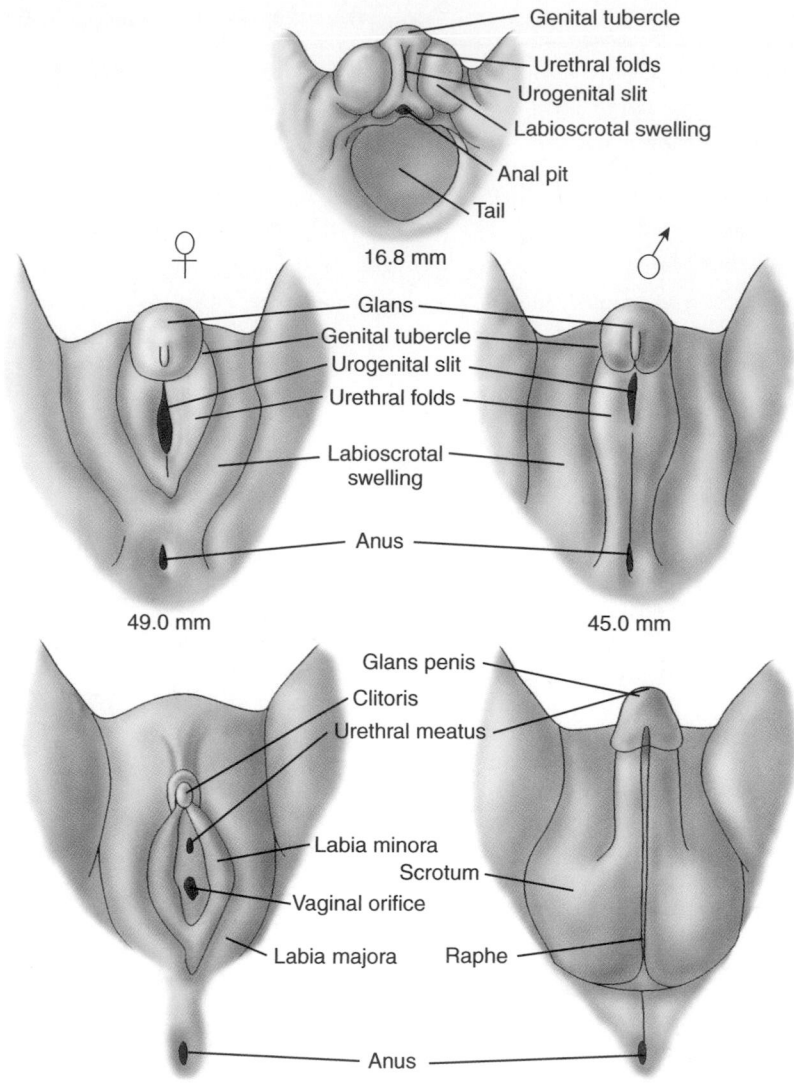

In the presence of a gene called *SRY* for sex-determining region on the Y gene on the Y chromosome, the primitive fetal gonad differentiates into a testis (Fig. 177-2). The testis secretes testosterone, which has direct effects (stimulating development of the wolffian ducts), but also is locally converted to dihydrotestosterone (DHT) by the 5α-reductase enzyme. DHT causes enlargement, rugation, and fusion of the labioscrotal folds into a scrotum; fusion of the ventral surface of the penis to enclose a penile urethra; and enlargement of the phallus with ultimate development of male external genitalia. Testicular production and secretion of müllerian-inhibitory substance cause the regression and disappearance of the müllerian ducts and their derivatives, such as the fallopian tubes and uterus. In the presence of testosterone, the wolffian ducts develop into the vas deferens, seminiferous tubules, and prostate.

The female phenotype develops unless specific *male* influences alter development. In the absence of *SRY*, an ovary spontaneously develops from the bipotential, primitive gonad. In the absence of fetal testicular secretion of müllerian-inhibitory substance, a normal uterus, fallopian tubes, and posterior third of the vagina develop out of the müllerian ducts, and the wolffian ducts degenerate. In the total absence of androgens, the external genitalia appear female.

A child with **ambiguous genitalia** may have a male karyotype or a female karyotype. In the female pseudohermaphrodite, the genotype is 46,XX, and the gonads are ovaries, but the external genitalia are virilized. In the male pseudohermaphrodite, the genotype is 46,XY, and the external genitalia are undervirilized. Reasons can include abnormal development of the testes; defects of sex steroid biosynthesis, including testosterone or DHT; or androgen receptor defects. On physical examination, it is essential to note where the urethral opening lies and whether there is fusion of the anterior portion of the labioscrotal folds. Endogenous excessive production of androgen (as in congenital adrenal hyperplasia [CAH]) in a female fetus between 9 and 13 weeks of gestation leads to ambiguous genitalia. If the vaginal opening is normal, and there is no fusion, but the clitoris is enlarged without ventral fusion of the ventral urethra, the patient had later exposure to androgens. A patient with a fully

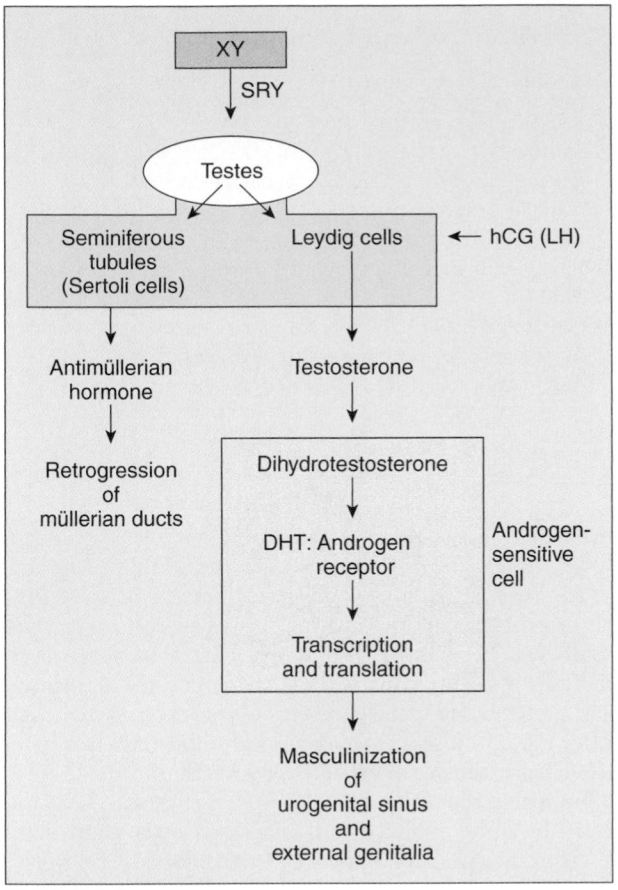

**FIGURE 177-2**

**A diagrammatic scheme of male sex determination and differentiation.** DHT, dihydrotestosterone; *SRY,* the gene for the testis-determining factor. *SRY* is the master gene controlling male sex differentiation, but there are many other genes and their products that control male and female sexual differentiation. (From Wilson JD, Foster DW [eds]: Williams Textbook of Endocrinology, 8th ed. Philadelphia, *WB Saunders*, 1992, p 918.)

formed scrotum, even if small, and a normally formed but small penis, termed a *microphallus,* must have had normal exposure to and action of androgen during 9 to 13 weeks of gestation.

## ABNORMAL SEXUAL DEVELOPMENT

### Virilization of the 46,XX Female (Female Pseudohermaphroditism)

Masculinization of the external genitalia of genotypic females (except for isolated enlargement of the clitoris, which can occur from later androgen exposure) is always caused by the presence of excessive androgens during the critical period of development (8–13 weeks of gestation) (Table 177-1). The magnitude of the changes reflects the quantity and duration of exposure to androgens. The degree of virilization can range from mild clitoral enlargement to the appearance of a *male* phallus with a penile urethra and fused scrotum with raphe. Congenital virilizing adrenal hyperplasia is the most common cause of ambiguous genitalia; it is most commonly the result of an enzyme deficiency that impairs synthesis of glucocorticoids, but

**TABLE 177-1 Causes of Virilization in the Female**

| Condition | Additional Feature(s) |
|---|---|
| P-450$_{c21}$ deficiency | Salt loss in some |
| 3β-Hydroxysteroid dehydrogenase deficiency | Salt loss |
| P-450$_{c11}$ deficiency | Salt retention/ hypertension |
| Androgenic drug exposure (e.g., progestins) | Exposure between 9 and 12 weeks of gestation |
| Mixed gonadal dysgenesis or mosaic Turner syndrome | Karyotype = 46,XY/45,X |
| True hermaphrodite | Testicular and ovarian tissue present |
| Maternal virilizing adrenal or ovarian tumor | Rare, positive history |

does not affect androgen production. The impaired cortisol secretion leads to adrenocorticotropic hormone (ACTH) hypersecretion, which stimulates hyperplasia of the adrenal cortex and excessive adrenal production of androgens (see Chapter 178).

### Inadequate Masculinization of the 46,XY Male (Male Pseudohermaphroditism)

Underdevelopment of the male external genitalia occurs because of a relative deficiency of testosterone production or action (Table 177-2). The penis is small, with various degrees of hypospadias (penile or perineal) and associated chordee or ventral binding of the phallus; unilateral, but more often bilateral, cryptorchidism may be present. The testes should be sought carefully in the inguinal canal or labioscrotal folds by palpation or ultrasound. Rarely a palpable gonad in the inguinal canal or labioscrotal fold represents a herniated ovary, or an ovotestis in true hermaphroditism. The latter patients have ovarian and testicular tissue and usually ambiguous external genitalia. Production of testosterone by a gonad implies that testicular tissue is present and that at least some cells carry the *SRY* gene.

Testosterone production can be reduced by specific deficiencies of the enzymes needed for androgen biosynthesis or by dysplasia of the gonads. In the latter, if müllerian-inhibiting substance production also is reduced, a rudimentary uterus and fallopian tubes are present. Enzyme defects in testosterone biosynthesis, which also block cortisol production, produce adrenal hyperplasia. Congenital gonadotropin deficiency may produce a normally formed but small penis (microphallus without hypospadias). Hypopituitarism with luteinizing hormone (LH) deficiency does not result in ambiguous genitalia because placental human chorionic gonadotropin (hCG) in the fetal circulation stimulates fetal gonadal testosterone synthesis during the critical 9 to 13 weeks of gestation to allow development of a normal male phallus. Later in gestation, fetal LH is needed to stimulate the testes to produce adequate androgen to enlarge the fetal penis. Hypopituitarism is often combined with deficiencies of growth

**TABLE 177-2  Causes of Inadequate Masculinization in the Male**

| Condition | Additional Feature(s) |
|---|---|
| P-450$_{scc}$ (StAR) deficiency | Salt loss |
| 3β-Hydroxysteroid dehydrogenase deficiency | Salt loss |
| P-450$_{c17}$ deficiency | Salt retention/hypokalemia/hypertension |
| Isolated P-450$_{c17}$ deficiency with 17,20-desmolase deficiency | Adrenal function normal |
| 17β-Hydroxysteroid oxidoreductase deficiency | Adrenal function normal |
| Dysgenetic testes | Possible abnormal karyotype |
| Leydig cell hypoplasia | Rare |
| Complete androgen insensitivity or testicular feminization | Female external genitalia, absence of müllerian structures |
| Partial androgen insensitivity | As above with ambiguous external genitalia |
| 5α-Reductase deficiency | Autosomal recessive, virilization at puberty |

StAR, steroid acute regulatory protein.

hormone (GH) and ACTH in neonatal hypopituitarism, causing neonatal hypoglycemia. Microphallus due to this cause responds to testosterone treatment, resulting in an enlargement of the penis.

The complete form of **androgen resistance** or **androgen insensitivity syndrome** is the most dramatic example of resistance to hormone action by defects in the androgen receptor. Affected patients have a **46,XY** karyotype, normally formed testes (usually located in the inguinal canal or labia majora), and feminine-appearing external genitalia with a short vagina and no internal müllerian structures. At the time of puberty, testosterone concentrations increase to normal or above normal male range. Because a portion of the testosterone is normally converted to estradiol in peripheral tissues and the estrogen cannot be opposed by the androgen, breast development ensues at the normal age of puberty without growth of pubic, facial, or axillary hair or the occurrence of menstruation. Gender identity and gender role are unequivocally **female**.

**5α-Reductase deficiency** presents at birth with predominantly female phenotype or with ambiguous genitalia, including perineoscrotal hypospadias. The defect is in 5α reduction of testosterone to its metabolite DHT. At puberty, spontaneous secondary male sexual development occurs, and the individual, if raised as a girl until this age, in most cases converts to a male gender identity and male gender role.

## APPROACH TO THE INFANT WITH GENITAL AMBIGUITY

The major goal is a rapid identification of any life-threatening disorders (salt loss and shock caused by the salt-losing form of CAH). The decision of female sex assignment can be rendered more complex by the realization that prenatal androgen exposure (in an individual without complete androgen resistance) causes a tendency toward a male gender identity and male gender role. Although the classic approach to sex assignment has been based on the feasibility of genital reconstruction and potential fertility rather than on karyotype or gonadal histology, the effects of prenatal androgen must be considered. And yet, it may be inappropriate to raise a female infant who is severely virilized from virilizing CAH as a male; in most reported cases, sex assignment and adult gender role remain

female and fertility can be retained because the internal organs are female. A 46,XY male with ambiguous genitalia and an extremely small phallus that does not increase in size with androgen therapy (partial androgen resistance) traditionally has been raised as a female because surgical construction of a fully functional phallus is difficult. Some of these patients frequently revert spontaneously to a male gender identity. Present management of ambiguous genitalia involves extensive open discussion with parents involving the biology of the infant and the likely prognosis. Treatment should be individualized and managed by a team including an experienced pediatric endocrinologist, urologist or gynecologist, and the primary care physician.

### Diagnosis

The first step toward diagnosis is to determine if the disorder represents virilization of a genetic female (androgen excess) or underdevelopment of a genetic male (androgen deficiency) (see Fig. 177-2). Inguinal gonads that are evident on palpation usually are testes and indicate that incomplete development of a male phenotype has occurred; this pattern is not consistent, and ovaries and ovotestes may feel similar. Similarly, absence of female internal genitalia (detected by ultrasound) implies that müllerian-inhibiting substance was present and secreted by fetal testes. Karyotype determination is only one of many factors in deciding the sexual identity for purposes of rearing; the *SRY* gene may be found on chromosomes other than the Y chromosome, and, conversely, a Y chromosome may lack an *SRY* gene (it may have been translocated to an X chromosome, leading to the development of a 46,XX male).

Statistically, most virilized females have CAH; 90% of these females have 21-hydroxylase deficiency. The diagnosis is established by measuring the plasma concentration of 17-hydroxyprogesterone and androstenedione (see Chapter 178), which typically is hundreds of times above the normal range. Other enzymatic defects also may be diagnosed by quantifying circulating levels of the adrenal steroid precursor proximal to the defective enzyme block.

Establishing an accurate diagnosis is more difficult in underdeveloped males. When certain types of adrenal hyperplasia coexist with defects in androgen production of the testes, excessive ACTH secretion elevates levels of specific adrenal steroid precursors substantially, allowing diagnosis. If the defect is restricted to testosterone biosynthesis, the measurement of testosterone and its precursors in the basal state and after stimulation by hCG may be required. Patients with normal levels of testosterone either have persistent androgen resistance or have had an interruption of normal morphogenesis of the genitalia. Abnormalities of the sex chromosomes may be associated with dysgenetic gonads, which may be associated with persistence of müllerian structures.

## Treatment

Treatment consists of replacing deficient hormones (cortisol in adrenal hyperplasia or testosterone in a child with androgen biosynthetic defects who will be raised as male), surgical restoration to make the individual look more appropriate for the gender of rearing, and psychological support of the whole family. Gonads and internal organs discordant for the gender of rearing are removed. Dysgenetic gonads with Y-genetic material always should be removed because **gonadoblastomas** or **dysgerminomas** may develop in the organ. Reconstructive surgery is usually by 2 years of age so that genital structure reflects gender of rearing. This recommendation for reconstructive surgery is controversial; some advocate that surgery not be performed in infancy or early childhood so that the child or young adolescent can be involved in the decision. A decision for gender of rearing is recommended from birth, however, and the knowledge that the intersexed person may change gender later on is shared with parents from the outset.

C H A P T E R  **178**

# Adrenal Gland Dysfunction

The adrenal gland consists of an outer cortex, responsible for the synthesis of steroids, and an inner medulla derived from neuroectodermal tissue, which synthesizes catecholamines. The *adrenal cortex* consists of three zones: an outer glomerulosa whose end product is the mineralocorticoid, aldosterone, which regulates sodium and potassium balance; a middle zone, the fasciculata, whose end product is cortisol; and an inner reticularis, which synthesizes sex steroids. The general scheme of these synthetic steps is shown in Figure 178-1.

Hypothalamic corticotropin-releasing hormone (CRH) stimulates the release of pituitary adrenocorticotropic hormone (ACTH, corticotropin), derived by selective processing from pro-opiomelanocortin. ACTH governs the synthesis and release of cortisol and adrenal androgens. Primary adrenal insufficiency or cortisol deficiency from any defect in the adrenal gland results in an oversecretion of ACTH; cortisol deficiency also may occur from ACTH (secondary) or CRH (tertiary) deficiency, causing

low serum ACTH concentrations and low cortisol. Endogenous (or exogenous) glucocorticoids feed back to inhibit ACTH and CRH secretion. The renin-angiotensin system and potassium regulate aldosterone secretion; ACTH has little effect on aldosterone production except in excess, when it may increase aldosterone secretion.

Steroids that circulate in the free form (not bound to cortisol-binding protein [transcortin]) may cross the placenta from mother to fetus, but ACTH does not. The placenta plays an important role in steroid biosynthesis in utero, acting as a metabolic mediator between mother and child. Because the fetal CRH-ACTH-adrenal axis is operational in utero, deficiencies in cortisol synthesis lead to excessive ACTH secretion. If a virilizing adrenal enzyme defect is present, such as 21-hydroxylase deficiency, the fetal adrenal gland secretes excess androgens, virilizing the fetus.

Normal variation of serum cortisol and ACTH levels leads to values that are high early in the morning and lower at night. This normal diurnal variation may not be established until the child is 1 to 4 years of age.

## ADRENAL INSUFFICIENCY

The **clinical manifestations** of inadequate adrenal function result from inadequate secretion or action of glucocorticoids, mineralocorticoids, or both (Table 178-1). In addition, in the case of enzyme defects that affect the gonad and the adrenal gland, overproduction or underproduction of potent androgens can occur, depending on the site of enzyme blockade (see Fig. 178-1). Progressive prenatal virilization of the external genitalia may occur in females; incomplete virilization may occur in males. Ambiguity of the external genitalia is a common manifestation of disordered fetal adrenal enzyme function. Precise *diagnosis* is essential for the prescription of appropriate therapy, long-term outlook, and genetic counseling. In patients with enzyme defects, an elevation in the precursor steroid is present proximal to the enzyme block and is metabolized through remaining normal alternate enzyme pathways, while a deficiency of steroids is present subsequent to the block.

The dominant clinical features of congenital adrenal mineralocorticoid deficiency are hyponatremia and hyperkalemia, usually developing by 5 to 7 days after birth but not usually immediately after birth. Vomiting, dehydration, and acidosis soon follow, as do hypotensive shock from glucocorticoid deficiency. Death may occur if the disorder remains undiagnosed and untreated. In females, the ambiguity of the external genitalia is an obvious clue that salt-losing congenital adrenal hyperplasia (CAH), or simple virilizing CAH, must be ruled out. Because these forms cannot be distinguished clinically, all presentations of ambiguous genitalia should involve evaluation for mineralocorticoid deficiency. In males, the most common form of CAH, 21-hydroxylase deficiency, does not cause abnormal genitalia. There may be hyperpigmentation of the scrotal skin, but this is a subtle sign. In all infants, the diagnosis of adrenal insufficiency may be overlooked or confused with pyloric stenosis. In pyloric stenosis, in contrast to salt-losing CAH, vomiting of stomach contents results in hypochloremia, serum potassium is normal or low, and alkalosis is present. This distinction may be lifesaving in preventing unnecessary investigations or inappropriate therapy.

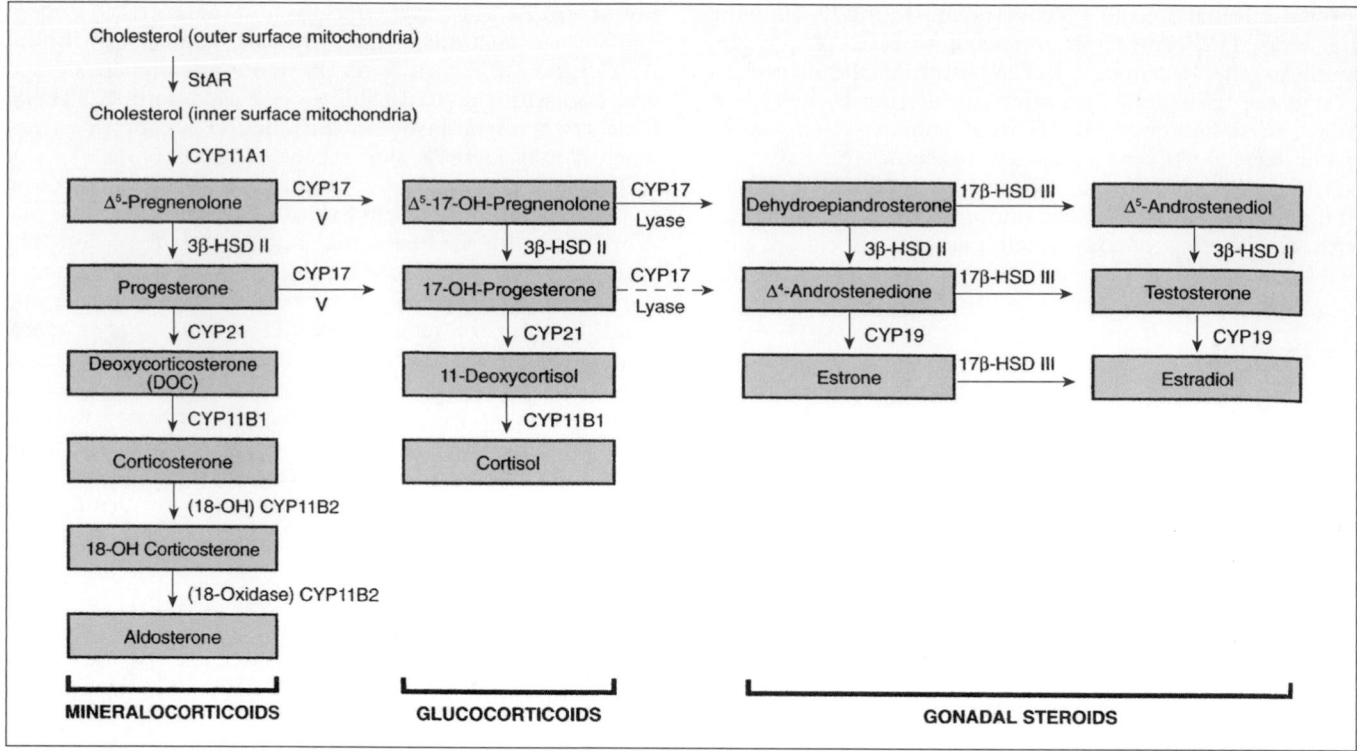

**FIGURE 178-1**

**Diagram of the steroid biosynthetic pathways and the biosynthetic defects that result in congenital hyperplasia.** The defect in patients with lipoid adrenal hyperplasia is not (except for one reported case) in the CYP11A1 (cholesterol side-chain cleavage) enzyme, but in StAR, the steroidogenic acute regulatory protein. This protein is involved in the transport of cholesterol from the outer mitochondrial membrane to the inner membrane, where the CYP11A1 enzyme is located. CYP11B1 (11β-hydroxylase) catalyzes 11β-hydroxylation of deoxcorticosterone and 11β-deoxycortisol primarily. CYP17 (17α-hydroxylase/17,20-lyase) catalyzes 17α-hydroxylation and splitting of the 17,20 bond, but for the latter it has preferential Δ⁵-17,20-lyase activity. CYP19 (aromatase) catalyzes the conversion of corticosterone to aldosterone. 3β-HSD I and 3β-HSD II, 3β-hydroxysteroid dehydrogenase/$Δ^{4,5}$-isomerase types I and II; CYP21 (P450$_{c21}$), 21-hydroxylase; 17β-HSD 3, 17β-hydroxysteroid dehydrogenase type 3. In the human, deletion of a homozygous null mutation of CYP11A (P450$_{ccc}$) is probably lethal in utero, but a heterogeneous mutation caused congenital lipoid adrenal hyperplasia. (From Melmed S, Polonsky K, Kronenberg H, Larsen R [eds]: Williams Textbook of Endocrinology, 10th ed. Philadelphia, *Elsevier*, 2003, p 917.)

Not all forms of adrenal hyperplasia present at birth; the spectrum of disorder ranges from severe, or classic, to mild, late-onset, or nonclassic. Milder forms may manifest in childhood, adolescence, or even young adulthood, not as glucocorticoid or mineralocorticoid deficiencies, but as androgen excess. In patients with congenital adrenal hypoplasia or adrenal hemorrhage, the secretion of all adrenal steroids is low. In contrast, CAH leads to a diagnostic steroid pattern in blood and urine (see Fig. 178-1). Deficiency of 21-hydroxylase is the most common form (95%) and serves as a paradigm for these disorders.

## 21-HYDROXYLASE DEFICIENCY

The incidence of classic 21-hydroxylase deficiency is about 1 in 12,000 among various white populations. A higher incidence occurs in Yupik Eskimos, Yugoslavians, and Ashkenazi Jews. Nonclassic CAH may occur with an incidence of 1 in 50 in certain populations. The gene for 21-hydroxylase lies on the short arm of chromosome 6; the genotype may be determined in a proband, permitting prenatal diagnosis in a subsequent pregnancy.

Deficient 21-hydroxylase activity (P-450$_{c21}$ deficiency) impairs the conversion of 17-hydroxyprogesterone to 11-deoxycortisol and, in the salt-losing form, of progesterone to deoxycorticosterone, a mineralocorticoid proximal in the pathway to the production of aldosterone. The decreased production of cortisol causes hypersecretion of ACTH, which stimulates the synthesis of steroids immediately proximal to the block and shunting of these to overproduction of androgens. The primary clinical manifestation is the virilization of the external genitalia of the affected female fetus, in whom the development of the uterus, ovaries, and fallopian tubes remains unaffected by the androgens. The degree of virilization varies, ranging from mild clitoromegaly to complete fusion of labioscrotal folds, with severe clitoromegaly simulating a phallus (see Chapter 177). A male infant with this defect appears normal at birth, although penile enlargement may be apparent thereafter. The deficiency in aldosterone, found in about 75% of patients, causes salt wasting with shock and dehydration until the diagnosis is established and appropriate treatment is given.

The treatment of 21-hydroxylase deficiency requires hydrocortisone, and fludrocortisone in the case of the

## TABLE 178-1  Clinical Manifestations of Adrenal Insufficiency

Cortisol deficiency
  Hypoglycemia
  Inability to withstand stress
  Vasomotor collapse
  Hyperpigmentation (in primary adrenal insufficiency with excess of adrenocorticotropic hormone)
  Apneic spells
  Muscle weakness, fatigue
Aldosterone deficiency
  Hyponatremia
  Hyperkalemia
  Vomiting
  Urinary sodium wasting
  Salt craving
  Acidosis
  Failure to thrive
  Volume depletion
  Hypotension
  Dehydration
  Shock
  Diarrhea
  Muscle weakness
Androgen excess or deficiency (caused by adrenal enzyme defect)
  Ambiguous genitalia in certain conditions

salt-losing form. Therapy must be adjusted throughout childhood at regular intervals. Overtreatment will cause growth stunting and weight gain (cushingoid features), whereas undertreatment will cause excessive height gain, skeletal advance, and early appearance puberty, ultimately jeopardizing adult height potential. Late-onset CAH is noted years after birth. Affected subjects have milder manifestations without ambiguous genitalia, but they do have acne, hirsutism, and, in girls, irregular menstrual cycles or amenorrhea. Late-onset CAH in girls may be confused with polycystic ovary disease.

**Biochemical diagnostic studies** show elevated levels of serum 17-OHP, the substrate for the defective 21-hydroxylase enzyme activity. In newborns with CAH, the values are elevated a hundredfold to a thousandfold. In late-onset CAH, an ACTH stimulation test is necessary to show an abnormally high response of 17-OHP. Serum cortisol and aldosterone levels (in salt losers) are low, whereas the testosterone level is elevated because it is derived from 17-OHP.

The goals of **treatment** are to achieve normal linear growth and bone age advancement. Long-term therapy consists of providing glucocorticoids at a dose of approximately 10 to 15 mg/m²/24 hours in three divided doses of oral hydrocortisone or its equivalent. Mineralocorticoid therapy for salt losers consists of fludrocortisone (Florinef) at a dose of 0.1 to 0.2 mg/24 hours often with sodium chloride supplementation in infancy and early childhood. Surgical correction of ambiguous external genitalia begins by 1 to 2 years of age. The adequacy of glucocorticoid replacement therapy is monitored by determining serum concentrations of adrenal precursors, including androstenedione and 17-OHP for 21-hydroxylase deficiency. In addition, the assessment of linear growth and skeletal age, by bone age determination, is required as a reflection of appropriate therapy. To avoid adrenal insufficiency, threefold higher doses of glucocorticoids are given during *stressful states*, such as febrile illnesses and surgery, and subcutaneous glucocorticoid (Solu-Cortef) is used in severe emergencies. Mineralocorticoid therapy is monitored with serum sodium and potassium and plasma renin activity levels. Prenatal treatment with dexamethasone to suppress fetal ACTH-induced androgen production can reduce or eliminate the ambiguity of the external genitalia in affected female fetuses, if begun at approximately 7 weeks of gestation; this remains experimental.

## OTHER ENZYME DEFECTS

Other enzyme defects are rare in contrast to 21-hydroxylase deficiency. In **11-hydroxylase deficiency**, the next most common cause of CAH, virilization occurs with salt retention and hypokalemia, as a result of the buildup of deoxycorticosterone (see Fig. 178-1), a potent mineralocorticoid. Hypertension develops as a result of excessive mineralocorticoid production. Table 178-2 summarizes the clinical and biochemical features of adrenal insufficiency in infancy.

## ADDISON DISEASE

Addison disease is a rare acquired disorder of childhood, usually associated with autoimmune destruction of the adrenal cortex. It is a form of primary adrenal insufficiency with absence of glucocorticoid and mineralocorticoid.

**Clinical manifestations** are hyperpigmentation, salt craving, postural hypotension, fasting hypoglycemia, anorexia, weakness, and episodes of shock during severe illness. Baseline and ACTH-stimulated cortisol values are subnormal, confirming the diagnosis; hyponatremia, hyperkalemia, and elevated plasma renin activity indicate mineralocorticoid deficiency. Addison disease may occur within the context of autoimmune polyglandular syndromes APS I and APS II. APS I includes hypoparathyroidism, mucocutaneous candidiasis, occasionally type 1 diabetes, and, often, hypothyroidism. Associated autoimmune disorders include oophoritis, pernicious anemia and malabsorption, chronic hepatitis, vitiligo, and alopecia. In contrast, APS II includes type 1 diabetes, and autoimmune thyroid disease. It is a genetically distinct entity. Other rare causes of adrenal insufficiency include congenital adrenal hypoplasia, some of the rarer causes of congenital adrenal hyperplasia, and conditions that affect the hypothalamus-pituitary, whether acquired, such as in craniopharyngioma, or iatrogenic, such as in irradiation for treatment of malignancy.

Replacement **treatment** with 10 to 15 mg/m²/24 hours of hydrocortisone is indicated, with supplementation during stress at three times the maintenance dosage or the use of subcutaneous glucocorticoid. The dose is titrated to allow a normal growth rate. Mineralocorticoid replacement with fludrocortisone is monitored by plasma renin activity and serum sodium and potassium determinations.

## TABLE 178-2 Clinical and Biochemical Features in Newborn Adrenal Insufficiency

| Feature | Ambiguous Genitalia | | Electrolyte Disturbance* | Serum Cortisol | Urine 11-Deoxycortisol | 17-OHP | DHEA | Aldosterone | 17-OHCS | 17-KS | Pregnanetriol |
| --- | --- | --- | --- | --- | --- | --- | --- | --- | --- | --- | --- |
| | Virilized Female | Undervirilized Male | | | | | | | | | |
| Hypoplasia | No | No | Severe | D | D | D | D | D | D | D | D |
| Hemorrhage | No | No | Moderate to severe | D | D | D | D | D | D | D | D |
| StAR deficiency | No | Yes | Severe | D | D | D | D | D | D | D | D |
| 3β-HSD | Yes | Yes | Severe | D | D | D | I | D | D | I | D |
| P-450$_{c21}$ deficiency | Yes | No | Absent to severe | D | D | I | I | D | D | I | I |
| Aldosterone synthesis block | No | No | Severe | Nl | Nl | Nl | Nl | D | Nl | Nl | Nl |
| Pseudohypoaldosteronism | No | No | Severe | Nl | Nl | Nl | Nl | I | Nl | Nl | Nl |
| P-450$_{c11}$ deficiency | Yes | No | None | D | I | Nl or I | Nl | D | I | I | Nl-sl I |
| P-450$_{c17}$ deficiency | No | Yes | † | D | Nl-D | D | D | Nl-D | D | D | D |
| Unresponsiveness to ACTH | No | No | † | D | Nl-D | Nl-D | Nl-D | Nl-D | D | D | Nl-D |

*Usually manifested after 5 days of age.

†High normal Na$^+$ and low normal to low K$^+$.

ACTH, adrenocorticotropic hormone; D, decrease; HSD, hydroxysteroid dehydrogenase; I, increase; Nl, normal; 17-KS, 17-ketosteroid; 17-OHCS, 17-hydroxycorticosteroid; StAR, steroid acute regulatory protein.

## CUSHING SYNDROME

Classic **clinical manifestations** of Cushing syndrome in children include progressive central or generalized obesity, marked failure of longitudinal growth, hirsutism, weakness, a nuchal fat pad (buffalo hump), acne, striae, hypertension, and, often, hyperpigmentation when ACTH is elevated. The most frequent cause is exogenous administration in the context of numerous conditions requiring long-term pharmacologic doses of glucocorticoids. Endogenous causes include adrenal adenoma, carcinoma, nodular adrenal hyperplasia, an ACTH-secreting pituitary microadenoma resulting in bilateral adrenal hyperplasia (Cushing disease), or an extremely rare ACTH-secreting tumor. A high-dose dexamethasone suppression test (20 μg/kg orally every 6 hours for 48 hours) suppresses glucocorticoid secretion in Cushing disease, but not in autonomous adrenal production of cortisol or in an ectopic ACTH-secreting tumor. Parenteral glucocorticoid therapy is necessary during and immediately after surgical treatment to avoid acute adrenal insufficiency.

**Treatment** of Cushing syndrome is directed to the etiology and may include excision of autonomous adrenal, pituitary, or ectopic ACTH-secreting tumors. Rarely, adrenalectomy or adrenal ablative agents (mitotane) are needed to control the symptoms.

## SUGGESTED READING

Arlt W, Allolio B: Adrenal insufficiency, *Lancet* 361:1881–1892, 2003.

Carel J-C, Léger J: Precocious puberty, *N Engl J Med* 358:2366–2377, 2008.

Chi C, Chong Lee H, Neely EK: Ambiguous genitalia in the newborn, *Neo Rev* 9:e78–e84, 2008.

Cowell KM: Focus on diagnosis: Type 2 diabetes mellitus, *Pediatr Rev* 29:289–292, 2008.

Cutler GB Jr, : Treatment of hypopituitary children, *J Pediatr* 144:415–416, 2004.

Devendra D, Liu E, Eisenbarth GS: Type 1 diabetes: Recent developments, *BMJ* 328:750–754, 2004.

Jospe N: Hyperthyroidism. In McInerny T, et al, editor: AAP Textbook of Pediatric Care.

Kliegman RM, Behrman RE, Jenson HB, et al: Nelson Textbook of Pediatrics, 18th ed, Philadelphia, 2007, *WB Saunders.*

Loscalzo ML: Turner syndrome, *Pediatr Rev* 29:219–227, 2008.

Misra M, Pacaud D, Petryk A, et al: Vitamin D deficiency in children and its management: review of current knowledge and recommendations, *Pediatrics* 122:398–417, 2008.

Roberts CGP, Landenson PW: Hypothyroidism, *Lancet* 363:793–802, 2004.

Rose SR, Vogiatzi MG, Copeland KC: A general pediatric approach to evaluating a short child, *Pediatr Rev* 26:410–420, 2005.

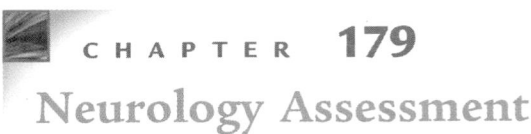

## CHAPTER 179

# Neurology Assessment

The process and interpretation of the neurologic examination varies with age. The newborn examination is unique with many transient and primitive reflex patterns, whereas the examination of an adolescent is similar to that of an adult.

## HISTORY

Gathering neurologic history follows the traditional medical model with two additions: the **pace** of the process and the **localization** of problem within the neuraxis. The pace or evolution of symptoms provides clues to the underlying nature of the disease process as symptoms may evolve in a **progressive**, **static**, or **episodic** fashion. Progressive symptoms may evolve suddenly or hyperacutely (seizures or stroke); acutely over minutes or hours (extradural hemorrhage); subacutely over days or weeks (brain tumor); or follow an indolent, slowly progressive course (hereditary neuropathies). Static neurologic abnormalities are observed in the first few months of life and do not change in character over time (cerebral palsy). They are often caused by congenital abnormalities of the brain or brain injury sustained during the prenatal or neonatal period. Intermittent attacks of recurrent, stereotyped episodes suggest epileptic or migraine syndromes. Episodic disorders are characterized by periods of symptoms, followed by partial recovery (demyelinating, autoimmune, and vascular diseases).

## PHYSICAL EXAMINATION

Because the brain and skin have the same embryonic origin (ectoderm), abnormalities of hair, skin, teeth, and nails are associated with congenital brain disorders (neurocutaneous disorders) such as neurofibromatosis (NF type 1) in which **café au lait macules** (flat, light brown areas of skin) are characteristic. **Adenoma sebaceum**, fibrovascular lesions that look like acne on the nose and malar face regions, is commonly seen in older children and adults with tuberous sclerosis.

The **head circumference** is measured in its largest occipitofrontal circumference and plotted against appropriate standard growth curves (see Chapter 5). **Microcephaly** and **macrocephaly** represent an occipitofrontal circumference 2 standard deviations (SDs) below or above the mean, respectively. Measurements are plotted over time and may show an accelerating pattern (hydrocephalus) or a decelerating pattern, indicating brain injury or degenerative neurologic disorder. The anterior fontanelle is slightly depressed and pulsatile when a calm infant is placed in the sitting position. A tense or bulging fontanelle may indicate increased intracranial pressure (ICP) but may be seen in a crying or febrile infant. Premature closure of one or more of the sutures (**craniosynostosis**) results in an unusual shape of the head. Abnormal shape, location, and condition of the face, eyes, nares, or ears are found in many genetic syndromes.

A careful **ocular examination** is an essential component of a complete neurologic assessment and should include a search for epicanthal folds, coloboma, conjunctival telangiectasias, or cataracts. A direct ophthalmoscopic examination assesses the optic disks and macula. A complete examination of the retina requires dilating the pupil and using an indirect ophthalmoscope.

Examination of the hands and feet reveals the presence of abnormal creases, polydactyly, or syndactyly (see Chapters 50 and 201). The neck and spine should be examined for midline defects that may be obvious (spina bifida with myelomeningocele) or subtle (cutaneous dimples, sinus tracts, tufts of hair, or subcutaneous lipomas). Kyphosis and scoliosis may result from abnormalities of the central or peripheral nervous system (see Chapter 202).

## NEUROLOGIC EXAMINATION OF A NEONATE

Because of the developmental immaturity of infants, the neurologic examination primarily assesses the function of the basal ganglia, brainstem, and more caudal structures and, because of the plasticity of the developing nervous system, the results of the examination should be used cautiously in predicting developmental outcome.

## Reflexes

Numerous **primitive reflexes**, many present at birth, are stereotyped motor responses that assess the functional integrity of the brainstem and basal ganglia (Table 179-1). They are symmetrical and disappear at 4 to 6 months of age, indicating the normal maturation of descending inhibitory cerebral influences (Moro reflex). The **grasp** and **rooting** reflexes are inhibited by maturation of frontal lobe structures but may reappear later in life with frontal lobe lesions. Other primitive reflexes emerge after the newborn period and indicate proper maturation of appropriate brain structures (**Landau, parachute reflexes**). Asymmetry or persistence of the primitive reflexes may indicate focal brain or peripheral nerve lesions.

## Posture

Posture is the position that a calm infant naturally assumes when placed supine. An infant at 28 weeks of gestation shows an extended posture. By 32 weeks, there is a slight trend toward increase in tone of the lower extremities and more lower extremity flexion. At 34 weeks, the lower extremities are flexed; the upper extremities are extended. The term infant flexes lower and upper extremities. **Recoil**, the liveliness with which an arm or leg springs back to its original position after passive stretching and release, is essentially absent in a small premature infant but is brisk at term.

## Movement and Tone

Spontaneous movements of a small premature infant are slow and writhing; those of a term infant are more rapid. The popliteal angle, heel-to-ear maneuver, scarf maneuver, and head control are used in assessing muscle tone and estimating gestational age (see Chapter 58).

## NEUROLOGIC EXAMINATION OF A CHILD

The purpose of the neurologic examination is to *localize* or identify the region within the neuraxis from which the symptoms arise. The **mental status examination** assesses the cerebral cortex. The **cranial nerve examination** evaluates the integrity of the brainstem. The **motor examination** evaluates upper and lower motor neuron function. The **sensory examination** assesses the peripheral sensory receptors and their central reflections. **Deep tendon reflexes** assess upper and lower motor connections. **Gait** assessment evaluates the motor system in a dynamic state for better functional assessment.

### TABLE 179-1 Central Nervous System (CNS) Reflexes of Infancy

| Reflex | Description | Age at Appearance | Age at Disappearance | Origin in CNS |
|---|---|---|---|---|
| Moro | Sudden head extension causes extension followed by flexion of the arms and legs | Birth | 4–6 mo | Brainstem vestibular nuclei |
| Grasp | Placing a finger in palm results in flexing of the infant's fingers, accompanied by flexion at elbow and shoulder | Birth | 4–6 mo | Brainstem vestibular nuclei |
| Rooting | Tactile stimulus about the mouth results in the infant's mouth pursuing the stimulus | Birth | 4–6 mo | Brainstem trigeminal system |
| Trunk incurvation | Stroking the skin along the edge of the vertebrae produces curvature of the spine with the apex opposite to the direction of the stroke | Birth | 4–6 mo | Spinal cord |
| Placing | Infant places foot on examining surface when dorsum of foot is brought into contact with the edge of the surface | Birth | 4–6 mo | Cerebral cortex |
| Asymmetrical tonic neck | With the infant supine, turning of the head results in ipsilateral extension of the arm and leg in a "fencing" posture | Birth | 4–6 mo | Brainstem vestibular nuclei |
| Parachute | The infant is suspended face down by the chest. When the infant is moved toward a table, the arms extend as if to protect itself. | 8–10 mo | Never | Brainstem vestibular nuclei |
| Landau | The infant is supported by the abdomen in prone position. The head will extend above the plane of the trunk with legs extended. When the examiner pushes the head into flexion, the legs drop into flexion. | 4–5 mo | 15 mo–2 yr | Brainstem |

See video demonstrations at: *http://library.med.utah.edu/pedneurologicexam/html/06month.html#14.*

## Mental Status Evaluation

**Alertness** is assessed in infants by observing spontaneous activities, feeding behavior, and visual ability to fix and follow the movement of objects. Response to tactile, visual, and auditory stimuli is noted. In circumstances of altered consciousness, the response to painful stimuli is noted. Observation of toddlers at play allows a nonthreatening assessment of developmentally appropriate skills. Older children can be tested for orientation to time, place, person, and purpose.

The best way to assess intellectual abilities is through language skills. **Language function** is receptive (understanding speech or gesture) and expressive (speech and use of gestures). Abnormalities of language resulting from disorders of the cerebral hemispheres are referred to as **aphasias**. Anterior, expressive, or *Broca aphasia* is characterized by sparse, nonfluent language. Posterior, receptive, or *Wernicke aphasia* is characterized by an inability to understand language. Speech is fluent but nonsensical. Global aphasia refers to impaired expressive and receptive language.

Many simple bedside measures exist to evaluate age-appropriate language and social skills (see Chapters 7 and 8). In addition to expressive and receptive language function, older children can be tested for reading, writing, numerical skills, fund of knowledge, abstract reasoning, judgment, humor, and memory.

## CRANIAL NERVE EVALUATION

The evaluation of cranial nerve function assesses the integrity of the brainstem but depends on the stage of brain maturation and the ability to cooperate. A colorful toy may capture a young child's attention and permit observation of cranial nerve function, coordination, and movements.

## Cranial Nerve I

The sense of smell can be assessed in verbal, cooperative children older than 2 years of age. Aromatic substances, such as perfumes and vanilla, should be used, not volatile substances (ammonia), which irritate the nasal mucosa.

## Cranial Nerve II

Full-term newborns in the quiet awake state follow a human face, a light in a dark room, or a large, opticokinetic strip. Visual acuity has been estimated to be 20/200 in newborns and 20/20 in infants 6 months old. Standard visual charts displaying pictures instead of letters assess visual acuity in toddlers. Peripheral vision is tested by surreptitiously bringing objects into the visual field from behind. A reduced pupillary reaction to light suggests lesions of the anterior visual pathways, including the retina, optic nerves, and chiasm. Unilateral optic nerve lesions are identified by the *swinging flashlight test*. Normally, both pupils constrict when a light shines in one eye. With an optic nerve problem, both pupils constrict when the light is directed into the normal eye. When the light is swung over to the abnormal eye, both pupils dilate inappropriately; this is called an *afferent pupillary defect* or **Marcus Gunn pupil**. Lesions of the posterior visual pathway, including the lateral geniculate, optic radiations, and occipital cortex, have normal pupillary light reactions, but are expressed by loss of visual fields.

## Cranial Nerves III, IV, and VI

These three cranial nerves control the movement of the eyes and are most easily examined with the use of a colorful toy to capture the child's attention. For infants too young to fix and follow, rotating the infant's head assesses oculocephalic vestibular reflexes (**doll's head maneuver**). The oculocephalic reflex is *uninhibited* when turning the head in one direction elicits an immediate movement of the eyes in the opposite direction. While normal in a newborn, in an older child, an uninhibited doll's head response indicates that the cortex is not functioning properly to inhibit the brainstem. The oculocephalic response is *incomplete* when the eyes do not move fully and conjugately in response to head turning. An incomplete response indicates dysfunction of the brainstem.

Abnormalities of these cranial nerves may cause diplopia (double vision). Cranial nerve III (oculomotor nerve) innervates the pupil; levator palpebrae superioris; medial, superior, and inferior recti; and inferior oblique muscles. Cranial nerve IV (trochlear nerve) innervates the superior oblique muscle. Cranial nerve VI (abducens nerve) innervates the lateral rectus muscle. Because cranial nerve VI has a long intracranial route within the subarachnoid space, failure of abduction of one or both eyes is a frequent but nonspecific sign of increased intracranial pressure (ICP).

Cranial nerve III controls the pupillary light reaction, which is present after 30 weeks of gestation. Lesions of the third cranial nerve produce a dilated, mydriatic pupil. Anticholinergic and sympathomimetic drugs dilate the pupil, and cholinergic, narcotic, and sedative drugs constrict the pupil. Third nerve lesions may be associated with incomplete eye movements. Interruption of the sympathetic innervation of the pupil and lid may produce **Horner syndrome** with meiosis, ptosis, and unilateral facial anhidrosis.

## Cranial Nerve V

The muscles of mastication can be observed as an infant sucks and swallows. The **corneal reflex** can be tested (cranial nerves V and VII) at any age. Facial sensation of light touch and pain can be determined with cotton gauze and pinprick. Facial sensation can be functionally assessed in an infant by gently brushing the cheek, which will produce the **rooting reflex** (the infant turns its head and neck with mouthing movement seeking to nurse).

## Cranial Nerve VII

Facial muscles are assessed by observing the face at rest, with crying, and with blinking. At older, cooperative ages, children can be asked to smile, blow out their cheeks, blink forcibly, and furrow their foreheads. Weakness of all muscles of the face, including the forehead, eye, and mouth, indicates a lesion of the ipsilateral facial nerve (**Bell's palsy**). If the weakness affects only the lower face and mouth, a contralateral lesion of upper motor neuron in the brain (tumor, stroke, abscess) must be considered because the upper third of the face receives bilateral cortical innervation.

## Cranial Nerve VIII

Lesions of cranial nerve VIII cause deafness, tinnitus, and vertigo. Alert neonates blink in response to a bell. Four-month-old infants turn their head and eyes to localize a sound stimulus. Hearing can be tested in a verbal child by whispering a word in one ear while covering or masking the opposite ear. Lesions of the vestibular component of cranial nerve VIII produce symptoms of vertigo, nausea, vomiting, diaphoresis, and nystagmus. Nystagmus is an involuntary beating eye movement with a rapid phase in one direction and a slow phase in the opposite direction. By convention, the direction of the nystagmus is defined by the fast phase and may be horizontal, vertical, or rotatory.

## Cranial Nerves IX and X

The gag reflex is brisk at all ages except the very immature neonate. An absent gag reflex suggests a lower motor neuron lesion of the brainstem, cranial nerves IX or X, neuromuscular junction, or pharyngeal muscles. Uvula deviation toward one side suggests palsy of cranial nerves IX or X on the opposite side. Weak, breathy, or nasal speech; weak sucking; drooling and inability to handle secretions; and gagging and nasal regurgitation of food are additional symptoms of cranial nerve X dysfunction.

## Cranial Nerve XI

Observing the infant's posture and spontaneous activity assesses the functions of the trapezius and sternocleidomastoid muscles. Head tilt and drooping of the shoulder suggest lesions involving cranial nerve XI. In later childhood, strength in these muscles can be tested directly and individually.

## Cranial Nerve XII

Atrophy and fasciculation of the tongue, usually indicating a lesion of the anterior horn cells (spinal muscular atrophy), can be observed at any age and are assessed most reliably when the infant is asleep. The tongue deviates toward the weak side in unilateral lesions.

# MOTOR EXAMINATION

## Power

Power in infants is assessed by observation of spontaneous movements and movements against gravity. Arm and leg movements should be symmetrical, seen best when the infant is held supine with one hand supporting the buttocks and one supporting the shoulders. The limbs should be lifted easily off the bed. Power is graded on a scale of declining function, as follows:

5. Normal
4. Weak but able to provide resistance
3. Able to move against gravity but not against resistance
2. Unable to move against gravity
1. Minimal movement
0. Complete paralysis

Strength in toddlers is assessed by observing functional abilities. The child should be able to reach high above his or her head, wheelbarrow walk, run, hop, easily go up and down stairs, and arise from the ground. Subtle asymmetry can be detected when the child extends his or her arms out in front with the palms upward and eyes closed. The hand on the weaker side cups and begins to pronate slowly (**pronator drift**). Cooperative children can undergo individual muscle strength testing. **Muscle fasciculations** indicate denervation from disease of the anterior horn cell or peripheral nerve.

## Tone

Tone represents the dynamic resistance of muscles to movement across a joint (stretch) or to gravity. Lower motor and cerebellar lesions produce decreased tone (**hypotonia**). Upper motor lesions produce increased tone (**spasticity**). In extrapyramidal disease, an increase in resistance is present throughout passive movement of a joint (**rigidity**).

## Bulk

Muscle bulk represents the volume of muscle tissue. In many lower motor neuron conditions (neuropathies or SMA [spinal muscle atrophy]), muscle bulk is diminished or atrophic. Excessive muscle bulk is seen in myotonia congenita and Duchenne muscular dystrophy (*pseudohypertrophy*).

## Coordination

Lack of coordination of movement is termed **ataxia**. The cerebellum and its associated pathways modulate volitional movement. If either the afferent (joint position senses) or efferent cerebellar connections (cerebellum through thalamus to cerebral cortex) are disturbed, the patient has ataxia. Truncal ataxia reflects disturbances of the midline cerebellar vermis (medulloblastoma, acute postinfectious cerebellar ataxia, or ethanol intoxication). Appendicular ataxia reflects disturbances of the ipsilateral cerebellar hemisphere (cystic cerebellar astrocytoma). Observation and functional analysis help assess coordination in infants and toddlers. Watching the child sit or walk assesses truncal stability. Exchanging toys or objects with the child permits assessment of intention tremor and dysmetria, signs of cerebellar dysfunction. Cooperative children can do repetitive finger or foot tapping to test rapid alternating movements. Cerebellar and corticospinal tract dysfunction produce slow, rapidly alternating movements.

## Gait

Watching a child creep, crawl, cruise or walk is the best global assessment for the motor and coordination systems (see Chapter 197). Subtle deficits in power, tone, or balance or subtle asymmetries may be observed. The toddler gait is normally wide-based and unsteady. The base of the gait narrows with age. By 6 years, a child is able to walk high on toes and heels and tandem walk (heel to toe). Cerebellar dysfunction results in a broad-based, unsteady gait accompanied by difficulty in executing turns. Corticospinal tract dysfunction produces a stiff, scissoring gait and toe walking. Arm swing is decreased, and the arm is flexed across the body. Extrapyramidal dysfunction produces a slow, stiff, shuffling gait with dystonic postures. A waddling gait occurs with hip weakness due to lower motor neuron disorders. A steppage gait results from weakness of ankle dorsiflexors (common peroneal palsy).

## Reflexes

**Deep tendon reflexes** can be elicited at any age. These reflexes are decreased in lower motor neuron diseases and increased in upper motor neuron disease. Clonus may be present in upper motor neuron disorders. **Babinski response**, or extensor plantar reflex, is an upward movement of the great toe and flaring of the toes on noxious stimulation of the side of the foot and is a sign of corticospinal tract dysfunction. This reflex is unreliable in neonates except when asymmetrical because the "normal" response at this age varies. The plantar response should consistently be flexor (toes down) after 18 months of age.

## SENSORY EXAMINATION

The sensory examination of newborns and infants is limited to observing the behavioral response to light touch or gentle sterile pinprick. Stimulation of the limb should produce a facial grimace. A spinal reflex alone may produce withdrawal movement of the limb. In a cooperative child, the senses of pain, touch, temperature, vibration, and joint position can be tested individually. The cortical areas of sensation must be intact to identify by touch an object placed in the hand (**stereognosis**) or a number written in the hand (**graphesthesia**) or to distinguish between two sharp objects applied simultaneously and closely on the skin (**two-point discrimination**).

## SPECIAL DIAGNOSTIC PROCEDURES

### Cerebrospinal Fluid Analysis

Analysis of cerebrospinal fluid (CSF) is essential when central nervous system (CNS) infection is suspected and provides important clues to other diagnoses (Table 179-2). Differentiating a hemorrhagic CSF caused by a traumatic lumbar puncture (LP) from a true subarachnoid hemorrhage may be difficult. In most cases of traumatic LP, the fluid clears significantly as the sequence of tubes are collected. Caution must be exercised before performing an LP to limit risk of cerebral herniation if there is clinical evidence of increased ICP (papilledema, depression of consciousness, or focal neurologic deficits). A computed

tomography (CT) scan should be performed before the LP if increased ICP is suspected. If increased ICP is present, it must be treated before an LP is performed.

### Electroencephalography

The electroencephalogram (EEG) records electrical activity generated by the cerebral cortex. EEG rhythms mature throughout childhood. There are three key features present: background, symmetry, and presence or absence of epileptiform patterns. The background varies with age, but there should be general symmetry between the background of the two hemispheres without a localized area of higher amplitude or slower frequencies (focal slowing). Fixed slow wave foci (1 to 3 Hz) delta rhythms

**TABLE 179-2  Analysis of Cerebrospinal Fluid (CSF)**

| CSF Finding | Normal CSF Values | |
|---|---|---|
| | **Newborn** | **>1 Month Old** |
| Cell count* | $10–25/mm^3$ | $5/mm^3$ |
| Protein | 65–150 mg/dL | <40 mg/dL |
| Glucose | >2/3 blood glucose *or* >40 mg/dL | >2/3 blood glucose *or* >60 mg/dL |

| CSF Change | Significance |
|---|---|
| Increased polymorphonuclear and decreased CSF glucose | Bacterial infection<br>Partially treated bacterial meningitis<br>Brain or parameningeal abscess<br>Parasitic infection<br>Leak of dermoid contents |
| Increased lymphocytes and decreased CSF glucose | Mycobacterial infection (tuberculosis)<br>Fungal infection<br>Carcinomatous meningitis<br>Sarcoidosis |
| Increased lymphocytes and normal CSF glucose | Viral meningitis<br>Post–infectious disease (ADEM)<br>Vasculitis |
| Increased CSF protein | Infection<br>Venous thrombosis<br>Hypertension<br>Spinal block (Froin syndrome)<br>Guillain-Barré syndrome<br>Meningeal carcinomatosis |
| Mild CSF pleocytosis | Tumor<br>Infarction<br>Multiple sclerosis<br>Subacute bacterial endocarditis |
| Bloody CSF | Subarachnoid hemorrhage<br>Subdural hemorrhage<br>Intraparenchymal hemorrhage<br>Hemorrhagic meningoencephalitis (group B streptococci, HSV)<br>Trauma<br>Vascular malformation<br>Coagulopathy |

*Cells should be lymphocytes.
ADEM, acute disseminated encephalomyelitis; HSV, herpes simplex virus.

suggest an underlying structural abnormality (brain tumor, abscess, or stroke). Bilateral disturbances of brain activity (increased ICP or metabolic encephalopathy) must be suspected when there is diffuse slow wave activity (delta frequency). Spikes, polyspikes, and spike-and-wave abnormalities, either in a localized region (focal) or distributed bihemispherically (generalized), indicate an underlying seizure tendency.

## Electromyography and Nerve Conduction Studies

Electromyography (EMG) and nerve conduction velocities (NCVs) assess abnormalities of the neuromuscular apparatus, including anterior horn cells, peripheral nerves, neuromuscular junctions, and muscles. Normal muscle is electrically silent at rest. Spontaneous discharge of motor fibers (**fibrillations**) or groups of muscle fibers (**fasciculation**) indicates denervation, revealing dysfunction of anterior horn cells or peripheral nerves. Abnormal muscle responses to repetitive nerve stimulation are seen with diseases of the neuromuscular junction, such as myasthenia gravis and botulism. The amplitude and duration of the muscle compound action potential are decreased in primary diseases of muscle. NCVs assess the transmission along peripheral nerves. NCVs are slowed in demyelinating neuropathies (Guillain-Barré syndrome). The amplitude of the signal is diminished in axonal neuropathies.

## Neuroimaging

Imaging the brain and spinal cord is accomplished using CT or magnetic resonance imaging (MRI). CT is quick and accessible for emergency purposes. MRI provides fine detail and, with different sequences, permits detection of subtle cerebral abnormalities, vascular anomalies, low-grade tumors, and ischemic changes. For a child with a head injury or sudden headache, cranial CT is the study of choice. For a child with new onset complex partial seizures, MRI is the study of choice. MRI may also provide excellent views of the entire spinal cord. Cranial ultrasonography is a noninvasive bedside procedure that can visualize the brain and ventricles of infants and young children with open fontanelles.

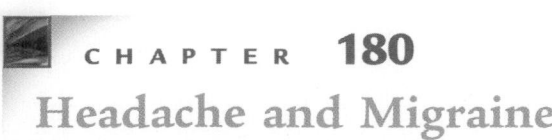

CHAPTER **180**

# Headache and Migraine

## ETIOLOGY AND EPIDEMIOLOGY

Headache is a common symptom in children and adolescents. Most are related to intercurrent viral illnesses and fever. Headache may be the first symptom of serious conditions (meningitis or brain tumors), so a systematic approach is necessary.

**Migraine** and **tension-type headache** are the most common causes of recurrent headaches in children and adolescents.

## CLINICAL MANIFESTATIONS

The temporal pattern of the headache must be clarified. Each pattern (acute, recurrent-episodic, chronic-progressive, and chronic-nonprogressive) has its own differential diagnosis (Table 180-1).

**Tension-type** headaches in children are the most common recurrent pattern of primary headache in children and adolescents. They are generally mild and do not disrupt the patient's lifestyle or activities. The pain is global and squeezing or pressing in character, but can last for hours or days. These headaches can be acute and related to environmental stresses or can be chronic and a symptom of underlying psychiatric illness, such as anxiety neurosis, hysterical neurosis, or depression. There is no nausea, vomiting, or photophobia.

**Migraine** frequently begins in childhood. Toddlers may be unable to verbalize the source of their discomfort and exhibit episodes of irritability, sleepiness, pallor, and vomiting. Migraine headaches are stereotyped attacks of frontal, bitemporal, or unilateral intense pounding or throbbing pain that are aggravated by activity and last 1 to 72 hours. Associated symptoms include nausea, vomiting, pallor, photophobia, phonophobia, and an intense desire to seek a quiet dark room for rest. A characteristic, but inconsistent symptom of childhood migraine is a visual aura that precedes the headache and persists for 15 to 30 minutes. The visual aura consists of spots, flashes, or lines of light that flicker in one or both visual fields. Migraine auras may also consist of brief episodes of unilateral or perioral numbness, unilateral weakness, or even vertigo that persist for hours, then resolve completely. Complex symptoms such as hemiparesis,

---

### TABLE 180-1 Four Temporal Patterns of Childhood Headache

**Acute**: Single episode of head pain without a history of such episodes. In adults, the "first and worst" headache raises concerns for aneurysmal subarachnoid hemorrhage, but in children, this pattern is commonly due to *febrile illness* related to upper respiratory tract infection.

**Acute recurrent**: Pattern of attacks of head pain separated by symptom-free intervals. Primary headache syndromes, such as *migraine or tension-type* headache, usually cause this pattern. Infrequently recurrent headaches are attributed to epileptic syndromes (e.g., benign occipital epilepsy), substance abuse, or recurrent trauma.

**Chronic progressive**: Most ominous of the temporal patterns—implies a gradually increasing frequency and severity of headache. The pathologic correlate is *increasing intracranial pressure*. Causes of this pattern include pseudotumor cerebri, brain tumor, hydrocephalus, chronic meningitis, brain abscess, and subdural collections.

**Chronic nonprogressive *or* chronic daily**: Pattern of frequent or constant headache. Chronic daily headache (CDH) generally is defined as ≥4-month history of ≥15 headaches/month, with headaches lasting ≥4 hours. Affected patients demonstrate normal findings on neurologic examination; psychological factors and great anxiety about possible underlying organic causes usually are interwoven.

monocular blindness, ophthalmoplegia, or confusion, accompanied by headache, warrant careful diagnostic investigations including neuroimaging, electroencephalogram (EEG), and appropriate metabolic studies.

## DIAGNOSTIC STUDIES

For a child with recurring headaches and symptom-free intervals with a normal neurologic examination, computed tomography (CT) or magnetic resonance imaging (MRI) is generally not necessary. Conversely, if the general physical or neurologic examinations are abnormal, cranial CT or MRI should be considered. Localized disturbances of function, alteration of consciousness, or a chronic progressive pattern may warrant imaging. Headaches that are most severe on awakening, awaken the patient from sleep, are exacerbated by coughing or bending, have acute onset without a previous history of headache, progressively worsening, or accompanied by persistent vomiting are all indications for neuroimaging. Headache with focal neurologic signs or evidence of increased intracranial pressure (papilledema) mandates immediate neuroimaging (Fig. 180-1).

## TREATMENT

The treatment of migraine requires an individually tailored regimen to address the frequency, severity, and disability produced by the headache. Intermittent or *symptomatic* analgesics are the mainstay for treatment of infrequent, intense episodes of migraine. Symptomatic therapy requires early administration of an analgesic (ibuprofen), rest, and sleep in a quiet, dark room. Administration of oral medication may be limited by nausea and vomiting.

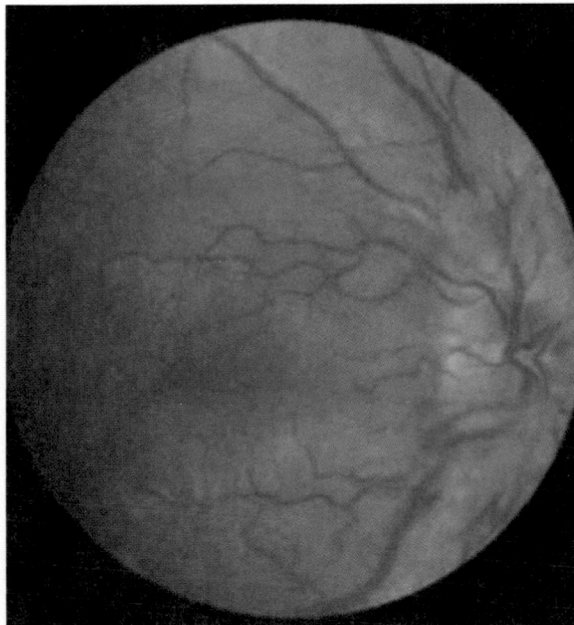

**FIGURE 180-1**

Papilledema with dilation of the vessels, obliteration of the optic cup, loss of disc margin, and hemorrhages around disc. (From Kliegman RE, Behrman, RM, Jenson HB [eds]: Nelson Textbook of Pediatrics, 18th ed. Philadelphia, *WB Saunders*, 2007 p 2107.)

The *triptan* agents, available in injectable, nasal spray, oral disintegrating, and tablet form, are serotonin receptor agonists that may alleviate migraine symptoms promptly.

Many children suffer with severe and frequent migraines that disrupt their daily lives. These children may require daily preventive agents to reduce both attack frequency and severity and also enhance the effectiveness of symptomatic medications (see Table 180-2). Before initiating daily medications, lifestyle modifications must be put into place to regulate sleep, establish routines including exercise, and identify any precipitating or aggravating influences, eliminating as many as possible (caffeine, stress, missed meals). Other treatment options include psychological support or counseling, stress management, and biofeedback. In addition to mild analgesics, treatment options for tension headaches include psychological support or counseling, biofeedback, antidepressants, and psychiatric intervention.

**TABLE 180-2  Treatment of Pediatric and Adolescent Migraine**

| Type of Treatment | Specific Measures/Agents |
|---|---|
| Biobehavioral | Regular sleep schedules |
| | Regular dietary schedule (avoid missing meals) |
| | Elimination of precipitating factors |
| | Reassurance |
| | Biofeedback |
| | Psychotherapy |
| Pharmacologic Acute therapy | Analgesics |
| |   Acetaminophen |
| |   Nonsteroidal anti-inflammatory drugs |
| |     Ibuprofen |
| |     Naproxen |
| | 5-Hydroxytryptamine agonists ("triptans") |
| |   Sumatriptan |
| |   Zolmitriptan |
| |   Rizatriptan |
| |   Almotriptan |
| |   Frovatriptan |
| |   Eletriptan |
| | Antiemetics |
| |   Metoclopramide |
| |   Promethazine |
| |   Ondansetron |
| Prophylactic therapy | Tricyclic antidepressants |
| |   Amitryptyline |
| | Cyproheptadine |
| | Anticonvulsants |
| |   Topiramate |
| |   Valproic acid |
| |   Levetiracetam |
| | β-Adrenergic blockers |
| |   Propranolol |
| | Calcium channel blockers |
| |   Verapamil |
| | Serotonin reuptake inhibitors |
| |   Fluoxetine |

# CHAPTER 181

# Seizures (Paroxysmal Disorders)

Paroxysmal disorders of the nervous system produce sudden, reversible changes in mental status or somatosensory function that tend to be stereotyped and repetitive in nature. They have a variable duration from seconds to minutes (rarely hours), end abruptly, and are followed by a gradual return to baseline. There may be a warning before (aura) or an altered state of awareness afterward (postictal state). The differential diagnosis of paroxysmal disorders includes **epileptiform disorders**, specifically seizures, and **nonepileptiform disorders** such as migraine, syncope, transient ischemic attack, paroxysmal dyskinesia, vertigo, hypoglycemia, breath-holding spells, tics, and conversion reactions (Table 181-1). A thorough medical history from the patient and primary witnesses is the most reliable tool for establishing the correct diagnosis.

The **electroencephalogram (EEG)** is the most useful neurodiagnostic test in distinguishing seizures from nonepileptic paroxysmal disorders. The EEG must be interpreted in the context of the clinical history because many normal children have epileptiform EEG patterns. Children with seizures may have normal EEGs between attacks. When the diagnosis is still unclear, more sophisticated EEGs with prolonged recordings with simultaneous video or ambulatory EEG monitoring of the patient in an attempt to capture a spell, may be necessary.

## ETIOLOGY AND EPIDEMIOLOGY

Seizures represent the abnormal and excessive discharging of the neuroglial network. A diverse group of disturbances of cerebral function or homeostasis can lead to seizures (Table 181-2). **Epilepsy** is defined as recurrent, unprovoked seizures. Epileptic seizures are generally classified

---

### TABLE 181-1 Paroxysmal Disorders of Childhood

Seizure disorders
Migraine and variants
  Paroxysmal torticollis
  Paroxysmal vertigo (benign)
Syncope and vasovagal events
  Breath-holding spells
Transient ischemic attack
Metabolic disorders
  Hypoglycemia
Sleep disorders
  Narcolepsy, cataplexy
  Night terrors
Paroxysmal dystonia or choreoathetosis
Shudder attacks
Pseudoseizures

---

### TABLE 181-2 Causes of Seizures

Perinatal conditions
  Cerebral malformation
  Intrauterine infection
  Hypoxic-ischemic*
  Trauma
  Hemorrhage*
Infections
  Encephalitis*
  Meningitis*
  Brain abscess
Metabolic conditions
  Hypoglycemia*
  Hypocalcemia
  Hypomagnesemia
  Hyponatremia
  Hypernatremia
  Storage diseases
  Reye syndrome
  Degenerative disorders
  Porphyria
  Pyridoxine dependency and deficiency
Poisoning
  Lead
  Cocaine
  Drug toxicity (see Chapter 45)
  Drug withdrawal
Neurocutaneous syndromes
  Tuberous sclerosis
  Neurofibromatosis
  Sturge-Weber syndrome
  Klippel-Trénaunay-Weber syndrome
  Linear sebaceous nevus
  Incontinentia pigmenti
Systemic disorders
  Vasculitis (CNS or systemic)
  SLE
  Hypertensive encephalopathy
  Renal failure
  Hepatic encephalopathy
Other causative disorders/conditions
  Trauma*
  Tumor
  Febrile*
  Idiopathic*
  Familial

*Common.
CNS, central nervous system; SLE, systemic lupus erythematosus.

---

into types on the basis of the electrical mechanism that arises from one region of the cortex (focal, partial, or localization-related) and seizures that arise from both hemispheres, simultaneously (generalized). The epileptic syndromes represent clinical entities wherein age, pattern of clinical event, EEG abnormality, natural history, and prognosis are distinctive (Table 181-3).

Partial or focal seizures constitute 40% to 60% of the classifiable epilepsies of childhood. Focal brain lesions (tumors, infarct, dysgenesis) may cause partial seizures,

| TABLE 181-3  Classification of Seizures and Epileptic Syndromes |
|---|

**PARTIAL SEIZURES**

Simple partial (consciousness not impaired)
  Motor signs
  Special sensory (visual, auditory, olfactory, gustatory, vertiginous, or somatosensory)
  Autonomic
Complex partial (consciousness impaired)
  Psychic (déjà vu, fear, and others)
  Impaired consciousness at onset
  Development of impaired consciousness
Secondarily generalized seizures
  Jacksonian seizures

**GENERALIZED SEIZURES**

Absence
  Typical
  Atypical
Tonic
Clonic
Tonic-clonic
Minor motor
  Atonic
  Myoclonic

**EPILEPTIC SYNDROMES**

Benign focal epilepsy (benign rolandic epilepsy, benign centrotemporal epilepsy)
Juvenile myoclonic epilepsy
Infantile spasms (West syndrome)
Lennox-Gastaut syndrome
Acquired epileptic aphasia (Landau-Kleffner syndrome)
Benign neonatal convulsions

but most partial seizures in children are due to genetic influences. Generalized tonic, clonic, and biphasic tonic-clonic seizures are common during childhood. Although it is often difficult to distinguish primary generalized tonic and clonic seizures from secondary generalized partial seizures on purely clinical grounds, this distinction is important. While the majority of children with primary generalized or partial onset epilepsy have a genetic basis for their seizures, brain lesions must be considered, especially when focal clinical or electrographic features are present. The presence of an aura indicates a focal origin of the attack. Young children often are unaware of an aura or focal onset of their seizure and caregivers frequently witness only the generalized aspects of the event.

Approximately 6% to 20% of epileptic children have typical generalized absence seizures (petit mal epilepsy). There is a 75% concordance rate in monozygotic twins, suggesting a genetic etiology. Approximately 40% to 50% of children with absence seizures have associated generalized convulsive seizures; 60% occur before and 40% occur after the onset of absence seizures.

Myoclonic, tonic, atonic, and atypical absence seizures compose 10% to 15% of childhood epilepsies. These seizures frequently are associated with underlying structural brain disease and are difficult to treat and classify. They often occur in combination with each other and with generalized tonic-clonic seizures. The peak age of occurrence of myoclonic absence seizures is within the first year. Status epilepticus can be the first ictal manifestation in patients with myoclonic features.

## CLINICAL MANIFESTATIONS

### Partial Seizures

Simple partial seizures arise from a specific anatomic focus. Clinical symptoms include motor, sensory, psychic, or autonomic abnormalities, but consciousness is preserved. Location and direction of spread of the seizure focus determine the clinical symptoms. Complex partial seizures are similar, but in addition, consciousness is impaired. When partial seizures spread to involve the whole brain and produce a generalized tonic-clonic seizure, they show secondary generalization (*jacksonian* seizures). Partial seizures that manifest only with psychic or autonomic symptoms can be difficult to recognize. **Uncinate seizures** arising from the medial temporal lobe manifest with an olfactory hallucination of an extremely unpleasant odor (burning rubber). **Gelastic seizures** originating from hypothalamic tumors are spells of uncontrolled laughter. Lip-smacking seizures arise from the anterior temporal lobe and episodes of macropsia, micropsia, altered depth perception, and vertigo from the posterior temporal lobe. Limbic temporal lobe discharges result in dreamlike states (déjà vu and bizarre psychic abnormalities). Episodic autonomic phenomena, such as fever, tachycardia, shivering, and increased gastrointestinal motility, may rarely be seizures of temporal lobe origin.

### Generalized Seizures

#### Generalized Tonic, Clonic, and Tonic-Clonic Seizures (Generalized Major Motor Seizures)

Tonic, clonic, and biphasic tonic-clonic seizures may occur alone or be associated with other seizure types. Typically the attack begins abruptly, but occasionally is preceded by a series of myoclonic jerks. During a tonic-clonic seizure, consciousness and control of posture are lost, followed by tonic stiffening and upward deviation of the eyes. Pooling of secretions, pupillary dilation, diaphoresis, hypertension, and piloerection are common. Clonic jerks follow the tonic phase, then the child is briefly tonic again. Thereafter, the child remains flaccid and urinary incontinence may occur. As the child awakens, irritability and headache are common. During an attack, the EEG shows repetitive synchronous bursts of spike activity followed by periodic paroxysmal discharges. Generalized tonic-clonic activity lasting longer than 20 minutes, or repeated seizures without restoration of consciousness for more than 30 minutes, is defined as **status epilepticus** and may lead to irreversible brain injury.

### Absence Seizures

Staring spells can be either primary generalized absence (petit mal) or complex partial seizures (temporal lobe epilepsy). The clinical hallmark of generalized absence seizures is a brief loss of environmental awareness accompanied by eye fluttering or simple automatisms, such as head bobbing and lip smacking. Seizures usually begin between 4 and 6 years of age. Neurologic examination and brain imaging are normal. The characteristic EEG patterns consist of synchronous **3-Hz spike-and-wave activity**. A clinical seizure can be provoked by **hyperventilation** or strobe light stimulation. Differentiating absence epilepsy from partial complex staring seizures can be difficult. Both seizure types are characterized by cessation of activity, staring, and alteration of consciousness and may include automatisms. The automatisms of partial complex seizures are usually more complicated and may involve repetitive swallowing, picking of the hands, or walking in nonpurposeful circles. Partial complex seizures are often followed by postictal confusion; absence seizures are not. Absence seizures are provoked by hyperventilation and usually last a few seconds; partial complex seizures occur spontaneously and usually last several minutes. Children may have dozens of absence seizures per day; children rarely have more than one or two partial complex seizures in a day. The distinction is important because the choice of anticonvulsant treatment is different.

## Myoclonic, Tonic, Atonic, and Atypical Absence Seizures

Atypical absence seizures manifest as episodes of impaired consciousness with automatisms, autonomic phenomena, and motor manifestations, such as eye opening, eye deviation, and body stiffening. The EEG shows slow spike-and-wave activity at 2 to 3 Hz. Myoclonus is a sudden jerk of all or part of the body; not all myoclonus is epileptic in nature. Nonepileptic myoclonus may originate in the basal ganglia, brainstem, or spinal cord. It may be benign, as in sleep myoclonus, or indicate serious disease. Myoclonic epilepsy usually is associated with multiple seizure types. The underlying illness producing myoclonic epilepsy may be developmental and static or progressive and associated with neurologic deterioration (neuronal ceroid lipofuscinosis). Myoclonic absence refers to the body jerks that commonly accompany absence seizures and atypical absence seizures.

## EPILEPTIC SYNDROMES

**Benign focal epilepsy**, also known as **rolandic epilepsy**, usually begins between ages 5 and 10 years. The incidence is 21 per 100,000, accounting for 16% of all afebrile seizures in children under 15 years of age. They are usually focal motor seizures involving the face and arm and tend to occur only during sleep or on awakening in more than half of patients. Symptoms commonly include abnormal movement or sensation around the face and mouth with drooling and a rhythmic guttural sound. Speech and swallowing are impaired. A family history of similar seizures is found in 13% of patients. The disorder is called benign because seizures usually respond promptly to anticonvulsant therapy; intellectual outcome and brain imaging are normal, and epilepsy resolves after puberty. Daily antiepileptic drug therapy may not be needed.

**Benign neonatal convulsions** are an autosomal dominant genetic disorder localized to chromosome 20. Generalized clonic seizures occur toward the end of the first week of life (*3-day fits* or familial 5-day fits). Response to treatment varies, but the outlook generally is favorable.

**Juvenile myoclonic epilepsy (of Janz)** occurs in adolescence and is an autosomal dominant disorder localized on chromosome 6 with variable penetrance. The patient may have absence, generalized tonic or clonic, and myoclonic seizures. The hallmark is morning myoclonus occurring predominantly within 90 minutes of awakening. Seizures usually resolve promptly with therapy with valproic acid, but therapy must be maintained for life.

**Infantile spasms (West syndrome)** are brief contractions of the neck, trunk, and arm muscles, followed by a phase of sustained muscle contraction lasting 2 to 10 seconds. The initial phase consists of flexion and extension in various combinations such that the head may be thrown either backward or forward. The arms and legs may be either flexed or extended. Spasms occur most frequently when the child is awakening from or going to sleep. Each jerk is followed by a brief period of relaxation, repeated multiple times in clusters of unpredictable and variable duration. Many clusters occur each day. The EEG during the waking state, **hypsarrhythmia**, is dramatically abnormal, consisting of high-voltage slow waves, spikes, and polyspikes accompanied by background disorganization. The peak age at onset is 3 to 8 months; 86% of infants experience the onset of seizures before age 1 year. When flexion of the thighs and crying are prominent, the syndrome may be mistaken for colic. Infantile spasms have a poor prognosis. The etiology is not determined in 40% of children. This idiopathic or "cryptogenic" group has a better response to therapy than the group with a clear etiology; 40% have a good intellectual outcome. Etiology is determined in 60% (Table 181-4). This symptomatic group responds poorly to anticonvulsant therapy and has a poor intellectual prognosis. **Tuberous sclerosis** is the most common recognized cause. Treatment options for infantile spasms include adrenocorticotropic hormone (ACTH), oral corticosteroids, benzodiazepines, valproic acid, and vigabatrin.

**Lennox-Gastaut syndrome** is an epileptic syndrome with variable age of onset. Most children present before age 5 years. Multiple seizure types, including atonic-astatic, partial, atypical absence, and generalized tonic, clonic, or tonic-clonic varieties characterize the disorder. Many children have underlying brain injury or malformations. These seizures usually respond poorly to treatment, but some patients have a good response to valproic acid.

**Astatic-akinetic** or **atonic seizures** have their onset between 1 and 3 years of age. The seizures last 1 to 4 seconds and are characterized by a loss of body tone, with falling to the ground, dropping of the head, or pitching forward or backward. A tonic component usually is associated. The seizures frequently result in repetitive head injury if the child is not protected with a hockey or football helmet. They are most frequent on awakening and on falling asleep; 50 or more daily seizures are usual. Children with astatic-akinetic seizures usually have developmental delay

| TABLE 181-4  Etiology of Infantile Spasms (West Syndrome) |
| --- |

Metabolic disorders
  Phenylketonuria
  Biotinidase deficiency
  Maple syrup urine disease
  Isovalericacidemia
  Ornithine accumulation
  Nonketotic hyperglycinemia
  Pyridoxine dependency
  Hypoglycemia
  Lipidosis
Developmental malformations
  Polymicrogyria
  Lissencephaly
  Schizencephaly
  Down syndrome and other chromosomal disorders
Aicardi syndrome
Organoid nevus syndrome
Neurocutaneous syndromes
  Tuberous sclerosis
  Sturge-Weber syndrome
Congenital infections
  Toxoplasmosis
  Cytomegalovirus
  Syphilis
Encephalopathies
  Post-asphyxia
  Post-traumatic
  Posthemorrhagic
  Postinfectious

and underlying brain abnormalities. **Tuberous sclerosis** is a frequent cause.

**Acquired epileptic aphasia (Landau-Kleffner syndrome)** is characterized by the abrupt loss of previously acquired language in young children. The language disability is an acquired cortical auditory deficit (auditory agnosia). Some patients develop partial and generalized epilepsy. The EEG is highly epileptiform in sleep, the peak area of abnormality often being in the dominant perisylvian region (language areas). It is unclear whether frequent temporal lobe seizures cause the language disability or whether unknown, perhaps inflammatory temporal lobe disease is responsible for the seizures and language loss.

**Rasmussen encephalitis** is a chronic, progressive focal inflammation of the brain and is of unknown origin. An autoimmune origin and focal viral encephalitis have been postulated. The usual age at onset is 6 to 10 years. The disease begins with focal, persistent motor seizure activity, including epilepsia partialis continua. Over months, the child develops hemiplegia and cognitive deterioration. EEG shows focal spikes and slow wave activity. Brain imaging studies are initially normal, then show atrophy in the involved area. Hemispherectomy has been the only successful therapy as measured by seizure eradication and prevention of cognitive deterioration, but permanent hemiparesis is an inevitable consequence.

## SPECIAL CONDITIONS

**Seizures** in the setting of fever may be caused by infections of the nervous system (meningitis, encephalitis, or brain abscess), unrecognized epilepsy triggered by fever, or **simple febrile convulsions**. The latter represents a common genetic predisposition to seizures in children between 6 months and 6 years that is precipitated by fever. They occur in 2% to 4% of children; most occur between ages 1 and 2 years (mean age 22 months). Simple febrile convulsions are generalized major motor seizures lasting less than 15 minutes that occur only once in a 24-hour period in a neurologically and developmentally normal child. If there are focal features, the seizures last longer than 15 minutes, the child has preexisting neurologic challenges, or the seizures occur multiple times within one febrile event, the seizure is referred to as a **complex** or **atypical febrile seizure**.

The prognosis of children with simple febrile convulsions is excellent. Intellectual achievements are normal. Many children have further febrile seizures, but the risk of subsequent epilepsy is no greater than that for the general population (approximately 1%). Febrile seizures recur in 30% to 50% of children who have their first febrile seizure before 1 year of age and in 28% of children who have their first seizure after 1 year of age. About 10% of children with febrile seizures have three or more recurrences. Children with complex febrile seizures have only a 7% risk of having further complicated febrile seizures. Factors that increase the risk for the development of epilepsy include abnormal neurologic examination or development, family history of epilepsy, and complex febrile seizures. The probability of developing epilepsy is 2% if one risk factor is present and 10% if two or three risk factors are present.

Because febrile seizures are brief and the outcome is benign, most children require no treatment. Rectal diazepam can be administered during a seizure to abort a prolonged event. Daily administration of phenobarbital or valproic acid prevents febrile seizures, but the potential for serious side effects limits the use of these agents. Intermittent treatment with oral diazepam three to four times per day during a febrile illness has shown variable effectiveness.

**Status epilepticus** is a neurologic emergency and is defined as ongoing seizure activity for greater than 20 minutes or repetitive seizures without return of consciousness for greater than 30 minutes. Status epilepticus can cause hypoxemia and decreased cortical perfusion resulting in irreversible brain injury. In 50% of children presenting with status epilepticus, there is no definable etiology, but in 50% of this group, status is triggered by fever. About 25% have an acute brain injury, such as purulent or aseptic meningitis, encephalitis, electrolyte disorder, or acute anoxia. Twenty percent have a history of brain injury or congenital malformation. Sudden cessation of anticonvulsant medication is another frequent cause. Overall the mortality rate of status epilepticus is less than 10% and is related to the etiology of the seizure pattern.

## IMMEDIATE TREATMENT

The first priority of treatment is to ensure an adequate airway and to assess the cardiovascular status (see Chapter 38). Oxygen is administered. If there is any doubt concerning the adequacy of the airway, the child should be intubated. An intravenous (IV) infusion should be started, and laboratory evaluation should be undertaken. Hypoglycemia and electrolyte abnormalities must be addressed. Several pharmacologic options exist for management of status epilepticus (Table 181-5). Initial management is usually with a benzodiazepine. Lorazepam (0.05-0.1 mg/kg), diazepam (0.1-0.3 mg/kg), and midazolam (0.2 mg/kg) all are effective agents. Diazepam distributes rapidly to the brain, but has a short duration of action. Alternatively, or even simultaneously, administration of either phenytoin (10-15 mg/kg) or fosphenytoin (10-20 mg/kg) at a rate of 1 mg/kg/min is effective. Phenytoin and fosphenytoin distribute more slowly but have a much longer duration of action. If the seizures persist with these measures, a continuous IV infusion of diazepam, loading dose of 10 to 20 mg/kg of phenobarbital, or IV valproic acid at a dose of 20 mg/kg is appropriate (see Table 181-5). If this approach is ineffective, preparations for general anesthesia are undertaken. While awaiting anesthesia, continuously infused diazepam or pentobarbital is recommended. When status epilepticus stops, maintenance therapy is initiated with the appropriate anticonvulsant.

**Pseudoseizures** may occur in children with hysteria or malingering. Children with genuine seizure disorders may, consciously or subconsciously, exhibit activity that simulates their own seizures. Although the clinical differentiation can be difficult, pseudoseizures differ from epileptic seizures in that movement is tremulousness or thrashing rather than true tonic-clonic activity. Verbalization and pelvic thrusting are seen more commonly in pseudoseizures; urinary and fecal continence is preserved, and injury does not occur. Pseudoseizures are more likely to be initiated or terminated by suggestion. An EEG performed during pseudoseizure activity does not show typical epileptiform patterns.

## LABORATORY AND DIAGNOSTIC EVALUATION OF SEIZURES

A complete laboratory evaluation of a child with the new onset of seizures includes a complete blood count; measurement of blood chemistries, including glucose, calcium, sodium, potassium, chloride, bicarbonate, urea nitrogen, creatinine, magnesium, and phosphorus; blood or urine toxicology screening; analysis of cerebrospinal fluid (CSF); and EEG and brain imaging (magnetic resonance imaging [MRI]). Neonates also may require testing for inborn errors of metabolism, blood ammonia, CSF glycine, lactate, and herpes simplex polymerase chain reaction; urine and stool culture (cytomegalovirus and enterovirus), and a clinical trial of pyridoxine. Analysis of CSF is not necessary if the patient is afebrile and has no other neurologic signs or if the history does not suggest a meningeal infection or subarachnoid hemorrhage. Children with **simple febrile seizures** who have recovered completely may require little or no laboratory evaluation other than studies necessary to evaluate the source of the fever.

**MRI** is superior to computed tomography (CT) in showing brain pathology, but in the emergency department setting, CT can be performed rapidly and shows acute intracranial hemorrhage more clearly than MRI. MRI is likely to be normal in patients with the primary generalized epilepsies, such as typical absence and juvenile myoclonic epilepsy. Lesions (tumors, arteriovenous malformations, cysts, strokes, gliosis, or focal atrophy) in 25% of other patients may be identified even when the clinical examination and EEG do not suggest focal features. Identification of some static lesions, such as cortical dysplasia, hamartoma, and mesial temporal sclerosis, may allow consideration of surgical correction of medically refractory epilepsy.

## LONG-TERM THERAPY

The decision to institute daily seizure medications for a first unprovoked seizure must be based on the likelihood of recurrence *balanced* against the risk of long-term drug therapy. Determination of the recurrence risk is based on the clinical history and results of neurodiagnostic testing. Absence seizures, infantile spasms, atypical absence seizures, and astatic-akinetic seizures are universally recurrent at the time of diagnosis, indicating the need for therapy. The overall risk of recurrence for children whose first seizure is generalized tonic-clonic is approximately 50%. It seems reasonable to wait for recurrence before therapy is instituted. An otherwise healthy child with a single unprovoked partial seizure with a normal neurodiagnostic evaluation, including a normal EEG, may have a recurrence risk of 25%. In such a case, it is reasonable to educate family members regarding first aid techniques for seizures and to withhold daily antiepileptic

---

**TABLE 181-5 Management of Status Epilepticus**

**STABILIZATION**

ABCs (airway, breathing, circulation)
ECG monitoring
Oxygen and pulse oximetry
Intravenous access
Immediate laboratory tests
   Glucose
   Basic metabolic panel—sodium, calcium, magnesium
   Antiepileptic drug levels
   Toxicology studies as appropriate

**PHARMACOLOGIC MANAGEMENT**

Benzodiazepine/(max rate of administration = 1 mg/min)
   Lorazepam 0.05-0.1 mg/kg
   Diazepam 0.2-0.5 mg/kg
   Midazolam 0.1-0.2 mg/kg
Fosphenytoin 10-20 mg/kg (phenytoin equivalents)
Phenobarbital 10-20 mg/kg
Valproic acid 20 mg/kg
General anesthesia

ECG, electrocardiogram.

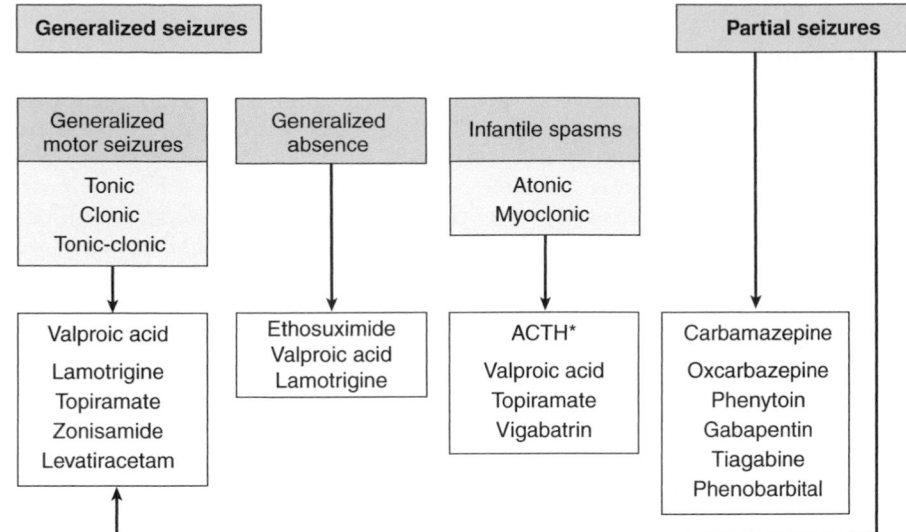

FIGURE 181-1

Treatment for epilepsy. ACTH, adrenocorticotropic hormone.*, for infantile spasms.

agents. Conversely a child with preexisting neurologic abnormality and an abnormal EEG may have a recurrence risk of 75%, in which case institution of a daily antiepileptic agent may be justified after the first seizure.

When treatment is initiated, the goal is to maintain an optimal functional state. Medication toxicity should be weighed against the risk of seizure itself. Initial drug selection is based on the mechanism of the seizure (Fig. 181-1). A single agent limits toxicity, contains cost, and improves compliance. Approximately 50% of children obtain satisfactory seizure control with the initial drug. If seizure control is not achieved with confirmed therapeutic anticonvulsant levels, addition of a second drug must be considered. When available, measuring anticonvulsant blood levels is helpful in adjusting medication and monitoring compliance, but the levels should be interpreted in light of the patient's clinical state. Antiepileptic drug levels should be drawn at trough, usually early in the morning before the morning doses. When hepatic or renal disease is present, drug binding is likely to be altered. In this instance, free and bound anticonvulsant levels can be helpful. Treatment is not necessary for benign febrile seizures.

The duration of anticonvulsant treatment varies with seizure type. Children with generalized tonic, clonic, and tonic-clonic seizures; absence seizures; and certain partial seizures may not require therapy for more than 2 to 4 years. The risk of recurrence is higher with partial complex seizures. Children with juvenile myoclonic epilepsy, progressive myoclonic epilepsy, atypical absence seizures, and Lennox-Gastaut syndrome usually require treatment for life. As a rule, children who are neurologically abnormal, have seizures that were initially difficult to control, and have persistently epileptiform EEGs are at highest risk for recurrence when therapy is discontinued.

General guidance for families with children with epilepsy is to be careful with heights, head injury, and swimming. Children with epilepsy have a greater risk of submersion accidents. This risk can be minimized by maintaining therapeutic anticonvulsant drug levels and by appropriate adult supervision.

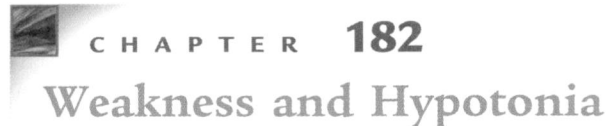

## CHAPTER 182
# Weakness and Hypotonia

## ETIOLOGY

The corticospinal tract and its neurons from the cerebral cortex through the spinal cord that control voluntary motor activity are known as the **upper motor neuron**. The anterior horn cells, their motor roots, peripheral motor nerves, neuromuscular junctions, and muscles represent the **lower motor neuron**. Maintenance of normal strength, tone, and coordination requires integrated communication between the motor nuclei of the cerebral cortex, spinal cord, cerebellum, brainstem, thalamus, basal ganglia, and motor cortex of the cerebrum. The cerebellum and basal ganglia facilitate volitional movement. The cerebellum provides dynamic feedback regarding joint position, and the basal ganglia modulate agonists and antagonistic muscle groups.

Dysfunction of the upper motor neuron causes loss of voluntary control, but not total loss of movement. Motor nuclei of the basal ganglia, thalamus, and brainstem have their own tracts that innervate anterior horn cells and produce simple or complex stereotyped patterns of movement. Damage of the spinal cord leaves simple, stereotyped reflex movements coordinated by local spinal reflexes below the level of the lesion intact. Destruction of the lower motor neuron leads to total absence of movement because it is the final common pathway producing muscle activity.

## CLINICAL MANIFESTATIONS

Weakness caused by upper motor neuron disease or corticospinal tract lesions is different in quality from weakness produced by the lower motor unit (Table 182-1).

**TABLE 182-1 Clinical Distinction between Upper Motor Neuron and Lower Motor Neuron Lesions**

| Clinical Sign | Upper Motor Neuron (Corticospinal Tract) | Lower Motor Neuron (Neuromuscular) |
|---|---|---|
| Tone | Increased (spastic) | Decreased |
| Reflexes | Increased | Decreased |
| Babinski reflex | Present | Absent |
| Atrophy | Absent | Possible |
| Fasciculations | Absent | Possible |

The corticospinal tract permits fine motor activity and is best tested by asking the patient to perform rapid alternating movements of the distal extremities. Mild dysfunction produces slowed, stiff motions. More severe dysfunction produces stiff, abnormal postures (spasticity) that do not respond to voluntary command. The posture in corticospinal tract disease consists of the forearm being flexed at the elbow and wrist and adducted close to the chest, with the leg extended and adducted. Disease of the lower motor unit produces progressive loss of strength with hypotonia and no abnormality of posture. Function is best tested by measuring the strength of individual muscle groups or, in a young child, by observing the ability to perform tasks requiring particular muscle groups (walk up or down stairs, arise from the ground, walk on toes or heels, raise the hands above the head, and squeeze a ball).

## DISEASE OF THE UPPER MOTOR NEURON

### Etiology and Epidemiology

Tumors, trauma, infections, demyelinating syndromes, infarction, metabolic diseases, and degenerative diseases may injure the corticospinal tract, producing an upper motor neuron pattern of weakness coupled with increased deep tendon reflexes, spasticity, and extensor plantar responses (Babinski sign).

### Clinical Manifestations

The distribution of weakness depends on the location of the lesion. A tumor in the left parietal region may produce a right hemiparesis. A brainstem glioma may produce a slowly progressive quadriparesis. Compression of the spinal cord in the thoracic region from a tumor, such as neuroblastoma or lymphoma, would produce a spastic paraparesis, affecting only the legs. A disorder of myelin synthesis, such as a leukodystrophy, would produce a progressive symmetrical quadriparesis.

## DISEASES OF THE SPINAL CORD

Acute spinal cord lesions, such as infarction or compression, may produce a **flaccid, areflexic paralysis** that mimics lower motor neuron disease. A child who exhibits an acute or subacute flaccid paraparesis is most likely to have either an acute cord syndrome or Guillain-Barré syndrome. The acute cord syndrome may be the result of transverse myelitis, a cord tumor, infarction, demyelination, or trauma. The hallmarks of spinal cord disease are a sensory level, a motor level, disturbance of bowel and bladder function, and local spinal pain or tenderness. **Transverse myelitis**, an acute postinfectious demyelinating disorder of the spinal cord, is treated with high-dose steroids. Trauma and tumors (neuroblastoma, lymphoma, sarcoma) compressing the spinal cord necessitate immediate neurosurgical management to preserve vital function.

## DISEASES OF THE LOWER MOTOR NEURON

Each anterior horn cell in the spinal cord and brainstem gives rise to a single myelinated axon that extends to muscle. The **lower motor unit** consists of the anterior horn cell, the peripheral nerve, the neuromuscular junction and the muscle. Neuromuscular disease affects any component of the lower motor neuron unit. The distribution of muscle weakness can point toward specific diseases (Table 182-2). Diseases may affect each component of the motor unit.

**TABLE 182-2 Topography of Neuromuscular Diseases**

| Location | Clinical Syndromes/Disorders |
|---|---|
| Proximal muscle weakness | Muscular dystrophy |
| | Duchenne |
| | Limb-girdle |
| | Dermatomyositis; polymyositis |
| | Kugelberg-Welander disease (late-onset spinal muscular atrophy) |
| Distal limb weakness | Polyneuropathy (Guillain-Barré syndrome) |
| | Hereditary motor sensory neuropathy I |
| | Hereditary motor sensory neuropathy II |
| | Myotonic dystrophy |
| | Distal myopathy |
| Ophthalmoplegia and limb weakness | Myasthenia gravis |
| | Botulism |
| | Myotonic dystrophy |
| | Congenital myotubular myopathy |
| | Miller Fisher variant of Guillain-Barré syndrome |
| Facial and bulbar weakness | Myasthenia gravis |
| | Botulism |
| | Polio |
| | Miller Fisher variant of Guillain-Barré syndrome |
| | Myotonic dystrophy |
| | Congenital myopathy |
| | Facioscapulohumeral dystrophy |

# DISEASES OF THE ANTERIOR HORN CELL

## Spinal Muscular Atrophy

### Etiology

Progressive degeneration of anterior horn cells is the key manifestation of spinal muscular atrophy (SMA), a genetic disease that may begin in intrauterine life or any time thereafter and may progress at a rapid or slow pace. The earlier in life the process starts, the more rapid the progression. Infants who are affected at birth or who become weak within the first several months of life usually progress to flaccid quadriplegia with bulbar palsy, respiratory failure, and death within their first year. This early severe form of the illness is called **Werdnig-Hoffmann disease**. A milder form of the illness, **Kugelberg-Welander syndrome**, begins in late childhood or adolescence with proximal weakness of the legs and progresses slowly over decades. Variants of SMA between these age extremes occur with unpredictable courses.

SMA is one of the most frequent autosomal recessive diseases, with a carrier frequency of 1 in 50. All types of SMA are caused by mutations in the survival motor neuron gene (*SMN1*). There are two almost identical copies, *SMN1* and *SMN2*, present on chromosome 5q13. Only homozygous absence of *SMN1* is responsible for SMA; homozygous absence of *SMN2*, found in about 5% of control subjects, has no clinical phenotype. The number of *SMN2* copies modulates the SMA phenotype.

### Clinical Manifestations

SMA may begin between 6 months and 6 years of age, may progress rapidly or slowly or may progress rapidly initially, then seemingly plateau. The clinical manifestations include progressive proximal weakness, decreased spontaneous movement, and floppiness. Atrophy may be marked. Head control is lost. With time, the legs stop moving altogether. The range of facial expression diminishes, and drooling and gurgling increase. The eyes remain bright, open, mobile, and engaging. Weakness is flaccid, with early loss of reflexes. **Fasciculations** (quivering of the lateral aspect of the tongue) are best identified by inspecting the mouth when the child is asleep. Infants have normal mental, social, and language skills and sensation. Breathing becomes rapid, shallow, and predominantly abdominal. In an extremely weak child, respiratory infections lead to atelectasis, pulmonary infection, and death.

### Laboratory and Diagnostic Studies

The level of creatine phosphokinase may be mildly elevated. The electromyelogram (EMG) shows fasciculations, fibrillations, positive sharp waves, and high-amplitude, long-duration motor units. Muscle biopsy specimens show grouped atrophy. The diagnosis is established by specific DNA probe for SMA.

### Treatment

No treatment for SMA exists. Symptomatic therapy is directed toward minimizing contractures, preventing scoliosis, aiding oxygenation, preventing aspiration, and maximizing social, language, and intellectual skills. Respiratory infections are managed early and aggressively with pulmonary toilet, chest physical therapy, oxygen, and antibiotics. The use or nonuse of artificial ventilation must be individualized for each patient in each stage of the illness.

# POLIOMYELITIS

**Poliomyelitis** is an acute enteroviral illness with prodromal vomiting and diarrhea associated with an aseptic meningitis picture during which the patient experiences the evolution of an **asymmetrical flaccid weakness** as groups of anterior horn cells become infected (see Chapter 101).

# PERIPHERAL NEUROPATHY

There are three principal peripheral nerve diseases in childhood:

Guillain-Barré syndrome
Hereditary motor sensory neuropathy (Charcot-Marie-Tooth disease)
Tick paralysis

Peripheral neuropathy produced by diabetes mellitus, alcoholism, chronic renal failure, amyloid, exposure to industrial or metal toxins, vasculitis (often as **mononeuritis multiplex**), or the remote effects of neoplasm is a common cause of weakness and sensory loss in adults but is rare in children.

## Guillain-Barré Syndrome

### Etiology

Guillain-Barré syndrome is a postinfectious autoimmune peripheral neuropathy that often occurs after a respiratory or gastrointestinal infection. Infection with *Campylobacter jejuni* is associated with a severe form of the illness.

### Clinical Manifestations

The characteristic symptoms are areflexia, flaccidity, and relatively symmetrical weakness beginning in the legs and ascending to involve the arms, trunk, throat, and face. Progression can occur rapidly, in hours or days, or more indolently, over weeks. Typically symptoms start with numbness or paresthesia in the hands and feet, then a *heavy*, weak feeling in the legs, followed by inability to climb stairs or walk. Deep tendon reflexes are absent even when strength is relatively preserved. Objective signs of sensory loss are usually minor compared with the dramatic weakness. Bulbar and respiratory insufficiency may occur rapidly. Close monitoring of respiratory function is essential. **Dysfunction of autonomic** nerves can lead to hypertension, hypotension, orthostatic hypotension, tachycardia, and other arrhythmias; urinary retention or incontinence; stool retention; or episodes of abnormal sweating, flushing, or peripheral vasoconstriction. This polyneuropathy can be difficult to distinguish from an acute spinal cord syndrome. Preservation of bowel and bladder function, loss of arm reflexes, absence of a sensory level, and lack of spinal tenderness would point more toward Guillain-Barré syndrome. A cranial nerve variant of Guillain-Barré syndrome called the **Miller Fisher variant** manifests with ataxia, partial ophthalmoplegia, and areflexia.

Porphyria and tick paralysis may simulate Guillain-Barré syndrome. Other causes of peripheral neuropathy include vasculitis, heredity, nutritional deficiency (vitamins $B_1$, $B_{12}$, and E), endocrine disorders, infections (diphtheria, Lyme disease), and toxins (organophosphate, lead).

The illness may resolve spontaneously; 75% of patients recover normal function within 1 to 12 months. Twenty percent of patients are left with mild to moderate residual weakness in the feet and lower legs. The mortality rate is 5%, and death is caused by autonomic dysfunction (hypertension-hypotension, tachycardia-bradycardia, and sudden death), respiratory failure, mechanical ventilation complications, cardiovascular collapse, or pulmonary embolism.

### Laboratory and Diagnostic Studies

The cerebrospinal fluid (CSF) in Guillain-Barré syndrome is often normal in the first days of the illness, but later in the disease shows elevated protein levels without significant pleocytosis. Nerve conduction velocity (NCV) and EMG may be normal early, but then show delay in motor NCV and decreased amplitude and temporal dispersion of the evoked compound motor action potential.

### Treatment

Children with moderate, severe or rapidly progressive weakness should be cared for in a pediatric intensive care unit (ICU). Pulmonary and cardiac functions are monitored continuously. Endotracheal intubation should be performed electively in patients who exhibit early signs of hypoventilation or accumulation of bronchial secretions. Therapy is symptomatic and rehabilitative and directed at blood pressure control and cardiac arrhythmia; nutrition, fluids, and electrolytes; pain control; prevention of complications (skin, cornea, and joints, infection); bowel and bladder management; psychological support; and communication therapy. Most patients are treated initially with **intravenous (IV) immunoglobulin** (total dose 1–2 g/kg given for 2 to 5 days). Plasma exchange and IV immunoglobulin are beneficial in rapidly progressive disease.

### Hereditary Motor Sensory Neuropathy (Charcot-Marie-Tooth Disease)

#### Etiology

Hereditary motor sensory neuropathy (HMSN), commonly called Charcot-Marie-Tooth disease, is a chronic, genetic polyneuropathy characterized by weakness and wasting of distal limb muscles. The most common form (Charcot-Marie-Tooth type 1A) is due to a duplication of DNA at 17p11.2-12, a region containing the peripheral myelin protein (*PMP 22*) gene. A deletion in this region gives rise to a much milder condition, known as hereditary neuropathy with liability to pressure palsies. An X-linked form of HMSN is caused by mutations of the gap junction protein, connexin 32. HMSN type II is a neuronal form with normal or mildly decreased NCV and no hypertrophic changes. Type I HMSN and type II HMSN are inherited as autosomal dominant traits with variable expressivity.

### Clinical Manifestations

Most often, complaints begin in the preschool years with **pes cavus deformity of the feet** and weakness of the ankles with frequent tripping (see Chapter 201). Examination shows high-arched feet, bilateral weakness of foot dorsiflexors, and normal sensation despite occasional complaints of paresthesia. Progression of HMSN is slow, extending over years and decades. Eventually, patients develop weakness and atrophy of the entire lower legs and hands and mild to moderate sensory loss in the hands and feet. Some patients never have more than a mild foot deformity, loss of ankle reflexes, and electrophysiologic abnormalities. Others in the same family may be confined to a wheelchair and have difficulties performing everyday tasks with their hands.

### Laboratory and Diagnostic Studies

HMSN type I is a demyelinating illness with severely decreased NCV and hypertrophic changes on nerve biopsy. Specific DNA testing is available for many forms of HMSN.

### Treatment

Specific treatment for HMSN is not available, but braces that maintain the feet in dorsiflexion can improve function measurably. Early surgery is contraindicated because progression of the disease destabilizes even a good repair.

### Tick Paralysis

Tick paralysis produces an acute lower motor neuron pattern of weakness clinically similar to Guillain-Barré syndrome. An attached female tick releases a toxin, similar to botulism, blocking neuromuscular transmission. Affected patients present with a severe generalized flaccid weakness, including ocular, papillary, and bulbar paralysis. A methodical search for an affixed tick, particularly in hairy areas, must be made in any child with acute weakness. Removal of the tick results in a prompt return of motor function.

## NEUROMUSCULAR JUNCTION DISORDERS

### Myasthenia Gravis

#### Etiology and Epidemiology

Myasthenia gravis is an autoimmune condition in which antibodies to the acetylcholine receptors at the neuromuscular junction block and, through complement-mediated pathways, damage the neuromuscular junction.

### Clinical Manifestations

Classic myasthenia gravis may begin in the teenage years with the onset of ptosis, diplopia, ophthalmoplegia, and weakness of extremities, neck, face, and jaw. Fluctuating and generally minimal symptoms are present on awakening in the morning and gradually worsen as the day progresses or with exercise. In some children, the disease never advances beyond ophthalmoplegia and ptosis (ocular myasthenia). Others have a progressive and potentially life-threatening illness that involves all musculature, including that of respiration and swallowing (systemic myasthenia).

## Diagnostic Studies

The diagnosis is confirmed with IV edrophonium chloride (Tensilon), which transiently improves strength and decreases fatigability. Antiacetylcholine receptor antibodies often can be detected in the serum. Repetitive nerve stimulation shows a decremental response at 1 to 3 Hz.

## Treatment

Treatment includes acetylcholine esterase inhibitors (pyridostigmine), thymectomy, prednisone, plasmapheresis, and immunosuppressive agents. When respiration is compromised, immediate intubation and ICU admission are indicated.

## Neonatal Transitory Myasthenia Gravis

A transitory myasthenic syndrome develops in 10% to 20% of neonates born to mothers with myasthenia gravis. Symptoms persist for 1 to 10 weeks (mean, 3 weeks). Almost all infants born to mothers with myasthenia have antiacetylcholine receptor antibody, but neither antibody titer nor extent of disease in the mother predicts which neonates have clinical disease. Symptoms and signs include ptosis, ophthalmoplegia, weak facial movements, poor sucking and feeding, hypotonia, and variable extremity weakness. The diagnosis is made by showing clinical improvement lasting approximately 45 minutes after intramuscular (IM) administration of neostigmine methylsulfate, 0.04 mg/kg. Treatment with oral pyridostigmine or neostigmine 30 minutes before feeding is continued until spontaneous resolution occurs.

## Congenital Myasthenic Syndrome

A variety of rare disorders of the neuromuscular junction have been reported that are not autoimmune mediated. The conditions manifest as hypotonic infants with feeding disorders and varying degrees of weakness. Some of the identified variants include abnormalities of the presynaptic region (familial infantile myasthenia), synaptic defects (congenital end plate acetylcholinesterase deficiency), or postsynaptic disorders (slow channel myasthenic syndrome).

# MUSCLE DISEASE

## Duchenne Dystrophy

### Etiology

Duchenne muscular dystrophy, a common sex-linked recessive trait (Xp21) appearing in 20 to 30 per 100,000 boys, results from absence of a large cytoskeletal protein called **dystrophin**. **Becker muscular dystrophy** arises from an abnormality in the same gene locus, resulting in abnormal dystrophin function with more indolent symptoms and later onset than Duchenne dystrophy.

### Clinical Manifestations

At about 2 to 3 years of age, boys develop an awkward gait and an inability to run properly. Some have an antecedent history of mild slowness in attaining motor milestones, such as walking and climbing stairs. Examination shows firm calf hypertrophy and mild to moderate proximal leg weakness with a hyperlordotic, waddling gait and inability to arise from the ground easily. The child typically arises from a lying position on the floor by using his arms to *climb up* his legs and body (**Gower sign**). Arm weakness is evident by 6 years of age, and most boys are confined to a wheelchair by 12 years of age. By age 16, little mobility of arms remains, and respiratory difficulties increase. Death is caused by pneumonia or congestive heart failure resulting from myocardial involvement.

### Laboratory and Diagnostic Studies

Serum creatine phosphokinase levels are always markedly elevated. Muscle biopsy shows muscle fiber degeneration and regeneration accompanied by increased intrafascicular connective tissue. Diagnosis is established by DNA probe for Duchenne muscular dystrophy. Prenatal diagnosis of both diseases is possible by genetic testing. Approximately one third of cases represent new mutations.

### Treatment

Supportive care includes physical therapy, bracing, proper wheelchairs, and prevention of scoliosis. A multidisciplinary approach is recommended. Steroid therapy (prednisone 0.75 mg/kg/day) is now instituted to slow the pace of the disease and delay motor disability.

## Other Forms of Muscular Dystrophy

**Limb-girdle dystrophy** is usually an autosomal recessive disease presenting with proximal leg and arm weakness. The genetic defect lies within one of the many muscle proteins that compose the muscle fiber plasma membrane cytoskeleton complex. The clinical manifestations are similar to those of Duchenne dystrophy, but are seen in an older child or teenager and progress slowly over years. By midadulthood, most patients are wheelchair bound.

**Facioscapulohumeral dystrophy** is usually an autosomal dominant disease presenting in teenagers. Genetic diagnosis is possible by finding a characteristic 4q35 deletion. The child has mild ptosis, a decrease in facial expression, inability to pucker the lips or whistle, neck weakness, difficulty in fully elevating the arms, scapular winging, and thinness of upper arm musculature. Progression is slow, and most patients retain excellent functional capabilities for decades.

## Myotonic Dystrophy

### Etiology and Epidemiology

Myotonic dystrophy is an autosomal dominant genetic disease caused by progressive expansion of a triplet repeat, GCT, on chromosome 19q13.2-13.3 in a gene designated myotonin protein kinase (*MP-PK*).

## Clinical Manifestations

Myotonia is a disorder of muscle relaxation. Patients grasp onto an object and have difficulty releasing their grasp, *peeling* their fingers away slowly. Myotonic dystrophy presents either at birth, with severe generalized hypotonia and weakness, or in adolescence, with slowly progressive facial and distal extremity weakness and myotonia. The adolescent type is the classic illness and is associated with cardiac arrhythmias, cataracts, male pattern baldness, and infertility in males (hypogonadism). The facial appearance is characteristic, with hollowing of muscles around temples, jaw, and neck; ptosis; facial weakness; and drooping of the lower lip. The voice is nasal and mildly dysarthric.

Some mothers with myotonic dystrophy give birth to infants with the disease who are immobile and hypotonic, with expressionless faces, tented upper lips, ptosis, absence of sucking and Moro reflexes, and poor swallowing and respiration. Often, weakness and atony of uterine smooth muscle during labor lead to associated hypoxic-ischemic encephalopathy and its sequelae. The presence of congenital contractures, clubfoot, or a history of poor fetal movements indicates intrauterine neuromuscular disease.

## Congenital Myopathies

### Etiology

Congenital myopathies (nemaline rod, central core, myotubular) are a group of congenital, often genetic, nonprogressive or slowly progressive myopathies characterized by abnormal appearance of the muscle biopsy specimen (Table 182-3).

### Clinical Manifestations

A child with a congenital myopathy is profoundly hypotonic with moderately diffuse weakness involving limbs and face. Associated conditions include congenitally dislocated hips, a high-arched palate, clubfoot, and contractures at hips, knees, ankles, or elbows secondary to intrauterine weakness. The attainment of motor milestones is moderately to severely delayed. The clinical course is either static or slowly progressive. Progressive kyphoscoliosis represents a significant problem in some children. Reflexes are diminished.

#### TABLE 182-3 Congenital Myopathies

Congenital structural myopathy
Central core
Nemaline rod
Centronuclear
Congenital fiber type of disproportion
Myotubular
Congenital muscular dystrophy
Miscellaneous types
Metabolic myopathies
Glycogen storage disease II (Pompe disease)
Carnitine metabolism abnormalities
Mitochondrial abnormalities
Endocrine myopathies
Thyroid myopathies

## Laboratory and Diagnostic Studies

Creatine phosphokinase levels may be mildly elevated. EMG may show a nonspecific *myopathic* pattern or may be normal. The definitive diagnosis is made by muscle biopsy showing nemaline rods, fiber-type disproportion, and central core changes.

## Dermatomyositis

### Etiology and Epidemiology

The etiology and epidemiology of dermatomyositis are discussed in Chapter 91.

### Clinical Manifestations

The clinical features include progressive proximal muscle weakness coupled with dermatologic features, including erythematous rash around the eyes (**heliotrope**) and plaques on the knuckles (**Gottron papules**) and on the extensor surfaces of the knees, elbows, and toes. Subcutaneous calcinosis is a late finding (see Chapter 91).

### Diagnostic Studies and Therapy

Myositis-specific autoantibodies may be identified in the serum. Diagnostic testing includes measurement of serum creatine phosphokinase levels, EMG, magnetic resonance imaging (MRI) of muscle, and muscle biopsy. See Chapter 91 for therapy.

## Metabolic Myopathies

**Glycogen storage disease type II** (Pompe disease) and muscle carnitine deficiency are discussed in Chapter 52. **Mitochondrial myopathies** are characterized by muscle biopsy specimens that display ragged red fibers, representing collections of abnormal mitochondria (see Chapter 57). Typical symptoms include hypotonia, ophthalmoplegia, and progressive weakness, but the phenotype of these disorders is broad. **Endocrine myopathies**, including hyperthyroidism, hypothyroidism, hyperparathyroidism, and Cushing syndrome, are associated with proximal muscle weakness. Hypokalemia and hyperkalemia produce fluctuating weakness (periodic paralysis) and loss of tendon jerks.

## Treatment of Neuromuscular Diseases

The major complications of neuromuscular disorders are the development of joint contractures, scoliosis, and pneumonia. Active range of motion exercises and bracing prevent and treat contractures, minimizing pain and maximizing function. Surgery to release contractures or to realign tendons is most helpful in nonprogressive or in very slowly progressive conditions. Kyphoscoliosis produces loss of function, disfigurement and, when severe, life-threatening decrease of ventilatory reserve. Prevention or delay in the development of these complications can be achieved by maintaining ambulation for as long as possible, ensuring a properly fitted wheelchair, bracing, and surgery. Pneumonia may be associated with thick secretions that are difficult to clear, progressive atelectasis, and respiratory failure. Anticipatory treatment with antibiotics, hospitalization, chest physical therapy, oxygen, and ventilatory support helps in most cases.

## Laboratory and Diagnostic Studies

See Table 182-4 and text for individual disorders.

## Malignant Hyperthermia

Patients with Duchenne muscular dystrophy, central core myopathy, and other myopathies are susceptible to the life-threatening syndrome of **malignant hyperthermia**. Malignant hyperthermia is manifested as a rapid increase of body temperature and $PCO_2$, muscle rigidity, cyanosis, hypotension, arrhythmias, and convulsions. This syndrome may occur during administration of muscle relaxants (succinylcholine) or inhalation agents such as halothane. Malignant hyperpyrexia can also occur in children without muscle disease as an autosomal dominant genetic disorder. A family history of unexplained death during operations is often noted. Diagnosis of idiopathic malignant hyperthermia is possible with genetic testing or the in vitro muscle contraction test. Excessive tonic contracture on exposure to halothane and caffeine in vitro indicates susceptibility. Treatment with IV dantrolene, sodium bicarbonate, and cooling is helpful.

## Neonatal and Infantile Hypotonia

The clinical distinction between upper and lower motor neuron disorders in infants is blurred because incomplete myelinization of the developing nervous system limits expression of many of the cardinal signs, such as spasticity. Neuromuscular and cerebral disorders may produce hypotonia in a young child or infant. The two critical clinical points are whether the child is weak and the presence or absence of deep tendon reflexes. Hypotonia and weakness coupled with depressed or absent reflexes suggest a neuromuscular disorder. A stronger child with brisk reflexes suggests an upper motor neuron source for the hypotonia.

## Hypotonia without Significant Weakness (Central Hypotonia)

Some infants who appear to move well when supine in their cribs are *floppy* when handled or moved. These infants are bright-eyed, have expressive faces, and can lift their arms and legs from the bed without apparent difficulty. When lifted, their heads flop, they *slip through* at the shoulders, do not stand upright, and form an *inverted* U in prone suspension (**Landau posture**). When placed prone as neonates, they may lie flat instead of having their arms and legs tucked underneath them. Passive tone is decreased, but reflexes are normal. This clinical picture may be associated with significant cerebral disease or may be a benign phenomenon that is outgrown.

**Prader-Willi syndrome** presents with severe neonatal hypotonia; severe feeding problems leading to failure to thrive; small hands and feet; and, in boys, small penis, small testicles, and cryptorchidism. Severe hyperphagia and obesity develop in early childhood. Approximately 60% to 70% of affected individuals have an interstitial deletion of paternal chromosome 15q11q13. Many other syndromes also present with severe neonatal floppiness and mental dullness (Table 182-5).

Infants who have a connective tissue disorder, such as **Ehlers-Danlos syndrome**, **Marfan syndrome**, or familial laxity of the ligaments, may exhibit marked passive hypotonia, *double jointedness*, and increased skin elasticity. They have normal strength and cognition and achieve motor and mental milestones normally. They have peculiar postures of their feet or an unusual gait.

Infants with **benign congenital hypotonia** typically exhibit the condition at 6 to 12 months old, with delayed gross motor skills. They are unable to sit, creep, or crawl, but have good verbal, social, and manipulative skills and an intelligent appearance. Strength appears normal, and the infants can kick arms and legs briskly and bring their toes to their mouths. The children display head lag, slip-through in ventral suspension, and floppiness of passive tone. The infant seems floppy from birth. The differential diagnosis includes upper and motor neuron disorders and connective tissue diseases. Extensive laboratory investigation is often unrevealing. Most of these children *catch up* to peers and appear normal by 3 years of age. Often, other family members have exhibited a similar developmental pattern.

## STROKE IN CHILDHOOD

### Etiology

Cerebrovascular infarction or hemorrhage is uncommon in children. The incidence is 2.5 to 10 per 100,000 children and is higher in neonates. A wide spectrum of conditions

---

### TABLE 182-4 Evaluation of Neuromuscular Disease

Complete medical history
Complete family history
Complete neurologic examination
Complete blood count with differential, ESR
Electrolytes, BUN, creatinine, glucose, calcium, phosphate, alkaline phosphatase, magnesium
Muscle chemistry studies: CK, aldolase
Metabolic studies: lactate, pyruvate
Chest radiograph
ECG
Stool: botulism culture and toxin testing, *Campylobacter* culture
CSF examination (protein, cells)
Tensilon test, neostigmine test, acetylcholine receptor antibody assay
EMG-NCV
Muscle biopsy
MRI of spinal cord

---

BUN, blood urea nitrogen; CK, creatine kinase; ECG, electrocardiogram; EMG, electromyography; ESR, erythrocyte sedimentation rate; MRI, magnetic resonance imaging; NCV, nerve conduction velocity [testing].

## TABLE 182-5 Approach to Differential Diagnosis in the Floppy Infant

### HYPOTONIA WITH WEAKNESS

*Awareness Intact*
Neuromuscular disease
  Spinal muscular atrophy*
  Myasthenic syndromes
  Congenital neuropathy or myopathy
Spinal cord disease (cervical cord trauma or compression)
  Tumor
  Spinal cord infarct
  Malformation
  Spina bifida
  Syringomyelia
*Consciousness Depressed*
Severe brain illness*
Structural (hydrocephalus)
Infectious
Metabolic (e.g., anoxia or hypoglycemia)
Intoxication through mother
  Magnesium sulfate
  Barbiturates
  Narcotics
  Benzodiazepines
  General anesthesia
Metabolic abnormality
  Hypoglycemia
  Kernicterus

### HYPOTONIA WITHOUT WEAKNESS

Acute systemic illness*
Mental retardation
Specific syndromes
  Down syndrome*
  Cerebrohepatorenal (Zellweger peroxisomal disorder)
  Oculocerebrorenal (Lowe syndrome)
  Kinky hair disease (Menkes syndrome—copper metabolism disorder)
  Neonatal adrenal leukodystrophy
  Prader-Willi syndrome
Connective tissue disorder
  Ehlers-Danlos syndrome
  Marfan syndrome
  Congenital laxity of ligaments
Nutritional-metabolic disease
  Rickets
  Renal tubular acidosis
  Celiac disease
  Biliary atresia
Congenital heart disease
Benign congenital hypotonia

*Common.

## TABLE 182-6 Causes of Stroke in Childhood

Cardiac or other embolic source
  Endocarditis
  Cyanotic congenital heart disease
  Valvular disease
  Patent foramen ovale
Infectious disorders
  Bacterial meningitis
  Encephalitis
  Chickenpox
Vasculitis or vasculopathy
  Arterial dissection—traumatic or spontaneous
Moyamoya disease
  Sickle cell anemia
  Neurofibromatosis
Vasculitis
Coagulopathies
*Hypocoagulation*
  Hemophilia, von Willebrand disease, thrombocytopenia
*Hypercoagulation*
  Factor V Leiden deficiency
  Protein C deficiency
  Protein S deficiency
  Antiphospholipid antibodies
  Antithrombin III deficiency
Sickle cell disease
Disseminated intravascular pathology
Head or neck trauma
  Carotid or vertebral dissections
  Atlantoaxial dislocation
Fibromuscular dysplasia
Atherosclerosis
Drugs or toxins
  Amphetamine, cocaine abuse
  Pregnancy/oral contraceptive pills
Hypertension
  Hemolytic uremic syndrome
  Nephrotic syndrome
Malignancy
  Carcinomatous meningitis
  Leukemic meningitis
  Chemotherapy (asparaginase)
Liver disease
Inborn error of metabolism
  Homocystinuria
Neonatal
  Emboli from dead twin
  Emboli from involuting umbilical vessels
  Polycythemia

can produce stroke in childhood (Table 182-6). The most common causes are congenital heart disease (cyanotic), sickle cell anemia, meningitis, and hypercoagulable states.

Heart disease and its complications (endocarditis) may give rise to thromboses in cerebral arteries or veins or to emboli in cerebral arteries. Cerebral venous and arterial thromboses occur in 1% to 2% of infants with unrepaired cyanotic congenital heart disease and probably are related to local congestion of blood flow, right-to-left cardiac shunting, and polycythemia. Predisposing factors include acute episodes of severe cyanosis, febrile illnesses, dehydration, hyperventilation, and iron deficiency anemia.

Sources of emboli include mural thrombi from poorly contracting cardiac chambers, bacterial or nonbacterial endocarditis, valvular disease, atrial myxoma, cardiac catheterization, and cardiac surgery. Septic emboli producing cerebral infarcts occur in 10% to 20% of patients who develop bacterial endocarditis.

## Clinical Manifestations

Cerebral embolization characteristically occurs without warning, produces its full deficit within seconds (hyperacute), and may be associated with focal deficits, seizures, sudden headache, and hemorrhagic infarction. The most common sources of cerebral emboli are the heart and the carotid artery. Cerebral thrombosis may be preceded by transient ischemic attacks that resolve completely. The deficits evolve over hours in a stepwise or stuttering progression. The sudden emergence of neurologic deficits implies cerebrovascular disease, and the site of occlusion is suggested by the neurologic deficits.

Occasionally a thorough evaluation of a child with a stroke fails to reveal the etiology. Angiography or magnetic resonance angiography may disclose the site of vascular occlusion, but the pathogenetic mechanism remains unknown. This condition is termed **acute hemiplegia of childhood**.

Congenital hemiplegia becomes apparent in infants 4 to 6 months old with decreased use of one side of the body, early *handedness*, or ignoring one side. CT reveals an area of encephalomalacia in the contralateral cerebral hemisphere. The details of the child's intrauterine, labor, delivery, and postnatal history often are unremarkable. Some neonates present with focal seizures. The timing of the injury is unknown, but the injury may represent an embolus from the fetal-placental unit.

## Diagnostic Tests and Imaging

If clinical assessment does not reveal the cause of the stroke, a complete laboratory investigation should be undertaken promptly based on suspected etiologies (see Table 182-6). On initial presentation, a non-contrast head CT scan is warranted, but acute, nonhemorrhagic stroke may not be seen on routine CT. More detailed investigation must include MRI and MRA (magnetic resonance angiography). Newer generations of MRI scan can detect an evolving stroke and patterns of ischemia by abnormal findings on diffusion-weighted images.

## Treatment

There is no treatment to repair the neurologic injury after the stroke, so prevention of future stroke must be the focus in children, if the etiology can be identified. The role of anticoagulants (IV heparin, subcutaneous low-molecular-weight heparin, and oral warfarin), platelet anti-aggregants (aspirin and dipyridamole), and thrombolysis via arterial or venous catheters for strokes that present *in evolution*, recurrent transient ischemic attacks, or ongoing cerebral embolization, appears to have some evidence of benefit despite significant risks.

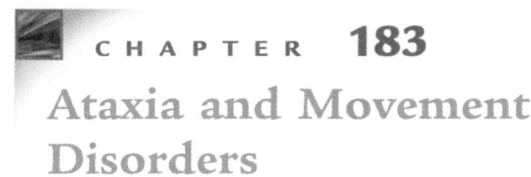

# CHAPTER 183
# Ataxia and Movement Disorders

## ETIOLOGY

Ataxia is an impairment of coordination or balance of voluntary movement. With few exceptions, this condition represents a disturbance of cerebellar pathways, including the cerebellar peduncles, spinocerebellar tract in the spinal cord, thalamic nuclei, and cortical reflections. The most common causes of acute ataxia in childhood are postinfectious acute cerebellar ataxia and drug intoxications. The **differential diagnosis** includes other disorders within the posterior fossa, such as tumors (medulloblastoma, ependymoma, cerebellar astrocytoma), multiple sclerosis, strokes, and hemorrhages. Other causes of recurrent or progressive ataxia, such as the paraneoplastic opsoclonus-myoclonus syndrome associated with neuroblastoma, inborn errors of metabolism, labyrinthine dysfunction, head trauma, epilepsy, postictal state, and migraine, can be difficult to diagnose and require special diagnostic testing for their identification. Congenital disorders also may produce chronic, nonprogressive ataxia (Table 183-1).

## CLINICAL MANIFESTATIONS

The usual symptoms are a broad-based, unsteady gait (truncal ataxia) and intention tremor or dysmetria. An intention tremor worsens as the arm approaches the target. Overshooting or undershooting of the target is termed **dysmetria** (abnormality of distance). Classically, these symptoms stem from disorders of the cerebellar pathways, but peripheral nerve lesions causing loss of proprioceptive inputs to the cerebellum (Miller Fisher variant of Guillain-Barré syndrome) may present with similar symptoms.

**Postinfectious acute cerebellar ataxia** may follow chickenpox, infectious mononucleosis, or a mild respiratory or gastrointestinal viral illness by about 1 week. The pathogenesis is uncertain and may represent either a direct viral infection of the cerebellum or an autoimmune response directed to the cerebellar white matter and precipitated by the viral infection. Symptoms begin abruptly, causing staggering and frequent falling. Symptoms can progress to difficulty with standing and sitting. Truncal ataxia may be the only symptom or dysmetria of the arms, dysarthria, nystagmus, vomiting, irritability, and lethargy may be present. Symptoms usually peak within 2 days, then stabilize and resolve over 1 to 2 weeks. Cerebrospinal fluid (CSF) examination sometimes shows a mild lymphocytic pleocytosis or mild elevation of protein content. Brain imaging is usually normal. No specific therapy is available except to prevent injury during the ataxic phase. Recovery is usually complete.

## TABLE 183-1 Causes of Ataxia

Neoplastic disease
  Medulloblastoma*
  Ependymoma
  Cystic cerebellar astrocytoma*
  Brainstem glioma
Paraneoplastic disease
  Neuroblastoma (opsoclonus-myoclonus-ataxia)
Infectious disorders
  Encephalitis
  Brainstem encephalitis
  Meningitis
Postinfectious disorders
  Acute cerebellar ataxia*
  Guillain-Barré syndrome (Miller Fisher variant)
Migrainous disorders
  Basilar migraine*
Trauma
  Cerebellar hemorrhage
  Cerebellar contusion
  Concussion
  Postconcussive syndrome*
Toxic ingestions*
  Antihistamines
  Ethanol
  Anticonvulsants
Vascular disorders
  Cerebellar hemorrhage or infarction
  Vertebral artery dissection
Demyelinative disorders
  Multiple sclerosis
  Acute disseminated encephalomyelitis
Structural or congenital disorders
  Cerebellar hypoplasia
  Vermal aplasia
  Dandy-Walker malformation
  Joubert syndrome
  Arnold-Chiari malformation
  Hydrocephalus
Hereditary ataxic disorders
  Episodic ataxia (acetazolamide-responsive)
  Friedreich ataxia
  Machado-Joseph disease
  Ramsay Hunt syndrome
  Spinocerebellar ataxia 1
  Spinocerebellar ataxia 2
  Ataxia-telangiectasia
  Marinesco-Sjögren syndrome
Metabolic disorders
  Metachromatic leukodystrophy
  Adrenoleukodystrophy
  Maple syrup urine disease
  Hartnup disease
  $GM_2$ gangliosidosis (juvenile)
  Refsum disease
  Vitamin E deficiency
  Leigh disease
  Wilson disease
  Abetalipoproteinemia
  Sea-blue histiocytosis

*Common.

## DRUG INTOXICATION

Overdosage with any sedative-hypnotic agent can produce acute ataxia and lethargy, but ataxia without lethargy usually results from intoxication with alcohol, phenytoin, or carbamazepine. It is important to ask whether anyone in the household (family or visitor) is taking anticonvulsant or antipsychotic medications. Treatment is supportive.

## POSTERIOR FOSSA TUMORS

Brain tumors are the second most common neoplasm in children. About 50% arise from within the posterior fossa. Tumors that arise in the posterior fossa or brainstem produce progressive ataxia with headache that may be acute or gradual in onset. There is a progressive worsening over days, weeks, or months. The ataxia and dysmetria may result from primary cerebellar invasion or from obstruction of the CSF pathways (aqueduct of Sylvius or fourth ventricle) with resultant hydrocephalus. The most common tumors in this region include medulloblastoma, ependymoma, cerebellar astrocytoma, and brainstem glioma.

## PARANEOPLASTIC OPSOCLONUS-MYOCLONUS SYNDROME

Rarely a neuroblastoma located in the adrenal medulla or anywhere along the paraspinal sympathetic chain in the thorax or abdomen is associated with degeneration of Purkinje cells and the development of severe ataxia, dysmetria, irritability, **myoclonus**, and **opsoclonus**. An immunologic reaction directed toward the tumor may be misdirected to also attack Purkinje cells and other neuronal elements. The myoclonic movements are irregular, lightning-like movements of a limb or the head. Opsoclonus is a rapid, multidirectional, conjugate movement of the eyes, which suddenly dart in random directions. The presence of this sign should prompt a vigorous search for an occult neuroblastoma, including urine testing for adrenergic metabolites (vanillylmandelic acid and homovanillic acid), chest x-ray, abdominal ultrasound, and magnetic resonance imaging (MRI) with contrast enhancement of the entire sympathetic chain. These tumors tend to be localized and curable by surgical resection. Treatment of paraneoplastic opsoclonus-myoclonus can be difficult, but immunotherapy with corticosteroids or intravenous immune globulin (IVIG) often relieves the acute neurologic symptoms; 64% of children are left with persistent cerebellar deficits, and 36% have intellectual deficits.

## INBORN ERRORS OF METABOLISM

Several rare inborn errors of metabolism can present with intermittent episodes of ataxia and somnolence. These include Hartnup disorder, branched chain ketoaciduria (maple syrup urine disease), multiple carboxylase deficiency (biotinidase deficiency), disorders of the urea cycle, and abnormalities of pyruvate metabolism.

## LABYRINTHINE DYSFUNCTION

Difficulty walking with a severe staggering gait is one manifestation of labyrinthine dysfunction, but the diagnosis usually is clarified by the associated symptoms of a severe sense of spinning dizziness (vertigo), nausea and vomiting, and associated signs of pallor, sweating, and nystagmus.

## MOVEMENT DISORDERS

Movement disorders or **dyskinesias** are a diverse group of entities associated with abnormal excessive, exaggerated, chaotic, or explosive movements of voluntary muscles. They are generally the result of abnormalities of the extrapyramidal system or the basal ganglia. Movement disorders in children are typically **hyperkinetic** patterns. The abnormal movements are activated by stress and fatigue and often disappear in sleep. They are typically diffuse and migratory (chorea), but may be isolated to specific muscle groups (segmental myoclonus, palatal myoclonus) and may not disappear in sleep.

**Chorea** is a hyperkinetic, rapid, unsustained, irregular, purposeless, nonpatterned movement. Muscle tone is decreased. Choreiform movement abnormalities may be congenital, familial, metabolic, vascular, toxic, infectious, or neoplastic in origin. The movements may occur alone or as part of a more extensive neurologic disorder (Sydenham chorea, Huntington chorea, cerebral palsy, Wilson disease, or reactions to toxins and drugs). Fidgety behavior, clumsiness, dysarthria, and an awkward gait may occur. The exact mechanism of dysfunction within the extrapyramidal system is unknown.

**Athetosis** is a hyperkinetic, slow, coarse, writhing movement that is more pronounced in distal muscles. Muscle tone may be increased. Athetosis is seen frequently in combination with chorea (choreoathetosis) and usually is present in conjunction with other neurologic signs. It may be seen in virtually all the disorders mentioned for chorea, but the most prominent cause is encephalopathy. Athetosis is a prominent feature of Hallervorden-Spatz disease, Wilson disease, and Pelizaeus-Merzbacher dystrophy. Many children with mixed forms of cerebral palsy have spasticity and choreoathetosis.

**Dystonia** is a hyperkinetic, sustained, slow, twisting motion (torsion spasm) that may progress to a fixed posture and can be activated by repetitive movement (action dystonia). It has many causes and associated neurologic signs. Dystonia usually begins in the legs when appendicular muscles are involved and in the neck or trunk when axial muscles are involved. Tardive dyskinesia usually is associated with antipsychotic drug use. Darting tongue movements, incessant flexion and extension of the distal muscles, standing and marching in place, and a perception of restlessness are common.

**Tremor** is a hyperkinetic, rhythmic, oscillatory movement caused by simultaneous contractions of antagonistic muscles. The amplitude and frequency are regular. In children, tremor is usually due to physiologic, familial, or cerebellar origin, but it may be seen in association with other disease processes (thyrotoxicosis, hypoglycemia, or Wilson disease) or drugs (bronchodilators, amphetamines, or tricyclic antidepressants).

**Myoclonus** is a hyperkinetic, brief flexion contraction of a muscle group, resulting in a sudden jerk. Myoclonus may be epileptic or nonepileptic. Nonepileptic myoclonus is distinguished from tremor in that it is a simple contraction of an agonist muscle, whereas tremor is a simultaneous contraction of agonist and antagonist muscles. Myoclonus is seen as a manifestation of various epilepsies and of infectious, toxic, and metabolic encephalopathies.

**Tics** are rapid, purposeless, involuntary, stereotyped movements and typically involve the face, eyes, shoulder, and arm. Most tic disorders in children are transient and not intrusive into the child's life, but often are a source of great parental anxiety. Occasionally, tics are *unmasked* by stimulant agents. Persistent motor tics (>12 months) in association with vocal tics are characteristic of **Tourette's syndrome**, a chronic tic disorder that usually begins before age 7 years. The prevalence is at least 5 in 10,000, with a male-to-female ratio of 4:1. The pathophysiology underlying tics is unknown, but a family history of tics is elicited in more than 50% of cases. The severity and pattern of the tics vary over months and years. Vocal tics begin later in the clinical course. The motor tics vary from muscle twitches (simple motor tic) and grunts (simple vocal tic) to complex stereotyped movement patterns (orchestrated movements). Co-morbid features, such as obsessive-compulsive disorder and attention-deficit/hyperactivity syndrome, may be present in half of children with Tourette's disorder (see Chapters 13 and 19). Tic disorders are clinical diagnoses, and neurodiagnostic studies have limited value. Many children with tic disorders or Tourette's syndrome are unperturbed by their tics and require no therapy. Others are quite disabled and may benefit from psychological support and pharmacologic therapy with α-adrenergic receptor agonists (clonidine) or neuroleptics (pimozide, haloperidol, risperidone). The natural history of Tourette's disorder is favorable; about two thirds of children experience a significant reduction of tics or complete remission.

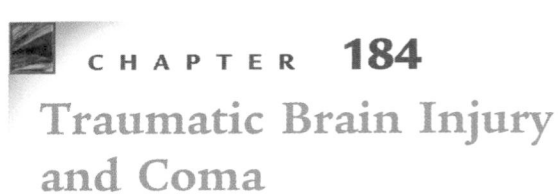

## CHAPTER 184

# Traumatic Brain Injury and Coma

Following head injury, children may have immediate depression of consciousness and neurologic deficits or may be completely alert without any immediate signs of neurologic injury. Most serious trauma results from motor vehicle crashes, sports, recreation-related injuries, and violence.

## PATIENTS WITH NEUROLOGIC DEFICITS

Victims of head trauma with neurologic deficits may arouse after the injury (lucid interval) and then undergo a depression of mental status or may remain unconscious from the moment of impact. Some progressively deteriorate and require immediate neurosurgical care (Table 184-1). Skull, cervical spine radiographs, and cranial computed tomography (CT) are obtained emergently.

**TABLE 184-1 Syndromes of Post-traumatic Intracranial Hemorrhage**

| Syndrome | Clinical and Radiologic Characteristics | Treatment |
|---|---|---|
| Epidural | Onset over minutes to hours<br>Uncal herniation with third nerve palsy and contralateral hemiparesis<br>Lens-shaped extracerebral hemorrhage compressing brain | Surgical evacuation or observation<br>Prognosis good |
| Acute subdural | Onset over hours<br>Uncal herniation<br>Focal neurologic deficits<br>Crescentic extracranial hemorrhage compressing brain | Surgical evacuation<br>Prognosis guarded |
| Chronic subdural | Onset over weeks to months<br>Anemia, macrocephaly<br>Seizures, vomiting<br>Crescentic, low-density mass on CT | Subdural taps or subdural shunt as necessary<br>Prognosis good |
| Intraparenchymal | Depressed consciousness<br>Focal neurologic deficits<br>Additional multiple contusions | Supportive care<br>Prognosis guarded |
| Subarachnoid | Stiff neck<br>Late hydrocephalus | Supportive care<br>Prognosis variable |
| Contusion | Focal neurologic deficits<br>Brain swelling with transtentorial herniation<br>CT findings: multifocal low-density areas with punctate hemorrhages | Medical treatment of elevated intracranial pressure*<br>Prognosis guarded |

*Mannitol, elevation of head of bed, diuresis, hyperventilation, steroids.
CT, computed tomography.

Children with cerebral contusion who survive the acute cerebral swelling may improve gradually or may remain vegetative. Maximal recovery may take weeks or months. Providing families with a prognosis can be challenging. Coma lasting for weeks after head trauma may be compatible with an ultimate good outcome, although the risk of late sequelae is significantly increased. Patients who remain in a vegetative state for months after head injury are unlikely to improve.

## Concussion

Concussion is a brief period of altered consciousness, lasting seconds to minutes, that occurs immediately after head trauma. Amnesia often follows concussion. **Retrograde amnesia** is the inability to remember events immediately before the trauma and may extend backward in time for minutes, hours, days, or weeks. Usually, retrograde memory is regained gradually, and permanent amnesia lasts only for the few minutes immediately before the injury. **Antegrade amnesia** is the inability to form new memories and is manifest by the incessant repeating of the same questions. The period of retrograde and antegrade amnesia usually correlates with the severity of the trauma, but may persist for hours or days.

The pathophysiology of concussion is thought to be a shearing phenomenon of white matter tracts as the brain undergoes torsional changes within the cranium, resulting in a temporary failure of axon conduction. If loss of consciousness is maintained for longer than 1 hour or if recovery of consciousness is slow and accompanied by focal neurologic deficits, the pathophysiology is likely to include contusion and laceration, which may lead to focal or generalized cerebral edema. Repeated concussions, especially within a short time frame (days or weeks) carry a significant risk of permanent brain injury (**second impact syndrome**). The summary statement of the 2nd International Conference on Concussion in Sport provides clear guidelines regarding return to full participation (Table 184-2).

**TABLE 184-2 Protocol for Return to Sport after Concussion**

Return to play after a concussion follows a stepwise process:
1. No activity, complete rest. Once the patient is asymptomatic, proceed to step 2.
2. Light aerobic exercise such as walking or stationary cycling; no resistance training.
3. Sport-specific exercise—for example, skating in hockey, running in soccer; progressive addition of resistance training at step 3 or 4.
4. Noncontact training drills.
5. Full-contact training after medical clearance.
6. Game play.

Modified from McCrory P, Johnston K, Meeuwisse W, et al: 2nd International Conference on Concussion in Sport, Prague 2004. *Clin J Sport Med* 15:2, 2005.

## Malignant Post-traumatic Cerebral Swelling

Occasionally, epidural, subdural, or intracranial hemorrhage or a rapid, life-threatening increase in intracranial pressure (ICP) develops unexpectedly in children who initially appear stable after head injury. The **Glasgow Coma Scale** is a valuable tool for monitoring the course of patients after trauma for signs of deterioration (see Chapter 42). Management includes ensuring an appropriate airway, breathing, and circulation. Emergent surgical intervention for decompression and drainage of the blood collection may be required. Increased ICP may require monitoring, placement of a ventricular drain, and aggressive medical management, including intubation and ventilation, osmotic therapy, and sedation.

**Transient neurologic disturbances** may develop a few minutes after head trauma and last for minutes to hours before clearing. The most common symptoms are cortical blindness and confusional states, but hemiparesis, ataxia, or any other neurologic deficit may appear. These symptoms may represent a trauma-triggered migraine in susceptible children, but care must be exercised to exclude intracranial pathology.

**Post-traumatic seizures** are divided into one of three patterns: impact seizures, early post-traumatic seizures, and late post-traumatic seizures. Impact seizures occur within seconds of the injury and are presumed to reflect a direct mechanical stimulation to the cortex. The prognosis is excellent, and likelihood of later epilepsy is negligible. Occasionally, pallid breath-holding spells can occur after head injury, mimicking impact seizures. Early post-traumatic seizures occurring within the first week of the head injury are likely the result of a localized area of cerebral contusion or edema. The long-term prognosis for these seizures is quite favorable. Late post-traumatic seizures arise more than a week after the trauma and most likely indicate an area of cortical gliosis or scarring that will be a source for long-term epilepsy. These patients often require long-term antiepileptic drug therapy.

**Drowsiness**, **headache**, and **vomiting** are common after head trauma. They are not, by themselves, of concern if consciousness is preserved, the clinical trend is one of improvement, and results of the neurologic examination are normal. Children are especially susceptible to somnolence after head trauma but should be easily arousable. If symptoms worsen or persist for more than 1 to 2 days, neuroimaging may be indicated to look for subdural hematoma or cerebral edema.

**Skull fractures** may be linear, diastatic (spreading the suture), depressed (an edge displaced inferiorly), or compound (bone fragments breaking the skin surface). Linear and diastatic fractures necessitate no treatment, but indicate trauma capable of producing an underlying hematoma. Small, depressed fractures have the same significance as linear fractures, but if the depression is more than 0.5 to 1 cm, surgical elevation of bone fragments and repair of associated dural tears are generally recommended. Compound fractures or penetrating injuries necessitate emergent surgical débridement but not prophylactic antibiotic therapy. Tetanus prophylaxis must be ensured. The risk of local brain contusion and early seizures is high.

Skull fractures may present with localized bogginess and pain; subcutaneous bleeding over the mastoid process (**Battle sign**) or around the orbit (**raccoon eyes**); blood behind the tympanic membrane (**hemotympanum**); or cerebrospinal fluid (CSF) leak from the nose (rhinorrhea) or ear (**otorrhea**). Rarely, a few weeks to months after linear skull fractures, a soft, pulsatile scalp mass is palpable. Radiographically the fracture edges are separated by a soft tissue mass that consists of fibrotic tissue and accumulated brain and meningeal tissue and, perhaps, a **leptomeningeal cyst**. The recommended treatment involves surgical excision of abnormal tissue and dural repair.

**CSF leak** occurs when a skull fracture tears adjacent dura, creating communications between the subarachnoid space and the nose, paranasal sinuses, mastoid air cells, or ear. Clear fluid that leaks from the nose or ear after head trauma is presumed to be CSF until proved otherwise. The presence of air within the subdural, subarachnoid, or ventricular space also indicates a dural tear and open communication between the nose or paranasal sinuses and brain. In most cases, the dura heals spontaneously when the patient's head is kept elevated. Patients with CSF leaks are at risk for the development of meningitis or extradural abscesses. If the leak persists or recurs or if meningitis develops, the dura is surgically repaired.

**Cranial nerve palsies**, secondary to a laceration or contusion of the cranial nerves, may result from a skull fracture and may be transitory or permanent. Longitudinal fracture of the petrous bone produces a conductive hearing loss and facial palsy, which begin hours after the injury and usually resolves spontaneously. Transverse petrous fractures produce sensorineural hearing loss and immediate facial palsy with a poor prognosis for spontaneous recovery. Disruption of the ossicular chain can cause hearing loss and may necessitate surgery. Vestibular disturbances, producing prolonged post-traumatic vertigo, are extremely common. Permanent loss of olfaction after a head injury is the result of a rupture of the thin olfactory nerves within the cribriform plate. Disruption of cranial nerves III, IV, and VI produces ophthalmoplegia, diplopia, and head tilt. Even seemingly minor head injuries can produce sixth nerve palsy with medial deviation of one eye.

**Cervical spine injuries** must be suspected in any unconscious child, especially if bruises are present on the head, neck, or back. In conscious children, findings of neck or back pain, burning or stabbing pains radiating to the arms, paraplegia, quadriplegia, or asymmetrical motor or sensory responses of arms or legs indicate spinal cord injury. Cervical spine injury (displaced or fractured vertebra) may result in complete transection of the cord with spinal shock, loss of sensation, and flaccid paralysis. A contused cord (without vertebral abnormality) may present in a similar manner. Any patient with a clinical or radiologic abnormality of the spine requires immediate spine and cardiopulmonary stabilization and neurosurgical consultation. The use of high-dose intravenous (IV) methylprednisolone in cases of spinal cord trauma is controversial but may improve the ultimate degree of recovery of function.

## Postconcussive Syndrome

Many children complain of headache, dizziness, forgetfulness, inability to concentrate, slowing of response time, mood swings, irritability, and other subtle aberrations of cerebral function for days or weeks after an uncomplicated concussion. These deficits resolve spontaneously, but may require weeks or months for full recovery. Children may require brief periods of special schooling, home tutoring, and reassurance.

### Evaluation and Treatment

Children who have been unconscious or have amnesia following a head injury should be evaluated in an emergency department. High-risk patients include those with persistent depressed or decreasing level of consciousness, focal neurologic signs, penetrating skull injury, or depressed skull fractures. These patients warrant care in a skilled trauma center and CT or magnetic resonance imaging (MRI) examination.

The observation period should increase with the severity of the injury and may include hospitalization even for children without neurologic deficits who have sustained a concussion. If the child appears well after several hours and is discharged home, parents should be instructed to call their physician for any change in alertness, orientation, or neurologic functioning. An increase in somnolence, headache, or vomiting is cause for concern and neuroimaging.

### Prognosis

Children with concussion without subsequent neurologic deficits have a favorable long-term prognosis, and late sequelae are rare. Children with moderate contusions usually make good recoveries even when neurologic signs persist for weeks. Long-term sequelae may include poor memory and slowing of motor skills or a generalized decrease in cognitive skills, behavioral alterations, and attention deficits. Language function, especially in a young child, frequently makes a good recovery. Rehabilitation programs with physical therapy, behavioral management, and appropriate education may be necessary. Poor prognostic signs include a Glasgow Coma Scale score of less than 4 on admission without improvement in 24 hours, absent pupillary light reflexes, and persistent extensor plantar reflexes. Extracranial trauma also contributes to the morbidity of these patients (aspiration pneumonia, acute respiratory distress syndrome, sepsis, and emboli).

## DISORDERS OF CONSCIOUSNESS

**Consciousness** represents awareness of self and environment (place and time). **Arousal** represents the system that initiates consciousness. Consciousness is mediated by the cerebral cortex, and arousal is mediated by the reticular activating system (RAS) extending from the mid pons through the midbrain and hypothalamus to the thalamus. **Coma** is a state of unresponsive unconsciousness and is caused by dysfunction of the cerebral hemispheres (bilaterally), the brainstem (herniation syndromes), or both simultaneously. Depression of consciousness may be acute, chronic, transitory, or recurring.

### Acute Disorders of Consciousness

Acute changes in consciousness vary in degree from mild lethargy and confusion to deep coma. In childhood, the most common causes of coma are infections, hypoxia-ischemia (cardiac arrest, near-drowning), intoxication, head trauma, and seizure-related, either a postictal state or, uncommonly, subclinical status epilepticus (Table 184-3).

### Assessment

Airway, breathing, and circulation are addressed first. Vital signs, including pulse oximetry, must be assessed. The most common cause of long-term morbidity in a patient with depressed consciousness is **hypoxia**. General physical examination searches for clues as to the cause of depressed consciousness, such as dehydration, unusual odors, needle tracts, trauma, or signs of organ system failure. Breathing patterns may provide important clues to the depth, localization, and etiology of the depressed consciousness. Some patterns of respiration have specific anatomic correlates such as **Cheyne-Stokes respiration**, central neurogenic hyperventilation, and gasping respiration. In Cheyne-Stokes respiration, a period of hyperventilation with a crescendo-decrescendo pattern alternates with a shorter period of apnea. Cerebral, thalamic, or hypothalamic modulation of respiration has been lost, but brainstem control is intact. This pattern also can be seen in patients with metabolic disorders, heart failure, or primary respiratory disease. A midbrain lesion yields **central neurogenic hyperventilation**, which consists of sustained rapid deep breathing. **Gasping** respirations are irregularly irregular and indicate dysfunction of the low brainstem-medulla. This pattern of respiration is ominous and usually is followed by terminal apnea.

The **Glasgow Coma Scale** (see Table 42-2) can be used to assess unresponsive patients regarding their best verbal responses, best motor response, and eye opening to stimulation with a score of 3 to 15 points. Depression of consciousness also can be documented (Table 184-4).

The detailed neurologic examination of a comatose patient focuses on the integrity of the brainstem (the location of the reticular activating system, which mediates arousal). Pupillary responses assess the midbrain function (Table 184-5). Eye movements are observed or elicited with the **doll's eye maneuver** (oculocephalic response) (see Chapter 179) or cold caloric stimulation (**oculovestibular response**). If the oculocephalic responses are not elicited or unclear, cold water is flushed into the external ear canal. In a conscious person, this maneuver elicits nystagmus to the opposite side and extreme vertigo with vomiting. In a comatose patient, cold water irrigation into the ear canal elicits a tonic eye deviation toward the ear irrigated if the brainstem is functioning. With complete loss of oculomotor function, the eyes remain in the center of the orbit regardless of any stimulation, indicating brainstem failure.

Body posture at rest and after noxious stimulation can indicate the anatomic level responsible for the alteration of consciousness. Mild depression may be manifested by

## TABLE 184-3  Causes of Coma and Diagnostic Approach

### CAUSES

Metabolic derangements
  Hypoglycemia
  Hyponatremia or its correction
  Hypernatremia or its correction
  Hyperosmolarity or its correction
  Hypercapnia
  Uremia
  Hyperammonemia
  Hepatic failure
  Reye syndrome
  Urea cycle enzyme deficiency
  Fatty acid acyl-coenzyme A dehydrogenase
    deficiency
  Methylmalonicaciduria
  Propionicaciduria
  Idiopathic hyperammonemia of prematurity
  Mitochondrial diseases
  Diabetes mellitus—ketoacidosis or hypoglycemia
  Lead intoxication
Hypertensive encephalopathy
Infection (see Table 179-2)
  Meningitis
  Encephalitis
  Brain abscess
  Toxic shock syndrome
  Cat-scratch disease
  Postinfectious (acute disseminated encephalomyelitis)
  Postimmunization syndrome (hypotonic-hyporesponsive
    spells)
Stroke
  Infarction
  Hemorrhage
  Subarachnoid hemorrhage
Trauma
  Shaken baby syndrome
  Epidural hemorrhage
  Subdural hemorrhage
  Subarachnoid hemorrhage
  Concussion
Hypoxia-ischemia
  Postdrowning
  Post–cardiopulmonary arrest
  Carbon monoxide intoxication
Neoplasm
  Brain tumor
Structural
  Hydrocephalus
Toxins
  Ethanol
  Narcotics
  Antihistamines
  Iron
  Acetaminophen
  Aspirin
  Recreational drugs
  Lead poisoning
  Drug intoxication or withdrawal
  Cerebral edema
Epilepsy
  Subclinical status epilepticus
  Postictal states
Migraine
Miscellaneous
  Gastrointestinal (intussusception)
  HUS-TTP
  Vasculitis (systemic lupus erythematosus)

### DIAGNOSTIC APPROACH

Glucose, $Na^+$, $K^+$, $Cl^-$, $CO_2$, BUN, creatinine, AST, ALT, PT, PTT, blood gases, ammonia, lead level, pyruvate, lactate, urinalysis, and urine amino and organic acids
CT, MRI, MRA, MRV, angiogram
CSF analysis
EEG
Blood and urine analyses for toxic substances

ALT, alanine aminotransferase; AST, aspartate aminotransferase; BUN, blood urea nitrogen; CSF, cerebrospinal fluid; CT, computed tomography; EEG, electroencephalogram; HUS-TTP, hemolytic uremic syndrome–thrombotic thrombocytopenic purpura; MRI/MRA/MRV, magnetic resonance imaging/angiography/venography; PT, prothrombin time; PTT, partial thromboplastin time.

## TABLE 184-4  Stages of Depressed Consciousness

| Stage | Manifestations |
| --- | --- |
| Lethargy | Sleepy, poor attention, fully arousable |
| Confusion | Poor orientation |
| Delirium | Agitated confusion, hallucinations, autonomic abnormalities (e.g., excess sweating, tachycardia, hypertension) |
| Obtundation | Arousable to noxious stimulation |
| Stupor | Arousable momentarily with noxious stimulation, localizes pain |
| Coma | Unarousable, does not localize pain |

a comfortable *sleeping* posture. Frequent spontaneous readjustments of position, yawns, and sighs are observed. Patients who lie in a flat, extended, unvarying position with eyes half-open exhibit a deeper coma. An asymmetrical posture suggests motor dysfunction of one side. Posture changes with noxious stimulation may indicate more serious neurologic conditions. **Decorticate posturing** consists of rigid extension of the legs and feet, flexion and supination of the arms, and fisting of the hands. It occurs when the midbrain and red nucleus control body posture without inhibition by diencephalon, basal ganglia, and cortical structures. **Decerebrate posturing** (rigid extension of legs, arms, trunk, and head with hyperpronation of lower arms) indicates pontine and vestibular

### TABLE 184-5  Effect of Coma-Producing Toxins on Pupillary Size

| Pupils Small | Pupils Large | Pupils Normal |
| --- | --- | --- |
| Narcotics (except meperidine) | Anticholinergics | Salicylates |
| Sedatives | Antihistamines | Acetaminophen |
| Barbiturates | Tricyclic antidepressants | |
| Alcohol | Phenothiazines | |
| Major tranquilizers | Glutethimide | |
| Phenothiazines | | |
| Cholinergic agonists | | |
| Organophosphate insecticides | | |
| Nicotine | | |
| Certain plants and mushrooms | | |

nucleus control of posture without inhibition from more rostral structures. These postures may be exhibited unilaterally or bilaterally, indicating equal or unequal dysfunction of the two sides of the brain.

## Etiology

Recognition of the pace or evolution of change in consciousness is an important clue to the etiology. A detailed history and physical examination usually provide sufficient clues to differentiate among the three major diagnostic categories producing coma: **metabolic** or **toxic**, **infectious**, and **structural**. In most clinical situations, the cause of coma is readily identified.

Metabolic derangements are common causes of disorders of consciousness. Disturbances of blood chemistries (glucose, sodium, calcium, bicarbonate, blood urea nitrogen [BUN], and ammonia) may produce depressed mental status. Metabolic causes of acute coma are suggested by spontaneous fluctuations in the level of consciousness, tremors, myoclonus, asterixis, visual and tactile hallucinations, and deep coma with preservation of pupillary light reflexes. Acute metabolic or toxic disorders usually produce a hypotonic, limp state, but hypertonia, rigidity, and decorticate and decerebrate posturing are observed sometimes in coma caused by hypoglycemia, hepatic encephalopathy, and short-acting barbiturates. A subacute course of somnolence progressing to deep, unarousable *sleep* (stupor) over hours suggests drug intoxication or organ system failure (kidney, liver) producing a metabolic encephalopathy. Care must be taken to investigate background medical conditions that may produce a decline in consciousness (diabetes mellitus, leukemia). Intoxication and ingestion are common causes of acute alteration of consciousness, and a thorough history must be taken to search for the offending agent (see Chapter 45).

Central nervous system (CNS) infection, such as meningitis or encephalitis, causes abrupt alteration of mental status. The presence of fever, petechiae, chills, and sweats suggests infection. Prodromal photophobia and pain on movement of the head or eyes are symptoms of meningeal irritation. Premonitory symptoms, such as abdominal pain, diarrhea, sore throat, conjunctivitis, cough, or rash, point toward viral encephalitis or a postinfectious syndrome as the cause of the altered consciousness.

Structural processes, such as hemorrhage, stroke, or acute hydrocephalus, are infrequent, sudden causes of depressed consciousness in children. If trauma or immersion injuries are suspected, neck manipulation should be avoided until the cervical spine films exclude vertebral fracture or subluxation. An evolution of headache and morning vomiting suggests increased ICP. A gradual fading of alertness or declining school performance over preceding weeks suggests an expanding intracranial mass, subdural effusion or hematoma, or chronic infection (tuberculous meningitis, human immunodeficiency virus [HIV]). A history of social and emotional difficulties, drug abuse, or depression raises concern for self-inflicted injury or toxic ingestion.

## Clinical Manifestations

Papilledema or paralysis of cranial nerves III or VI in a patient with depressed consciousness is strong evidence of elevated ICP, a medical and neurosurgical emergency. A progressive loss of consciousness accompanied by a characteristic progression of motor, oculomotor, pupillary, and respiratory signs (Table 184-6) indicates incipient transtentorial herniation. *Uncal herniation* implies the mesial temporal lobe is shifting across the tentorial edge, producing a unilateral third nerve palsy and contralateral hemiparesis. Medical therapy (hyperventilation, osmotic agents, steroids) must be instituted, emergency cranial CT performed, and urgent neurosurgical consultation obtained.

Deprivation of oxygen to the brain, caused by either deficient oxygen in the blood (hypoxemia) or deficient delivery of blood to the brain (ischemia), impairs consciousness (Table 184-7). Severe ischemia produces loss of

### TABLE 184-6  Progression of Stages and Anatomic Levels of Transtentorial Central Herniation

| Signs | Thalamus | Midbrain | Medulla* |
| --- | --- | --- | --- |
| Consciousness | Confusion; stupor | Coma | Coma |
| Respirations | Sighs; Cheyne-Stokes type | Central neurogenic hyperventilation | Gasping; absent |
| Pupils | Small, reactive | 3–5 mm, fixed | Unreactive |
| Extraocular movements | Roving; uninhibited | Incomplete, dysconjugate | Absent |
| Motor response | Spastic; decorticate | Decerebrate | Flaccid |

*Uncal herniation with unilateral oculomotor nerve palsy or hemiplegia is another sign of severe increased intracranial pressure.

**TABLE 184-7 Causes of Hypoxia and Ischemia**

**HYPOXIA (DECREASED OXYGEN LEVELS)**

*$Po_2$ Decreased*
Pulmonary disease
Cardiac disease; right-to-left shunt
Hypoventilation
Exogenous (e.g., drowning, choking, suffocation)
Neuromuscular disease
Central respiratory drive decreased
*$Po_2$ Normal—Decreased Oxygen Content*
Severe anemia
Carbon monoxide poisoning
Methemoglobinemia

**ISCHEMIA (DECREASED PERFUSION)**

Cardiac disease (decreased cardiac output)
Myocardial infarction
Arrhythmia
Valvular disease
Pericarditis
Pulmonary embolism
Hypotension, shock
Hanging, strangulation
Extensive cerebrovascular disease

consciousness within seconds and permanent brain damage within a few minutes. Deterioration in functioning may occur for several hours after a severe hypoxic-ischemic insult. The development of circulatory failure from anoxic cardiac injury, disseminated intravascular coagulation, or cerebral edema may compound the initial injury.

The prognosis of cerebral hypoxic-ischemic injury is extremely variable in children. Short duration of coma (hours to 1 to 2 days) and intact brainstem function on hospital admission indicate a favorable prognosis. The most common permanent neurologic sequelae are spasticity, ataxia, choreoathetosis, parkinsonian syndrome, intention or action myoclonus, memory loss, visual agnosia, and impairments of learning and attention. Improvement can occur for several months to 1 year after the insult. Treatment involves physical therapy, occupational therapy, rehabilitative services, and education.

**Primary subarachnoid hemorrhage** usually is caused by rupture of a saccular **berry aneurysm** of one of the major cerebral arteries in the circle of Willis. These aneurysms are presumed to result from localized developmental defects in the arterial walls and are associated with cystic kidney disease and coarctation of the aorta. Aneurysmal hemorrhage is uncommon in childhood. The usual clinical manifestations are the sudden onset of intense headache followed by collapse and loss of consciousness. Focal neurologic deficits vary, but nuchal rigidity almost invariably is present. Treatment should take place in an intensive care unit (ICU) and consists of bed rest, sedation, and therapy to eliminate vascular spasm until surgical or endovascular elimination of the aneurysm is feasible.

Postinfectious syndromes (**acute disseminated encephalomyelitis**) closely resemble episodes of viral meningoencephalitis, but are the consequence of acute multifocal, immunologically mediated demyelination rather than of direct viral invasion of the brain. Fever, stiff neck, depression of consciousness, and focal neurologic deficits occur a few days after a benign systemic viral syndrome. The course is variable, but most children recover without sequelae within a few days to weeks. Systemic viral infection seems to trigger the syndrome by an unknown mechanism. These syndromes were first described after measles, mumps, rubella, and chickenpox and after vaccination against smallpox and rabies.

## Laboratory and Diagnostic Imaging

**Head CT** remains the preferred imaging technique in emergency situations because it can be performed rapidly and accurately identifies acute hemorrhages, large space-occupying lesions, edema, and shifts of the midline. The initial head CT scan is done without contrast material to identify blood and calcifications. Contrast material can be administered to identify inflammatory and neoplastic lesions. Several metabolic derangements (hepatic encephalopathy, Reye syndrome, hyponatremia, lead encephalopathy, trauma, treatment of diabetic ketoacidosis, and global or multifocal hypoxic-ischemic injury) may give rise to severe elevations of ICP without producing recognizable CT abnormalities. Lumbar puncture (LP) in a patient with impending transtentorial herniation should be avoided.

**Examination of the CSF** may establish the cause of the alteration of consciousness. Appropriate neuroimaging should be performed to ensure that no added injury is inflicted with LP. The presence of red blood cells in the cerebrospinal fluid (CSF) suggests primary subarachnoid hemorrhage, parenchymal hemorrhage, or hemorrhagic infection (herpes simplex virus, group B streptococcus, *Neisseria meningitidis*). White blood cells in the CSF usually denote infectious meningitis or meningoencephalitis, but may also be associated with subacute bacterial endocarditis, vasculitis, carcinomatous meningitis, or a parainfectious syndrome.

## Treatment

The etiology of coma determines the treatment. Ingestions may necessitate gastric lavage, charcoal administration, forced diuresis, dialysis, or specific antidotes (see Chapter 45). Infections are treated with appropriate antibiotics or antiviral agents (Chapter 95). Structural brain lesions may necessitate surgical excision or medical treatment of increased ICP.

## Prognosis

The outcome of coma relates to many variables, including the etiology. Intoxication carries a good prognosis, whereas hypoxia carries a bad prognosis. Other prognostic factors include the duration of coma and the age of the patient (children have a better outcome than adults). The Glasgow Coma Scale on admission also projects outcome. Complete recovery from traumatic coma of several days' duration is possible in children; however, many survivors of severe coma are left in a persistent vegetative state or with severe neuropsychiatric disability.

## Brain Death

Brain death means irreversible cessation of all cortical and brainstem functions. Guidelines that are generally accepted as death for children and adolescents exclude neonates (Table 184-8). In certain clinical situations, demonstration of a total absence of cerebral blood flow on four-vessel intracranial angiography or nuclide brain scanning may be required as definitive confirmation of brain death. Application of brain death criteria is particularly problematic in premature and newborn infants.

## Transient, Recurrent Depression of Consciousness

Episodic alteration or depression of consciousness with full recovery is usually due to seizure, migraine, syncope, or metabolic abnormality (hypoglycemia). Consciousness can be impaired during **seizures** or in the postictal state. Nonconvulsive status epilepticus (generalized or partial complex) can directly impair consciousness for extended periods. Some patients may have a prolonged postictal state after an unrecognized seizure.

Basilar artery or **confusional migraine** attacks can last hours and be accompanied by agitation, ataxia, cortical blindness, vertigo, or cranial nerve palsies. Headache may precede or follow the neurologic signs.

**TABLE 184-8 Guidelines for Determination of Brain Death***

Two physicians must be present
The treating physician must be a board-eligible or board-certified neurologist, neurosurgeon, internist, pediatrician, surgeon, or anesthesiologist
Body temperature $\geq 33°C$
No confounding drug intoxication (e.g., presence of barbiturates at higher than therapeutic levels)
No spontaneous movements, communication, or interaction with the environment
No supraspinal response to externally applied stimuli (pain, touch, light, sound)
Absence of brainstem reflexes including:
  Pupillary light
  Oculocephalic
  Oculovestibular
  Corneal
  Oropharyngeal—gag
  Tracheal—cough
Apnea test (includes at least a 10-minute period of preoxygenation with 100% oxygen) allowing the $Paco_2$ to increase to >60 mm Hg, with no spontaneous breaths
Electrocerebral silence on electroencephalogram
Absence of cerebral perfusion (e.g., on nuclear perfusion scan)

All of the criteria listed should be present on multiple examinations at least 6 to 24 hours after the onset of coma and apnea. There must be documented absence of drug intoxication (including sedatives and neuromuscular blocking agents), hypothermia, and cardiovascular shock. A cause of coma sufficient to account for the loss of brain function should be established.

**Syncope** is one of the most common causes of abrupt, episodic loss of consciousness. Neurocardiogenic syncope, cardiac arrhythmia, or an obstructive cardiomyopathy can cause recurrent episodes of loss of consciousness. Two thirds of children with syncope have irregular, myoclonic movements as they lose consciousness (anoxic seizures). Children with unexplained syncope require a complete cardiac examination (see Chapter 140).

Metabolic derangements, particularly **hypoglycemia**, give rise to episodes of lethargy, confusion, seizures, or coma. Autonomic symptoms, such as anxiety, excess sweating, tremulousness, and hunger, often herald attacks. A typical spell may be aborted by ingesting orange juice or other sugar-containing solutions. Several other metabolic disorders cause recurrent bouts of **hyperammonemia** (see Chapter 53). Symptoms include nausea, vomiting, lethargy, confusion, ataxia, hyperventilation, and coma.

## INCREASED INTRACRANIAL PRESSURE

### Etiology

When the cranial sutures are fused, the skull becomes a rigid container enclosing a fixed volume, including the brain (80–85%), CSF (10–15%), and blood (5–10%). The exponential relationship between the volume within a closed container and pressure results in a massive increase in ICP as intracranial volume increases. The brain accommodates increased ICP initially by expelling CSF and blood from the intracranial compartment into the spinal subarachnoid space. When the limits of this accommodation are reached, the brain itself begins to shift in response to the continuing elevation of ICP. The brain shifts across the dural extensions (falx cerebri, tentorium cerebelli) or skull barriers are called **herniations** and may occur under the falx, through the tentorial notch, or into the foramen magnum. Supratentorial masses produce a downward transtentorial herniation. Infratentorial masses produce foramen magnum herniation. Unilateral frontal masses produce transfalcial herniation. Transtentorial herniation is more likely to occur with a unilateral hemispheric lesion than with diffuse supratentorial brain swelling. Transtentorial and foramen magnum herniations are immediately life-threatening and indicate critically increased ICP (Table 184-9). Herniation sequences also compress vascular supply, leading to infarction of vital thalamic and brainstem structures. Withdrawal of CSF in the thecal sac can change pressures between the intracranial compartments promoting brainstem shifts and herniations. The causes of increased ICP can be categorized broadly as follows: mass lesion, hydrocephalus, and brain swelling (Table 184-10).

**Mass lesions (brain abscess or tumor)** may produce increased ICP not only by virtue of large size, but by blockage of CSF pathways, blockage of venous outflow, or production of cerebral edema. This vasogenic edema is produced by leakage of plasma proteins and fluid through a damaged blood-brain barrier at the level of the endothelial cell. Brain abscesses usually present as mass lesions, producing focal neurologic signs and increased ICP. Symptoms of infection, including fever, malaise, anorexia, and stiff neck, may be subtle or absent. Brain edema around

**TABLE 184-9 Herniation Syndromes**

| Location | Etiology | Description | Clinical Finding(s) |
|---|---|---|---|
| **Transtentorial** | | | |
| Unilateral (uncal) | Tumor<br>Stroke<br>Hemorrhage<br>Abscess<br>Unilateral edema | Temporal lobe structures shift below tentorium compressing midbrain, cranial nerve III, and PCA | Hemiparesis<br>Enlarged pupil<br>Coma |
| Bilateral (central) | Cytotoxic edema<br>Anoxia<br>Trauma | Downward displacement of both temporal lobes compressing the diencephalons and midbrain | Posture—decorticate, decerebrate<br>Pupils—small, reactive<br>Respirations—Cheyne-Stokes |
| Cerebellar | Diffuse mass lesions<br>Cerebellar mass lesions<br>Diffuse CNS edema | *Upward* movement, midbrain compression<br>*Downward* movement, medulla through foramen | Pupils dilated<br>Respiration irregular<br>Coma<br>Cranial nerve palsies<br>Apnea<br>Bradycardia<br>Death |

PCA, posterior cerebral artery.

**TABLE 184-10 Causes of Increased Intracranial Pressure**

| Imaging Abnormality* | No Definable Imaging Abnormality |
|---|---|
| *Mass Effect* | Idiopathic intracranial hypertension (pseudotumor cerebri) |
| Hydrocephalus | Intracranial venous sinus thrombosis |
| Infarction with edema | Drugs |
| Hemorrhage |   Vitamin A, retinoic acid |
| Tumor |   Tetracycline, nalidixic acid |
| Abscess | Endocrinologic disturbance |
| Cyst | Withdrawal of long-term steroid administration |
| Inflammatory mass | Addison disease |
| *Diffuse Edema* | Hypoparathyroidism |
| Hypoxic-ischemic injury | Obesity in women with menstrual irregularities |
| Trauma | Iron deficiency anemia |
| Infection | Catch-up growth in infants with malnutrition (e.g., cystic fibrosis) |
|   Meningitis | High-altitude brain edema |
|   Encephalitis | |
| Hypertension | |
| Metabolic derangement or toxin | |
|   Hyponatremia | |
|   Diabetic ketoacidosis | |
|   Dialysis dysequilibrium syndrome | |
|   Reye syndrome | |
|   Fulminant hepatic encephalopathy | |
|   Pulmonary insufficiency with hypercarbia | |
|   Lead intoxication | |

*By computed tomography or magnetic resonance imaging.

an abscess is usually severe and extends into the surrounding white matter. The diagnosis of brain abscess is suspected in children with chronic cardiac or pulmonary disease that may embolize infected material to their brains. Caution must be exercised before LP in a patient with a brain abscess because the risks of transtentorial herniation are high as a result of the extensive unilateral white matter edema.

**Hydrocephalus** usually produces a slowly evolving syndrome of increased ICP extending over weeks or months. Enlarging ventricles and interstitial edema in the periventricular white matter exert pressure. The edema is created by transudation of CSF through the ependymal barrier. CSF is an ultrafiltrate of plasma, continuously produced by the choroid plexus within the lateral, third, and fourth ventricles. The normal volume of CSF is approximately 50 mL in neonates and 150 mL in adults. CSF flows from the lateral ventricles through the intraventricular foramen of Monro to the third ventricle. It then passes through the cerebral aqueduct to the fourth ventricle. CSF exits the fourth ventricle from the single midline foramen of Magendie and the two lateral foramina of Luschka. Subarachnoid flow occurs superiorly to the cisterns of the brain and inferiorly to the spinal subarachnoid space. Absorption of CSF is accomplished predominantly by the arachnoid villi, microtubular invaginations into the large dural sinuses which are most concentrated along the superior sagittal sinus.

Hydrocephalus is due to the obstruction of CSF flow anywhere along its course (Table 184-11). **Obstructive hydrocephalus** is caused by a block before the CSF flows to the subarachnoid space, usually within the fourth ventricle or at the level of the aqueduct. Impairment of CSF flow within the subarachnoid space or impairment of absorption is known by the misnomer ***communicating hydrocephalus***, where there is actually extraventricular obstruction of CSF flow (external hydrocephalus). Hydrocephalus caused by overproduction of CSF without true obstruction is seen in choroid plexus papillomas, which account for 2% to 4% of childhood intracranial tumors and manifest in early infancy.

Ventricular distention and increased ICP cause the clinical manifestations of hydrocephalus. Dilation of the lateral ventricles results in stretching of the corticopontocerebellar and corticospinal pathways, which sweep around the lateral margins of these ventricles to reach the cerebral peduncles. This stretching results in ataxia and spasticity that initially are most marked in the lower extremities because the leg fibers are closest to the ventricles. Distention of the third ventricle may compress the hypothalamic regions and result in endocrine dysfunction. The optic nerves, chiasm, and tracts also are in proximity to the anterior third ventricle, and visual dysfunction results when these structures are compressed. Dilation of the cerebral aqueduct compresses the surrounding periaqueductal vertical gaze center, causing paresis of upward gaze (sunsetting eyes or **Parinaud syndrome**). Manifestations of increased ICP may evolve slowly when obstruction is not complete and there is time for transependymal absorption of CSF into the veins, or rapidly when obstruction is abrupt and complete (as in subarachnoid hemorrhage), and compensation cannot occur.

The **treatment** of hydrocephalus may be medical or surgical, depending on the etiology. After subarachnoid hemorrhage or meningitis, the flow or absorption of

---

**TABLE 184-11  Causes of Hydrocephalus**

| Pathogenic Mechanism | Etiologic Disorder/Condition |
|---|---|
| Obstruction of CSF pathways | Intraventricular foramina (Monro) obstruction |
| |    Parasellar mass (e.g., craniopharyngioma, germinoma, pituitary tumor) |
| |    Intraventricular tumor (e.g., ependymoma) |
| |    Tuberous sclerosis |
| | Aqueduct of Sylvius (cerebral aqueduct) obstruction |
| |    Aqueductal stenosis |
| |    Midbrain or pineal region tumor |
| |    Postinfectious or postinflammatory |
| |    Posthemorrhagic |
| | Impaired flow from the fourth ventricle foramina of Luschka and Magendie |
| |    Basilar impression |
| |    Platybasia |
| | Dandy-Walker malformation |
| | Arnold-Chiari malformation |
| | Congenital bone lesions of the cranial base |
| |    Achondroplasia, rickets |
| Overproduction of CSF | Choroid plexus papilloma |
| Defective reabsorption of CSF (e.g., extraventricular obstruction or communicating hydrocephalus) | Hypoplasia of the arachnoid villi |
| | Postinfectious or posthemorrhagic (destruction of arachnoid villi or subarachnoid fibrosis) |
| | Superior sagittal sinus occlusion (preventing absorption of CSF) |

CSF, cerebrospinal fluid.

CSF may be transiently impaired. In this circumstance, the use of agents, such as acetazolamide to decrease CSF production, may be beneficial. Surgical management consists of removing the obstructive lesion or placing a shunt or both. A shunt consists of polyethylene tubing extending usually from a lateral ventricle to the peritoneal cavity (**ventriculoperitoneal shunt**). Shunts carry the hazards of infection (*Staphylococcus epidermidis* or *Corynebacterium*) or sudden occlusion with signs and symptoms of acute hydrocephalus.

**Diffuse brain swelling** in an acutely ill child usually results from hypoxic-ischemic injury, trauma, infection, metabolic derangement, or toxic ingestion. Hypoxic-ischemic injury produces cytotoxic edema, which consists of swelling of neurons, glia, and endothelial cells because of damage to the cellular metabolic machinery.

**Bacterial meningitis** may produce increased ICP by blockage of CSF pathways, toxic cerebral edema, increase in cerebral blood flow, or multifocal cerebral infarctions (see Chapter 100). Most children with bacterial meningitis can undergo LP safely because the brain swelling is diffuse and distributed evenly throughout the brain and spinal CSF compartments. A few patients with meningitis show transtentorial herniation, however, within a few hours of LP. Focal neurologic signs, poorly reactive pupils, and a tense fontanelle are contraindications to LP in an infant or child with suspected bacterial meningitis. Bacterial meningitis is a common *benign* cause of increased ICP, but herniation does *not* occur. Patients do not appear critically ill. They exhibit a daily debilitating headache associated with diplopia, abducens palsy, and papilledema. Brain imaging studies are usually normal. This syndrome has been associated with the ingestion of certain drugs (tetracycline). Level of consciousness should be assessed frequently within the first 12 hours after LP. If the pupils dilate, or other evidence of increased ICP becomes evident, immediate treatment must be undertaken and may be lifesaving.

**Idiopathic intracranial hypertension (pseudotumor cerebri)** is a *benign* cause of increased ICP, usually with normal brain imaging. Patients exhibit a daily debilitating headache associated with diplopia, abducens palsy, and papilledema. The syndrome has been associated with ingestion of drugs (tetracycline vitamin A, oral contraceptive agents), endocrine disturbances (thyroid disease, Addison disease), chronic sinopulmonary diseases, and intracranial venous sinus thrombosis. Most commonly, this condition is idiopathic and affects children who are otherwise well except for being overweight. The diagnosis rests upon direct measurement of ICP with a monometer during lumbar puncture. After the diagnosis is established after appropriate neuroimaging and documentation of an elevated opening pressure with LP, idiopathic intracranial hypertension gradually resolves over several weeks or months. **Treatment** options, including serial LPs, acetazolamide or other diuretic, or a short course of corticosteroids, are generally effective. Infrequently, chronic papilledema from persistent pseudotumor cerebri produces visual impairment, and more aggressive management is required (optic nerve fenestration) to preserve visual function.

## Clinical Manifestations

The symptoms and signs of increased ICP include headache, vomiting, lethargy, irritability, sixth nerve palsy, strabismus, diplopia, and papilledema. Infants who have an open fontanelle usually do not develop papilledema or abducens palsy. Specific signs of increased ICP in infants consist of a bulging fontanelle, suture diastasis, distended scalp veins, a persistent downward deviation of the eyes (*sunsetting*), and rapid growth of head circumference. Specific signs of increased ICP in the infratentorial compartment (posterior fossa) include stiff neck and head tilt.

Focal neurologic deficits reflect the site of the lesion that is producing the increased ICP and may include hemiparesis from supratentorial lesions and ataxia from infratentorial lesions. The major specific sign of critically increased ICP is dilation and poor reactivity of one or both pupils. The **Cushing triad** of elevated blood pressure, decreased pulse, and irregular respirations is a late sign of critically elevated ICP.

## Laboratory and Diagnostic Studies

The cause of increased ICP is determined by brain imaging with either CT or MRI. CT is rapid, readily available, and provides clear visualization of an acute hemorrhage. Mass lesions, hydrocephalus, and trauma are easily recognized. Diffuse brain swelling produced by hypoxic-ischemic injury, meningitis, encephalitis, metabolic abnormalities, or toxins may be more difficult to recognize.

## Treatment

The treatment of acute increased ICP should be carried out in an intensive care setting with vigilant attention to vital signs and continuous monitoring. The patient's response to specific interventions must be carefully assessed. Immediate endotracheal intubation and hyperventilation produces the most rapid reduction in ICP by cerebral vasoconstriction, leading to decreased cerebral blood volume. Mannitol (0.25–1 g/kg) or 3% saline may be used acutely to produce an osmotic shift of fluid from the brain to the plasma. A ventricular catheter is used to remove CSF and to monitor the ICP continuously. Pentobarbital-induced coma reduces pressure by severely suppressing cerebral metabolism and cerebral blood flow. Acetazolamide and furosemide may transiently decrease CSF production. Acute interventions, such as hyperventilation, osmotic therapies, and barbiturates, can have negative impacts on systemic and cerebral perfusion, so must be used judiciously.

All treatments for increased ICP are temporary measures intended to prevent herniation until the underlying disease process either is treated or resolves spontaneously. Timely intervention can reverse cerebral herniation. A complete neurologic recovery is possible even after clear signs of transtentorial or foramen magnum herniation have begun. When these signs are completed, however, with bilaterally dilated, unreactive pupils, absent eye movements, and flaccid quadriplegia, recovery is no longer possible.

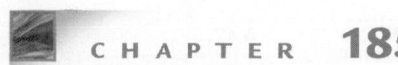

CHAPTER **185**

# Neurodegenerative Disorders (Childhood Dementia)

Children typically acquire developmental milestones in a variable but predictable sequence (see Chapter 7). Rarely, children present with stagnation of development or frank loss of previously acquired skills. These entities are referred to as neurodegenerative disorders.

Primary degenerative diseases of the nervous system are usually hereditary or metabolic processes. Their onset is often insidious with gradual progression over weeks, months, or years. Typically, they are symmetrical in their manifestations. Symptoms may target either gray matter structures or white matter tracts.

## ACQUIRED ILLNESSES MIMICKING DEGENERATIVE DISEASES

Children with poorly controlled epilepsy may be continuously in either an ictal or a postictal state. They may appear stuporous. The antiepileptic regimen may be contributing to the lack or loss of developmental abilities. Antiepileptic drugs that are sedating or affect mood, memory, motivation, or attention may contribute to school failure. Use of high doses or multiple anticonvulsants may compound this problem. Readjustment of medications or achievement of better control returns the child to his or her previous level of functioning.

Other chronic drug use or overuse (sedatives, tranquilizers, anticholinergics) can bring about progressive mental confusion, lethargy, and ataxia (see Chapter 45). Intoxications with metals, such as lead, may cause chronic learning difficulties or may present acutely with irritability, listlessness, anorexia, and pallor, progressing to fulminant encephalopathy. Vitamin deficiency of thiamine, niacin, vitamin $B_{12}$, and vitamin E can produce encephalopathy, peripheral neuropathy, and ataxia. Congenital and acquired hypothyroidism impairs intelligence and retards developmental progress. Unrecognized congenital hypothyroidism produces irreversible damage if it is not treated immediately after birth (see Chapter 175).

Structural brain diseases, such as hydrocephalus and slowly growing tumors, may mimic dementia. Certain indolent brain infections, such as rubeola (measles causing subacute sclerosing panencephalitis), rubella (German measles), syphilis, prion disease, and some fungi, cause mental and neurologic deterioration over months and years. Congenital human immunodeficiency virus (HIV) infection causes failure of normal development and regression of acquired skills.

Emotional disorders, such as depression and severe psychosocial deprivation in infancy, can give rise to apathy and failure to attain developmental milestones (see Chapter 21). Children with autism spectrum disorder may go through a phase of developmental stagnation or disintegration at about 12 to 18 months of age after a period of early normal milestones. Depression in older children can lead to blunting of affect, social withdrawal, and poor school performance, which raise the question of encephalopathy and dementia.

## HEREDITARY AND METABOLIC DEGENERATIVE DISEASES

Degenerative diseases may affect gray matter (**neuronal degenerative disorders**), white matter (**leukodystrophies**), or specific, focal regions of the brain. Many white and gray matter degenerative illnesses result from enzymatic disorders within subcellular organelles, including lysosomes, mitochondria, and peroxisomes. Disorders of lysosomal enzymes typically impair metabolism of brain sphingolipids and gangliosides. These enzyme deficiencies have classic patterns of expression (Niemann-Pick disease, Gaucher disease, Tay-Sachs disease). The same enzymatic deficiency may produce unusual clinical syndromes that differ greatly from the classic patterns. The age at onset, rate of progression, and neurologic signs may vary. For this reason, any patient with a degenerative neurologic condition of unknown cause should have leukocytes or skin fibroblasts harvested for measurement of a standard battery of lysosomal, peroxisomal, and mitochondrial enzymes (see Chapters 56 and 57).

**Gray matter degeneration (neuronal degeneration)** is characterized early by **dementia** and **seizures**. This group of gray matter disorders, which cause slowly progressive loss of neuronal function, is separated into disorders with and disorders without accompanying hepatosplenomegaly. Most are autosomal recessive traits except for Hunter syndrome (sex-linked recessive), Rett syndrome (sex-linked dominant), and the mitochondrial encephalopathies (nuclear or mitochondrial DNA defects).

### Gray Matter Degenerative Diseases with Visceromegaly

**Mucopolysaccharidoses** are caused by defective lysosomal hydrolases resulting in the accumulation of mucopolysaccharides within lysosomes. Abnormally large amounts are excreted in the urine. The clinical manifestations include dwarfism, kyphoscoliosis, coarse facies, hepatosplenomegaly, cardiovascular abnormalities, and corneal clouding. Neurologic involvement is seen in mucopolysaccharidosis types I H (**Hurler syndrome**), II (**Hunter syndrome**), III (**Sanfilippo syndrome**), and VII. Children with Hurler syndrome, the most severe of these illnesses, appear normal during the first 6 months of life, then develop the characteristic skeletal and neurologic features. Mental deficiency, spasticity, deafness, and optic atrophy are progressive. Hydrocephalus frequently occurs because of obstruction to CSF flow by thickened leptomeninges.

**Mucolipidosis II** (I-cell disease), **mucolipidosis III**, **GM$_1$ gangliosidosis**, **fucosidosis**, and **mannosidosis** resemble Hurler syndrome clinically but do not exhibit excess excretion of mucopolysaccharides and involve different disorders in lysosomal hydrolases. The diagnosis is confirmed by analysis of enzymes in white blood cells, serum, and skin fibroblasts.

Classic **Niemann-Pick disease** is caused by a deficiency of the enzyme sphingomyelinase. Sphingomyelin accumulates in foam cells of the reticuloendothelial system of the liver, spleen, lungs, and bone marrow. It also distends neurons of the brain. Intellectual retardation and regression, myoclonic seizures, hypotonia, hepatosplenomegaly, jaundice, and sometimes retinal cherry-red spots are noted within the first year of life. The diagnosis is confirmed by finding foam cells in the bone marrow and sphingomyelinase deficiency in leukocytes and skin fibroblasts.

Although the most common form of **Gaucher disease** is an indolent illness of adults, there is a rapidly fatal infantile form featuring severe neurologic involvement caused by deficiency of the enzyme glucocerebrosidase. Glucoceramide accumulates in the liver, spleen, and bone marrow. The characteristic neurologic signs are neck retraction, extraocular palsies, trismus, difficulty swallowing, apathy, and spasticity. Gaucher cells are found in bone marrow, and the level of serum acid phosphatase is increased.

locus), the late infantile form (NCL2) is pepstatin-resistant proteinase deficiency (gene at the 11p15.5 locus), and the original juvenile form (NCL3) is a defect in a gene (locus 16p11.2-12.3) whose product, the NCL3 protein, still lacks functional characterization. The clinical features are dementia, retinal degeneration, and severe myoclonic epilepsy. Visceral symptoms, despite the presence of the storage process, are absent. The disease may present at any age.

**Mitochondrial diseases** represent a clinically heterogeneous group of disorders that fundamentally share a disturbance in oxidative phosphorylation (adenosine triphosphate [ATP] synthesis) (see Chapter 57). Abrupt symptoms are often manifest concurrent with periods of physiologic stress such as febrile illness or fasting. Specific genetic diagnoses are often difficult to identify because clinical features are pleotropic within individual defects, overlap between different defects, and because analysis of mitochondrial protein function is technically demanding. Specific syndromes include **MELAS** (*m*itochondrial myopathy, *e*ncephalopathy, *l*actic *a*cidosis, and *s*troke-like episodes); **MERRF** (*m*yoclonus, *e*pilepsy, and *r*agged *r*ed *f*ibers), which includes dementia, hearing loss, optic nerve atrophy, ataxia, and loss of deep sensation; and **NARP** (*n*europathy, *a*taxia, and *r*etinitis *p*igmentosa).

## Gray Matter Degenerative Disease without Visceromegaly

**Tay-Sachs disease** (GM$_2$ gangliosidosis) is caused by deficiency of hexosaminidase A and results in the accumulation of GM$_2$ ganglioside in cerebral gray matter and cerebellum. Infants are normal until 6 months of age, when they develop listlessness, irritability, hyperacusis, intellectual retardation, and a retinal cherry-red spot. The ganglion cells of the retina and macula are distended with ganglioside and appear as a large area of white surrounding a small red fovea that is not covered by ganglion cells. Within months, blindness, convulsions, spasticity, and opisthotonos develop.

**Rett syndrome** is a common neurodevelopmental disorder affecting only females with onset at about 1 year of age. It is characterized by the loss of purposeful hand movements and communication skills; social withdrawal; gait apraxia; stereotypic repetitive hand movements that resemble washing, wringing, or clapping of the hands; and acquired microcephaly. The illness plateaus for many years before seizures, spasticity, and kyphoscoliosis develop. The etiology is a mutation on an X chromosome gene coding for a transcription factor called *methyl-CpG-binding protein 2*. The exact phenotype is influenced by whether the mutation is missense or truncating and on the pattern of X chromosome inactivation in the individual patient.

**Neuronal ceroid lipofuscinosis** is a family of genetic diseases characterized histologically by the accumulation of autofluorescent hydrophobic proteins and esterified dolichol lipopigments in lysosomes. The original infantile form of neuronal ceroid lipofuscinosis (NCL1) is palmitoyl protein thioesterase deficiency (gene at the 1p32

## Degenerative Diseases of the White Matter (Leukodystrophies)

The prominent signs of diseases affecting primarily white matter are spasticity, ataxia, optic atrophy, and peripheral neuropathy. Seizures and dementia are late manifestations. Life expectancy ranges from months to a few years.

**Metachromatic leukodystrophy** is an autosomal recessive lipidosis caused by deficiency of arylsulfatase. Demyelination of the CNS and peripheral nervous system occurs. Children present between 1 and 2 years of age with stiffening and ataxia of gait, spasticity, optic atrophy, intellectual deterioration, absent reflexes, up-going toes, increased CSF protein, and slowing of motor nerve conduction velocity.

**Krabbe disease** (globoid cell leukodystrophy) is an autosomal recessive lipidosis caused by a deficiency of galactocerebrosidase. It begins at 6 months of age and includes extreme irritability, macrocephaly, hyperacusis, and seizures. Demyelination of the CNS and peripheral nervous system results in upper and lower motor neuron signs.

**Adrenoleukodystrophy** is a sex-linked, recessively inherited disorder associated with progressive central demyelination and adrenal cortical insufficiency (see Chapter 178). It is caused by an impaired capacity of a subcellular organelle, the peroxisome, to degrade saturated unbranched very long chain fatty acids, particularly hexacosanoate (C26:0). The most common presentation occurs in boys in early school years who develop subtle behavioral changes and intellectual deterioration, followed by cortical visual and auditory deficits and a stiff gait. Later, spastic quadriparesis, coma, and seizures supervene. Symptomatic adrenocortical insufficiency with fatigue, vomiting, and hypotension develops in 20% to 40% of patients, usually at the same time as the neurologic illness. The disease can present with slowly progressive paraplegia in young men, which is called adrenomyeloleukodystrophy. The diagnosis is established by finding an elevated hexacosanoate level in plasma lipids and typical abnormalities of neuroimaging.

## Degenerative Diseases with Focal Manifestations

Some neurodegenerative disorders have predilections to target specific regions or systems within the neuraxis, producing symptoms referable to the affected region. Ataxia indicates disease of the cerebellum or spinocerebellar pathways. Abnormalities of extraocular movement or respiration indicate disease of the brainstem. Choreoathetosis or dystonia indicates disease of the motor basal ganglia. Paraplegia indicates disease of the spinal cord. Hereditary degenerative diseases can cause ataxia (see Table 183-1).

### Cerebellar Pathways

**Friedreich ataxia** is a relentlessly progressive, autosomal recessive disorder that manifests in the early teenage years with ataxia, dysmetria, dysarthria, pes cavus, hammer toes, diminished proprioception and vibration, diminished or absent reflexes, up-going toes, kyphoscoliosis, nystagmus, and a hypertrophic cardiomyopathy. It is caused by a homozygous GAA expansion of 120 to 1700 trinucleotide repeats of the first intron of the frataxin gene on chromosome 9. The GAA repeats are unstable on transmission. The size of the GAA expansion determines the frequency of cardiomyopathy and loss of reflexes in the upper limbs.

**Ataxia-telangiectasia** is an autosomal recessive genetic disorder of DNA repair that produces a neurologic disorder, immunologic deficiency, lymphoid malignancy, and gonadal dysgenesis (see Chapter 73). The basic pathologic defect is an inability to respond properly to homologous double-stranded DNA breaks by either DNA repair or induction of apoptosis due to a lack of the ATM protein (a DNA-binding protein kinase related to kinases involved in cell cycle progression and response to DNA damage). The ATM gene is a large gene on 11q22-23. Most mutations of the gene are unique and nonsense. Most patients are compound heterozygotes. In 80% of cases, a genetic diagnosis can be made by failure to detect the ATM protein on Western blot.

The neurologic symptoms manifest between 1 and 2 years of age with progressive ataxia, dystonia, chorea, swallowing difficulty, poor facial movements, and severe abnormalities of saccadic and pursuit eye movements. Most characteristically, patients develop oculomotor apraxia, a disorder in which the child visually tracks by making head movements to compensate for the inability to generate saccadic eye movements. Intellect is preserved. Patients are wheelchair bound in childhood. The external hallmark of the disease, **conjunctival telangiectasia**, does not manifest until about 5 years of age. Telangiectases also develop on the ear, malar face, neck, elbows, knees, hands, and feet. In addition, prematurely gray hair and

atrophic skin develop in patients. Recurrent sinopulmonary infections are a problem in some patients from infancy. Thirty percent of patients die of lymphoreticular cancers. Laboratory clues to the diagnosis include elevation of blood alpha-fetoprotein levels and depression of blood IgA and circulating T-cell levels. Patients with IgA deficiency are at risk of anaphylaxis after blood transfusion that includes IgA. There is presently no therapy for the disease or its symptoms.

**Lesch-Nyhan syndrome** is a sex-linked recessive disorder caused by deficiency of hypoxanthine-guanine phosphoribosyltransferase, leading to the formation of excess uric acid. Infants appear normal until late in the first year of life, when they exhibit psychomotor retardation, choreoathetosis, spasticity, and severe self-mutilation. These patients never achieve ambulation. Gouty arthritis and renal calculi with renal failure occur. Hyperuricemia and renal complications are treated with allopurinol, a xanthine oxidase inhibitor, but no effective treatment for the neurologic disease is available.

**Wilson disease** is a treatable, degenerative condition that exhibits signs of cerebellar and basal ganglia dysfunction. It is an autosomal recessive inborn error of copper metabolism. Serum ceruloplasmin levels are low. Abnormal copper deposition is found in the liver, producing cirrhosis; in the peripheral cornea, producing a characteristic green-brown (Kayser-Fleischer) ring; and in the CNS, producing neuronal degeneration and protoplasmic astrocytosis. Neurologic symptoms characteristically begin in the early teenage years with dysarthria, dysphasia, drooling, fixed smile, tremor, dystonia, and emotional lability. MRI shows abnormalities of the basal ganglia. Treatment is with a copper-chelating agent, such as oral penicillamine.

### Brainstem

**Subacute necrotizing encephalomyelopathy**, or Leigh disease, is a neuropathologically defined, degenerative inherited CNS disease primarily involving the periaqueductal region of the brainstem, caudate, and putamen. Symptoms usually begin before 2 years of age and consist of hypotonia, feeding difficulties, respiratory irregularity, weakness of extraocular movements, and ataxia. Blood and CSF lactate and pyruvate levels are elevated. Different disorders of mitochondrial function can produce this clinical syndrome. Decreased pyruvate carboxylase or pyruvate dehydrogenase activity, biotinidase deficiency, and cytochrome *c* oxidase deficiency have been identified as causative in some cases. Vitamin therapies have been attempted but with little success except in children with biotinidase deficiency. Many degenerative encephalopathies defy diagnosis despite extensive laboratory analysis. The diagnosis of leukodystrophy usually can be made confidently on the basis of extensive cerebral white matter changes on CT or MRI. The diagnosis of hereditary or metabolic gray matter encephalopathy, when histologic and biochemical studies are normal, is much less secure. Acquired lesions (infectious, inflammatory, vascular, or toxic) are difficult to exclude completely. Brain biopsy is not likely to be helpful, unless specific lesions are shown on neuroimaging.

## CHAPTER 186

# Neurocutaneous Disorders

The skin, teeth, hair, nails, and brain are derived embryologically from ectoderm. Abnormalities of these surface structures may indicate abnormal brain development. The term **phakomatosis** means *mother spots* or *birthmarks* and refers to tuberous sclerosis and neurofibromatosis. Not all of the so-called neurocutaneous disorders have characteristic cutaneous lesions, however, and not all are of ectodermal origin. Neurofibromatosis, tuberous sclerosis, Sturge-Weber disease, von Hippel–Lindau disease, and ataxia-telangiectasia are the most common of the more than 40 neurocutaneous disorders.

## NEUROFIBROMATOSIS

### Etiology

There are two distinct genetic types of neurofibromatosis. **Neurofibromatosis type 1 (NF1)**, also known as von Recklinghausen disease, is an autosomal-dominant disorder with an incidence of approximately 1 in 3000. It is caused by mutations of the *NF1* gene, located at chromosome 17q11.2 and coding for a tumor suppressor gene, neurofibromin. Spontaneous new mutations occur in 30% to 50% of cases. Neurofibromin is a major negative regulator of a key signal transduction pathway in cells, the Ras pathway, which transmits mitogenic signals to the nucleus. Loss of neurofibromin leads to increased levels of activated Ras (bound to guanosine triphosphate [GTP]) and increased downstream mitogenic signaling. Somatic mosaicism, in which an abnormality in one copy of the *NF1* gene is present in some cells but not others, indicates a postzygotic mutation, and is called **segmental neurofibromatosis**. NF2 is an autosomal-dominant disorder with an incidence of 1 in 33,000. Half the cases have no family history. The *NF2* gene is a tumor suppressor gene on chromosome 22 that codes for a protein called *merlin*. Merlin is similar to a family of proteins that serve as links between integral membrane proteins and the cytoskeleton and are involved in Rho-mediated signal transduction.

### Clinical Manifestations

The cardinal features of neurofibromatosis are café au lait spots, axillary freckling, cutaneous neurofibromas, and iris hamartomas (Lisch nodules). **Café au lait spots** are present in more than 90% of patients who have NF1 (Fig. 186-1). They typically appear in the first few years of life and increase in number and size over time. The presence of six or more spots larger than 5 mm suggests the diagnosis. **Lisch nodules** also increase in frequency with age and are present in more than 90% of adults who have NF1. Approximately 25% of children exhibit these iris nodules.

**Neurofibromas** are composed of various combinations of Schwann cells, fibroblasts, mast cells, and vascular

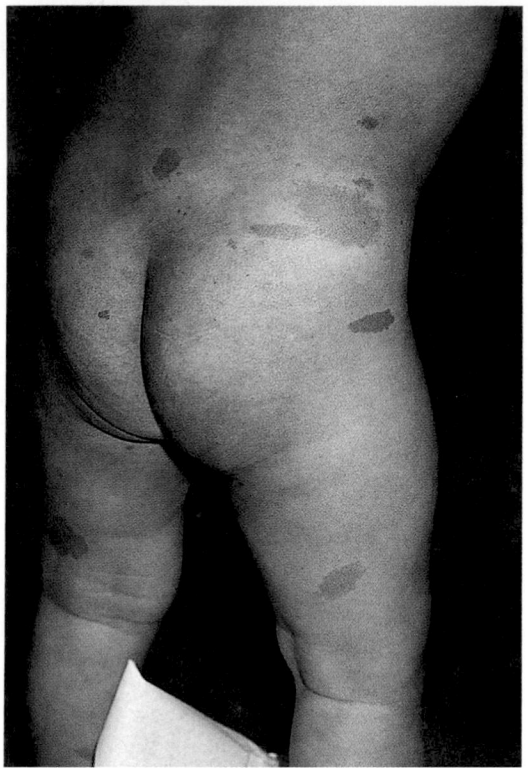

**FIGURE 186-1**

Café au lait macules. (From Kliegman RE, Behrman RE, Jenson HB [eds]: Nelson Textbook of Pediatrics, 18th ed. Philadelphia, *WB Saunders*, 2007 p 2680.)

elements. Dermal neurofibromas are nearly universal and consist of discrete, small, soft lesions that lie within the dermis and epidermis and move passively with the skin. They rarely cause any symptoms. Plexiform neurofibromas are large, occasionally nodular, subcutaneous lesions that lie along the major peripheral nerve trunks. They often cause symptoms including pain, weakness, and invasion of adjacent viscera or spinal cord. Sarcomatous degeneration may occur. Surgical treatment is attempted, but results are often unsatisfactory. Other tumors that occur in NF1 are optic nerve gliomas, astrocytomas of brain and spinal cord, and malignant peripheral nerve tumors.

NF2 predisposes patients to multiple intracranial and spinal tumors, including bilateral acoustic schwannomas, schwannomas of other cranial and spinal nerves, meningiomas, and gliomas. Peripheral nerve tumors, including schwannomas and neurofibromas, are uncommon. The average life span is less than 40 years. Posterior capsular or cortical cataracts are common, but Lisch nodules, café au lait spots, and axillary freckling are not features of the disease.

Common complications are learning disability, scoliosis, macrocephaly, headache, and optic gliomas. Other skeletal complications include sphenoid wing dysplasia and cortical thinning of the long bones with pseudarthrosis. Systemic complications, including peripheral nerve malignancy, pheochromocytoma, renovascular hypertension, and epilepsy, are individually rare. Hyperintense lesions on T2-weighted magnetic resonance images (hamartomas) in the basal ganglia, internal capsule, thalamus, cerebellum, and brainstem are common and distinctive for the disease. They are benign and disappear in adulthood. The average life expectancy of patients with NF1 may be reduced by 10 to 15 years, and malignancy is the most common cause of death. Genetic and psychological counseling are important components of care for this chronic disorder.

## TUBEROUS SCLEROSIS

### Etiology

Tuberous sclerosis, an autosomal dominant disorder, is characterized by hamartomas in many organs, especially the brain, eyes, skin, kidneys, and heart. The incidence is 1 in 10,000 births. Two thirds of cases are sporadic and thought to represent new mutations. Germline mosaicism is uncommon, but explains how parents who apparently do not have the disease can have multiple children with tuberous sclerosis. Mutations, affecting either of the presumed tumor suppressor genes *TSC1* (chromosome 9) or *TSC2* (chromosome 16), cause tuberous sclerosis. The *TSC1* and *TSC2* genes encode distinct proteins, hamartin and tuberin, which are widely expressed in the brain. These proteins may interact as part of a cascade pathway that modulates cellular differentiation, tumor suppression, and intracellular signaling. Tuberin has a GTPase-activating, protein-related domain that may contribute to a role in cell cycle passage and intracellular vesicular trafficking. Somatic loss or intragenic mutation of the corresponding wild-type allele is seen in the associated hamartomas. Among sporadic tuberous sclerosis cases, mutations in *TSC2* are more frequent and often accompanied by more severe neurologic deficits.

### Clinical Manifestations

The classic clinical features are facial angiofibromas (**adenoma sebaceum**), mental retardation, and epilepsy. Less than 50% of patients with tuberous sclerosis exhibit all three features. Other major signs are ungual fibromas, retinal hamartomas, hypopigmented macules, shagreen patches, renal angiomyolipoma, cardiac rhabdomyoma, brain tubers, and brain subependymal nodules and astrocytomas. Facial angiofibromas do not develop until 2 to 5 years of age, but hypomelanotic macules, called **ash-leaf spots**, are present in infancy and best detected with a Wood lamp under ultraviolet light. **Shagreen patches** are elevated, rough plaques of skin with a predilection for the lumbar and gluteal regions that develop in late childhood or early adolescence. Cardiac rhabdomyomas are largest during prenatal life and infancy and are rarely symptomatic. Occasionally, they may cause arrhythmias or cardiac outflow obstruction. Renal angiomyolipomas may undergo malignant transformation and are the most common cause of death in adults with tuberous sclerosis.

Tubers in the cerebral cortex are areas of cerebral dysplasia that, in combination with other microscopic areas of abnormal development, are responsible for the symptoms of mental retardation and epilepsy. Subependymal nodules are hamartomas that may mutate into a growth phase and become subependymal giant cell astrocytomas causing obstruction of cerebrospinal fluid (CSF) outflow and hydrocephalus. These brain lesions can be detected directly by magnetic resonance imaging (MRI). Computed tomography (CT) shows periventricular calcifications within the nodule, especially around the foramen of Monro. Specific DNA probes for *TSC1* and *TSC2* are available.

Tuberous sclerosis is one of the most common causes of infantile spasms. These children often develop intractable epilepsy, with myoclonic, atonic, partial, and grand mal seizures; mental retardation; autism; and hyperactivity.

## STURGE-WEBER SYNDROME

The Sturge-Weber syndrome is characterized by angiomas of the leptomeninges overlying the cerebral cortex in association with an ipsilateral facial port-wine nevus that, at the least, covers part of the forehead and upper eyelid. The nevus may have a much more extensive and even bilateral distribution. This nevus flammeus is an ectasia of superficial venules, not a hemangioma, because it has no endothelial proliferation. Ocular defects of Sturge-Weber syndrome include glaucoma and hemangiomas of the choroid, conjunctiva, and episclera. Glaucoma is present in 30% to 50% of patients and may be progressive. Sturge-Weber syndrome is sporadic and not genetic.

The most common associated neurologic abnormality is seizures. Seizures develop because of ischemic injury to the brain underlying the meningeal angiomas. Angiomas, most commonly located in the posterior parietal, posterior temporal, and anterior occipital lobes, consist of thin-walled veins within the pia mater. They produce venous engorgement and presumably stasis within the involved areas. Positron emission tomography has shown hypoperfusion and hypometabolism in these areas. In some children with Sturge-Weber syndrome, progressive ischemia of the underlying brain develops, resulting in hemiparesis, hemianopia, intractable focal seizures, and dementia. Calcium is detectable in the gyri of the brain underlying the angioma, and, as the intervening sulci are spared, the radiologic picture of *tram track* or *railroad track* calcifications is seen in about 60% of cases. Many children with Sturge-Weber syndrome are intellectually normal, and seizures are well controlled with standard anticonvulsants. Hemispherectomy has been proposed for infants whose seizures begin early in life and are difficult to control. Intellectual and motor outcome seems improved, but the surgical risks of the procedure are considerable. Laser surgery is the most promising therapeutic option for cosmetic management of the facial nevus flammeus. Expert ophthalmologic management of glaucoma and choroidal hemangiomas is required.

# Congenital Malformations of the Central Nervous System

The precursor of the nervous system is the neural plate of the embryonic ectoderm, which develops at 18 days of gestation. The neural plate gives rise to the neural tube, which forms the brain and spinal cord, and the neural crest cells, which form the peripheral nervous system, meninges, melanocytes, and adrenal medulla. The neural tube begins to form on day 22 of gestation. The rostral end forms the brain, and the caudal region forms the spinal cord. The lumen of the neural tube forms the ventricles of the brain and the central canal of the spinal cord. Most brain malformations can be produced by a variety of injuries occurring during a vulnerable period of gestation. Precipitating factors include chromosomal, genetic, and metabolic abnormalities; infections (toxoplasmosis, rubella, cytomegalovirus, herpes); and exposure to irradiation, certain drugs, and maternal illness during pregnancy.

## CONGENITAL ANOMALIES OF THE SPINAL CORD

### Etiology and Clinical Manifestations

Defective closure of the caudal neural tube at the end of week 4 of gestation results in anomalies of the lumbar and sacral vertebrae or spinal cord called **spina bifida**. These anomalies range in severity from clinically insignificant defects of the L5 or S1 vertebral arches to major malformations of the spinal cord that lies uncovered by skin or bone on the infant's back. The latter severe defect, called a **meningomyelocele**, results in total paralysis, loss of sensation in the legs and incontinence of bowel and bladder. In addition, affected children usually have an associated **Arnold-Chiari malformation** of the brainstem that may result in hydrocephalus and weakness of face and swallowing. In a **meningocele**, the spinal canal and cystic meninges are exposed on the back but the underlying spinal cord is anatomically and functionally intact. In **spina bifida occulta**, the skin of the back is apparently intact, but defects of the underlying bone or spinal canal are present. These defects include tethering of the cord to a thick filum terminale, a lipoma or dermoid cyst, or a tiny epithelial tract extending from the skin surface to the meninges. A small dimple or tuft of hair may be present over the affected vertebra. Patients with spina bifida occulta may have difficulties controlling bowel or bladder, weakness and numbness in the feet, and recurrent ulcerations in the areas of numbness. Bladder dysfunction may result in repeated episodes of urinary tract infections, reflux nephropathy, and renal insufficiency. An epithelial tract may predispose to recurrent episodes of meningitis.

### Diagnostic Studies

Meningomyelocele in the fetus is suggested by an elevated **alpha-fetoprotein** in the mother's blood and confirmed by ultrasound examination and high concentrations of alpha-fetoprotein and acetylcholinesterase in the amniotic fluid.

## TREATMENT AND PREVENTION

Neonates with meningomyelocele must undergo operative closure of the open spinal defects and treatment of hydrocephalus by placement of a ventriculoperitoneal shunt. Toddlers and children with lower spinal cord dysfunction require physical therapy and bracing of the lower extremities and intermittent bladder catheterization. Children with meningomyelocele who do not have associated brain anomalies are likely to have normal intelligence.

The spina bifida malformation can be prevented in many cases by **folate** administration to the pregnant mother. Because the defect occurs so early in gestation, all women of childbearing age are advised to take oral folic acid daily.

### Diastematomyelia

In diastematomyelia, a bone spicule or fibrous band divides the spinal cord into two longitudinal sections. An associated lipoma that infiltrates the cord and tethers it to the vertebrae may be present. Symptoms include weakness and numbness of the feet and urinary incontinence. Reflexes in the feet are diminished or absent. Surgical treatment to free the cord prevents further neurologic deterioration and may improve preexisting symptoms.

## CRANIAL DEFECTS

Defective closure of the rostral neural tube produces anencephaly or encephaloceles. Neonates with anencephaly have a rudimentary brainstem or midbrain, but no cortex or cranium. This is a rapidly fatal condition. Patients with encephalocele usually have a skull defect and exposure of meninges alone or meninges and brain. Occasionally the defect can produce protrusion of frontal lobe into the nose without a noticeable skull or skin defect. The recurrence risk in subsequent pregnancies for either cranial or spinal neural tube defects is 10%. Within a family, an anencephalic birth may be followed by the birth of a child affected with a lumbosacral meningomyelocele. The inheritance of neural tube defects is polygenic.

## CONGENITAL MALFORMATIONS OF THE BRAIN

### Macrocephaly and Microcephaly

Macrocephaly represents a head circumference above the 97th percentile and may be the result of **macrocrania** (increased skull thickness), **hydrocephalus** (enlargement of the ventricles), or **megalencephaly** (enlargement of the brain). Diseases of bone metabolism or hypertrophy of the bone marrow resulting from hemolytic anemia cause macrocrania. Megalencephaly may be the result of an embryologic disorder causing abnormal proliferation of brain tissue (neurofibromatosis, tuberous sclerosis, Sotos syndrome, Riley-Smith syndrome, and hemimegalencephaly) or accumulation of abnormal metabolic substances (Alexander disease, Canavan disease, Tay-Sachs disease, and mucopolysaccharidoses).

Microcephaly represents a head circumference below the 3rd percentile. Myriad syndromes and metabolic disorders are associated with microcephaly, some of which are hereditary (Table 187-1). In most instances, a small head circumference is a reflection of a small brain. Brain growth is rapid during the perinatal period, and any insult (infectious, metabolic, toxic, or vascular disorder) sustained during this period or early infancy is likely to impair brain growth and result in microcephaly. Rarely a small head is the result of premature closure of one or more skull sutures called **craniosynostosis**. This diagnosis is readily made by the abnormal shape of the skull. **Microcephaly vera** is an autosomal recessive disorder that produces severe hypoplasia of the frontal regions of the brain and skull. These children are severely mentally retarded. As a rule, macrocephaly and microcephaly raise a concern about cognitive ability, but head circumference alone should never be used to establish a prognosis for intellectual development.

**Holoprosencephaly** represents varying degrees of failure of the primary cerebral vesicle to divide and expand laterally and often is associated with midline facial defects (hypotelorism, cleft lip, and cleft palate). This anomaly may be isolated or associated with a chromosomal or genetic disorder. The prognosis for infants with severe holoprosencephaly is uniformly poor. Children with trisomy 13 characteristically have varying degrees of holoprosencephaly.

**Hydrocephalus** represents enlargement of the ventricular system. In all types of congenital hydrocephalus, the degree of ventricular enlargement correlates roughly with outcome, but examples of neonates treated for severe hydrocephalus who then have normal development are well known. Children with congenital hydrocephalus often have associated defects in the closure of the neural tube.

**Hydranencephaly** is a condition in which the brain presumably develops normally, but then is destroyed by an intrauterine, probably vascular, insult. The result is virtual absence of the cerebrum with an intact skull. The thalamus, brainstem, and some occipital cortex are present. The child may have a normal appearance but does not achieve developmental milestones.

Many malformations result from the failure of normal migration of neurons from the periventricular germinal matrix zone to the cortical surface at 1 to 5 months of gestation. Multiple malformations may exist in the same patient. Neurologic development with all of these anomalies, described subsequently, varies and depends on the type and extent of the malformations.

**Schizencephaly** is characterized by symmetrical bilateral clefts within the cerebral hemispheres that extend from the cortical surface to the ventricular cavity. Clinical manifestations include severe mental and motor retardation. Some children have unilateral schizencephaly manifested by hemiparesis and mild mental impairment.

| TABLE 187-1 Causes of Microcephaly |
|---|
| **PRIMARY MICROCEPHALY** |
| Microcephaly vera |
| Chromosomal disorders |
|   Trisomy 21 |
|   Trisomy 13 |
|   Trisomy 18 |
|   5p– |
|   Angelman syndrome |
|   Prader-Willi syndrome |
| Central nervous system (CNS) malformation |
|   Holoprosencephaly |
|   Encephalocele |
|   Hydranencephaly |
| CNS migrational disorder |
|   Lissencephaly |
|   Schizencephaly |
|   Pachygyria |
|   Micropolygyria |
|   Agenesis of the corpus callosum |
| Sex-linked microcephaly syndromes |
|   Smith-Lemli-Opitz syndrome |
|   Cornelia de Lange syndrome |
|   Seckel dwarfism syndrome |
|   Cockayne syndrome |
|   Rubinstein-Taybi syndrome |
|   Hallermann-Streiff syndrome |
| **SECONDARY (ACQUIRED) MICROCEPHALY** |
| Infections (congenital) |
|   Rubella |
|   Cytomegalovirus |
|   Toxoplasmosis |
|   Syphilis |
|   Human immunodeficiency virus (HIV) |
| Infections (noncongenital) |
|   Meningitis |
|   Encephalitis |
| Stroke |
| Toxic |
|   Radiation exposure—fetal |
|   Fetal alcohol syndrome |
|   Maternal phenylketonuria |
| Hypoxic-ischemic or other severe brain injury |
|   Periventricular leukomalacia |
| Systemic disease |
|   Chronic cardiac or pulmonary disease |
|   Chronic renal disease |
|   Malnutrition |
| Craniosynostosis totalis |

There are three major patterns of cortical migration defects. **Lissencephaly** indicates smooth brain with absence of sulcation. The normal six-layered cortex does not develop. Affected children have seizures and profound developmental retardation. This anomaly most commonly is part of a genetic or chromosomal disorder. In **pachygyria**, the gyri are few in number and too broad. In **polymicrogyria**, the gyri are too many and too small. Sometimes pachygyria and polymicrogyria affect an entire hemisphere, producing enlargement of that hemisphere and a clinical syndrome of severe, medically intractable seizures that begin in early infancy. Hemispherectomy is required to stop the seizures. Gray matter heterotopias are abnormal islands within the central white matter of neurons that have never completed the migratory process.

**Agenesis of the corpus callosum** may be partial or complete and may occur in an isolated fashion or in association with other anomalies of cellular migration. **Dandy-Walker malformation** is diagnosed on the basis of the classic triad: complete or partial agenesis of the vermis, cystic dilation of the fourth ventricle, and enlarged posterior fossa. There may be associated hydrocephalus, absence of the corpus callosum, and neuronal migration abnormalities. Intelligence may be normal or impaired, depending on the degree of associated cerebral neuronal defects.

**Megalencephaly**, or large brain, is diagnosed by finding a large head with radiographically normal-appearing intracranial contents. Most often this is a familial trait of no clinical significance. Sometimes it is associated with disorders of neuronal migration and a clinical syndrome of developmental retardation. Neurofibromatosis and Sotos syndrome (cerebral gigantism) are two genetic syndromes associated with megalencephaly and sometimes with mental retardation. Megalencephaly is also a feature of numerous metabolic diseases that produce a progressive, degenerative encephalopathy.

# PSYCHOMOTOR RETARDATION

## Mental Retardation

See Chapter 10.

## Chromosomal Disorders

Many chromosomal abnormalities, such as **trisomy 21**, are associated with mental retardation (see Chapter 49). The most common form of familial mental retardation, affecting 1 in 1250 males, is the **fragile X syndrome**. The syndrome is caused by expansion of a trinucleotide repeat, CGG, and abnormal methylation of a CpG island of the *FMR-1* gene at chromosome position Xq27.3. The features are varying degrees of mental retardation, autistic behavior, large ears, macro-orchidism, and an elongated, narrow face. Females may be affected, but usually not as severely as males.

Two other syndromes associated with mental retardation are caused by deletions of the same region of the long arm of chromosome 15. **Angelman syndrome** is caused by the loss of the maternal allele and is manifested by severe mental retardation, intractable seizures, tremulousness, a characteristic facies, and a happy external demeanor. **Prader-Willi syndrome** is caused by the loss of the paternal allele and is manifested by severe hypotonia and feeding difficulties in infancy, cryptorchidism, small hands and feet, mild mental retardation, and almond-shaped eyes. The difference in phenotype, depending on loss of the maternal or paternal allele, supports the genetic phenomenon of **imprinting**.

**SUGGESTED READING**

Avner JR: Altered states of consciousness, *Pediatr Rev* 27:331–338, 2006.

Filiano JF: Neurometabolic diseases in the newborn, *Clin Perinatol* 33:411–479, 2006.

Klein CJ: The inherited neuropathies, *Neurol Clin* 25:173–207, 2007.

Kliegman RM, Behrman RE, Jenson HB, et al: Nelson Textbook of Pediatrics, 18th ed, Philadelphia, 2007, *WB Saunders*.

Lewis DW: Pediatric migraine, *Pediatr Rev* 28:43–53, 2007.

Major P, Thiele EA: Seizures in children: Determining the variation, *Pediatr Rev* 28:363–371, 2007.

Walker WO, Johnson CP: Mental retardation: Overview and diagnosis, *Pediatr Rev* 27:204–212, 2006.

SECTION 25

# DERMATOLOGY

**Valerie B. Lyon**

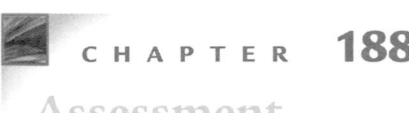

CHAPTER **188**

## Assessment

Approximately one of three Americans of any age has at least one recognizable skin disorder at any time. The most common cutaneous diseases encountered in community settings, in relative order of frequency, are dermatophytosis, acne vulgaris, seborrheic dermatitis, atopic dermatitis (eczema), verrucae (warts), tumors, psoriasis, vitiligo, and infections such as herpes simplex and impetigo. In children attending pediatric dermatology clinics, atopic dermatitis, impetigo, tinea capitis, acne vulgaris, verrucae vulgaris, and seborrheic dermatitis account for most diagnoses.

### HISTORY

The age of the patient, onset, duration, progression, associated cutaneous symptoms (pain, pruritus), and associated systemic signs or symptoms (fever, malaise, weight loss) are important clues. Obtaining an accurate description of the **original lesion** improves diagnostic accuracy. Over-the-counter remedies may alter the appearance of a rash dramatically. Patients often do not consider a topical antibiotic or anti-itch medication as *treatment*. Thus, it is important to probe deeply with related questions in the history. Other important information includes a history of allergies, environmental exposure, travel history, previous treatment, and family history.

### PHYSICAL EXAMINATION

A careful examination of the skin requires a visual and a tactile assessment. Examination of the skin over the entire body must be performed systematically. Mucous membranes, hair, nails, and teeth, all of ectodermal origin, also may be involved in cutaneous disorders and should be assessed.

### COMMON MANIFESTATIONS

A descriptive nomenclature of skin lesions helps with generating a differential diagnosis and also with communication between health care providers. Determination of the primary and secondary nature of the lesion is the cornerstone of dermatologic diagnosis. A **primary lesion** is defined as the basic lesion that arises de novo and is most characteristic of the disease process (Table 188-1 and Fig. 188-1). A primary lesion is unaltered by time or external factors such as medication applied, secondary infection, or physical manipulation (e.g., scratching). Frequently, only rare primary lesions exist on a patient at the time of presentation; most of the lesions are secondary. A search for the primary lesion often proves worthwhile and focuses the differential diagnosis to a category of lesion that is specific for the underlying diagnosis. On occasion, two different types of primary lesions may be present. In most cases, **secondary lesions** are the residue, or result, of the effects of the primary lesion, and may be created by scratching or secondary infection and may be seen in the absence of a primary lesion (Table 188-2).

The color, texture, configuration, location, and distribution of the lesion should be recorded. A localized or grouped eruption may suggest a cutaneous infection, whereas widespread, symmetrical involvement of extensor surfaces may suggest a primary skin disorder, such as psoriasis. Herpesvirus lesions are usually grouped lesions. Annular lesions may suggest Lyme disease, syphilis, and fungal infections. Lesions on mucous membranes are usually short-lived, and lesions in thick-skinned areas, such as the palms and soles, may be particularly difficult to characterize. Characteristic cutaneous signs of many systemic diseases are listed in Table 188-3.

### INITIAL DIAGNOSTIC EVALUATION AND SCREENING TESTS

A thorough history and physical examination are usually sufficient for diagnosis because of the visibility of the skin. Screening tests may be indicated based on the history and physical examination findings. It is usually unnecessary

## TABLE 188-1  Primary Skin Lesions

| Lesion | Description |
|---|---|
| Macule | Flat, well-circumscribed lesion <1 cm in diameter distinguished from surrounding skin by color only, with variable size and shape, which may be erythematous, pigmented, or purpuric |
| Patch | Similar to macule, but >1 cm in diameter |
| Papule | Elevated, circumscribed solid lesion <1 cm in diameter, which may be scaly or ulcerated or may become pustular |
| Plaque | Similar to papule, but >1 cm in diameter |
| Nodule | Large, palpable papule that extends 2 cm deep into the dermis or subcutaneous tissue |
| Tumor | Similar to nodule, but extends >2 cm into the dermis or subcutaneous tissue |
| Vesicle | Small, fluid-filled (usually clear or straw-colored) epidermal lesion <1 cm in diameter |
| Bulla | Similar to vesicle, but >1 cm in diameter, which may be flaccid or tense, reflecting depth within the skin |
| Purpura | Macule resulting from extravasated blood into the skin; does not blanch with pressure |
| Petechia | Small, red-to-purple circumscribed macule resulting from extravasated blood measuring a few millimeters in diameter |
| Ecchymosis | Larger, hemorrhagic patch or plaque resulting from extravasated blood |
| Palpable purpura | Papule resulting from extravasated blood; characteristic of leukocytoclastic vasculitis, which may occur in various conditions, including infection, collagen vascular disorders, serum sickness, and drug eruptions |
| Pustule | Papule that contains purulent exudate (pus), which may have an initial papular phase and often is surrounded by erythema |
| Wheal (hive) | Transient, rounded or flat-topped edematous plaque; varies greatly in size and may have an annular or gyrate configuration |
| Telangiectasia | Collection of small superficial red blood vessels |
| Milia | Superficial, white, small epidermal keratin cysts |
| Comedo | Plug of keratin and sebum within the orifice of a hair follicle, which can be open (whitehead) or closed (blackhead) and is the characteristic lesion of acne vulgaris |
| Cyst | Papule or nodule with an epidermal lining composed of fluid or solid material |

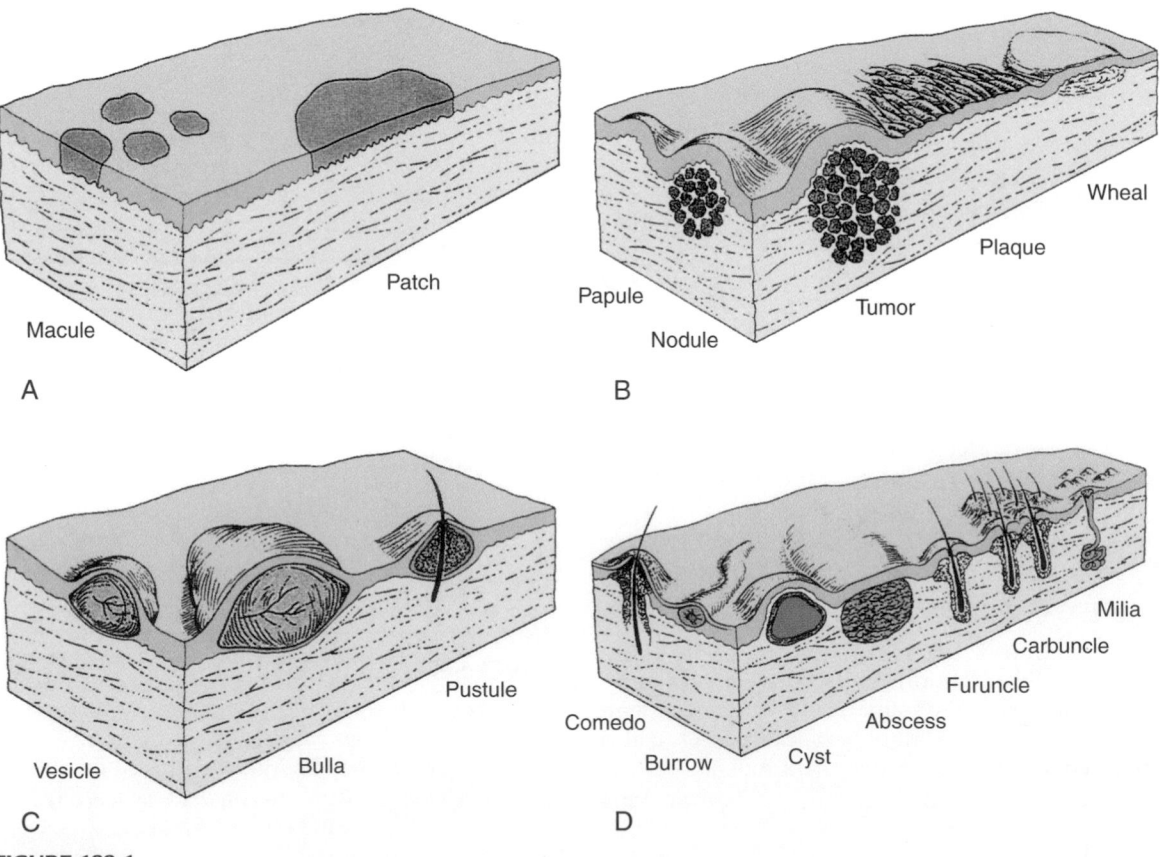

**FIGURE 188-1**

**Morphology of primary skin lesions. A**, Macules are flat and nonpalpable. **B**, Papules are palpable, elevated, and solid. **C**, Vesicles are palpable, elevated, and fluid-filled. **D**, Special primary lesions. (From Swartz MH: Textbook of Physical Diagnosis: History and Examination. Philadelphia, *WB Saunders*, 1989.)

**TABLE 188-2 Secondary Skin Lesions**

| Lesion | Description |
|---|---|
| Scale | Results from abnormal keratinization; may be fine or sheetlike |
| Crust | Dried collection of serum and cellular debris |
| Erosion | Moist, shallow epidermal depression with loss of the superficial epidermis |
| Ulcer | Circumscribed, depressed, focal loss of entire epidermis into dermis; heals with scarring |
| Atrophy | Shallow depression that results from thinning of epidermis or dermis |
| Scar | Thickened, firm, and discolored collection of connective tissue that results from dermal damage; initially pink, but lightens with time |
| Sclerosis | Circumscribed or diffuse hardening of skin; usually forms in a plaque |
| Lichenification | Accentuated skin lines/markings that result from thickening of the epidermis |
| Excoriation | Superficial linear erosion that is caused by scratching |
| Fissure | Linear break within the skin surface that usually is painful |

**TABLE 188-3 Characteristics of Cutaneous Signs of Systemic Diseases**

| Disease | Age at Onset | Skin Lesions | Distribution |
|---|---|---|---|
| Systemic lupus erythematosus | Any | Erythematous patches; palpable purpura; livedo reticularis; Raynaud phenomenon; thrombocytopenic and nonthrombocytopenic purpura | Photodistribution; malar |
| Discoid lupus | Adolescents | Annular, scaly plaques; atrophy; dyspigmentation | Photodistribution |
| Neonatal lupus erythematosus | Newborn to 6 months | Annular, erythematous, scaly plaques | Photodistribution; head/neck |
| Juvenile dermatomyositis | Any | Erythematous-to-violaceous, scaly macules; discrete papules overlying knuckles | Periocular, face; shoulder girdle; extensor extremities; knuckles; palms |
| Henoch-Schönlein purpura | Children and adolescents | Purpuric papules and plaques | Buttocks; lower extremities |
| Kawasaki disease | Infants, children | Erythematous, maculopapular-to-urticarial plaques; acral and groin erythema, edema, and desquamation | Diffuse |
| Inflammatory bowel disease | Children and adolescents | Aphthae; erythema nodosum; pyoderma gangrenosum; thrombophlebitis | Oral ulcers; perianal fissures |
| Sweet syndrome | Any | Infiltrated erythematous, edematous plaques | Diffuse |
| Graft-versus-host disease | Any | Acute: erythema; papules; vesicles; bullae | Head and neck; palms/soles; diffuse |
| Hypersensitivity | Any | Erythema; urticarial macules and plaques | Diffuse reaction |
| Serum sickness–like reaction | Any | Edematous, purpuric plaques | Acral; diffuse |

to perform laboratory or imaging studies. Initial tests that may be indicated include potassium hydroxide (KOH) examination for fungi and dermatophytes, skin scrapings for scabies, Gram stain for bacterial infections, cytologic examination (Tzanck test) for herpesvirus and varicella-zoster virus infection, and Wood light examination for the yellowish gold fluorescence of tinea versicolor.

The most definitive dermatologic test is a skin biopsy, which is required only occasionally. The biopsy specimen can be accomplished by punch biopsy, a simple, relatively painless procedure. Other definitive tests useful to diagnose underlying diseases with cutaneous manifestations include patch testing of suspected allergens, dark-field examination for syphilis, and blood tests.

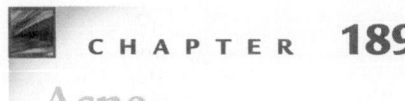

CHAPTER **189**

# Acne

## ETIOLOGY

**Acne vulgaris** (or acne) is a chronic inflammatory disorder of pilosebaceous units that affects areas with the greatest concentration of sebaceous glands, such as the face, chest, and back. The pathogenesis of acne is multifactorial. Gender, age, genetic factors, and environment are all major contributing factors. Stress may trigger acne, possibly by affecting hormone levels. There is no evidence linking chocolate, candy, or fried foods to acne.

The **primary event** in all acne lesions (inflammatory and noninflammatory) is the development of the **microcomedo**, which results from the obstruction of the sebaceous follicle with lamellated keratin, increased sebum production from sebaceous glands, and overgrowth of normal skin flora, leading to pilosebaceous occlusion and enlargement. Androgens are a potent stimulus of the sebaceous gland. The subsequent inflammatory component and pustule formation results from proliferation of *Propionibacterium acnes*, coagulase-negative staphylococci, and the yeast *Malassezia furfur*. The pathogenesis of acne thus involves three components: increased sebum production, hyperkeratosis, and bacterial infection. Effective treatment focuses on minimizing these factors.

## EPIDEMIOLOGY

Acne is the most common skin disorder in adolescents, occurring in 85% of teenagers. The incidence is similar in both sexes, although boys often are more severely affected. Acne may begin as early as 8 years of age and even earlier in patients treated with systemic corticosteroids.

## CLINICAL MANIFESTATIONS

Superficial plugging of the pilosebaceous unit with keratinous material, lipid, and bacteria results in noninflammatory small (2–3 mm) **open (blackhead)** and **closed (whitehead) comedones**. Comedones, superficial lesions that are the earliest lesion of acne, are typically found over the nose, chin, and central forehead. An open comedo is less likely to become inflammatory than a closed comedo. Rupture of a comedo into adjacent dermis induces a neutrophilic inflammatory response and development of inflammatory **papules** and **pustules** in the same distribution. Larger (1–3 cm), skin-colored or red cysts and nodules represent deeper plugging and usually are found over the cheeks, around the nose, and on the back. Increased and persistent inflammation, especially with **cystic acne** and rupture of a deep cyst, increases the risk of scarring.

**Neonatal acne** occurs in about 20% of normal newborns at 2 to 4 weeks of age and is thought to be a response to maternal androgens. The primary lesions are pinpoint, red, inflammatory closed comedones found on the lateral cheeks and forehead and occasionally on the chest or back. These lesions usually resolve spontaneously over months; mild topical keratolytic agents can be used. **Neonatal cephalic pustulosis** consists of papules or papulopustules on the face and may have *Malassezia* present. These lesions are treated with topical antifungal preparations. Neonatal acne must be differentiated from more common and benign cutaneous disorders presenting in newborns, such as milia or **miliaria rubra (prickly heat)**. Laboratory studies and imaging studies are not necessary to diagnose acne. The diagnosis of acne is usually not difficult because of the characteristic and chronic lesions.

## TREATMENT

The mainstays of treatment of acne are topical keratolytic agents and topical antibiotics. Creams, lotions, gels, foams, ointments, and solutions are available. Gels and solutions are commonly used as acne skin is generally greasier and these agents tend to be drying, but they have the tendency to be irritating and therefore should not be combined with drying soaps (salicylic acid washes). Creams are a preferable first choice when available because they are more easily tolerated.

The keratolytic agents (2.5–10% benzoyl peroxide, 2% salicylic acid, 20% azelaic acid, 0.025–0.1% tretinoin, 0.1% adapalene, 0.05–0.1% tazarotene) produce superficial desquamation and, subsequently, relieve follicular obstruction. They are a mainstay of first-line therapy. There is a direct relationship between the potency of the keratolytic cream or gel and the degree of associated irritation.

The topical retinoids (tretinoin, adapalene, tazarotene) are based on the vitamin A molecule and promote decreased keratin production, decreased sebum production, and are anti-inflammatory and antibacterial. Thus, they can be the most effective when used as monotherapy or in combination with benzoyl peroxide therapy for second-line treatment in cases of persistent acne. Several topical antibiotics (2% erythromycin, 1% clindamycin, 2.2% tetracycline) are available but are not as effective as monotherapy.

Oral antibiotics (tetracycline, erythromycin) should be combined with a topical retinoid for deeper cystic lesions. Combination therapy, typically for 8 to 12 weeks, results in significantly faster and greater clearing of acne than with antimicrobial therapy alone, which is not recommended. Tetracyclines are the most effective antibiotics because of their significant anti-inflammatory activity. A first generation tetracycline is a good choice because of its relative lack of potential adverse effects. All tetracyclines may cause photosensitivity; thus, sunscreen should be prescribed with them to minimize this adverse effect.

For recalcitrant or severe nodulocystic acne, oral isotretinoin (1 mg/kg/day for a 20-week period) may be instituted. Isotretinoin, an oral analog of vitamin A, normalizes follicular keratinization, reduces sebum production, and decreases 5α-dihydrotestosterone formation and androgen receptor–binding capacity. It has an approximately 80% response rate but has a high incidence of adverse effects and should be used only by physicians familiar with all of the potential adverse effects. Isotretinoin therapy requires careful patient selection, pretreatment counseling, and monthly laboratory monitoring. It is **teratogenic** and must not be used immediately before or during pregnancy.

## COMPLICATIONS

Although not associated with a high degree of clinical morbidity, acne has significant and frequently devastating effects on an adolescent's body image and self-esteem. There may be little correlation between severity and psychosocial impact.

## PROGNOSIS

Classically, acne lasts 3 to 5 years although some individuals may have disease for 15 to 20 years. Only early treatment with isotretinoin may alter the natural course of acne. Acne lesions often heal with temporary postinflammatory erythema and hyperpigmentation. Depending on the severity, chronicity, and depth of involvement, pitted, atrophic, or hypertrophic scars may develop. **Cystic acne** has the highest incidence of scarring because rupture of a deep cyst induces the greatest inflammation. In susceptible individuals, scarring may follow pustular or even comedonal acne.

## PREVENTION

Greasy hair and cosmetic preparations should be avoided because they exacerbate preexisting acne. There are no effective means for preventing acne and little evidence that diet is associated with acne. Repetitive cleansing with soap and water or use of astringents or abrasives removes only surface lipids. Their use makes the skin appear less oily but does not prevent formation of microcomedones; their use may be damaging because of the irritation and dryness they cause.

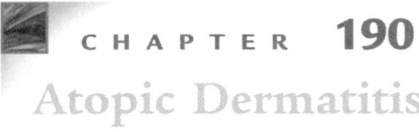

CHAPTER **190**

# Atopic Dermatitis

## ETIOLOGY

Atopic dermatitis is a chronic inflammatory disease with no known cure. It is a form of eczema associated with significant psychosocial morbidity and decreased health-related quality of life. For many affected individuals, atopic dermatitis is the skin manifestation of atopy accompanied by asthma and allergic rhinitis. Affected individuals may have only one or two manifestations of atopy; up to one quarter of affected individuals have no other forms of atopy. Genetics and environmental factors play a role. Genes for atopic dermatitis have been linked to many chromosomes including loci that control inflammation, as well as to single gene disorders, suggesting genetic polymorphism.

Inflammatory mediators involved include predominantly T helper cells, with the $T_H2$ pathway implicated early in acute lesions and a $T_H1$ predominance found in chronic lesions. Langerhans cells, IgE, and eosinophils play a prominent role, as well as many other inflammatory mediators. Two forms of atopic dermatitis have been proposed recently: an atopic form (also called extrinsic) and a nonatopic (intrinsic) form, because some individuals show no sensitizations to common allergens. The conditions behave similarly.

## EPIDEMIOLOGY

Atopic dermatitis is the most common skin disease in children, with an estimated prevalence of up to 20% of children. Only 1% to 2% of adults manifest disease. In addition to genetic factors, an environmental influence contributes. Atopic dermatitis occurs more frequently in urban areas and in higher socioeconomic classes and less frequently in rural areas. Prevalence is lower in areas where industrial pollution is less and where eosinophil-mediated infections such as helminthic infections are endemic.

Patients generally have a family history of atopy. Children with atopic dermatitis are predisposed to the development of allergy and allergic rhinitis, referred to as the *atopic march*. Asthma develops in up to half of children with atopic dermatitis, and allergic rhinitis even more frequently. Food sensitivities are commonly associated with atopic dermatitis.

## CLINICAL MANIFESTATIONS

Atopic dermatitis manifests with a defective skin barrier, reduced innate immune responses, and exaggerated immune responses to allergens and microbes. Clinically, this leads to characteristic skin lesions with inflammation and increased skin infections. A chronic, relapsing course is typical. Pruritus and skin hyper-reactivity manifest with characteristic erythematous skin lesions. Foods, allergens, infections, irritants, extremes of temperature, and lack of humidity can exacerbate the condition as well as scratching or rubbing. Triggers are somewhat variable from individual to individual.

Characteristic locations vary with the age of the patient. Infantile eczema typically affects the face and extensor surfaces of the extremities and is often generalized. Childhood lesions predominate in flexural surfaces (antecubital and popliteal fossae), wrists, ankles, hands, and feet (Fig. 190-1). The adult phase occurs after puberty and manifests in the flexural areas including the neck as well as predominant involvement on the face, dorsa of the hands, fingers and toes, and the upper arms and back. Generalized xerosis is commonly found in all stages. The condition generally remits in adulthood.

Characteristic lesions of atopic dermatitis are erythematous plaques with ill-defined borders and overlying hyperkeratosis. Lesions can be secondarily excoriated or have an overlying crusting that is yellow or hemorrhagic. Weeping may be present in acute stages. Lichenification is found in older lesions. Formation of fissures is common in both acute and chronic lesions. Papular lesions may also occur. The formation of vesicles is associated with intensely inflammatory lesions. Regardless of the stage, hypo- and hyperpigmentation can be seen, representing transient changes. Atopic dermatitis is not usually scarring unless secondary features become severe (e.g., infection or physical manipulation [scratching]).

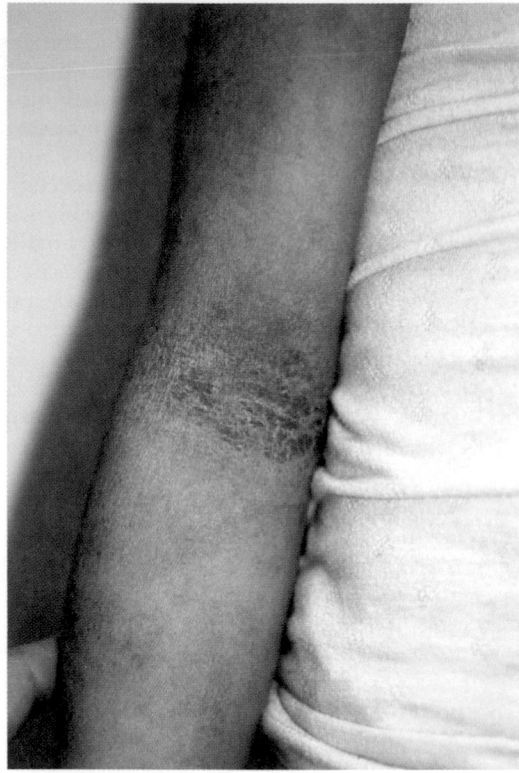

**FIGURE 190-1**

Atopic dermatitis (arm).

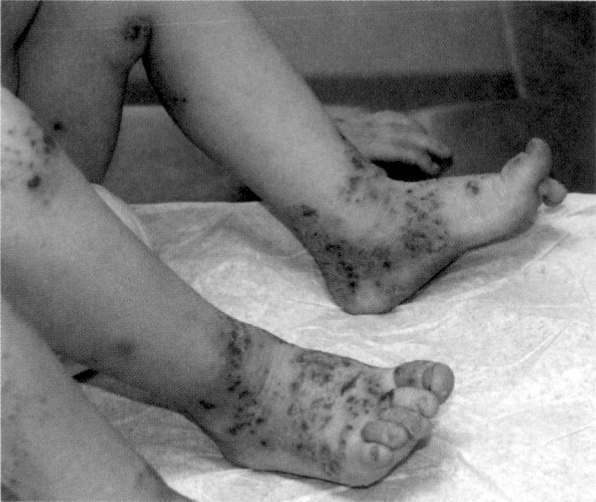

**FIGURE 190-2**

Atopic dermatitis with *Staphylococcus superinfection*.

Secondary bacterial infection, most commonly with *Staphylococcus aureus* or less commonly with *Streptococcus pyogenes*, is frequently present. Patients are at increased risk for infections with cutaneous viruses, such as herpes simplex virus or varicella virus, and can develop disseminated skin infections with viruses such as herpes simplex virus (eczema herpeticum), varicella-zoster virus, smallpox virus (eczema vaccinatum), and *Molluscum contagiosum*. Atopic skin is more susceptible to fungal infections as well. Signs of concomitant infection include acute worsening of disease in an otherwise well-controlled patient, resistance to standard therapy, fever, and presence of pustules, fissures, or exudative or crusted lesions (Fig. 190-2). Eczema herpeticum can be life threatening.

## LABORATORY AND IMAGING STUDIES

Diagnosis of atopic dermatitis is based on clinical signs and symptoms. Skin biopsy findings are generally characteristic but not exclusively diagnostic and can overlap with other skin conditions. Peripheral blood eosinophilia and elevated IgE levels can be found but are not specific. Skin testing or measurement of specific IgE antibody levels can detect sensitization to inhalant allergens. Skin tests should be interpreted with caution in patients with active skin lesions as false positive findings occur.

## DIFFERENTIAL DIAGNOSIS

The differential diagnosis of atopic dermatitis is extensive, but the history of a relapsing pruritic condition in the setting of atopy and skin lesions in a characteristic distribution is typical.

The lesions of seborrheic dermatitis have circumscribed and well-defined borders, and the scale or hyperkeratosis, when present, is thicker, greasy, and yellowish. Their distribution is different than that of atopic dermatitis. Occasionally the two conditions coexist.

Psoriasis tends to localize on the elbows and knees, the pretibial areas, and scalp. The lesions of psoriasis on exposed surfaces are salmon color at the base with an overlying hyperkeratosis that is much thicker with silver coloration. They are generally very well demarcated, oval or round, thick plaques.

Contact dermatitis has a distribution limited to one area of the body corresponding to the contact with the allergen. The lesions generally make bizarre, linear, square, or angulated shapes corresponding to the source. **Nickel dermatitis** is common and results from contact sensitization to nickel in metals. It occurs in characteristic locations, such as the periumbilical area (where metal from pants snaps rubs against skin); on the ear lobule or inferior to the auricle on the neck (where earrings contact skin); circumferentially around the neck (necklaces); and under rings or wristbands. Patients with atopic dermatitis can have concomitant contact dermatitis as well.

## TREATMENT

Ideal therapy for atopic dermatitis includes three main components: avoidance of triggers of inflammation, use of topical anti-inflammatory medication to affected areas of skin when needed, and frequent, liberal use of bland emollients to restore the skin barrier. Control of pruritus and infection should be considered on an individual basis. If topical therapy and these measures are inadequate, systemic therapy with immunosuppressive agents or ultraviolet light therapy may be indicated.

Common triggers of inflammation in atopic dermatitis include rubbing or scratching, contact with saliva or foods that are acidic, soaps and detergents, fabric softeners, wool or other harsh materials, bubble baths and other products with fragrances that contact the skin, sweat, highly chlorinated pools, low humidity, tobacco smoke, dust mites, animal dander, grass pollens, and molds. Exposure to these triggers should be limited whenever possible. Infections that are unrelated to skin disease can also exacerbate atopic dermatitis.

A daily short bath with warm but not hot water is generally advisable followed by immediate application of emollients and medications before evaporative loss is allowed to occur. Some controversy surrounds the frequency of bathing as there are some advocates of limiting bathing for these patients to less than once daily. Additional information for patients and families can be found at the website of the National Eczema Association for Science and Education (http://www.nationaleczema.org).

Food allergy is commonly seen in patients with atopic dermatitis and can contribute to clinical exacerbations of disease. More frequently, skin manifestations occur independent of the food allergy exacerbation. Eggs, milk, nuts, wheat, and fish are the most commonly implicated food allergens. Egg allergy may be of particular relevance. Excessively restrictive diets should be avoided.

**Topical corticosteroids** are the mainstay of anti-inflammatory therapy for atopic dermatitis and are used intermittently as needed on affected areas. Only mild to moderately potent preparations should be used in children and on areas of thinner skin such as the face, genital, and intertriginous areas. Topical corticosteroids should be used in conjunction with adequate skin care, such as avoiding triggers of inflammation and frequent application of emollients. The goal is to limit the need for anti-inflammatory medications and thereby avoid potential for adverse effects with prolonged use or frequent application to large body surface areas. Different therapeutic schemes have been recommended, including monotherapy or combination therapy with nonsteroidal anti-inflammatory medications (topical calcineurin inhibitors). Monotherapy schemes with topical corticosteroids may involve early use of moderate potency corticosteroids for more rapid improvement followed by tapering to less potent corticosteroids. Early lesions and lesions in anatomic areas with thinner skin (face, genitals, axillae, antecubital and popliteal fossae) respond more readily to lower potency topical corticosteroid preparations than do chronic, thicker lesions and lesions in areas of thicker skin (hands and feet). It is important to individualize the topical corticosteroid treatment regimen.

Hundreds of topical corticosteroids are available and are classified according to strength from I to VII. Class I is the highest potency and class VII is the lowest potency. Potency varies according to the steroid molecule (active ingredient) and, for a given ingredient, strength can vary according to relative concentration and vehicle base. Class I steroids are generally avoided in young children. Classes I and II steroids are avoided in areas of thinner skin or enhanced penetration. Inadvertent or purposeful enhanced penetration occurs in areas of natural occlusion (flexures such as axillae and groin), with external occlusion (diapers or bandages), in areas of open skin (excoriations), and with heat or hydration. Use of wet wraps with lower strength topical corticosteroid application takes advantage of this principle of heat and hydration for enhanced penetration for recalcitrant lesions.

Corticosteroids are available in different vehicles. In general, ointments are very effective because of their occlusive nature and they are very well tolerated. Creams may be slightly less effective for a given steroid ingredient, but may be more cosmetically acceptable for older patients or in warmer climates. Lotions may have more preservatives that can cause irritation and are generally less potent. Sprays, foams, solutions, and gels can be especially useful for hair-bearing areas, and can be very potent. Sprays, solutions, and gels can be particularly irritating when applied to atopic skin and should generally be avoided on areas of open skin. Twice-daily application of corticosteroids is recommended.

Topical **calcineurin inhibitors** (also referred to as topical immune modulators) have been recently introduced in the therapy for atopic dermatitis and include topical tacrolimus and pimecrolimus. They can be effective for mild to moderate atopic dermatitis, and can be helpful adjunctive agents in severe atopic dermatitis. These agents selectively inhibit T-cell proliferation by inhibiting calcineurin and subsequent phosphatase activity, which normally lead to production of inflammatory mediators and T-cell proliferation. There is no potential for skin atrophy. Thus, these agents are particularly useful in face or neck or genital lesions. These agents can be particularly helpful as monotherapy or, anecdotally, when used in combination with corticosteroid therapy. Many different application schemes have been advocated. They are currently approved for intermittent therapy as second-line treatments for mild to moderate atopic dermatitis. Long-term studies, combined with other modalities for treatment, are under way.

Topical antibiotic therapy as monotherapy for atopic dermatitis is ineffective. Some improvement can be seen because of the natural moisturizing properties of topical antibiotics and treatment of the exacerbating infection. They are more effective when combined with topical anti-inflammatory treatment.

Topical extract of coal tar can be used as an effective anti-inflammatory medication for atopic dermatitis and can be compounded in low concentrations with an emollient vehicle base. Cosmetic inelegance with staining and odor, as well as potential for irritation, limits its use. Tar is also mutagenic.

Antihistamines are useful adjunctive therapy, especially during flares. Sedating antihistamines are generally prescribed in low doses for nighttime use (one fourth of the total dose), improving itching and the sleeplessness that can be related to scratching during the night. Additional daytime doses can be added on an individual basis when needed, but are infrequently necessary. Nighttime dosing of nonsedating oral antihistamines may be more advantageous for school-age children when drowsiness is not desirable.

Systemic corticosteroids are indicated for short-term administration for cases of severe disease and may be appropriate in selected rare cases when adequate topical therapy failed or is being instituted. Systemic corticosteroid courses should be adequately tapered and used in conjunction with an appropriate atopic skin care regimen. Rebound flare of atopic dermatitis is common following withdrawal of corticosteroids and should be anticipated to avoid misinterpretation of the natural disease severity. Long-term and frequent repeated courses should be avoided to prevent adverse effects.

Systemic cyclosporine (up to 5 mg/kg/day) can be effective therapy for atopic dermatitis in severe cases. It can be tapered once disease is controlled and is typically used on a longer-term basis (5–12 months) to produce remission. Ultraviolet light therapy (UVB, narrow band UVB, UVA, or UVA1) can be used alternatively in moderate to severe cases in older children. Typically, light therapy is administered two to three times weekly until improvement is seen, and then is tapered or discontinued once the acute flare has resolved. Requirements for frequent office visits, ability to cooperate with standing in a light box while wearing protective goggles, and risk of long-term skin damage, including the potential for skin cancer development with excessive UV light exposure, prevent more frequent use of light therapy in children.

## COMPLICATIONS

An increased tendency toward bacterial, viral, and fungal skin infections is due to an impaired skin barrier and results from changes in the stratum corneum, lipid metabolism in the epidermis, a decrease in innate immune proteins in the skin, as well as maladaptive secondary immune responses.

Superinfection with *S. aureus* is the most common secondary skin infection found in atopic dermatitis. Group A streptococcus infection is also common. Infection manifests with pustules, erythema, crusting, scabbing, flare of disease, or lack of response to adequate anti-inflammatory therapy. Localized lesions can be treated with topical mupirocin. Widespread and generalized lesions require systemic therapy, most commonly with a first-generation cephalosporin, such as cephalexin. Erythromycin and azithromycin can also be effective unless patients are colonized with a macrolide-resistant strain of *S. aureus*. Methicillin-resistant *S. aureus* infection manifests with deeper, more inflammatory skin lesions. Diagnosis is confirmed by culture and treatment guided by antimicrobial susceptibilities. Treatment should include concomitant atopic skin care routine to treat active areas of inflammation, restore the skin barrier, and avoid triggers of inflammation. Although secondary skin infection with *S. aureus* is common, progression to cellulitis or septicemia is unusual. Colonization and infection worsens inflammation in atopic dermatitis by promoting resistance to topical corticosteroids, superantigen activation in susceptible individuals, and production of IgE antistaphylococcal antibodies.

**Eczema herpeticum** (Kaposi's varicelliform eruption) is one of the potentially serious infectious complications in atopic dermatitis. After herpes simplex virus (HSV) infection and an incubation period of 5 to 12 days, an eruption of multiple, pruritic vesiculopustular lesions occurs in a disseminated pattern. Characteristic lesions are umbilicated vesicles and pustules and punctuate hemorrhagic crusts that coalesce in groups that are discontinuously distributed over the skin and surrounded by inflammation (Fig. 190-3). Irritability, anorexia, and fever can also be seen. Systemic and central nervous system disease have been reported. Bacterial superinfection of eroded areas of

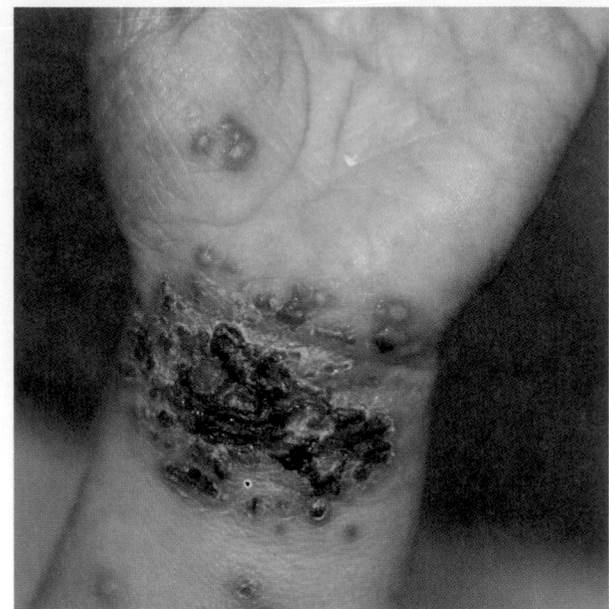

**FIGURE 190-3**

Eczema herpeticum (hand).

the skin often occurs. Diagnosis can be made rapidly from a scraping from the skin lesion stained with Giemsa or Wright's stain (**Tzanck test**), though these are not highly sensitive. These stains allow microscopic visualization of the presence of multinucleated giant cells indicative of herpes simplex virus or varicella-zoster virus infection. Vesicle fluid can also be sent for rapid direct fluorescent antibody testing or for culture for virus confirmation. Polymerase chain reaction (PCR) detection for herpes simplex virus DNA from fluid is also available. Laboratory confirmation of infection is important because similar clinical manifestations can occur with bacterial infections.

Complications from topical corticosteroid therapy include local development of acne, hypopigmentation, and hypertrichosis. Atrophy, telangiectasia, or striae can result from misuse of corticosteroids (too high potency or application for longer than appropriate). Glaucoma and cataract formation have been reported in association with chronic topical corticosteroid use. Hypothalamic-pituitary adrenal axis suppression can occur with high potency steroid use or chronic use of low potency topical corticosteroids to large body surface areas. In general, topical corticosteroids should be applied only to affected areas, discontinued when no longer needed, and used in conjunction with appropriate atopic skin care regimens that lessen the need for topical steroid therapy. Rotational or combination therapy with nonsteroidal anti-inflammatory agents can limit application of corticosteroids preventing adverse effects.

The psychosocial impact of the condition can be significant. There is often disfigurement, lack of sleep from restlessness and pruritus resulting in irritability and fatigue, and limitations on participations in sports. Significant time, as well as financial strain, are involved in caring for a child with atopic dermatitis. Thus, management should address these potential issues and provide adequate anticipatory guidance.

## PROGNOSIS

Atopic dermatitis frequently remits during childhood and is much less common after puberty. The condition is generally most severe and widespread in infancy and early childhood. Relapse of disease in adults can occur and commonly manifests as face or hand dermatitis. Frequently adults have generalized dry skin and are aware that their skin is sensitive to many over-the-counter preparations. Patients with atopic dermatitis can also develop asthma and allergic rhinitis. Asthma is more commonly associated with more severe skin disease.

## PREVENTION

Individual flares of atopic dermatitis can be prevented by avoiding triggers of inflammation and can be lessened with frequent emollient application. Recent evidence shows that breastfeeding for at least 4 months, compared with feeding formula made with intact cow's milk protein, prevents or delays the occurrence of atopic dermatitis (as well as cow's milk allergy and wheezing) in early childhood. For infants with a parent or sibling with atopic disease and who are not exclusively breastfed for 4 to 6 months, there is modest evidence that the onset of atopic disease, and especially atopic dermatitis, may be delayed or prevented by the use of extensively hydrolyzed casein-based formulas. There is insufficient evidence that soy-based formulas, delaying the introduction of complementary foods beyond 4 to 6 months of age, or other dietary intervention prevents the development of atopic disease. There is no convincing evidence that women who avoid peanuts or other foods during pregnancy or while breastfeeding lower their child's risk of allergies.

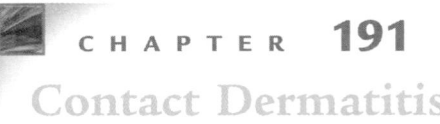

## CHAPTER 191
## Contact Dermatitis

## ETIOLOGY AND EPIDEMIOLOGY

Inflammation in the top layers of the skin, caused by direct contact with a substance, is divided into two subtypes: contact irritant dermatitis and contact allergic dermatitis. **Contact irritant dermatitis** is common and observed after the skin surface is exposed to an irritating chemical or undergoes repeated exposure to a substance that dries the skin. **Allergic contact dermatitis** is a cell-mediated immune reaction. The antigens, or haptens, involved in allergic contact dermatitis readily penetrate the epidermis and are bound by Langerhans cells, the antigen-presenting cells of the skin. The hapten is presented to T lymphocytes, and an immune cascade follows.

Contact diaper dermatitis is a common problem that affects approximately 10% of infants between birth and 2 years of age.

## CLINICAL MANIFESTATIONS

Contact irritant dermatitis is characterized by ill-defined red patches and plaques with secondary scales (Fig. 191-1). The eruption is localized to skin surfaces that are exposed to the irritant. Irritant diaper dermatitis is distributed in the perianal region and on the buttocks, areas that are exposed repeatedly to urine and feces. Contact irritant dermatitis is also observed frequently on the dorsal surfaces of the hands in patients who repeatedly wash their hands with an irritating soap.

Contact allergic dermatitis is usually an acute and sometimes severe reaction that is limited to exposed sites. The initial lesions are bright red, pruritic patches, often in linear or sharply marginated bizarre configurations. Within the patches are clear vesicles and bullae with serosanguineous drainage (Fig. 191-2). Signs and symptoms of the disease may be delayed for 7 to 14 days after exposure if the patient has not been sensitized previously. On reexposure, symptoms begin within hours and are usually more severe. The eruption may persist for weeks.

## LABORATORY AND IMAGING STUDIES

The diagnosis is established by clinical presentation and history of exposure to a recognized irritant or allergen. *Candida* dermatitis can be confirmed, if necessary, by a potassium hydroxide preparation of skin scrapings to identify the presence of budding yeast.

## DIFFERENTIAL DIAGNOSIS

The distribution and appearance of the dermatitis and a detailed exposure history are the most useful diagnostic tools. Involvement of the lower legs and distal arms suggests exposure to plants of the *Rhus* species (poison ivy or poison oak), especially when linear configurations of lesions are present. Dermatitis of the ears (earrings), wrist (bracelet or watch), or periumbilical region (buckle of jeans or pants) suggests a metal allergy to nickel. Distribution on the dorsal surfaces of the feet indicates a shoe allergy, usually to dyes, rubber, or leather. Topical antibiotics (neomycin) and fragrances (soaps, perfumes, cosmetics) are frequent causes of allergic contact dermatitis.

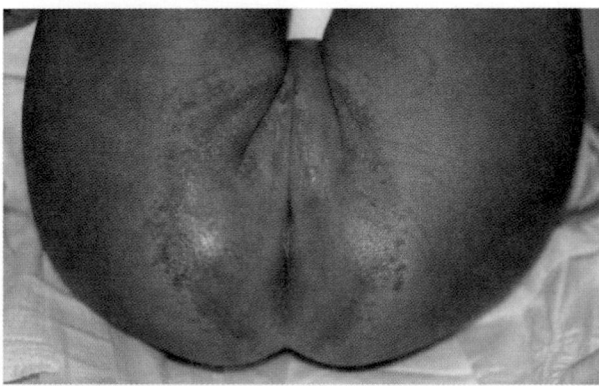

**FIGURE 191-1**

Irritant diaper dermatitis.

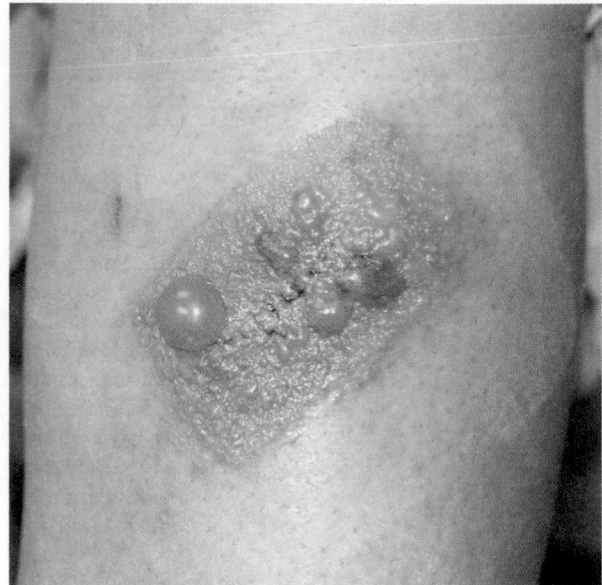

**FIGURE 191-2**

Allergic contact dermatitis to tincture of benzoin.

Diaper rashes caused by *Candida* are quite common. Contact irritant dermatitis primarily affects the prominent, exposed surfaces, whereas *Candida* primarily affects intertriginous areas. The two are frequently present simultaneously, as secondary *Candida* infection may complicate irritant dermatitis.

Psoriasis, seborrheic dermatitis, and Langerhans cell histiocytosis can present with an erythematous rash in the diaper area. Referral to a dermatologist should be considered for any child with severe rash or with diaper rash that does not respond to conventional therapy.

## TREATMENT

Topical steroids are effective in treatment of allergic and irritant contact dermatitis. High potency steroids may be necessary for severe reactions of allergic contact dermatitis. Oral antihistamines or oral corticosteroids may be required to control itching.

Treatment of candidal diaper dermatitis consists of topical nystatin cream or ointment, clotrimazole 1% cream, or miconazole 2% ointment. Concurrent oral thrush should be treated with nystatin oral suspension or topically applied gentian violet. Lesions associated with significant inflammation can be treated adjunctively with a short course (1–2 days) of topical 1% hydrocortisone. Hydrocortisone 2.5% is frequently used in addition to topical antifungal therapy to treat the irritant component of the diaper dermatitis when present concomitantly.

## COMPLICATIONS

Inflamed skin, especially macerated skin, is prone to injury from friction and to bacterial or candidal superinfection. *Candida albicans* is present in 70% of cases of diaper dermatitis.

## PREVENTION

It is controversial whether diaper rash is more frequent with use of absorbent disposable diapers or with cloth diapers. Occlusion, such as with plastic pants, should be avoided because it predisposes the skin to maceration. Every effort should be made to identify the trigger of contact dermatitis because re-exposure often leads to increasingly severe reactions.

 CHAPTER **192**

# Seborrheic Dermatitis

## ETIOLOGY

Seborrheic dermatitis is a common, chronic inflammatory disease that has different clinical presentations at different ages. Areas prone to seborrheic dermatitis include the scalp and scalp margins, eyebrows, base of eyelashes, nasolabial folds, external auditory canals, and posterior auricular folds. Seborrheic dermatitis classically presents in infants as **cradle cap** or dermatitis in the **intertriginous** areas of the axillae, groin, anticubital and popliteal fossae and umbilicus, and is seen in adolescents as **dandruff**. Genetic and environmental factors influence the onset and clinical course, which parallels the distribution, size, and activity of sebaceous glands, although their role is uncertain. *Malassezia furfur* may play a causative role.

## CLINICAL MANIFESTATIONS

Seborrheic dermatitis in infants presents as **cradle cap**, which may begin during the first month and persist during the first year of life. It is usually asymptomatic other than the appearance. Cradle cap describes the thick, waxy, yellow-white scaling and crusting of the scalp with greasy adherent scale (Fig. 192-1). It is usually prominent on the vertex of the skull, but it may be diffuse. A greasy, scaly, erythematous, nonpruritic papular dermatitis may extend to the face, posterior auricular folds, and diaper area and may involve the entire body. Diaper and intertriginous areas can have sharply demarcated erythematous patches with yellowish, greasy, or waxy-appearing scale. Significant erythema may be present, particularly if the eruption spreads onto the face and torso. Hypopigmentation may persist after the inflammation has faded. The eruption is usually asymptomatic, which helps differentiate it from infantile atopic dermatitis, which is pruritic.

Classic seborrheic dermatitis during adolescence usually is localized to the scalp and intertriginous areas and may include blepharitis and involvement of the external auditory canals. **Dandruff** is a fine, white, dry scaling of the scalp with minor itching. Scalp changes vary from diffuse, brawny scaling to focal areas of thick, oily, yellow crusts with underlying erythema. Pruritus may be minimal or severe. Seborrheic plaques on the extremities are pink with hyperkeratosis. The borders are frequently demarcated to a greater extent than plaques of atopic dermatitis.

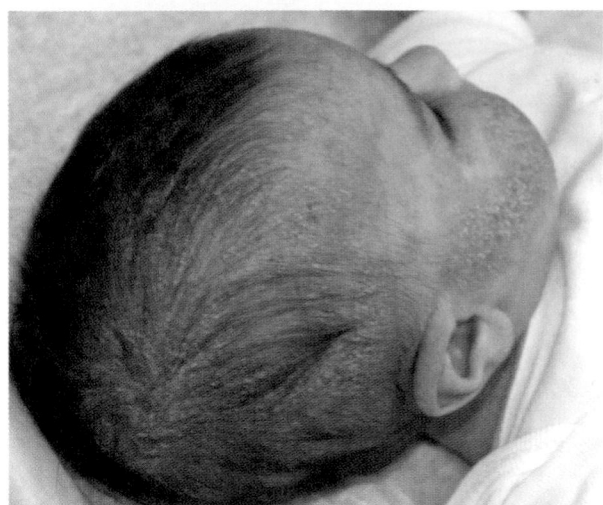

**FIGURE 192-1**

Seborrheic dermatitis (cradle cap).

## LABORATORY AND IMAGING STUDIES

Laboratory studies and imaging studies are not necessary to diagnose cradle cap or dandruff. Atypical or resistant cases should have fungal cultures and potassium hydroxide studies for *Trichophyton tonsurans* (see Chapter 98).

## DIFFERENTIAL DIAGNOSIS

The differential diagnosis includes atopic dermatitis, cutaneous fungal infections, pityriasis rosea, psoriasis, secondary syphilis, and drug eruption. Intractable, severe generalized seborrheic dermatitis suggests histiocytosis. Intractable seborrheic dermatitis, accompanied by chronic diarrhea and failure to thrive, suggests Leiner disease or acquired immunodeficiency syndrome (AIDS). Pityriasis rosea has a peak age of onset in adolescence, and commonly manifests with distribution in a **Christmas tree** pattern on the back. Psoriasis is characterized by thick silvery scale and most commonly manifests on the extensor surfaces of the extremities.

## TREATMENT

Minor amounts of scale of seborrheic dermatitis can be removed easily by frequent shampooing. For all ages, daily shampooing with zinc pyrithione (Head & Shoulders, DHS Zinc), selenium sulfide 1% to 2.5%, or salicylic acid (T-Sal) can treat scalp scale. Seborrheic dermatitis with inflamed lesions responds rapidly to treatment with low potency steroids two to four times daily for 3 to 5 days. Wet compresses should be applied to the moist or fissured plaques before application of the corticosteroid ointment.

The response to treatment is usually rapid. Secondary bacterial infection can occur but is uncommon. Intractable disease and other complications warrant further evaluation for other etiologies.

## PROGNOSIS

Cradle cap is self-limited and resolves during the first year of life. Seborrheic dermatitis does not cause permanent hair loss. Continued use of an antiseborrheic shampoo is often required for control of dandruff.

## PREVENTION

Frequent shampooing, especially with early signs of seborrheic dermatitis, may help prevent progression.

## OTHER PAPULOSQUAMOUS DERMATITIS

**Pityriasis rosea** is a benign, self-limited eruption that may occur at any age, with peak incidence during adolescence. A solitary 2 to 5 cm, pink, round patch that often has a hint of central clearing, the so-called **herald patch**, is the first manifestation of the eruption. The herald patch typically is found on the breast, lower torso, or proximal thigh and is often misdiagnosed as fungal or eczematous in origin. One to 2 weeks later, multiple 0.5 to 2 cm, oval to oblong, red or tan (*fawn*-colored) macules with a fine, bran-like scale erupt on the torso and proximal extremities in a characteristic arrangement parallel to skin tension lines (*Christmas tree pattern*). Papular and papulovesicular variants may be seen in infants and young children. Rarely the eruption may have an inverse distribution involving the axillae and groin. Usually the condition is asymptomatic, but mild prodromal symptoms may be present with the appearance of the herald patch; pruritus is present in 25% of cases. The eruption lasts 4 to 14 weeks, with gradual resolution. Residual hyperpigmentation or hypopigmentation can take additional months to clear. The etiology is unknown. Treatment is unnecessary. Pruritus can be managed with oral antihistamines, phototherapy, and low potency topical corticosteroids.

**Psoriasis** is a common papulosquamous condition characterized by well-demarcated, erythematous, scaling papules and plaques. Psoriasis occurs at all ages, including infancy, with onset of 30% of cases during childhood. The disease is characterized by a chronic and relapsing course, although spontaneous remissions can occur. Infections, stress, trauma, and medications may cause disease exacerbations. The disease tends to worsen during the fall and winter, probably secondary to decreased humidity. Various subtypes of psoriasis exist. The most common variety is **plaque-type psoriasis (psoriasis vulgaris)**, which can be localized or generalized. The lesions consist of round, well-demarcated, red plaques measuring 1 to 7 cm with **micaceous scale**, which is distinctive in its thick, silvery appearance with pinpoint bleeding points revealed on removal of the scales (**Auspitz sign**). The lesions of psoriasis have a distinctive distribution involving the extensor aspect of the elbows and knees, posterior occipital scalp, periumbilical region, lumbosacral region, and intergluteal cleft. Children often have facial lesions involving the upper inner aspect of the eyelids. Nail plate involvement is common and includes pitting, onycholysis, subungual hyperkeratosis, and *oil staining* (reddish brown subungual macular discoloration). Guttate (numerous small plaques diffusely distributed on the torso), erythrodermic (erythematous papules and plaques coalescing and covering large body surface areas), and pustular forms may occur.

The foundation of therapy is topical corticosteroids. Treatment of psoriasis with oral systemic corticosteroids can induce pustular psoriasis and should be avoided. Because of the risk of atrophy, striae, and telangiectases, especially when potent fluorinated corticosteroid preparations are administered long-term, the goal is to use the least potent corticosteroid. Topical calcipotriene, a vitamin D analog, is a useful adjuvant to topical corticosteroids. Phototherapy with ultraviolet (UV) light can be useful as secondary therapy in older children. Generalized erythrodermic psoriasis and pustular psoriasis may necessitate systemic treatments with other immune suppressives (methotrexate, cyclosporine). More selective immune modulating agents such as tumor necrosis factor antagonists are now available. Goeckerman therapy involves simultaneous UVB irradiation and tar.

CHAPTER **193**

# Pigmented Lesions

## DERMAL MELANOSIS (MONGOLIAN SPOT)

The most frequently encountered pigmented lesion is dermal melanosis (mongolian spot), which occurs in 70% to 96% of African-American, Asian, and Native American infants and in approximately 5% of white infants. This is a heritable, developmental lesion caused by entrapment of melanocytes in the dermis during their migration from the neural crest into the epidermis. Although most of these lesions are found in the lumbosacral area, they also occur at other sites such as the buttocks, flank, extremities, or, rarely, the face (Fig. 193-1). The lesion is macular and gray-blue, lacks a sharp border, and may cover an area greater than 10 cm in length. Most lesions gradually disappear during the first few years of life; aberrant lesions in unusual sites are more likely to persist. Dermal melanosis has been associated with cleft lip, spinal meningeal tumor, and melanoma, but is usually a benign finding.

## CAFÉ AU LAIT MACULES

Café au lait spots are pigmented macules with smooth borders, which may be present in a newborn but tend to develop during childhood (Fig. 193-2). They range in color from very light brown to a chocolate brown. Up to five café au lait macules are found in 1.8% of newborns and 25% to 40% of normal children and have no significance. Children with six or more café au lait macules (0.5 cm in diameter or > 1.5 cm in diameter after puberty), especially when accompanied by **freckling** in the flexural creases, should be evaluated carefully for additional stigmata of neurofibromatosis type 1. Axillary and inguinal freckles represent tiny café au lait macules. Café au lait spots and axillary freckling are usually the first cutaneous lesions to appear in a patient with neurofibromatosis; other signs include the presence of Lisch nodules on the

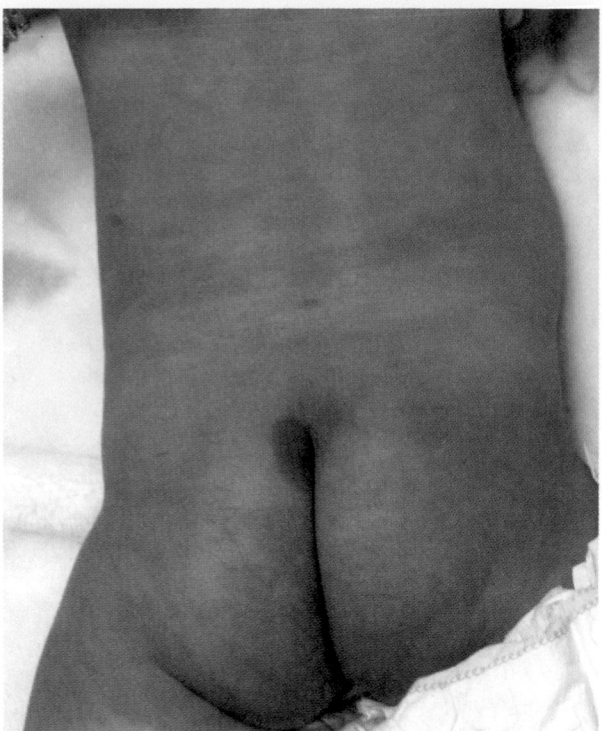

**FIGURE 193-1**

Dermal hypermelanosis (back).

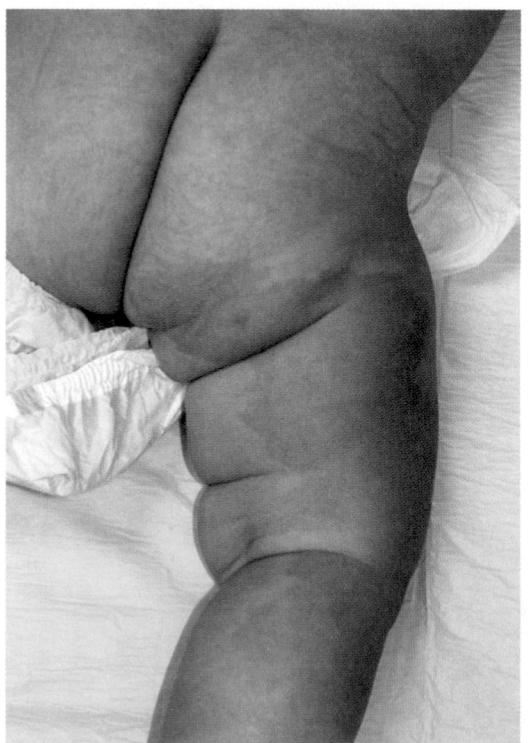

**FIGURE 193-2**

Café au lait spots (leg).

iris, optic glioma, or neurofibromas. Two or more characteristic features are required to establish the diagnosis of neurofibromatosis. Other disorders also associated with café au lait macules include the other forms of neurofibromatosis, McCune-Albright syndrome, multiple lentiginosis/LEOPARD syndrome, Noonan syndrome, and Russell-Silver syndrome.

## CONGENITAL MELANOCYTIC NEVI

Approximately 1% to 2% of newborns have melanocytic nevi. Smaller lesions (as opposed to giant pigmented nevi) are flat or slightly elevated plaques, often with an oval or lancet configuration. Most lesions are dark brown; scalp lesions may be red-brown at birth. The pigmentation within an individual lesion is often variegated or speckled with an accentuated epidermal surface ridge pattern (Fig. 193-3). Textural changes, deeper pigmentation, and elevation help to differentiate these lesions from café au lait macules. Thick, dark, coarse hair frequently is associated with congenital melanocytic nevi (Fig. 193-4). These lesions vary in site, size, and number, but are most often solitary. Histologically, they are characterized by the presence of nevus cells in the dermis; most have nevus cells extending into the deeper dermis. The lesions pose a slightly increased risk for the development of malignant melanoma, usually developing during adulthood. Thus, many dermatologists advise removal of the lesions before or near the time of puberty. Periodic evaluation of the lesion for surface changes and associated symptoms should be performed in those who elect observation. Excisional

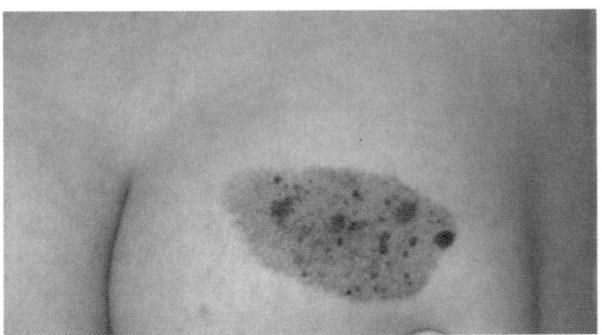

**FIGURE 193-3**

Congenital melanocytic nevus (buttock).

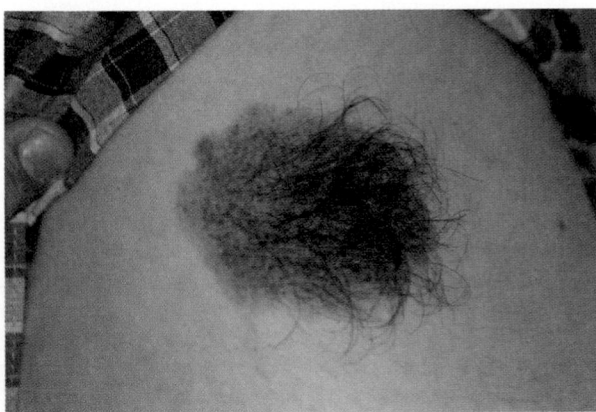

**FIGURE 193-4**

Hairy congenital nevus.

biopsy is indicated in instances in which malignant change is suspected. The differential diagnosis of brown color and various other color birthmarks is listed in Table 193-1.

## CONGENITAL GIANT MELANOCYTIC NEVI

Giant congenital nevi are defined as nevi that would be approximately 20 cm in length in adulthood, but smaller in a newborn (approximately 5–12 cm). These nevi may occupy 15% to 35% of the body surface, most commonly involving the trunk or head and neck region. The pigmentation often is variegated from light brown to black. The affected skin may be smooth, nodular, or leathery. Prominent, dark hypertrichosis is often present. Numerous smaller (1–5 cm) light brown patches (**satellite nevi**) are diffusely distributed. **Malignant melanoma** develops in the nevus in approximately 2% to 10% of affected patients over a lifetime. Because of the incidence of malignant degeneration, extensive deformity, and the intense pruritus that may accompany these lesions, staged surgical excision usually is attempted. The use of tissue expansion techniques has greatly improved the capability for surgical removal of large lesions.

**Neurocutaneous melanosis** is the presence of melanocytes in the central nervous system (CNS) (leptomeninges) that is rarely associated with giant congenital melanocytic nevi in an axial distribution. Affected patients may have hydrocephalus and seizures from melanocyte hyperplasia or frank CNS melanoma. In symptomatic patients, death results during early childhood.

## POSTINFLAMMATORY HYPERPIGMENTATION

Hyperpigmentation may be secondary to any inflammatory process in the skin. Postinflammatory hyperpigmentation is characterized by a hyperpigmented macule with ill-defined borders located in an area of previous skin inflammation. The hyperpigmentation resolves spontaneously, but can last for weeks to months. Lesions on the lower extremities are slower to resolve. No treatment is necessary, but reassurance is often helpful.

## ACQUIRED NEVI

Acquired melanocytic nevi or **moles** are common skin lesions. Melanocytic nevi may occur at any age; however, the lesions seem to develop most rapidly in prepubertal children and teenagers. Melanocytic nevi are well-delineated, round-to-oval, brown papules. Lesions are most common on the face, chest, and upper torso. Family history, skin type, and sun exposure are considered major risk factors. Irregular pigmentation, rapid growth, bleeding, and a change in configuration or borders suggest signs of malignant degeneration. Surgical excision and histologic examination are indicated for moles that have such features or are changing.

**Malignant melanoma** is rare in childhood; however, there is an alarming increase in incidence in adolescence. Education of parents and children regarding the risks of sun exposure, appropriate sun protection, and observation of changes in moles that are suggestive of malignancy is important.

**TABLE 193-1 Common Birthmarks**

| Color/Lesion | Birthmark | Location | Other Features |
|---|---|---|---|
| Brown/macule or patch | Café au lait macule | Variable, trunk | Associated with neurofibromatosis |
| Brown (<20 cm)/plaque | Congenital melanocytic nevus | Scalp, trunk | Possible increased risk of melanoma |
| Brown (>20 cm)/plaque | Giant melanocytic nevus | Trunk most common | 3–7% risk of melanoma, neurocutaneous melanosis |
| Brown–"flesh-colored"/ plaque | Epidermal nevus | Variable, trunk and neck | |
| Red/patch | Port-wine stain (nevus flammeus) | Variable, face most common | Associated with Sturge-Weber syndrome |
| Red/papule or plaque | Hemangioma | Variable, head and neck most common | Facial lesions (beard distribution) associated with airway lesions |
| Red-purple/plaque | Lymphatic malformation | Variable, trunk, proximal leg | Often has a vesicular appearance |
| Gray-blue/patch | Dermal melanosis (mongolian spot), nevus of Ito | Buttocks, lower trunk | Usually resolves spontaneously |
| | Nevus of Ota | Forehead and eyelids | Ocular pigmentation |
| | Nevus of Ito | Posterior shoulder | |
| Blue/nodule | Dermoid cyst | Scalp, face, neck | May connect to CNS if midline |
| Blue-purple/nodule | Cephalohematoma | Scalp | |
| Blue-purple/plaque | Venous malformation | Variable | Enlarges slowly over time |
| Yellow-orange/plaque | Nevus sebaceus | Scalp, face, neck | Basal cell carcinoma may arise within lesion |
| Yellow-orange/nodule | Congenital juvenile xanthogranuloma | Trunk | |
| Yellow-brown/papule or nodule | Mastocytoma | Variable | May become urticarial or blister |
| Hypertrichosis/plaque | Congenital melanocytic nevus | Scalp, trunk | |
| | Smooth muscle hamartoma | Trunk | |
| Hypertrichosis/tumor | Plexiform neurofibroma | Trunk most common | Associated with neurofibromatosis |
| White/patch | Nevus anemicus | Variable | |
| | Nevus depigmentosus | Variable | |

CNS, central nervous system.

Biopsy is indicated for any of the following:

Any lesion that is symptomatic (itching, bleeding, change in shape or color) for more than 2 weeks
Any lesion that continues to grow out of proportion to the growth of the child
Any nodular lesion that is growing
Something growing under a nail

CHAPTER **194**

# Hemangiomas and Vascular Malformations

**Birthmark** is a term that describes congenital anomalies of the skin. It should not be used as a definitive diagnosis because congenital skin lesions vary greatly in their appearance and prognosis (see Table 193-1).

Vascular lesions can be divided into two major categories: hemangiomas and vascular malformations. **Hemangiomas** are benign tumors resulting from proliferation of cells of the vascular endothelium and are characterized by a growth phase, marked by endothelial proliferation and hypercellularity, and by an involutional phase. Vascular malformations, however, are developmental defects derived from the capillary, venous, arterial, or lymphatic vessels. In contrast to hemangiomas, vascular malformations remain relatively static; growth is commensurate with growth of the child and there is no involution. Differentiating between these two entities is important because they have different prognoses and clinical implications.

## HEMANGIOMAS

Hemangiomas are the most common soft tissue tumors of infancy, occurring in approximately 5% to 10% of 1-year-old infants. True hemangiomas are characterized by a growth phase followed by a longer regression phase. Hemangiomas are heterogeneous; their appearance is dictated by the depth and location in the skin and by the stage of evolution. In newborns, hemangiomas may originate as a pale white macule with threadlike telangiectasia (superficial component). When the tumor proliferates, it assumes its most recognizable form as a bright red, slightly elevated, noncompressible plaque to a very elevated tumorlike growth

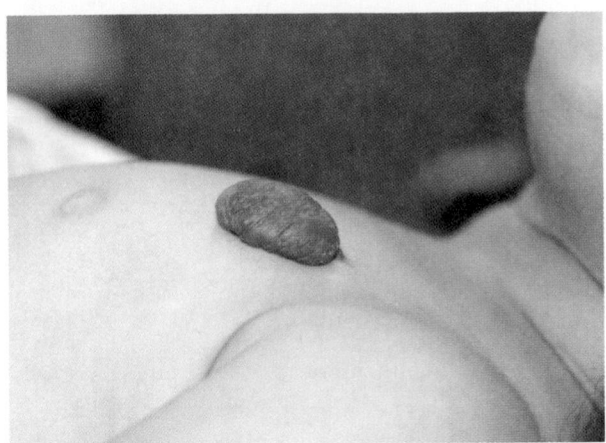

**FIGURE 194-1**

Hemangioma (chest).

(Fig. 194-1). Hemangiomas that lie deeper in the skin are soft, warm masses with a slightly bluish discoloration (deeper component). Frequently, hemangiomas have both a superficial and a deep component. They range from a few millimeters to several centimeters in diameter and are usually solitary; 20% involve multiple lesions. Hemangiomas occur predominantly in females (3:1) and have an increased incidence in premature infants. Approximately 55% are present at birth; the rest develop in the first weeks of life. Superficial hemangiomas reach their maximal size by 6 to 8 months, but deep hemangiomas may grow for 12 to 14 months. They then undergo slow, spontaneous resolution, which takes 3 to 10 years.

Despite the benign nature of most cutaneous hemangiomas, there may be the risk of functional compromise or permanent disfigurement depending on the location and extent. Ulceration, the most frequent complication, can be painful and increases the risk of infection, hemorrhage, and scarring.

**Periorbital hemangiomas** pose considerable risk to vision (amblyopia) and should be monitored carefully. Amblyopia can result from the hemangioma, causing obstruction of the visual axis or pressure on the globe, resulting in astigmatism. If there is any concern, the patient should have urgent evaluation by an ophthalmologist Treatment may be indicated to prevent blindness. Hemangiomas involving the ear may decrease auditory conduction, which ultimately may cause speech delay. Multiple cutaneous (diffuse hemangiomatosis) and large facial hemangiomas may be associated with visceral hemangiomas. **Subglottic hemangiomas** manifest as hoarseness and stridor; progression to respiratory failure may be rapid. Approximately 50% of affected infants have associated cutaneous hemangiomas; *noisy breathing* in an infant with a cutaneous hemangioma involving the chin, lips, mandibular region, and neck warrants direct visualization of the airway. Symptomatic airway hemangiomas develop in more than 50% of infants with extensive facial hemangiomas in the *beard* distribution. Hemangiomas in a segmental distribution, rather than a localized distribution, have a higher risk of complications.

Extensive cervicofacial hemangiomas may be associated with multiple anomalies, including *p*osterior fossa malformations, *h*emangiomas, *a*rterial anomalies, *c*oarctation of aorta and cardiac defects, and *e*ye abnormalities (**PHACE syndrome**). **Lumbosacral hemangiomas** suggest an occult spinal dysraphism with or without anorectal and urogenital anomalies. Imaging of the spine is indicated in all patients with midline cutaneous hemangiomas in the lumbosacral area.

Most hemangiomas do not necessitate medical intervention and involute spontaneously; however, if complications arise and treatment is warranted, oral systemic corticosteroids are the mainstay of therapy. Areas frequently associated with complications include periocular region, lip, nasal tip, beard, face (large facial lesions), groin, and buttocks.

## Pyogenic Granuloma

A pyogenic granuloma is an acquired, benign vascular tumor of toddlers and young children that occurs on the face in the periocular region and on the oral mucosa, hands, fingers, proximal upper extremity, and shoulders. Initially the lesions appear to be inconsequential as pink-red papules that often appear after minor trauma. The lesions can grow rapidly over a period of weeks to months to produce a bright red, vascular, often pedunculated papule measuring 2 to 10 mm. The lesions often have the appearance of granulation tissue and are very friable. When traumatized, these lesions may bleed profusely, often requiring emergent medical attention. Surgical excision is the most definitive treatment option, and pulsed dye laser can be useful for very small lesions.

## Port-Wine Stain (Nevus Flammeus)

Port-wine stains (nevus flammeus) are malformations of the superficial capillaries of the skin. These lesions are present at birth and should be considered permanent developmental defects. Port-wine stain lesions may be only a few millimeters in diameter or may cover extensive areas, occasionally involving half the body surface. They do not proliferate after birth; any apparent increase in size is caused by growth of the child. A port-wine stain may be localized to any body surface but facial lesions are the most common. They are pink-red, sharply demarcated macules and patches in infancy (Fig. 194-2). With time, they darken to a purple or *port-wine* color and may develop a pebbly or slightly thickened surface. Dilated vascular channels may form within the lesions and become symptomatic. More superficial vascular blebs may bleed. The most successful treatment modality in use is the pulsed dye laser, which can result in 80% to 90% improvement in these lesions after a series of treatment sessions and can avoid future complications associated with vascular dilation. Treatment is more effective if undertaken in infancy. Overgrowth of underlying bone can occur and is frequently seen with facial lesions. Affected patients often need maxillofacial intervention from malalignment that develops.

Most port-wine stains occur as isolated defects and do not indicate systemic malformations. Rarely, they may suggest ocular defects or specific neurocutaneous syndromes. **Sturge-Weber syndrome** (encephalotrigeminal angiomatosis) consists of a facial port-wine stain, usually in the cutaneous distribution of the first branch of the

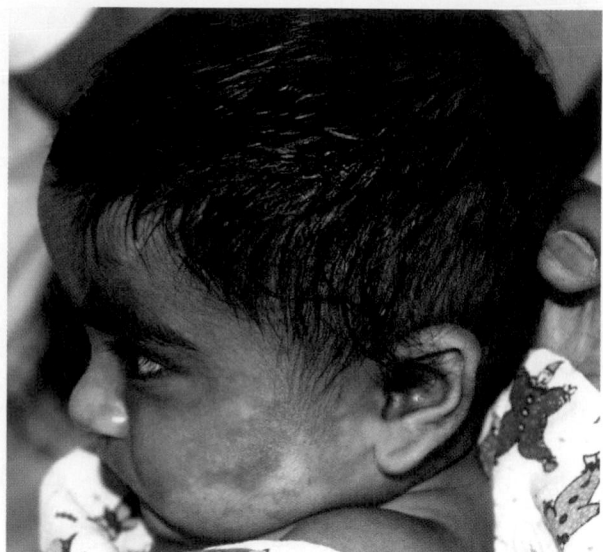

**FIGURE 194-2**

Port-wine stain (face).

trigeminal nerve; leptomeningeal angiomatosis; mental retardation; seizures; hemiparesis contralateral to the facial lesions; and ipsilateral intracortical calcification. Ocular manifestations are frequent and include buphthalmos, glaucoma, angioma of the choroid, hemianoptic defects, and optic atrophy. Anticonvulsant therapy and neurosurgical procedures have been of value in some patients. Glaucoma can occur in association with port-wine stains located on the eyelid, even in the absence of Sturge-Weber syndrome, and these patients need life-long monitoring of ocular pressures.

**Klippel-Trénaunay-Weber** syndrome is characterized by the triad of cutaneous capillary and venous malformations (usually a port-wine stain), venous varicosities, and hyperplasia of the soft tissues—and often bone—of the involved area. The lower limb is most commonly affected.

### Transient Macular Stains (Salmon Patches)

Transient macular stains (salmon patches, stork bite, angel's kiss) are variants of nevus flammeus that are present in 70% of normal newborns. They are red, irregular, macular patches resulting from dilation of dermal capillaries and usually are found on the nape of the neck, the eyelids, and the glabella. Most of the facial lesions fade by 1 year of age, but lesions on the neck may persist for life. Surveys of adult populations confirm the persistence of the nuchal lesions in approximately 25% of the population.

### EPIDERMAL NEVI/NEVUS SEBACEOUS

Epidermal nevi are a group of lesions that are found in the neonatal period. Most consist of an overgrowth of keratinocytes that often have an identifiable differentiation toward one of the cutaneous appendages. They vary considerably in size, clinical appearance, histologic characteristics, and evolution, depending on topographic location. Lesions occurring in sites normally rich in sebaceous glands (the scalp) may look like sebaceous nevi, whereas others that are found in areas where the epidermis is thick (the elbow) look primarily warty in nature. Unlike port-wine stains, these lesions don't progress and are not associated with elevated intraocular pressure or intracranial vascular lesions.

The most common type of epidermal nevus in a newborn is the nevus sebaceous, which is a hairless, papillomatous, yellow or pink, slightly elevated plaque on the scalp, forehead, or face. These lesions have a characteristic shape, often being oval or lancet-shaped. The lesions tend to thicken over time, especially during and after puberty, and are easily irritated with trauma. Because there is a significant incidence of basal cell epithelioma in these head or neck lesions after puberty, they are often removed surgically.

## CHAPTER 195

# Erythema Multiforme, Stevens-Johnson Syndrome, and Toxic Epidermal Necrolysis

Erythema multiforme (EM minor), Stevens-Johnson syndrome (SJS) (EM major), and toxic epidermal necrolysis (TEN) are acute hypersensitivity reactions characterized by cutaneous and mucosal necrosis. These disorders may represent a continuum of a clinical spectrum ranging from the well-localized lesions of EM to the serious and life-threatening extensive desquamation of TEN. These syndromes represent a T cell–mediated hypersensitivity reaction to a precipitating cause, usually infectious organisms or drugs. Infectious agents are associated more closely with eruptions of EM minor and SJS, whereas drugs are implicated with the more severe reactions of TEN. The differential diagnosis of vesiculobullous eruptions is listed in Table 195-1.

### ERYTHEMA MULTIFORME MINOR

EM minor is a common, self-limiting, acute hypersensitivity syndrome characterized by the abrupt onset of 1 to 3 cm, oval or round, deep red, well-demarcated, flat macules with a dusky gray or bullous center. Some of the lesions have a wheal-like appearance; in contrast to urticaria, these are fixed and represent epidermal cell necrosis rather than the transient tissue edema of urticaria. The classic **target lesion** consists of three concentric rings; the outermost is red, the intermediate is white, and the center is a dusky red or blue. If blistering occurs, it is mild and involves less than 10% of the body surface area. Mucous membrane involvement tends to be minimal and affects no more than one mucosal surface. Cutaneous lesions are symmetrical and involve the upper extremities, with the dorsal hands, palms, and extensor surfaces most commonly involved.

## TABLE 195-1 Vesiculobullous Eruptions

| Entity | Clinical Clues |
|---|---|
| **INFECTIOUS** | |
| *Bacterial* | |
| Staphylococcal scalded skin syndrome | Generalized, tender erythema |
| | Nikolsky sign |
| | Occasionally associated with underlying infection such as osteomyelitis, septic arthritis, pneumonia |
| | Desquamation, moist erosions observed |
| | More common in children younger than 5 years of age |
| Bullous impetigo | Localized benign staphylococcal scalded skin syndrome |
| *Viral* | |
| Herpes simplex | Grouped vesicles on erythematous base |
| | May be recurrent at same site—lips, eyes, cheeks, hands |
| | Reactivated by fever, sunlight, trauma, stress |
| | Positive Tzanck smear, herpes simplex virus culture |
| Varicella | Crops of vesicles on erythematous base ("dewdrops on rose petal") |
| | Highly contagious |
| | May see multiple stages of lesions simultaneously |
| | Associated with fever |
| | Positive Tzanck smear, varicella-zoster virus culture |
| Herpes zoster | Grouped vesicles on erythematous base limited to one or several adjacent dermatomes |
| | Usually unilateral |
| | Burning, pruritus |
| | Positive Tzanck smear, varicella-zoster culture |
| | Thoracic dermatomes most commonly involved in children |
| Hand-foot-mouth syndrome (coxsackievirus infection) | Prodrome of fever, anorexia, sore throat |
| | Oval blisters in acral distribution, usually few in number |
| | Shallow oval oral lesions on erythematous base |
| | Highly infectious |
| | Peak incidence in late summer and in fall |
| **HYPERSENSITIVITY** | |
| Erythema multiforme major (Stevens-Johnson syndrome) | Prodrome of fever, headache, malaise, sore throat, cough, vomiting, diarrhea |
| | Involvement of two mucosal surfaces, usually seen as hemorrhagic crusts on lips |
| | Target lesions progress from central vesiculation to extensive epidermal necrosis; may have sheets of denuded skin |
| | Associated with infections and drugs |
| Toxic epidermal necrolysis | Possible extension of erythema multiforme major involving >30% of body surface |
| | Severe exfoliative dermatitis |
| | Older children and adults |
| | Frequently related to drugs (e.g., sulfonamides, anticonvulsants) |
| | Nikolsky sign |
| **EXTRINSIC** | |
| Contact dermatitis | Irritant or allergic |
| | Distribution dependent on the irritant or allergen |
| | Distribution helpful in establishing diagnosis |
| Insect bites | Occur occasionally following flea or mosquito bites |
| | May be hemorrhagic bullae |
| | Often in linear or irregular clusters |
| | Very pruritic |
| Burns | Irregular shapes and configurations |
| | May be suggestive of abuse |
| | Range in severity from first- to third-degree, bullae with second- and third-degree injuries |
| Friction | Usually on acral surfaces |
| | May be related to footwear |
| | Often activity-related |

*Continued*

| TABLE 195-1 Vesiculobullous Eruptions—cont'd | |
|---|---|
| Entity | Clinical Clues |
| **MISCELLANEOUS** | |
| Urticaria pigmentosa | Positive Darier sign |
| | Frequently hyperpigmented |
| | Usually manifests during infancy |
| | Dermatographism commonly seen |
| Miliaria crystallina | Clean, 1- to 2-mm superficial vesicles occurring in crops, rupture spontaneously |
| | Intertriginous areas, especially neck and axillae |
| Hereditary: epidermolysis bullosa, incontinentia pigmenti, epidermolytic hyperkeratosis | |
| Autoimmune: linear IgA disease, bullous pemphigoid, dermatitis herpetiformis | |

From Nopper AJ, Rabinowotz RG: Rashes and skin lesions. In Kliegman RM (ed): Practical Strategies in Pediatric Diagnosis and Therapy. Philadelphia, *WB Saunders*, 1996.

EM minor is less severe than SJS and accounts for nearly 80% of EM cases. Most EM cases in children are precipitated by herpes simplex virus infection and may recur with each episode of inapparent herpes infection. A positive clinical history of herpes labialis is obtained in 50% of cases. Herpes simplex virus DNA is detected in 80% of children with EM, suggesting that it is the primary cause of EM minor in children. Symptomatic treatment is usually sufficient. Oral antihistamines help suppress pruritus, stinging, and burning. The use of systemic corticosteroids is controversial and usually not indicated. Children with recurrent lesions associated with documented herpes simplex virus infections may be candidates for prophylactic oral acyclovir. The prognosis is excellent, with most lesions lasting no more than 2 weeks. Healing occurs without scarring.

## STEVENS-JOHNSON SYNDROME (ERYTHEMA MULTIFORME MAJOR)

Stevens-Johnson syndrome is a severe, life-threatening, blistering hypersensitivity reaction. It is usually preceded by a febrile respiratory illness 1 to 14 days before the onset of cutaneous lesions. Involvement of at least two mucous membrane surfaces is required for diagnosis and is a distinguishing characteristic from EM minor. Children have extreme irritability, anorexia, and fever. The upper and lower lips are swollen and bright red with erosions and hemorrhagic crusts. Erosions of the tongue, buccal mucosa, and gingival margin may be seen. The eyelids are usually swollen. Early in the disease process, there is bilateral conjunctival injection; however, this usually progresses to conjunctival erosions. There may be erosions of the vaginal or perianal mucosa. Urogenital, esophageal, and tracheal surfaces may be involved in the most severe cases. The extent of skin involvement varies. There may be mucosal lesions only or a combination of mucosal and skin lesions. Red macules and target-like lesions appear suddenly and tend to coalesce into large patches, with a predominant distribution over the face and trunk. Skin lesions evolve rapidly into bullae and areas of necrosis. The extent of epidermal detachment is 10% to 20% of the body surface area.

Drugs and *Mycoplasma pneumoniae* infections are the most common causes of SJS in children. Herpes simplex virus seems to have no role in the pathogenesis of SJS. Other precipitating factors are other viral infections, bacterial infections, syphilis, and deep fungal infections. The most common drugs implicated are nonsteroidal anti-inflammatory drugs (NSAIDs), followed by sulfonamides, anticonvulsants, penicillins, and tetracycline derivatives.

SJS occurs in children 2 to 18 years old and seems to be more common in younger patients than EM. The diagnosis of SJS is clinical; there are no diagnostic tests. Confusion with Kawasaki disease and bacterial toxin-mediated diseases (scarlet fever, toxic shock syndrome, and staphylococcal scalded skin syndrome) may occur. Patients with Kawasaki disease have conjunctival injection and hyperemia of the mucous membranes. Necrosis of the mucosal surfaces does not occur; blistering, erosions, and severe crusting are not observed. The mucosal changes of staphylococcal scalded skin syndrome are minor, and frank erosions are not present. The blistering of the skin is superficial and involves larger areas of the face and intertriginous regions. Other rheumatologic disorders usually can be excluded by their chronic, less abrupt course.

SJS is a serious illness with a 5% to 15% mortality rate. Discontinuation of the offending agent, pain management, and supportive care are the mainstays of therapy. Children with severe intraoral pain, resulting in poor oral intake, often require prolonged hospitalization. Parenteral or nasogastric feeding should be instituted early to accelerate the healing process. Careful fluid management and monitoring of electrolytes are essential. Skin cultures for potential infections should be performed. Appropriate parenteral antibiotics should be given if warranted. Use of systemic corticosteroids has not been shown to be beneficial and may increase risk of morbidity and death.

The most common serious long-term sequelae of SJS involve ocular complications. Keratitis, corneal ulcerations, uveitis, severe conjunctivitis, and panophthalmitis may occur, leading to partial or complete blindness. Emergent ophthalmology consultation with close follow-up is essential.

## TOXIC EPIDERMAL NECROLYSIS

TEN is a severe, life-threatening condition characterized by extensive skin necrosis equivalent to a second-degree burn. It is on the same clinical spectrum with SJS, and patients who present with SJS may progress to TEN. It is distinguished from EM minor and SJS by greater body surface area involvement (>30%) and massive, sheetlike denudation of skin (Fig. 195-1). Typically, more than 50% of the body surface area is affected. Individual lesions of TEN overlap with lesions of EM, but are more abrupt in occurrence and evolution. Intraepidermal blistering is suggested by the **Nikolsky sign**, which is elicited by slight pressure along the skin and demonstrates an absence of cohesion between the keratinocytes of the superficial epidermis so that the separated layers easily slip laterally with minimal pressure. The children have exquisite pain of their skin and appear toxic. The dusky redness rapidly progresses into sheetlike peeling of the entire epidermis, leaving deep erosions.

Nonsteroidal anti-inflammatory drugs, particularly ibuprofen and naproxen, are the most common precipitating factors. Sulfonamides, anticonvulsants, penicillins, and tetracyclines also have been reported to cause TEN. Infections can be associated with the development of TEN.

TEN is a severe disease with a mortality rate of 30% to 50%. Supportive care with aggressive fluid and electrolyte management, wound care, and pain control results in decreased morbidity and mortality rates. Superinfection and respiratory failure are the major causes of death. Severely affected children may benefit from the wound care expertise of a burn unit. The use of systemic corticosteroids is controversial and is thought to increase the risk of infection and decrease wound healing. Intravenous immunoglobulin and cyclosporine have been used with encouraging results; controlled studies have not been performed.

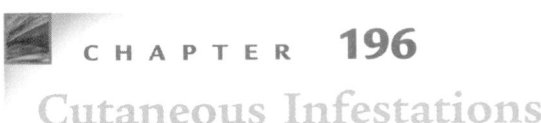

## CHAPTER 196
# Cutaneous Infestations

Arthropods are common in the environment. Although many can bite or sting humans, only a few infest humans. Arachnids (mites) are the most common, parasitizing humans and animals by burrowing into the skin and depositing eggs within the skin.

## SCABIES

### Etiology and Epidemiology

Scabies is caused by the mite *Sarcoptes scabiei*. The female mite burrows into the epidermis and deposits her eggs, which mature in 10 to 14 days. The disease is highly contagious because infested humans do not manifest the typical signs or symptoms for 3 to 4 weeks, facilitating transmission. An immunocompetent person with scabies typically harbors 10 to 20 mites.

Scabies is the most common human infestation, affecting at least 300 million persons worldwide.

### Clinical Manifestations

The clinical presentation varies depending on the age of the patient, duration of infestation, and immune status of the patient. Severe and paroxysmal itching is the hallmark, with complaints of itching that is frequently worse than the eruption would suggest. Most children exhibit an eczematous eruption composed of red, excoriated papules and nodules. The classic linear papule or burrow is often difficult to find. Distribution is the most diagnostic finding; the papules are found in the axillae, umbilicus, groin, penis, instep of the foot, and web spaces of the fingers and toes (Fig. 196-1). Infants infested with scabies have diffuse erythema, scaling, and pinpoint papules. Pustules and vesicles are much more common in infants and are found in the axillae and groin and on the palms and soles. The face and scalp usually are spared in adults and older children, but these areas are usually involved in infants. Nodular lesions may occur on the trunk, axillary regions, or genitalia and can represent active infection or prolonged hypersensitivity lesions following resolution of infestation. Chronic lesions may develop a malodorous, scaly crust. Immunocompromised or neurologically impaired persons may develop a severe form of the disease known as **Norwegian** or **crusted scabies**, with infestation of 2 million live mites at one time.

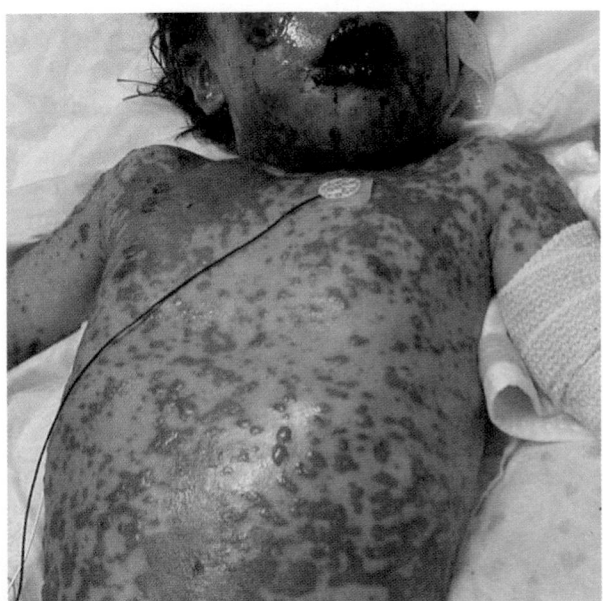

**FIGURE 195-1**

Toxic epidermal necrolysis (chest and abdomen).

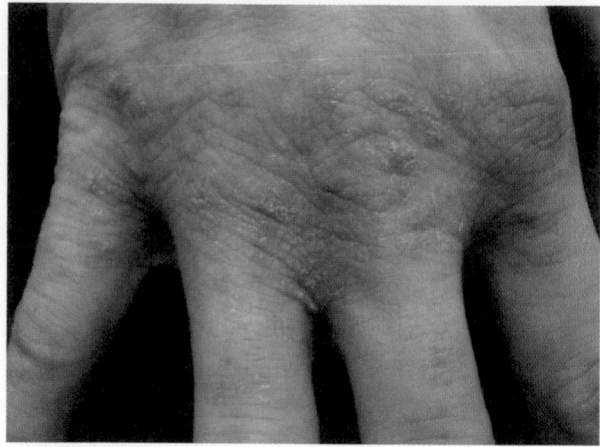

**FIGURE 196-1**

Scabies (hand).

## Laboratory and Imaging Studies

The diagnosis of scabies can be confirmed by microscopic visualization of the mite, eggs, larvae, or feces in scrapings of papules or burrows examined under oil immersion. Skin biopsy is rarely necessary but may be useful if lesions have become nodular.

The diagnosis of scabies should be considered in any child with severe itching. A thorough search for an infested contact should be undertaken.

## Treatment

Curative treatment is achieved by a 12-hour (overnight) application of permethrin 5% cream applied to the entire body, which may be repeated 1 week later if necessary. Gamma benzene hexachloride should be avoided in young children because of a small risk of central nervous system (CNS) toxicity. Parents and all caregivers should be treated simultaneously. Itching persists for 7 to 14 days after the mites have been killed and may continue for up to 6 weeks. Bed linens, towels, pajamas, and clothes worn for the previous 2 days before treatment should be machine-washed in hot water and machine-dried using high heat. Heat is the most effective scabicide. Items that are not washable may be dry-cleaned or placed in a sealed plastic bag for 7 days.

## Complications and Prognosis

Secondary bacterial infection may occur but is uncommon. Scabies can be much more severe among immunocompromised persons. In contrast to the pediculoses, scabies is not a vector for infections.

Pruritus may persist for 7 to 14 days after successful therapy because of a prolonged hypersensitivity reaction, which does not indicate treatment failure. Inadequate treatment or reinfestation should be suspected if new lesions develop after treatment.

## Prevention

The family should be educated about the mode of scabies transmission. Mites live only a short time off the body and extensive fumigation is not necessary.

## PEDICULOSES

### Etiology

Three species of lice infest humans: *Pediculus humanus capitis*, the **head louse**; *Pthirus pubis*, the **pubic louse** or **crab louse**; and *Pediculus humanus humanus*, (also known as *Pediculus humanus corporis*), the **body louse**. Lice are wingless insects 2 to 4 mm in length that cannot fly or jump. Transmission usually occurs by direct contact with the head of another infested individual. Indirect spread through contact with fomites or personal belongings, such as hairbrushes, combs, or caps, is much less frequent.

Pediculosis differs from scabies infestation in that the louse resides on the hair or clothing and intermittently feeds on the host by piercing the skin. The *bite* causes small urticarial papules and itching. Head lice live close to the skin and may live for 30 days, depositing 100 to 400 eggs as **nits** on hair shafts, usually within 6 mm of the scalp.

### Epidemiology

Head lice are seen most frequently in early school-age children. Head lice infestations are unrelated to hygiene and are not more common among children with long hair or with dirty hair. It is estimated that 6 to 12 million persons in the United States and 1% to 3% of persons in developed countries are infested with head lice each year. In the United States, head lice infestation is rare among African Americans and may be more common in girls, which is attributed to their tendency to play more closely with one another than boys do.

Pubic lice are transmitted by sexual contact. Their presence in children may be a sign of child abuse. Body lice are firm evidence of poor hygiene, such as infrequent washing and clothing changes.

### Clinical Manifestations

Itching, if present, is the primary symptom. Pediculosis capitis usually causes pruritus behind the ears or on the nape of the neck or a crawling sensation in the scalp. Pediculosis pubis usually causes mild to severe pruritus in the groin. Eyelash involvement in children may cause crusting and blepharitis. Pediculosis corporis causes pruritus that, because of repeated scratching, may result in lichenification or secondary bacterial infection. Excoriations and crusting, with or without associated regional lymphadenopathy, may be present.

### Laboratory and Imaging Studies

No laboratory or imaging studies are necessary.

### Differential Diagnosis

Infestation with the head louse may be asymptomatic and has little morbidity. The diagnosis can be confirmed by visualizing a live louse. A fine-toothed comb to trap lice is more effective than simply looking at the hair. Wet combing is more time-consuming, but dry combing produces static that may propel the lice away from the comb.

Nits represent the outer casing of the louse ova. Viable nits have an intact operculum (cap) on the nonattached end and a developing louse within the egg. **Brown nits** located on the proximal hair shaft suggest active infestation. **White nits** located on the hair shaft 4 cm or farther from the scalp indicate previous infestation. Because nonviable nits can remain stuck in the hair for weeks to months after an infestation has resolved, many children with nits do not have active lice infestation.

### Treatment

The treatment of head lice is controversial because of resistance to many established options. Over-the-counter permethrin (1%) and pyrethrin-based products (0.17–0.33%) are the first choices of therapy. Because 20% to 30% of eggs may survive one treatment, a second treatment should be applied in 7 to 10 days. The prevalence of drug resistance has not been determined. Malathion (0.5%) lotion may be used as an alternative for resistant cases.

Everyone in the family should be checked for head lice and treated if live lice are found to reduce the risk of reinfestation. Bed linens, towels, pajamas, and clothes worn for the previous 2 days before treatment should be machine-washed in hot water and machine-dried using high heat. Items that are not washable may be dry-cleaned or placed in a sealed plastic bag for 2 weeks. Brushes and combs should be soaked in dish detergent or rubbing alcohol for 1 hour. Rugs, furniture, mattresses, and car seats should be vacuumed thoroughly.

The finding of active lice infestation indicates their presence for 1 month or more. Manual removal of nits after treatment is not necessary to prevent spread. Children treated for head lice should return to school immediately after completion of the first effective treatment or first wet combing, regardless of the presence of remaining nits. There is no evidence that *no nit* or *nit-free* policies reduce transmission of head lice. If required for return to school, nit removal is best achieved by wetting the hair and combing with a fine-toothed metal comb.

### Complications

Excoriations can become secondarily infected with skin bacteria, usually *Staphylococcus* and *Streptococcus*. The body louse functions as a vector for potentially serious infectious diseases, including **epidemic typhus**, caused by *Rickettsia prowazekii*; **louse-borne relapsing fever**, caused by *Borrelia recurrentis*; and **trench fever**, caused by *Bartonella quintana*. These louse-borne infections are rare in the United States. In contrast to body lice, head lice and pubic lice are not associated with transmission of other infections.

### Prognosis and Prevention

Pediculicide treatment along with appropriate disinfestation measures of fomites is highly effective. Reinfestation from untreated contacts or fomites, especially for pediculosis corporis, is more likely than primary treatment failure.

Families, school nurses, and other health care professionals need to be educated about the mode of transmission and precise diagnosis before treatment of contacts is instituted. There is no evidence that group screening is effective.

## SUGGESTED READING

Callen J, Chamlin S, Eichenfield LE, et al: A systematic review of the safety of topical therapies for atopic dermatitis, *Br J Dermatol* 156:203–221, 2007.

Eichenfield LE, Esterly NB, Frieden IJ: Textbook of Neonatal Dermatology, 2nd ed, Philadelphia, 2008, *WB Saunders*.

Oranje A, Harper J, Prose N: Textbook of Pediatric Dermatology, 22nd ed, Hoboken, NJ, 2006, *John Wiley*.

Paller AS, Mancini AJ: Hurwitz Clinical Pediatric Dermatology, 3rd ed, Philadelphia, 2006, *WB Saunders*.

Palmer CM, Lyon VB: Stepwise approach to topical therapy for atopic dermatitis, *Clin Pediatr* 47:423–434, 2008.

Sundine MJ, Wirth GA: Hemangiomas: An overview, *Clin Pediatr* 46:206–221, 2007.

CHAPTER 197

# Orthopedics Assessment

To care for the pediatric patient, one must understand the growth and development of the musculoskeletal system as well as common orthopedic terms (Table 197-1). Practitioners should recognize common mechanisms for congenital and acquired orthopedic disorders (Table 197-2).

## GROWTH AND DEVELOPMENT

The ends of the long bones contain a much higher proportion of cartilage in the skeletally immature patient than an adult (Figs. 197-1 and 197-2). The high cartilage content allows for a unique vulnerability from trauma and infection (particularly in the metaphysis).

The physis is responsible for the longitudinal growth of the long bones. Articular cartilage allows the ends of the bone to enlarge and accounts for growth of smaller bones, such as the tarsals. The periosteum can provide circumferential growth. Trauma, infection, nutritional deficiency (rickets), inborn errors of metabolism (mucopolysaccharidoses), and other metabolic disorders (renal tubular acidosis, hypothyroid) may affect each of the growth processes and produce distinct aberrations.

## DEVELOPMENTAL MILESTONES

Neurologic maturation, marked by achievement of developmental motor milestones, is important for normal musculoskeletal development (see Section 2). A neurologic disorder may cause a secondary musculoskeletal abnormality (e.g., extremity contractures in Duchenne muscular dystrophy). Thus, normal motor development must be included in the definition of a normal musculoskeletal system.

| TABLE 197-1 Common Orthopedic Terminology | |
|---|---|
| Abduction | Movement away from midline |
| Adduction | Movement toward or across midline |
| Apophysis | Bone growth center that has a muscular insertion but is not considered a growth plate (*example*: tibial tubercle) |
| Arthroscopy | Surgical exploration of a joint using an arthroscope |
| Arthroplasty | Surgical reconstruction of a joint |
| Arthrotomy | Surgical incision into a joint; an "open" procedure |
| Deformation | Changes in limb, trunk, or head due to mechanical force |
| Dislocation | Displacement of bones at a joint |
| Equinus | Plantar flexion of the forefoot, hindfoot, or entire foot |
| Femoral anteversion | Increased angulation of the femoral head and neck with respect to the frontal plane |
| Malformation | Defect in development that occurs during fetal life (*example*: syndactyly) |
| Osteotomy | Surgical division of a bone |
| Pes cavus | High medial arch of the foot |
| Pes planus | Flat foot |
| Rotation, internal | Inward rotation (toward midline) |
| Rotation, external | Outward rotation (away from midline) |
| Subluxation | Incomplete loss of contact between two joint surfaces |
| Tibial torsion | Rotation of the tibia in an internal or external fashion |
| Valgus/valgum | Angulation of a bone or joint in which the apex is toward the midline (*example*: knock-knee) |
| Varus/varum | Angulation of a bone or joint in which the apex is away from the midline (*example*: bowlegs) |

**TABLE 197-2  Mechanisms of Common Pediatric Orthopedic Problems**

| Category | Mechanism | Example(s) |
|---|---|---|
| | **CONGENITAL** | |
| Malformation | Teratogenesis before 12 weeks of gestation | Spina bifida |
| Disruption | Amniotic band constriction | Extremity amputation |
| | Fetal varicella infection | Limb scar/atrophy |
| Deformation | Leg compression | Developmental dysplasia of the hip (DDH) |
| | Neck compression | Torticollis |
| Dysplasia | Abnormal cell growth or metabolism | Osteogenesis imperfecta |
| | | Skeletal dysplasias |
| | **ACQUIRED** | |
| Infection | Pyogenic-hematogenous spread | Septic arthritis, osteomyelitis |
| Inflammation | Antigen-antibody reaction | Systemic lupus erythematosus |
| | Immune mediated | Juvenile rheumatoid arthritis |
| Trauma | Mechanical forces, overuse | Child abuse, sports injuries, unintentional injury, fractures, dislocations, tendinitis |
| Tumor | Primary bone tumor | Osteosarcoma |
| | Metastasis to bone from other site | Neuroblastoma |
| | Bone marrow tumor | Leukemia, lymphoma |

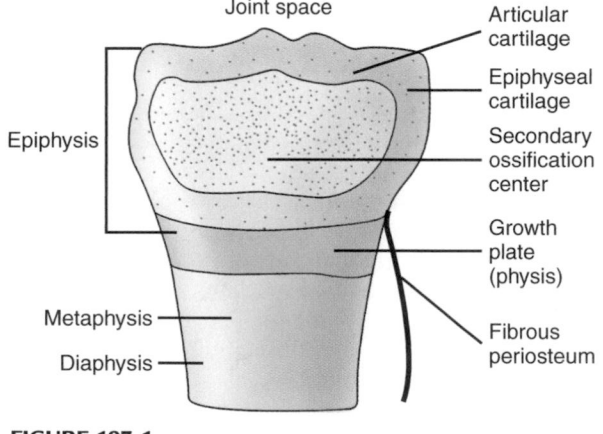

**FIGURE 197-1**

Schematic of long bone structure.

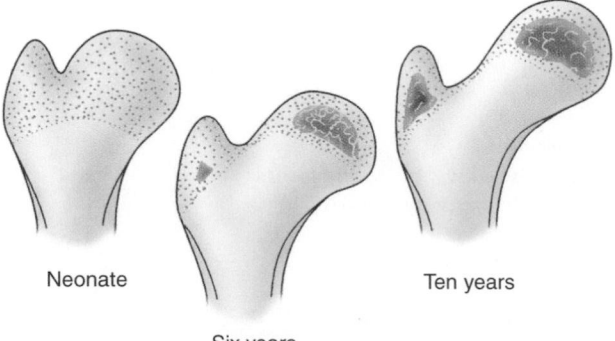

**FIGURE 197-2**

The ends of long bones at various ages. Lightly stippled areas represent cartilage composition, whereas heavily darkened areas are zones of ossification. (From Tachjidan MO: Congenital Dislocation of the Hip. New York, *Churchill Livingtone*, 1982, p 105.)

## Infants

The in utero position of the fetus produces joint and muscle contractures that can affect the angular and torsional alignment (temporary or permanent) of the skeletal system, especially of the lower extremity (Fig. 197-3). The newborn's hips are externally rotated. Pes planus and genu varum are common. Infants are usually born with a flexed posture. These contractures usually decrease to neutral within the first 4 to 6 months. The foot is often flat and *tucked under* at birth; the ankle will be inverted and the forefoot is adducted when compared with the hindfoot. The lateral border of the foot must straighten out, even with dorsiflexion, to be considered secondary to in utero positioning.

The head and neck may also be distorted by in utero positioning. The spine and upper extremities are less likely to be affected. By the age of 3 to 4 years, the effects of in utero positioning have usually resolved.

## Gait

Normal gait has a stance phase and swing phase; each leg should have symmetrical timing with each phase. The stance phase represents 60% of the gait and begins with foot contact (usually the heel strike) and ends with the toe-off. During the swing phase (40%), the foot is off the ground. The gait cycle is the interval between stance phases on the same limb.

Toddlers will generally walk independently by 18 months of age. Their broad-based gait is usually inconsistent and is characterized by short, rapid steps and does not have the reciprocal arm swing. Gait coordination improves over time and a normal gait is usually achieved by the time a child enters elementary school. An excessively clumsy 3- or 4-year-old should spark concerns for muscular dystrophy.

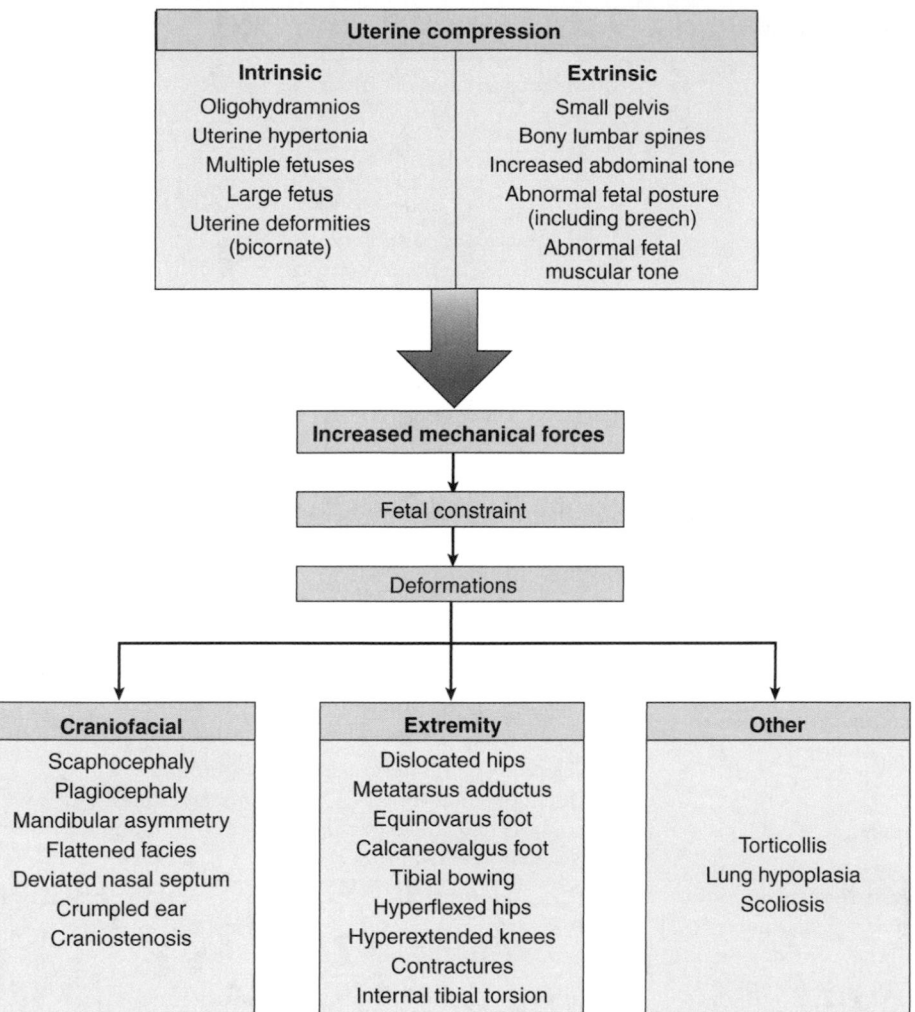

**FIGURE 197-3**

Deformation abnormalities resulting from uterine compression.

## The Limping Child

The differential diagnosis for a limping child is often categorized by age and painful or painless limp (Table 197-3). An **antalgic gait** is a painful limp; the stance phase and stride of the affected limb are shortened to decrease the discomfort of weight bearing on the affected limb. The **Trendelenburg gait** has a normal stance phase, but excessive swaying of the trunk. The gluteus medius muscle stabilizes the pelvis during the stance phase, preventing the pelvis from dropping toward the leg in swing phase. Trauma or weakness of the gluteal muscles is a common cause of painless limp. **Waddling gait** refers to a bilateral decrease in function of the gluteus muscles.

| **TABLE 197-3  Differential Diagnosis of Limping in Children** | |
| --- | --- |
| **Age Group** | **Diagnostic Considerations** |
| Early walker: 1 to 3 years of age | *Painful Limp* |
| | Septic arthritis and osteomyelitis |
| | Transient monarticular synovitis |
| | Occult trauma ("toddler's fracture") |
| | Intervertebral diskitis |
| | Malignancy |
| | *Painless Limp* |
| | Developmental dysplasia of the hip |
| | Neuromuscular disorder |
| |    Cerebral palsy |
| | Lower extremity length inequality |

*Continued*

**TABLE 197-3 Differential Diagnosis of Limping in Children—cont'd**

| Age Group | Diagnostic Considerations |
|---|---|
| Child: 3 to 10 years of age | *Painful Limp*<br>Septic arthritis, osteomyelitis, myositis<br>Transient monarticular synovitis<br>Trauma<br>Rheumatologic disorders<br>  Juvenile rheumatoid arthritis<br>Intervertebral diskitis<br>Malignancy<br>*Painless Limp*<br>Developmental dysplasia of the hip<br>Legg-Calvé-Perthes disease<br>Lower extremity length inequality<br>Neuromuscular disorder<br>    Cerebral palsy<br>    Muscular dystrophy (Duchenne) |
| Adolescent: 11 years of age to maturity | *Painful Limp*<br>Septic arthritis, osteomyelitis, myositis<br>Trauma<br>Rheumatologic disorder<br>Slipped capital femoral epiphysis: acute; unstable<br>Malignancy<br>*Painless Limp*<br>Slipped capital femoral epiphysis: chronic; stable<br>Developmental dysplasia of the hip: acetabular dysplasia<br>Lower extremity length inequality<br>Neuromuscular disorder |

**Toe walking** is a common complaint in early walkers. Any child older than 3 years of age who still toe walks should be evaluated by a physician. Although it may result from habit, a neuromuscular disorder (cerebral palsy, tethered cord), Achilles tendon contracture (heel cord tightness), or a leg-length discrepancy may be present.

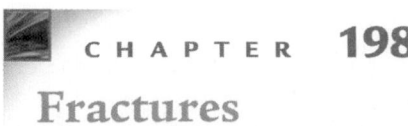

# CHAPTER 198

# Fractures

Fractures account for 10% to 15% of all childhood injuries. The anatomic, biomechanical, and physiologic differences in children account for unique fracture patterns and management. Fracture terminology helps describe fractures (Table 198-1).

The pediatric skeleton has a higher proportion of cartilage and a thicker, stronger, and more active periosteum capable of producing a larger callus more rapidly than in an adult. The thick periosteum may decrease the rate of displaced fractures and stabilize fractures after reduction. Because of the higher proportion of cartilage, the

skeletally immature patient can withstand more force before deformation or fracture than adult bone. As children mature into adolescence, the rate of healing slows and approaches that of adults.

## PEDIATRIC FRACTURE PATTERNS

### Buckle Fractures

The buckle or torus fracture occurs after compression of the bone; the bony cortex does not truly break. These fractures will typically occur in the metaphysis and are stable fractures that heal in approximately 4 weeks with immobilization. A common example is a fall onto an outstretched arm causing a buckle fracture in the distal radius.

**Complete fractures** occur when both sides of bony cortex are fractured. This is the most common fracture and may be classified as comminuted, oblique, transverse, or spiral, depending on the direction of the fracture line.

**Greenstick fractures** occur when a bone is angulated beyond the limits of plastic deformation. The bone fails on the tension side and sustains a bend deformity on the compression side. The force is insufficient to cause a complete fracture (Fig. 198-1).

**Bowing fractures** demonstrate no fracture line evident on radiographs, but the bone is bent beyond its limit of plastic deformation. This is not a true fracture, but will heal with periosteal reaction.

| TABLE 198-1 Useful Fracture Terminology | |
|---|---|
| Complete | The bone fragments separate completely |
| Incomplete | The bone fragments are still partially joined |
| Linear | Referring to a fracture line that is parallel to the bone's long axis |
| Transverse | Referring to a fracture line that is at a right angle to the bone's long axis |
| Oblique | Referring to a fracture line that is diagonal to the bone's long axis |
| Spiral | Referring to a twisting fracture (can be associated with child abuse) |
| Comminution | A fracture that results in several fragments |
| Compaction | The bone fragments are driven into each other |
| Angulation | The fragments have angular malalignment |
| Rotation | The fragments have rotational malalignment |
| Shortening | The fractured ends of the bones overlap |
| Open | A fracture in which the bone has pierced the skin |

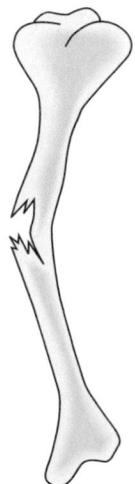

**FIGURE 198-1**

**The greenstick fracture is an incomplete fracture.** (Modified from White N, Sty R: Radiological evaluation and classification of pediatric fractures. *Clin Pediatr Emerg Med* 3:94–105, 2002.)

## Epiphyseal Fractures

Fractures involving the growth plate constitute about 20% of all fractures in the skeletally immature patient. These fractures are more common in males (2:1 male-female ratio). The peak incidence is 13 to 14 years in boys and 11 to 12 years in girls. The distal radius, distal tibia, and distal fibula are the most common locations.

Ligaments frequently insert onto epiphyses. Thus traumatic forces to an extremity may be transmitted to the physis, which is not as biomechanically strong as the metaphysis, so it may fracture with mechanisms of injury that may cause sprains in the adult. The growth plate is most susceptible to torsional and angular forces.

Physeal fractures are described using **Salter-Harris classification**, which allows for prognostic information regarding premature closure of the growth plate and poor

functional outcomes. The higher the type number, the more likely the patient will have complications. There are five main groups (Fig. 198-2):

Type I – transverse fracture through the physis, growth disturbance is unusual

Type II – fracture through a portion of the physis and metaphysis, most common type of Salter-Harris fracture (75%)

Type III – fracture through a portion of the physis and epiphysis into the joint that may result in complication because of intra-articular component and because of disruption of the growing or hypertrophic zone of the physis

Type IV – fracture through the metaphysis, physis, and epiphysis with a high risk of complication

Type V – a crush injury to the physis with a poor functional prognosis

Types I and II fractures can often be managed by closed reduction and do not require perfect alignment. A major exception is the type II fracture of the distal femur which is associated with a poor outcome unless proper anatomic alignment is obtained. Types III and IV fractures require anatomic alignment for successful treatment. Type V fractures can be difficult to diagnose and often result in premature closure of the physis.

## MANAGEMENT OF PEDIATRIC FRACTURES

The majority of pediatric fractures can be managed with closed methods. Some fractures need closed reduction to improve alignment. Approximately 4% of pediatric fractures require internal fixation. Patients with open physes are more likely to require internal fixation if they have one of the following fractures:

Displaced epiphyseal fractures
Displaced intra-articular fractures
Fractures in a child with multiple injuries
Open fractures
Unstable fractures

The goal of internal fixation is to improve and maintain anatomic alignment. This is usually done with Kirschner wires, Steinmann pins, and cortical screws with subsequent external immobilization in a cast until healing is satisfactory. After healing, the hardware is frequently removed to prevent incorporation into the callus and prevent physeal damage.

External fixation without casting is often necessary for pelvic and open fractures. Fractures associated with soft tissue loss, burns, and neurovascular damage benefit from external fixation.

## SPECIAL CONCERNS

### Remodeling

Fracture remodeling occurs because of a combination of periosteal resorption and new bone formation. Many pediatric fractures do not need perfect anatomic alignment for proper healing. Younger patients have greater potential

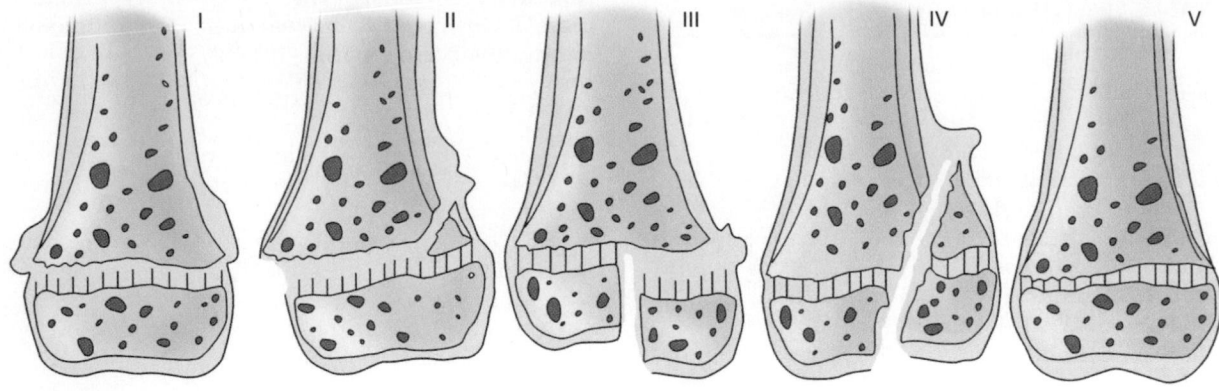

**FIGURE 198-2**

**The types of growth plate injury as classified by Salter and Harris.** See text for descriptions of types I to V. (From Salter RB, Harris WR: Injuries involving the epiphyseal plate. *J Bone Joint Surg Am* 45:587, 1963.)

for fracture remodeling. Fractures that occur in the metaphysis, near the growth plate, may undergo more remodeling. Fractures angulated in the plane of motion also remodel very well. Intra-articular fractures, angulated or displaced diaphyseal fractures, rotated fractures, and fracture deformity not in the plane of motion, tend not to remodel as well.

## Overgrowth

Overgrowth occurs in long bones as the result of increased blood flow associated with fracture healing. Femoral fractures in children younger than 10 years of age will frequently overgrow 1 to 3 cm. This is the reason end-to-end alignment for femur and long bone fractures may not be indicated. After 10 years of age, overgrowth is less of a problem, so end-to-end alignment is recommended.

## Progressive Deformity

Fractures and injuries to the physis can result in premature closure. If it is a partial closure, the consequence may be an angular deformity. If it is a complete closure, limb shortening may occur. The most commonly affected locations are the distal femur and tibia, and the proximal tibia.

## Neurovascular Injury

Fractures and dislocations may damage adjacent blood vessels and nerves. The most common location is the distal humerus (**supracondylar fracture**) and the knee (dislocation and physeal fracture). It is necessary to perform and document a careful neurovascular examination distal to the fracture (pulse, sensory, and motor function).

## Compartment Syndrome

Compartment syndrome is an orthopedic emergency that results from hemorrhage and soft tissue swelling within the tight fascial compartments of an extremity. This can result in muscle ischemia and neurovascular compromise unless it is surgically decompressed. The most common sites are the lower leg (tibial fracture) and arm (supracondylar fracture).

Affected patients have severe pain and decreased sensation in the dermatomes supplied by the nerves located in the compartment. Swollen and tight compartments and pain with passive stretching are present. This can happen underneath a cast and may actually occur when a cast is applied too tightly. It is important to educate all patients with fractures on the signs of ischemia and ensure they realize it is an emergency.

## Toddler's Fracture

This is an oblique fracture of the distal tibia without a fibula fracture. There is often no significant trauma. Patients are usually 1 to 3 years old, but can be as old as 6 and present with limping and pain with weight bearing. There may be minimal swelling and pain. Initial radiographs do not always show the fracture; if symptoms persist, a repeat x-ray in 7 to 10 days may be helpful.

## Child Abuse

Child abuse must always be considered in the differential diagnosis of a child with fractures, especially in those younger than 3 years (see Chapter 22). Common fracture patterns that should increase the index of suspicion include multiple fractures in different stages of radiographic healing, spiral fractures of the long bones (forcible twisting of extremity), metaphyseal corner fractures (shaking), fractures too severe for the history, or fractures in nonambulatory infants.

When there is concern for child abuse, the child should have a full evaluation, which may include admission to the hospital. A thorough and well-documented physical examination should focus on soft tissue injuries, the cranium, and a funduscopic examination for retinal hemorrhages or detachment. A skeletal survey or a bone scan may be helpful in identifying other fractures.

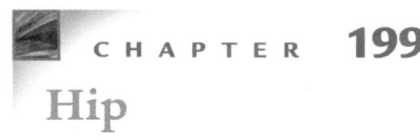

CHAPTER 199

# Hip

The hip is a ball (femoral head) and socket (acetabulum) joint that is important for skeletal stability. The femoral head and acetabulum are interdependent for normal growth and development. The femoral neck and head, which contain the capital femoral epiphysis, are intra-articular. The blood supply to this region is unique because the blood vessels are extraosseous and lie on the surface of the femoral neck, entering the epiphysis peripherally. Thus, the blood supply to the femoral head is vulnerable to trauma, infection, and other causes that may increase intra-articular pressure. Damage to the blood supply can lead to **avascular necrosis**.

## DEVELOPMENTAL DYSPLASIA OF THE HIP

In developmental dysplasia of the hip (DDH), the hips at birth are usually not dislocated, but *dislocatable*, so the term congenital hip dysplasia or dislocation is not appropriate. The femoral head and acetabulum develop from the same mesenchymal cells; by 11 weeks' gestation, the hip joint is formed. There are two types of DDH: teratologic and typical:

**Teratologic dislocations** occur early in utero and are usually associated with neuromuscular disorders (spina bifida, arthrogryposis).

**Typical dislocations** occur in the neurologically normal infant and can occur before or after birth.

The true incidence of DDH is unknown, but it may be as high as 1.5 cases per 1000 infants.

### Etiology

Newborn infants have ligamentous laxity and, if significant enough in the hip, there may be spontaneous dislocation and reduction of the femoral head. Persistence of this spontaneous pattern can lead to pathologic changes, such as flattening of the acetabulum, muscle contractures which limit motion, and joint capsule tightening. The left hip is affected three times as often as the right hip, possibly due to in utero positioning.

Physiologic risk factors for DDH include a generalized ligamentous laxity, perhaps from maternal hormones that are associated with pelvic ligament relaxation (estrogen and relaxin). Female infants are at higher risk (9:1); 20% of all patients with DDH have a positive family history.

Other risk factors include breech presentation, first-born child (60%), oligohydramnios, and postnatal infant positioning. In breech presentations, the fetal pelvis is situated in the maternal pelvis, which can increase hip flexion and limit overall fetal hip motion, causing further stretching of the already lax joint capsule and exposing the posterior aspect of the femoral head. This abnormal position then alters the relationship between the acetabulum and femoral head, causing abnormal acetabular development. Postnatal positioning of the hips in a tight swaddle with the hips adducted and extended can displace the hip joint.

Congenital muscular torticollis (15–20% of cases) and metatarsus adductus (1–10%) are associated with DDH. An infant with either of these two conditions necessitates a careful examination of the hips.

### Clinical Manifestations

Every newborn requires a screening physical examination for DDH; further evaluation through at least the first 18 months of life is part of the physical examination for toddlers. DDH evolves over time, so the examination may change as the patient ages. The examination starts with inspection for asymmetrical thigh and gluteal folds with the hips and knees flexed. A relative shortening of the femur with asymmetrical skin folds is a positive **Galeazzi sign** and indicates DDH. Range of motion should be assessed with the pelvis stabilized and the patient supine on the examining table, not in the parent's lap (Fig. 199-1). Hip abduction

**FIGURE 199-1**

**Hip abduction test**. Place the infant supine, flex the hips 90 degrees, and fully abduct the hips. Although the normal abduction range is broad, hip disease should be suspected in any patient who lacks more than 30 to 45 degrees of abduction. (From Chung SMK: Hip Disorders in Infants and Children. Philadelphia, *Lea & Febiger*, 1981, p 69.)

ABDUCTION TEST

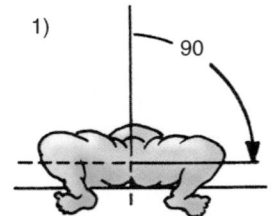

1) 90

Normal at birth to 1 month of age

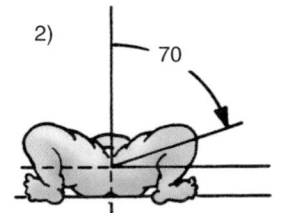

2) 70

Often normal, 1 to 9 months of age

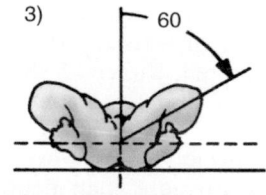

3) 60

Suspected significant limitation

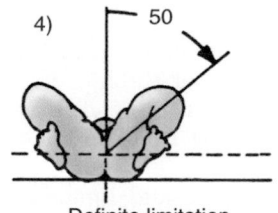

4) 50

Definite limitation

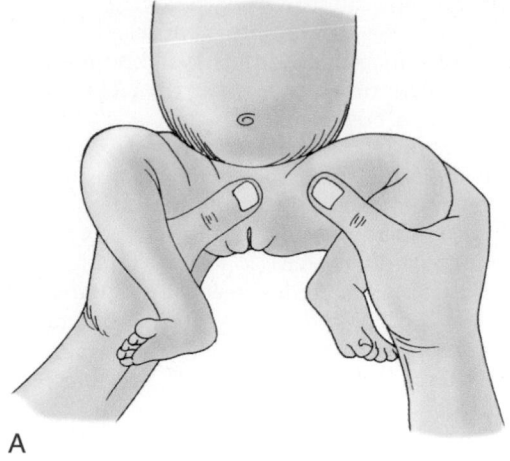

A

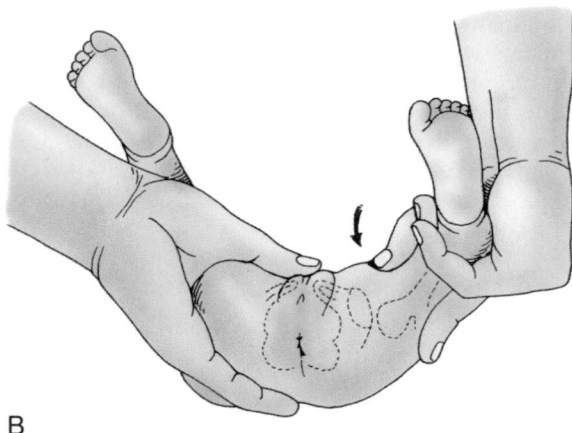

B

**FIGURE 199-2**

**Barlow (dislocation) test.** Reverse of Ortolani test. If the femoral head is in the acetabulum at the time of examination, the Barlow test is performed to discover any hip instability. **A,** The infant's thigh is grasped as shown and adducted with gentle downward pressure. **B,** Dislocation is palpable as the femoral head slips out of the acetabulum. Diagnosis is confirmed with the Ortolani test.

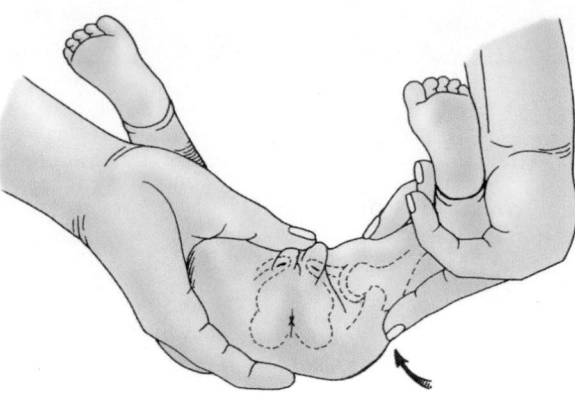

**FIGURE 199-3**

**Ortolani (reduction) test.** With the infant relaxed and content on a firm surface, the hips and knees are flexed to 90 degrees. The hips are examined one at a time. The examiner grasps the infant's thigh with the middle finger over the greater trochanter and lifts the thigh to bring the femoral head from its dislocated posterior position to opposite the acetabulum. Simultaneously the thigh is gently abducted, reducing the femoral head in the acetabulum. In a positive finding, the examiner senses reduction by a palpable, nearly audible *clunk.*

should easily reach or exceed 75 degrees and hip adduction should reach 30 degrees. Limitations may indicate contractures associated with DDH especially decreased abduction.

The **Barlow test** attempts to dislocate an unstable hip (Fig. 199-2). The examiner should stabilize the infant's pelvis with one hand and grasp the abducted and flexed thigh in the other hand. The hip should be flexed to 90 degrees. Next, begin to adduct the hip, while applying a posterior force to the anterior hip. A hip that can be dislocated in this method is readily felt (clunk feeling) and is a positive test. It may reduce spontaneously once the posterior force is removed, or the examiner may need to perform the Ortolani test.

The **Ortolani test** may reduce a dislocated hip (Fig. 199-3). The examiner should stabilize the pelvis and hold the leg in the same method as for the Barlow test. The infant's hip should be in 90 degrees of flexion. Abduct the hip while applying anterior pressure to the posterior thigh. A positive test is the palpable reduction of the dislocation, which may be felt (clunk) and heard (audible click). After 2 months of age, the hip may develop muscular contractures, preventing positive Ortolani tests.

These tests should be performed with only gentle force and done one hip at a time. The examiner may need to do them multiple times, as they can be difficult to interpret. It can be very difficult to diagnose bilateral DDH because of the symmetry found on examination. With time, it becomes easier to differentiate between normal hip clicks and the abnormal clunks associated with dislocation. A click may occur from breaking the surface tension of the hip joint or snapping gluteal tendons.

Older children with unrecognized DDH may present with limping. A patient with increased lumbar lordosis and a waddling gait may have an unrecognized bilateral DDH.

## Radiographic Evaluation

Because the femoral head does not begin to ossify until 4 to 6 months of age, plain radiographs can be misleading until patients are older. Ultrasound is used for initial evaluation of infants with DDH. Ultrasonography is necessary for all infants with a positive family history or breech presentation.

## Treatment

The treatment of DDH is individualized and depends on the child's age at diagnosis. The goal of treatment is a stable reduction that results in normal growth and development of the hip. If DDH is suspected, the child should be sent to a pediatric orthopedist.

The Pavlik harness is an effective treatment up to 6 months of age. It provides hip flexion to just over 90 degrees and limits adduction to no more than neutral. This positioning redirects the femoral head toward the acetabulum. The hip should be reduced within 1 to 2 weeks of beginning the Pavlik harness, although the infant will need more time in the device. If the hips are not reduced during the initial weeks, then the patient will need surgical intervention or casting. The Pavlik harness is successful in treating approximately 95% of dysplastic or subluxated hips, and 80% successful for treatment of true dislocations.

Children over 6 months or those that have failed a Pavlik harness should undergo closed reduction using a hip spica cast, which is usually done under general anesthesia; reduction is confirmed by computed tomography (CT) or magnetic resonance imaging (MRI). If closed reduction fails, open reduction is indicated. Patients over 18 months of age may require a pelvic osteotomy.

## Complications

The most important and severe complication of DDH is iatrogenic avascular necrosis of the femoral head. This can occur from excessive flexion or abduction during positioning of the Pavlik harness or hip spica cast. Infants under 6 months of age are at highest risk. Pressure ulcers can occur with prolonged casting. Redislocation or subluxation of the femoral head and residual acetabular dysplasia can occur.

## TRANSIENT MONOARTICULAR SYNOVITIS

Transient synovitis, also known as **toxic synovitis**, is a common cause of limping in children. It is a diagnosis of exclusion, because **septic arthritis** and **osteomyelitis** of the hip must be excluded (see Chapters 117 and 118).

## Etiology and Epidemiology

The etiology of transient synovitis is uncertain, but possible causes are viral illness and hypersensitivity. Approximately 70% of children diagnosed with transient synovitis have an upper respiratory tract viral infection in the preceding 7 to 14 days. Biopsies have revealed nonspecific synovial hypertrophy. Hip joint aspirations, when necessary, are negative for bacterial culture or signs of bacterial infection.

The mean age at onset is 6 years, with a range of 3 to 8 years. It is twice as common in male children.

## Clinical Manifestations and Evaluation

The patient or family will describe an acute onset of pain in the groin/hip, anterior thigh, or knee. Irritation of the obturator nerve can cause referred pain in the thigh and knee when the pathology is at the hip. Patients with transient synovitis are often afebrile, walk with a painful limp, and have normal to minimally elevated white blood cell count and erythrocyte sedimentation rate compared with bacterial diseases of the hip (Table 199-1). Table 197-3 lists the differential diagnosis of a limping child.

Anteroposterior and frog-leg radiographs of the hip are usually normal. Ultrasonography may reveal a small joint effusion. A bone scan may help differentiate transient synovitis from a septic process.

**TABLE 199-1 Differences Between Bacterial Infection and Transient Synovitis**

| Bacterial Infection* | Transient Synovitis |
|---|---|
| Septic arthritis | |
| Osteomyelitis of hip | |
| Fever—temperature >38.5 ° C | Afebrile |
| Leukocytosis | Normal WBC count |
| ESR >20 mm/hour | Normal ESR and CRP |
| Refusal to walk | Painful limp |
| Hip held in external rotation, abduction, and flexion | Hip held normally |
| Severe pain and tenderness | Moderate pain and mild tenderness |

CRP, C-reactive protein; ESR, erythrocyte sedimentation rate; WBC, white blood cell.
*Examples: Septic arthritis, osteomyelitis of hip.

## Treatment

The mainstay of treatment is bed rest and minimal weight bearing until the pain resolves. Nonsteroidal anti-inflammatory medication is usually sufficient to decrease pain. Limiting strenuous activity and exercise for 1 to 2 weeks following recovery is helpful. Follow-up will help ensure that there is no deterioration. Lack of improvement necessitates further evaluation for more serious disorders.

## LEGG-CALVÉ-PERTHES DISEASE

## Etiology and Epidemiology

Legg-Calvé-Perthes disease (LCPD) is idiopathic **avascular necrosis** (osteonecrosis) of the capital epiphysis of the femoral head. The etiology is unclear, but it is likely caused by an interruption of the blood supply to the capital femoral epiphysis. There may be an associated hypercoagulability state (factor V Leiden).

LCPD commonly presents in patients 3 to 12 years of age, with a mean age of 7 years. It is four to five times more common in boys. Approximately 20% of patients have bilateral involvement.

## Clinical Manifestations

Patients may not present for several weeks because of minimal discomfort; the classic presentation is a child with an atraumatic, painless limp. There may be mild or intermittent hip/groin, anterior thigh, or knee pain. Decreased internal rotation and abduction with some discomfort, thigh muscle spasm, and anterior thigh muscular atrophy may be present. Patients have delayed bone age.

## Radiologic Evaluation

Anteroposterior and frog-leg radiographs of both hips are usually adequate for diagnosis and management. It is necessary to document the extent of the disease and follow its progression. MRI and bone scan are helpful to diagnose early LCPD.

## Treatment and Prognosis

LCPD is usually a self-limited disorder that should be followed by a pediatric orthopedist. Initial treatment focuses on pain control and restoration of hip range of motion. The goals of treatment are prevention of complications, such as femoral head deformity and secondary osteoarthritis.

**Containment** is important in treating LCPD; the femoral head is contained inside the acetabulum, which acts like a mold for the capital femoral epiphysis as it reossifies. Nonsurgical containment uses abduction casts and orthoses, while surgical containment is accomplished with osteotomies of the proximal femur and pelvis.

The short-term prognosis is determined by the magnitude of the femoral head deformity after healing has completed. It is improved by early diagnosis, good follow-up, and compliance with the treatment plan. Older children and children with a residual femoral head deformity are more likely to develop osteoarthritis (OA). The incidence of OA in patients who developed LCPD after 10 years of age is close to 100%; it is negligible in children with onset before 5 years of age. Patients between 6 and 9 years of age have a risk of OA of less than 40%.

## SLIPPED CAPITAL FEMORAL EPIPHYSIS

### Etiology and Epidemiology

Slipped capital femoral epiphysis (SCFE) is a common adolescent hip disorder that is an orthopedic emergency. The incidence is 10.8 per 100,000, and it is slightly higher in males. African-American and Hispanic populations are at higher risk. Approximately 20% of patients with SCFE will have bilateral involvement at presentation, and another 20% to 40% may progress to bilateral involvement. The average age is 10 to 16 years, with a mean of 12 years in boys and 11 years in girls. Additional risk factors for SCFE include obesity, trisomy 21, and endocrine disorders (hypothyroid, pituitary tumor, growth hormone deficiency).

## Classification

SCFE is classified as stable or unstable. Unstable patients refuse to ambulate. Stable patients have an antalgic gait. SCFE can also be characterized as acute (symptoms less than 3 weeks) or chronic (symptoms over 3 weeks). Acute-on-chronic SCFE is seen when more than 3 weeks of symptoms are accompanied by an acute exacerbation of pain and difficulty/inability to bear weight.

## Clinical Manifestation

The presentation is variable, based on severity and type of slip. Patients will often report hip or knee pain, limp or inability to ambulate, and decreased hip range of motion. There may or may not be a traumatic event. Any knee pain should trigger an examination of the hip, as hip pathology can cause referred pain to the anterior thigh and knee along the obturator nerve. The patient usually holds the affected extremity in external rotation. As the hip is flexed, it will progressively externally rotate. There is usually a limitation of internal rotation, but there may also be a loss of flexion and abduction. If the patient can bear weight, it is typically an antalgic gait with the affected leg in external rotation. It is important to examine both hips to determine bilateral involvement.

## Radiologic Evaluation

Anteroposterior and frog-leg radiographs are indicated. Patients with known SCFE or with a high index of suspicion should not undergo frog-leg lateral radiographs. Instead, a cross table lateral radiograph reduces the risk of iatrogenic progression. The earliest sign of SCFE is widening of the physis without slippage (**preslip condition**). Klein's line (Fig.199-4) is helpful in assessing the anteroposterior radiograph for SCFE. The slippage can be classified radiographically as type I (0–33% displacement), type II (34–50%), or type III (>50%). The likelihood of complications increases with degree of displacement.

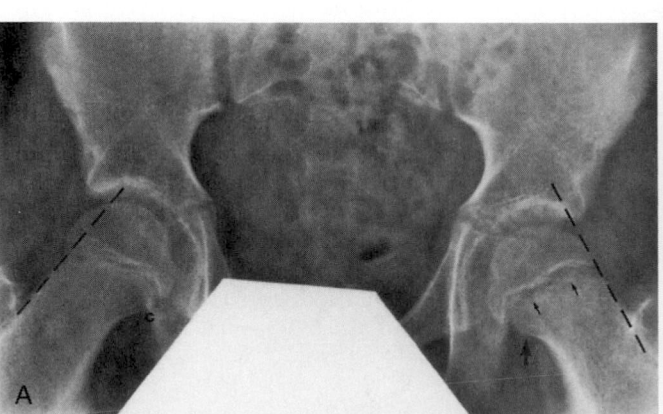
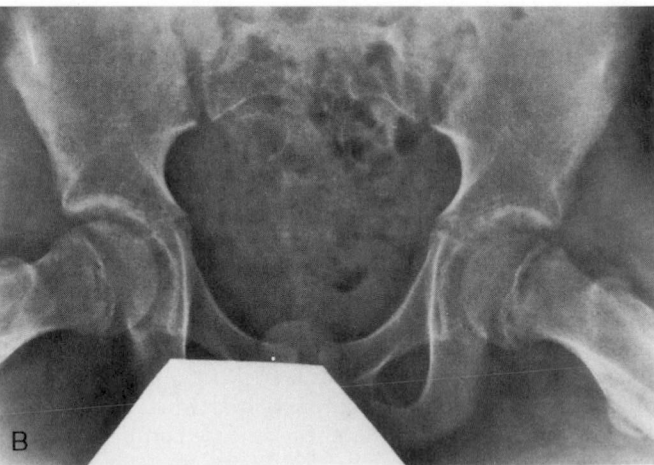

**FIGURE 199-4**

**Slipped capital femoral epiphysis (SCFE). A,** Anteroposterior radiograph reveals a widened physis (*small arrows*) and decreased height of the epiphysis on the left. In addition, there is loss (*large arrow*) of the Capener triangle (*c*) (normal double density of the medial metaphysis superimposed on the posterior acetabular rim on right) and an abnormal lateral femoral neck line (normal on right). **B,** Frog, lateral view confirms the inferomedial position of the SCFE. (From Blickman H: Pediatric Radiology, The Requisites, 2nd ed. St. Louis, *Mosby*, 1998, p 244.)

## Treatment

Patients with SCFE should be immediately made non-weight bearing and referred to a pediatric orthopedist. The goal is to prevent further slippage, enhance physeal closure, and minimize complications, which is usually accomplished with internal fixation in-situ with a single cannulated screw. More severe cases may require osteotomy or bone graft epiphysiodesis to realign the femur. There is controversy surrounding the prophylactic fixation of the nonaffected side. Assessment for endocrine disorders is important, particularly in children outside the range of 10 to 16 years of age.

## Complications

The two most serious complications of SCFE are **chondrolysis** and **avascular necrosis**. Chondrolysis is destruction of the articular cartilage. It is associated with more severe slips and with intra-articular penetration of operative hardware. This can lead to severe osteoarthritis (OA) and disability. Avascular necrosis occurs when there is a disruption of the blood supply to the capital femoral epiphysis. This usually happens at the time of injury, but may occur during forced manipulation of an unstable slip. Avascular necrosis may occur in up to 50% of unstable SCFEs and may lead to OA.

# CHAPTER 200

# Lower Extremity and Knee

Torsional (in-toeing and out-toeing) and angular (physiologic bowlegs and knock knees) variations in the legs are common reasons that parents seek medical attention for their child. Most of these concerns are physiologic and resolve with normal growth. It is important to understand the natural history in order to reassure the family and to identify nonphysiologic disorders that necessitate further intervention. Physiologic disturbances are referred to as variations, and pathologic disturbances are called deformities.

## TORSIONAL VARIATIONS

The femur is internally rotated (anteversion) at birth about 30 degrees, decreasing to about 10 degrees at maturity. The tibia begins with up to 30 degrees of internal rotation at birth and can decrease to a mean of 15 degrees at maturity.

Torsional variations should not cause a limp or pain. Unilateral torsion should raise the index of suspicion for a neurologic (hemiplegia) or neuromuscular disorder.

## In-Toeing

### Femoral Anteversion

Internal femoral torsion or femoral anteversion is the most common cause of in-toeing in children 2 years or older (Table 200-1). It is at its worst between 4 and 6 years

| TABLE 200-1 Common Causes of In-Toeing and Out-Toeing | |
|---|---|
| **In-Toeing** | **Out-Toeing** |
| Internal femoral torsion or anteversion | External femoral torsion |
| Internal tibial torsion | External tibial torsion |
| Metatarsus adductus | Calcaneovalgus feet |
| Talipes equinovarus (clubfoot) | Hypermobile pes planus (flatfoot) |
| Developmental dysplasia | Slipped capital femoral epiphysis |

of age, and then resolves. It occurs twice as often in girls. Many cases are associated with generalized ligamentous laxity. The etiology of femoral anteversion is likely congenital, and is common in individuals with abnormal sitting habits such as *W-sitting*.

**Clinical Manifestations.** The family may give a history of W-sitting, and there may be a family history of similar concerns when the parents were younger. The child may have *kissing kneecaps* due to increased internal rotation of the femur. While walking, the entire leg will appear internally rotated, and with running the child may appear to have an *egg-beater* gait where the legs flip laterally. The flexed hip will have internal rotation increased to 80 to 90 degrees (normal 60–70 degrees) and external rotation limited to about 10 degrees. Radiographic evaluation is usually not indicated.

### Internal Tibial Torsion

This is the most common cause of in-toeing in a child *younger* than 2 years old. When it is the result of in utero positioning, it may be associated with metatarsus adductus.

**Clinical Manifestations.** The child will present with a history of in-toeing. The degree of tibial torsion may be measured using the **thigh-foot angle** (Fig. 200-1). The patient lies prone on a table with the knee flexed to 90 degrees. The long axis of the foot is compared with the long axis of the thigh. An inwardly rotated foot represents a negative angle and internal tibial torsion. Measurements should be done at each visit to document improvement.

### Treatment of In-toeing

The mainstay of management is identifying patients who have pathologic reasons for in-toeing and reassurance and follow-up to document improvement for patients with femoral anteversion and internal tibial torsion. It can take 7 to 8 years for correction, so it is important to inform families of the appropriate timeline. Braces (Denis Browne splint) do not improve these conditions. The lack of improvement by 2 years of age for children with internal tibial torsion should result in referral to a pediatric orthopedist. Approximately 1% to 2% of all patients with in-toeing will need surgical intervention due to functional disability or cosmetic appearance.

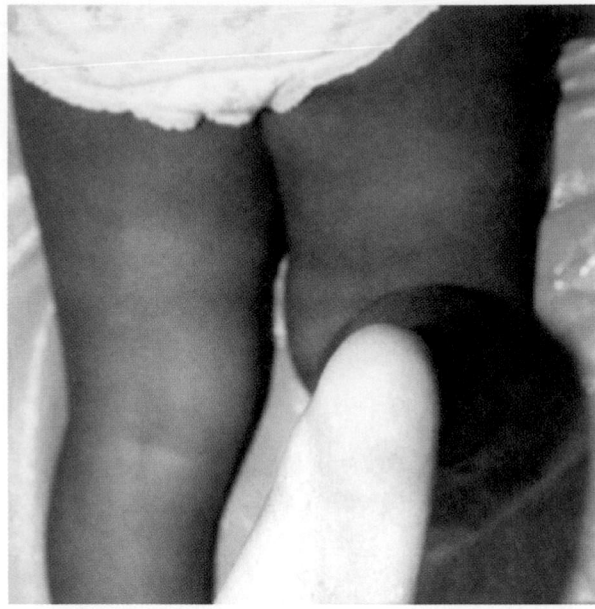

**FIGURE 200-1**

**Thigh-foot angle measurement**. The thigh-foot angle is useful for assessment of tibial torsion. The patient lies prone, with knees flexed to 90 degrees. The long axis of the thigh is compared to the long axis of the foot to determine the thigh-foot angle. Negative angles are associated with internal tibial torsion, and positive angles are associated with external tibial torsion.

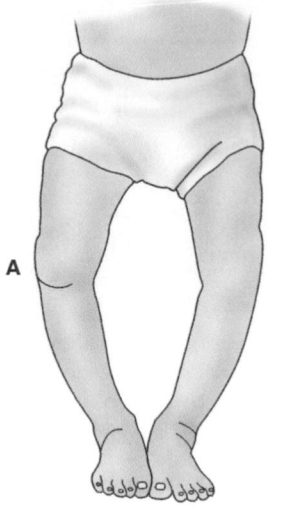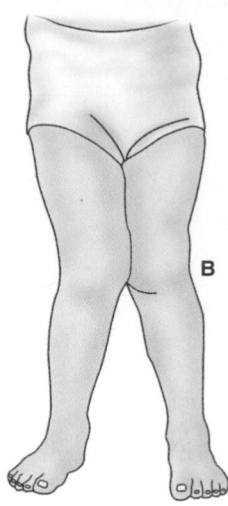

**FIGURE 200-2**

**Bowleg and knock-knee deformities. A,** Bowleg deformity. Bowlegs are referred to as varus angulation (genu varum) because the knees are tilted away from the midline of the body. **B,** Knock-knee or valgus deformity of the knees. The knee is tilted toward the midline. (From Scoles P: Pediatric Orthopedics in Clinical Practice. Chicago, *Year Book Medical Publishers*, 1982, p 84.)

## Out-Toeing

### External Tibial Torsion

External tibial torsion is the most common cause of out-toeing and may be associated with a calcaneovalgus foot (see Chapter 201). This is often related to in utero positioning. It may improve over time, but because the tibia rotates externally with age, external tibial torsion can worsen. It may be an etiologic factor for patellofemoral syndrome, especially when combined with femoral anteversion. Treatment is usually observation and reassurance, but patients with dysfunction and cosmetic concerns may benefit from surgical intervention.

## ANGULAR VARIATIONS

The majority of the patients that present with knock-knees (**genu valgum**) or bowlegs (**genu varum**) are normal (Fig. 200-2). Infants are born with maximum genu varum. The lower extremity straightens out around 18 months of age. Children typically progress to maximal genu valgum around 4 years. The legs are usually straight to a slight genu valgum in adulthood.

It is important to inquire about family history and assess overall height. A child who is 2 standard deviations (SDs) below normal with angular deformities may have skeletal dysplasia. Dietary history should be obtained, as rickets (see Chapter 31) may cause angular deformities. For genu valgum, following the intermalleolar distance (distance between the two tibial medial malleoli with the knees touching) is used. Measurement of the intercondylar

distance (the distance between the medial femoral condyles with the medial malleoli touching) is used for genu varum. These measurements track improvement or progression. When obtaining radiographs, it is important to have the patella, not the feet, facing forward. In the child with external tibial torsion, having the feet facing forward gives the false appearance of bowlegs.

## Genu Valgum

Physiologic knock-knees are most common in 3- to 4-year-olds and usually resolve between 5 and 8 years of age. Patients with asymmetrical genu valgum or severe deformity may have underlying disease causing their knock-knees (e.g., renal osteodystrophy, skeletal dysplasia). Treatment is based on reassurance of the family and patient. Surgical intervention may be indicated for severe deformities, gait dysfunction, pain, and cosmesis.

## Genu Varum

Physiologic bowlegs are most common in children older than 18 months with symmetrical genu varum. This will generally improve as the child approaches 2 years of age. The most important consideration for genu varum is differentiating between physiologic genu varum and Blount disease (tibia vara).

## Tibia Vara (Blount Disease)

Tibia vara is the most common pathologic disorder associated with genu varum. It is characterized by abnormal growth of the medial aspect of the proximal tibial epiphysis, resulting in a progressive varus deformity. Blount disease is classified according to age of onset:

Infantile (1–3 years)
Juvenile (4–10 years)
Adolescent (>11 years)

Late onset Blount disease is less common than infantile disease. The cause is unknown, but it is felt to be secondary to growth suppression from increased compressive forces across the medial knee.

## Clinical Manifestations

Infantile tibia vara is more common in African Americans, females, and obese patients. Many patients were early walkers. Nearly 80% of patients with infantile Blount disease have bilateral involvement. It is usually painless. The patients will often have significant internal tibial torsion and lower extremity leg-length discrepancy. There may also be a palpable medial tibial metaphyseal beak.

*Late onset* Blount disease is more common in African Americans, males, and patients with marked obesity. Only 50% have bilateral involvement. The initial presentation is usually painful bowlegs. Late onset Blount disease is usually not associated with palpable metaphyseal beaking, significant internal tibial torsion, or significant leg length discrepancy.

## Radiologic Evaluation

Weight-bearing anteroposterior and lateral radiographs of both legs are necessary for the diagnosis of tibia vara. Fragmentation, wedging, and beak deformities of the proximal medial tibia are the major radiologic features of infantile Blount disease. In late onset Blount disease, the medial deformity may not be as readily noticeable. It can be very difficult to tell the difference between physiologic genu varum and infantile Blount disease on radiographs in the patient younger than 2 years of age.

## Treatment

Once the diagnosis of Blount disease is confirmed, treatment should begin immediately. The use of orthotics to unload the medial compressive forces can be done in children younger than 3 years of age with a mild deformity. Compliance with this regimen can be difficult. Nonoperative management of more severe Blount disease is contraindicated.

Any patient older than 4 years should undergo surgical intervention. Patients with moderate to severe deformity and patients that fail orthotic treatment also require surgical intervention. Proximal tibial valgus osteotomy with fibular diaphyseal osteotomy is the usual procedure performed.

## LEG-LENGTH DISCREPANCY

Leg-length discrepancy (LLD) is common and may be due to differences in the femur, tibia, or both bones. The differential diagnosis is extensive, but common causes are

| TABLE 200-2 | Common Causes of Leg-Length Discrepancy |
|---|---|
| Congenital | Coxa vara |
| | Clubfoot |
| | Hypoplasia |
| Developmental | Developmental dysplasia of the hip (DDH) |
| | Legg-Calve-Perthes disease (LCPD) |
| Neuromuscular | Hemiplegia |
| | Disuse secondary to developmental delay |
| Infectious | Physeal injury secondary to osteomyelitis |
| Tumors | Fibrous dysplasia |
| | Physeal injury secondary to irradiation or neoplastic infiltration |
| | Overgrowth |
| Trauma | Physeal injury with premature closure |
| | Malunion (shortening of extremity) |
| | Overgrowth of healing fracture |
| Syndrome | Neurofibromatosis |
| | Beckwith-Wiedemann syndrome |
| | Klippel-Trénaunay syndrome |

listed in Table 200-2. The majority of the lower extremity growth comes from the distal femur (38%) and the proximal tibia (27%).

## Measuring Leg-Length Discrepancy

Clinical measurements using bony landmarks (anterior superior iliac spine to medial malleolus) are inaccurate. The **teloradiograph** is a single radiograph of both legs that can be done in very young children. The **orthoradiograph** consists of three slightly overlapping exposures of the hips, knees, and ankles. The **scanogram** consists of three standard radiographs of the hips, knees, and ankles with a ruler next to the extremities. A **computed tomography (CT) scanogram** is the most accurate measure of LLD. Distal radiography with computer assisted measurement is the most accurate method. The measured discrepancy is followed using Moseley and Green-Anderson graphs.

## Treatment

Treating LLD is complex. The physician must take into account the estimated adult height, discrepancy measurements, skeletal maturity, and the psychological aspects of the patient and family. LLD greater than 2 cm usually requires treatment. Shoe lifts can be used, but they will often cause psychosocial problems for the child and may make the shoes heavier and less stable. Surgical options include shortening of the longer extremity, lengthening of the shorter extremity, or a combination of the two procedures. Discrepancies less than 5 cm are treated by epiphysiodesis (surgical physeal closure) of the affected side, while discrepancies greater than 5 cm are treated by lengthening.

# KNEE

The knee joint is constrained by soft tissues rather than the usual geometric fit of articulating bones. The medial and lateral collateral ligaments as well as the anterior and posterior cruciate ligaments maintain knee stability. Weight and force transmission can cross articular cartilage and the meniscus. The patellofemoral joint is the extensor mechanism of the knee and a common site of injury in the adolescent (Fig. 200-3).

Knee effusion or swelling is a common sign of injury. When the fluid accumulates rapidly after an injury, it is usually a hemarthrosis (blood in the joint) and may indicate a fracture, ligamentous disruption (often of the anterior cruciate ligament, ACL), or meniscus tear. Unexplained knee effusion may occur with arthritis (septic, Lyme disease, viral, postinfectious, juvenile idiopathic arthritis, systemic lupus erythematosus). It may also occur as a result of overactivity and hypermobile joint syndrome (ligamentous laxity). An aspiration and laboratory evaluation of unexplained effusion can help expedite a diagnosis.

## Discoid Lateral Meniscus

Each meniscus is normally semilunar in shape; rarely the lateral meniscus will be disc shaped. A normal meniscus is attached at the periphery and glides anteriorly and posteriorly with knee motion. The discoid meniscus is less mobile, and may tear more easily. When there is inadequate posterolateral attachment, the discoid meniscus can displace anteriorly with knee flexion, causing an audible click. Most commonly, patients will present in late childhood or early adolescence after an injury with knee pain and swelling. The anteroposterior radiographs can show widening of the lateral femoral condyle; magnetic resonance imaging (MRI) can confirm the diagnosis. Treatment is usually arthroscopic excision of tears and reshaping of the meniscus.

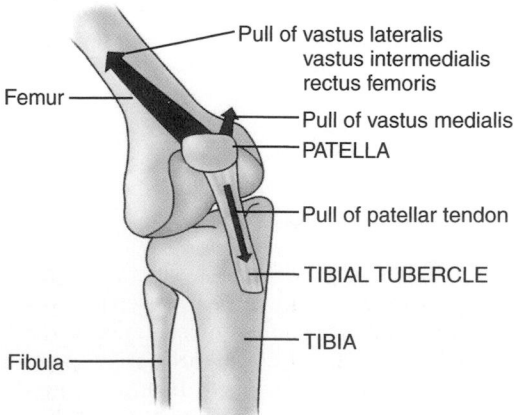

**FIGURE 200-3**

**Diagram of the knee extensor mechanism.** The major force exerted by the quadriceps muscle tends to pull the patella laterally out of the intercondylar sulcus. The vastus medialis muscle pulls medially to keep the patella centralized. (Modified from Smith JB: Knee problems in children. *Pediatr Clin North Am* 33:1439, 1986.)

## Popliteal Cyst

A popliteal cyst (**Baker cyst**) is commonly seen in the middle childhood years. The cause is the distension of the gastrocnemius and semimembranous bursa along the posteromedial aspect of the knee by synovial fluid. In adults, Baker cysts are associated with meniscus tears. In childhood, the cysts are usually painless and benign. They often spontaneously resolve, but it may take several years. Knee radiographs are normal. The diagnosis can be confirmed by ultrasound. Treatment is reassurance, since surgical excision is indicated only for progressive cysts or cysts that cause disability.

## Osteochondritis Dissecans

Osteochondritis dissecans (OCD) most commonly involves the knee. It occurs when an area of bone adjacent to the articular cartilage suffers a vascular insult and separates from the adjacent bone. It most commonly affects the lateral aspect of the medial femoral condyle. Patients may complain of knee pain or swelling. The lesions can be seen on anteroposterior, lateral, and tunnel view radiographs. MRI can be helpful in determining the extent of the injury. In young patients with intact articular cartilage, the lesion will often revascularize and heal with rest from activities. The healing process may take several months and requires radiographic follow-up to document healing. With increasing age, the risk for articular cartilage damage and separation of the bony fragment increase. Older patients are more likely to need surgical intervention. Any patient with a fracture of the articular cartilage will not improve without surgical intervention.

## Osgood-Schlatter Disease

Osgood-Schlatter disease is a common cause of knee pain at the insertion of the patellar tendon on the tibial tubercle. The stress from a contracting quadriceps muscle is transmitted through the developing tibial tubercle, which can cause a microfracture or partial avulsion fracture in the ossification center. It usually occurs after a growth spurt and is more common in boys. The age at onset is typically 11 years for girls and 13 to 14 years for boys.

Patients will present with pain during and after activity as well as have tenderness and local swelling over the tibial tubercle. Radiographs may be necessary to rule out infection, tumor, or avulsion fracture.

Rest and activity modification are paramount for treatment. Pain control medications and icing may be helpful. Lower extremity flexibility and strengthening exercise programs are important. Some patients may require immobilization. The course is usually benign, but symptoms frequently last 1 to 2 years. Complications can include bony enlargement of the tibial tubercle and avulsion fracture of the tibial tubercle.

## Patellofemoral Disorders

The patellofemoral joint is a complex joint that depends on a balance between restraining ligaments of the patella, muscular forces around the knee, and alignment for normal function. The interior surface of the patella has a V-shaped bottom which moves through a matching groove in the femur called the trochlea. When the knee is flexed, the patellar ligaments and the majority of the muscular forces pulling through the quadriceps tendon move the patella in a lateral direction. The vastus medialis muscle counteracts the lateral motion, pulling the patella toward the midline. Problems with function of this joint usually result in anterior knee pain.

**Idiopathic anterior knee pain** is a common complaint in adolescents. It is particularly prevalent in adolescent female athletes. Previously, this was referred to as chondromalacia of the patella, but this term is incorrect as the joint surfaces of the patella are normal. It is now known as **patellofemoral pain syndrome** (PFS). The patient will present with anterior knee pain that worsens with activity, going up and down stairs, and soreness after sitting in one position for an extended time. There is usually no associated swelling. The patient may complain of a grinding sensation under the kneecap. Palpating and compressing the patellofemoral joint with the knee extended elicits pain. The patient may have weak hip musculature or poor flexibility in the lower extremities. Radiographs are rarely helpful but may be indicated to rule out other diagnoses such as osteochondritis dissecans.

Treatment is focused on correcting the biomechanical problems that are causing the pain. This is usually done using an exercise program emphasizing hip girdle and vastus medialis strengthening with lower extremity flexibility. Anti-inflammatory medication, ice, and activity modifications may also be helpful. Persistent cases should be referred to an orthopedist or sports medicine specialist.

One must exclude **recurrent patellar subluxation** and **dislocation** when evaluating a patient with PFS. Acute traumatic dislocation will usually cause significant disability and swelling. Recurrent episodes may not have the degree of swelling, loss of motion, and difficulty weight bearing seen in an initial dislocation. Patients with recurrent episodes often have associated ligamentous laxity, genu valgum, and femoral anteversion. The initial treatment is nonoperative and may involve a brief period of immobilization, followed by an aggressive physical therapy program designed to strengthen the quadriceps and improve function of the patellofemoral joint. Continued subluxation or dislocation is failure of this treatment plan and surgical repair is usually necessary.

CHAPTER **201**

# Foot

In newborns and non–weight bearing infants, the difference between posturing and deformity is important. Posturing is the habitual position the infant holds the foot; passive range of motion is normal. Deformity produces an appearance similar to posturing, but passive motion is restricted. Most pediatric foot disorders are painless. Foot pain is more common in older children (Table 201-1).

| TABLE 201-1 Differential Diagnosis of Foot Pain by Age | |
|---|---|
| **Age Group** | **Diagnostic Considerations** |
| 0 to 6 years | Poor-fitting shoes |
| | Fracture |
| | Puncture wound |
| | Foreign body |
| | Osteomyelitis |
| | Cellulitis |
| | Juvenile idiopathic arthritis |
| | Hair tourniquet |
| | Leukemia |
| 6 to 12 years | Poor-fitting shoes |
| | Trauma (fracture, sprain) |
| | Juvenile idiopathic arthritis |
| | Puncture wound |
| | Sever disease |
| | Accessory tarsal navicular |
| | Hypermobile flatfoot |
| | Oncologic (Ewing sarcoma, leukemia) |
| 12 to 18 years | Poor-fitting shoes |
| | Stress fracture |
| | Trauma (fracture, sprain) |
| | Foreign body |
| | Ingrown toenail |
| | Metatarsalgia |
| | Plantar fasciitis |
| | Achilles tendonopathy |
| | Accessory ossicles (navicular, os trigonum) |
| | Tarsal coalition |
| | Avascular necrosis of metatarsal (Freiberg infarction) or navicular (Kohler disease) |
| | Plantar warts |

## CLUB FOOT (TALIPES EQUINOVARUS)

A clubfoot deformity involves the entire leg, not just the foot. It affects 1 in 1000 newborns and is bilateral in one half of the cases. The tarsals in the affected foot are hypoplastic; the talus is most affected. The muscles of the limb are hypoplastic because of the abnormal tarsal interactions, which leads to a generalized limb hypoplasia, mainly affecting and shortening the foot. There is usually atrophy of the calf musculature.

### Etiology

Family history is important. Club foot can be congenital, teratologic, or positional. Congenital clubfoot (75% of all cases) is usually an isolated abnormality. Teratologic clubfoot is associated with a neuromuscular disorder, such as myelomeningocele, arthrogryposis, or other syndromes. Positional clubfoot is a normal foot that was held in the deformed position in utero.

## Clinical Manifestations

The diagnosis is seldom confused with other disorders (Fig. 201-1). The presence of clubfoot should prompt a careful search for other abnormalities. The infant will have hindfoot equinus and varus, forefoot adduction, and varying degrees of rigidity. All are secondary to the abnormalities of the talonavicular joint. Calf atrophy and foot shortening are more noticeable in older children.

## Radiologic Evaluation

In infants, radiographs and advanced imaging are rarely necessary for assessment since their tarsals have incomplete ossification. The navicular ossifies at about 3 years of age for girls and 4 years for boys. As children age, radiographs can be used to follow the tibial calcaneal and lateral talocalcaneal angles and to assess navicular positioning.

## Treatment

The goal of treatment is to correct the deformity and preserve mobility. Nonoperative treatment involves the Ponseti method of serial casting. The Ponseti method also relies on a percutaneous tenotomy of the Achilles tendon to help correct the equinus deformity.

About 20% of patients will require an anterior tibialis tendon transfer in early childhood. Rarely, more aggressive surgical procedures may need to be done. Complications of untreated clubfoot include severe disability. Complications of treated clubfoot include recurrence and stiffness.

# METATARSUS ADDUCTUS

Metatarsus adductus is the most common foot disorder in infants. It is characterized by a convexity of the lateral foot (Fig. 201-2) and is caused by in utero positioning. It is bilateral in half of the cases. Occurring equally in boys and girls, it is more common in first-born children due to the smaller primigravid uterus. Two percent of infants with metatarsus adductus have **developmental dysplasia** of the hip.

## Clinical Manifestations

The forefoot is adducted and sometimes supinated, but the midfoot and hindfoot are normal. The lateral border of the foot is convex, while the medial border is concave. Ankle dorsiflexion and plantar flexion are normal. With the midfoot and hindfoot stabilized, the deformity can be pushed beyond a neutral position (into abduction). Older children may present with an in-toeing gait.

## Treatment

True metatarsus adductus resolves spontaneously over 90% of the time without treatment, so reassurance is all that is needed. Metatarsus adductus that does not improve within 2 years needs evaluation by a pediatric orthopedist. Persistent cases may benefit from serial casting or bracing, and potentially surgery. Many feel that it is acceptable to live with the deformity because it is not associated with a disability.

It is important to differentiate between metatarsus adductus, **metatarsus varus**, and **skewfoot**. Metatarsus varus looks like metatarsus adductus, but it is an uncommon rigid deformity that will need serial casting. Skewfoot is an uncommon deformity that is characterized by hindfoot plantar flexion, midfoot abduction, and forefoot adduction, giving the foot a Z or serpentine appearance. This needs to be managed very carefully with serial casting and surgery to help reduce the risk of disability in adulthood.

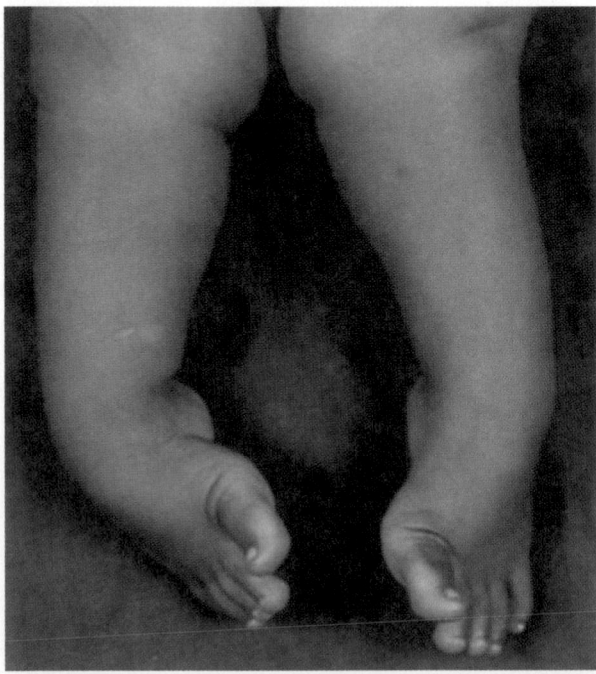

**FIGURE 201-1**

**Clinical picture demonstrating clubfoot deformity.** (From Kliegman RM, Behrman, RE, Jenson HB, et al: Nelson's Textbook of Pediatrics, 18th ed. Philadelphia, *WB Saunders*, 2007, p 2778.)

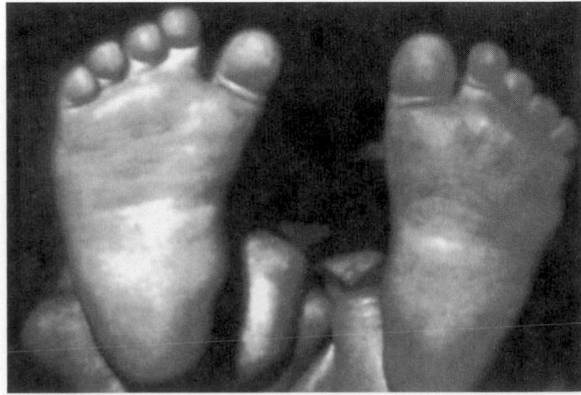

**FIGURE 201-2**

**Clinical picture of metatarsus adductus with a normal foot on opposite side.** (From Kliegman RM, Behrman, RE, Jenson HB, et al: Nelson's Textbook of Pediatrics, 18th ed. Philadelphia, *WB Saunders*, 2007, p 2777.)

## CALCANEOVALGUS FOOT

The calcaneovalgus foot is another common foot disorder in newborns that is secondary to in utero positioning. It is characterized by a hyperdorsiflexed foot with forefoot abduction and heel valgus. It is usually unilateral. The appearance may be quite severe dorsiflexion, but it is not a rigid deformity like congenital vertical talus. Simulated weight-bearing radiographs may be necessary for questionable diagnoses. The calcaneovalgus foot will appear normal or have minimal hindfoot valgus.

This disorder requires no treatment beyond reassurance. Parents can be taught passive stretching exercises for their infant's foot. Most affected infants realign by 2 years.

## HYPERMOBILE PES PLANUS (FLEXIBLE FLATFOOT)

Hypermobile or pronated feet are seen in 15% of adults. The child with flatfeet is usually asymptomatic and has no activity limitations. Newborn and toddler flatfoot is the result of ligamentous laxity and fat in the medial longitudinal arch. This is called **developmental flatfoot** and usually improves by 6 years of age. In older children, flatfoot is typically the result of generalized ligamentous laxity, and there is often a positive family history. Hypermobile flatfoot can be thought of as a normal variant.

### Clinical Manifestations

In the non-weight bearing position, the older child with a flexible flatfoot will have a medial longitudinal arch. When weight bearing, the foot pronates (arch collapse) with varying degrees of hindfoot valgus. Subtalar motion (essentially all ankle motion except plantar and dorsiflexion) is normal. Any loss of subtalar motion may indicate a rigid flatfoot, which can be related to tarsal coalition, neuromuscular disorders (cerebral palsy), and heel cord contractures. Radiographs of hypermobile flatfeet are usually not indicated.

### Treatment

Hypermobile pes planus cannot be diagnosed until after 6 years of age; prior to that, it is developmental pes planus. Reassurance that this is a normal variant is very important. Patients who are symptomatic with activity may require education on proper, supportive footwear, orthotics/arch supports, and heel cord stretching.

## TARSAL COALITION

Patients with tarsal coalition will usually present with a **rigid** flatfoot (loss of inversion and eversion at the subtalar joint). Coalition is produced by a congenital fusion or failure of segmentation of two or more tarsal bones. The attachment may be fibrous, cartilaginous, or osseus. Tarsal coalition can be unilateral or bilateral and will often become symptomatic in early adolescence. The most common forms of tarsal coalition are **calcaneonavicular** and **talocalcaneal**.

### Clinical Manifestations

The patient will usually present with hindfoot pain, which may radiate laterally due to peroneal muscle spasm. Symptoms are exacerbated by sports, and young athletes can present with frequent *ankle sprains*. There is a familial component. Pes planus is usually present in both weight bearing and non–weight bearing positions. There is usually a loss of subtalar motion, and passive attempts at joint motion may produce pain.

### Radiologic Evaluation

Anteroposterior, lateral, and oblique radiographs should be obtained, but they may not always clearly identify the disorder. The oblique view often identifies the calcaneonavicular coalition. Computed tomography (CT) is the gold standard for diagnosis of tarsal coalition. Even patients with obvious calcaneonavicular coalition on plain radiographs should have a CT scan to rule out a second coalition.

### Treatment

Coalitions that are asymptomatic (the majority) do not need treatment. Nonoperative treatment for patients with pain consists of cast immobilization for a few weeks and foot orthotics. The symptoms will often return, necessitating surgery. Surgical excision of the coalition and soft tissue interposition to prevent reossification can be very effective.

## CAVUS FOOT

Cavus foot is characterized by increased height of the medial longitudinal arch (**high arch**) and frequently hindfoot varus. It can be classified as physiologic or neuromuscular. Most patients with physiologic cavus foot are asymptomatic. A thorough neurologic examination on all patients with a cavus foot is important. Patients with painful high arches have a high risk of neurologic (tethered cord) and neuromuscular disease, and there is a strong association with **Charcot-Marie-Tooth disease**, a familial neuropathy. The underlying disorder should be treated first. Nonoperative treatment using orthotics is usually not helpful. Progressive, symptomatic cavus foot will likely need surgical reconstruction.

## IDIOPATHIC AVASCULAR NECROSIS

**Kohler disease** (tarsal navicular) and **Freiberg disease** (head of the second metatarsal) are uncommon and due to avascular necrosis. Patients will present with pain at the affected site with activity and weight bearing. Infection, fracture, and neoplasm should be excluded. Treatment consists of immobilization and activity restriction. The majority of the patients will improve upon subsequent revascularization and re-formation of bone.

## SEVER DISEASE (CALCANEAL APOPHYSITIS)

Sever disease is common cause of heel pain among active young people. The mean age of presentation for girls is about 9 years of age and for boys about 11 to 12 years. Approximately 60% of cases are bilateral. Sever disease is caused by the forces of the calf musculature through the Achilles tendon at the calcaneal apophysis, causing microfracture. As the child ages and the apophysis begins to close, the pain disappears.

## Clinical Manifestations

The common presentation is a young athlete who develops heel pain with activity which decreases with rest. There is rarely swelling, but there may be limping associated with Sever disease. The child will have pain to palpation of the posterior calcaneus and often tight heel cords. Radiographs are rarely indicated, but with persistent pain they should be done to exclude infection or tumor.

## Treatment

Activity modification, icing, and anti-inflammatory medications can be helpful. A program designed to improve heel cord flexibility and overall ankle strength may decrease symptoms. Heel elevation using heel wedges or heel cups can be helpful.

## TOE DEFORMITIES

**Curly toes** are the most common deformity of the lesser toes. The fourth and fifth toes are most commonly affected. Curly toes are characterized by flexion at the proximal interphalangeal joint with lateral rotation of the toe. It is caused by contractures of the flexor digitorum brevus and longus tendons. About 25% to 50% of curly toes will spontaneously resolve by 3 to 4 years of age. Persistent deformity may be treated by surgical tenotomy.

**Polydactyly** (extra toes) are usually found on the initial newborn physical examination. When the extra toe is adjacent to the fifth toe, and attached by only a stalk of soft tissue or skin, simple ligation or amputation is effective. When the deformity involves the great toe or middle toes, or when the extra digit has cartilage or bone, delayed surgical intervention is indicated. **Syndactyly** (fusion of toes) is more common than polydactyly. It is usually a benign cosmetic problem. Both syndactyly and polydactyly may be associated with malformation syndromes (Table 201-2).

**TABLE 201-2  Disorders Associated with Syndactyly and Polydactyly**

| Polydactyly | Syndactyly |
|---|---|
| Ellis-van Creveld syndrome | Apert syndrome |
| Rubinstein-Taybi syndrome | Carpenter syndrome |
| Carpenter syndrome | de Lange syndrome |
| Meckel-Gruber syndrome | Holt-Oram syndrome |
| Polysyndactyly | Orofaciodigital syndrome |
| Trisomy 13 | Polysyndactyly |
| Orofaciodigital syndrome | Fetal hydantoin syndrome |
|  | Laurence-Moon-Biedl syndrome |
|  | Fanconi pancytopenia |
|  | Trisomy 21 |
|  | Trisomy 13 |
|  | Trisomy 18 |

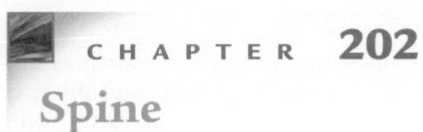

CHAPTER **202**

# Spine

## SPINAL DEFORMITIES

A simplified classification of the common spinal abnormalities, scoliosis and kyphosis, is presented in Table 202-1.

**TABLE 202-1  Classification of Spinal Deformities**

| SCOLIOSIS |
|---|
| *Idiopathic* |
| Infantile |
| Juvenile |
| Adolescent |
| *Congenital* |
| Failure of formation |
|   Wedge vertebrae |
|   Hemivertebrae |
| Failure of segmentation |
|   Unilateral bar |
|   Bilateral bar |
| Mixed |
| *Neuromuscular* |
| Neuropathic diseases |
| Upper motor neuron |
|   Cerebral palsy |
|   Spinocerebellar degeneration |
|     Friedreich ataxia |
|     Charcot-Marie-Tooth disease |
|   Syringomyelia |
|   Spinal cord tumor |
|   Spinal cord trauma |
| Lower motor neuron disease |
|   Myelodysplasia |
|   Poliomyelitis |
|   Spinal muscular atrophy |
| Myopathic diseases |
|   Duchenne muscular dystrophy |
|   Arthrogryposis |
|   Other muscular dystrophies |
| *Syndromes* |
| Neurofibromatosis |
| Marfan syndrome |
| *Compensatory* |
| Leg-length inequality |
| **KYPHOSIS** |
| Postural roundback |
| Scheuermann disease |
| Congenital kyphosis |

Adapted from the Terminology Committee of the Scoliosis Research Society, 1975.

## Clinical Manifestations

Most patients will present for evaluation of an asymmetrical spine, which is usually pain free. A complete physical examination is necessary for any patient with a spinal deformity, because the deformity can indicate an underlying disease.

The back is examined from behind (Fig. 202-1). First the levelness of the pelvis is assessed. Leg-length discrepancy produces pelvic obliquity, which often results in **compensatory scoliosis**. When the pelvis is level, the spine is examined for symmetry and spinal curvature with the patient

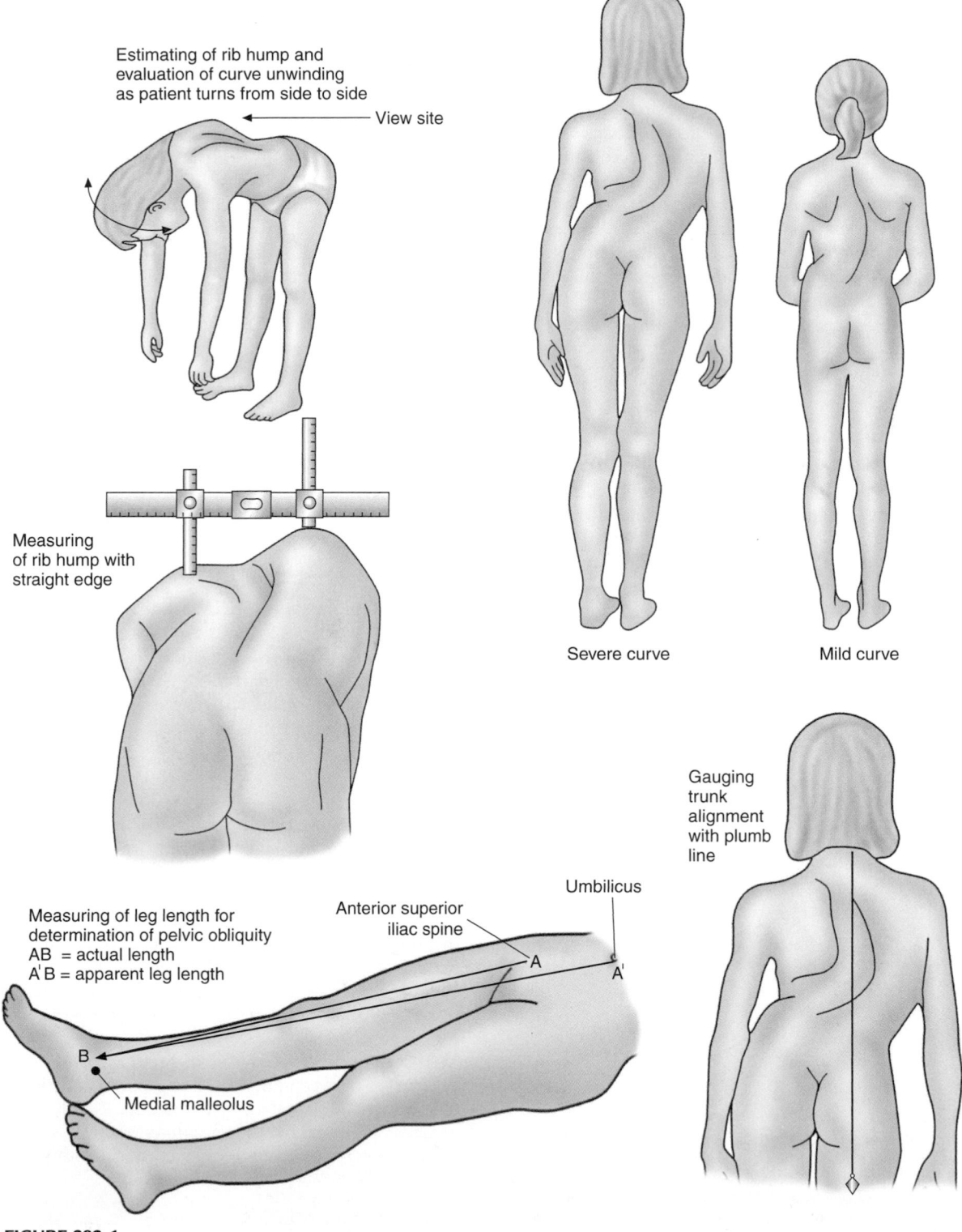

**FIGURE 202-1**

Clinical evaluation of a patient with scoliosis.

upright. Cutaneous lesions (hemangioma, skin dimple, or hair tuft) should be noted. The spine should be palpated for areas of tenderness.

The patient is then asked to bend forward with the hands directed between the feet (**Adams forward bend test**). The examiner should inspect for asymmetry in the spine. The presence of the hump in this position is the hallmark for scoliosis. The area opposite the hump is usually depressed, which is due to spinal rotation. Scoliosis is a rotational malalignment of one vertebra on another, resulting in rib elevation in the thoracic spine and paravertebral muscle elevation in the lumbar spine. With the patient still in the forward flexed position, inspection from the side can reveal the degree of roundback. A sharp forward angulation in the thoracolumbar region indicates a **kyphotic deformity**. It is important to examine the skin for café au lait spots (**neurofibromatosis**), hairy patches, and nevi (**spinal dysraphism**). Abnormal extremities may indicate skeletal dysplasia, whereas heart murmurs can be associated with Marfan syndrome. It is essential to do a full neurologic examination to determine whether the scoliosis is idiopathic or secondary to an underlying neuromuscular disease, and to assess whether the scoliosis is producing any neurologic sequelae.

## Radiologic Evaluation

Initial radiographs should include a posteroanterior and lateral standing film of the entire spine. The iliac crests should be visible to help determine skeletal maturity. The degree of curvature is measured from the most tilted or end vertebra of the curve superiorly and inferiorly to determine the Cobb angle (Fig. 202-2).

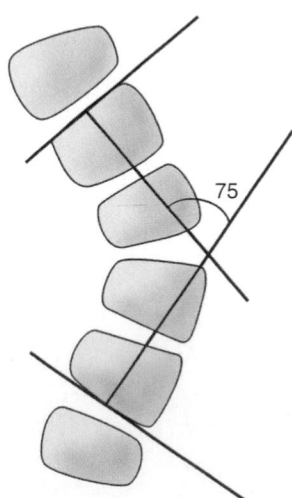

**FIGURE 202-2**

**Cobb method of scoliotic curve measurement.** Determine which are the end vertebrae of the curve: They are at the upper and lower limits of the curve and tilt most severely toward the concavity of the curve. Draw two perpendicular lines, one from the bottom of the lower body and one from the top of the upper body. Measure the angle formed. This is the accepted method of curve measurement according to the Scoliosis Research Society. Curves of 0 to 20 degrees are mild; 20 to 40 degrees, moderate; and greater than 40 degrees, severe.

## SCOLIOSIS

Alterations in normal spinal alignment that occur in the anteroposterior plane are termed scoliosis. Most scoliotic deformities are idiopathic. Scoliosis may also be congenital, neuromuscular, or compensatory from a leg-length discrepancy.

### Idiopathic Scoliosis

#### Etiology and Epidemiology

Idiopathic scoliosis is the most common form of scoliosis. It occurs in healthy, neurologically normal children. Approximately 20% of patients have a positive family history. The incidence is slightly higher in girls than boys, and the condition is more likely to progress and require treatment in females. There is some evidence that progressive scoliosis may have a genetic component as well.

Idiopathic scoliosis can be classified in three categories: **infantile** (birth to 3 years), **juvenile** (4–10 years), and **adolescent** (>11 years). Idiopathic adolescent scoliosis is the most common cause (80%) of spinal deformity. The right thoracic curve is the most common pattern. Juvenile scoliosis is uncommon, but may be under-represented because many patients do not seek treatment until they are adolescents. In any patient younger than 11 years of age, there is a greater likelihood that their scoliosis is not idiopathic. The prevalence of an intraspinal abnormality in a child with congenital scoliosis is approximately 40%.

#### Clinical Manifestations

Idiopathic scoliosis is a painless disorder 70% of the time. A patient with pain requires a careful evaluation. Any patient presenting with a left-sided curve has a high incidence of intraspinal pathology (syrinx or tumor). Evaluation of the spine with magnetic resonance imaging (MRI) is indicated in these cases.

#### Treatment

Treatment of idiopathic scoliosis is based on the skeletal maturity of the patient, the size of the curve, and whether the spinal curvature is progressive or nonprogressive. Initial treatment for scoliosis is likely observation and repeat radiographs to assess for progression. No treatment is indicated for nonprogressive deformities. The risk factors for curve progression include gender, curve location, and curve magnitude. Girls are five times more likely to progress than boys. Younger patients are more likely to progress than older patients.

Typically curves under 25 degrees are observed. Progressive curves between 20 and 50 degrees in a skeletally immature patient are treated with bracing. A radiograph in the orthotic is important to evaluate correction. Curves greater than 50 degrees usually require surgical intervention.

### Congenital Scoliosis

Abnormalities of the vertebral formation during the first trimester may lead to structural deformities of the spine

**Congenital scoliosis**

**Closed vertebral types**
(MacEwen classification)

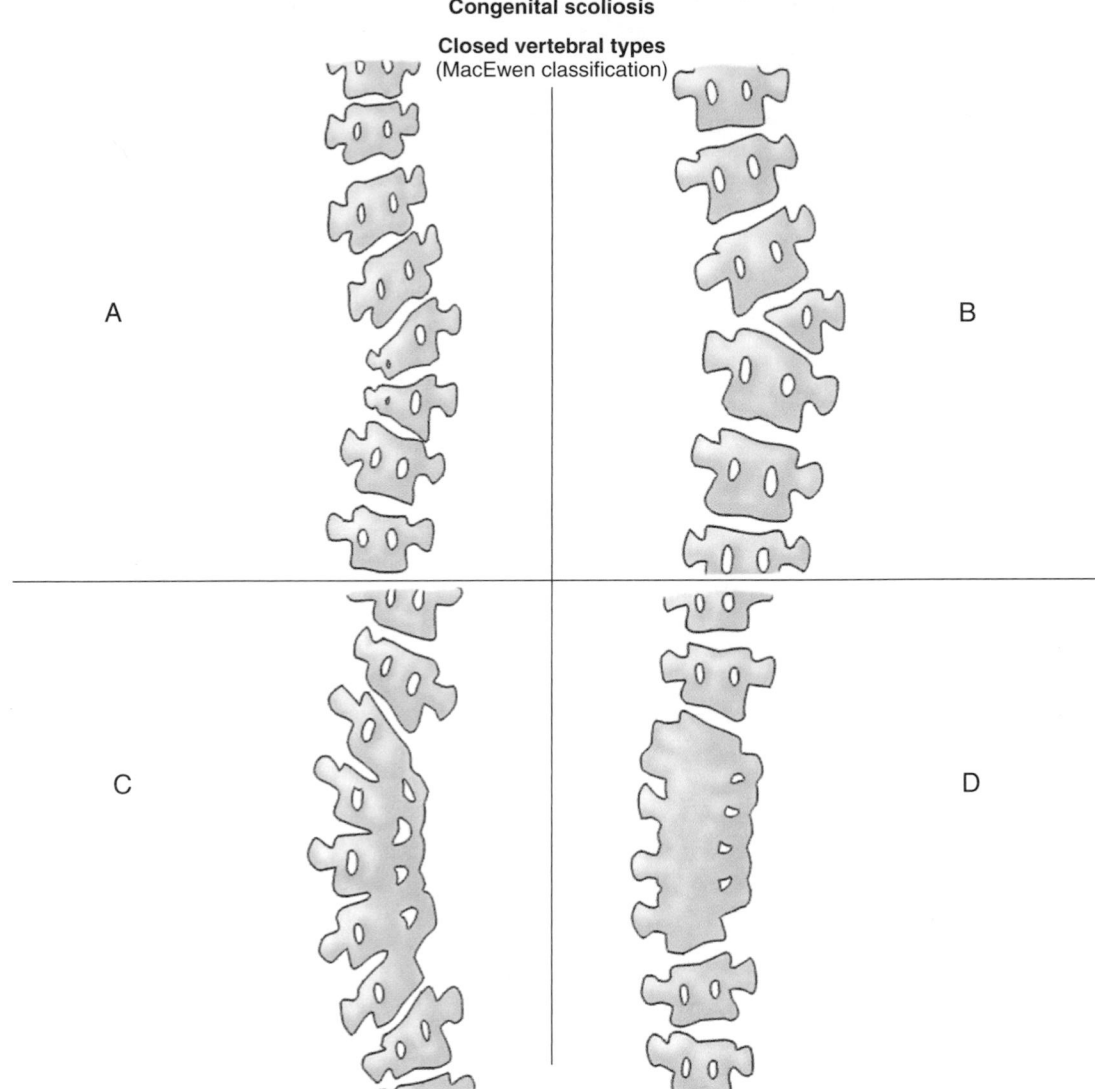

**FIGURE 202-3**

**Types of closed vertebral and extravertebral spinal anomalies that result in congenital scoliosis. A,** Partial unilateral failure of formation (wedge vertebra). **B,** Complete unilateral failure of formation (hemivertebra). **C,** Unilateral failure of segmentation (congenital bar). **D,** Bilateral failure of segmentation (block vertebra).

that are evident at birth or early childhood. Congenital scoliosis can be classified as follows (Fig. 202-3):

Partial or complete failure of vertebral formation (wedge vertebra or hemivertebrae)
Partial or complete failure of segmentation (unsegmented bars)
Mixed

Over 60% of patients have other associated abnormalities, such as VACTERL association (*v*ertebral defects, imperforate *a*nus, *c*ardiac anomalies, *t*racheoesophageal fistula, *r*enal anomalies, *l*imb abnormalities like radial agenesis) or Klippel-Feil syndrome. Renal anomalies occur in 20% of children with congenital scoliosis, with renal agenesis being the most common; 6% of children have a silent, obstructive uropathy suggesting the need for evaluation with ultrasonography. Congenital heart disease

occurs in about 12% of patients. **Spinal dysraphism** (tethered cord, intradural lipoma, syringomyelia, diplomyelia, and diastematomyelia) occurs in approximately 20% of children with congenital scoliosis. These disorders are frequently associated with cutaneous lesions on the back and abnormalities of the legs and feet (e.g., cavus foot, neurologic changes, calf atrophy). MRI is indicated in evaluation of spinal dysraphism.

The risk of spinal deformity progression in congenital scoliosis is variable and depends on the growth potential of the malformed vertebrae. A unilateral unsegmented bar typically progresses, but a block vertebra has little growth potential. About 75% of patients with congenital scoliosis will show some progression that continues until skeletal growth is complete, and about 50% will require some type of treatment. Progression can be expected during periods of rapid growth (before 2 years and after 10 years).

**Treatment** of congenital scoliosis hinges on early diagnosis and identification of progressive curves. Orthotic treatment is not helpful in congenital scoliosis. Early spinal surgery should be performed once progression has been documented. This can help prevent major deformities. Patients with large curves that cause thoracic insufficiency should undergo surgery immediately.

## Neuromuscular Scoliosis

Progressive spinal deformity is a common and potentially serious problem associated with many neuromuscular disorders, such as cerebral palsy, Duchenne muscular dystrophy, spinal muscular atrophy, and spina bifida. Spinal alignment must be part of the routine examination for a patient with neuromuscular disease. Once scoliosis begins, progression is usually continuous. The magnitude of the deformity depends on the severity and pattern of weakness, whether the underlying disease process is progressive and the amount of remaining musculoskeletal growth. Nonambulatory patients have a higher incidence of spinal deformity than ambulatory patients. In nonambulatory patients, the curves tend to be long and sweeping, produce pelvic obliquity, involve the cervical spine, and also produce restrictive lung disease. If the child cannot stand, then a supine anteroposterior radiograph of the entire spine, rather than a standing posteroanterior view, is indicated.

The goal of **treatment** is to prevent progression and loss of function. Nonambulatory patients are more comfortable and independent when they can sit in their wheelchair without external support. Progressive curves can impair sitting balance, which affects quality of life. Orthotic treatment is usually ineffective in neuromuscular scoliosis. Surgical intervention is necessary in most cases with frequent fusion to the pelvis.

## Compensatory Scoliosis

Adolescents with a leg-length discrepancy (Chapter 200) may have a positive screening examination for scoliosis. When examining the patient before correcting the pelvic obliquity, the spine curves in the same direction of the obliquity. However, with identification and correction of their pelvic obliquity, the curvature should resolve, and treatment should be directed at the leg-length discrepancy. Thus, it is important to distinguish between a structural and compensatory spinal deformity.

# KYPHOSIS

Kyphosis refers to a roundback deformity or to increased angulation of the thoracic or thoracolumbar spine in the sagittal plane. Kyphosis can be postural, structural (Scheuermann kyphosis), or congenital.

## Postural Roundback

Postural kyphosis is secondary to poor posture. It is voluntarily corrected in the standing and prone positions. The patient may also have increased lumbar lordosis.

Radiographs are usually unnecessary if the kyphosis fully corrects. If not, radiographs will reveal no vertebral abnormalities. Treatment, if needed, is aimed at improving the child's posture.

## Scheuermann Kyphosis

Scheuermann disease is the second most common cause of pediatric spinal deformity. It occurs equally in males and females. The etiology is unknown, but there may be hereditary factors. Scheuermann kyphosis is differentiated from postural roundback on physical examination and by radiographs.

A patient with Scheuermann disease cannot correct the kyphosis with standing or lying prone. When viewed from the side in the forward flexed position, patients with Scheuermann disease will have an abrupt angulation in the mid to lower thoracic region (Fig. 202-4), and patients with postural roundback show a smooth, symmetrical contour. In both conditions, lumbar lordosis is increased. However, half of the patients with Scheuermann disease will have atypical back pain, especially with thoracolumbar kyphosis. The **classic radiologic findings** of Scheuermann kyphosis include the following:

Narrowing of disk space
Loss of anterior height of the involved vertebrae producing wedging of 5 or more degrees in at least three consecutive vertebrae
Irregularities of the vertebral endplates
Schmorl nodes

**Treatment** of Scheuermann kyphosis is similar to idiopathic scoliosis. It is dependent on the degree of deformity, skeletal maturity, and the presence or absence of pain. Nonoperative treatment begins with bracing. Surgical fusion is done for patients who have completed growth, have a severe deformity, or who have intractable pain.

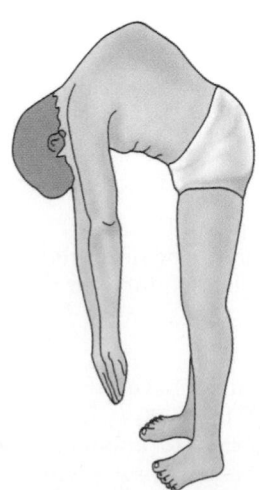

**FIGURE 202-4**

**Note the sharp break in the contour of a child with kyphosis.** (From Behrman RE: Nelson Textbook of Pediatrics, 14th ed. Philadelphia, *WB Saunders*, 1992.)

## Congenital Kyphosis

Congenital kyphosis is a failure of the formation of all or part of the vertebral body (with preservation of posterior elements) or failure of anterior segmentation of the spine, or both. Severe deformities are found at birth and tend to progress rapidly. Progression will not cease until the end of skeletal growth. A progressive thoracic spine deformity may result in paraplegia. This complication is most often associated with failure of vertebral body formation. When indicated, treatment is often surgical.

## TORTICOLLIS

### Etiology and Epidemiology

Torticollis is usually first identified in newborns because of a head tilt. Torticollis is usually secondary to a shortened sternocleidomastoid muscle (muscular torticollis). This may result from in utero positioning or birth trauma. Acquired torticollis may be related to upper cervical spine abnormalities or central nervous system pathology (mass lesion). It can also occur in older children during a respiratory infection (potentially secondary to lymphadenitis) or local head or neck infection, and may herald psychiatric diagnoses.

### Clinical Manifestations and Evaluation

Infants with muscular torticollis have the ear tilted toward the clavicle on the ipsilateral side. The face will look upward toward the contralateral side. There may be a palpable swelling or fibrosis in the body of the sternocleidomastoid shortly after birth, which is often the precursor of a contracture. Congenital muscular torticollis is associated with skull and facial asymmetry (**plagiocephaly**) and developmental dysplasia of the hip.

After a thorough neurologic examination, anteroposterior and lateral radiographs should be obtained. The goal is to rule out a nonmuscular etiology. A computed tomography (CT) scan or MRI of the head and neck is necessary for persistent neck pain, neurologic symptoms, and persistent deformity.

### Treatment

Treatment of muscular torticollis is aimed at increasing the range of motion of the neck and correcting the cosmetic deformity. Stretching exercises of the neck can be very beneficial for infants. Surgical management is indicated if patients do not improve with adequate stretching exercises in physical therapy. Postoperative physical therapy is needed to decrease the risk of recurrence. Treatment in patients with underlying disorders should target the disorder.

## BACK PAIN IN CHILDREN

### Etiology and Epidemiology

Back pain in the pediatric population should always be approached with concern. In contrast to adults, in whom back pain is frequently mechanical or psychological, back pain in children may be the result of organic causes, especially in preadolescents. Back pain lasting longer than a week requires a detailed investigation. In the pediatric population, approximately 85% of children with back pain for greater than 2 months have a specific lesion: 33% are post-traumatic (spondylolysis, occult fracture), 33% developmental (kyphosis, scoliosis), and 18% have an infection or tumor. In the remaining 15%, the diagnosis is undetermined.

### Clinical Manifestations and Management

The history must include the onset and duration of symptoms. The location, character, and radiation of pain are important. Neurologic symptoms (muscle weakness, sensory changes, and bowel or bladder dysfunction) must be reviewed. Past history and family history should be obtained, with a focus on back pain, rheumatologic disorders, and neoplastic processes. The review of systems should include detailed questions on overall health, fever, chills, recent weight loss, and recent illnesses. Physical examination should include a complete musculoskeletal and neurologic evaluation. Spinal alignment, range of motion, areas of tenderness, and muscle spasm should be noted. Red flags for childhood back pain include persistent or increasing pain, systemic findings (e.g., fever, weight loss), neurologic deficits, bowel or bladder dysfunction, young age (under 4 is strongly associated with tumor), night waking, pain that restricts activity, and a painful left thoracic spinal curvature.

Anteroposterior and lateral standing films of the entire spine with bilateral oblique views of the affected area should be obtained. Secondary imaging with bone scan, CT scan, or MRI may be necessary for diagnosis. MRI is very useful for suspected intraspinal pathology. Laboratory studies, such as a complete blood count, erythrocyte sedimentation rate (ESR), C-reactive protein (CRP), and specialized testing for juvenile idiopathic arthritis and ankylosing spondylitis, may be indicated.

The differential diagnosis of pediatric back pain is extensive (Table 202-2). Treatment depends on the specific diagnosis. If serious pathology has been ruled out and no definite diagnosis has been established, an initial trial of physical therapy with close follow-up for reevaluation is recommended.

## SPONDYLOLYSIS AND SPONDYLOLITHESIS

### Etiology and Epidemiology

Spondylolysis is a defect in the pars interarticularis. Spondylolithesis refers to bilateral defects with anterior slippage of the superior vertebra on the inferior vertebra. The lesions are not present at birth, but about 5% of children will have the lesion by 6 years of age. It is most common in adolescent athletes, especially those involved in sports that involve repetitive back extension. Classically, this was an injury seen in gymnasts and divers. However, with increased intensity and year-round sports, the incidence is increasing. Football interior lineman (extension while blocking), soccer players (extension while shooting), and basketball players (extension while rebounding) are

**TABLE 202-2 Differential Diagnosis of Back Pain**

### INFECTIOUS DISEASES

Diskitis (most common before the age of 6 years)
Vertebral osteomyelitis (pyogenic or tuberculous)
Spinal epidural abscess
Pyelonephritis
Pancreatitis

### RHEUMATOLOGIC DISEASES

Juvenile idiopathic arthritis
Reiter syndrome
Ankylosing spondylitis
Psoriatic arthritis
Inflammatory bowel disease

### DEVELOPMENTAL DISEASES

Scheuermann kyphosis
Scoliosis (left thoracic)
Spondylolysis
Spondylolithesis

### TRAUMATIC AND MECHANICAL ABNORMALITIES

Hip and pelvic abnormalities (sacroiliac joint dysfunction)
Herniated nucleus pulposus (intervertebral disk)
Overuse injuries (facet syndrome)
Vertebral stress fractures (spondylolysis, spondylolithesis)
Vertebral compression fracture (steroid, sickle cell anemia)
Upper cervical spine instability (Atlantoaxial instability)

### NEOPLASTIC DISEASES

Primary vertebral tumors (osteogenic sarcoma)
Metastatic tumor (neuroblastoma)
Primary spinal tumor (astrocytoma)
Bone marrow malignancy (leukemia, lymphoma)
Benign tumors (eosinophilic granuloma, osteoid osteoma)

### OTHER

Conversion disorder
Juvenile osteoporosis

examples of athletes at higher risk. The most common location of spondylolysis is L5, followed by L4.

Spondylolithesis is classified according to the degree of slippage:

Grade 1: less than 25%
Grade 2: 25% to 50%
Grade 3: 50% to 75%
Grade 4: 75% to 99%
Grade 5: complete displacement

The most common location of spondylolithesis is L5 on S1.

## Clinical Manifestations

Patients will often complain of an insidious onset of low back pain persisting over 2 weeks. The pain tends to worsen with activity and with extension of the back and improves with rest. There may be some radiation of pain to the buttocks. A loss of lumbar lordosis may occur due to muscular spasm. Pain is present with extension of lumbar spine and with palpation over the lesion. Patients with spondylolithesis may have a palpable *step off* at the lumbosacral area. A detailed neurologic examination should be done, especially because spondylolithesis can have nerve root involvement.

## Radiologic Evaluation

Anteroposterior, lateral, and oblique radiographs of the spine should be obtained. The oblique views may show the classic *Scotty dog* findings associated with spondylolysis. The lateral view will allow measurement of spondylolithesis. Unfortunately, plain radiographs do not regularly reveal spondylolysis, so secondary imaging may be needed. A bone scan and CT scan can be helpful with diagnosis of spondylolysis. MRI may be required in patients with neurologic deficits.

## Treatment

### Spondylolysis

Painful spondylolysis requires activity restriction. Bracing is controversial but may help with pain relief. Patients benefit from an aggressive physical therapy plan to improve lower extremity flexibility and increase core strength and spinal stability. It is most beneficial to begin with flexion exercises and progress to extension exercises as tolerated. There is evidence that some patients with an acute spondylolysis can achieve bony union and that these patients have a decreased incidence of low back pain and degenerative change in the low back as they age when compared with spondylolysis patients with nonunion. Rarely, surgery is indicated for intractable pain and disability.

### Spondylolithesis

Patients with spondylolithesis require periodic evaluation for progression of their slippage. Treatment of spondylolithesis is based on grading.

Grade 1: Same treatment as spondylolysis. Failure of nonoperative management may lead to surgical fusion.
Grade 2: Reasonable to try nonoperative management, but if the slippage is progressing, surgical intervention may be needed. Any patient with neurologic symptoms requires surgical intervention.
Grades 3 to 5: Spinal fusion is usually required to prevent further slippage or damage.

## DISKITIS

Diskitis is an intervertebral disk space infection that does not cause associated vertebral osteomyelitis (see Chapter 117). The most common organism is *Staphylococcus aureus*. The infection can occur at any age but is more common in patients under 6 years of age.

## Clinical Manifestations

Children may present with back pain, abdominal pain, pelvic pain, irritability, and refusal to walk. Fever is an inconsistent symptom. The child typically holds the spine in a straight or stiff position, generally has a loss of lumbar lordosis due to paravertebral muscular spasm, and refuses to flex the lumbar spine. The white blood cell count is normal or elevated, but the ESR is usually high.

## Radiologic Evaluation

Radiographic findings vary according to the duration of symptoms prior to diagnosis. Anteroposterior, lateral, and oblique radiographs of the lumbar or thoracic spine will typically show a narrow disk space with irregularity of the adjacent vertebral body end plates. In early cases, bone scan or MRI may be helpful, because they will be positive before findings are noticeable on plain radiographs. MRI can also be used to differentiate between diskitis and the more serious condition of vertebral osteomyelitis.

## Treatment

Intravenous antibiotic therapy is the mainstay of treatment. Blood cultures may occasionally be positive and identify the infectious agent. Aspiration and needle biopsy are reserved for children who are not responding to empirical antibiotic treatment. Symptoms should resolve rapidly with antibiotics, but intravenous antibiotics should be continued for 1 to 2 weeks, and be followed by 4 weeks of oral antibiotics. Pain control can be obtained with medications and temporary orthotic immobilization of the back.

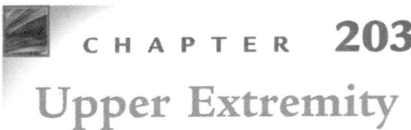

# CHAPTER 203
# Upper Extremity

## SHOULDER

The shoulder actually comprises four joints:

Glenohumeral joint (commonly referred to as the shoulder joint)
Acromioclavicular joint
Sternoclavicular joint
Scapulothoracic joint

The glenohumeral joint has minimal geometric stability because the relatively small glenoid fossa articulates with the proportionately larger head of the humerus. The low level of intrinsic stability allows for a large range of motion. The rotator cuff muscles help give the glenohumeral joint more stability, but they need normal contact of the glenohumeral joint to be successful. The scapulothoracic movement also expands the range of motion of the shoulder, but like the glenohumeral joint, it requires strong, coordinated musculature to function efficiently.

## Sprengel Deformity

Sprengel deformity is the congenital elevation of the scapula. There are varying degrees of severity; it is usually unilateral. There is restricted scapulothoracic motion (especially with abduction) so most of the shoulder motion is through the glenohumeral joint. There is usually associated hypoplasia of the parascapular muscles. Webbing of the neck and low posterior hairline can be associated problems. There is an association with congenital syndromes, such as Klippel-Feil anomaly, so a thorough history and examination are necessary. Mild forms with a cosmetic deformity and mild loss of shoulder motion do not need surgical correction. Severe forms may have a bony connection (omovertebral) between the scapula and lower cervical spine. Moderate and severe forms may need surgical repositioning of the scapula in early childhood to improve comesis and function.

## Brachial Plexus Injuries

**Obstetric brachial plexus palsy** is discussed in Section 11. **Brachial plexopathy** is an athletic injury, commonly referred to as a **stinger** or **burner**. The symptoms are often likened to a *dead arm*. There is pain (often burning), weakness, and numbness in a single upper extremity. There are three mechanisms of injury:

Traction caused by lateral flexion of the neck away from the involved upper extremity
Direct impact to the brachial plexus at Erb's point
Compression caused by neck extension and rotation toward the involved extremity

Symptoms are always unilateral and should resolve within 15 minutes. It is paramount to assess the cervical spine for serious injury. Bilateral symptoms, lower extremity symptoms, persistent symptoms, or recurrent injury are all signs of more serious disease and may need a more extensive workup and cervical spine stabilization. Athletes may return to activity if there are no red flags on history or physical examination and the athlete has full pain-free range of motion and strength in the neck and affected extremity.

## Glenohumeral Dislocation

Shoulder dislocation is uncommon in childhood, but becomes more frequent in adolescence. The younger the patient is at presentation, the more likely the patient will have recurrent dislocation. Anterior dislocation is the most common. When a patient sustains a dislocation, it is imperative to assess neurovascular status of the affected extremity. If there is compromise, then reduction is urgent to prevent further complications. Patients will need radiographs to assess for fractures of the glenoid (Bankhart lesion) and humeral head (Hill-Sachs lesion). Most patients will require a brief period of protection in a sling or shoulder immobilizer, as well as pain control. As symptoms resolve, a gentle range of motion program, followed by an aggressive strengthening program, should be done. Unfortunately, recurrence occurs in nearly 90% of athletes participating in contact sports, so orthopedists are considering surgical intervention early rather than awaiting further dislocation.

## Proximal Humeral Epiphysitis

Proximal humeral epiphysitis is commonly referred to as Little Leaguer's shoulder. It occurs in children who participate in overhead (tennis, volleyball) and throwing sports, particularly baseball pitchers. It usually occurs in 9- to 14-year-old boys. It is a stress injury that potentially can be a fracture (epiphysiolysis) of the proximal humeral physis. Most patients present with pain when throwing, which can last for a few days afterward. There may be tenderness to palpation over the proximal humerus, but if the athlete has been resting for a few days, the examination may be normal. Radiographs should include comparison views to assess the physis. There may be widening of the proximal humeral physis in the affected arm, or the films may be normal. Treatment is rest from the offending activity, followed by an exercise program designed to improve strength in the shoulder muscles. Pitchers should also be encouraged to follow youth pitching guidelines published at www.littleleague.org.

## Overuse Injuries

The incidence of overuse injuries is increasing due to increased opportunities for athletic participation, but also due to higher levels of intensity during sports. Overuse injuries are inflammatory responses in tendons and bursae that are subjected to repetitive motions and trauma (e.g., rotator cuff tendonopathy in swimmers). These injuries are uncommon in children, but may be seen in adolescents. It is important to rule out bony injury, such as physeal fractures and apophysitis, before making the diagnosis of a soft tissue overuse injury. Many of the overuse injuries in the shoulder, such as rotator cuff tendonopathy, are secondary to joint laxity.

The patient will often present with discomfort over the affected area that worsens with activity. Physical examination usually reveals tenderness to palpation and often weakness of the associated muscles due to pain. It is important to assess for glenohumeral stability. Radiographs may be indicated for acute trauma or when symptoms are not improving. Treatment consists of activity modification, icing, anti-inflammatory medication, and a physical therapy program aimed at strengthening, flexibility, and improving posture.

## ELBOW

The elbow consists of three articulations:

Ulnar-humeral joint
Radial-humeral joint
Proximal radioulnar joint

Collectively, these joints produce a hinge-type joint that allows for supination (palm up) and pronation (palm down) positioning of the hand. The elbow has excellent geometric stability, and the musculature around the elbow primarily produces flexion and extension.

## Radial Head Subluxation

Radial head subluxation is more commonly known as **nursemaid's elbow**. Because the radial head is not as bulbous in infants and young children, the annular ligament that passes around it can partially slip off the radial head with traction across the elbow (Fig. 203-1). The subluxation is usually caused by a quick pull on the extended elbow when a child is forcefully lifted by the hand or when the child falls while holding hands with an adult. After a subluxation, the child usually holds the hand in a pronated position and will refuse to use the hand or move the elbow. Moving the hand into the supinated position while applying pressure to the radial head will usually reduce the injury. Usually, radiographs are not necessary unless reduction cannot be obtained or there is concern for fracture (swelling and bruising). Once the injury is reduced, the child will begin using the arm again without complaint. Parents should be educated about the mechanism of injury and encouraged to avoid that position. There is a high rate of recurrence for this injury. The problem generally resolves with maturation, but some children with high recurrence rates may benefit from casting or, rarely, surgical intervention.

## Panner Disease

Panner disease is an osteochondritis of the capitellum (lateral portion of distal humeral epiphysis) that occurs spontaneously in late childhood. Clinical features include elbow pain, decreased range of motion, and tenderness to palpation over the capitellum. Radiographs reveal fragmentation of the capitellum. Treatment is activity restriction and follow-up radiographs to demonstrate spontaneous reossification of the capitellum over several months. There is usually no need for further treatment or imaging studies. This is not to be confused with osteochondritis dissecans of the capitellum, which usually will occur in adolescents involved with throwing sports.

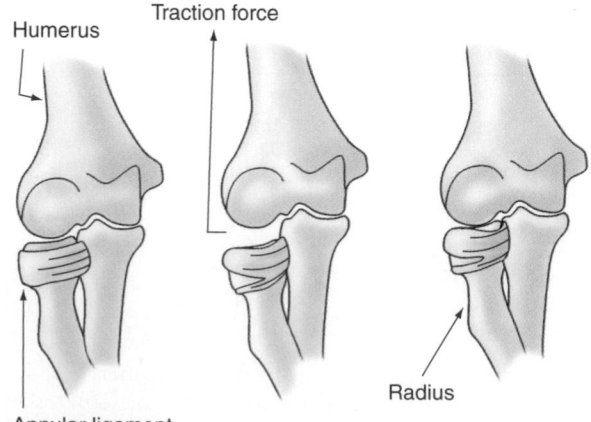

**FIGURE 203-1**

**Nursemaid's elbow.** The annular ligament is torn when the arm is pulled. The radial head moves distally, and when traction is discontinued, the ligament is carried into the joint. (From Rang M: Children's Fractures. Philadelphia, *JB Lippincott*, 1974, p 121.)

## Throwing Injuries

The elbow is especially vulnerable to throwing injuries in the skeletally immature athlete. These occur from excessive and repetitive tension forces across the radial aspect of the elbow and compression forces across the lateral aspect of the elbow. These injuries are commonly known as **Little Leaguer's elbow**.

While this injury is most common in baseball players who throw frequently (pitcher, catcher, third base, and shortstop), it also occurs in football quarterbacks and tennis players. Patients will usually complain of pain over the medial elbow with throwing that may last for a few days afterward. There may be associated swelling and lateral or posterior elbow pain. Radiation of pain may be secondary to ulnar neuritis. There is often a flexion contracture of the elbow when compared to the opposite side. Palpation of the medial epicondyle, radial head, capitellum, lateral epicondyle, and olecranon process often reveals tenderness. Ulnar (medial) collateral ligament stability should be assessed. Radiographs should include the contralateral elbow for comparison. Radiographic findings in Little Leaguer's elbow can vary and may include normal anatomy, medial humeral epicondyle apophyseal avulsion fracture, osteochondritis dissecans of the capitellum, radial head abnormalities, and foreign bodies in the elbow. MRI is often a useful tool to provide more information.

Treatment depends on the underlying diagnosis, but always includes pain control and rest from activity. Athletes with bony changes should be followed by a sports medicine specialist or pediatric orthopedist. *Classic Little Leaguer's elbow* refers to medial humeral epicondyle apophysitis. These athletes benefit from rest, ice, anti-inflammatory medication, and a physical therapy program aimed at upper body strengthening. Throwing mechanics and the pitching guidelines published by Little League Baseball/Softball should be reviewed with these players. Switching players to a lower throwing position (e.g., first base) after rehabilitation, to avoid pitching for the remainder of the season, is often recommended.

## WRIST AND HAND

Multiple small joints, a delicately balanced intrinsic muscle system, a powerful extrinsic muscle system, dense sensory innervation, and specialized skin combine to make the hand a highly mobile and sensitive yet powerful anatomic part. The extrinsic muscles originate in the forearm and the intrinsic muscles are located in the hand and coordinate small, delicate movements. The movements of opening the hand, extending and spreading the fingers, and then clenching the hand into a fist requires coordinated function of the intrinsic and extrinsic muscles. Tenderness of direct palpation of the bones raises the concern for fracture. **Scaphoid fracture** is the most common carpal bone fracture in the pediatric population. It requires immobilization in a thumb spica cast, while displaced fractures require surgical intervention. **Salter-Harris fractures of the distal radius** are also very common. In young gymnasts, there is increased risk for injury at the distal radial physis from repetitive impact and upper extremity weight bearing. This is commonly called **gymnast's wrist**

and requires absolute rest from impact and weight bearing to prevent premature closure of the growth plate.

**Ganglion cysts** are synovial fluid-filled cysts about the wrist. The most common location is the dorsum of the wrist near the radiocarpal joint, followed by the volar radial aspect of the wrist. The defect is in the joint capsule, which allows synovial fluid into the soft tissues with wrist use, where it can become walled off with fibrous tissue. Often, in skeletally immature patients, the process is benign and disappears over time. Large ganglion cysts or cysts that are painful and interfere with function may require more aggressive therapy. Aspiration and steroid injection into the cyst may be helpful, but many will recur. Surgical excision will remove the tract that attaches to the wrist joint, so it is usually curative.

## Finger Abnormalities

**Polydactyly** (extra digits) occurs in simple and complex varieties (see Table 201-2). Skin tags and digit remnants that occur near the metacarpophalangeal joint of the fifth digit and thumb that do not have palpable bones or possess voluntary motion are simple varieties. These may be excised or ligated in the nursery. Complex deformities should be referred to a pediatric orthopedist for amputation. **Syndactyly** (fused digits) are concerning because of the possibility of shared structures and the tethering effects on bone growth (see Table 201-2). All patients with syndactyly should be referred for treatment options.

**Trigger thumb** and **trigger finger** are secondary to isolated thickening of the flexor tendons. As the thickened nodule enlarges, it may catch in a bent position, then snap or *trigger* straight as it passes through the first pulley that anchors the tendon. Ultimately, as it enlarges, it cannot pass through at all and produces a flexion deformity at the interphalangeal joints. The nodule may be palpable near the metacarpophalangeal joint. These children should be referred for surgical correction.

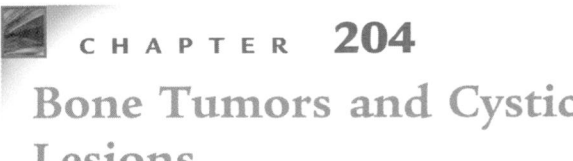

# CHAPTER 204

# Bone Tumors and Cystic Lesions

Benign bone tumors and cystic lesions are common in childhood. Some represent fibrous dysplasia, and others are benign bone cysts (unicameral) or benign bone tumors (osteoid osteoma). Subacute osteomyelitis (**Brodie abscess**) and eosinophilic granulomas are lesions not associated with abnormal bone or cartilage growth. Some of these lesions can produce pain, limp, and pathologic fractures. Others can be incidental findings on radiographs. The prognosis is usually excellent. A brief differential diagnosis of bone tumors and their management is listed in Table 204-1. Malignant bone tumors are discussed in Section 21.

**TABLE 204-1  Benign Bone Tumors and Cysts**

| Disease | Characteristics | Radiographic Findings | Treatment | Prognosis |
| --- | --- | --- | --- | --- |
| Osteochondroma (osteocartilaginous exostosis) | Common; distal metaphysis of femur, proximal humerus, proximal tibia; painless, hard, nontender mass | Bony outgrowth, sessile or pedunculated | Excision, if symptomatic | Excellent; malignant transformation rare |
| Multiple hereditary exostoses | Osteochondroma of long bones; bone growth disturbances | As above | As above | Recurrences |
| Osteoid osteoma | Pain relieved by aspirin; femur and tibia; found predominantly in boys | Dense sclerosis surrounds small radiolucent nidus, <1 cm | As above | Excellent |
| Osteoblastoma (giant osteoid osteoma) | As above, but more destructive | Osteolytic component; size >1 cm | As above | Excellent |
| Enchondroma | Tubular bones of hands and feet; pathologic fractures, swollen bone; Ollier disease if multiple lesions are present | Radiolucent diaphyseal or metaphyseal lesion; may calcify | Excision or curettage | Excellent; malignant transformation rare |
| Nonossifying fibroma | Silent; rare pathologic fracture; late childhood, adolescence | Incidental radiographic finding; thin sclerotic border, radiolucent lesion | None or curettage with fractures | Excellent; heals spontaneously |
| Eosinophilic granuloma | Age 5–10 years; skull, jaw, long bones; pathologic fracture; pain | Small, radiolucent without reactive bone; punched-out lytic lesion | Biopsy, excision rare; irradiation | Excellent; may heal spontaneously |
| Brodie abscess | Insidious local pain; limp; suspected as malignancy | Circumscribed metaphyseal osteomyelitis; lytic lesions with sclerotic rim | Biopsy; antibiotics | Excellent |
| Unicameral bone cyst (simple bone cyst) | Metaphysis of long bone (femur, humerus); pain, pathologic fracture | Cyst in medullary canal, expands cortex; fluid-filled unilocular or multilocular cavity | Curettage; steroid injection into lesion | Excellent; some heal spontaneously |
| Aneurysmal bone cyst | As above; contains blood, fibrous tissue | Expands beyond metaphyseal cartilage | Curettage, bone graft | Excellent |

# SUGGESTED READING

Abbassian A: The limping child: A clinical approach to diagnosis, *Br J Hosp Med (London)* 68:246–250, 2007.

Benjamin HJ, Briner WW: Little league elbow, *Clin J Sport Med* 15:37–40, 2005.

Carson S: Pediatric upper extremity injuries, *Pediatr Clin North Am* 53:41–67, 2006.

Dixit S, DiFiori JP, Burton M, et al: Management of patellofemoral pain syndrome, *Am Fam Physician* 75:194–202, 2007.

Herring JA: Tachdjian's Pediatric Orthopedics, 4th ed, Philadelphia, 2007, *WB Saunders*.

Kliegman RM, Behrman RE, Jenson HB, et al: Nelson Textbook of Pediatrics, 18th ed, Philadelphia, 2007, *WB Saunders*.

Lehmann CL, Arons RR, Loder RT, et al: The epidemiology of slipped capital femoral epiphysis: An update, *J Pediatr Orthop* 26:286–290, 2006.

McCleary MD, Congeni JA: Current concepts in the diagnosis and treatment of spondylolysis in young athletes, *Curr Sports Med Rep* 6:62–66, 2007.

Shipman SA, Helfand M, Moyer VA, et al: Screening for developmental dysplasia of the hip: A systemic literature review for the U.S. Preventive Services Task Force, *Pediatrics* 117:e557–e576, 2006.

Staheli LT: Practice of Pediatric Orthopedics, 2nd ed, Philadelphia, 2006, *Lippincott Williams & Wilkins*.

Wenger DR, Pring ME, Rang M: Rang's Children's Fractures, 3rd ed, Philadelphia, 2005, *Lippincott Williams & Wilkins*.

Note: Page numbers followed by *f* indicate figures and those followed by *t* indicate tables.